Tobacco

Science, policy, and public health

Tobacco
Science, policy, and public health

SECOND EDITION

Edited by

Peter Boyle

Nigel Gray

Jack Henningfield

John Seffrin

Witold A. Zatoński

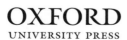

OXFORD
UNIVERSITY PRESS

OXFORD
UNIVERSITY PRESS

Great Clarendon Street, Oxford OX2 6DP

Oxford University Press is a department of the University of Oxford.
It furthers the University's objective of excellence in research, scholarship,
and education by publishing worldwide in

Oxford New York

Auckland Cape Town Dar es Salaam Hong Kong Karachi
Kuala Lumpur Madrid Melbourne Mexico City Nairobi
New Delhi Shanghai Taipei Toronto

With offices in

Argentina Austria Brazil Chile Czech Republic France Greece
Guatemala Hungary Italy Japan Poland Portugal Singapore
South Korea Switzerland Thailand Turkey Ukraine Vietnam

Oxford is a registered trade mark of Oxford University Press
in the UK and in certain other countries

Published in the United States
by Oxford University Press Inc., New York

British Library Cataloguing in Publication Data
Data available

Library of Congress Cataloging in Publication Data
Tobacco : science, policy, and public health / edited by Peter Boyle ... [et al.].—2nd ed.
        p. ; cm.
    Rev. ed. of: Tobacco and public health : science and policy. 2004.
    Includes bibliographical references and index.
    ISBN 978–0–19–956665–5
1. Tobacco—Toxicology. 2. Tobacco use—Health aspects. 3. Tobacco use—Government policy.
I. Boyle, P. (Peter) II. Tobacco and public health.
    [DNLM: 1. Tobacco Use Disorder—complications. 2. Public Policy. 3. Tobacco WM 290 T6284 2010]
    RA1242.T6T62 2010
    362.29'6—dc22

Typeset in Minion by Glyph International, Bangalore, India
Printed in Great Britain
on acid-free paper by
CPI Antony Rowe, Chippenham, Wiltshire

ISBN 978–0–19–956665–5

10 9 8 7 6 5 4 3 2 1

Preface

C. Everett Koop

At the turn of the last century, public health interventions and medical breakthroughs were beginning to radically curb many forms of disease and premature death (CDC 1999a). It was also a time in which lung cancer was so rare that surgeons travelled to witness and learn from the few operations performed to save the lives of those afflicted (Kluger 1996; Wynder 1997). It was, of course, the dawn of the twentieth century. It was also a time in which an outgrowth of the cottage tobacco industry was metastasizing into one of the largest companies in the United States (Corti 1931; Taylor 1984; White 1988). That company was the American Tobacco Company, and it came to rival US Steel and Standard Oil as an economic and political powerhouse in the first few two decades of the twentieth century (Taylor 1984; White 1988). In the decades to follow, it would come to be rivalled by no industry and no war in terms of destruction of human life. By the end of the twentieth century the offspring of this company, which I will collectively refer to as 'Big Tobacco', were selling enough cigarettes to kill more than 400 000 people annually in the US and 5 million worldwide (Garrett *et al.* 2001). On current course, the global trajectory will increase to 10 million deaths per year early in the twenty-first century and will cost the lives of nearly one half of the world's 1.1 billion cigarette smokers (World Bank 1999; World Health Organization 2008a). In fact tobacco is the leading preventable cause of death and a risk factor in six of the eight leading causes of death worldwide (World Health Organization 2008a).

These statistics can become numbing by their almost incomprehensible magnitude. So it becomes important to frame the challenge and our focus constructively. When I became the United States' spokesperson for AIDS in the early years of the epidemic, I said we were fighting a disease and not the people who have it. For tobacco use, however, I have to say that we are fighting the diseases of tobacco and the purveyors of the products who knowingly have spread disease, disability, and death throughout the world. We should not ostracize those who have been harmed the most, namely, tobacco-addicted persons, but rather should work with them to reduce their risk of disease and to prevent the further spread of this deadly affliction.

Insofar as the vector that spreads the disease is Big Tobacco, the major challenge is to isolate and contain it. This will not be easy. Big Tobacco enjoys unparalleled protections from legal recourse, and possesses enormous political influence and economic power that it is willing to use to undermine public health efforts (Hilts 1996; Orey 1999; Kessler 2000). In addition, it sells a highly addictive product that, ironically, makes many of its most debilitated consumers its strongest supporters (Taylor 1984; Kluger 1996; Givel and Glantz 2001). By way of contrast, there are probably few malaria afflicted persons who would fight for their 'right' to continue to be exposed to the mosquitoes spreading these disease, nor are HIV afflicted persons lobbying for the right of other persons to wilfully afflict others with the disease, but there is a 'smokers rights' movement which must be appropriately addressed and hopefully recruited to the side of public health.

The enormity and complexity of the public health assault demands a broad and sophisticated public health response. I would like to take this opportunity to briefly comment on what I believe should be our vision for health, and how we can achieve it. I will begin with a few additional comments on how we got to this place in the epidemic because understanding these issues is crucial whenever addressing the problem.

Historical perspective

Tobacco use and addiction have existed for centuries, and there surely was resultant death and disease (Corti 1931; US DHHS 1989). However, tobacco-based mass destruction of life around the planet was only possible with the emergence of multinational companies capable of daily making and distributing billions of units of the most destructive of all forms of tobacco – the cigarette. Further, the modern cigarette has extraordinary toxic and addictive capability: its increasingly smooth and alkaline smoke both enabled and required inhalation of the toxins deep into the lungs to maximize nicotine absorption.

In the early days of the industry's growth, tobacco manufacturing and selling might have appeared to be a legitimate form of consumer product development and marketing. There were, however, two important distinctions between legitimate consumer marketing and the tobacco industry that were not generally recognized until decades after the industry was well entrenched into the economic, political, and cultural framework of many countries. The first distinction was clearly appreciated by the first modern cigarette marketers. This was that, following a few occasions of smoking, many cigarette smokers would come to be as addicted to their daily fix of tobacco as other drug addicts become to their form of narcotic, and the industry discovered that nicotine was critical to this process (US DHHS 1988; Slade *et al.* 1995; Hurt and Robertson 1998; Kessler 2000). The second distinction was that cigarette smoking carried a substantial risk of lung cancer, as discovered in the pioneering studies of Richard Doll, Alton Ochsner, Ernst Wynder, and others in the 1950s (Wynder 1997).

The cigarette companies hid much of their knowledge of the addiction issue and disputed the possibility that cigarette smoking was addictive until recently (Sharfstein 1999; Kessler 2000; Henningfield *et al.* 2006). The industry addressed the lung cancer issue head on in the press with their *Frank Statement to Cigarette Smokers*, published in major newspapers in 1954. In this statement, Big Tobacco disputed the link between cigarette smoking and lung cancer, accepted an interest in people's health as a basic responsibility, and pledged to cooperate closely with public health experts, among other long ago broken promises. Such strategies enabled Big Tobacco to buy time, buy influence over politicians, buy exemptions of their products from consumer product laws intended to minimize unnecessary harms from other products, and even to buy questionable science in an effort to undermine or at least complicate interpretation of the science which damned their products (Taylor 1984; White 1988; Kluger 1996; Hilts 1996; Hirschhorn 2000; Hirschhorn *et al.* 2000).

In the 1960s, the US Federal Trade Commission (FTC) tried to provide consumers with a means of selecting presumably less toxic products and cigarette companies with an incentive to make such products. The Commission adopted a cigarette testing method originally developed by the American Tobacco Company (Bradford *et al.* 1936), and later recognized as the FTC method for measuring tar and nicotine levels (National Cancer Institute 1996, 2001). Big Tobacco responded by developing creative methods to circumvent the test in order to enable consumers to continue to readily expose themselves to high levels of tar and nicotine with 'elastic' cigarette designs, and then to thwart efforts to constructively revise the testing methods (National Cancer Institute 1996, 2001; Wilkenfeld *et al.* 2000). The FTC method was codified internationally as the International Standards Organization (ISO) method and Big Tobacco globally extended its deadly game of deception of its consumers, and obfuscation of efforts to provide meaningful information about the nicotine and toxin deliveries of its products (World Health Organization 2001; Bialous and Yach 2001).

It was not until the 1990s that the American Cancer Society (Thun and Burns 2001) and National Cancer Institute (1996) recognized that the intended benefits of so-called 'reduced tar' or 'light' cigarettes were virtually nonexistent, and that the marketing of these products may have actually impaired public health by undermining tobacco use prevention and cessation efforts (Stratton *et al.* 2000; National Cancer Institute 2001; Wilkenfeld et al. 2000). By 1996, the US Federal Trade Commission recognized that its cigarette testing method, which provided a presumed objective basis for categorizing cigarettes as light and low tar, was flawed and needed revision; the Food and Drug Administration (FDA) concurred (National Cancer Institute 1996; Food and Drug Administration 1995, 1996). But there was no strong regulatory oversight over tobacco, and apparently no clear regulatory authority over this issue and it was not until 2008 that the FTC finally rescinded the method and with very strong words: 'Our action today ensures that tobacco companies may not wrap their misleading tar and nicotine ratings in a cloak of government sponsorship. Simply put, the FTC will not be a smokescreen for tobacco companies' shameful marketing practices' (Federal Trade Commission 2008). The FDA, with its new found authority to regulate tobacco will now have the charge to develop methods of communicating tobacco product ingredients, risks, and exposure levels in a meaningful way to consumers. Globally, the World Health Organization has made clear that the ISO cigarette test method is flawed and must be replaced (WHO 2002).

Hopefully armed with the WHO Framework Convention on Tobacco Control (FCTC), such misleading testing and labelling will be abolished worldwide and replaced with meaningful testing and communications. This is vital if we are to reverse the course of the tobacco epidemic. We can never let history repeat itself. As Big Tobacco, and small tobacco companies, attempt to entice us with the false promises of their new generations of so-called reduced risk products (Slade 2000; Fairclough 2000), we must be at least as sceptical as we would of pharmaceutical and food products sold on the basis of their health claims (explicit or implied). *Scientific proof to the satisfaction of an empowered agency such as the Food and Drug Administration* must be the gold standard for reduced risk or other health claims made by the tobacco industry throughout the world. This standard should apply to claims including those implied through the use of terms such 'reduced risk'. Meeting the standard should be required prior to the marketing of any new brand of cigarettes and any new type of tobacco product with such claims.

My vision for tobacco and health in the twenty-first century

My vision for the future is simple and achievable: To improve global health by drastically reducing the risk of disease and premature death in existing tobacco users and by severing the pipeline of tomorrow's tobacco users. I turn your attention to a figure (Fig. 1) developed by the World Bank (1999) projecting mortality from the twentieth century to 2050. This figure illustrates the grim current course. What gives us hope for the future is the powerful effect of reducing disease by smoking cessation. The benefit would be apparent within a few years because there is a dramatic reduction in risk of heart disease evident within 1–2 years of smoking cessation. I believe it is within our reach to do much better than the effect predicted by the World Bank but the public health community will need to marshal powerful political allies or the impact will be much less than that projected in the figure. We need to make it as easy to get treatment for tobacco addiction as it is to get the disease.

In addition to the dramatic impact of smoking cessation, is the delayed but powerful beneficial effect of preventing initiation. It is delayed because the main increase in mortality does not begin until about age 50. Therefore, the effect of prevention will be apparent about 30–50 years later, the age at which smoking caused diseases begin to escalate dramatically. Here again I am not satisfied with a goal of 50% reduction of initiation, because I think we can do better. If we look at the results of tobacco prevention and cessation efforts in California and Massachusetts during the

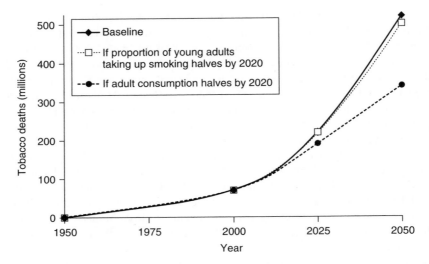

Figure 1 Projecting mortality from the twentieth century to 2050.

1990s we see that smoking initiation and prevalence can be reduced, and it is reasonable to predict even stronger results if the efforts and expenditures were more commensurate with the magnitude of the health problem caused by tobacco (CDC 1999b; CDC 2000). I also would point out that Fig. 1 shows only premature mortality. It does not include the important and more rapid benefits of preventing initiation in terms of projected missed days of school, and lost work productivity due to diseases that may not be life threatening, but can be debilitating and account for unnecessary suffering. Of course, the greatest effect on smoking prevalence in the near and long term would be from the simultaneous reduction of initiation and increase in cessation that could have synergistic effects (Farkas *et al.* 1999). Regulation of tobacco products has the potential to further contribute to prevention and cessation efforts as I discuss further on.

One of the most important loci for preventing initiation and fostering cessation early in the trajectory of addiction is the family. My vision for twenty-first century tobacco control includes the family as a vital potential asset in breaking the cycle of tobacco addiction. My own professional practice and interests are derived from my own family roots, and fortunately it was a family that did not support tobacco use. Many other youth are not so fortunate. We need to engage family health practitioners and counsellors to treat tobacco use as importantly as they urge the use of sanitary practices with food and water, good general hygiene, immunization, wearing seatbelts, and protection from mosquitoes in malaria-plagued regions. It is not just to discourage smoking among the children; parents must be encouraged to quit smoking and their efforts supported with treatment because this is a powerful force in reducing the uptake of smoking in their children. Parents must not allow smoking in the home, because such smoking not only sends a message to children that smoking is all right, such secondhand exposure contributes to asthma and other respiratory disease and is a leading cause of sudden infant death syndrome. Smoking also contributes to the cycle of poverty and deprivation as the smoker diverts vital family resources to support this deadly addiction (WHO 2004).

I believe my vision is possible because we already have the science foundation to support substantial progress. We know enough to predict significant reductions in risk through substantial increases in smoking cessation (World Bank 1999; US DHHS 1989). We have treatments, both behavioural and pharmacological, that can help people quit smoking at far less cost per person and far greater cost-benefit than treatment costs of many of the diseases caused by tobacco (World Bank 1999; Cromwell *et al.* 1997). We know that prevention of initiation of tobacco use can be accomplished with comprehensive educational programmes that increase awareness of the harms, decrease access, and increase the point of purchase costs through increased tobacco taxes (FDA 1995, 1996; Kessler *et al.* 1996; Chaloupka *et al.* 2001; Bachman *et al.* 2002). We have a solid scientific foundation to move forward and to make considerable progress in the US and globally (WHO 2001).

Realizing the vision

I have already touched upon some of the elements that will be critical to realize my vision for the twenty-first century and many other potential features are discussed in this volume. At this point, I would like to make some general observations that I think are particularly important to focus our efforts on so that we may achieve our goals.

First, we have to understand that we are fighting disease and Big Tobacco, not cigarette smokers. We have to isolate and contain Big Tobacco interests in the interest of health. We have to fight for the resources to support the science that is yet needed and to support the application of its lessons to protect those who do not use tobacco products, to serve those who are addicted, and those who will yet become addicted. We need to work to keep our political leaders on the right path, or the powerful interests of Big Tobacco will surely steer them wrongly.

As I have written before, we will have to channel outrage to ensure that, from local communities to the global community, we do not become complacent. Our tasks will consume all the energy we can muster (Koop 1998a). Consider that on the backs of the approximately 50 million smokers in the United States alone, lawsuit settlements generated a potential monetary pipeline approaching 10 billion US dollars per year for 25 years. But across the nation, the percentage of these funds that is being used to contain Big Tobacco, to prevent initiation, and to treat the addicted is in the single digits. The decisions to divert the vast majority of those funds have been unconscionably wrong and I continue to wonder at the relative absence of outrage at this fact (Koop 1998a, b). Perhaps I should not be surprised because, as I have reviewed previously secret documents from Big Tobacco, I have seen that this is not only an evil industry, it is also one that has ensnared its potential political, regulatory, and legal adversaries as tightly as it has the consumers of its products.

Moving forward will require us to build linkages to isolate and contain Big Tobacco. The linkages we need are many and varied. Global, country, community, and organizational linkages are needed to coordinate policy and political efforts. Linkages among research, education, and service are important to maximize their yield.

In addition to linkages, there is much about the process of initiation and maintenance of tobacco addiction that needs to be considered if we are to more effectively prevent and treat it. We need to consider racial, gender, age-related, cultural, and philosophical issues to prevent tobacco use just as Big Tobacco exploits these same characteristics to initiate the use of its products. We need to appreciate the fact that once exposed to the pernicious effects of tobacco-delivered nicotine, the structure and function of the brain begins to change such that tobacco use is not a simple adult choice. It is, in part, a behavioural response to deeply entrenched physiological drives created by years of daily exposure to nicotine during the years of adolescent neural plasticity. This means that tobacco users will need education to guide their decisions and, often, treatment support, to act upon them. Addiction to tobacco-delivered nicotine should be considered the primary disease to which the major causes of morbidity and premature mortality are secondary. We should treat it no less seriously than we treat consequences such as lung cancer and heart disease, because treatment of addiction may help avoid the subsequent need for treatment of lung cancer and heart disease. In fact, such efforts will support prevention because the children of parents who quit smoking are half as likely to initiate and twice as likely to try quitting if they have already begun (Farkas *et al.* 1999).

Our prevention and containment messages need to move people to action. Decades of research show that perception of harm is a major determinant of use and addiction to drugs ranging from tobacco to cocaine and marijuana (Bachman *et al.* 2002). Messages that generate emotion convey information about the harms that are meaningful to the targeted populations, and messages that challenge the myths that have been foisted upon the public by Big Tobacco need to become as ubiquitous as Big Tobacco's lies. More than 'tobacco kills', we need consumer-tested messages to ensure that every individual understands that using tobacco impairs quality of life. Similarly, policy-makers should care about reduced productivity and economic viability of the workforce, if not the economics of tobacco-caused disease (Warner 2000).

Our efforts to communicate the relevant reasons for freedom from tobacco will be countered by Big Tobacco, and we must resolve to never again let its false and misleading statements go unanswered. We need a strong voice to ensure that policy-makers know the truth about the tobacco products of today and tomorrow. We are beginning to see the twenty-first century version of 'low tar' cigarettes from the tobacco industry – new products with even stronger allusions to reduced risk with even less precedent upon which to base policy and reaction. We must not forget the lessons of the twentieth-century products and product promotions that were intended, by Big Tobacco, to address smokers concerns even as they perpetuated the pipeline of death and disease (Kessler 2000). The release of the tobacco industry documents has been a treasure trove for tobacco control advocates and policy-makers alike. It is tantamount to cracking the genetic code of the malaria carrying mosquito or the operational plans of an illicit drug smuggling ring. This inside knowledge does not make our course of actions as clear or as easy as we would like, but it provides a sobering view of what we are up against and what kinds of challenges we face.

Although the major global killers are major brands of cigarettes from multinational tobacco companies, we have seen how small companies and local tobacco product makers are important contributors to the tobacco epidemic, as we have seen documented so well in the South East Asia Nations (India Ministry of Health and Family Welfare 2004), and increasingly in many forms including the powerful emergence of roll-your own tobacco products, in Germany, waterpipe use on college campuses throughout the world as well as the Middle Eastern Region (WHO 2005, 2006); and increasingly, all manner of unregulated nicotine delivery systems whose contaminants we have no present way of even knowing. These new forms of products include lozenges from tobacco companies, nicotine liquids and gels, and electronic nicotine delivery systems commonly sold as 'electronic cigarettes' in shopping malls throughout the United States, and by proliferation retail vendors and the Internet globally (WHO 2006, 2008b). It is sobering how fast such products have emerged and proliferated just since the publication of the first edition of this book in 2004. All tobacco products and all forms of nicotine delivery must be subject to regulation nationally and globally. Marketing must not be allowed to undermine tobacco prevention and cessation efforts nor should the products contribute to death and disease through their own toxic effects or by enabling perpetuation of tobacco use in individuals who use them when smoking and other forms of tobacco use are prohibited.

Getting the message out

I would like to propose a strategy for ensuring that public perceptions will begin to reflect the truth about tobacco. The experience in California and elsewhere has shown that effective public education strategies can mobilize action and reduce smoking (Balbach and Glantz 1998). To be effective however, *we need to know who the public is, how the public can use our expertise, and what the public should know.*

Who?

The public is a diverse patchwork of cultures, each with special languages, values, norms, and expectations. I propose that at least one-third of our strategic planning and daily endeavours be devoted to understanding cultural diversity, protecting human dignity, and helping each 'public' develop its own means to become free of tobacco disease.

How?

We can take as a starting point that the information and emotions held by consumers with respect to tobacco products are heavily derived from explicit advertising and implicit purchasing of good will by Big Tobacco, such as its 'philanthropic' efforts to sponsor sporting events, entertainment, charities, and, in some countries, public street signs and traffic signals. Following well-accepted principles of advertising, our message must be simple, consistent, pervasive, repetitious, and delivered through many sources. It must be framed so that it is interesting and relevant to the intended listeners. Although our motivation may be to reverse the course of death and disease, our message should be upbeat and provide hope and opportunity, not death and disease.

We must engage all manner of organizations that provide for society and its well-being. Even as the tobacco industry has attempted to subvert various organizations, we must reclaim them to serve humanity and to help disseminate messages of freedom from tobacco and its attendant diseases. There can be no place for turf wars or divisive exercise if we are to maximize effectiveness. Unity should be the watchword from the level of local community organizations to the WHO. To reach the diversity of smokers, we must enlist the support of a diversity of organizations as measured by culture, ethnicity, and even those with entirely different purposes ranging from religious organizations to hobby industries to the entertainment industry.

What?

We need more focused themes that can be effectively communicated. The public needs to know that good health and quality of life are taken away by tobacco and are achieved through its avoidance. The public needs to know that the so-called economic benefits of tobacco to society are naught and that stronger economic health at the individual and national level is possible without tobacco. The public needs to know that commercial speech in the form of advertising is appropriately held to standards of truth and scientific proof, even within the context of freedom of speech. The public needs honest information about the ingredients and design features of their products presented in a regulated manner so that, under the guise of full disclosure, the industry is not given new tools to promote their products (Gray 2006, 2009; WHO 2007). Finally, the public needs to know that the tobacco industry does not represent business as usual. Big Tobacco has stepped beyond the bounds of all but the most unethical of business practices. This has been evident though the disclosure of previously secret documents and through litigation by State Attorneys General in the United States and elsewhere.

A place for harm reduction?

Much of public health can be viewed as efforts to reduce disease prevalence and severity by reducing exposures to pathogens, and by treating those exposed. In principle, this approach could be applied to reduce the death and disability caused by tobacco in ongoing tobacco users. This has been discussed elsewhere with respect to tobacco (Food and Drug Law Institute 1998; Warner *et al.* 1998; Stratton *et al.* 2000; Henningfield and Fagerstrom 2001; Warner 2001) and in this volume. It is certainly among the most controversial elements among potential strategies for reducing the risk of death and disease in tobacco users who, despite our best efforts, will be unable to completely abstain from tobacco. We should not ignore their plight any more than the plight of the person who has contracted a tobacco caused disease. After all, their volitional control over their tobacco use may be little different than their volitional control over the expression of cancer in their bodies. Furthermore, if we can reduce their risk of disease despite aspects of their behaviour that we cannot control are we not better off, both as a global community, and as individuals? Here again, I draw upon my experience with the HIV epidemic in the United States. Before we were even certain that a virus was the etiological culprit, I, as the nation's Surgeon General, advocated strategies to reduce the spread of the disease, strategies ranging from the use of condoms to drug abuse treatment. Despite our best efforts, we could not eliminate risky sex or drug abuse, but we were able to reduce the spread of the disease by reducing the risk of transmission (Bullers 2001).

The problem with harm reduction approaches is that many pose theoretical benefits to a few individuals along with real and theoretical risks to many others. This was the experience with smokeless tobacco products in the United States in which a relative few recalcitrant cigarette smokers may have switched from cigarettes to snuff, incurring theoretical (but as yet uncertain) disease reduction; while at the same time a new epidemic of smokeless tobacco use exploded on the backs of young boys who happened to be athletes (US DHHS 1986). In this domain, I concur with the general conclusions of the Institute of Medicine report which concluded, in essence, that although there is great potential to reduce disease by harm reduction methods, none have yet been studied adequately to allow their promotion, and those promoted by tobacco companies in particular, carry substantial risks of worsening the total public health picture by undermining prevention and cessation (Stratton et al. 2000). This is also an area in which our science needs to be substantially expanded because, at present, the main body of knowledge pertaining to the potential health effects of tobacco product design and ingredients manipulations seems to reside within Big Tobacco. They are a proven unreliable source of complete and accurate information. In the future we cannot be held hostage to such a state of affairs. If there is a place for harm reduction, it should be within a regulated framework that holds health, and not monetary profit, at the forefront and with planning for not only the short-term consequences, but the mid-term and long-term, looking toward the twenty-second century and beyond (Fiore and Baker 2009; Gray 2009; Gray et al. 2005; Gray and Henningfield 2004; Zeller *et al.* 2009).

Concluding comments

I have a vision for public health that is optimistic and realistic. In my lifetime, I have seen the rise and fall of epidemics and I have come to believe that well-intentioned men and women, motivated by a will to serve, and guided by science, can control disease and eradicate plagues. Unlike other epidemics, the disease of tobacco addiction and its many life-threatening accompaniments has an important ally in Big Tobacco. But no form of institutionalized evil can perpetuate itself for long when the truth about its intentions and methods becomes known. Therefore, it is realistic to believe that we will turn the tide on this epidemic. We will isolate and contain Big Tobacco and we will see the decline of tobacco-caused disease and disability. We have the foundation to make tobacco-caused disease history, and the dawn of the next century a time that once again will see lung cancer a relative rarity.

Greed has never been considered a virtue, but greed that flourishes at the expense of the destruction of millions of lives a year has stepped over a line in personal morality and ethics. Such greed is infectious and pervasive and in the tobacco industry extends into the realm of stockholders, as evidenced by the fact that those who hold large portfolios of investments such as colleges, universities, pension plants, etc, by keeping investments in tobacco stock, have convinced themselves that the rules of the marketplace override separation from evil if a profit is to be made. President Reagan called the Soviet Union, 'the evil empire' and President George W. Bush referred to Iraq, Iran, and North Korea, as 'the axis of evil'. Yet these entities to whom evils were attributed didn't kill 400 000 of US citizens or millions of our global brethren each year. The evil empire is Big Tobacco and unlike military and political enemies who say, 'I intend to kill you if I can', Big Tobacco disguised its evil with the invitation to light up and become alive with pleasure.

There are those who believe we can negotiate with Big Tobacco, and others who believe that the only way to bring Big Tobacco to its knees is to destroy it as it presently exists. I question whether the first aforementioned tactic will ever work, but with due diligence, the second tactic might work under carefully orchestrated circumstances. In days of yore, when military combatants protected themselves with suits of armour, combat was at close quarters, and frequently hand-to-hand. You destroyed your enemy by finding the chink in his armour and through it you thrust your spear, shot your arrow, or guided your sword or your dagger.

Isn't it time that public health people united, studied the armour of Big Tobacco carefully, found the chinks therein, and acted accordingly? The tobacco enemy is big, powerful, extraordinarily wealthy, and has learned to practice its deceitful ways over half a century, but the one thing they do not have on their side is righteousness. I do believe that in the long run Big Tobacco can be brought to its knees with the combined righteous outrage of the citizens of the world. This will require those diverse supporters of tobacco control and public health to work together despite differences of opinion over strategies that in some cases are healthy, and in any case will persist.

There is a joke that public health professionals tend to unite by 'circling the wagons and shooting in'. I think this represents the approach and anticipates the consequences of recent debates over harm reduction, regulation, and other issues that have replaced civil and potentially constructive discourse and debate with sloganeering and questions of morality and purpose of those who disagree. Such energy should be channelled constructively into guiding, and not undermining, some potentially powerful assets. These include WHO FCTC, which is coming into force and which the United States needs to ratify (WHO 2009a). It includes consensus-building, such as occurred through the Strategic Dialogue process addressing harm reduction in the United States (Zeller et al. 2009). It includes an emerging global tobacco product testing network established by the WHO (WHO 2009b).

In the United States, our newest asset in tobacco control, hardly imaginable just a few years ago, is the regulatory authority granted to the United States FDA over tobacco. Like any act of Congress this one is not perfect but it has the tools to reduce the addictiveness of tobacco products by reducing (albeit not eliminating entirely) nicotine to non-addictive levels, and by the reduction or elimination of other ingredients and emissions. It will ban the use of candy-like flavourings and could lead to the elimination of substances including menthol, chocolate and other additives that appear to contribute to tobacco use, addiction, and disease. It has the potential to make ever clearer to every user of tobacco just how deadly and addictive the products are. This could be a powerful asset to prevention and cessation efforts. But the FDA will need to be guided by a constant input from public health scientists and other health professionals. I am encouraged by the statement of the new leadership at FDA that the agency will keep its role as contributor to public health as its foremost driving force (Hamburg and Sharfstein 2009). Such focus will be vital if the FDA's regulation of tobacco is to realize its potential in tobacco control. I urge my public health colleagues, nationally and globally, to help FDA achieve that laudable goal by keeping FDA well informed of the consequences of its regulation, desired and undesired.

Of course none of this will be easy and we do not have all the answers to the questions before us. Never has so deadly an epidemic been so well protected by intertwined commercial and political interests. But never has so deadly a commercial empire faced so many assaults on so many fronts. I do believe in the ultimate triumph of right over wrong. The tobacco industry has been blatantly and reprehensibly wrong for much of the twentieth century and is attempting to extend that record into thetwenty-first, but it will not succeed. Now that the truth has leaked out through documents, through research, and through testimony in the courtroom, the clock cannot be turned back and their denials will not hold. Good people will not allow the lies to stand, nor the destructive course to be stayed. Good and dedicated people need to work together, from the voluntary workers in the charitable organizations, to the public health leaders, and to many leading politicians who increasingly are refusing to take tobacco money and are willing to stand up for public health. The challenge will not be easy but the there is a public health path and I predict that many will follow it.

As a doctor and as the nation's Surgeon General, I learned to be guided by scientific truth even as I was motivated by basic principles of justice and service to humanity. My appraisal of the state of the science confirms that reducing tobacco-caused disease is an achievable goal, and that continued research can be the supportive companion of our public health efforts. When the history of the twenty-first century is written, I believe it will be observed that its dawn was the beginning of the end for Big Tobacco and its diseases, and that by its end, lung cancer was once again relegated to the status of a rare disease.

Acknowledgement

I thank Jack E. Henningfield for his assistance in development of this manuscript.

References

Bachman, J.G., O'Malley, P.M., Schulenberg, J.E., Johnston, L.D., Bryant, A.L., and Merline, A.C. (2002). *The Decline of Substance Abuse in Young Adulthood*. Mahwah, New Jersey: Lawrence Erlbaum Associates, Publishers.

Balbach, E.D. and Glantz, S.A. (1998). Tobacco control advocates must demand high-quality media campaigns: the California experience. *Tobacco Control*, 7:397–408.

Bialous, S.A. and Yach, D. (2001). Whose standard is it, anyway? How the tobacco industry determines the International Organization for Standardization (ISO) standards for tobacco and tobacco products. *Tobacco Control*, 10:96–104.

Bradford, J.A., Harlan, W.R., and Hanmer, H.R. (1936). Nature of cigarette smoke. Technic of experimental smoking. *Industrial Engineering and Chemistry*, 28:836–839.

Bullers, A.C. (2001). Living with AIDS – 20 years later. *FDA Consumer*, November to December (www.fda.gov/fdac/features/2001/601_aids.html).

Centers for Disease Control and Prevention. (1999a). Ten great public health achievements – United States, 1900–1999. *Morbidity and Mortality Weekly Report*, 48(12):241–243.

Centers for Disease Control and Prevention. (1999b). *Best practices for comprehensive tobacco control programs, August*.

Centers for Disease Control and Prevention. (2000). Declines in lung cancer rates – California, 1988–1997. *Morbidity and Mortality Weekly Report*, 49(47):1066–1069.

Chaloupka, F.J., Wakefield, M., and Czart, C. (2001). Taxing tobacco: the impact of tobacco taxes on cigarette smoking and other tobacco use. In R.L. Raabin, S.D. Sugarman (Eds), *Regulating Tobacco* (pp.39–71). New York, NY: Oxford University Press.

Cromwell, J., Bartosch, W.J., Fiore, M.C., Hasselblad, V., and Baker, T. (1997). Cost-effectiveness of the clinical practice recommendations in the AHCPR guideline for smoking cessation. *Journal of the American Medical Association*, **278**:1759–1766.

Corti, C. (1931). *A History of Smoking*. London: George G. Harrap & Co. Ltd.

Fairclough, G. (2000). Smoking's next battleground. *Wall Street Journal*, B1&B4.

Farkas, A.J., Distefan, J.M., Choi, W.S., Gilpin, E.A., and Pierce, J.P. (1999). Does parental smoking cessation discourage adolescent smoking?. *Preventive Medicine*, **28**:213–218.

Federal Trade Commission. (2008). FTC rescinds guidance from 1966 on statements concerning tar and nicotine yields, (Accessed 15 June 2009 http://www.ftc.gov/opa/2008/11/cigarettetesting.shtm).

Fiore, M.C. and Baker, TB. (2009). Stealing a march in the 21st century: accelerating progress in the 100-year war against tobacco addiction in the United States. *American Journal of Public Health*, **99**: 1170–1175.

Food and Drug Administration. (1995). Regulations restricting the sale and distribution of cigarettes and smokeless tobacco products to protect children and adolescents; proposed rule analysis regarding FDA's jurisdiction over nicotine-containing cigarettes and smokeless tobacco products; notice. *Federal Register*, **60**:41314–41792.

Food and Drug Administration. (1996). Regulations restricting the sale and distribution of cigarettes and smokeless tobacco to protect children and adolescents; final rule. *Federal Register*, **61**:44396–45318.

Food and Drug Law Institute. (1998). Special Issue. Tobacco dependence: innovative regulatory approaches to reduce death and disease. *Food and Drug Law Journal*, **53**(Supplement):1–137.

Garrett, B.E., Rose, C.A., and Henningfield, J.E. (2001). Tobacco addiction and pharmacological interventions. *Expert Opinion in Pharmacotherapy*, **2**:1545–1555.

George, T.P. and O'Malley, S.S. (2004). Current pharmacological treatments for nicotine dependence. *Trends in Pharmacological Sciences*, **25**:42–48.

Givel, M.S. and Glantz, S.A. (2001). Tobacco lobby political influence on US state legislatures in the 1990s. *Tobacco Control*, **10**:124–134.

Henningfield, J.E. and Fagerstrom, K.O. (2001). Swedish match company, Swedish snus and public health: a harm reduction experiment in progress?. *Tobacco Control*, **10**:253–257.

Gray, N. (2006). The consequences of the unregulated cigarette. *Tobacco Control*, **15**:405–408.

Gray, N. (2009). Global tobacco control policy. In P. Boyle, N. Gray, J. Henningfield, J. Seffrin, and W. Zatonski (Eds) *Tobacco and Public Health: Science and Policy*. Oxford University Press, Oxford, Present Edition.

Gray, N.J. and Henningfield, J.E. (2004). A long-term view of harm reduction. *Nicotine and Tobacco Research*, **6**:759–764.

Gray, N., Henningfield, J.E., Benowitz, N.L., Connolly, G.N., Dresler, C., Fagerstrom, K.O., *et al.* (2005). Toward a comprehensive long term nicotine policy. *Tobacco Control*, **14**:161–165.

Hamburg, M.A. and Sharfstein, J.M. (2009). The FDA as a public health agency. *The New England Journal of Medicine*, **360**:2493–2495.

Henningfield, J.E., Rose, C.A., and Zeller, M. (2006). Tobacco industry litigation position on addiction: continued dependence on past views. *Tobacco Control*, **15**(Supplement IV):iv27–iv36.

Hilts, P.J. (1996). *Smokescreen: The Truth Behind the Tobacco Industry Cover*-Up. Reading, Massachusetts: Addison-Wesley Publishing Company.

Hirschhorn, N. (2000). Shameful science: four decades of the German tobacco industry's hidden research on smoking and health. *Tobacco Control*, **9**:242–247.

Hirschhorn, N, Bialous, S.A., and Shatenstein, S. (2000). Phillip Morris' new scientific initiative: an analysis. *Tobacco Control*, **10**:247–252.

Hurt, R.D. and Robertson, C.R. (1998). Prying open the door to the tobacco industry's secrets about nicotine: the Minnesota Tobacco Trial. *Journal of the American Medical Association*, **280**:1173–1181.

India Ministry of Health and Welfare. (2004). In K.S. Reddy and P.C. Gupta (Eds) *Report on Tobacco Control in India*. New Delhi, Ministry of Health and Welfare.

Kessler, D.A. (2000). *A Question of Intent: a Great American Battle with a Deadly Industry*. New York, NY: Public Affairs.

Kessler, D.A., Witt, A.M., Barnett, P.S., Zeller, M.R., Natanblut, S.L., Wilkenfeld, J.P., *et al.* (1996). The Food and Drug Administration's regulation of tobacco products. *New England Journal of Medicine*, **335**:988–994.

Kluger, R. (1996). *Ashes to Ashes*. New York: Alfred A. Knopf.

Koop, C.E. (1998a). The tobacco scandal: where is the outrage?. *Tobacco Control*, **7**:393–396.

Koop, C.E. (1998b). Don't forget the smokers. *Washington Post*, Sunday, March 8, C7.

National Cancer Institute. (1996). *The FTC cigarette test method for determining tar, nicotine, and carbon monoxide yields of US cigarettes: report of the NCI expert committee. Smoking and tobacco control monograph No.7*. Bethesda, MD: US Department of Health and Human Services, National Institutes of Health, National Cancer Institute.

National Cancer Institute. (2001). *Risks associated with smoking cigarettes with low*-machine *measured yields of tar and nicotine. Smoking and Tobacco Control Monograph No. 13*. Bethesda, MD: US Department of Health and Human Services, National Institutes of Health, National Cancer Institutes, NIH Pub. No. 02-5074.

Orey, M. (1999). *Assuming the Risk: The Mavericks, the Lawyers, and the Whistle-Blowers Who Beat Big Tobacco*. New York: Little, Brown and Company.

Sharfstein, J. (1999). Blowing smoke: how cigarette manufacturers argued that nicotine is not addictive. *Tobacco Control*, **8**:210–213.

Slade, J. (2000). Innovative nicotine delivery devices from tobacco companies. In R. Ferrence, J. Slade, R. Room, and M. Pope (Eds) *Nicotine and Public Health*. (pp. 209–228). Washington, D.C.: American Public Health Association.

Slade, J., Bero, L.A., Hanauer, P., Barnes, D.E., and Glantz, S.A. (1995). Nicotine and addiction. The Brown and Williamson documents. *Journal of the American Medical Association*, **274**:225–233.

Stratton, K., Shetty, P., Wallace, R., and Bondurant, S. (Eds) (2000). *Clearing the Smoke: Assessing the Science Base for Tobacco Harm Reduction*. Washington, D.C.: National Academy Press.

Taylor, P. (1984). *The Smoke Ring*. New York: Pantheon Books.

Thun, M.J. and Burns, D.M. (2001). Health impact of 'reduced yield' cigarettes: a critical assessment of the epidemiological evidence. *Tobacco Control*, **10**(Supplement):i4–11.

US Department of Health and Human Services. (1986). *The Health Consequences of Using Smokeless Tobacco. A Report of the Advisory Committee to the Surgeon General*. Washington, DC: US Department of Health and Human Services, NIH Publication No. 86-2874.

US Department of Health and Human Services. (1988). *The Health Consequences Of Smoking: Nicotine Addiction. A Report of the Surgeon General*. Washington, DC: US Department of Health and Human Services, DHHS Publication No. (CDC) 88-8406.

US Department of Health and Human Services. (1989). *Reducing the Health Consequences of Smoking: 25 Years of Progress. A Report of the Surgeon General*. Washington, DC: US Department of Health and Human Services, DHHS Publication No. (CDC) 89-8411.

Warner, K.E. (2000). The economics of tobacco: myths and realities. *Tobacco Control*, **9**:78–89.

Warner, K.E. (2001). Reducing harm to smokers: methods, their effectiveness, and the role of policy. In R.L. Raabin and S.D. Sugarman (Eds.), *Regulating Tobacco* (pp.111–142). New York, NY: Oxford University Press.

Warner, K.E., Peck, C.C., Woosley, R.L., Henningfield, J.E., and Slade, J. (1998). Preface to Tobacco dependence: innovative regulatory approaches to reduce death and disease. *Food and Drug Law Journal*, **53**(Supplement):1–16.

Wilkenfeld, J., Henningfield, J.E., Slade, J., Burns, D., and Pinney, J.M. (2000). It's time for a change: cigarette smokers deserve meaningful information about their cigarettes. *Journal of the National Cancer Institute*, **92**:90–92.

White, L.C. (1988). *Merchants of Death*. New York: Beech Tree Books.

World Bank. (1999). *Curbing the Epidemic: Governments and the Economics of Tobacco Control*. Washington, DC: World Bank.

World Health Organization. (2001). *Advancing Knowledge on Regulating Tobacco Products*. Geneva: World Health Organization.

World Health Organization. (2002). Scientific Advisory Committee on Tobacco Product Regulation (SACTob) Recommendation on Health Claims derived from ISO/FTC Method to Measure Cigarette Yield. Geneva: World Health Organization.

World Health Organization. (2004). Tobacco and Poverty: A Vicious Circle, Geneva, World Health Organization, (Accessed 15 June 2009 at http://www.who.int/tobacco/communications/events/wntd/2004/en/wntd2004_brochure_en.pdf).

World Health Organization. (2005). Advisory Note Waterpipe Smoking: Health Effects, Research Needs and Recommended Actions by Regulators. Geneva: World Health Organization.

World Health Organization and reviewed and approved through WHO process as an official WHO report. (2006). *Tobacco: Deadly in Any Form or Disguise*, World No Tobacco Day Monograph, WHO, Geneva, (Accessed 15 June 2009 at http://www.who.int/tobacco/communications/events/wntd/2006/Tfi_Rapport.pdf).

World Health Organization. (2007). The Scientific Basis of Tobacco Product Regulation; Report of a WHO Study Group (TobReg). WHO Technical Report Series, No. 945, Geneva.

The MPOWER package. (2008a). Geneva, World Health Organization.

World Health Organization. (2008b). Draft abbreviated advisory of the WHO Study Group on Tobacco Product Regulation (WHO TobReg) concerning electronic nicotine delivery systems (ENDS).

World Health Organization. (2009a). WHO Tobacco Framework Convention on Tobacco Control. Geneva, World Health Organization, (Accessed 15 June 2009 at http://www.who.int/fctc/en/index.html).

World Health Organization. (2009b). Global Tobacco Laboratory Network (TobLabNet) combating the tobacco epidemic. Geneva, World Health Organization, (Accessed 15 June 2009 at http://www.who.int/tobacco/global_interaction/toblabnet/pr_meeting_rio/en/index.html).

Wynder, E.L. (1997). Tobacco as a cause of cancer: Some reflections. *American Journal of Epidemiology*, **146**:687–694.

Zeller, M., Hatsukami, D., Backinger, C., Benowitz, N., Biener, L., Burns D., *et al.* (2009). The strategic dialogue on tobacco harm reduction: a vision and blueprint for action in the United States. *Tobacco Control*, doi:10.1136/tc.2008.027318.

Foreword

We, Peter Boyle, Jack Henningfield, John Seffrin, and Witold A. Zatoński wish to dedicate this book to our co-editor Nigel Gray.

We believe that Nigel Gray is a remarkable man who has made a remarkable contribution to Tobacco Control. Things that we take for granted today, notably the international tobacco movement, were not feasible or popular only a few decades ago. Nigel's contribution to making Tobacco an international issue was fundamental and is encapsulated in the following text found on the web site of the Minnesota Tobacco documents (Document RP4006STMNRED/0007&fn=2023625049-Philip Morris Web Site) and is a biography written for Philip Morris (apparently in 1984).

Nigel Gray MB BS FRACP

It is the Australian, Dr Gray, who appears to have done more than any other individual to bring to bring the anti-tobacco movement together in an international sense, to exert pressure on governments and other influential bodies. Active in the Australian anti-smoking movement since before 1970, the experience with organising the voluntary work of the Victorian Anti Cancer Council clearly showed both the potential and the limits of national volunteer organisations (see his speech at the third World Conference). Starting with the seminal 'Workshop on Smoking and Lung Cancer' in 1976 (which was the first time Gray, Daube, Bjartveit, Ramstrom and Masironi met together in a formal sense), he therefore began to work with and through the UICC as a flexible and single minded international organisation, setting in motion the chain of events which has led to the formation of an International Liaison Group on Smoking and Health with himself as Chairman. The UICC workshops were his idea, and also the Programme on Smoking and Cancer, with what are virtually regional co-ordinators for specific areas; he edited the first and second editions of "Guidelines for Smoking Control". He has done his share of speaking at meetings, of course, but his special contribution is to organise the integration of the disparate elements of the anti-tobacco movement into the most organic whole that it could be, short of being one big centralised body.

Today society benefits greatly from the protection given to non-smokers, the help given to smokers to quit smoking and the assistance available to stop young persons taking up the smoking habit. Laws now are enacted in many countries regarding many aspects of Tobacco Control but this was not the case when Nigel Gray set out to energize and coordinate the international community.

Nigel Gray has had a glorious career and has made a major contribution. He originally is an MBBS, trained in infectious disease, but has received a number of Honorary degrees since (LLD is a Doctor of Law and he has received two of these from Melbourne and Monash Universities). He was awarded the Order of Australia (AO) which is the second highest civilian award from the Australian Government. His major career contributions have been: Director Anti Cancer Council of Victoria 1968–1995; Chairman UICC Tobacco Project/program 1974–1990—organized 70 workshops, mostly in developing countries; President UICC 1994–1998; Architect of Victorian Tobacco Act 1987—originated the idea of hypothecating/earmarking taxes for Health purposes; Deputy Chair Victorian Health Promotion Foundation 1988–1995, where he successfully advocated spending tobacco taxes for health. He was awarded the Luther Terry Award for Tobacco

Control in Chicago in August 2000. In addition he has been a remarkable source of advice and experience in the composition of the European Tobacco Directive, which has been the inspiration for many anti-tobacco laws throughout Europe.

There are very few individuals that can be said to have led successful Public Health movements but certainly Nigel falls into this elite category. Quite simply, there are many people alive today who would otherwise no longer be with us but for the inspirational work of Nigel Gray.

Contents

Contributors

Maribel Almonte
Cancer Research UK Centre for Mathematics,
Statistics and Epidemiology, Wolfson Institute of Preventive Medicine,
Queen Mary University of London, Barts & The London School of Medicine and Dentistry, London, UK

Amanda Amos
Professor of Health Promotion,
UK Centre for Tobacco Control Studies,
Public Health Sciences,
Divison of Community Health Sciences,
University of Edinburgh, UK

Neal L. Benowitz
University of California,
San Francisco, USA

Douglas Bettcher
Director, Tobacco Free Initiative,
World Health Organization,
Geneva, Switzerland

Paolo Boffetta
International Agency for Research on Cancer,
Lyon, France

Jillian Boreham
Senior Research Fellow,
Clinical Trial Service Unit,
Nuffield Department of Clinical Medicine,
Oxford, UK

Ron Borland
The Cancer Council Victoria,
Australia

Peter Boyle
International Prevention Research Institute,
Lyon, France

David M. Burns
Professor Emeritus of Family and Preventive Medicine,
UCSD School of Medicine,
Del Mar, USA

Carrie M. Carpenter
Harvard School of Public Health,
Division of Public Health Practice,
Boston, USA

Simon Chapman
Professor of Public Health,
University of Sydney, Australia

Zhen-Ming Chen
Director, China Program,
Clinical Trial Service Unit,
Nuffield Department of Clinical Medicine,
Oxford, UK

K. Michael Cummings
Roswell Park Cancer Institute,
Buffalo, USA

Jack Cuzick
Cancer Research UK Centre for Mathematics,
Statistics and Epidemiology,
Wolfson Institute of Preventive Medicine,
Queen Mary University of London,
Barts & The London School of Medicine and Dentistry,
London, UK

Richard A. Daynard
Northeastern University School of Law,
Boston, USA

Mirjana V. Djordjevic
Tobacco Control Research Branch,
Behavioral Research Program,
Division of Cancer Control and Population Sciences, National Cancer Institute,
Bethesda, USA

Richard Doll*
Emeritus Professor of Medicine & Honorary
Member, Cancer Studies Unit,
Nuffield Department of Medicine,
Radcliffe Infirmary,
Oxford, UK

Geoffrey Ferris Wayne
Harvard School of Public Health,
Division of Public Health Practice,
Boston, USA

Graham G. Giles
Cancer Epidemiology Centre,
The Cancer Council Victoria,
Australia

Edward Giovannucci
Harvard School of Public Health,
Departments of Nutrition and Epidemiology;
and Channing Laboratory,
Department of Medicine, Brigham and
Women's Hospital and Harvard Medical
School, Boston, USA

Nigel Gray
Honorary Senior Associate,
Cancer Council Victoria,
Australia

Prakash C. Gupta
Director, Healis - Sekhsaria Institute for
Public Health,
Mumbai, India

Allan Hackshaw
Deputy Director,
Cancer Research UK & University College
London Cancer Trials Centre,
London, UK

Dorothy Hatsukami
Masonic Cancer Center,
Department of Psychiatry,
University of Minnesota,
Minneapolis, USA

Stephen S. Hecht
Masonic Cancer Center,
University of Minnesota, USA

S. J. Henley
Department of Epidemiology and
Surveillance Research,
American Cancer Society,
Atlanta, USA

Jack E. Henningfield
Johns Hopkins University School of
Medicine, and Pinney Associates,
Maryland, USA

David Hill
Anti-Cancer Council of Victoria,
Australia

Dietrich Hoffmann
American Health Foundation,
New York, USA

Ilse Hoffmann
American Health Foundation,
New York, USA

Crystal N. Holick
Department of Epidemiology,
Harvard School of Public Health,
Boston, USA

Richard Hurt
Professor of Medicine,
Mayo Clinic Nicotine Dependence Center,
Mayo Clinic,
Rochester, USA

Konrad Jamrozik
Professor of Primary Care Epidemiology,
Imperial College of Science,
Technology and Medicine,
London, UK

Il Soon Kim
Korean Associations of Smoking and Health,
Seoul, Republic of South Korea

Yong-Ik Kim
Department of Health Policy and
Management,
Seoul National University College
of Medicine,
Seoul, Republic of South Korea

* It is with regret that we report the death of Sir
Richard Doll since the publication of the first
edition.

C. Everett Koop
Senior Scholar,
C. Everett Koop Institute,
Dartmouth College,
Hanover, USA

Lynn T. Kozlowski
Department of Biobehavioral Health,
Penn State University, USA

Carlo La Vecchia
Istituto di Ricerche Farmacologiche
"Mario Negri", Milan, Italy

Areti Lagiou
Faculty of Health Professions,
Athens Technological Educational Institute,
Greece

Qing Lan
Division of Epidemiology and Genetics,
National Cancer Institute,
Bethesda, USA

Jin Soo Lee
Research Institute and Hospital,
National Cancer Center,
Goyang, Republic of South Korea

Jong-Koo Lee
Korea Center for Disease Control
and Prevention,
Seoul, Republic of South Korea

Maria Leon-Roux
Lifestyle and Cancer Group,
International Agency for Research on Cancer,
Lyon, France

Fabio Levi
Registres Vaudois et Neuchâtelois des
Tumeurs, Institut universitaire de médecine
sociale et preventive,
Centre Hospitalier Universitaire Vaudois,
Lausanne, Switzerland

Albert B. Lowenfels
Professor of Surgery,
New York Medical College,
New York, USA

Vera Luiza da Costa e Silva
Senior Public Health Consultant,
Rio de Janeiro, Brazil

Judith Mackay
Senior Advisor,
World Lung Foundation, and
Director, Asian Consultancy on
Tobacco Control,
Kowloon,
Hong Kong

Patrick Maisonneuve
Division of Epidemiology and
Biostatistics,
European Institute of Oncology,
Milan, Italy

Marta Mańczuk
Division of Epidemiology and
Cancer Prevention,
Center and Institute of Oncology,
Warsaw, Poland

Raman Minhas
Technical Officer, WHO Tobacco Free
Initiative,
World Health Organization,
Geneva, Switzerland

Eva Negri
Istituto di Ricerche Farmacologiche
"Mario Negri",
Milan, Italy

Richard J. O'Connor
Department of Biobehavioral Health,
Penn State University, USA

Dae-Kyu Oh
The Health Promotion Bureau at the
Ministry of Health,
Welfare, Gender Equality and Family,
Seoul, Republic of South Korea

Patricia H. Owens
Department of Epidemiology and
Public Health,
Yale University School of Medicine,
New Haven, USA

Mark Parascandola
Epidemiologist,
Tobacco Control Research Branch,
National Cancer Institute,
Bethesda, USA

Jae-Gahb Park
Cancer Research Institute and Cancer
Research Center,
Seoul National University,
Seoul, Republic of South Korea

Ji Won Park
Research Institute and Hospital,
National Cancer Center,
Goyang, Republic of South Korea

Richard Peto
Clinical Trial Service Unit and
Epidemiological Studies Unit (CTSU),
Radcliffe Infirmary,
Oxford, UK

John P. Pierce
Professor of Cancer Research and
Associate Director for Cancer Prevention
and Control, UCSD Cancer Center,
California, USA

Cecily S. Ray
Research Fellow, Healis - Sekhsaria Institute
for Public Health, Mumbai, India

Robyn L. Richmond
School of Public Health and
Community Medicine,
The University of New South Wales,
Kensington, Australia

Harvey A. Risch
Department of Epidemiology and
Public Health,
Yale University School of Medicine,
New Haven, USA

Channing Robertson
Department of Chemical Engineering,
Stanford University, USA

Thomas E. Rohan
Department of Epidemiology and
Population Health,
Albert Einstein College of Medicine,
New York, USA

Jonathan M. Samet
Department of Preventive Medicine and the
USC Institute for Global Health,
Keck School of Medicine,
University of Southern California, USA

Hong-Gwan Seo
Research Institute and Hospital,
National Cancer Center,
Goyang, Republic of South Korea

Anne Szarewski
Cancer Research UK Centre
for Mathematics,
Statistics and Epidemiology, Wolfson
Institute of Preventive Medicine,
Queen Mary University of London,
Barts & The London School of
Medicine and Dentistry,
London, UK

Paul D. Terry
Department of Epidemiology,
Rollins School of Public Health,
Emory University, Atlanta, USA

Michael J. Thun
Department of Epidemiology and
Surveillance Research,
American Cancer Society, Atlanta, USA

Dimitrios Trichopoulos
Department of Epidemiology,
Harvard School of Public Health,
Boston, USA
Bureau of Epidemiologic Research,
Academy of Athens, Greece

Melanie Wakefield
Director and NHMRC Principal
Research Fellow,
Centre for Behavioural Research in Cancer,
The Cancer Council Victoria, Australia

Elisabete Weiderpass
Department of Medical Epidemiology and
Biostatistics,
Karolinska Institutet, Stockholm,
Sweden and The Cancer
Registry of Norway,
Oslo, Norway

John Wise
Laboratory of Environmental and
Genetic Toxicology,
Bioscience Research Institute,
University of Southern Main,
Portland, USA

David Zaridze
Director, Institute of Carcinogenesis,
N.N. Blokhin Russian Cancer
Research Center,
Moscow, Russia

Witold A. Zatoński
Director and Professor in the Division of
Epidemiology and Cancer Prevention,
Center and Institute of Oncology;
Founder and President of the Health
Promotion Foundation,
Warsaw, Poland

Bing Zhang
Department of Epidemiology and
Biostatistics,
McGill University,
Montreal, Canada

Yawei Zhang
Department of Epidemiology and
Public Health,
Yale University School of Medicine,
New Haven, USA

Tongzhang Zheng
Associate Professor,
Department of Epidemiology and
Public Health,
Yale School of Medicine,
New Haven, USA

Nicholas Zwar
School of Public Health and
Community Medicine,
The University of New South Wales,
Kensington, Australia

Abbreviations

AAA	Abdominal aortic aneurysm
AC	Adenocarcinoma
ACO	Adenocarcinoma of the oesophages
ACS	American Cancer Society
AKR	Aldo-keto reductase
ALTS	ASCUS and LSIL Triage Study
AMI	Acute myocardial infarction
ANCCA	Asian National Cancer Center Alliance
APA	The American Psychiatric Association
ARCI	Addiction Research Centre Inventory
ASH	Action on Smoking and Health
BaA	Benz(a)anthracene
BaP	Benzo(a)pyrene
BAT	British America Tobacco
BMI	Body mass index
BO	Barrett's oesophagus
BPDE	Anti-7,8-dihydroxy-9,10-epoxy-7,8,9,10-tetrahydrobenzo[a]pyrene
CAD	Coronary artery disease
CDC	Centers for Disease Control
CDCP	Centers for Disease Control and Prevention
CEDAW	Conference on Women and the Convention to Eliminate All Forms of Discrimination Against Women
CeVD	Cerebrovascular disease
CHD	Coronary heart disease
CI	Confidence interval
CIMP	CpG island methylator phenoptype
CIN	Cervical intraepithelial neoplasia
CIS	Carcinoma in situ
CO	Carbon monoxide
COLD	Chronic obstructive lung disease
COMT	Catechol O-methyl transferase
COP	Conference of the Parties
COPD	Chronic obstructive pulmonary disease
CORESTA	Centre De Cooperation Pour Les Recherches Scientifiques Relative Au Taba
COX	Cyclooxygenase
CPP	Conditioned place preference
CPS	Cancer Prevention Study
CSC	Cigarette smoke condensates
CVD	Cardiovascular disease
CYP1A1	Cytochrome P-450 1A1
DATI	Dopaminergic transporter
DBH	Dopamine β-hydroxylase
DHEAS	Dehydroepiandrosterone
DMBA	7,12-dimethylbenz[a]anthracene
DRR	Direct reversal repair
DSM	Diagnostic and statistical manual
DVT	Deep vein thrombosis
EPHX1	Epoxide hydrolase
EPIC	European prospective investigation into cancer
ESPN	Entertainment and Sports Programming Network
ETS	Environmental tobacco smoke
EU	European Union
FCTC	Framework Convention of Tobacco Control
FCV	Flue Cured Virginia
FDA	Food and Drug Administration
FHIT	Fragile histidine triad
FISH	Fluorescent *in situ* hybridization
FSH	Follicle-stimulating hormone
FTC	Federal Trade Commission
FTND	Fagerström test for tobacco dependence
FTQ	Fagerström tolerance questionnaire
FUBYAS	First usual brand adult smoker
GC	Gas chromatography
GC–MS	Gas chromatography–mass spectrometry
GC–MS/MS	Gas chromatography–tandem mass spectrometry
GNP	Gross national product
GPG	Global Public Good
GRAS	Generally regarded as safe
GSTs	Glutathione S-transferases

GYTS	Global youth tobacco survey
Hb	Haemoglobin
HBSC	Health Behaviour in School-Aged Children Survey
HEA	Health Education Authority
1-HOP	1-Hydroxypyrene
HIV	Human Immunodeficiency virus
HPB	4-Hydroxy-1-(3-pyridyl)-1-butanone
HPLC	High-performance liquid chromatography
HPV	Human papillomavirus
HRT	Hormone replacement therapy
HSC	Human smoking conditions
HSV	Herpes simplex virus
IARC	International Agency for Research on Cancer
IC	Intermittent claudication
ICD	International Classification of Diseases
ICMR	Indian Council for Medical Research
IHD	Ischaemic heart disease
ILO	International Labour Organization
INB	Intergovernmental Negotiation Body
IPCS	International programme on clinical safety
ISO	International Standards Organization
KASH	Korean Association of Smoking & Health
LC-MS/MS	liquid chromatography-tandem mass spectrometry
LH	Luteinizing hormone
LLETZ	Large loop excision of the transformation zone
MBG	Morphine-Benzedrine group scale
MDPH	Massachusetts Department of Public Health
7-methyl-dG	7-Methyldeoxyguanosine
MGMT	O^6-methylguanine DNA methyl-transferase
MMP-1	Matrein metalloproteinase-1 gene
MRFIT	Multiple risk factor intervention trial
MS	Mainstream smoke OR mass spectrometry
MSA	Master Settlement Agreement
MSI	Microsatellite instability
MUS	Marlboro UltraSmooth

nAChRs	Nicotinic acetylcholine receptors
NATs	N-acetyl transferase
NCC	National Cancer Center
NDMA	N-nitrosodimethylamine
NER	Nucleotide excision repair
NHMRC	National Health and Medical Research Council
NNAL	4-(methylnitrosamino)-1-(3-pyridyl)-1-butanol
NNK	4-(methylnitrosamino)-1-(3-pyridyl)-2-butanone
NNN	N'-nitrosonornicotine
NOx	Nitrogen oxides (NO, NO_2, and N_2O)
NPYR	N-nitrosopyrrolidine
NRT	Nicotine replacement therapy
NSDNC	Nocturnal sleep-disturbing nicotine craving
NSSO	National Sample Survey Organisation
OC	Oesophageal cancer
OECD	Organization for Economic Collaboration and Development
2-OEH1	2-Hydroxyestrone
16α-OEH1	16α-Hydroxyestrone
OTC	Over-the-counter
PAD	Peripheral arterial disease
PAHs	Polycyclic polynuclear aromatic hydrocarbons
PAR	Population attributable risk
PCR	Polymerase chain reaction
PCSS	Perter community stroke study
PE	Pulmonary embolism
PG	Propylene glycol
PlCH	Primary intracerebral haemorrhage
POB	Pyridyloxobutyl
POMS	Profile of mood state
POS	Point of sale
PREPs	Potential reduced-exposure products
QTL	Quantitative trait loci
RR	Relative risk
RT	Reconstituted tobacco
s.c.	Subcutaneous
SACTob	Scientific Advisory Committee on Tobacco Product Regulation
SAH	Subarachnoid haemorrhage
SCC	Squamous cell carcinoma

SCCO	Squamous cell carcinoma of the oesophagus	TNCO	'Tar', nicotine, and carbon monoxide
SCENIHR	Scientific Committee on Emerging and Newly Identified Health Risks	TPLP	Tobacco products liability project
SHBG	Sex-hormone binding globulin	*trans-anti-*BaP-tetraol	$r\text{-}7,t\text{-}8,9,c\text{-}10$-tetrahydroxy-7,8,9,10-tetrahydrobenzo[a]pyrene
SHS	Secondhand smoke		
SIDS	Sudden infant death syndrome	TSNAs	Tobacco-specific N-nitrosamines
SS	Sidestream smoke	UICC	International union against cancer
SSA	Sub-Saharan Africa	VNAs	Volatile N-nitrosamines
ST	Smokeless tobacco	WCOO	World tobacco product
SUCCEED	Study to Understand Cervical Cancer Early Endpoints and Determinants	WHA	World Health Assembly
		WHO FCTC	WHO Framework Convention on Tobacco Control
TAMA	Tobacco Association of Malawi	WHO	World Health Organization
TCOG	Taiwan Cooperative Oncology Group	XPA	Xeroderma pigmentosum group A
		XPC	Xeroderma pigmentosum group C
TEAM	Total exposure assessment methodology	YAS	Young adult smoker
		YSP	Youth smoking prevention
TFI	Tobacco Free Initiative		
TIA	Transient cerebral ischaemic attack		

Preamble to the second edition

When the first edition was published in 2004 the editors thought that the science was substantially mature, that policy was on a stable course, and thus a definitive text might have a 'shelf-life' of a decade. That was not quite so. The science of tobacco caused disease, tobacco products themselves, and tobacco control policy have advanced rapidly. We have tried to encompass as much as possible in this new text and we believe that we have an outstanding compendium of the state of the science and policy as we enter the second decade of the twenty-first century. Almost all the original chapters have been updated except for a few occasions when authors (notably Sir Richard Doll) are no longer with us or other factors have interfered, and several new chapters reflect what can only be considered major breakthroughs in science and policy since 2004.

Policy has moved extraordinarily quickly. Public smoking restrictions, increased tobacco product taxes, stronger regulation of marketing – even in the cinema from Hollywood to Bollywood tobacco cessation treatment access are spreading further and faster than we imagined possible. The concept that regulation of the products themselves could emerge as powerful forces in tobacco control efforts focused on prevention, cessation, and disease control was just beginning to receive serious thought at the turn of the century. Consider that the WHO Framework Convention on Tobacco Control was still an evolving document as we worked on the first edition. It came into force with astounding speed and broad acceptance and is now being implemented by most parties to the United Nations, together representing more than 80% of the world population. There now exists a global tobacco product testing laboratory network of approximately 30 organizations collaborating to assist policy and regulation by monitoring the evolution of tobacco products. In the United States, the Food and Drug Administration has been granted powerful authority and extensive professional and financial resources to control tobacco products: the repercussions of which will surely be felt globally as it begins to limit or ban certain ingredients of special concern and evaluate new products.

Yet much is yet to be done as is also documented in this volume. We still face and enormous adversary in the tobacco industry and public health experts are frequently stymied by the powerful economic, political, and social forces manipulated by the industry. For comparison, whereas the battle against major infectious diseases was won over about a decade in the 1950s, in part, by identification and control of vectors of disease spread, we have waited one half century for health authorities to finally begin to exert control over the major vectors of the spread of tobacco diseases since their identification in the 1950s and 1960s. Of course tuberculosis and other diseases were not spread by powerful commercial organizations with the capacity to sell products everywhere on the planet. No one was selling tuberculosis, whereas tobacco companies successfully defended their 'right' to sell cancer, heart, and lung disease with their powerful engines financed by people they had addicted. Although many higher income nations have begun to successfully curtail tobacco industry political influence and marketing, the industry continues its relentless push into every sector of lower income nations. But here too, hope abounds as new assets such as growing ubiquitous and inexpensive internet communications enable speedy unveiling of the sociopathic tricks of the industry in even the poorest and most isolated of regions.

So much has been accomplished but so much is still to be done.

We have made every effort to develop this book as a practical and useful asset to all in tobacco control from basic scientists to epidemiologists to regulators and policy-makers. Much has changed in the text apart from the updates of well-know facts covering the various diseases. Sections on product design factors and addiction are new and the process of carcinogenesis as currently understood is elegantly described and updated. There is a new focus on marketing; its relation to tobacco chemistry; a modern and comprehensive coverage of cessation; on harm reduction; on advocacy; the merits of evaluation; the effectiveness of policies; and on regulatory efforts mediated through WHO. There is more discussion of continuing events in the major areas of tobacco use exemplified by Eastern Europe, China, and India, with a vignette on tobacco control in the Republic of South Korea – as an example of change in a country with a short history in this field.

It is hoped that students of all the health-related disciplines will be assisted by the book and that it will provide a reference point for all those with an interest in what remains one of the world's greatest continuing public health challenges.

Peter Boyle,
Nigel Gray,
Jack Henningfield,
John Seffrin,
Witold A. Zatoński
2 September 2009

Chapter 1

Evolution of knowledge of the smoking epidemic

Richard Doll

Introduction

Tobacco was grown and used widely in North, Central, and South America for two to three millennia before being introduced to Europe at the end of the fifteenth century. Its use was promoted initially for medicinal purposes, for the treatment of a variety of conditions from cough, asthma, and headaches to intestinal worms, open wounds, and malignant tumours, when it was prescribed to be chewed, taken nasally as a powder, or applied locally.

The use of tobacco for pleasure was discouraged by Church and State and it was not until the end of the sixteenth century that it came to be smoked widely in Europe, at first in pipes in Britain, where it was popularized by Sir Walter Raleigh. Here it became so common that by 1614 there are estimated to have been some 7000 retail outlets in London alone (Laufer 1924). Attempts to ban its use for recreational purposes were made in Austria, Germany, Russia, Switzerland, Turkey, India, and Japan, but prohibition was invariably flouted and control by taxation came to be preferred. This eventually proved to be such an important source of revenue that, in 1851, Cardinal Antonelli, Secretary to the Papal States, ordered that the dissemination of anti-tobacco literature was to be punished by imprisonment (Corti 1931).

Gradually, the way in which tobacco was most commonly used changed. By the end of the seventeenth century, its use as nasal snuff had spread from France, largely replacing pipe smoking. This practice remained common until a century later, when it, in turn, began to be replaced by the smoking of cigars, which had long been smoked in a primitive form in Spain and Portugal. By then cigarettes were already being made in South America and their use had spread to Spain, but it was not until after the Crimean War that they began to be at all widely adopted. They were made fashionable in Britain by officers returning from the Crimea, and by the end of the nineteenth century cigarettes had begun to replace cigars. Consumption in this form increased rapidly during the First World War, and by the end of the Second World War cigarettes had largely replaced all other tobacco products in most developed countries.

By this time, smoking had become so much the norm for men that, in Britain, some 80 per cent were regular smokers and some doctors even offered a cigarette to patients who came to consult them, to put them at their ease. Women began to smoke in large numbers much later, except in New Zealand, where, by the end of the nineteenth century, Maori women were commonly smoking pipes. Then, in the 1920s, women began to smoke cigarettes, at first in the USA and then in Britain, where the practice gained popularity during the Second World War, as an increasing proportion of women began to work outside the home and have an independent income. However, in many other developed countries, women have begun to smoke in large numbers only in the past few decades.

The reason for the swing to cigarettes

The important change in the use of tobacco, for its impact on health, was the swing to cigarettes. This was brought about by two industrial developments. The first was a new method of curing tobacco. With the old method, the smoke that had come from pipes and cigars was alkaline, irritating, and difficult to inhale. However, the nicotine in it was predominantly in the form of a free base which could be absorbed across the oral and pharyngeal mucosa. Blood levels of nicotine could consequently be high and addiction was readily produced; but only small amounts of other constituents were absorbed. The new method, called flue-curing, was introduced in North Carolina in the mid-nineteenth century (Tilley 1948). It exposed the leaf to high temperatures and increased its sugar content, which caused the pH of the smoke to be acid. In this environment, the nicotine was predominantly in the form of salts and was dissolved in smoke droplets, which were less irritating than the free base and easier to inhale. With each inhalation there was a rapid rise in the level of nicotine in the blood, which was perceived in the brain, and was particularly satisfying to the addict, but other constituents of the smoke were also absorbed and distributed throughout the body.

The second development was mechanical: namely, the introduction of cigarettemaking machines. One was patented in 1880, and was eventually adapted by the Duke family to work so efficiently that 120 000 cigarettes of good quality could be produced every 10 hours by one machine, the equivalent of the production of about 100 unassisted workers. As a result, the price fell and a mass market became feasible.

The impact of tobacco on health

Until cigarette smoking became common, very little evidence of harmful effects was detected—for the good reason that relatively little harm was probably caused. One harmful effect, which was first suggested more than 200 years ago (Sömmering 1795), was the production of cancer of the lip. In the course of the nineteenth century, on the basis of clinical series in France (Bouisson 1859), Germany (Virchow 1863–7), and the United Kingdom (Anon 1890), additional consequences were linked to smoking, such as the production of cancers of the tongue and other parts of the mouth. These findings, are now simply explained because we know that these cancers can be produced at least as easily by the smoking of pipes and cigars as by the smoking of cigarettes. However, little attention was paid to these effects by clinicians, who characterized cancer of the lip as the result of smoking clay pipes, which was a custom of agricultural workers. When, as a medical student in the mid-1930s, I asked the senior surgeon at my teaching hospital whether he thought pipe smoking or syphilis was a cause of cancer of the tongue, he replied that he didn't know, but that the wise man should certainly avoid the combination of the two.

However, one disease was unequivocally attributed to tobacco, and taught as being so: namely, tobacco amblyopia. It was described by Beer in 1817, and occurred in heavy pipe-smokers in combination with malnutrition. It was probably caused by the cyanide in smoke not being detoxified because of a deficiency of vitamin B12 (Heaton *et al.* 1958). The disease is no longer seen, at least in developed countries.

The early impact of cigarette smoking

With the advent of the twentieth century, several new diseases began to be associated with smoking: first, intermittent claudication, which was described by Erb in 1904 and then, in 1908, a rare form of peripheral vascular disease affecting relatively young people, which Buerger called thrombo-angiitis obliterans, and which has subsequently been named after him. It is now recognized that both diseases were made much more common by smoking, with the latter almost limited to smokers, but neither reached the epidemic proportions that two other, relatively new, diseases achieved in the next few decades.

One of these was coronary thrombosis or, as we would now prefer to say,myocardial infarction. It was first described at autopsy in 1876 (Hammer 1878), although it had certainly occurred earlier, and it was not diagnosed in life until 1910, when it was diagnosed by Herrick (1912) in Chicago. Subsequently it was reported progressively more often every year for four or five decades. As early as 1920, Hoffman, an American statistician, linked the increase in coronary thrombosis with the increasing consumption of cigarettes. Several clinical studies of the relationship between the disease and smoking were published, but the findings were confused, and no substantial evidence was obtained until 1940, when English *et al.* reported finding an association in the records of the Mayo Clinic. Their findings led them to conclude that the smoking of tobacco probably had 'a more profound effect on younger individuals owing to the existence of relatively normal cardiovascular systems, influencing perhaps the earlier development of coronary disease'. However, they eschewed reference to causation, because the subject would be controversial, adding perceptively that 'Physicians are not yet ready to agree on this important subject'. That cigarette smoking played a part in the increasing incidence of the disease was eventually clearly demonstrated. The association was not close enough for it to have been the only cause of the increase, or even probably the most important, and, unlike the other disease that burst into medical prominence in the first half of the twentieth century, the full explanation of its rapid increase is still a matter for debate (Doll 1987).

The other disease was, of course, cancer of the lung. Until then it had been thought to be exceptionally rare. A small cluster of cases in tobacco workers in Leipzig had led Rottmann to suggest, in 1898, that the disease might be caused by the inhalation of tobacco dust. The first suggestion that it might be due to smoking was not made until 14 years later, by Adler (1912), who noted that, although the disease was still rare, it appeared to have become somewhat less so in the recent past. Many people were subsequently struck by the parallel increase in the consumption of cigarettes and the incidence of the disease and by the frequency with which patients with lung cancer described themselves as heavy smokers, several even ventured to suggest that the two were related (Tylecote 1927; Lickint 1929; Hoffman 1931; Arkin and Wagner 1936; Fleckseder 1936; Ochsner and de Bakey 1941). However, few believed it. Koch's postulates, which were taught as criteria for determining causality, could not be satisfied, as one required the agent to be present in every case of the disease and cases certainly occurred in non-smokers. Moreover, pathologists generally failed to produce cancer experimentally by the application of tobacco tar to the skin of animals. Only Roffo (1931), in Argentina, succeeded in doing so, and his results were discounted in the United Kingdom and the United States because he had produced the tar by burning the tobacco at unrealistically high temperatures. However, diagnostic methods had certainly improved, notably the widespread use of radiology and bronchoscopy, and the idea that the increase in the incidence of the disease was an artefact of improved diagnosis came to be widely believed.

Three case-control studies that were carried out in Germany and The Netherlands between 1939 and 1948 should have focused attention on smoking, as all three suggested, albeit on rather inadequate grounds (Doll 2001), that smoking was a possible cause of lung cancer. However, the war distracted attention from the German literature (Müller 1939; Schairer and Schöniger 1943), and the Dutch paper (Wassink 1948) was published in Dutch and not noticed widely for several years. Outside Germany, smoking was still commonly regarded as having only minor effects as late as 1950, and inside Germany, where chronic nicotine poisoning had been thought to produce effects in nearly every system, the reaction against the Nazis brought with it a reaction against their antagonism to tobacco—for propaganda against the use of tobacco had been a major plank in the public health policy of the Nazi government (on the grounds that it damaged the national germ plasm and that addiction to it detracted from obedience to the Führer) (Proctor 1999).

The 1950 watershed

Then in 1950, five case-control studies were published in the United Kingdom (Doll and Hill 1950) and the United States (Levin *et al.* 1950; Mills *et al.* 1950; Schrek *et al.* 1950; Wynder and Graham 1950), with much larger numbers of cases and, in some, so refined a technique, that Bradford Hill and I were able to conclude that 'cigarette smoking is a factor, and an important factor, in the production of carcinoma of the lung' (Doll and Hill 1950). The results were given wide publicity, but the conclusion was not widely believed. Medical scientists had as yet to appreciate the power of epidemiology in unravelling the aetiology of non-infectious disease. Statisticians had failed to recognize the implication of such high relative risks as those estimated from the findings, and argued that the association with smoking might be due to confounding with some other factor that was the true cause of the disease. Fisher (1957), of international statistical fame, thought that the lack of an association with inhaling in our first report was a major difficulty, and preferred the idea that some genetic factor caused both the disease and the individual to want to smoke, while Berkson (1955), a leading medical statistician at the Mayo Clinic, argued that the cases and the controls, not being random samples of the population, might have been subject to selection bias. The tobacco industry was consequently able to present the findings as controversial. However, Scientific curiosity had been aroused, a great deal of research was initiated, and government departments were forced to consider the implications of the findings for the practice of public health.

Acceptance of evidence of harm

Further evidence was clearly needed if the scientific world was to accept that cigarette smoking was the cause of the lung cancer epidemic, which was, by then, spreading in all developed countries, and this was rapidly produced. Cohort studies were begun in which people who had provided information about their smoking habits were followed to see the extent to which their habits predicted mortality. One such study obtained information from 34 000 male doctors in the United Kingdom, and showed, within 3 years, that mortality from lung cancer was proportional to the amount smoked—as predicted by the case-control studies—and suggested that there might also be a similar, although less marked, relationship with coronary thrombosis (Doll and Hill 1954). Another study, based on larger numbers in the United States, gave similar results, and found that, under 65 years of age, the mortality from coronary thrombosis among men who smoked 20 or more cigarettes a day was twice that of non-smokers (Hammond and Horn 1954). In the larger study in the United States, the results were much clearer for coronary heart disease than for lung cancer. This was because the switch to cigarette smoking occurred on a mass scale later in North America than it did in the United Kingdom, and it takes several decades of smoking before the risk of cancer is high, whereas less time is required to produce a major risk of coronary disease.

Meanwhile, laboratory workers had shown that tobacco tar, appropriately produced, contained polycyclic aromatic hydrocarbons that were known to be carcinogenic (Cooper and Lindsay 1955), and that the tar could cause cancer on the skin of mice if applied regularly for months on end (Wynder *et al.* 1953; Doll 1998). As a consequence of these results, in 1957 the Medical Research Council was able to advise the British government that cigarette smoking was the cause of the increased incidence of lung cancer. Similar conclusions were reached, over the next 3 years, by a study group on Smoking and Health (1957) appointed jointly by the US National Cancer and Heart Institute and the US Public Health Service (Burney 1959), and by specially appointed committees in The Netherlands and Sweden, and the World Health Organization (see Doll 1998).

Impact on total mortality

A few years later, when the Royal College of Physicians (1962), in England, and the Surgeon General (1964), in the United States, issued reports on smoking, it had become clear that its total impact was greater than had at first been conceived, and that the incidence of more diseases might be affected. With the passage of time, more and more diseases were found that were linked in some way to smoking. The total number now believed to be caused in part by smoking is at least 35, 22 of which can be recognized in the cohort study of British doctors and in the massive study of a million men and women subsequently undertaken by the American Cancer Society (Table 1.1). Other harmful effects caused in part by smoking are listed in Table 1.2. These are mostly relatively

Table 1.1 Principal diseases caused in part by smoking

Disease	Ratio of mortality rates in continuing cigarette smokers and lifelong non-smokers		
	British doctors 1951–91[a]	US population 1984–91[b]	
	Men	Men	Women
Cancers of mouth, pharynx, and larynx	24.0	11.4	6.9
Cancers of the oesophagus	7.5	5.6	9.8
Cancers of the lung	14.9	23.9	14.0
Cancers of the pancreas	2.2	2.0	2.3
Cancers of the bladder	2.3	3.9	1.8
Ischaemic heart disease	1.6	1.9	2.0
Hypertension	1.4	2.4	2.6
Myocardial degeneration	2.0		
Pulmonary heart disease	∞[c]	2.1	2.1
Other heart disease	–		
Aortic aneurysm	4.1	6.3	8.2
Peripheral vascular disease	–	9.7	5.7
Arteriosclerosis	1.8	2.7	3.0
Cerebrovascular disease	1.5	1.9	2.2
Chronic bronchitis and emphysema	12.7	17.6	16.2
Pulmonary tuberculosis	2.8	–	–
Asthma[d]	2.2	1.3	1.4
Pneumonia	1.9	2.5	1.7
Other respiratory disease	1.6		
Peptic ulcer	3.0	4.6	4.0
All causes	1.8	2.5	2.1

[a] Doll et al. (1994).
[b] C. Heath Jr and M. Thun, personal communication.
[c] No death was reported in British doctors who were lifelong non-smokers.
[d] Continuing cigarette smokers and ex-cigarette smokers combined, as asthma may cause smokers to stop smoking.

Table 1.2 Other conditions caused in part by smoking

Cancer of lip	Crohn's disease
Cancer of nose	Osteoporosis
Cancer of stomach	Periodontitis
Cancer of kidney pelvis	Tobacco amblyopia
Cancer of kidney body	Age-related macular degeneration
Myeloid leukaemia	Reduced fecundity
Reduced growth of fetus	

rare and less lethal, and evidence relating to them has often had to be obtained from case-control studies or surveys, or, occasionally, from cohort studies in which special enquiries have been made about the condition of interest. That so many conditions are affected by smoking should not be surprising, as tobacco smoke contains some 4000 different chemicals and many of the diseases are caused by similar mechanisms.

Even the 35 smoking-related diseases mentioned above do not complete the list, because a few others that are primarily associated with smoking through confounding are also probably caused by it in part, including cancer of the liver (Doll 1996) and death from conflagration—two doctors in our study, for example, set fire to themselves by smoking in bed.

Of course, confounding does account for some of the excess mortality from all causes of death. However, detailed investigation has shown that the amount is relatively small and, in some populations, may not exist at all, for confounding can operate in both directions, and certainly does in elderly populations in countries in which there is a high mortality from ischaemic heart disease. Here, confounding with alcohol both causes the excess for cirrhosis of the liver and reduces the mortality from ischaemic heart disease.

It now appears that the excess mortality from smoking is greater than was long suspected, for it has increased with time, as the smoking epidemic has matured and old people have come to be smoking cigarettes throughout their smoking lives. This is shown by the data in Table 1.3 from both the British doctors' study, which has continued for over 40 years with periodic updates on changes in smoking habit, and the studies of the American public carried out by the American Cancer Society over two different periods. Regular cigarette smoking since youth is now seen to double mortality, on average, throughout middle and old age, so that 1 in 4 smokers die prematurely as a result of their habit in middle age (now defined as from 35 to 74 years) and 1 in 4 die similarly in old age.

Table 1.3 Cigarette smokers compared with Lifelong non-smokers: change in all-cause mortality in men

British doctors[a]	Period	1951–71	1971–91
	Relative risk	1.6	2.1
American Public[b]	Period	1959–65	1982–86
	Relative risk	1.8	2.3

[a] Doll et al. (1994)
[b] Surgeon General (1989).

The epidemic that the world is now facing is not, in truth, a smoking epidemic so much as a cigarette epidemic, for the small effect of smoking pipes and cigars that gave rise to so little concern in the nineteenth century has continued to be relatively small. For example, in our study of British doctors, the mortality of pipe and cigar smokers who had never smoked cigarettes was only 9 per cent greater than that of lifelong non-smokers (Doll and Peto 1976). This represents a material increase in all-cause mortality, certainly, but one qualitatively different from that of cigarette smoking, and it is only the effect of the latter that I shall consider further.

The spread of the epidemic

Two things about the epidemic are clear. First, the number of manufactured cigarettes consumed has increased astronomically, from near zero in 1880 to some 5700 billion a year worldwide in the mid-1990s, since when there has been a very slight decrease (Proctor 2001). Secondly, the increase in cigarette smoking occurred at different rates, at different periods, in each sex, in different countries. Even within developed countries, to which the increase was initially confined, the differences were substantial.

Developed countries

Detailed consumption rates of different tobacco products in 22 developed countries have been brought together by Nicolaides-Bouman *et al.* (1993) from the time of the earliest record to 1985. The three highest and three lowest rates of consumption of manufactured cigarettes by adults, averaged over the decade 1920–29, are shown in Table 1.4, together with the corresponding age-standardized mortality rates for lung cancer in 1955, some 30 years later, to allow for a sufficiently long period of exposure to produce an appreciable effect. That lung cancer was more common when manufactured cigarettes were taken up early is clear, but the correlation is not close. This is hardly surprising, because many factors affect the incidence of the disease other than the one examined in Table 1.4: the changes in cigarette consumption over the intervening period, the distribution of consumption by sex and age, the characteristics of the cigarettes, the way they are smoked, the amount of tobacco consumed in hand-rolled cigarettes and in other tobacco products, which are not without hazard, and, it appears, the local diet, which may modify the quantitative effect of a given number of cigarettes (see Darby *et al.* 2001).

In order to determine the extent of the proportion of the total threat to mortality caused by smoking, a method for estimating the mortality attributable to cigarette smoking that is not dependent on statistics for tobacco consumption was suggested by Peto *et al.* (1992). It is worth describing in some detail as so much depends on it. In brief, Peto *et al.* used the excess mortality from lung cancer over that observed in non-smokers in the American Cancer Society's massive

Table 1.4 Manufactured cigarette consumption in 1920s and lung cancer mortality in 1955

Country	Mean number of cigarettes smoked daily by adults, 1920–29	Lung cancer
Finland	3.6	89
Greece	3.4	57
UK	3.0	109
Sweden	0.8	16
Norway	0.7	11
Portugal	<0.7	11

Table 1.5 Categories of disease used by Peto *et al.* (1992)

Lung cancer	
Upper aerodigestive cancers	Vascular diseases
Other cancers	Cirrhosis of liver
Chronic obstructive pulmonary disease	Other medical causes
Other respiratory diseases	Non-medical causes

second cancer prevention study, as an indication of the extent to which the population had been exposed to tobacco products in the past. This is justified for developed countries because, whenever data are available, the mortality from lung cancer in lifelong non-smokers has been found to be low, approximately the same in each country, and not to have changed over time. However, the same method cannot be used directly to estimate the effects of smoking on mortality from other diseases, as the rates for other diseases in non-smokers vary considerably, and smoking interacts with other causes in a complex way that is nearer multiplicative than additive. Peto *et al.* (1992) consequently divided other causes into eight broad categories (Table 1.5) and used the second cancer prevention study's data as an indication of the *proportional* excess mortality for each broad cause group to be associated with the corresponding *absolute* excess of lung cancer in each 5-year age group. However, to be on the safe side (that is, to under-, rather than to overestimate the mortality attributable to smoking) they excluded all deaths in two categories (cirrhosis and non-medical causes) and all deaths under 35 years of age in all categories, even though some deaths in both groups were attributable to smoking, and then *halved* the estimated excess proportion for each of the remaining six categories. This last, it should be noted, is not as extreme as halving the number of excess deaths, for it has little effect on the number of deaths attributable to tobacco when the relative risks are high; reducing it, for example, by only 10 per cent if the relative risk is ninefold.

The trends in the proportions of mortality consequently attributed to smoking between 1955 and 1995 are shown in Table 1.6 (the data for 1995 were projected from the trend between 1980 and 1985, but have been found to be generally reliable). They are given separately for men and women, and for the United Kingdom, the United States, and all developed countries, the latter

Table 1.6 Trends in per cent mortality attributed to smoking: selected populations

Sex	Country	Year				
		1955	1965	1975	1985	1995
M	UK	27	35	36	34	27
M	USA	14	20	26	28	29
M	OECD	12	19	23	25	25
M	Former socialist	15	22	24	29	32
F	UK	3.0	5.9	9.8	14	17
F	USA	0.3	2.0	7.1	14	22
F	OECD	0.5	1.7	3.9	7.4	12
F	Former socialist	1.3	2.0	3.0	3.7	5.2

being divided into the Organization for Economic Collaboration and Development (OECD) countries, and former socialist economies. The highest percentage of mortality attributed to smoking was in men in the United Kingdom in 1975; since when the proportion has dropped by a quarter and is now less than that in the United States. The OECD countries, as a group, had slightly lower proportions than the United States and the proportion stabilized after 1985. In the former socialist economy countries, the percentage has increased progressively, and in 1995 was approaching the maximum previously recorded in the United Kingdom. In women the proportions have generally been much lower, but in 1995 were approaching the figures for men, in both the United Kingdom and, most notably, the United States of America. In all four categories the increase in female mortality has been progressive and in the United States and many parts of the United Kingdom lung cancer has now displaced cancer of the breast from its position as the leading cause of death from cancer in women.

Developing countries

For the developing countries there are few quantitative data, apart from those for China, where cigarette consumption per adult increased from about 1 per day in 1952, to 10 per day in 1992. Two studies are particularly revealing. One, a case-control study of a million deaths in men and women in 98 parts of China, both urban and rural, obtained information about the deceased persons' smoking habits and compared those of men and women who died of cancer, respiratory disease, and vascular disease with those of men and women who died of other diseases, postulated not to be due to smoking (Liu *et al.* 1998). The other, a cohort study of a quarter of a million men aged over 40, in 45 selected representative areas, provided mortality rates by smoking habit over a 5–6-year period (Niu *et al.* 1998). Both led to the conclusion that about 12 per cent of deaths in middle-aged and elderly men were attributable to smoking, while the case-control study provided the much lower figure, of 2–3 per cent, in women, few of whom, outside the big towns, had been smoking for long. However, the pattern of mortality was different from that in the developed world, with a much smaller proportion of attributable deaths due to ischaemic heart disease and lung cancer, and a greater proportion due to stroke, chronic obstructive pulmonary disease, and cancers of the oesophagus, stomach, and liver.

Future expectations

What then of the future? For China it is relatively easy to predict, for the prevalence of smoking and attributable mortality are reproducing what was observed in the United States 40 years previously, where cigarette consumption per adult had been 1 per day in 1910 and 10 per day in 1950, and the risk of premature death in smokers, attributable to smoking, increased from 1 in 4 in the early 1960s, to 1 in 2 in the 1980s. For Chinese men who began smoking before they were 20 years old, after the revolution in 1949, the risk is already 1 in 4 and must be expected to become 1 in 2 in 20 years time. Two-thirds of men now become smokers before 25 years of age and, if present patterns continue, about 100 million of the 300 million Chinese males now under 30 years of age will be killed by tobacco. However, the number of female deaths attributable to smoking in the future may be relatively small, as, contrary to what has happened in the West, progressively fewer women have been starting to smoke, and the prevalence for those born between 1950 and 1964 is now only 1–2 per cent.

For the developing world as a whole, Peto and Lopez (1990) estimated that, in the 1990s, there were already likely to have been 1 million deaths per year attributable to tobacco, against approximately 2 million in the developed world. However, in many parts, the prevalence of smoking in men, like that in China, already exceeds 50 per cent, although, again, the female prevalence is relatively low. We also know that in India, for example, where tuberculosis has become a major cause of death, the impact of smoking on that disease is to increase the incidence of clinical cases and double the fatality, as it was in the developed world 40 years ago. However, in many countries there is still major mortality from causes unrelated to tobacco, such as other infectious diseases and trauma, much greater than in the developed world, so that the *proportion* of persistent smokers eventually killed by the habit may be a third, rather than the half suggested by the North American, British, and, indeed, also the Chinese, data. Therefore, perhaps only about 250 million of the 800 million young people who, according to current patterns, will be smokers in early adult life will be killed by the habit. The majority of the deaths will not, of course, occur for some decades, when smoking has been prolonged and the chronic diseases of middle age become common; but in two or three decades the total toll must be expected to be about 10 million deaths a year worldwide, of which some 7 million will be in what are now the developing countries (Peto *et al.* 1996).

The benefit of stopping smoking

If the prevalence of smoking stays as it is, the death toll of tobacco in the first half of the twenty-first century will be tremendous, but it does not have to be. For the prevalence can be reduced and with it, some years later, the mortality from lung cancer and from all other tobacco-related diseases. This is illustrated for lung cancer by the findings in our recent study of the disease in Devon and Cornwall (Peto *et al.* 2000) and in our study of British doctors, in which we found that survival was improved whatever the age at which smoking was stopped. With the numbers we had, survival was indistinguishable from that of lifelong non-smokers when smoking was stopped under 35 years of age (corresponding, in our study, to less than 10 years continued smoking), and longer than that of continuing smokers even if smoking was stopped only after 65 years of age (Doll *et al.* 1994).

I believe, therefore, that with adequate education of the public, for which both doctors and the media must take responsibility, and with the support of government in increasing taxation on tobacco and prohibiting the promotion of the habit, we may see the current predictions materially reduced.

Acknowledgement

I am grateful to the Royal College of Physicians of Edinburgh for permission to reproduce here, under a new title with minor changes and additions, the text of a lecture I gave at the College in October 2001, which has been published in the College Proceedings (*Journal of the Royal College of Physicians of Edinburgh* 2002, **32**, 24–30).

References

Adler, I. (1912). *Primary malignant growths of the lung and bronchi*. Longmans Green and Co., London.

Anon (1890). Cancer and smoking. *British Medical Journal*, **1**, 748.

Arkin, A. and Wagner, D.H. (1936). Primary carcinoma of the lung. *Journal of the American Medical Association*, **106**, 587–91.

Beer, G.J. (1817). Lehre von den Augenkrankheiten, Vol. II, Vienna. (Cited by Duke-Elder, W. S. D. *Textbook of Ophthalmology*, Vol. 3, p. 3009. Henry Kimpton, London).

Bouisson, E.F. (1859). Du cancer buccal chez les fumeurs. *Montpelier Medical Journal*, **2**, 539–99 and **3**, 19–41.

Buerger, L. (1908). Thrombo-angiitis obliterans: a study of the vascular lesions leading to presenile spontaneous gangrene. *American Journal of the Medical Sciences*, **136**, 567–80.

Cooper, R.L. and Lindsay, A.J. (1955). 3-4 Benzpyrene and other polycyclic hydrocarbons in cigarette smoke. *British Journal of Cancer*, **9**, 442–4.

Darby, S., Whitley, E., Doll, R., Key, T., and Silcocks, P. (2001). Diet, smoking and lung cancer: a casecontrol study of 1000 cases and 1500 controls in South-West England. *British Journal of Cancer*, **84**, 728–35.

Doll, R. (1987). Major epidemics of the twentieth century: from coronary thrombosis to AIDS. *Journal of the Royal Statistical Society, Series A*, **150**, 373–95.

Doll, R. (1996). Cancers weakly related to smoking. *British Medical Bulletin*, **52**, 35–49.

Doll, R. (1998). Uncovering the effects of smoking: historical perspective. *Statistical Methods in Medical Research*, **7**, 87–117.

Doll, R. (2001). Commentary: lung cancer and tobacco consumption. *Intertnational Journal of Epidemiology*, **30**, 30–1.

Doll, R. and Hill, A.B. (1950). Smoking and carcinoma of the lung. Preliminary report. *British Medical Journal*, **2**, 739–48.

Doll, R. and Hill, A.B. (1954). The mortality of doctors in relation to their smoking habits. A preliminary report. *British Medical Journal*, **1**, 1451–5.

Doll, R. and Peto, R. (1976). Mortality in relation to smoking: 20 years' observations on male British doctors. *British Medical Journal*, **2**, 1525–36.

Doll, R., Peto, R.,Hall, E.,Wheatley, K., and Gray, R. (1994). Mortality in relation to consumption of alcohol: 13 years' observations on male British doctors. *British Medical Journal*, **309**, 911–18.

English, J.P.,Willius, F.A., and Berkson, J. (1940). Tobacco and coronary disease. *Journal of the American Medical Association*, **115**, 1327–9.

Erb,W. (1904). Ueber dysbasia angiosclerotica ('intermittierendes Hinken'). *Münchener med Woch*, **51**, 905–8.

Fleckseder, R. (1936). Ueber den Bronchialkrebs und einiger seiner Entstehungsbedigungen. *Münchener medizin Wochenschr*, **83**, 1585–8.

Hammer, A. (1878). Ein fall von thrombotischen Verschlusse einer des Kranzarterien des Herzens. *Wein med Wchnschr*, **28**, 97–102.

Hammond, E.C. and Horn, D. (1954). The relationship between human smoking habits and death rates: a follow-up study of 187,766 men. *Journal of the American Medical Association*, **155**, 1316–28.

Heaton, J.M., McCormick, A.J.A., and Freeman, A.G. (1958). Tobacco amblyopia. A clinical manifestation of vitamin B12 deficiency. *Lancet*, **2**, 286–90.

Herrick, J.B. (1912). Clinical features of sudden obstruction of the coronary arteries. *Journal of the American Medical Association*, **59**, 2015–20.

Hoffman, F.L. (1920). Recent statistics of heart disease with special reference to its increasing incidence. *Journal of the American Medical Association*, **74**, 1364–71.

Hoffman, F.L. (1931). Cancer and smoking habits. *Annals of Surgery*, 50–67.

Laufer, B. (1924). *Introduction of tobacco into Europe*. Field Museum of Natural History, Chicago.

Lickint, F. (1929). Tabak und Tabakrauch als ätiologischer Faktor des Carcinoms. *Zeitschrift für Krebsforsch*, **30**, 349–365.

Liu, B.Q., Peto, R., Chen, Z.M., Boreham, J., Wu,Y.P., Li, J.Y., *et al.* (1998). Emerging hazards in China: proportional mortality studies of one million deaths. *British Medical Journal*, **317**, 1411–22.

Medical Research Council (1957). Tobacco smoking and cancer of the lung. *British Medical Journal*, **1**, 1523.

Müller, F. H. (1939). Tabakmissbrauch und lungencarcinoma. *Zeitschrift für Krebsforsch*, **49**, 57–85.

Nicolaides-Bouman, A., Wald, N., Forey, B., and Lee, P. (1993) *International smoking statistics*. Oxford University Press, Oxford.

Niu, S.-R., Yang, G.-H., Chen, Z.-M., Wang, J.-L., Wang, G.-H., He, X.-Z., *et al.* (1998). Emerging tobacco hazards in China: 2. Early mortality results from a prospective study. *British Medical Journal*, **317**, 1423–4.

Ochsner, A. and De Bakey, M. (1941). Carcinoma of the lung. *Archives of Surgery*, **42**, 209–58.

Peto, R. and Lopez, A.D. (1990).Worldwide mortality from current smoking patterns:WHO consultative group on statistical aspects of tobacco-related mortality. In: *Tobacco and health 1990: The global war*, (ed. B. Durston and K. Jamrozik). Proceedings of the 7th World Conference on Tobacco and Health, April, Perth, Western Australia.

Peto, R., Lopez, A., Boreham, J., Thun, M., and Heath, C. (1992). Mortality from tobacco in developed countries: indirect estimation from national vital statistics. *Lancet*, **339**, 1268–78.

Peto, R., Darby, S., Deo, H., Silcocks, P.,Whitley, E., and Doll, R. (2000). Smoking, smoking cessation and lung cancer in the UK since 1950: combination of national statistics with two case-control studies. *British Medical Journal*, **321**, 323–9.

Proctor, R.N. (1999). *The Nazi war on cancer*. Princeton University Press, Princeton.

Proctor, R.N. (2001). Tobacco and the global lung cancer epidemic. *Nature Reviews*, **1**, 82–6.

Roffo, A.H. (1931). Durch Tabak beim Kaninchen entwickeltes Carcinom. *Zeitschrift für Krebsforsch*, **33**, 321–32.

Rottmann, H. (1898). *Über primäre lungencarcinoma*. Inaugural dissertation, Universität Würzburg.

Royal College of Physicians of London (1962). *Smoking and health*. Pitman Medical Publishing, London.

Schairer, E. and Schöniger, E. (1943). Lungenkrebs und Tabakverbrauch. *Zeitschrift für Krebsforsch*, **54**, 261–9.

Sömmering, S.T. (1795). De morbis vasorum absorbentium corporis humani. (Cited by Clemmesen, J. (1965). *Statistical studies in malignant neoplasms. I. Review and results*. Munksgaard, Copenhagen).

Surgeon General (1964). *Smoking and health. Report of the Advisory Committee to the Surgeon General of the Public Health Service*. US Department of Health, Education and Welfare, Public Health Services, US Government Printing Office,Washington, DC.

Surgeon General (1989). *Reducing the health consequences of smoking: 25 years of progress. Report of the Surgeon General, 1989*. US Department of Health and Human Services, Maryland.

Tilley, N.W. (1948). *The Bright-tobacco industry, 1860–1929*. University of North Carolina Press, Chapel Hill.

Tylecote, F.E. (1927). Cancer of the lung. *Lancet*, **2**, 256–7.

Virchow, R.L. (1863 7). *Die krankhaften Geschwülste*. A. Hirschwald, Berlin.

Wassink,W.F. (1948). 'Onstaansvoorwasrden voor Longkanker'. *Ned Tijdschr Geneesk*, **92**, 3732–47.

Wynder, E.L., Graham, E.A., and Croninger, A.B. (1953). Experimental production of carcinoma with cigarette tar. Part I. *Cancer Research*, **13**, 855–64.

Chapter 2

The great studies of smoking and disease in the twentieth century

Michael J. Thun and S. J. Henley

Introduction

Much of what is known about the harm caused by tobacco use was learned from large prospective epidemiologic studies conducted during the second half of the twentieth century in the United Kingdom and United States. To understand why these studies were so important in documenting the deleterious effects of smoking, one must appreciate the pervasive grip that tobacco, particularly cigarette smoking held on the United Kingdom and its former Western colonies at the close of World War II. The culture of cigarettes was sustained not only by nicotine addiction and by the political and economic power of the tobacco industry, but also by the symbols and imagery with which advertising had imbued it and by prevailing social norms. How could an apparently ordinary behaviour practiced by so many people with so little evidence of acute toxicity prove to have such severe chronic effects?

Sir Richard Doll, a pioneer of tobacco epidemiology, has examined the history of scientific and social factors that ultimately led to the recognition of the carcinogenicity and pathogenicity of smoking [1]. Before his death in 2005, he noted that the medical evidence of the adverse health effects of tobacco accumulated for 200 years before it was generally accepted in the late 1950s that smoking caused lung cancer [1]. By the late 1970s it was established that smoking caused many other diseases as well. He cites three factors that contributed to the strength of resistance against the idea that smoking was a major cause of lung cancer: 'the ubiquity of the habit, which was as entrenched among male doctors and scientists as among the rest of the adult male population and had dulled the collective sense that tobacco might be a major threat to health', the novelty of the epidemiological techniques, particularly as applied to non-infectious diseases, and 'the primacy given to Koch's postulates in determining causation', since criteria had not yet been developed to assess the causation of chronic diseases such as cancer.

This chapter examines the contributions of several large prospective studies conducted over the second half of the twentieth century to our understanding of the health hazards of tobacco use. The designation 'Great Studies' is used to refer to prospective studies that were particularly informative about tobacco during this interval. It does not imply that other studies have not been equally important for understanding health scourges other than tobacco, or that all of the really important questions about tobacco have been answered. There is a continuing need for large cohort studies to understand and limit the progression of the tobacco pandemic as it evolves in different cultures with varying background disease profiles, cofactors, and patterns of usage.

Background

Two aspects concerning the historical use of tobacco in Europe help to explain the surprisingly low level of scientific scrutiny regarding its adverse health effects until the mid-twentieth century.

First, for approximately four hundred years after the introduction of tobacco into Europe by Spanish explorers returning from the New World in the late fifteenth century, most tobacco usage involved pipe or cigar smoking or use of snuff or chewing tobacco rather than cigarettes. The historical review by Doll notes that these products were widely used, first for medicinal purposes and then for pleasure [1]. Tobacco was periodically denounced by critics such as James VI of Scotland (who later became James I of England), who published the tract entitled 'A Counterblaste to Tobacco' in 1603. Attempts to ban its use in Japan, Russia, Switzerland, and parts of Germany were unsuccessful, however, and for the most part anti-tobacco movements through the nineteenth century emphasized undesirable moral and social consequences of addiction rather than documented evidence of adverse health effects [1]. Medical concern about carcinogenicity was limited to a few case reports of pipe smokers who developed cancer of the lip, tongue, or oral cavity [2–5]. These were not taken very seriously, however, and according to Doll were commonly attributed to the heat of the clay pipe stem rather than to any carcinogenic component of the smoke [1].

Beginning in the late nineteenth century, a series of technological innovations resulted in the rise of manufactured cigarettes and transformation of tobacco use [6]. The invention of safety matches in the late 1800s made it possible to smoke tobacco more frequently throughout the day in diverse settings. The development of machines to mass-produce and package cigarettes inexpensively allowed the cigarette to displace more expensive or cumbersome products such as cigars and pipes. New strains of tobacco and new curing processes were patented that produced less irritating smoke that could be inhaled more deeply than the smoke from traditional tobacco products. Whereas the nicotine released by older products such as cigars, pipes, roll-your own cigarettes, chewing tobacco, and snuff was highly alkaline and could be absorbed in ionized form through the oropharyngeal mucosa, nicotine released from the newer strains of tobacco was un-ionized and had to be inhaled to provide efficient absorption through the trachea and large bronchi. Deeper inhalation increased the surface area exposed to tobacco smoke. These changes in cigarette design were coupled, in the early twentieth century, with mass advertising campaigns to glamorize smoking of particular brands of cigarettes [6]. Free cigarettes were distributed in military rations to allied soldiers in World Wars I and II.

Collectively, these changes caused a large increase in the number of people smoking manufactured cigarettes, greater daily consumption of cigarettes, and a much greater surface area of tissues exposed to the carcinogens in tobacco smoke. A dramatic increase in cigarette smoking occurred first among men in the United Kingdom and United States and later among women. In Britain, nearly 70% of men and over 40% of women between the ages of 25 and 59 currently smoked cigarettes by mid-century [7]. In the United States, 57% of men and 28% of women reported current cigarette smoking in 1955, the time of the first national survey [8]. Despite widespread smoking, little scientific attention was paid to the negative health effects of cigarettes before the mid-twentieth century. Rottman had reported a small cluster of lung cancer among tobacco workers in Leipzig in 1898 [9]. Several correlation studies noted the statistical association between the rise in cigarette consumption and the increasing population rates of lung cancer in men [10–15]. Raymond Pearl described reduced longevity in smokers, based on family history records at the Johns Hopkins School of Hygiene [16]. Several small case-control studies of smoking and lung cancer published before 1950 [17–19] found a higher percentage of smokers among patients with lung cancer than with other diseases. A series of skin-testing experiments in rabbits were either negative [20, 21] or demonstrated some increase in skin tumours [22, 23] after prolonged contact with tar extracts from cigarettes. The tumorigenicity of tobacco extracts appeared to be less than that of coal tar, however, and the interpretation of animal experiments was complicated by controversy about the temperature at which the tar was extracted from tobacco for the animal experiments compared to the typical burning conditions in a cigarette [1]. Only in Germany were doctors and the Nazi political authorities concerned about the potential cardiovascular and reproductive toxicity of 'nicotinism', which was not at the time based on sound scientific evidence [1].

It was the extraordinary rise in lung cancer that began early in the twentieth century among men in the United Kingdom and later among men in other countries and subsequently women that finally drew serious attention to the hazards of smoking [24, 25]. Lung cancer had hitherto been a rare disease. The increase in the age-standardized death rate from lung cancer had begun among men in England and Wales by 1912 and accelerated sharply after World War I [24]. The number of lung cancer deaths recorded per year in England and Wales increased approximately fifteen-fold over the 25-year period between 1922 and 1947, far in excess of the increase in the size or longevity of the population. In the United States, where cigarette smoking began later and vital statistics data on mortality did not become available for most of the nation until 1930, the age-adjusted lung cancer death rate increased approximately five-fold from 1930 to the mid-1940s [26].

For some years it was debated whether the apparent increase in lung cancer incidence and death rates represented a true increase in occurrence or merely an artefact of improved diagnosis. Sceptics noted that several technologies introduced beginning in the 1920s could have increased recognition of previously undiagnosed disease [1]. These included the widespread introduction of chest x-rays in the United Kingdom in the 1920s, bronchograms in the 1930s, and bronchoscopy in the 1950s. Open chest surgery became practicable following improvements in anaesthesia during World War II [1]. The introduction of sulfapyridine in 1938 reduced mortality from pneumonia that had previously been lethal in the early stages of lung cancer, allowing cases to live long enough to be diagnosed. Nevertheless, the continued increase in lung cancer over several decades and its more frequent diagnosis in men than women made it increasingly unlikely that improved diagnosis could explain the entire increase [1].

Five case-control studies published in 1950

The publication in 1950 of five case-control studies reporting an association between smoking and lung cancer [24, 25, 27–29] provoked sudden interest among the medical and scientific communities on the potential health hazards of tobacco use. The two studies that drew the most attention were the British study by Doll and Hill [24] and an American study by Wynder and Evarts [25]. These were considerably larger than were earlier case-control studies of smoking and lung cancer [17–19], had higher response rates, and defined smoking more precisely. The association between smoking and lung cancer was very strong in the largest case-control studies in Britain (OR = 14) [24] and the United States (OR = 6.6) [25]; even the study by Schrek et al. that showed the weakest association had an odds ratio of 1.8 [28].

Although the case-control studies suggested that cigarette smoking was an important cause of lung cancer, the results were viewed as provocative rather than conclusive. Scientists were initially uncertain of the utility of case-control studies for studying chronic conditions such as cancer, since the methods had been developed for infectious diseases [1]. Some epidemiologists questioned whether smokers with lung cancer were more likely to be hospitalized because of cough, perhaps introducing selection bias [30] or whether the control group might be biased by cultural factors related to smoking [31]. Cuyler Hammond, of the American Cancer Society noted that the studies 'disagree so markedly in their measurement of the size of that relationship' that one could not tell whether the relationship is of 'major clinical interest' or 'of academic interest only' [32]. In retrospect, it seems likely that some of this variation may have arisen from including in the control series patients hospitalized for diseases that later proved to be smoking-attributable.

In any case, epidemiologists agreed that sound evidence was essential, given the high prevalence of smoking and the social and economic implications of the results.

The need for cohort studies

Doll and Hill realized that the simplest way to attempt to replicate the findings of the case-control studies, using a different methodology, was to obtain information on the individual smoking habits of a large number of people and to follow them to determine whether an individual's smoking habits predicted the risk of developing disease [1]. Such cohort studies would need to be large so that they could provide a sufficient number of events to be informative within a reasonable time period. They would need to collect questionnaire information on smoking behaviour, since such information was not then (and is not now) routinely collected on vital statistics records. In turn, the cohort studies would provide several important advantages over case-control studies. They could examine the relationship between smoking and many different endpoints, not just a single disease. This was important, because more than 70% of deaths caused by smoking result from diseases other than lung cancer [33]. The comparison group in cohort studies could be defined as lifelong non-smokers, thus avoiding the problem of including patients with other smoking-attributable diseases in the control group. Finally, cohort studies are intuitively more understandable than are case-control studies, because they reflect the desired temporal sequence in which exposure precedes disease.

The earliest cohort studies

The two earliest cohort studies of tobacco use and mortality were the British Doctors' Study, begun in the United Kingdom in 1951 [34, 35], and the Hammond Horn or Nine-State Study, initiated by the American Cancer Society (ACS) in 1952 [31, 36]. Both of these were designed to facilitate enrolment and follow-up of large populations. For instance, the physicians who participated in the British Doctors' Study were identified from the Medical Register of the United Kingdom and followed through the Registrars General, the British Medical Association and the General Medical Council [35]. The information on clinical diagnoses and cause of death was thought to be more accurate for doctors than for the general population. Similarly, the extensive network of local volunteers for ACS provided an extraordinary human resource to enrol and help to follow large prospective epidemiological studies in the United States [26]. Both the ACS cohorts and the British Doctors' Study provided effective conduits for disseminating information about the adverse effects of tobacco use. Publicity about the studies caused many doctors in the United Kingdom and United States to stop smoking, well ahead of the general public.

British Doctors' Study

In 1951, a questionnaire on smoking habits was sent to all British doctors included in the Medical Register. Of the 41 024 replies received, 40 701 were sufficiently complete to be utilized [34]. The 34 494 men and 6 207 women included in the follow-up comprised 69% and 60% of men and women respectively in the Registry. Further questionnaires about changes in smoking habits were sent in 1957 to men, in 1960 to women, and in 1966 and 1972 to all participants. On each occasion, approximately 97% of the doctors responded. The analyses defined lifelong non-smoking as never having smoked as much as one cigarette per day or quarter ounce of other forms of tobacco for as much as one year. A preliminary report was published by Doll and Hill in 1954 [34], and a second report in 1956 [35]. Results from the 10-year follow-up of male doctors was published in 1964 [37], the 20-year follow-up (through October 1971) for men in 1976 [38], and the 22-year follow-up for women in 1980 [39]. Results from the 40-year follow-up were published in 1994 [40] and the final report on the 50-year follow-up in 2004 [41].

Hammond Horn (the Nine-State Study)

The Hammond Horn Study began in October, 1952, when over 22 000 ACS volunteers distributed a questionnaire to ten white men, aged 50–69 years, whom he or she knew well [36]. A total of 204 547 men in nine states participated. Patterns of cigarette, cigar, and pipe smoking were similar in the Hammond Horn cohort to those in a representative survey of US males in 1955 [8]. Study participants were enrolled from among the friends, neighbours, and acquaintances of local volunteers and thus resembled the socio-demographic characteristics of the volunteers. A higher percentage were graduates of high school or college, and were more affluent than the general US population. After exclusions, a cohort of 187 783 men was followed from 1952 through 1955. A total of 11 783 deaths (6.2%) occurred during an average of 44 months of follow-up, with 1.1% of the cohort being lost to follow-up. Death certificates were collected for all reported deaths and further information was collected from the physician, hospital, or tumour registry whenever cancer was mentioned [42]. Preliminary results from the first 20 months of follow-up were published in 1954 [36]. Final results were published in 1958 for total mortality [42] and for specific causes of death [43]. The Hammond Horn Study was ended after 44 months of follow-up.

Early findings from the British Doctors' and Hammond Horn studies

Preliminary results from both the British Doctors' and the Hammond Horn studies were published in 1954. The British cohort demonstrated a statistically significant and steady increase in lung cancer occurrence among smokers, although this was based on only 36 lung cancers. The age standardized rate increased from 0.00 per 1 000 among the 3 093 non-smokers, to 1.14 per 1 000 among the 5 203 men recorded as smoking 25 g or more of tobacco daily. A similar but less steep rise was seen in mortality from coronary thrombosis, from a rate of 3.89 in non-smokers, to 5.15 in the heaviest smokers. In the Hammond Horn Study, men with a history of regular cigarette smoking had a substantially higher death rate from all causes (based on 4 854 deaths), from coronary heart disease (1 328 deaths), and from lung cancer (167 deaths) than men who had never smoked regularly.

A second report from the British Doctors' Study was published in 1956 on the basis of 84 confirmed cases of lung cancer. This too demonstrated a steady increase in the annual death rate from lung cancer with increasing amount smoked [35]. The annual death rate in men who smoked at least 25 g (approximately 25 cigarettes) per day was 1.66 per thousand, over 20 times the death rate of the non-smokers (0.07 per thousand). Greater cigarette consumption was also associated with higher death rates from chronic bronchitis, peptic ulcer, and pulmonary tuberculosis, although the trend was statistically significant only for chronic bronchitis.

Of interest is that the principal investigators of the earliest cohort studies did not initially expect that cigarette smoking would prove to be the cause of the increasing lung cancer in the United Kingdom and United States. When Doll first began work on the British case-control study in 1948, he suspected that 'motor cars and the tarring of roads' were a more likely explanation than cigarette smoking [44]. Both Doll and Hill were impressed by the results of the case-control study, however, and in their 1950 publication concluded that, 'smoking is a factor, and an important factor, in the production of carcinoma of the lung' [24]. Hammond and Horn, who initially smoked, remained sceptical of the earlier case-control studies that associated lung cancer with cigarette smoking. When they began the first ACS cohort study, they considered it equally plausible that automotive exhaust, dust from tarred roads, and/or air pollution from coal and oil furnaces might be partly or wholly responsible [31, 32]. However the results of their Nine-State Study [36, 42, 43] persuaded Hammond and Horn to stop smoking and to focus ACS attention on tobacco use as an important cause of cancer and other diseases.

Growing scientific consensus

Sufficient scientific evidence had accumulated by the late 1950s that at least six scientific consensus groups concluded that cigarette smokers had higher lung cancer death rates than non-smokers. These expert reviews were convened by health ministries in the United Kingdom. [45], United States [46], Canada [47], Sweden [48], and the Netherlands [49] and by cancer societies in Denmark, Norway, and Finland [50]. The evidence at the time included early reports from the cohort studies [34, 35, 42, 43, 51], additional case-control data [52–59] and experimental evidence that prolonged application of condensates of tobacco smoke induced skin cancer in rabbits and mice [60–65].

Counterarguments to the idea that smoking caused lung cancer grew increasingly implausible in the face of the evidence that had accumulated by the late 1950s. The hypothesis proposed by R.A. Fisher that some underlying constitutional factor predisposed smokers to both smoking and lung cancer [66–69] did not explain the temporal increase in lung cancer in the population, nor the decrease in lung cancer in persons who stopped smoking. Berkson's contention that the hospital-based case-control studies were biased by the differential affects of illness on enrolment [30] was countered by the stability of the association between smoking and lung cancer during longer follow-up of the British Doctors' Study [35]. The lack of specificity whereby smoking was associated with multiple diseases [70] was also not considered strong evidence against causation, because of the complex mixture of chemicals in tobacco smoke [1].

The scientific consensus that tobacco smoking caused lung cancer became even stronger after 1960 with the publication of reports from the World Health Organization [71], the Royal College of Physicians of London [72], and the Advisory Committee to the US Surgeon General [50]. In 1962 the Royal College of Physicians concluded, 'Cigarette smoking is a cause of lung cancer and bronchitis and probably contributes to the development of coronary heart disease.... It delays healing of gastric and duodenal ulcers'. The 1964 Report of the Advisory Group to the Surgeon General in the US [50] was particularly influential, according to Doll, because of its thoroughness and because its members had been individually vetted by the tobacco industry to exclude those who had publicly expressed views on the topic [1]. On the basis of an independent analyses of 7 published and unpublished prospective studies and review of 29 retrospective studies of smoking and health, the Report stated, 'Cigarette smoking is associated with a 70 percent increase in the age-specific death rates of males and to a lesser extent with increased death rates of females.' It concluded,

> Cigarette smoking is causally related to lung cancer in men; the magnitude of the effect of cigarette smoking far outweighs all other factors. The data for women, although less extensive, point in the same direction. A relationship exists between cigarette smoking and emphysema, but it has not been established that this relationship is causal: Male cigarette smokers have a higher death rate from coronary artery disease than non-smoking males. Although the causative role of cigarette smoking in deaths from coronary disease is not proven, the Committee considers it more prudent from the public health viewpoint to assume that the established association has causative meaning than to suspend judgment until no uncertainty remains. [50]

After 1964 there was no serious scientific controversy about whether smoking caused lung cancer. The official scepticism of the tobacco industry was maintained as a legal and political strategy rather than a consequence of any genuine scientific debate, as revealed later through disclosure of internal documents [73]. Many important scientific questions remained, however, concerning other deleterious effects of tobacco use, the magnitude of the problem, and the potential benefits of cessation and other possible interventions.

Additional cohort studies

Among the seven cohort studies considered by the 1964 Report to the Surgeon General [50] were two that, like the British Doctors Study, were of sufficient size and duration to qualify as 'Great Studies'. These were the US Veterans' Study, begun by the National Institutes of Health and US Veteran's Administration in 1954, and Cancer Prevention Study I, a second large cohort study initiated by the American Cancer Society, in 1959 [74].

The US Veterans' (Dorn) Study

In September 1954, the US Veterans' Administration contacted 293 958 men who served in the armed forces at any time between 1917 and 1940 and who held US government Life Insurance policies [75]. Subjects were mainly white men of the middle and upper social classes. A total of 248 195 men (response rate 85% after two mailings) returned a questionnaire on their smoking habits. Vital status of these veterans was followed until death by tracking life insurance claims to the Veterans Administration or termination of the policy for other reasons. Supplemental information was obtained on deceased persons from certifying physicians or hospitals. Results from the Veterans Study were published in 1958 [76], 1959 [77], 1966 [75], 1990 [78], and 1995 [79]. A total of 192 756 deaths occurred during 26-year follow-up from 1954 to 1980.

Cancer Prevention Study I (CPS-I)

Between October 1959 and February 1960, volunteers for the ACS in 25 states recruited more than one million subjects from among their friends, neighbours, and acquaintances to complete a four-page questionnaire [80, 81]. Known as Cancer Prevention Study I (CPS-I) or the 25 State Study, the cohort was substantially larger than Hammond Horn Study and included women as well as men [80, 82]. Enrolment was by family; all family members over 30 years of age were requested to fill out detailed questionnaires on smoking behaviour [74]. For the 1 045 087 subjects with usable questionnaire information, vital status was determined annually through the volunteers. Updated information on smoking was obtained every 2 years. Approximately 1% of subjects were lost during the first 6 years of follow-up, through September 1965 [81]. Three states were then dropped from the study [83] and follow-up in the remainder was 98.4 9% complete through September 1971, and 92.8% through September 1972 [82]. Death certificates were obtained from state or local authorities, and, when cancer was mentioned, further information was sought from physicians.

Several other large cohort studies initiated after 1960 examined the deleterious effects of tobacco in women and in other geographic regions and time periods. These are described briefly below.

Swedish Study

In 1963, questionnaires about smoking were mailed to a national probability sample of 55 000 Swedish adults, aged 18 through 69 years [84]. The response rate was 69%. Information on smoking status was collected in 1963. Mortality follow-up over the ensuing 10 years was conducted through linkage with the national death registry. The results for 10 years of follow-up were published in 1975 [84] and for longer follow-ups in 1987 [85] and 1997 [86].

Japanese Six Prefecture Cohort Study

In late 1965, 142 857 women and 122 261 men, aged 40 years and older were interviewed in 29 health districts in Japan [87, 88]. The study group comprised between 91% and 99% of adults of this age in the districts represented, which were distributed throughout six prefectures. Information on tobacco smoking, diet, alcohol consumption, occupation, and marital status was obtained by interview at enrolment. After 6 years, a second interview of 3 728 randomly selected women showed that the percentage of smokers had decreased only slightly (from 10.4% to 9.7%). A record linkage system was established for annual follow-up. During 16 years of follow-up, 51 422 deaths occurred. Until recently, the Hiriyama cohort was unique in being the only large prospective study of smoking and mortality among Asians.

Nurses' Health Study I

A cohort of 121 700 30–55-year-old female nurses was assembled in the United States in 1976. At enrolment and periodically thereafter, the nurses completed a mailed questionnaire on risk factors for cancer and heart disease. Much of the exposure information concerned nutritional factors, yet the cohort has been very informative about the effects of smoking and smoking cessation on many health endpoints in women [89, 90].

Kaiser Permanente Study

Between 1979 and 1986, the Kaiser Permanente Medical Care Program obtained baseline information about tobacco smoking from 36 035 women and 24 803 men aged 35 years or older [91]. Participants in the programme make up about 30% of the population in the areas it serves. Follow-up through 1987 identified 1 098 deaths among all women. The study provides the only published data on premature death associated with cigarette smoking among African-American women.

Cancer Prevention Study II (CPS-II)

The third large prospective study, begun by the ACS, was called Cancer Prevention Study II (CPS-II). Begun in 1982, it is a prospective mortality study of nearly 1.2 million adults, 30 years of age and older, drawn from the entire population of the United States. Like CPS-I it included more than 50% women. Enrolment into the study was accomplished by completing a brief confidential mailed questionnaire addressing alcohol and tobacco use, diet and other factors affecting mortality. Deaths were ascertained from month of enrolment through 1988 by personal inquiries by ACS volunteers at 2-year intervals. Follow-up after 1988 has continued through linkage with the National Death Index. Analyses of smoking and mortality have largely been restricted to the first 6 years of follow-up, since information on tobacco use was not updated after enrolment. By 1988, 2% of the cohort were lost to follow-up and 0.2% could not be followed because personal identifiers provided were insufficient for linkage to the National Death Index. By 1991, 12% of the cohort had died and death certificates were obtained for 98% of the deceased. Participants in CPS-II were more likely to be white (93%), married (81%), middle class and educated (high school graduates or above 85.6%) than the general population of the United States.

Contributions of later cohort studies

Continuing follow-up of the original cohorts and the initiation of new large cohort studies proved essential to the scientific consensus that smoking caused a multiplicity of diseases besides lung cancer. One advantage of cohort studies was their ability to examine many endpoints simultaneously.

Initially this invoked criticism of the lung cancer hypothesis in that Berkson argued that smoking was associated with so many different diseases that none of the associations were interpretable [30, 70]. However, the relative risk for lung cancer was 10.8 among all cigarette smokers, compared to non-smokers, in the seven cohort studies analysed by the 1964 Advisory Committee to the Surgeon General [50] and was 24 among heavy cigarette smokers in the British Doctors Study [35]. While the relative risk estimates were lower for death from laryngeal cancer (RR = 5.4) and chronic bronchitis (RR = 6.1) than was the association with lung cancer, they nevertheless persuaded the 1964 Advisory Committee to conclude that cigarette smoking caused lung cancer, laryngeal cancer, and chronic bronchitis in men [50].

Early consensus groups were more cautious in interpreting the relationship of smoking with various cardiovascular diseases and other conditions. The 1964 Report to the Surgeon General noted that 'Male cigarette smokers have a higher death rate from coronary artery disease than non-smoking males, but it is not clear that the association has causal significance' (RR = 6.1) [50]. The median relative risk for death from coronary heart disease in male smokers compared to non-smokers was 1.7 (range 1.5–2.0) in the cohort studies reviewed in 1964. However, by 1967, a later Surgeon General Report concluded, 'The convergence of many types of evidence – epidemiological, experimental, pathological and clinical – strongly suggests that cigarette smoking can cause death from coronary heart disease' [92]. The language attributing causation became progressively stronger over time, as results from the Framingham Study and other cardiovascular cohorts confirmed that smoking, hypertension, and increased cholesterol were all strong and independent risk factors [93].

With prolonged follow-up, the cohort studies included many more cases and/or deaths from less common conditions and more detailed analyses of diseases attributable to smoking. By 1989, the US Surgeon General had designated 14 disease categories that contribute to smoking-attributable deaths in the United States [94]. These included coronary heart disease, hypertensive heart disease, cerebrovascular lesions, aortic aneurism (non-syphilitic), ulcer (gastric, duodenal, jejunal), influenza and pneumonia, bronchitis and emphysema, cancers of the lip-oral cavity-and pharynx, esophagus, pancreas, larynx, lung, kidney, and bladder and other urinary organs [94]. An updated review by the International Agency for Research on Cancer (IARC) in 2002 refined this list by including cancers of the naso-, oro-, and hypopharynx, nasal cavity and paranasal sinuses, stomach, liver, kidney (parenchyma as well as renal pelvis), ureter, uterine cervix, and bone marrow (myeloid leukaemia) [95].

Besides contributing to the inventory of diseases officially designated as being caused by smoking, the cohort studies also reveal how the epidemic changed and evolved over time. This progression is particularly evident in the increase in lung cancer death rates that occurred among women smokers in the two ACS cohorts during the last 50 years, [96, 97], and by the growing disparity in overall survival rates between smokers and non-smokers from the first to the second half of the British Doctors' Study [40, 98].

Figure 2.1 illustrates the death rate from lung cancer among women who smoked cigarettes, within 5-year age intervals, for four time periods between 1960 and 1986. Lung cancer mortality increased enormously in women smokers over the 26-year period. Not shown in Fig. 2.1 is that the death rate from lung cancer remained essentially constant over this interval among women who had never smoked [97, 99]. Consequently, the relative risk associated with current cigarette smoking in women increased from approximately two in 1960–1964 to nearly 11 in 1982–1986. The protracted increase in lung cancer among women smokers contradicted the hypothesis of the early 1950s, that women might be less susceptible than men to the adverse effects of smoking, and refuted the theory proposed by R.A. Fisher that the absence of increasing lung cancer among women smokers in the 1950s was evidence that smoking did not cause lung cancer [68]. Instead, it

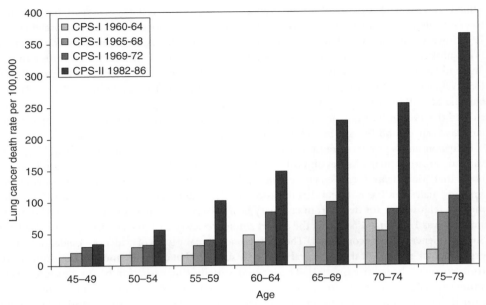

Figure 2.1 Age-specific lung cancer death rates among women who currently smoked cigarettes when enrolled in CPS-I and CPS-II.
Data from Garfinkel L and Stellman SD. Smoking and lung cancer in women: Findings from a prospective study. Cancer Research 1988;48:6951–6955.

supported Doll's prediction [100], that as successive birth cohorts of women smoked more intensively from earlier ages, their lung cancer risk would approach that of male smokers.

An analogous picture of the progression of the epidemic is apparent in the widening gap in overall survival between cigarette smokers and lifelong non-smokers from the first to the second half of the British Doctors' Study. Figure 2.2 illustrates the probability of survival to various ages beyond 40 years among male British Doctors who never smoked tobacco or who currently smoked cigarettes during the first or second 20-year interval of follow-up [40]. During both time periods, the percentage surviving was higher among men who had never smoked than among those who smoked regularly. The percentage surviving to age 70 was 58% among current cigarette smokers and 76% among lifelong non-smokers in the interval 1951–1971, and 60% and 83% in follow-up from 1971 to 1991. Furthermore, the median difference in overall survival between smokers and non-smokers widened over time, from 5 years in 1951–1971 to 7 years in 1971–91. The difference widened largely because improvements in survival affected never-smokers more than smokers.

Contributing to the increase in lung cancer mortality among female smokers, and to the widening disparity in survival between smokers and non-smokers was a generational shift towards initiating cigarette smoking at younger ages. Successive birth cohorts of both male and female smokers began smoking regularly earlier in adolescence [101]. The relationship between early age of initiation and lung cancer risk is illustrated in Fig. 2.3, showing the lung cancer death rate (per 100 000) among men, age 55–64 in the US Veterans Study [75]. Men who began smoking earlier at an earlier age have higher death rates from lung cancer at a given level of smoking than men who initiated smoking later. The difference in risk is seen for both 'moderate' (10–20 cigarettes per day) and 'heavy' smokers (21–39 cigarettes per day). This analysis cannot differentiate whether the higher lung cancer rate in persons who begin smoking early reflects longer duration of smoking or greater vulnerability of the immature lung to the carcinogenicity of smoke, since the two

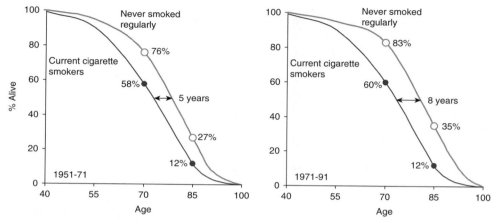

Figure 2.2 Survival after age 35 among cigarette smokers and non-smokers in first half (left) and second half of the British Doctors' Study (right). For ages 35–44 rates for the whole study are used in both halves since little information on these is available from the second half.
Reproduced from Doll R, Peto R, Wheatley K, Gray R, Sutherland I. Mortality in relation to smoking: 40 years' observations on male British doctors. BMJ 1994:309:901–911 (with permission from the BMJ Publishing Group).

factors are inseparably correlated in current smokers of the same age. However, Fig. 2.3 does illustrate that earlier age of initiation is a strong predictor of higher lung cancer risk.

Finally, the cohort studies demonstrate the substantial benefit of smoking cessation in preventing much of the increased mortality caused by continued smoking. Figure 2.4 illustrates the cumulative probability of death from lung cancer, conditional on survival from other conditions, during 7-year follow-up of CPS-II in relation to age, sex, and smoking status. The highest risk is

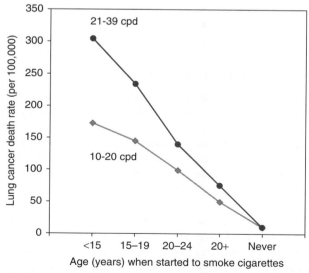

Figure 2.3 Relationship between age of starting regular cigarette smoking in early adult life and lung cancer death rates at age 55–64 for US male veterans, 1954–62. Data presented separately for heavy and moderate smokers.
Source: Kahn D. The Dorn study of smoking and mortality among US veterans. Report on eight and one-half years of observation. Natl Cancer Inst Monogr. 1966;19:1–125.

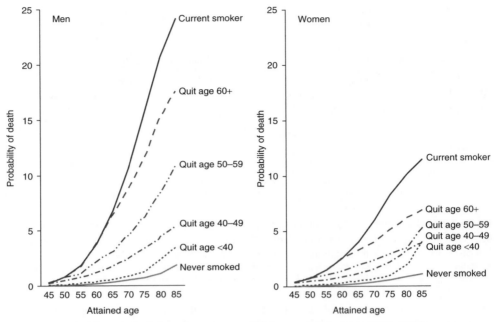

Figure 2.4 Probability of death from lung cancer: CPS-II men and women, 1984–1991.

seen in men and women who actively smoked cigarettes at the time of enrolment into the study in 1982. Their cumulative risk equals 24% and 11% in men and women respectively by age > 85. The lowest risk of lung cancer is seen in men and women who have never smoked regularly. The risk is intermediate among men and women who have quit smoking at various ages, prior to enrolment in the study, and decreases the earlier the age of quitting. Persons who stop smoking avoid much of the dramatic further increase in risk incurred by those who continue.

Continuing need for cohort studies

It is important to note that there is a continuing need for cohort studies to monitor the course of the pandemic in other countries and to improve strategies for ending tobacco dependence. Not all of the important questions have been answered. There is still much to learn about the nature and treatment of addiction, the phenomenon that obligates continues smoking for most adults. This is very important for the 43.1 million Americans [102] and over 1.2 billion people worldwide [103] who are addicted to tobacco use. Most of the attention of cohort studies in the past has been directed at understanding the disease burden caused by smoking, not at developing or testing interventions.

Furthermore, the diseases that tobacco use causes differ somewhat in different countries, depending on background risks of diseases that either compete with or interact with smoking. For example, much of the disease burden caused by tobacco in the United States and other Western countries involves cardiovascular diseases, because of the high background rate of these conditions. The same is not true in China, where a much higher proportion of the burden involves chronic obstructive pulmonary disease [104], or in India, where the most common disease by which smoking causes premature death is tuberculosis [105].

Summary and conclusions

Beginning in the early 1950s, large cohort studies played a major role in helping to identify the multitude of adverse health effects caused by tobacco use, particularly manufactured cigarettes. They demonstrated that the harmful effects applied to women as well as men [106], that cigarettes with low machine-measure tar and nicotine were no less hazardous with respect to lung cancer than filter-tip 'regular' tar cigarettes [107] and that the burden of disease caused by smoking increased over time as smokers initiated regular cigarette smoking at progressively earlier ages. Large cohort studies will continue to be important for monitoring the course of the epidemic as it evolves in different cultures and for sustaining the political resolve to end it.

References

1. Doll, R. (1998). Uncovering the effects of smoking: historical perspective. *Stat Methods Med Res*, 7:87–117.

2. Bouisson, E. (1859). Du cancer buccal chez les fumeurs. *Montpelier Medical Journal*, 2:539–99 and 1859; 3:19–41.

3. Anonymous. (1890). Cancer and smoking. *Br Med J*, 1:748.

4. Hoffman, F. (1927). *Cancer and Overnutrition:* Prudential Press.

5. Lombard, H. and Doering, C. (1928). Cancer studies in Massachusetts. 2. Habits, characteristics and environment of individuals with and without cancer. *N Engl J Med*, 198:481–7.

6. Slade, J. (1993). Nicotine delivery devices. In: Orleans C, Slade J, eds. *Nicotine Addiction, Principles and Management*. New York: Oxford University Press, pp. 3–23.

7. Peto, R., Darby, S., Deo, H., Silcocks, P., Whitley, E., and Doll, R. (2000). Smoking, smoking cessation and lung cancer in the UK since 1950: combination of national statistics with two case-control studies. *BMJ*, 321:323–9.

8. Haenszel, W., Shimkin, M., and Miller, H. (1956). Tobacco smoking patterns in the United States. In: Public Health Monograph Number 45. PHS Pub. No. 463. Public Health Service. Washington, D.C.: U.S. Government Printing Office.

9. Rottmann, H. (1898). Uber primare lungencarcinoma [Inaugural-dissertation]. Wurzburg: Universitat Wurzburg.

10. Tylecote, F. (1927). Cancer of the lung. *Lancet*, 2:256–7.

11. Lickint, F. (1929). Tabac und tabakrauch ais atiologischer factor des carcinoma. *Zeitschrift fur Krebsforschung*, 30:349–65.

12. Fleckseder, R. (1936). Uber den bronchialkrebs und einiger seiner entstehungsbedigungen. *Munchener Medizinische Wochenschrift*, 83:1585–88.

13. Adler, I. (1912). *Primary Malignant Growths of The Lung and Bronchi*. London: Longmans Green.

14. Hoffman, F. (1931). Cancer and smoking habits. *Ann Surg*, 93:50–67.

15. Arkin, A. and Wagner, D. (1936). Primary carcinoma of the lung. *JAMA*, 106:587–91.

16. Pearl, R. (1938). Tobacco smoking and longevity. *Science*, 87:216–7.

17. Muller, F. (1939). Tabakmissbrauch und lungencarcinoma. *Zeitschrift fur Krebsforschung*, 49:57–85.

18. Schairer, E. and Schioninger, E. (1943). Lungenkrebs und tabakverbrauch. *Zeitschrift fur Krebsforschung*, 54:261–69.

19. Wassink, W. (1948). Onstanvoorwarden voor Longkanker. *Nederlands Tijdschrift voor Geneeskunde (Amsterdam)*, 92:3732–47.

20. Leitch, A. (1928). Experimental production of tumours by other methods. In: *Fifth Annual Report of the British Empire Cancer Campaign*. London: British Empire Cancer Campaign, p. 26.

21. Passey, R. (1929). Cancer of the lung. In: *Sixth Report of British Empire Cancer Research Campaign*. London: British Empire Cancer Campaign, p. 85.

22. Roffo, A. (1931). Durch Tabak beim Kaninchen entwickeltes Carcinom. *Zeitschrift fur Krebsforschung*, **33**:321–2.

23. Cooper, E., Lamb, F., Sanders, E., and Hirst, E. (1932). The role of tobacco-smoking in the production of cancer. *J Hyg (Lond)*, **32**:293–300.

24. Doll, R. and Hill, A. (1950). Smoking and carcinoma of the lung: preliminary report. *Br Med J*, **2**:739–48.

25. Wynder, E. and Graham, E. (1950). Tobacco smoking as a possible etiologic factor in bronchogenic carcinoma: a study of six hundred and eighty-four proved cases. *J Am Med Assoc*, **143**:329–36.

26. Thun, M., Calle, E., Rodriguez, C., and Wingo, P. (2000). Epidemiological research at the American Cancer Society. *Cancer Epidemiol Biomark Prev*, **9**:861–8.

27. Levin, M., Goldstein, H., and Gerhardt, P. (1950). Cancer and tobacco smoking: a preliminary report. *J Am Med Assoc*, **143**:336–8.

28. Schrek, R., Baker, L., Ballard, G., and Dolgoff, S. (1950). Tobacco smoking as an etiologic factor in disease. I. Cancer. *Cancer Res*, **10**:49–58.

29. Mills, C. and Porter, M. (1950). Tobacco smoking habits and cancer of the mouth and respiratory system. *Cancer Res*, **10**:539–42.

30. Berkson, J. (1955). The statistical study of association between smoking and lung cancer. *Proceedings of the Staff Meetings of the Mayo Clinic*, **30**:319–48.

31. Hammond, E. (1953). Possible etiologic factors in lung cancer. In: Sixty-Second Annual Meeting of the Association of Life Insurance Medical Directors of America; 1953; New York: Press of Recording and Statistical Corporation, p. 3–7.

32. Hammond, E. and Horn, D. (1952). Tobacco and lung cancer. *CA Cancer J Clin*, **2**:97–8.

33. CDC. (2002). Annual smoking-attributable mortality, years of potential life lost, and economic costs – United States, 1995–1999. *MMWR*, **51**:300–3.

34. Doll, R. and Hill, A. (1954). The mortality of doctors in relation to their smoking habits. A preliminary report. *Br Med J*, **1**:1451–5.

35. Doll, R. and Hill, A. (1956). Lung cancer and other causes of death in relation to smoking. A second report on the mortality of British doctors. *Br Med J*, **2**:1071–81.

36. Hammond, E. (1954). Smoking in relation to lung cancer – a follow-up study. *Connecticut State Med J*, **18**:3–11.

37. Doll, R. and Hill, A. (1964). Mortality in relation to smoking: ten years' observations of British doctors. *Br Med J*, **1**:1399–1410, 1460–7.

38. Doll, R. and Peto, R. (1976). Mortality in relation to smoking: 20 years' observations on male British doctors. *Br Med J*, **2**:1525–36.

39. Doll, R., Gray, R., Hafner, B., and Peto, R. (1980). Mortality in relation to smoking: 22 years' observations on female British Doctors. *Br Med J*, i:967–71.

40. Doll, R., Peto, R., Wheatley, K., Gray, R., and Sutherland, I. (1994). Mortality in relation to smoking: 40 years' observations on male British doctors. *BMJ*, **309**:901–11.

41. Doll, R., Peto, R., Boreham, J., and Sutherland, I. (2004). Mortality in relation to smoking: 50 years' observations on male British doctors. *Br Med J*.

42. Hammond, E. and Horn, D. (1958). Smoking and death rates-report on forty-four months of follow-up of 187,783 men. I. Total mortality. *JAMA*, **166**:1159–72.

43. Hammond, E, and Horn, D. (1958). Smoking and death rates-report on forty-four months of follow-up of 187,783 men. II. Death rates by cause. *JAMA*, **166**:1294–308.

44. Doll, R. (1998). The first reports on smoking and lung cancer. In: *Ashes to ashes: the history of smoking and health*. Lock S, Reynolds L, and Tansey E, eds. Clio Medica, pp. 130–42.

45 Medical Research Council (1957). Tobacco smoking and cancer of the lung. *Br Med J*, **1**:1523.

46. Burney, L. (1959). Smoking and lung cancer: a statement of the Public Health Service. *JAMA*, **171**:1829–37.

47. National Cancer Institute of Canada (1958). Lung cancer and smoking. *Can Med Assoc J*, **79**:566–8.

48. Swedish Medical Research Council (1958). Statement to the King, May 12.

49. Netherlands Ministry of Social Affairs and Public Health (1957). Roken en longkanker. *Nederlands Tijdschrift voor Geneeskunde (Amsterdam)*, **101**:459–64.

50. U.S. Public Health Service (1964). Smoking and Health. Report of the Advisory Committee to the Surgeon General of the Public Health Service. Washington, DC: U.S. Department of Health, Education, and Welfare, Public Health Service, Center for Disease Control.

51. Hammond, E. and Horn, D. (1954). The relationship between human smoking habits and death rates. *JAMA*, **155**:1316–28.

52. Doll, R. and Hill, A. (1952). Study of aetiology of carcinoma of the lung. *Br Med J*, **2**:1271–86.

53. Kouloumies, M. (1953). Smoking and pulmonary carcinoma. *Acta Radiology (Stockholm)*, **30**:255–60.

54. Linckint, F. (1953). 2. Statistische Voraussetzungen zur Klarung der Tabakrauchatiologie des Lungenkrebses. In: Atiologie und Prophylaxe des Lungenkrebses. Leipzig: Theodor Steinkopff, p. 76–102.

55. Gsell, O. (1954). Carcinome bronchique et tabac. *Medical Hygiene*, **12**:429–31.

56. Randig, K. (1954). Untersuchungen zur atiologie des bronchialkarzinomas. *Off Gesundheitsdienst*, **16**:305–13.

57. Kreyberg, L. (1955). Lung cancer and tobacco smoking in Norway. *Brit J Cancer*, **9**:495–510.

58. Schwartz, D. and Denoix, P. (1957). L'enquete Francais sur l'etiologie du cancer broncho-pulmonaire. Role de tabac. *Semaine des Hospitaux de Paris*, **33**:3630–43.

59. Segi, M., Fukushima, L., Fujisako, S., Kurihara, M., Saito, S., Atano, K., *et al.* (1957). An epidemiological study on cancer in Japan. *Gann*, **48**:1–63.

60. Wynder, E., Graham, E., and Croninger, A. (1953). Experimental production of carcinoma with cigarette tar. Part I. *Cancer Res*, **13**:855–64.

61. Wynder, E., Graham, E., and Croninger, A. (1955). Experimental production of carcinoma with cigarette tar. Part II. *Cancer Res*, **15**:445–8.

62. Engelbreth-Holm, J. and Ahlmann, J. (1957). Production of carcinoma in St/Eh mice with cigarette tar. *Acta Microbiol Acad Sci Hung Pathalogical Microbiology Scandinavia*, **41**:267–72.

63. Guerin, M. and Cuzin, J. (1957). Action carcinogene du goudron de fumée de cigarette sur le peau de souris. *Bulletin of the Association of France Cancer*, **44**:387–408.

64. Sugiura, K. (1956). Experimental production of carcinoma in mice with cigarette smoke tar. *Gann*, **47**:243–4.

65. Croninger, A., Graham, E., and Wynder, E. (1958). Experimental production of carcinoma with cigarette tar. Part V. *Cancer Res*, **18**:1263–71.

66. Fisher, R. (1957). Dangers of cigarette smoking. *BMJ*, **2**:43.

67. Fisher, R. (1958). Cancer and smoking. *Nature*, **182**:596.

68. Fisher, R. (1958). Lung cancer and cigarettes? *Nature*, **182**:168.

69. Fisher, R. (ed.) (1959). *Smoking: the cancer controversy. Some attempts to assess the evidence.* Edinburgh: Oliver and Boyd.

70. Berkson, J. (1958). Smoking and lung cancer: some observations on two recent reports. *J Am Stat Assoc*, **53**:28–38.

71. World Health Organization (1960). Epidemiology of cancer of the lung. Report of a study group. *World Health Organization Technical Report Series* 192. Geneva: World Health Organization.

72. Royal College of Physicians of London (1962). *Smoking and health.* London: Pitman Medical.

73. Glantz, S., Slade, J., Bero, L., Hanauer, P., and Barnes, D. (1996). Looking through a keyhole at the tobacco industry. In: Glantz, S., Slade, J., Bero, L., Hanauer, P., and Barnes, D. (eds) *The Cigarette Papers*, p. 1–24. Berkeley, CA: University of California Press.

74. Hammond, E. and Garfinkel, L. (1961). Smoking habits of men and women. *J Natl Cancer Instit*, **27**:419–42.

75. Kahn, H. (1966). The Dorn study of smoking and mortality among U.S. veterans: report on eight and one-half years of observation. In: Haenszel, W. (ed.) Monograph 19, Epidemiological Study of Cancer

and Other Chronic Diseases. Bethesda, MD: U.S. Department of Health, Education, and Welfare, Public Health Service, National Cancer Institute, p. 1–126.

76. Dorn, H. (1958). The mortality of smokers and nonsmokers. In: *Proc Soc Stat Sect Amer Stat Assn*, pp. 34–71.

77. Dorn, H. (1959). Tobacco consumption and mortality from cancer and other diseases. *Public Health Rep*, **74**:581–93.

78. Hsing, A., McLaughlin, J., Hrubec, Z., Blot, W., and Fraumeni, J. (1990). Cigarette smoking and liver cancer among US veterans. *Cancer Causes Control*, **1**:217–21.

79. Chow, W., McLaughlin, J., Hrubec, Z., and Fraumeni, J. (1995). Smoking and biliary tract cancer in a cohort of US Veterans. *Br J Cancer*, **72**:1556–8.

80. Hammond, E. (1964). Smoking in relation to mortality and morbidity: findings in first thirty-four months of follow-up in a prospective study started in 1959. *J Natl Cancer Inst*, **32**:1161–88.

81. Hammond, E. (1966). Smoking in relation to the death rates of one million men and women. In: Haenszel, W. (ed). Epidemiologic Approaches to the Study of Cancer and Other Chronic Diseases. *Natl Cancer Inst Monogr 19*. Rockville, MD: US Department of Health, Education, and Welfare, pp. 127–204.

82. Garfinkel, L. (1985). Selection, follow-up and analysis in the American Cancer Society prospective studies. *Monogr Natl Cancer Inst*, **67**:49–52.

83. Hammond, E. and Seidman, H. (1980). Smoking and cancer in the United States. *Prev Med*, **9**:169–73.

84. Cederlof, R., Friberg, L., Hrubec, Z., and Lorich, U. (1975).*The Relationship of Smoking and Some Social Covariables to Mortality and Cancer Morbidity*. Stockholm, Sweden: Department of Environmental Hygiene, The Karolinska Institute.

85. Carstensen, J., Pershagen, G., and Eklund, G. (1987). Mortality in relation to cigarette and pipe smoking: 16 years' observation of 25,000 Swedish men. *J Epidemiol Community Health*, **41**:166–72.

86. Nordlund, L., Carstensen, J., and Pershagen, G. (1997). Cancer incidence in female smokers: a 26-year follow-up. *Int J Cancer*, **73**:625–8.

87. Hirayama, T. (1990). Life-style and mortality. A large-scale census-based cohort study in Japan. In: *Contributions to Epidemiology and Statistics*. Basel: Karger.

88. Akiba, S. and Hirayama, T. (1990). Cigarette smoking and cancer mortality risk in Japanese men and women – results from reanalysis of the six-prefecture cohort study data. *Environ Health Perspect*, **87**:19–26.

89. Kawachi, I., Colditz, G., Stampfer, M., Willett, W., Manson, J., Rosner, B., *et al.* (1997). Smoking cessation and decreased risks of total mortality, Stroke, and coronary heart disease incidence among women: a prospective cohort study. In: Samet, J. (ed.) *National Cancer Institute, Smoking and Tobacco Control*, Monograph 8: Changes in Cigarette-Related Disease Risks and Their Implication for Prevention and Control. Washington, DC: National Institute of Health, p. 531–65.

90. U.S. Department of Health and Human Services. (2001). *Women and Smoking: A Report of the Surgeon General*. Atlanta, Georgia: U.S. Department of Health and Human Services, Centers for Disease Control and Prevention, National Center for Chronic Disease Prevention and Health Promotion, Office on Smoking and Health.

91. Friedman, G., Tekawa, I., Sadler, M., and Sidney, S. (1997). Smoking and mortality: the Kaiser Permanente experience. *Natl Cancer Inst Monogr*, **97**:472–99.

92. U.S. Public Health Service. (1967). *The Health Consequences of Smoking. A Public Health Review: 1967.* Washington, DC: U.S. Department of Health, Education, and Welfare, Public Health Service, Center for Disease Control.

93. Kannell, W., Dawber, T., and McNamara, P. (1966). Detection of the coronary-prone adult: the Framingham study. *J Iowa Med Soc*, **56**:26–34.

94. U.S. Department of Health and Human Services. (1989). *Reducing the Health Consequences of Smoking: 25 Years of Progress. A Report of the Surgeon General*. Rockville, MD: U.S. Department of Health and Human Services, Public Health Service, Centers for Disease Control, Center for Chronic Disease Prevention and Health Promotion, Office on Smoking and Health.

95. IARC. (2002). IARC monographs on the evaluation of the carcinogenic risk of chemicals to humans: tobacco smoke and involuntary smoking. International Agency for Research on Cancer. http://193.52.164.11/htdocs/monographs/vol83/02-involuntary.html ed. Lyon: International Agency for Research on Cancer;.

96. Garfinkel, L. and Stellman, S. (1988). Smoking and lung cancer in women: findings in a prospective study. *Cancer Res*, **48**:6951–5.

97. Thun, M., Day-Lally, C., Meyers, D., Calle, E., Flanders, W., Namboodiri, M, *et al.* (1997). Trends in tobacco smoking and mortality from cigarette use in Cancer Prevention Studies I (1959 through 1965) and II (1982 through 1988). In: Shopland, D., Burns, D., Garfinkel, L., and Samet, J., (eds) National Cancer Institute. Changes in Cigarette-related Disease Risks and Their Implication for Prevention and Control. Smoking and Tobacco Control Monograph No. 8. Bethesda, MD: U.S. Department of Health and Human Services, National Institutes of Health, National Cancer Institute, NIH Pub No. 97–4213;. pp. 305–82.

98. Doll, R., Peto, R., Boreham, J., and Sutherland, I. (2000). Smoking and dementia in male British doctors: prospective study. *Br Med J*, **320**:1097–102.

99. Garfinkel L. (1981). Time trends in lung cancer mortality among nonsmokers and a note on passive smoking. *J Natl Cancer Instit*, **66**:1061–6.

100. Doll, R., Gray, R., Hafner, B., and Peto, R. (1980). Mortality in relation to smoking: 22 years' observations on female British doctors. *Brit Med J*, **280**:967–71.

101. Anderson, C.M., Burns, D.M., Major, J.M., Vaughn, J.W., and Shanks, T.G. (2002). Canges in adolescent smoking behaviors in sequential birth cohorts. In: Burns, D., Amacher, R., and Ruppert, W. (eds) *Changing Adolescent Smoking Prevalence*. Bethesda, MD: U.S. Department of Health and Human Services, National Institutes of Health, National Cancer Institute, p. 141–55.

102. CDC. (2008). Cigarette smoking among adults – United States, 2007. *MMWR Morb Mortal Wkly Rep*, **57**:1221–1226.

103. Corrao, M., Guindon, G., Sharma, N., and Shokoohi, D. (2000). *Tobacco Control: Country Profiles*. Atlanta, GA: American Cancer Society.

104. Liu, B.Q., Peto, R., Chen, Z.M., Boreham J, Wu, Y.P., Li, J.Y., *et al.* (1998). Emerging tobacco hazards in China: 1. Retrospective proportional mortality study of one million deaths. *BMJ*, **317**(7170): 1411–22.

105. Jha, P., Gajalakshmi, V., Gupta, P.C., Kumar, R., Mony, P., Dhingra, N., *et al.* (2006). Prospective study of one million deaths in India: rationale, design, and validation results. *PLoS Med*, **3**(2):e18.

106. US DHHS. (2001). Women and smoking: a report of the Surgeon General. Rockville, MD: US Department of Health and Human services, p.673.

107. Harris, J., Thun, M., Mondul, A., and Calle, E. (2004). Cigarette tar yields in relation to lung cancer mortality in the Cancer Prevention Study-II prospective cohort, 1982–1988. *BMJ*, **328**:72–6.

Chapter 3

Dealing with health fears: cigarette advertising in the United States in the twentieth century

Lynn T. Kozlowski and Richard J. O'Connor

Since the beginning of the twentieth century, cigarette advertising in the United States has been largely an effort to deal with the health fears related to smoking. Three main techniques have been used: reassurance, misdirection of attention, and inducements to be brave in the face of fear. Others have also considered the history of cigarette advertising and carried out content analyses (Warner 1985; McCaullife 1988; Pollay 1989; Ringold and Calfee 1989; Cohen 1992). This chapter depends on this earlier work and is an extension of an earlier paper on the topic (Kozlowski 2000). Note that we focus on advertising in the United States – similar themes have been examined in Canadian advertising (see Pollay 2002).

Background

In the 1890s, leading tobacco companies became organized in a large commercial conglomerate (Heimann 1960). By 1910, the large majority of tobacco products sold in the United States were sold by this group. This monopoly was prosecuted under the Sherman Anti-trust Act and, as a result, was broken up into separate companies in 1911. When the R. J. Reynolds Tobacco Company became a separate company again, as part of this action, it was given no established cigarette brand as part of the settlement (Tilley 1985); Richard Joshua Reynolds responded by creating a new brand. Earlier, he had been successful with a burley-based pipe tobacco blend called Prince Albert, and soon developed a new cigarette brand that made heavy use of burley tobacco in the blend (Heimann 1960). Camel was introduced in 1913 as a cheaper cigarette with a milder, novel taste. Backed by a national advertising campaign, sales of Camel cigarettes rose from 1 145 000 cigarettes shipped in the first year, to 2 255 310 000 in 1915, 11 923 640 000 in 1917, and 31 424 218 000 in 1924 (Tilley 1985). It was the leading cigarette of the period. Three national cigarette brands dominated cigarette sales for the first 50 years of the twentieth century: Camel (R. J. Reynolds), Lucky Strike (American Tobacco), and Chesterfield (Liggett and Myers).

The risks of smoking were known

Many smokers at that time were likely to have been aware of health concerns about tobacco. In the late 1800s and early 1900s, the Anti-Cigarette League, under the direction of Lucy Page Gaston, helped spread the word about the dangers of cigarettes (Tate 1999). States had even placed bans on cigarettes. See Tate (1999) for a detailed account of anti-smoking activities, many directed specifically at the dangers to health of cigarette smoking (cf. Robert 1967). There were also widespread concerns in the newspapers about possible impurities, adulterants, and dirty conditions involved in cigarette making (see Young 1917).

President Ulysses S. Grant died a very public death due to throat cancer, and Patterson (1989) has argued that this death of a famous cigar smoker contributed greatly to fear of tobacco-caused cancer in the United States around the turn of the century. A prevailing theory of cancer during the early twentieth century held that cancers were caused by 'irritation' (Patterson 1989). This model proposed that excessive use of tobacco irritated the linings of the throat and mouth, eventually leading to cancerous growths. ('Moderate' tobacco use was viewed as not especially dangerous, even if definitions of moderate and excessive were far from clear – see Young 1917). At this time, cigarettes were a small fraction of the market, and excessive pipe and cigar use were implicated in oral cancers; lung cancer was virtually unheard of at the time (Patterson 1989). Since cigarettes were so mild they could be inhaled, they could be positioned as the obviously safer form of tobacco use (Kozlowski 1982).

During the first few decades of the twentieth century, few laws or guidelines impeded the marketing of cigarettes or the claims that could be made about them. Manufacturers were free to say just about anything they wanted. Once restrictions were enacted, manufacturers could not directly claim safety or healthfulness of their products. Therefore, they had to use alternative routes (within the bounds of the restrictions) to convince customers that smoking was less dangerous than critics claimed. The claims made by manufacturers about cigarettes might be seen both as what was most advantageous for manufacturers to say, and what consumers most desired to hear: cigarettes are safe, and you can continue to smoke. Over the years, the messages have been varied; reassurance, misdirection of attention, and inducements to be brave in the face of fear are three themes that recur repeatedly.

Reassurance

This theme attacks the health issue straight on, offering ways to smoke 'safely'. Various technical 'innovations' over the years have been advertised as 'health protection'. Reassurance marketing began early – consider the text of a 1932 advertisement for Lucky Strike:

> Do you inhale? What's there to be afraid of? 7 out of 10 inhale knowingly—the other 3 do so unknowingly.
>   Do you inhale? Lucky Strike meets the vital issue fairly and squarely ... for it has solved the vital problem. Its famous purifying process removes certain impurities that are concealed in even the choicest, mildest tobacco leaves. Luckies created that process. Only Luckies have it!

> (cited in Brecher *et al.* 1963)

It later proclaims: 'IT'S TOASTED! *Your protection against irritation, against cough*' (as cited in Brecher *et al.* 1963). This advertisement sets Lucky Strike apart from other cigarettes as purer and safer to inhale. What supposedly sets 'Luckies' apart is their special processing, which removes unspecified impurities (a technical 'innovation'). Other ads at the time touted cigarettes as so healthful athletes could smoke them without affecting their performance (see Lewine 1970).

Filter tips and the 'tar derby'

The introduction of the filter tip, and the concomitant 'tar derby', is one of the best examples of reassurance marketing. Beginning in the 1950s, concern began to appear about the tar content of cigarettes and its relationship to disease (e.g. Wynder and Graham 1950; Doll and Hill 1952). Although manufacturers have argued that the introduction of filter tips was only circumstantially related to health concerns (e.g. Tilley 1985), recently revealed industry documents tell a different story. Ernest Pepples, Vice-President and General Counsel for Brown and Williamson Tobacco, noted in 1976 that 'the manufacturers' marketing strategy has been to overcome and *even to make marketing use of* the smoking/health connection [emphasis added]' (as cited in Glantz *et al.* 1996).

Pepples wrote that the smoker had abandoned regular (unfiltered cigarettes) because of health concerns, and that '… the "tar derby" in the United States resulted from industry efforts to cater to the public's concern and to attract consumers to the new filtered brands' (as cited in Glantz *et al.* 1996).

Filters, although they appeared as early as the 1930s, did not begin to become popular until the 1950s. During this time, filters made of paper, asbestos, and cellulose acetate, among other materials, were attached to cigarettes. Kents were promoted as the 'greatest health protection in cigarette history' (an ironic claim given the Micronite filter contained asbestos). Other manufacturers were making similar claims regarding the health benefits of their filters (see Table 3.1).

At the height of the tar derby of the late 1950s, the United States Congress held a hearing on false and misleading advertising of filter-tip cigarettes (False and Misleading Advertising 1957), now known as the Blatnik report (Tilley 1985; see Kozlowski 2000 for discussion). During the hearing, the then Federal Trade Commission (FTC) chairman, Sechrest, testified about the Cigarette Advertising Guides developed by his agency (15 September 1955). The Guide specifically prohibited health or physical claims, forbade linking filters to such claims, and eliminated false testimonials. All this seems to have been a legitimate effort to eliminate the most far-fetched health claims. Chairman Sechrest noted that: 'Prior to the issuance of the guides, cigarette advertising generally involved health claims. Since their issuance, the theme of all such advertising, including that of filter tips, has centered around *taste and flavor*' (False and Misleading Advertising 1957, p. 304). This is a key concept, for the FTC's guide stated quite clearly, '…*Nothing contained in these guides is intended to prohibit the use of any representation, claim, or illustration relating solely to taste, flavor, aroma, or enjoyment* [emphasis added]'.

By 1956, the most egregious health claims had vanished, and statements regarding taste and flavour proliferated. In 1960, the industry and the FTC concluded an agreement to eliminate tar information from advertising. In 1964, the Surgeon-General's Report was released (USDHEW 1964),

Table 3.1 Advertising slogans from the tar derby era[a]

Kent (one of the first lower tar and nicotine cigarettes)	1952	'No other cigarette approaches such a degree of health protection and taste satisfaction.' 'Because this filter is exclusive with KENT, it is possible to say that no other cigarette offers smokers such a degree of health protection and taste satisfaction.'
L&M	1953	'… Alpha Cellulose. Exclusive to L&M Filters, and entirely pure and harmless to health'.
	1954	'L&M Filters are Just What the Doctor Ordered!'
Parliament	1952	'… like millions today, you are turning to filter cigarettes for pleasure plus protection … it's important that you know the Parliament Story'.
Philip Morris	1954	'The cigarette that takes the FEAR out of smoking!'
Viceroy	1951	'*Filtered* cigarette smoke is better for your health.'
	1953	'New King-Size Viceroy gives *Double*-Barreled Health Protection … is safer for throat, safer for lungs than any other king-size cigarette'.

Note

[a] The slogans come from various sources, including: Lewine (1970), Harris (1978), Sobel (1978), Mullen (1979), and Glantz *et al.* (1996).

reporting a dose–response relationship between number of cigarettes and disease. This report was seen to encourage using filter cigarettes, as well as those with less tar.

During the 1960s, both the American Cancer Society and *Reader's Digest* criticized the loss of tar information in cigarette advertising. The FTC maintained that any claims had to be supported by objective evidence, and so they began to seek input on devising a standardized test for tar and nicotine content (for a review, see Peeler 1996). FTC Commissioner Sechrest was worried that standardized testing might lead consumers to say, 'I want the one with the least tar' (False and Misleading Advertising 1957, p. 303), which might be a health issue. In 1966, the FTC announced that tar and nicotine statements were not considered health claims, and instituted its cigarette testing programme the following year. This opened the door for manufacturers to develop a cigarette that could make health claims implicitly, rather than explicitly: the Light cigarette.

Light cigarettes

Light cigarettes were the natural extension of the tar derby of the 1950s. Since tar was linked to lung cancer, the most dreaded smoking-related disease, smokers would naturally be attracted to products that reduced tar to lower and lower levels. So, lower tar cigarettes were reassuring, particularly when combined with a consoling name such as 'Light' that implied fewer toxins and purity at the same time (more on this point later).

Several design changes can reduce standard tar and nicotine numbers (for a review, see Kozlowski *et al.* 2001). Probably the most important is filter ventilation (Kozlowski *et al.* 1998a). This introduces air into the mainstream smoke, diluting it and reducing standard machine measurements. However, filter ventilation does not necessarily reduce the amounts of tar and nicotine delivered to smokers, in that smokers are able to compensate for the dilution, primarily by taking bigger puffs, or by blocking the vents with their lips or fingers (Kozlowski and Pillitteri 1996; Kozlowski and O'Connor 2002). For brands with less than 60% ventilation, small increases in puff volume will adequately compensate for the dilution, while for heavily ventilated brands (greater than 60%), vent blocking is more important for compensation.

The Light cigarette increased in popularity in the 1970s, when Light versions of established brands began to appear, and smokers began to switch from 'Full-Flavor' to 'Light' brands (National Cancer Institute 2001). The sales-weighted average tar yield dropped from 21.6 mg in 1968 to 12.0 mg in 1997, a 44.4% decline. See the recent National Cancer Institute (2001) monograph on Lights for a more detailed overview of the product and its epidemiology.

The Light cigarette took full advantage of the allowable advertising claims (Glantz *et al.* 1996). Internal memos from the time show that these products were marketed precisely to keep smokers who were concerned about their health from quitting by offering them a 'safer' smoke. One Brown and Williamson employee wrote:

> All work in this area [communications] should be directed towards providing consumer reassurance [emphasis in original] about cigarettes and the smoking habit ... by claiming low deliveries, by the perception of low deliveries and by the perception of 'mildness'. Furthermore, the advertising for low delivery or traditional brands should be constructed in ways so as not to provoke anxiety about health, but to alleviate it, and enable the smoker to feel assured about the habit and confident in maintaining it over time.

> (Short 1977)

Amercian Tobacco (Carlton) and R. J. Reynolds (Now) competed for the lowest yield cigarette, and positioned these brands as having the lowest recorded tar and nicotine levels (even though the hard-pack versions that measured the lowest were generally unavailable in stores; Pollay and Dewhirst 2001). Now was described as a 'break-through' (1980, as cited in Pollay and Dewhirst 2001), while Carlton advertisements claimed that 'Latest U.S. Gov't Laboratory test confirms, of all cigarettes: Carlton is lowest' (1985, as cited in Pollay and Dewhirst 2001). In 1980, Brown and Williamson introduced Barclay, a cigarette they promoted as '99 per cent Tar Free' (as cited in Pollay and Dewhirst 2001). However, this cigarette employed a unique ventilation system that was subject to easy compensation, so much so that Brown and Williamson's competitors sued to stop the cigarette's low-tar claim (FTC v. Brown and Williamson 1985). A campaign for True cigarettes was explicit about reassurance: 'Considering all I'd heard [presumably about smoking and health], I decided to either quit or smoke True. I smoke True' (as cited in Pollay and Dewhirst 2001). This sort of advertisement allowed smokers to conclude that some cigarettes were a reasonable alternative to quitting, and indeed many smokers were lulled into a false sense of security by Lights (National Cancer Institute 2001).

A secondary effect of ventilation is that it makes the smoke actually taste 'lighter'. That is, even though smokers are very likely not getting less tar and nicotine per cigarette, each puff tastes lighter than a puff of equivalent yield on a regular cigarette (Kozlowski and O'Connor 2002). In national surveys, smokers note that Lights do taste lighter (e.g. Kozlowski *et al.* 1998*b*), and industry studies note that adding ventilation can significantly reduce smokers' ratings of 'irritation', 'impact', and increase ratings of 'mildness' (Anderson 1979; Hirji 1980; Philip 1989).

To sell lower tar cigarettes to a public used to higher tar brands, manufacturers had to convince the public that the new cigarettes would offer the same satisfaction or great taste that their old cigarettes did, but still be less dangerous. However, the advertisements also had to deal with issues of lighter taste and satisfaction. Consider a 1972 Vantage advertisement:

Anyone who's old enough to smoke is old enough to make up his own mind.

By now, as an adult, you must have read and heard all that's been written and said for and against cigarettes. And come to your own conclusions … if you like to smoke and have decided to continue, we'd like to tell you a few facts about a cigarette you might like to continue with …

Vantage gives you real flavor like any high 'tar' and nicotine cigarette you ever smoked, without the high 'tar' and nicotine. And since it is the high 'tar' and nicotine that many critics seem most opposed to, even they should have some kind words for Vantage. We don't want to mislead you.

Vantage is not the lowest 'tar' and nicotine cigarette. But, it is the lowest 'tar and nicotine cigarette you'll enjoy smoking. It has only 12 milligrams 'tar' and 0.9 mg nicotine. With anything lower, you'd have to work so hard getting taste through the filter that you'd end up going back to your old brand…

(Reynolds 1972)

This advertisement promises that the cigarette will: (1) deliver less tar and nicotine (implicitly healthier); and, at the same time, (2) still deliver good taste. This doubly reassures the smoker that he can continue to smoke, with reduced health risk but without losing the taste and pleasure he enjoys. It implies that health advocates who say tar and nicotine are dangerous might have 'kind words' for Vantage. The 'work so hard' phrase acknowledges that compensatory smoking can require significant effort, but reassures the smoker that Vantage will not be like that. Other brands have been marketed using similar tactics (see Table 3.2).

Reassurance marketing resurfaced with the advent of Potential Reduced Exposure Products (PREPs). Take, for example, advertising for Omni™ cigarettes:

NEW! Omni.™ Reduced Carcinogens. Premium Taste. Introducing the first premium cigarette created to significantly reduce carcinogenic PAH's, nitrosamines, catechols, and organics, which are the major causes of lung cancer in smokers.

(Vector Tobacco 2001)

What happens to a [picture of cigarette] when you reduce carcinogens? You get a really good tasting smoke. The only cigarette to significantly reduce carcinogens that are among the major causes of

Table 3.2 Selected slogans for Light cigarette brands, 1970s to 1990s.

Merit	
1980	Merit Wins Taste Honors. Research establishes low tar MERIT as proven taste alternative to high tar smoking. [20610112428][a]
1992	Merit introduces surprising flavor at only 1 mg tar. [20610071836][a]
1996	(Merit) Yes! Yes, you can switch down from full flavor and still get satisfying taste. [206100073377][a]
True	
1974	New. True 100's. Lower in both tar and nicotine than 98% of all other 100's sold. [502293758][b]
1974	Is new True 100 lower in tar than your 100? Tests for tar and nicotine by US Gov't Method prove it. New True 100 mm is lowest in both tar and nicotine of all these leading 100 mm cigarettes [lists several brands]. [502293760][b]
Vantage	
1971	(Vantage). You don't cop out. We don't cop out. You demand good taste. But want low 'tar' and nicotine. Only Vantage gives you both.[c]
Triumph	
1980	TRIUMPH BEATS MERIT! Triumph, at less than half the tar, preferred over Merit. Taste the UMPH! in Triumph at only 3 mg tar.[c]
Barclay	
1981	Barclay. 99% Tar Free. The pleasure is back.[c]
Winston Lights	
1976	Most low 'tar' cigarettes have no taste. A lot of new cigarettes give you low 'tar' and nicotine numbers. But I can't taste numbers. What I can taste is Winston Lights. I get lower 'tar' and nicotine. But I still get real taste. And real pleasure. For me, Winston Lights are for real. [515222693][b]
Kent Golden Lights	
1976	Kent Golden Lights. As low as you can go and still get good taste and smoking satisfaction ... Kent Golden Lights. Tastes so good, you won't believe the numbers. [500331489][b]

Note

[a] Available at: http://www.pmadarchive.com
[b] Available at: http://www.rjrtdocs.com
[c] As cited in National Cancer Institute (2001).

lung cancer. The only one to still deliver premium taste. The only one to finally give smokers a real reason to switch. Only Omni.™

(Vector Tobacco 2002)

The advertisements feature disclaimers, in smaller type, noting that reductions in carcinogens are not proven to make a cigarette safer. Still, the offer of 'reduced carcinogens at a premium taste' is likely to be very reassuring to the health-concerned smoker. These advertisements resemble early 'tar derby' ads by making a nearly explicit health claim, small-print disclaimers notwithstanding.

Reassurance marketing took different forms over time, but all of them aimed to keep smokers smoking by encouraging them to believe that smoking was less dangerous. The addition of filters and their aggressive marketing, followed by the introduction of Lights, fostered the notion that cigarettes were getting safer without needing to say so directly. Smokers were doubly reassured that their cigarettes were giving them less deadly tar, but would still taste good enough to keep them satisfied, and the lighter taste of Lights helped convince smokers that Lights were safer for them.

Misdirection of attention

Reassurance marketing can go only so far to convince consumers to keep smoking. Misdirection of attention, as an advertising theme, only indirectly engages the health issue. Instead of directly confronting the health issue with reassurance, advertising simply focuses on other attributes of the product that are consistent with reduced risk. From the earliest days, cigarettes were promoted for their mildness and for their ability to satisfy. Table 3.3 lists slogans from the first decades of the twentieth century. Note the prominence of the 'mild' theme.

To understand how misdirection of attention can work to deflect health concerns, one must understand how words can relate to one another. Kozlowski (2000) has described how 'hyponomy', or the hierarchical organization of words under broader concepts, relates to cigarette advertising. By mentioning 'mild', for example, one can extend its meaning in several directions, following the hyponymic branches. Antonyms such as 'harsh' can come to mind, as well as concepts such as 'good', 'safe', 'not irritating'. Crucial hyponyms of 'good' are 'pleasantness' and 'safety'. Basically, positive terms such as 'pleasantness', 'mildness', 'tastiness', or 'mellowness' evoke 'goodness', which is a hyponym for 'healthful'. If something is 'mild', 'mellow', or 'Light', it is unlikely to be 'unhealthful'. The health issue does not need to be engaged directly, because evoking the semantic networks associated with taste and satisfaction can be enough to influence the consumer's thinking that the cigarette isn't so bad.

Some words or phrases, called tropes, are used in a non-literal way that still carries important meaning (Bloom 1975). In the current case, 'light', 'smooth', 'mild' are all tropes that carry meanings for consumers: less irritating, less risky, less deadly. Those in the industry, and their

Table 3.3 Selected cigarette advertising slogans, early twentieth century[a].

1929	[Chesterfield] 'MILD … and yet THEY SATISFY'
1929	[Lucky Strike] '20,679 physicians have confirmed the fact that Lucky Strike is less irritating in the throat than other cigarettes'
1936	[Philip Morris] '… tests proved conclusively that after changing to Philip Morris, every case of irritation due to smoking cleared completely or definitely improved'
1937	[Camel] 'They're so mild and never make my throat harsh or rough'
1938	[Viceroy] 'Viceroy's filter neatly checks the throat-irritants in tobacco … Safer smoke for any throat. Inhale without discomfort'
1943	[Viceroy] '… filtering the flavor and aroma of the world's finest tobaccos into the smoothest of blends and checking OUT resins, tar and throat irritants that can spoil the EVENNESS of smoking enjoyment!'
1946	[Camel] 'More Doctors Smoke Camels Than Any Other Cigarette'

Note

[a] The slogans come from various sources, including: Lewine (1970), Harris (1978), Sobel (1978), Mullen (1979), and Glantz *et al.* (1996).

supporters, often claim that Light labels are justified because Lights actually deliver less tar to machines than 'full-flavors'. However, humans do not smoke like machines. Smokers generally believe that tar numbers reflect what they are inhaling, and that lower tar cigarettes are safer (see Rickert *et al.* 1989; Giovino *et al.* 1996). Surveys of American smokers show that 39% (*n* = 360) of Light and 58% (*n* = 218) of Ultra-light smokers state that *they smoke their brands to reduce the risks of smoking* (Kozlowski *et al.* 1998*b*). Borland *et al.* (2004) found that 51% of US smokers in 2002 believed Light cigarettes offered a health benefit over regular cigarettes. Indeed, most Marlboro Lights smokers in another survey believed incorrectly that lower tar, light, and ultra-light cigarettes were less harmful compared with higher tar, full-flavoured cigarettes, and only 11% of Marlboro Lights smokers knew that the tar delivery of a light cigarette was equivalent to a full-flavoured cigarette (Cummings *et al.* 2004). A Light cigarette, to the consumer, must seem similar to Light ice cream, or Light beer – indicating that they are actually ingesting less of something (fat or calories in the cases of ice cream and beer, tar in the case of cigarettes). The meaning of *Light* as 'lower standard tar yield' is only a 'technical truth' that should not carry assumptions about reduced risk [cf. *P. Lorillard Co.*v. *FTC* (1950)]. *Light* is also a trope referring to 'more pure' and 'not as dangerous' (and literally, 'not heavy'). It makes implicit health and safety claims. Groups in both the United States and Canada called for a ban on Light descriptors (National Cancer Institute 2001; Ministerial Advisory Council on Tobacco Control 2002). These calls were incorporated in the World Health Organization's Framework Convention on Tobacco Control, which specifies a ban on 'misleading descriptors' of cigarette brands (Article 11).

> Each Party shall, within a period of three years after entry into force of this Convention for that Party, adopt and implement, in accordance with its national law, effective measures to ensure that:
> (a) tobacco product packaging and labelling do not promote a tobacco product by any means that are false, misleading, deceptive or likely to create an erroneous impression about its characteristics, health effects, hazards or emissions, including any term, descriptor, trademark, figurative or any other sign that directly or indirectly creates the false impression that a particular tobacco product is less harmful than other tobacco products. These may include terms such as 'low tar', 'light', 'ultra-light', or 'mild'.
>
> (FCTC Article 11)

Bills to grant the Food and Drug Administration authority over US tobacco regulation have contained similar restrictions. Consistent with the FCTC, the European Union banned the terms Light and Mild in 2004, and Canada and Australia followed suit in 2006. However, manufacturers have substituted words such as 'smooth', 'fine', and 'finesse' (King and Borland, 2005). These may have trope functions similar to light and mild to the extent that they evoke beliefs about health and safety. Manufacturers have also employed colour names such as silver and blue, which capitalize on perceptions of these colours as being 'lighter' and 'healthier' as substitute descriptors. And, Borland and colleagues (2008) have found that removing the descriptors in the United Kingdom did not resolve misperceptions of the safety of Light/Mild cigarettes, indicating that more intervention is necessary to correct these false beliefs.

Inducements to bravery

A third way advertisers can encourage smokers to keep smoking is to help them identify with being a risk-taker. Without acknowledging the risks of smoking, advertising creates an image of smoking that encompasses bravery, risk taking, and other positive images. The best known, and most successful, of these campaigns has been the cowboy of Philip Morris' Marlboro brand (the world's best-selling brand).

Marlboro advertisements generally have little text, but contain strong imagery. Marlboro print ads often involve obviously dangerous activities, such as bronco-riding or roping horses. By linking smoking with such activities, smoking is acknowledged as dangerous, but possessing similar dangers to those encountered by the Marlboro cowboy in his life. These images have been extended to Marlboro Lights (1970s) and Marlboro Ultra Lights (1990s). Consider an advertisement for Marlboro Lights (Philip Morris 1976): 'The spirit of Marlboro in a low tar cigarette'. This text is accompanied by a painting of the Marlboro cowboy riding with horses, seemingly travelling rather quickly. Marlboro Lights and Ultra Lights might be seen as cigarettes for the cowboy who might be concerned for his health, but not so concerned that he would give up his exciting life style, or his favourite smoke.

R.J. Reynolds has used similar themes to market Camel Filters and Camel Lights. In the late 1970s and early 1980s, male smokers were variously seen sitting around camp-fires with mountains in the background (Pollay Collection, Camel 19.13), canoeing (Pollay Archive, Camel 16.16), whitewater rafting (Pollay Collection, Camel 26.14), driving Jeeps up mountains (Pollay Collection, Camel 34.15), and arm wrestling (Pollay Collection, Camel 10.01) (advertisements available in the Richard W. Pollay Twentieth Century Tobacco Advertisement Collection at http://www.tobacco.org/ads/?tdo_code=pollay_ads). Tag lines proclaimed 'Share a new adventure' and 'Where a man belongs'. During the Joe Camel promotion, Joe was depicted water skiing (Pollay Collection, Camel 20.14), riding motorcycles (Pollay Collection, Camel 35.15), windsailing (Pollay Collection, Camel 20.13), and driving race cars (Pollay Collection, Camel 20.19). He was even seen in a bombadier jacket with fighter jets behind him (Pollay Collection, Camel 27.14). Clearly these images are meant to set the Camel smoker apart as adventurous and masculine – someone willing to take on the risks of smoking.

Consumer perception and types of persuasion

The *raison d'être* of advertising is to convince consumers to buy and use a particular product, often by convincing them that it is the right thing to do (for an overview, see Jones 1998). People generally want to believe the 'right' thing (Cacioppo *et al.* 1996). That is, people do not like to be wrong. Advertisements that present messages aimed at persuading individuals are likely to be consciously processed by consumers. But argument also invites evaluation. Consumers then have the opportunity to consider what is being said, what points are being made, what arguments are being advanced, and who the source is. This is known as the 'central route to persuasion' (cf. Petty *et al.* 1983). Advertisements that rely on reassurance generally follow this route. When a message contains no arguments, however, a 'peripheral route to persuasion' is involved (cf. Petty *et al.* 1983). Little conscious scrutiny is involved: the attractiveness of the images and positive feelings become influential. Ads that rely on misdirection of attention or inducement to bravery involve peripheral persuasion heavily. A claim that a cigarette is Light or Mild or Smooth is not something for which objective evidence can be produced. Similarly, imagery alone is not subject to evaluation in the same way as a claim of 'great taste, less tar'. When an advertisement makes the case that cigarette X is not as dangerous, central processing is engaged. Consumers may or may not be persuaded by the information provided. However, when a cowboy sits alone in the desert smoking a cigarette, the heart and mind process the imagery and are unencumbered by conscious information processing.

An overall effect of the FTC's advertising guidelines, which were enacted to prevent cigarette makers from making specific (unsupportable) claims, was to encourage advertising based on subtle implications and symbolism related to taste and satisfaction (Kozlowski 2002). However, since 'health protection' messages may remind the consumer that their health needed protection (i.e. cigarettes are dangerous), eliminating health claims may have benefited manufacturers. Making use of semantic networks allows manufacturers to imply safety without ever having to say the word. This also has the added benefit of not needing objective evidence – for example, the smokers' own judgement, that the cigarette tastes lighter, can be enough to substantiate the claim. By using the peripheral route of persuasion, manufacturers run less risk of consumers rejecting the message by evaluation, because the Marlboro cowboy is unevaluable – he simply is. Consumers can accept or reject new charcoal filters, exclusive blends, and even claims about better taste, but Joe Camel the fighter pilot, and the name Merit Ultra Light are much harder to dismiss.

Advertising since the Master Settlement Agreement

The Master Settlement Agreement (MSA), entered into by 47 states' attorneys general and the major cigarette manufacturers, set new guidelines for advertising, primarily aimed at reducing appeals to children. Billboards, product placements, and advertisements in magazines with large youth readership were banned (National Association of Attorneys General 2002). However, the agreement did not address the crucial advertising issues discussed in this chapter (National Association of Attorneys General 2002). The Marlboro cowboy is alive and well. Omni implies that its cigarettes are safer. Only recently have counter-marketing efforts begun to correct consumers' misapprehensions surrounding Light cigarettes (e.g. Kozlowski *et al.* 1999, 2000; Shiffman *et al.* 2001*a*, *b*; Bansal *et al.* 2004). Both Brown and Williamson and Philip Morris, perhaps responding to such counter-marketing, added disclaimers to their listings of FTC test results in advertising: Brown and Williamson: 'Actual deliveries will vary based on how you hold and smoke your cigarette'; Philip Morris: 'The amount of 'tar' and nicotine you inhale will vary depending on how you smoke the cigarette'.

Because the MSA made no provisions for the advertising themes discussed in this chapter, manufacturers remain free to use health fears to market their products. However, the tide appears to have turned in the legal realm. In her ruling in the DOJ lawsuit, Judge Gladys Kessler ordered the industry to conduct corrective advertising on the issue of Light cigarettes (Kessler 2006); this ruling has been stayed by the US Court of Appeals for the District of Columbia. In November 2008, the FTC rescinded its guidance on the use of machine yields in advertising (FTC 2008). In December 2008 the US Supreme Court ruled that the Federal Cigarette Labelling and Advertising Act does not bar or pre-empt lawsuits in state courts under consumer fraud statutes (Vicini 2008).

Conclusions

Cigarette advertising in the United States since the beginning of the twentieth century has been an enterprise in reducing health fears around smoking. Advertisements have relied on three basic themes. Some ads reassure smokers that (1) new developments are making cigarettes safer, and (2) these developments will not remove the flavour and enjoyment from smoking. Others use tropes and semantic networks to imply safety without actually making explicit health claims. A third class of ads uses imagery to convince smokers that smoking might be risky, but is worth the risk. By allowing imagery and claims based on taste, regulators opened the door for manufacturers to subtly suggest that cigarettes were becoming less dangerous and that consumers could continue to smoke.

References

Anderson, P. (1979). HTI test of production Marlboro 85 versus Marlboro 85, Model '1' with 10% dilution and no reduction in tar delivery. Philip Morris. Available at: http://www.pmdocs.com (Bates Number 2040077052).

Bansal, M.A., Cummings, K.M., Hyland, A., Bauer, J.E., Hastrup, J.L., and Steger, C. (2004). Do smokers want to know more about the cigarettes they smoke? Results from the EDUCATE study. *Nicotine Tob Res.* Dec 6(Suppl 3):S289–302.

Bloom, H. (1975). *A Map of Misreading.* Oxford University Press, Oxford.

Borland, R., Fong, G.T., Yong, H,H., Cummings, K.M., Hammond, D., King, B, *et al.* (2008). What happened to smokers' beliefs about light cigarettes when 'light/mild' brand descriptors were banned in the UK? Findings from the International Tobacco Control (ITC) Four Country Survey. *Tob Control.* Aug 17(4):256–62.

Borland, R., Yong, H.H., King, B., Cummings, K.M., Fong, G.T., Elton-Marshall. T., *et al.* (2004). Use of and beliefs about light cigarettes in four countries: findings from the International Tobacco Control Policy Evaluation Survey. *Nicotine Tob Res.* Dec 6(Suppl 3):S311–21.

Brecher, R., Brecher, E., Herzog, A., Goodman, W., and Walker, G. (ed.) (1963). The consumers union report on smoking and public interest. Consumers Union, Mount Vernon, New York.

Cacioppo, J.T., Petty, R.E., Feinstien, J.A., Blair, W., and Jarvis, G. (1996). Dispositional differences in cognitive motivation: the life and times of individuals varying in need for cognition. *Psychological Bulletin,* **119**:197–253.

Cohen, J.B. (1992). Research and policy issues in Ringold and Calfee's treatment of cigarette health claims. *Journal of Public Policy and Marketing,* **11**: 82–6.

Cummings, K.M., Hyland, A., Bansal, M.A., and Giovino, G.A. (2004). What do Marlboro Lights smokers know about low-tar cigarettes? *Nicotine Tob Res.* Dec; 6(Suppl 3):S323–32.

Doll, R. and Hill, A.B. (1952). A study of the aetiology of carcinoma of the lung. *British Medical Journal,* 1271–82.

False and Misleading Advertising (Filter-tip cigarettes) (1957). Hearings before a subcommittee of the Committee on Government Operations, House of Representatives, 85th Congress, First Session, (18–26 July). John A. Blatnik, chair.

Federal Trade Commission (2008). Rescission of FTC Guidance Concerning the Cambridge Filter Method. Federal Register: December 8, (Volume 73, Number 236) pp 74500–505. Available at http://www.ftc.gov/os/2008/11/P944509cambridgefiltermethodfrn.pdf

FTC v. Brown and Williamson Tobacco Corporation (1985). 580. SUPP 981 (D.C.C., 1983), 778F.2d 35 (D.C.CIR. 1985).

Giovino, G.A., Tomar, S.L., Reddy, M.N., Peddicord, J.P., Zhu, B.P., Escobedo, L.G., *et al.* (1996). Attitudes, knowledge and beliefs about low-yield cigarettes among adolescents and adults. In: The FTC cigarette test method for determining tar, nicotine, and carbon monoxide yields of U.S. cigarettes: report of the NCI Expert Committee, pp. 39–57. National Cancer Institute, US Department of Health and Human Services, Bethesda, Maryland.

Glantz, S.A., Slade, J., Bero, L.A., Hanauer, P., and Barnes, D.E. (1996). *The cigarette papers.* University of California Press, Berkeley.

Harris, R.W. (1978). *How to keep on smoking and live.* St. Martin's Press, New York.

Heimann, R.K. (1960). *Tobacco and Americans.* McGraw-Hill, New York.

Hirji, T. (1980). Effects of paper permeability, filtration, and tip ventilation on deliveries, impact, and irritation. British American Tobacco. Available at http://www.bw.aalatg.com (Bates Number 650331009).

Jones, J.P. (ed.) (1998). *How advertising works: the role of research.* Sage, Thousand Oaks, California.

Kessler, G. (2006). Amended Final Opinion. United State of America v. Philip Morris USA *et al.* Civil Action No. 99-2496 (GK). 17 August Available at http://www.usdoj.gov/civil/cases/tobacco2/amended%20opinion.pdf

King, B. and Borland, R. (2005). What was 'light' and 'mild' is now 'smooth' and 'fine': new labelling of Australian cigarettes. *Tob Control,* Jun;**14**(3):214–5.

Kozlowski, L.T. (1982). The determinants of tobacco use: Cigarettes in the context of other forms of tobacco use. *Canadian Journal of Public Health,* **73**:236–41.

Kozlowski, L.T. and O'Connor, R.J. (2002). Filter ventilation is a defective design because of lighter taste, bigger puffs, and blocked vents. *Tobacco Control,* **11**(Suppl. 1):i40–i50.

Kozlowski, L.T. and Pillitteri, J.L. (1996). Compensation for nicotine by smokers of lower yield cigarettes. In *The FTC cigarette test method for determining tar, nicotine, and carbon monoxide yields of U.S.*

cigarettes: report of the NCI Expert Committee. National Cancer Institute, US Department of Health and Human Services, Bethesda, Maryland.

Kozlowski, L.T., Mehta, N.Y., Sweeney, C.T., Schwartz, S.S., Vogler, G.P., Jarvis, M.J., *et al.* (1998a). Filter ventilation and nicotine content of tobacco in cigarettes from Canada, the United Kingdom, and the United States. *Tobacco Control*, **7**(4):369–75.

Kozlowski, L.T, Goldberg, M.E., Yost, B.A., White, E.L., Sweeney, C.T., and Pillitteri, J.L. (1998b). Smokers' misperceptions of light and ultra-light cigarettes may keep them smoking. *American Journal of Preventive Medicine*, **15**:9–16.

Kozlowski, L.T., Goldberg, M.E., Sweeney, C.T., Palmer, R.F., Pillitteri, J.L., Yost, B.A., *et al.* (1999). Smoker reactions to a 'radio message' that light cigarettes are as dangerous as regular cigarettes. *Nicotine and Tobacco Research*, **1**:67–76.

Kozlowski, L.T., Yost, B., Stine, M.M., and Celebucki, C. (2000). Massachusetts' advertising against light cigarettes appears to change beliefs and behavior. *American Journal of Preventive Medicine*, **18**(4):339–42.

Kozlowski, L.T. (2000). Some lessons from the history of American tobacco advertising and its regulations in the 20th century. In: R. Ferrence, J. Slade, R. Room, and M. Pope, *Nicotine and Public Health*. Washington DC: American Public Health Association.

Kozlowski, L.T., O'Connor, R.J., and Sweeney, C.T. (2001). Cigarette design. In: *Risks associated with smoking cigarettes having low machine*-measured *levels of tar and nicotine*. Smoking and Tobacco Control Monograph, No. 13. US Department of Health and Human Services, National Institutes of Health, National Cancer Institute, Bethesda, Maryland.

Lewine, H. (1970). *Good-bye to all that*. McGraw-Hill, New York.

Lorillard, P. Co. v. FTC (1950). 6140, US Court of Appeals, 4th Circuit, 29 December, pp. 52–9.

McCaullife, R. (1988). The FTC and the effectiveness of cigarette advertising regulations. *Journal of Public Policy and Marketing*, **7**:49–64.

Ministerial Advisory Council on Tobacco Control (2002). *Putting an End to the Deception: Proceedings of the International Expert Panel on Cigarette Descriptors*. Ottawa, ON: Canadian Council for Tobacco Control.

Mullen, C. (1979). *Cigarette pack art*. Totem Books, Toronto.

National Association of Attorneys General (2002). Multistate settlement with the tobacco industry. Available at: http://www.tobacco.neu.edu/Extra/multistate_settlement.htm.

National Cancer Institute (2001). *Risks associated with smoking cigarettes having low machine-measured levels of tar and nicotine*. Smoking and Tobacco Control Monograph, No. 13. US Department of Health and Human Services, National Institutes of Health, National Cancer Institute, Bethesda, Maryland.

Patterson, J.T. (1989). *The dread disease: Cancer and modern American culture*. Harvard University Press, Cambridge, Massachusetts.

Peeler, C.E. (1996). *Cigarette testing and the Federal Trade Commission: a historical overview. The FTC cigarette test method for determining tar, nicotine, and carbon monoxide yields of U.S. cigarettes*. Smoking and Tobacco Control Monograph, No. 7. Bethesda, MD: National Cancer Institute.

Petty, R.E., Cacioppo, J.T., and Schumann, D. (1983). Central and peripheral routes to advertising effectiveness: The moderating role of involvement. *Journal of Consumer Research*, **10**:135–46.

Philip Morris (1976). Advertisement for Marlboro Lights cigarettes. Available at http://www.pmadarchive.com (Bates Number 2061015726).

Philip Morris (1989). Korea product tests. Philip Morris. Available at http://www.pmdocs.com (Bates Number 2504034439).

Pollay, R.W. (1989). Filters, flavor… flim-flam, too! On 'health information' and policy implications in cigarette advertising. *Journal of Public Policy and Marketing*, **8**:30–9.

Pollay, R.W. and Dewhirst, T. (2001). Marketing cigarettes with low machine measured yields. In:*National Cancer Institute, Risks Associated with Smoking Cigarettes with Low Machine-Measured Yields of Tar and Nicotine*. Bethesda, MD: National Cancer Institute.

Pollay, R.W. (2002). *How cigarette advertising works: Rich imagery and poor information.* Tobacco Research Unit, Special Report Series, June 2002, Toronto, Ontario.

Reynolds, R.J. (1972). *Advertisement for Vantage cigarettes.* Available at http://www.rjrtdocs.com (Bates Number 502612052).

Rickert, W.S., Robinson, J.C., and Lawless, E. (1989). Limitations to potential uses for data based on the machine smoking of cigarettes: Cigarette smoke contents. In: N. Wald and P. Froggatt (ed.) *Nicotine, smoking and the low tar programme,* pp. 85–99. Oxford University Press, New York.

Ringold, D.J. and Calfee, J.E. (1989). The informational content of cigarette advertising: 1926–1986. *Journal of Public Policy and Marketing,* **8**:1–23.

Robert, J.C. (1967). *The story of tobacco in America.* The University of North Carolina Press, Chapel Hill.

Shiffman, S., Pillitteri, J.L., Burton, S.L., Rohay, J.M., and Gitchell, J.G. (2001a). Effect of health messages about 'Light' and 'Ultra Light' cigarettes on beliefs and quitting intent. *Tobacco Control,* **10**(Suppl 1): i24–i32.

Shiffman, S., Burton, S.L., Pillitteri, J.L., Gitchell, J.G., Di Marino, M.E., Sweeney, C.T. *et al.* (2001b). Test of 'Light' cigarette counter-advertising using a standard test of advertisingeffectiveness. *Tobacco Control,* **10**(Suppl 1):i33–i40.

Short, P.L. (1977). *Smoking and health item 7: The effect on marketing.* BATCO, April 14. (Minnesota Exhibit 030).

Sobel, R. (1978). *They satisfy: The cigarette in American life.* Doubleday, New York.

Tate, C. (1999). *Cigarette Wars: The Triumph of the Little White Slaves.* Oxford: Oxford University Press.

Tilley, N.M. (1985). *The R.J. Reynolds Tobacco Company.* The University of North Carolina Press, Chapel Hill.

US Department of Health, Education, and Welfare (1964). *Smoking and health: Report of the advisory committee to the Surgeon General of the Public Health Service, 1964.* Public Health Publication, No. 1103. US Public Health Service, Washington DC.

Vector Tobacco (2001). Advertisement for Omni cigarettes. *Parade,* 23 December.

Vector Tobacco (2002). Advertisement for Omni cigarettes. *Playboy,* June.

Vicini, J. (2008). Court rules against Altria on Light cigarettes. Reuters, 16 December. Available at http://www.reuters.com/article/domesticNews/idUSTRE4BE4RL20081216?sp=true

Warner, K.E. (1985). Tobacco industry response to public health concern: A content analysis of cigarette ads. *Health Education Quarterly,* **12**:115–27.

Wynder, E.L. and Graham, E. (1950). Tobacco smoking as a possible etiologic factor in bronchiogenic carcinoma: a study of 684 proven cases. *Journal of the American Medical Association,* **143**:329–36.

Young, W.W. (1917). *The Story of the Cigarette.* New York: D. Appleton & Company.

Chapter 4

Market manipulation: how the tobacco industry recruits and retains smokers

Melanie Wakefield

The tobacco industry has been spectacularly successful in marketing its products over a long period of time. Marketing and trade publications attest to the success of tobacco advertising campaigns, with the Marlboro Man being labelled by *Advertising Age* as the top icon of the twentieth century. Advertising campaigns for cigarette brands such as Marlboro, Benson & Hedges, Winston, Camel, and Lucky Strike have garnered positions in the top 100 list of all advertising campaigns (Advertising Age 2005). A distinguishing feature of tobacco industry marketing is that, rather than relying on traditional avenues such as television, radio and print media, a full range of advertising and promotional opportunities has been used.

To appreciate the breadth of tobacco marketing, it is important to understand the nested relationships between mass media advertising, marketing communications, consumer marketing, and stakeholder marketing (NCI 2008). Figure 4.1 shows that each level of these media communications from 1 through 4 represents a broader and more indirect level of marketing efforts, as well as a more powerful one. Although the ultimate impact of media efforts may be felt most clearly by direct consumer response to advertising or marketing communications, interventions at the stakeholder level often have broad-reaching effects on promotional efforts, social attitudes towards an issue or product, or even policies and regulation.

Mass media advertising includes so-called 'measured media' such as advertising on television, radio, cinema, magazines, newspapers, and billboards for which syndicated marketing research services estimate audience exposure. Other marketing communications include tobacco sponsorship, tobacco packaging, and point-of-sale promotions, as well as a host of sampling and brand-stretching strategies. Broader consumer marketing efforts include issues such as pricing and product design, discussed elsewhere in this volume (see Chapter 9). Finally, at the broadest level, stakeholder marketing includes corporate social responsibility programmes, youth smoking prevention programmes, and other relationship-building programmes.

To provide context for these strategies, the chapter first examines the gradual move by tobacco companies from measured media towards other marketing communications. The chapter then focuses on two tobacco marketing communications of prime importance – point-of-sale marketing and tobacco packaging. The final section of the chapter considers corporate social responsibility programmes and youth smoking prevention programmes, which have emerged as traditional avenues for advertising have been closed, or have threatened to be limited by tobacco control legislation or legal agreements.

From traditional advertising to other communications

As evidence has grown about the serious health consequences of tobacco use, tobacco control efforts have sought to limit the abilities of tobacco companies to market their products. In the

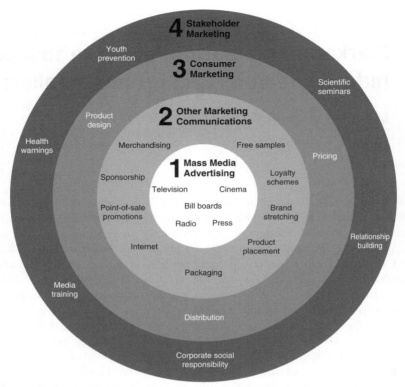

Figure 4.1 The role of the media in promoting and reducing tobacco use.
Source: Tobacco Control Monograph No. 19. Bethesda, MD: US Department of Health and Human Services, National Institutes of Health, National Cancer Institute. NIH Pub. No 07-6242. (p6). Available at: http://cancercontrol.cancer.gov/tcrb/monographs/19/index.html Reproduced with permission from: National Cancer Institute (2008).

main, tobacco companies have largely anticipated, or at least stayed in step with, the way in which tobacco control policies and actions attempt to limit their tobacco promotion efforts and have accordingly evolved their strategies. When one marketing channel has been closed or limited, tobacco companies have been adept in creating or using different strategies to promote tobacco products and pro-tobacco ideas. For example, in the United States, from 1940 to 2005, the tobacco industry spent about US$250 billion on cigarette advertising and promotion, averaging more than US$10 million per day (NCI 2008, p. 119). In 2005, the industry spent just over US$13.5 billion, or US$37 million per day. Over time, the percentage of expenditures dedicated to measured media declined dramatically from 82% in 1970 to almost nil in 2005. Correspondingly, the percentage of marketing expenditures dedicated to promotional activities (price discounts, promotional allowances, coupons, retail value-added promotions) increased during the same period from 18% to almost 100% (NCI 2008, p. 120).

These shifts in marketing expenditures reflect the tobacco industry's response to tobacco advertising being banned on US television and radio in the 1970s (NCI 2008) and on billboards in the United States 1998 as part of the Master Settlement Agreement (Wakefield *et al.* 2002a). The predominance of price discounts, accounting for three-quarters of cigarette marketing expenditures in the United States is a highly effective marketing tool, given smokers' sensitivity to cigarette prices, especially those who are young or in otherwise vulnerable population groups such as low-income groups, less educated people, and minority populations (USDHHS 2000). The price elasticity of demand for cigarettes is −0.3 to −0.5, meaning that a 10% increase in price will reduce overall cigarette consumption by 3–5% (USDHHS 2000). Efforts to reduce population smoking by increasing the price of cigarette through tobacco tax increases, are being undermined by tobacco companies in countries such as the United States, where price discounting tobacco promotions are still permitted.

A recent review by the National Cancer Institute concluded that the total weight of evidence from multiple types of studies, conducted by investigators from different disciplines, and using data from many countries, demonstrates a causal relationship between tobacco advertising and promotion and increased tobacco use (NCI 2008). The review also included econometric studies which have examined the impact of marketing bans on tobacco consumption, concluding that comprehensive bans reduce tobacco consumption. However, non-comprehensive restrictions were generally found to induce an increase in expenditures for advertising in 'non-banned' media and for other marketing activities, which offset the effects of the partial ban so that any net change in consumption is minimal or undetectable (NCI 2008).

Point-of-sale tobacco marketing

Cigarette pack displays and associated retail advertising are a key component of point-of-sale (POS) marketing and tobacco companies pay a premium to ensure prime placement within stores and superior positioning of their brands relative to others (Feighery *et al.* 2003). It has been demonstrated that widespread retail tobacco advertising can influence and distort adolescents' perceptions regarding popularity, use and availability of tobacco. Experimental research has shown that adolescents exposed to retail tobacco advertising perceived significantly easier access to cigarettes than a control group (Henriksen *et al.* 2002). Advertising exposure also influenced perceptions about smoking prevalence, peer approval for smoking and support for tobacco control policies (Henriksen *et al.* 2002). Further research has shown that adolescents who reported at least weekly exposure to retail tobacco marketing were more likely to have experimented with smoking (Henriksen *et al.* 2004) and that in-store branded tobacco advertising and promotion are strongly associated with choice of cigarette brands by adolescents (Wakefield *et al.* 2002b).

The presence of tobacco in stores alongside everyday items such as confectionery, soft drinks, and magazines helps to create a sense of familiarity with tobacco products. This familiarity may act to de-emphasize the serious health consequences of tobacco consumption and increase youth perceptions of the prevalence of smoking, as well as their perceived access to tobacco products (Lee *et al.* 2004). The presence of tobacco products in neighbourhood retail outlets conveys to young people that tobacco use is desirable, socially acceptable, and prevalent in society (Feighery *et al.* 1998).

Retail tobacco marketing restrictions have to date primarily eliminated branded tobacco advertising and promotions. In countries with such restrictions, such as Canada, New Zealand, and Australia, POS cigarette pack displays have evolved into prominent 'power walls' of carefully coordinated colourful packs (Fraser 1998; Carter *et al.* 2003; Dewhirst 2004). According to industry documents, tobacco companies use cigarette pack displays in order to maintain prominence for their brands in the face of restrictions on retail marketing (Wakefield *et al.* 2002c; DiFranza *et al.* 2002; Lavack and Toth 2006; Pollay 2007). For example, US tobacco companies circumvented self-service display bans by furnishing enclosed acrylic displays to showcase their products (Lee *et al.* 2001). In-store displays increase sales of other consumer products (Curhan 1974; Chevalier 1976, 1985; Wilkinson *et al.* 1982; Blattberg and Neslin 1989). A study of purchase choices made by approximately 4 000 shoppers in 14 US cities found that product displays were associated with a greater likelihood of unplanned (rather than planned) purchases (Inman and Winer 1998). Furthermore, unplanned purchases were more likely when displays were located near the cash register, or at the end of shopping aisles, than in the middle of an aisle.

The tobacco industry's increasing reliance on POS marketing in countries with traditional tobacco advertising bans means that there is a profusion of smoking cues in most convenience stores, petrol stations and supermarkets, with cigarette pack displays positioned near the cash register for maximum salience (Feighery et al. 2003). Even without accompanying branded tobacco advertising, the presence of cigarette pack displays has been shown to influence youth and current smokers. For example, an experimental study randomly allocated over 600 Australian ninth-grade students to view a photograph of a typical convenience store POS which had been digitally manipulated to show either cigarette advertising and pack displays, pack displays only, or no cigarettes (Wakefield et al. 2006a). Students then completed a self-administered questionnaire. Compared to the no cigarette condition, students exposed to the cigarette display condition thought it would be easier to purchase cigarettes from the pictured store and were more easily able to recall cigarette brand names, both factors associated with increased likelihood of smoking uptake.

The extent to which these cigarette displays act as cues to purchase cigarettes was examined in a population survey involving 526 smokers in the Australian state of Victoria. When shopping for items other than cigarettes, 25.2% said they at least sometimes purchased cigarettes on impulse as a result of seeing the cigarette display (Wakefield et al. 2008a). Thirty-eight per cent of smokers who had tried to quit in the past 12 months, and 33.9% of 67 recent quitters (who had quit in the past year), experienced an urge to buy cigarettes as a result of seeing the retail cigarette display. One in five smokers trying to quit and one in eight recent quitters avoided stores where they usually bought cigarettes in case they might be tempted to purchase them. In addition, nearly one-third of smokers (31.4%) thought the removal of cigarette displays from stores would make it easier for them to quit. This study suggested that POS cigarette displays act as cues to smoke, even among those not explicitly intending to buy cigarettes, and those trying to avoid smoking.

This suggests that effective POS marketing restrictions should include elimination of cigarette displays, requiring cigarettes to be stored out of sight. Such legislation has already been implemented in Thailand and most Canadian provinces, and legislation is awaiting implementation in several Australian states.

The cigarette pack as brand image

In the face of more comprehensive restrictions on tobacco advertising and promotion, tobacco packaging itself has become a key vehicle for communicating brand image (NCI 2008). Through the use of colour, fonts, images, and trademarks, cigarette packs project a brand image that says something about the user of the product. Commonly referred to as a 'badge product', the user often associates with the identity and personality of the brand image (Wakefield et al. 2002c; Hammond 2007). Unlike most other consumer products, cigarette packs remain with users once opened and are repeatedly displayed in social situations, thereby serving as a direct form of mobile advertising for the brand.

In countries such as Australia where traditional forms of advertising are banned, packaging now serves as a key vehicle for tobacco marketing. Accordingly, Australian tobacco companies have experimented with producing more colourful and varied packs, as well as designs to pique curiosity. For example, British American Tobacco (BAT) Australia experimented with its trademark design on packs of Benson and Hedges and Winfield cigarettes in 2002–2003 (Wakefield and Letcher 2002) and introduced split Dunhill packs (so-called 'kiddie packs') in 2006 (Chapman 2007; Anonymous 2006), by which two low-consumption smokers could more easily procure and split apart a single pack for their own use. Some brands have also begun to incorporate the colour schemes of graphic health warnings into the overall colour and design of the entire pack, causing the warnings to become less salient since they blend in with the overall pack design (Kylie Lindorff, Quit Victoria, personal communication, July 2008).

Tobacco industry research has shown that the design of a cigarette pack can not only generate powerful images about the type of person who might typically smoke the brand, but also provide cues about the sensory perceptions of the smoke which may be expected from a particular cigarette. For example, given identical cigarettes to try, men and women rated the sensory experience of smoking a cigarette differently depending on the brand name given to the cigarette, with women rating the attributes of the smoke more positively when assigned a feminine brand name, and males rating it more positively if it had a masculine brand name (Freedman and Dipple 1978). Similarly, sensory perceptions of cigarettes can be manipulated simply by changing the colour or shade of colour on a pack, through a process called 'sensation transfer'. Package testing for Camel Filter cigarettes revealed that increasing the amount of white space on the pack, and lightening brown colour tones reduced the perception of the cigarette's strength when the cigarette was smoked (Etzel 1979). Research conducted by Philip Morris USA also indicated strong sensation transfer effects when testing identical Marlboro Ultra light cigarettes, placed in either a blue or red pack. Although the cigarettes were exactly the same, those placed in the red packs were perceived to be 'harsher' than those in blue packs, while cigarettes in the blue packs were rated as 'too mild', 'not easy drawing' and 'burned too fast' (Isaacs 1981).

In recognition of the importance of cigarette packaging in the marketing of tobacco, proposals to introduce 'plain' cigarette packaging have emerged, whereby packs would be stripped of colours, brand imagery, corporate logos, and trademarks and manufacturers would be permitted to print only the brand name in a mandated size, font, and location, in addition to required health warnings and other legally mandated information such as toxic constituents, tax-seals, or pack contents (Cunningham and Kyle 1995; Freeman *et al.* 2008). In their review, Freeman and colleagues (Freeman *et al.* 2008) conclude that trademark laws and international trade laws do not preclude mandating the removal of brand design elements on tobacco packs and that plain packaging could and should be pursued under the FCTC.

In a recent Australian study of 813 adult smokers, researchers used an internet online method to expose smokers to either a branded cigarette pack or one of three plain pack version, each of which has been increasingly stripped of branding design elements, after which respondents completed ratings of the pack (Wakefield *et al.* 2008b). Compared to current cigarette packs with full branding, cigarette packs that displayed progressively fewer branding design elements were perceived increasingly unfavourably in terms of smokers' appraisals of the packs, the smokers who might smoke such packs, and the inferred experience of smoking a cigarette from these packs. For example, cardboard brown packs with the number of enclosed cigarettes displayed on the front of the pack and featuring only the brand name in small standard font at the bottom of the pack face were rated as significantly less attractive and popular than original branded packs. Smokers of these plain packs were rated as significantly less trendy/stylish, less sociable/outgoing and less mature than smokers of the original pack. Finally, compared with original packs, smokers inferred that cigarettes from these plain packs would be less rich in tobacco, less satisfying and of lower quality tobacco.

These results imply that plain packaging policies that remove most brand design elements are likely to be most successful in removing cigarette brand image associations. With a likely acceleration in the rate of comprehensive restrictions on tobacco advertising and promotion as countries strive to meet their responsibilities under the Framework Convention on Tobacco Control (FCTC) (World Health Organization 2005a), tobacco packaging will assume even greater importance internationally as a promotional vehicle for driving brand image (Hammond 2007).

Stakeholder marketing: tobacco company youth smoking prevention programmes

Youth smoking prevention programmes run by the tobacco industry began emerging in the United States in the 1980s. A review of tobacco industry documents made public under the terms of legal settlements show that the focus and timing of these programmes were commenced at least in part as a response to mounting public concern about industry marketing practices and as a strategy to forestall legislation or regulation that would restrict tobacco industry activities (Landman *et al.* 2002). A confidential Tobacco Institute presentation that Landman *et al.* (2002) surmised was written around 1982–1983 and suggests:

> The potential positive outcomes of adopting programs of this nature [socially responsible programs] may be…a more sophisticated understanding by government regulators of the needs/behaviours of our industry. For example, a program to discourage teens from smoking (an adult decision) might prevent or delay further regulation of the tobacco industry.

(Tobacco Institute undated)

Tobacco industry youth smoking efforts have tended to focus on parental and peer influences on youth smoking, general decision-making and life skills, and issues around youth access to tobacco, especially the notion that under-age smoking is 'illegal'. It is notable that the youth smoking prevention activities and education programmes developed and supported by the tobacco industry tend to ignore the influence of tobacco advertising and promotion on youth smoking uptake, the importance of parents not smoking or quitting to provide non-smoking role models for their children, and explanation about tobacco addiction and serious smoking-related illnesses. The tobacco industry's youth smoking prevention activities fall broadly into five main categories: family involvement self-help booklets, school-based smoking prevention programmes, programmes to prevent youth access to tobacco, mass media campaigns advocating that youth should not smoke, and community-based programmes for youth (Sussman 2002).

Mass media campaigns have perhaps been the highest profile and most costly initiative of all tobacco company youth smoking prevention efforts. In the late 1990s, two tobacco companies launched televised mass-media campaigns focusing on youth smoking prevention in the United States. In 1998, Philip Morris launched a campaign consisting of several television and magazine advertisements aimed at youth with the slogan 'Think. Don't smoke' (Sussman 2002) and the campaign ran until 2002. The target audience for the 'Think. Don't smoke' campaign, according to Philip Morris, was youth aged 10–14 (Sussman 2002). In 1999, Philip Morris launched a campaign with the slogan, 'Talk. They'll Listen,' focused on parental responsibility for talking to children about smoking (Sussman 2002) and this campaign ran until late 2006. On 4 April 2005, in the Department of Justice lawsuit, Howard Willard, Senior Vice President Youth Smoking and Corporate Responsibility at Philip Morris, described the amount of money Philip Morris has committed to youth smoking prevention since 1998: 'Our budget has fluctuated from year to year, but on average, we have spent $100 million a year over the last 6 years in the department. The expenditures from 1998 to 2004 total $657 million.' (Willard 2005). On its website, Philip Morris indicates it has spent 'over $1 billion on youth smoking prevention efforts' (www.philipmorrisuse.com/en/our_inititatives/ysp.asp accessed 30 June 2008).

Between 1999 and 2004, Lorillard's prevention advertisements with the 'Tobacco Is Whacko, if You're a Teen' slogan appeared widely in teen magazines and on cable television, including the most popular shows for adolescents on Entertainment and Sports Programming Network (ESPN), MTV, and Warner Brothers stations (Landman *et al.* 2002). The budget for this campaign was about $13 million (Farrelly *et al.* 2003) Eventually, Lorillard replaced its advertisements aimed at youth with advertisements targeting parents. Formerly known as 'Take 10', the subsequent Lorillard prevention campaign featured the slogan, 'Parents. The best thing between kids and cigarettes.' On its website, Lorillard indicates it has spent over $80 million on youth smoking prevention efforts (http://www.lorillard.com/index.php?id=5 accessed 30 June 2008).

Studies of youth responses to tobacco company-sponsored youth smoking prevention advertising have most often focused on ratings of individual ads in a forced exposure setting, compared with ratings of public health-sponsored antitobacco ads. In these studies, youth are exposed individually or in a group setting to a series of ads and then complete questionnaire ratings of each advertisement immediately after viewing it (e.g. Henriksen and Fortmann 2002; Wakefield *et al.* 2005; Donovan *et al.* 2006). Some studies also required youth to select the advertisement they perceived to be most effective or to complete post-exposure measures of smoking-related beliefs, attitudes, and intentions (e.g. Pechmann and Riebling 2006; Henriksen *et al.* 2006) and others added follow-up measures of recall and cognitive processing of the advertisements (e.g. Terry-McElrath *et al.* 2005). Of the seven forced exposure studies conducted to date, all demonstrate that tobacco company-sponsored youth smoking prevention advertisements perform poorly in terms of new learning, perceived effectiveness, and influence on intention to smoke, by comparison with many public health-sponsored antitobacco advertisements. The studies generally show that these poor ratings are not a function of the advertisements being sponsored by tobacco companies per se; rather they are a reflection of the messages delivered in them. Consistent with their other youth smoking prevention efforts, both Philip Morris and Lorillard have limited their youth smoking prevention messages to emphasizing social themes, such as making a choice about smoking among peers and within the family, or presenting the short-term benefits of not smoking.

Forced exposure studies of advertising effects are helpful for assessing immediate reactions to individual advertisements and short-term influences on smoking-related beliefs and intentions, but they do not reflect the usual television-viewing environment with all of its contextual distractions of television programmes, other competing advertising and variable attention on the part of the viewer. In addition, forced exposure studies cannot assess the effects of cumulative exposure to campaign messages over time. By comparison, naturalistic exposure studies of media campaign effects attempt to assess the effects of media campaigns when viewed in the usual viewing environment and do so with more population-representative samples of participants. In these studies, exposure to advertising is usually measured by asking if participants can recall seeing any antitobacco advertisements in a specified period and, if so, having them describe it they recall, in order to generate a measure of confirmed recall (Biener 2002; Farrelly *et al.* 2002; 2008; Davis *et al.* 2007). However, one study employed gross rating points as an advertising exposure measure (Wakefield *et al.* 2006b).

Three groups of naturalistic exposure studies of tobacco company media campaign effects have been conducted in the United States. The first, conducted in Massachusetts in 1999, found in a population survey that among adolescents aged 14–17 years who had recalled seeing particular ads in the past 30 days, the Philip Morris' 'Think. Don't Smoke' youth smoking prevention advertisements and Massachusetts advertisements that did not discuss illness were rated as significantly less effective than those featuring the serious health consequences of smoking (Biener 2002). These effects were more pronounced among youth aged 16–17 years than those aged 14–15 years. The second group of studies used a telephone survey of a nationally representative sample of US adolescents aged 12–17 to compare youth who recalled Legacy 'truth' advertisements with those who recalled who reported seeing any one of the 'Think. Don't Smoke' Philip Morris youth smoking prevention advertisements. In the first report from this study conducted ten months after the launch of the 'truth' campaign, youth who recalled the 'Think. Don't Smoke' ads were significantly less likely than unexposed peers to have increased intentions to smoke in future, whereas confirmed recall of the legacy campaign was associated with reduced intentions to smoke (Farrelly *et al.* 2002). In addition, youth who recalled the 'Think. Don't Smoke' campaign were less likely to agree with statements, such as 'cigarette companies deny that cigarettes cause disease,' and 'I would like to see cigarette companies go out of business' (Farrelly *et al.* 2002). In subsequent reports using eight cross-sectional telephone surveys over a three-year period, exposure to additional Philip Morris advertisements reinforced these attitudes (Farrelly *et al.* 2008). Unlike exposure to 'truth' ads, which were associated with reduced perceptions of the prevalence of smoking in the three-year study, recall of 'Think. Don't Smoke' was unrelated to perceived smoking prevalence (Davis *et al.* 2007). Because the data from this second group of studies are cross-sectional, an alternate interpretation is that adolescents who already held more favourable opinions about cigarette companies and more strongly intended to smoke were more attentive to Philip Morris advertisements and therefore were more likely to recall them.

The third naturalistic exposure study was conducted with over 100 000 students (8th, 10th, and 12th graders) who completed the Monitoring the Future school-based surveys from 1999 to 2002, where smoking beliefs, intentions and behaviour comprised the study outcomes (Wakefield *et al.* 2006b). Unlike previous studies, this study measured advertising exposure using gross rating points for each type of advertising campaign in the four months preceding the surveys in the media markets in which the schools were located. Two tobacco company campaigns evaluated in this study included youth-directed smoking prevention advertising ('Think. Don't Smoke' and 'Tobacco is Whacko if You're a Teen') and the Philip Morris parent-directed campaign called 'Talk. They'll Listen'. Models for the variables associated with behaviour, attitude, and intention controlled for demographic and other personal data, region, the real price of cigarettes, a smoke-free air index, and exposure to public health-sponsored antitobacco advertising. The analyses discerned that greater exposure to industry-sponsored youth-directed advertising was associated with stronger intentions to smoke among 8th graders, but was unrelated to other outcomes for 8th graders and 10–12th graders. However, exposure to the tobacco industry's parent-directed campaign advertising was associated with lower perceived harm from smoking, stronger approval of smoking, stronger intentions to smoke in future and a higher likelihood of smoking in the past month for 10th and 12th graders.

Wakefield and colleagues cite theories in developmental psychology to explain these findings (Wakefield *et al.* 2006b). As adolescents mature, they consider themselves more independent and less reliant on their parents. Thus, messages aimed at parents as authority figures invite rejection by older adolescents.

In court testimony, Philip Morris witnesses have stressed the seriousness of their efforts in trying to reduce smoking among youth by pointing to the amount of funding allocated to youth smoking prevention. Increases in funding, however, have tended to coincide with increases in tobacco litigation cases (Wakefield *et al.* 2006c). Despite the sophisticated naturalistic exposure methods available for determining the effectiveness of advertising campaigns, the considerable funding of their youth smoking prevention programmes, and from the companies' insistence on the seriousness of their efforts, it is notable that tobacco companies have used very weak methods of programme evaluation. In court testimonies from 1992 to 2003, company witnesses focused on advertising reach as a measure of effectiveness (e.g. 90% of 10- to 14-year-olds had seen the advertisements) and on qualitative data (Wakefield *et al.* 2006c). Although Philip Morris withdrew its television advertising campaign after the Wakefield *et al.* (2006b) study was published, it still cites its own weak evaluation data to suggest that its 'Talk. They'll Listen' campaign had beneficial effects. (http://www.philipmorrisusa.com/en/cms/Responsibility/Helping_Reduce_Underage_Tobacco_Use/Our_Focus_Areas/Parent_Communications/default.aspx)

The tobacco industry gains many benefits from its youth smoking prevention initiatives. First, it is seen to be doing something about the issue by the public, by legislators and by judges and members of juries. Thus, these programmes are important for promoting pro-tobacco industry attitudes, underlining their considerable public relations value. Such positive attitudes could serve to limit the industry's legal liability and make it easier for the industry's views to be heard on issues concerning tobacco legislation and regulation. More favourable impressions of tobacco companies among youth themselves could serve to keep the door open for taking up smoking in future (e.g. Thrasher *et al.* 2006; Wakefield *et al.* 2006b). Second, the tobacco industry has been able to use the relationships it has forged through its youth smoking prevention programmes to learn of and lobby against proposed tobacco control legislation that would reduce tobacco sales (Forster and Wolfson 1998). Third, it is able to use these youth smoking prevention efforts to argue for diverting tobacco control funding from demonstrably effective strategies with mass reach (Mandel *et al.* 2006). Fourth, investment in youth smoking prevention programmes means that tobacco companies can now freely admit to monitoring youth smoking in order to develop their programmes (Mandel *et al.* 2006). A fifth benefit for the tobacco industry, if only from the viewpoint of preserving its future customer base, is that for some of its programmes, older teens demonstrate reactance to the tobacco industry programme message that tobacco use is for adults only, thereby leading to a greater likelihood of youth smoking uptake (Donovan *et al.* 2006; Henriksen *et al.* 2006; Wakefield *et al.* 2006b).

The World Health Organization Tobacco-Free Initiative recommends that government and non-government organizations avoid partnering with tobacco industry youth smoking prevention programmes because the programmes have been proven ineffective and are used to leverage governments to opt for weaker legislation (World Health Organization 2005b). While there is no good evidence that tobacco industry-sponsored youth smoking prevention efforts have been effective in reducing youth smoking, there is plenty of evidence that the tobacco industry has used its youth smoking prevention efforts in ways that permit the tobacco industry to preserve its ability to freely market tobacco products.

References

Advertising Age. (2005). The advertising century. *Advertising Age.* http://adage.com/century

Anonymous. (2006). Cigarette split pack defeated. *Daily Telegraph*, 18 November, Sydney, Australia.

Biener, L. (2002). Anti-tobacco advertisements by Massachusetts and Philip Morris: what teenagers think. *Tob Control* 11(Suppl II):ii43–6.

Blattberg, R.C., and Neslin, S.A. (1989). Sales promotion: the long and short of it. *Marketing Letters* 1:87–97.

Carter, S.M. (2003). New frontier new power: the retail environment in Australia's dark market. *Tob Control* 12(suppl III):iii95–101.

Chapman, S. (2007). Australia: British American Tobacco 'addresses' youth smoking. *Tob Control* 16:2–3.

Chevalier, M. (1976). Substitution patterns as a result of display in the product category. *J Retailing* 51:65–72.

Chevalier, M. (1985). Increase in sales due to in-store display. *J Marketing Res* 12:426–31.

Cunningham, R., and Kyle, K. (1995). The case for plain packaging. *Tob Control* 4:50–86.

Curhan, R.C. (1974). The effects of merchandising and temporary promotional activities on the sales of fresh fruits and vegetables in supermarkets. *J Marketing Res* 11:286–94.

Davis, K.C., Nonnemaker, J.M., and Farrelly, M.C. (2007). Association between national smoking prevention campaigns and perceived smoking prevalence among youth in the United States. *J Adol Health* 41:430–6.

Dewhirst, T. (2004). POP goes the power wall? Taking aim at promotional strategies utilised at retail. *Tob Control* **13**:209–10.

DiFranza, J.R., Clark, D.M., and Pollay, R.W. (2002). Cigarette package design: opportunities for disease prevention. *Tob Induced Dis* **1**:97–109.

Donovan, R.J., Jalleh, G., and Carter, O.B.J. (2006). Tobacco industry smoking prevention advertisements' impact on youth motivation for smoking in the future. *Social Mark Q* **12**(2):3–13.

Etzel, E. (1979). Consumer research proposal: Camel Filter revised packaging Test Study. RJ Reynolds. 2 March 1979. Bates No. 500566627/6632. Available at: http://legacy.library.ucsf.edu/ Accessed 7 July 2008.

Farrelly, M.C., Healton, C.G., Davis, K.C., Messeri, P., Hersey, J.C., and Haviland, M.L. (2002). Getting to the truth: evaluating national tobacco countermarketing campaigns. *Am J Public Health* **92**(6): 901–07.

Farrelly, M.C., Niederdeppe, J., and Yarsevich, J. (2003). Youth smoking prevention mass media campaigns: past, present, and future directions. *Tob Control* **12**(suppl 1): i35–i47.

Farrelly, M.C., Davis, K.C., Duke, J., and Messeri, P. (2008). Sustaining 'truth': changes in youth tobacco attitudes and smoking intentions after 3 years of a national antismoking campaign. *Health Educ Res* Advance Access published 17 January 2008 doi:10.1093/her/cym087

Feighery, E., Borzekowski, D.L.G., Schooler, C., and Flora J. (1998). Seeing, wanting, owning: the relationship between receptivity to tobacco marketing and smoking susceptibility in young people. *Tob Control* **7**: 123–8.

Feighery, E.C., Ribisl, K.M., Clark, P.I., and Haladjian, H.H. (2003). How tobacco companies ensure prime placement of their advertising and products in stores: interviews with retailers about tobacco company incentive programmes. *Tob Control* **12**:184–8.

Forster, J.L., and Wolfson, M. (1998). Youth access to tobacco: policies and politics. *Ann Rev Public Health* **19**:203–35.

Fraser, T. (1998). Phasing out point-of-sale tobacco advertising in New Zealand. *Tob Control* **7**:82–4.

Freedman, H.H., and Dipple, W.S. (1978). The effect of masculine and feminine brand names on the perceived taste of a cigarette. *Decision Sciences* **9**:467–71.

Freeman, B., Chapman, S., and Rimmer, M. (2008). The case for plain packaging of tobacco products. *Addiction* **103**:580–90.

Hammond, D. (2007). FCTC Article 11: Tobacco packaging and labelling: a review of evidence. University of Waterloo, Canada, November 2007. Available at: http://www.cctc.ca/cctc/EN/tcrc/books/tcmonograph.2007-12-19.7863543963 Accessed 7 July 2008.

Henriksen, L., Flora, J.A., Feighery, E., and Fortmann, S.P. (2002). Effects on youth of exposure to retail tobacco advertising. *J Appl Soc Psychol* **32**:1771–89.

Henriksen, L., Feighery, E.C., Wang, Y., and Fortmann, S.P. (2004). Association of retail tobacco marketing with adolescent smoking. *Am J Public Health* **94**:2081–3.

Henriksen, L., and Fortmann, S.P. (2002). Young adults' opinions of Philip Morris and its television advertising. *Tob Control* **11**:236–40.

Henriksen, L., Dauphinee, A.L., Wang, Y., and Fortmann, S.P. (2006). Industry sponsored anti-smoking ads and adolescent reactance: test of a boomerang effect. *Tob Control* **15**:13–18.

Inman, J.J., and Winer, R.S. (1998). Where the rubber meets the road: a model of in-store consumer decision-making. Marketing Science Institute, Working Paper 98–112. Accessed 14 June 2007. Available at: http://www.msi.org/publications/publication.cfm?pub=502

Isaacs, J. (1981). Identified HTI test of Marlboro Ultra Lights in a blue pack vs. Marlboro Ultra Lights in a red pack. Philip Morris, USA, July 1981. Bates No. 2047387079/7089. Available at: http://legacy.library.ucsf.edu/ Accessed 7 July 2008.

Landman, A., Ling, P.M., and Glantz, S.A. (2002). Tobacco industry youth smoking prevention programs: protecting the industry and hurting tobacco control. *Am J Public Health* **92**:917–30.

Lavack, A.M., and Toth, G. (2006). Tobacco point of purchase promotion: examining tobacco industry documents. *Tob Control* **15**:377–84.

Lee, R.E., Feighery, E.C., Schleicher, N.C., and Halvorson, S. (2001). The relation between community bans of self-service tobacco displays and store environment and between tobacco accessibility and merchant incentives. *Am J Public Health* **91**:2019–21.

Lee, R.G., Taylor, V.A., and McGetrick, R. (2004). Toward reducing youth exposure to tobacco messages: examining the breadth of brand and nonbrand communication. *J Health Commun* **9**:461–79.

Mandel, L.L., Bialous, S.A., and Glantz S.A. (2006). Avoiding 'truth': tobacco industry promotion of Life Skills Training. *J Adol Health* **39**:868–79.

National Cancer Institute. (2008). The role of the media in promoting and reducing tobacco use. Tobacco Control Monograph No. 19. Bethesda, MD: US Department of Health and Human Services, National Institutes of Health, National Cancer Institute. NIH Pub. No 07-6242. Available at: http://cancercontrol.cancer.gov/tcrb/monographs/19/index.html

Pechmann, C., and Riebling, E.T. (2006). Antismoking advertisements for youths: an independent evaluation of health, counter-industry, and industry approaches. *Am J Public Health* **96**(5):906–13.

Pollay, R. (2007). More than meets the eye: on the importance of retail cigarette merchandising. *Tob Control* **16**:270–4.

Sussman, S. (2002). Tobacco industry youth smoking prevention programming: a review. *Prev Sci* **3**(1):57–67.

Terry-McElrath, Y., Wakefield, M., Ruel, E., Balch, G., Emery, S., Szczypka, G. *et al.* (2005). The effect of anti-smoking advertisement executional characteristics on youth comprehension, appraisal, recall and engagement. *J Health Commun* **10**:127–43.

Thrasher, J.F., Niederdeppe, J.D., Jackson, C., and Farrelly, M.C. (2006). Using anti-tobacco industry messages to prevent smoking among high-risk adolescents. *Health Educ Res* **21**:325–37.

United States Department of Health and Human Services. (2000). Reducing tobacco use: a report of the Surgeon-General. Atlanta: US Department of Health and Human Services, Centers for Disease Control and Prevention, National Center for Chronic Disease Prevention and Health Promotion, Office on Smoking and Health. http://www.cdc.gov/tobacco/data_statistics/sgr/sgr_2000/index.htm

Wakefield, M., Balch, G.I., Ruel, E.E., Terry-McElrath, Y., Szczypka, G., Flay, B. *et al.* (2005). Youth responses to anti-smoking advertisements from tobacco-control agencies, tobacco companies and pharmaceutical companies. *J Appl Soc Psych* **35**(9):1894–911.

Wakefield, M., and Letcher, T. (2002). My pack is cuter than your pack. *Tob Control* **11**:154–6.

Wakefield, M., Germain, D., Durkin, S., and Henriksen, L. (2006a). An experimental study of effects on schoolchildren of exposure to point-of-sale cigarette advertising and pack displays. *Health Educ Res* **21**:338–47.

Wakefield, M., Germain, D., and Durkin, S. (2008a). How does increasingly plainer cigarette packaging influence adult smokers' perceptions about brand image? An experimental study. *Tobacco Control* doi:10.1136/tc.2008.026732.

Wakefield, M., McLeod, K., and Perry, C. (2006c). 'Stay away from them until you're old enough to make decision': tobacco company testimony about youth smoking initiation. *Tob Control* **15** (Suppl IV):iv44–53.

Wakefield, M., Morley, C., Horan, J.K., and Cummings, K.M. (2002c). The cigarette pack as image: new evidence from tobacco industry documents. *Tob Control* **11**(Suppl I):i73–i80.

Wakefield, M., Germain, D., and Henriksen, L. (2008b). The effect of retail cigarette pack displays on impulse purchase. *Addiction* **103**:322–8.

Wakefield, M.A., Ruel, E.E., Chaloupka, F.J., Slater, S.J., and Kaufman, N.J. (2002b). Association of point-of-purchase tobacco advertising and promotions with choice of usual brand among teenage smokers. *J Health Commun* **7**:113–21.

Wakefield, M., Terry-McElrath, Y., Emery, S., Saffer, H., Chaloupka, F., Szczypka, G. *et al.* (2006b). Effect of televised, tobacco company-funded smoking prevention advertising on youth smoking-related beliefs, intentions, and behavior. *Am J Public Health* **96**(12):2154–60.

Wakefield, M.A., Terry-McElrath, Y.M., Chaloupka, F.J., Barker, D.C., Slater, S.J., Clark, P.I. *et al.* (2002a). Tobacco industry marketing at the point-of-purchase after the 1998 MSA billboard advertising ban. *Am J Public Health* **92**(6):937–9.

Wilkinson, J.B., Mason, B., and Paksoy, C.H. (1982). Assessing the impact of short-term supermarket strategy variables. *J Marketing Res* **19**:72–86.

Willard, H. (2005) Senior Vice President, Youth Smoking Prevention and Corporate Responsibility, Philip Morris. Trial Testimony. United States of America v. Philip Morris. Case No. 99-CV-2496(GK). United States District Court for the District of Columbia. 9, www.altria.com/download/pdf/media_doj_livewitness_willard_04042005.pdf

World Health Organisation. (2005a). WHO Framework Convention on Tobacco Control. Available at: http://www.who.int/fctc/en/ Accessed 7 July 2008.

World Health Organization. (2005b). *Building Blocks for Tobacco Control: A Handbook*. Geneva, Switzerland: WHO. Available at: http://www.who.int/tobacco/resources/publications/tobaccocontrol_handbook/en/

Chapter 5

In their own words: an epoch of deceit and deception

Channing Robertson and Richard Hurt

Prologue

'Of all animals, man is the only one that lies'

Mark Twain

In 1847 Philip Morris opened a London shop selling hand-rolled Turkish cigarettes. It was not until 1907 that Philip Morris was re-incorporated and by 1919 had created an American-owned company Philip Morris, Ltd. Though Philip Morris is the dominant brand today, the American tobacco story actually begins in Virginia in the 1880s when James Buchanan 'Buck' Duke took over his father's tobacco company, a producer of chewing and smoking tobacco, and declared, 'I'm going in the cigarette business.' This he did by hiring workers to roll cigarettes, that being the state-of-the-art production methodology. In 1880 an enterprising 21-year-old Virginian, James Albert Bonsack, was granted a patent for a mechanical cigarette-rolling machine. In 1883, 27-year-old Buck Duke leased the Bonsack machine and with that emerged the mass production of cigarettes. They became affordable to more people and their use extended to all regions of the country. Buck Duke grew his American Tobacco Company into a monopoly. It was broken up by the federal government in 1911. Four new companies took hold: the American Tobacco Company, Liggett and Myers, RJ Reynolds, and P Lorillard. The introduction of the first 'modern' cigarette, Camels, by RJ Reynolds in 1914 caused a rapid increase in the per capita consumption of cigarettes in the United States that would not peak until 1964. Camel for the first time used a blend of three types of tobacco and its sales grew as a result of a mass marketing and media campaign to capture customers. The American Tobacco Company countered with a similarly formulated Lucky Strike as did Liggett and Myers with a reformulated Chesterfield. Philip Morris introduced its namesake brand, Philip Morris, which proved very popular. In the early 1930s Marlboro was introduced by Philip Morris as a women's brand. Marlboro was reintroduced in the 1960s as a man's brand and the rest of that story transformed the cigarette industry. By the 1930s, cigarettes were America's favoured form of tobacco and that continues today.

Cigarette smoking became a common practice and the industry grew rapidly through the depression, two world wars, and the Korean War. Actors and actresses could be seen smoking on the big screen and doctors appeared in magazine advertisements, some even placed in medical journals, attesting to the merits of one brand over another.

Then, during the period 1950–1953, dark clouds began to form on the horizon. Wynder and his colleagues published articles linking smoking to cancer.[1,2] These events were the triggers that led to the tobacco industry engaging in nearly a half century of lies, deceit, cover-up, and smoke-and-mirrors obfuscation. Indeed, Philip Morris spent considerable time and effort to pursue and manipulate Wynder to legitimize its own corporate positions on cigarettes and health.[3] As the twentieth century came to a close, the world was coming to terms with an industry whose product, when used as intended, led directly to immense and immeasurable pain and suffering and premature death among its consumers.

In recent years, the World Health Organization (WHO) has identified tobacco product control as one of its highest priorities. Indeed, the WHO Framework Convention on Tobacco Control is the first global public health treaty, which now has over 160 signators, one of which unfortunately is not the United States of America, the site of the origin of the 'modern' cigarette.

Rather than paraphrase, interpret or 'spin' the events of the past 60 years, it is far more sobering and powerful to have the tobacco industry speak to us, in their own words, about their strategies and plans for duping their customers and promoting abject disregard for the public health and trust.

This story needs no commentary. It is self-evident.

Cigarettes: adverse health effects

...and in the beginning

For decades the tobacco industry publically denied that adverse health effects, in particular cancers, were associated with cigarette smoking or exposure to secondhand tobacco smoke.

In response to the Wynder studies, the American Tobacco Company, RJ Reynolds, Philip Morris, the US Tobacco Company, P Lorillard, and the Brown & Williamson Tobacco Corporation created the Tobacco Institute Research Committee (TIRC) – later known as the Council for Tobacco Research (CTR) – to provide 'public relations' assistance in dealing with the 'health scare'. On 4 January 1954 the TIRC ran a full-page promotion in more than 400 newspapers aimed at 43 million Americans. It was entitled 'A Frank Statement to Cigarette Smokers'. Here in its entirety is the text of the first stone placed in a grand foundation of lies and misrepresentations on which a house of cards would be built over the next 50 years:[4]

> Recent reports on experiments with mice have given wide publicity to a theory that cigarette smoking is in some way linked with lung cancer in human beings.
>
> Although conducted by doctors of professional standing, these experiments are not regarded as conclusive in the field of cancer research. However, we do not believe results are inconclusive, should be disregarded or lightly dismissed. At the same time, we feel it is in the public interest to call attention to the fact that eminent doctors and research scientists have publicly questioned the claimed significance of these experiments.
>
> Distinguished authorities point out:
> 1. That medical research of recent years indicates many possible causes of lung cancer.
> 2. That there is no agreement among the authorities regarding what the cause is.
> 3. That there is no proof that cigarette smoking is one of the causes.
> 4. That statistics purporting to link cigarette smoking with the disease could apply with equal force to any one of many other aspects of modern life. Indeed the validity of the statistics themselves is questioned by numerous scientists.
>   We accept an interest in people's health as a basic responsibility, paramount to every other consideration in our business.
>   We believe the products we make are not injurious to health.
>   We always have and always will cooperate closely with those whose task it is to safeguard the public health.

For more than 300 years tobacco has given solace, relaxation, and enjoyment to mankind. At one time or another during those years critics have held it responsible for practically every disease of the human body. One by one these charges have been abandoned for lack of evidence.

Regardless of the record of the past, the fact that cigarette smoking today should even be suspected as a cause of a serious disease is a matter of deep concern to us.

Many people have asked us what we are doing to meet the public's concern aroused by the recent reports. Here is the answer:

1. We are pledging aid and assistance to the research effort into all phases of tobacco use and health. This joint financial aid will of course be in addition to what is already being contributed by individual companies.

2. For this purpose we are establishing a joint industry group consisting initially of the undersigned. This group will be known as Tobacco Industry Research Committee.

3. In charge of the research activities of the Committee will be a scientist of unimpeachable integrity and national repute. In addition there will be an Advisory Board of scientists disinterested in the cigarette industry. A group of distinguished men from medicine, science, and education will be invited to serve on this Board. These scientists will advise the Committee on its research activities.

This statement is being issued because we believe the people are entitled to know where we stand on this matter and what we intend to do about it.

While the Frank Statement raised false doubts and charted a course for actions and behaviour for decades to come during which the tobacco industry challenged and refuted the existence of causal effects between smoking and adverse health effects, tobacco companies were saying something much different behind their closed doors. Here, provided in chronological order, is the industry commentary, some public, but most secret.

The 1950s

'Studies of clinical data tend to confirm the relationship between heavy and prolonged tobacco smoking and incidence of cancer of the lung.'[5]

'You can see why the Parliament filter mouthpiece gives you maximum protection. You're so smart to smoke Parliaments.'[6]

'...there still isn't a single shred of substantial evidence to link cigarette smoking and lung cancer directly.'[7]

'There is only one problem – confidence, and how to establish it; public assurance, and how to create it.... .And, most important, how to free millions of Americans from the guilty fear that is going to arise deep in their biological depths – regardless of any pooh poohing logic – every time they light a cigarette.'[8]

'Boy, wouldn't it be wonderful if our company was the first to produce a cancer-free cigarette? What we could do to the competition!'[9]

'...if we can eliminate or reduce the carcinogenic agent in smoke we will have made real progress.'[10]

'I state that in our considered opinion there is no proof at all that smoking causes lung cancer and much to suggest that it cannot be the cause.'[11]

'Cigarette smoking is compatible with normal health, and even heavier-than-average cigarette smoking is compatible with better-than-average mortality rates, according to a scientific report presented before the Southern Medical Association.'[12]

'As a result of several statistical surveys, the idea has arisen that there is a causal relation between ZEPHYR *(code for cancer)* and tobacco smoking, particularly cigarette smoking. Various hypothesis have been propounded one of which is that "tobacco smoke contains a substance or substances which may cause ZEPHYR."'[13,14]

'[n]o substance has been found in tobacco smoke known to cause cancer in human beings.'[15]

'With one exception the individuals with whom we met believed that smoking causes lung cancer; if by "causation" we mean any chain of events which leads finally to lung cancer and which involves smoking as an indispensable link.'[16]

'The cigarette industry has not changed its mind. Our position was and is based on the fact that scientific evidence does not support the theory that there is anything in cigarette smoke known to cause human lung cancer... . [The Tobacco Institute] believes that the health of the people is more important than dividends for any industry.'[17]

'Evidence is building up that heavy smoking contributes to lung cancer.'[18]

'... intestinal fortitude to jump on the other side of the fence admitting that cigarettes are hazardous. "Just look what a wealth of ammunition would be at his disposal" to attack the other companies who did not have safe cigarettes.'[19]

The 1960s

'Our basic position in the cigarette controversy is subject to the charge, and may be subject to a finding, that we are making false or misleading statements to promote the sale of cigarettes.'[20]

'There are biologically active materials present in cigarette smoking. These are

a) cancer causing

b) cancer promoting

c) poisonous

d) stimulating, pleasurable and flavourful.'[21]

'... which will take 7–10 years because it will require a major research effort, because carcinogens are found in practically every class of compounds in smoke.'[22]

'What would be the effect on this company of not publishing these data now, but being required at some future date to disclose such data, possibly in the unfavourable atmosphere of a lawsuit? ...It is recommended that the Company's management recognise that many members of its Research Department are intensely concerned about the cigarette smoke-health problem and eager to participate in its study and solution.'[23]

'When the health question was first raised we had to start by denying it at the PR *(public relations)* level. But by continuing that policy we had got ourselves into a corner and left no room to manoeuvre. In other words, if we did get a breakthrough and were able to improve our product we should have to about face, and this was practically impossible at the PR level.'[24]

'I have no wish to be tarred and feathered, but I would suggest the industry might serve itself on several fronts if it voluntarily adopted a package legend such as 'excessive use of this product may be injurious to health of susceptible persons' ...This is so controversial a suggestion – indeed shocking – that I would rather not try to anticipate the arguments against it in this note but reserve my defence.'[25]

'[P]eople sometimes forget that there are good reasons why the theories about smoking and health problems are in dispute, and are often questioned by responsible scientists.... [T]he original theory about smoking and lung cancer – the theory that smoke was a direct, contact carcinogen – has virtually been abandoned.'[26]

'Many distinguished scientists are of the opinion that it has not been established that smoking causes disease.'[27]

'There exists no definite proof that smoking cigarettes causes lung cancer or any other dreaded disease.'[28]

'Many nitrosamines [substances in tobacco smoke] have been shown to be carcinogenic for different organs in several species of animals. As nitrosamines are formed by the reaction of oxides of nitrogen with secondary amines, it is possible that cigarette smoke could contain nitrosoanabasine and nitrosonornicotine. Nitroanabasine, which is a derivative of the carcinogenic nitrosopiperidine, has now produced many tumors of the esophagus when given orally to rats.'[29]

'The main power on the smoking and health situation undoubtedly rest with the lawyers...the U.S. cigarette manufacturers are not looking for means to reduce the long-term activity of cigarettes.'[30]

'We don't accept the idea that there are harmful agents in tobacco.'[31]

'We have reason to believe that in spite of gentleman's [sic] agreement from the tobacco industry in previous years that at least some of the major companies have been increasing biological studies within their own facilities.'[32]

'Because known carcinogens are produced from such a wide variety of organic materials during the process of pyrolysis, it is most unlikely that a completely safe form of tobacco smoking can be evolved.'[33]

'The long-range purpose of Project 0107 has been to provide information which would be of use in developing cigarettes which have less tendency to cause lung cancer in smokers than do cigarettes presently available. The evidence linking cigarette smoking with lung cancer is of three types: (1) statistical studies on humans showing that, other factors being held constant, there is a positive correlation between the number of cigarettes smoked and the incidence of lung cancer; (2) studies on mice and other animals showing that cigarette smoke is a carcinogen both in skin painting experiments and by other methods of application; and (3) chemical studies in which compounds of known carcinogenic activity were isolated from cigarette smoke.'[34]

'[C]igarettes will most likely be implicated as one of the causative agents in these diseases [emphysema and bronchitis]'.[35]

'[G]ross lung pathology can be induced by smoking cigarettes'.[36]

'(the Harrogate research report might) ...concede a significant causal relation between the use of tobacco and cancer of the lung.... [W]e would hope to be afforded the opportunity of consulting with the people on your side concerning the way Harrogate's work is presented, admittedly with the hope of "slanting" the report.'[37]

The tobacco industry knew 'of no valid scientific evidence demonstrating that either "tar" or nicotine is responsible for any human illness'.[38]

'Doubt is our product since it is the best means of competing with the "body of fact" that exists in the mind of the general public. It is also a means of establishing a controversy.'[39]

'No case against cigarette smoking has ever been made despite millions spent on research …The longer these tests go on, the better our case becomes.'[40]

'The most important type of story is that which casts doubt in the cause and effect theory of disease and smoking. Eye-grabbing headlines were needed and "should strongly call out the point – Controversy! Contradiction! Other Factors! Unknowns!"'[41]

'We would like the public to be fully informed.'[42]

'[O]ur basic position in the cigarette controversy is subject to the charge, and may be subject to a finding, that we are making false or misleading statements to promote the sale of cigarettes.'[43]

'[T]he cause of cancer in humans, including the cause of cancer of the lung, is unknown.'[44]

'[T]he concept that cigarette smoking is the cause of the increase in lung cancer and emphysema is a colossal blunder.'[45]

'The scientist who has been associated with more research in tobacco and health than any other person [Clarence Cook Little, Executive Director of CTR] declared today that there is no demonstrated causal relationship between smoking and any disease. The gaps in knowledge are so great that those who dogmatically assert otherwise – whether they state that there is or is not such a causal relationship – are premature in judgment. If anything, the pure biological evidence is pointing away from, not toward, the causal hypothesis… .

Statistical associations between smoking and lung cancer, based on study of those two factors alone, are not proof of causal relationship in the opinion of most epidemiologists.'[46]

'No scientist has produced clinical or biological proof that cigarettes cause the diseases they are accused of causing… . We are not going to knuckle under to the Times or anybody else who tries to force us to accept a theory which, in the opinion of men who should know, is half baked.'[47]

The 1970s

'We believe that the Auerbach work proves beyond all reasonable doubt that fresh whole cigarette smoke is carcinogenic to dog lungs and therefore it is highly likely that it is carcinogenic to human lungs … the results of the research would appear to us to remove the controversy regarding the causation of the majority of human lung cancer … to sum up we are of the opinion that the Auerbach's work proves beyond reasonable doubt the causation of lung cancer by smoke.'[48]

'While in the past it has seemed good sense for the industry to contest the validity of all the evidence against smoking (and may still be necessary to avoid damages in lawsuits), there is little doubt that the inflexibility of this attitude is beginning to create in some countries hostility and even contempt for the industry among intelligent, fair-minded doctors … it is thought that we should reconsider our basic answer on causation.'[49]

'I do not believe it has been scientifically established that cigarette smoking causes human disease.'[50]

'It has been stated that CTR is a program to find out about the "truth about smoking and health." What is truth to one is false to another. CTR and the Industry have publicly and frequently denied what others find as "truth". Let's face it. We are interested in evidence which we believe denies the allegations that cigarette smoking causes disease.'[51]

'We do not believe that cigarettes are hazardous; we don't accept that.'[52]

'It is our opinion … that the repeated assertion without conclusive proof that cigarettes cause disease – however well-intentioned – constitutes a disservice to the public.'[53]

'It was abundantly clear, for example, as a result of our recent visit to the USA that manufacturers are concentrating on the low TPM [total particulate matter] and nicotine segment in order to create brands with distinctive product features which aim, in one way or another, to reassure the consumer that these brands are relatively more "healthy" than orthodox blended cigarettes like Viceroy, Marlboro and Winston.'[54]

'For nearly twenty years, this industry has employed a single strategy to defend itself on three major fronts – litigation, politics and public opinion.

While the strategy was brilliantly conceived and executed over the years in helping us win important battles, it is only fair to say that it is not – nor was it intended to be – a vehicle for victory. On the contrary, it has always been a holding strategy, consisting of

- creating doubt about the health charge without actually denying it
- advocating the public's right to smoke, without actually urging them to take up the practice
- encouraging objective scientific research as the only way to resolve the question of health hazard.

In the cigarette controversy, the public – especially those who are present and potential supporters (e.g. tobacco state congressmen and heavy smokers) – must perceive, understand, and believe in evidence to sustain their opinions that smoking may not be the causal factor.
… there are millions of people who would be receptive to a new message, stating,
Cigarette smoking may not be the health hazard that the anti-smoking people say it is *because other alternatives are at least as possible.*' [emphasis in original][55]

'I believe it will not be possible indefinitely to maintain the rather hollow "we are not doctors" stance and that, in due course, we shall have to come up in public with a more positive approach towards cigarette safety.'[56]

'Before concluding my remarks on product acceptance, I want to return to the element of psychologic acceptance and discuss another component of this element which I will call "Health Psychology." Clearly the consumer is concerned about smoking and health and is convinced in varying degrees that smoking is a possible deterrent to his health. Presently, this factor is of active interest to R&D since it has been used to an advantage in marketing both the Kent and True brands.'[57]

'I share MCA's overall conclusion that the switching study confirms the rightness of our five year plan; focusing company effort against smokers' health concerns … Low T&N brands seem to be satisfying smokers' intellectual T&N concerns.'[58]

'Very few smokers claim to know the tar and nicotine levels of their brand … . On the other hand all smokers like to think of their brand as having no more than average levels and probably less … . However, the i[m]pression of "average or less" is probably required for a successful [brand] entry.'[59]

'People believe that cigarettes low in tar and nicotine have different "tobacco" ingredients and different kinds of filters than other cigarettes—the tobacco is milder or a special mild blend, perhaps treated to remove tar and nicotine, perhaps mixed with additives or fillers, perhaps cured differently—or maybe just more loosely packed … . Those who smoke low tar and nicotine cigarettes generally do so because they believe such cigarettes are 'better for you'.'[60]

'Health concerns are the usual reasons for switching to a low T&N [tar and nicotine] brand. Such cigarettes are "better for you" – milder and less irritating (now) as well as less likely to cause serious problems (later) … . To many SHF [super-high-filtration] smokers, a low T&N cigarette represents a compromise smoke between a more satisfying smoke and not smoking at all … . Most 'health oriented' smokers exhibit an openness to changing their cigarette brand on safety as well as other grounds. To deal with this ambivalence, they rationalize (e.g., "I may be better off smoking"), they compromise (turning to "milder" or lower tar and nicotine cigarettes; trying to smoke less), and they temporize ("I'll quit when things quiet down around here").'[61]

'This research indicates a number of directions for approaching the "health-oriented" cigarette market with viable new, improved and optimized product/marketing concepts' and outlines a way of "Targeting to Health-Oriented Market Segments."' [62]

'[A]s for the lack of research on the 'harmful' effects of smoking, the fact is there is good reason to doubt the culpability of cigarette smoking in coronary heart disease.'[63]

'The (smoking) habit can never be safe …'[64]

'Is it morally permissible to develop a safe method for administering a habit forming drug when, in so doing, the number of addicts will increase?'[65]

'Cigarettes have never been proven to be unsafe.'[66]

'Rationalization through modifying smoking behavior is a feasible means of conflict reduction … . One way of reducing the conflict within the smoker is to deny, devalue or otherwise rationalize the health argument. The four modes of potential conflict reduction discussed so far rely on either a fatalistic disposition to health or a faith in "safer" smoking, or a denial of anti-smoking information.'[67]

'[I]t has not been established that smoking causes any human disease.'[68]

'No conclusive clinical or medical proof of any cause-and-effect relationship between cigarette smoking and disease has yet been discovered.'[69]

The 1980s

'It is simply incorrect to say, "There is still no scientific proof that smoking causes ill-health."'[70]

'The industry has retreated behind impossible demands for 'scientific proof' whereas such proof has never been required as a basis for action in the legal and political fields … It may therefore be concluded that for certain groups of people smoking causes the incidence of certain diseases to be higher than it would otherwise be … A demand for scientific proof is always a formula for inaction and delay and usually the first reaction of the guilty.'[71]

'The company's position on causation is simply not believed by the overwhelming majority of independent observers, scientists and doctors …The industry is unable to argue satisfactorily for its own continued existence, because all arguments eventually lead back to the primary issue of causation, and at this point our position is unacceptable …our position on causation, which we have maintained for some twenty years in order to defend our industry is in danger of becoming the very factor which inhibits our long term viability … . On balance, it is the opinion of this department that … we should now move to position B, namely, that we acknowledge 'the probability that smoking is harmful to a small percentage of heavy smokers'… . By giving a little we may gain a lot. By giving nothing we stand to lose everything.'[72]

'[C]igarette smoking has not been scientifically established to be a cause of chronic diseases, such as cancer, cardiovascular disease, or emphysema.'[73]

'…the evidence is irrefutable that the companies were aware by 1954 of the early epidemiologic studies and the 1953 Wynder-Graham mouse skin painting study (linking cigarettes and lung cancer).'[74]

'From an historical perspective, the adoption of filters in the late 1940s and early 1950s was probably not animated by a desire to lower deliveries. Advertising claims to the contrary aside, earlier filtered cigarettes had deliveries equal to or in excess of their unfiltered cousins.'[75]

'The intent and effect … [of] low tar, low gas, charcoal filters, all natural or ultra low tar cigarettes … . was to derogate from the warning or awareness of the health hazard and to reassure the smoker in his decision to continue smoking.'[76]

When asked whether smoking causes lung cancer, Dawson stated, '[i]t's not a yes and it's not a no … . We're not going to tell anyone that smoking is good for them. We're not going to tell them that smoking is bad for them. It may be, it may not be.'[77]

'all the links that have been established between smoking and certain diseases are based on statistics. What that means is that the causative [sic] relationship has not yet been established.'[78]

'The view that smoking causes specific diseases remains an opinion or a judgment, and not an established scientific fact.'[79]

The 1990s

'Ultra lights smokers: Can you get at least 50% less tar and nicotine and still get flavor in a cigarette? Now you can.'[80]

'Despite all the research going on, the simple and unfortunate fact is that scientists do not know the cause or causes of the chronic diseases reported to be associated with smoking … '[81]

'It has been argued for several years that low tar and ultra low tar cigarettes are not really what they are claimed to be … the argument can be constructed that ULT advertising is misleading to the smoker.'[82]

'I'm a scientist who says: 'It's about time they quit this charade. I'm sick and tired of the way they distort and ignore the science. It's time for them to tell the truth … They had a responsibility early on to tell what their own researchers were finding out. Instead, they ignored it and made a mockery of it. I think it's time for the tobacco industry to say: This stuff kills people. We know that. Smoke at your own risk.'[83]

'Philip Morris does not believe cigarette smoking is addictive.'[84]

'[T]here's a health risk with smoking and disease,' but that it 'hasn't been proven that it [smoking] causes lung cancer.'[85]

'We have no internal research which proves that smoking causes lung cancer or other diseases or, indeed that, smoking is addictive.'[86]

'We have been taking note of public health concerns by developing "lighter" products, but we cannot promote these products as "safer"cigarettes because we simply don't have sufficient understanding of all the chemical processes to do so.'[87]

'I'm unclear in my own mind whether anyone dies of cigarette smoking-related diseases.'[88]

'We don't believe it's ever been established that smoking is the cause of disease'.[89]

'I'm not aware that RJ Reynolds has ever warned consumers about the health effects of compensation.'[90]

'It's not scientifically established that smoking by itself causes disease.'[91]

'There is an overwhelming medical and scientific consensus that cigarette smoking causes lung cancer, heart disease, emphysema, and other serious disease in smokers.'[92]

Into the twenty-first century

'Our main problem appears to be the notion that "the technology exists to make cigarettes which are appreciably less lethal and that many tobacco companies appear to be looking for any excuse not to use it." The technology does not exist, despite the impression given by the patent record or Star Scientific. It will not exist. We should tone down future expectations. Firstly, it is not ethical and secondly we shall be asked to explain our failures at some point in the future.'[93]

'For one of our tobacco companies to commission this study *(AD Little Report concluding that smokers save the state money – by dying early)* was not just a terrible mistake, it was wrong. All of us at Philip Morris, no matter where we work, are extremely sorry for this. No one benefits from the very real, serious and significant diseases caused by smoking. We understand the outrage that has been expressed and we sincerely regret this extraordinarily unfortunate incident. We will continue our efforts to do the right thing in all our businesses, acknowledging mistakes when we make them and learning from them as we go forward.'[94]

Smoking poses 'significant health risks and may contribute to certain diseases in some people'.[95]

'PM USA agrees with the overwhelming medical and scientific consensus that cigarette smoking causes lung cancer, heart disease, emphysema and other serious diseases in smokers. Smokers are far more likely to develop serious diseases, like lung cancer, than non-smokers. There is no safe cigarette.'[96]

'To reduce the health effects of cigarette smoking, the best thing to do is to quit.'[97]

'Brand descriptors or terms such as 'Light,' 'Ultra Light,' 'Medium' and 'Mild' do NOT mean safe, safer or less harmful. These terms are used as descriptors of strength of taste and flavor.'[98]

'Public health officials have concluded that secondhand smoke from cigarettes causes disease, including lung cancer and heart disease, in non-smoking adults, as well as causes conditions in children such as asthma, respiratory infections, cough, wheeze, otitis media (middle ear infection) and Sudden Infant Death Syndrome.'[99]

'Our guiding principles and beliefs…

At R.J. Reynolds Tobacco Company we operate our business in a responsible manner that best balances the desires of our many stakeholders. Our Guiding Principles and Beliefs seek to reflect the interests of shareholders, consumers, employees, and other stakeholders. In particular,

R.J. Reynolds is committed to addressing the issues regarding the use of and harm associated with tobacco products in an open and objective manner.

Here's what we believe:

Tobacco Use & Health...

+ Cigarette smoking is a leading cause of preventable deaths in the United States. Cigarette smoking significantly increases the risk of developing lung cancer, heart disease, chronic bronchitis, emphysema and other serious diseases and adverse health conditions.

+ The risk for serious diseases is significantly affected by the type of tobacco product and the frequency, duration and manner of use.

+ No tobacco product has been shown to be safe and without risks. The health risks associated with cigarettes are significantly greater than those associated with the use of smoke-free tobacco and nicotine products.

+ Nicotine in tobacco products is addictive but is not considered a significant threat to health.

+ It is the smoke inhaled from burning tobacco which poses the most significant risk of serious diseases.

+ Quitting cigarette smoking significantly reduces the risk for serious diseases.

+ Adult tobacco consumers have a right to be fully and accurately informed about the risks of serious diseases, the significant differences in the comparative risks of different tobacco and nicotine-based products, and the benefits of quitting. This information should be based on sound science.

+ Governments, public health officials, tobacco manufacturers and others share a responsibility to provide adult tobacco consumers with accurate information about the various health risks and comparative risks associated with the use of different tobacco and nicotine products.

Tobacco Consumers...

+ Individuals should consider the conclusions of the U.S. Surgeon General, the Centers for Disease Control and other public health and medical officials when making decisions regarding smoking.

+ The best course of action for tobacco users concerned about their health is to quit. Adults who continue to use tobacco products should consider the reductions of risks for serious diseases associated with moving from cigarettes to the use of smoke-free tobacco or nicotine products.

+ Minors should never use tobacco products and adults who do not use or have quit using tobacco products should not start.

+ Adults who smoke should avoid exposing minors to secondhand smoke, and adult smokers should comply with rules and regulations designed to respect the rights of other adults.

Harm Reduction...

+ Reducing the diseases and deaths associated with the use of cigarettes serves public health goals and is in the best interest of consumers, manufacturers and society. Harm reduction should be the critical element of any comprehensive public policy surrounding the health consequences of tobacco use.

+ Significant reductions in the harm associated with the use of cigarettes can be achieved by providing accurate information regarding the comparative risks of tobacco products to adult tobacco consumers, thereby encouraging smokers to migrate to the use of smoke-free tobacco and nicotine products, and by developing new smoke-free tobacco and nicotine products and other actions.

♦ Governments, public health officials, manufacturers, tobacco producers and consumers should support the development, production, and commercial introduction of tobacco leaf, and tobacco and nicotine-based products that are scientifically shown to reduce the risks associated with the use of existing tobacco products, particularly cigarettes.

Adult tobacco consumers should have access to a range of commercially viable tobacco and nicotine-based products.'[100]

'Along with the pleasures of smoking there are real risks of serious diseases such as lung cancer, respiratory disease and heart disease, and for many people, smoking is difficult to quit.'[101]

'Smoking is a cause of various serious and fatal diseases, including lung cancer, emphysema, chronic bronchitis and heart diseases.'[102]

'All cigarettes are dangerous and smoking can cause serious diseases, including lung cancer.'[103]

'As part of the March 1997 settlement agreements, Liggett Group publicly acknowledged that cigarette smoking causes disease and is addictive.'[104]

Nicotine the drug: addiction, manipulation, free-basing, dosage, and delivery

For decades the tobacco industry publically denied that nicotine was a drug or that it was addictive.

The 1950s

'To reduce the nicotine per cigarette as much as possible and thus satisfy the trend of consumer demand … might end in destroying the nicotine habit in a large number of consumers and prevent it ever being acquired by new smokers.'[105]

The 1960s

'It's fortunate for us that cigarettes are a habit they can't break.'[106]

'Experiments of Hippo have led to a great increase in our knowledge of the effects of nicotine … . Smoking demonstrably is a habit based on a combination of psychological and physiological pleasure, and it also has strong indications of being an addiction. It differs in important features from addiction to other alkaloid drugs, but yet there are sufficient similarities to justify stating that smokers are nicotine addicts.' [107]

'[I]t should also create addiction in the same relative amounts.'[108]

'… smoking is a habit of addiction … nicotine is … a very fine drug'.[109]

'As a result of these various researches, we now possess a knowledge of the effects of nicotine far more extensive than exists in published scientific literature … . We believe that we have found possible reasons for addiction in two other phenomena that accompany steady absorption of nicotine. Experiments have so far only been carried out with rats, but with these it is found that certain rats become tolerant to repeated doses and after a while show the usual nicotine reactions but only on a very diminished scale … . Supposing the tranquilizing action of nicotine can be tracked down in this way, then these reactions will be compared in the case of rats who have never had nicotine, or alternatively have become addicted to it. Subsequent similar measurements will be made on human nonsmokers and on addicted smokers'.[110]

'What we need to know above all things is what constitutes the hold of smoking, that is, to understand addiction …'[111]

'Moreover, nicotine is addictive. We are, then, in the business of selling nicotine, an addictive drug effective in the release of stress mechanisms.'[112]

'Nicotine is by far the most characteristic single constituent in tobacco, and the known physiological effects are positively correlated with smoker response … . I think that we can say even now that we can regulate, fairly precisely, the nicotine and sugar levels to almost any desired level management might require. Of this I am confident'.[113]

'There seems no doubt that the "kick" of a cigarette is due to the concentration of nicotine in the bloodstream which it achieves, and this is a product of the quantity of nicotine in the smoke and the speed of transfer of that nicotine from the smoke to the bloodstream.'[114]

'It would appear that the increased smoker response is associated with nicotine reaching the brain more quickly … . On this basis, it appears reasonable to assume that the increased response of a smoker to the smoke with a higher amount of extractable nicotine [not synonymous with but similar to free base nicotine] may be either because this nicotine reaches the brain in a different chemical form or because it reaches the brain more quickly'.[115]

'It may be useful, therefore, to look at the tobacco industry as if for a large part its business is the administration of nicotine (in the clinical sense).'[116]

'Smoking is an addictive habit attributable to nicotine and the form of nicotine affects the rate of absorption by the smoker.'[117]

'… selling a nicotine effect, not fighting it'.[118]

'I would be more cautious in using the pharmic-medical model – do we really want to tout cigarette smoke as a drug? It is, of course, but there are dangerous FDA implications to having such conceptualization go beyond these walls.'[119]

'The primary motivation for smoking is to obtain the pharmacological effect of nicotine. In the past, we at R&D have said that we're not in the cigarette business, we're in the smoke business. It might be more pointed to observe that the cigarette is the vehicle of smoke, smoke is the vehicle of nicotine, and nicotine is the agent of a pleasurable body response.'[120]

The 1970s

'… we are in a nicotine rather than a tobacco industry'.[121]

'Increasing the pH of a medium in which nicotine is delivered increases the physiological effect of the nicotine by increasing the ratio of free base to acid salt form, the free base form being more readily transported across physiological membranes. We are pursuing this project with the eventual goal of lowering the total nicotine present in smoke while increasing the physiological effect of the nicotine which is present, so that no physiological effect is lost on nicotine reduction.'[122]

'[i]n designing any cigarette product, the dominant specification should be nicotine delivery'.[123]

'In a sense, the tobacco industry may be thought of as being a specialized, highly ritualized and stylized segment of the pharmaceutical industry. Tobacco products, uniquely, contain and deliver nicotine, a potent drug with a variety of physiological effects … . Thus a tobacco product is, in essence, a vehicle for delivery of nicotine, designed to deliver the nicotine in a generally acceptable and attractive form. Our Industry is then based upon design, manufacture and sale of attractive dosage forms of nicotine, and our Company's position in our Industry is determined by our ability to produce dosage forms of nicotine which have more overall value, tangible or intangible, to the consumer than those of our competitors ... . If nicotine is the *sine qua non* of tobacco products and tobacco products are recognized as being attractive dosage forms of nicotine, then it is logical to design our products – and where possible, our advertising – around nicotine delivery rather than 'tar' delivery or flavour ... . If, as proposed above, nicotine is the *sine qua non* of smoking, and if we meekly accept the allegations of our critics and move toward reduction or elimination of nicotine from our products, then we shall eventually liquidate our business. If we intend to remain in business and our business is the manufacture and sale of dosage forms of nicotine, then at some point we must make a stand.'[124]

'... more precisely define the minimum amount of nicotine required for 'satisfaction' in terms of dose levels, dose frequency, dosage form and the like'.[125]

'... [s]tudy means for enhancing nicotine satisfaction via synergists, alteration of pH, or other means to minimize dose level and maximize desired effects'.[126]

'What we should really make and sell would be the proper dosage form of nicotine with as many other built-in attractions and gratifications as possible – that is, an efficient nicotine delivery system with satisfactory flavor, mildness, convenience, cost, etc.'[127]

'I believe that for the typical smoker nicotine satisfaction is the dominant desire, as opposed to flavor and other satisfactions.'[128]

'More precisely define the minimum amount of nicotine required for 'satisfaction' in terms of dose levels, dose frequency, dosage form, and the like. This would involve biological and other experiments.'[129]

'No one has ever become a cigarette smoker by smoking cigarettes without nicotine.'[130]

'The majority of conferees would accept the proposition that nicotine is the active constituent of cigarette smoke ... . The cigarette should be conceived not as a product but as a package. The product is nicotine. Think of the cigarette pack as a storage container for a day's supply of nicotine ... . Think of the cigarette as a dispenser for a dose unit of nicotine ... . Think of a puff of smoke as the vehicle of nicotine ... . Smoke is beyond question the most optimized vehicle of nicotine and the cigarette the most optimized dispenser of smoke'.[131]

'Smoking is fairly irrational like other drug dependencies. If there is a positive side to smoking, and I think there is, it is not easy for the smoker to articulate. He "votes with his feet" and continues with this irrational act.'[132]

'Monkeys can be trained to inject themselves with nicotine for its own sake, just as they will inject other dependence-producing drugs e.g. opiates, caffeine, amphetamine, cocaine ... The absorption of nicotine through the lungs is as quick as the junkie's "fix."'[133]

'Addiction – Some emphasis is now being placed in the habit-forming capacities of cigarette smoke. To some extent the argument revolving around "free choice" is being negated on the grounds of addiction. The threat is that this argument will increase significantly and lead to further restrictions on product specifications and greater danger in litigation.'[134]

'... cigarettes allow people to self-administer nicotine and at a self-determined rate'.[135]

'Nearly all regular smokers are nicotine dependent.'[136]

'Methods which may be used to increase smoke pH and/or nicotine "kick" include: (1) increasing the amount of (strong) burley in the blend, (2) reduction of casing sugar used on the burley and/or blend, (3) use of alkaline additives, usually ammonia compounds, to the blend, (4) addition of nicotine to the blend, (5) removal of acids from the blend, (6) special filter systems to remove acids from or add alkaline materials to the smoke, and (7) use of high air dilution filter systems. Methods 1–3, in combination, represent the Philip Morris approach, and are under active investigation.'[137]

'In essence, a cigarette is a system for delivery of nicotine to the smoker in attractive, useful form.'[138]

'Still, with an old style filter, any desired additional nicotine "kick" could be easily obtained through pH regulation.'[139]

'Whatever the characteristics of cigarettes as determined by smoking machines, the smoker adjusts his pattern to deliver his own nicotine requirements.'[140]

'However, as additional evidence of the addictive qualities of smoking, those who tried to quit, both male and female, admitted great difficulties in overcoming the psychological and/or the physiological urge or craving to smoke.'[141]

'If tobacco were to be placed under a Food and Drug law, classification of tobacco under the food section would be acceptable, but classification of tobacco as a drug should be avoided at all costs.'[142]

'In summary, it appears that most workers who are not directly concerned with the tobacco industry use the terms addiction or dependence rather than habituation and can be considered quite correct in doing so. If cigarette smoking is as addictive as the evidence suggests, it is not surprising that antismoking campaigns are so ineffective …'[143]

'Compromisers' *were defined as those* 'heavily addicted' *smokers who have made* 'many attempts to quit.'[144]

'The smoker profile data reported earlier indicated that Marlboro Lights cigarettes were not smoked like regular Marlboros. There were differences in the size and frequency of the puffs, with larger volumes taken on Marlboro Lights by both regular Marlboro smokers and Marlboro Lights smokers. In effect, the Marlboro 85 smokers in this study did not achieve any reduction in the smoke intake by smoking a cigarette (Marlboro Lights) normally considered lower in delivery.'[145]

'Nicotine is an important aspect of "satisfaction", and if the nicotine delivery is reduced below a threshold "satisfaction" level, then surely smokers will question more readily why they are indulging in an expensive habit.'[146]

'If the desired goal is defined to be increased nicotine yield in the delivered smoke, there appear to be only two alternatives: either increase the absolute yield of delivered nicotine, or increase the pH, which increases the "apparent" nicotine content without changing the absolute amount.'[147]

'The consensus of opinion derived from a review of the literature on the subjects indicates that the most probable reason for the addictive properties of the smoke is the nicotine.'[148]

'In smoking the effect produced on the human body is ascribable to nicotine.'[149]

'Without any question, the desire to smoke is based on the effect of nicotine on the body.'[150]

'The pH also relates to the immediacy of the nicotine impact. As the pH increases, the nicotine changes its chemical form so that it is more rapidly absorbed by the body and more quickly gives a "kick" to the smoker.'[151]

'To the extent that [he is] an addict, he is probably smoking to keep nicotine or one of its active metabolites at some optimal level. If, then, the heavy smoker does switch to low nicotine brands, he may very well end up smoking more cigarettes and taking more puffs of each.'[152]

'... market an ADDICTIVE PRODUCT in an ETHICAL MANNER'.[153]

'... have FREE NICOTINE as opposed to BOUND'.[154]

'... communicate pleasure of higher nicotine W/O using word'.[155]

'How to increase free to bound nicotine in smoke – *masking additive* gets the attention W/O pain of free nicotine.'[156]

'Should we market cigarettes intended to reassure the smoker that they are safer without assuring ourselves that indeed they are so or are not less safe? For example, should we "cheat" smokers by "cheating" League Tables? [League tables are the British equivalent of the FTC ratings of cigarette delivery of tar and nicotine.] If we are prepared to accept that government has created league tables to encourage low delivery cigarette smoking and further if we make league tables claims as implied health claims – or allow health claims to be so implied – should we use our superior knowledge of our products to design them so that they give low league table positions but higher deliveries on human smoking? Are smokers entitled to expect that cigarettes shown as lower delivery in league tables will in fact deliver less to their lungs than cigarettes shown higher?'[157]

'If she is able to demonstrate, as she anticipates, no withdrawal effects of nicotine, we will want to pursue this with some vigor. If, however, the results with nicotine are similar to those gotten with morphine and caffeine, we will want to bury it.'[158]

'[P]roducts *must* provide the appropriate levels of *nicotine* ...'[159]

'Opiates and nicotine may be similar in action.'[160]

'We accept the fact that nicotine is habituating.'[161]

'There is a relationship between nicotine and the opiates.'[162]

'... the problem of addiction via nicotine [is] increasing'.[163]

'We think that most smokers can be considered nicotine seekers, for the pharmacological effect of nicotine is one of the rewards that come from smoking. When the smoker quits, he foregoes his accustomed nicotine. The change is very noticeable, he misses the reward, and so he returns to smoking.'[164]

'If the industry's introduction of acceptable low-nicotine products does make it easier for dedicated smokers to quit, then the wisdom of the introduction is open to debate.'[165]

'Very few consumers are aware of the effects of nicotine, i.e., its addictive nature and that nicotine is a poison.'[166]

'It appears that we have sufficient expertise available to "build" a lowered mg tar cigarette which will deliver as much "free nicotine" as a Marlboro, Winston, or Kent without increasing the total nicotine delivery above that of a "Light" product.'[167]

'It is obvious that such a tremendous sales gain of "cigarette substitutes" is done at the expense of normal, conventional cigarettes, and there lies all the danger in the near future for the very survival of [the] Tobacco Industry, because these "cigarette substitutes" are unable to make smokers addicts to tobacco. The present smokers of "cigarette substitutes" are the future smoker quitters.'[168]

'The suspected relationship between free nicotine concentration and smoke impact implies that we could create an ultra low tar cigarette that produces much more impact than its delivery would suggest.'[169]

'We are searching explicitly for a socially acceptable addictive product involving: …'[170]

'… the high profits additionally associated with the tobacco industry are directly related to the fact that the customer is dependent upon the product'.[171]

The 1980s

'It has been suggested that cigarette smoking is the most addictive drug. Certainly large numbers of people will continue to smoke because they can't give it up. If they could they would do so. They can no longer be said to make an adult choice.'[172]

'It appears that we have sufficient expertise available to 'build' a lowered mg tar cigarette which will deliver as much 'free nicotine' as a Marlboro, Winston or Kent without increasing the total nicotine delivery above that of a "Light" product. There are products already being marketed which deliver high percentage "free nicotine" levels in smoke, i.e. Merit, Now.'[173]

'[D]etermine the minimum level of nicotine that will allow continued smoking. We hypothesize that below some very low nicotine level, diminished physiological satisfaction cannot be compensated for by psychological satisfaction. At this point, smokers will quit or return to higher T&N brands.'[174]

'Any action on our part, such as research on the psychopharmacology of nicotine, which implicitly or explicitly treats nicotine as a drug, could well be viewed as a tacit acknowledgment that nicotine is a drug. Such acknowledgment, contend our attorneys, would be untimely.'[175]

'Our attorneys, however, will likely continue to insist upon a clandestine effort in order to keep nicotine the drug in low profile.'[176]

'The psychopharmacology of nicotine is a highly vexatious topic. It is where the action is for those doing fundamental research on smoking, and from where most likely will come significant scientific developments profoundly influencing the industry. Yet it is where our attorneys least want us to be, for two reasons. It is important to have these two reasons expressed and distinguished from one another. The first reason is the oldest and most implicit in the legal strategy employed over the years in defending corporations within the industry from the claims of heirs and estates of deceased smokers: "We within the industry are ignorant of any relationships between smoking and disease. Within our laboratories no work is being conducted on biological systems." That posture has moderated considerably as our attorneys have come to acknowledge that the original carte blanche avoidance of all biological research is not required in order to plead ignorance about any pathological relationship between smoke and smoker.' [177]

'PM sells cigarettes. Cigarettes deliver nicotine.'[178]

'If even only some smokers smoke for the nicotine effect (I personally believe most regular smokers do), then in today's climate we would do well to have a low TPM [total particulate matter] and CO [carbon monoxide] delivering cigarette that can supply adequate nicotine.'[179]

'BAT should learn to look at itself as a drug company rather than as a tobacco company.'[180]

'This is another aspect of the smoking and health issue which cannot be overlooked. Unlike dangerous sports and other high risk activities (except the drinking of alcohol) smoking is addictive/habituative in addition to being an additional risk and many smokers would like to give up the habit if they could.'[181]

'This program includes both behavioral effects as well as chemical investigation. My reason for this high priority is that I believe the thing we sell most is nicotine.'[182]

'Shook, Hardy [Shook, Hardy, and Bacon, LLP, is a Kansas City, Mo, law firm that directed legal strategy for the tobacco industry] reminds us, I'm told, that the entire matter of addiction is the most potent weapon a prosecuting attorney can have in a lung cancer/cigarette case. We can't defend continued smoking as "free choice" if the person was "addicted." '[183]

'I feel reasonably certain that it should not be too difficult to find prominent experts in the area of addiction who would write a "position paper", clearly showing that smoking is not an "addictive drug".'[184]

'The nature of possible compensation phenomena in relation to highly ventilated cigarettes was discussed at length. It was noted that we have very little data on the long-term consequences of smoking behavior patterns following switching to low tar products … . It was agreed that efforts should not be spent on designing a cigarette which, through its construction, denied the smoker the opportunity to compensate or oversmoke to any significant degree.'[185]

'… current research is directed toward increasing the nicotine levels while maintaining or marginally reducing the tar deliveries'.[186]

'Cigarettes are not just habit forming – the body builds up a requirement for them. Twenty million smokers cannot do without their weed. Take the example of a man going to work in the morning. It's pouring with rain. There are six cars already parked outside the shop. So, there are at least 90 yards to walk back. Would he stop for a newspaper? Would he get out for a Kit Kat? The answer is probably No, but he would stop for his fags, because he is addicted to cigarettes. And while he is buying a pack, he takes a morning paper and a Kit Kat.'[187]

'Overall, the evidence shows that Belair smokers are extremely addicted to smoking and they know it.'[188]

'Smokers of brands in Viceroy's competitive set are more addicted to smoking than smokers in general.'[189]

'… with regard to addiction, there is absolutely no proof that cigarettes are addictive'.[190]

'If delivery levels are reduced too quickly or eventually to a level which is so low that the nicotine is below the threshold of pharmacological activity then it is possible that the smoking habit would be rejected by a large number of smokers … . The simple answer would seem to be to offer the smoker a product with comparatively high nicotine deliveries so that with a minimum of effort he could take the dose of nicotine suitable to his immediate needs.'[191]

'Nicotine is the most pharmacologically active constituent in tobacco smoke and is probably the most usual factor responsible for maintaining the smoking habit …'[192]

'… addicted to smoking and often wished they never started'.[193]

'… heavily addicted to smoking. To run out of cigarettes would be a real problem for them … from the moment they wake up they smoke'.[194]

RJR '… cannot be comfortable marketing a product which most of our consumers would do without if they could'.[195]

'Nicotine is the addicting agent in cigarettes.'[196]

'Based on the results of studies similar to those summarized above, it has been stated that low – "tar" smokers use their cigarettes differently than smokers of higher – "tar" products. Different "usage" includes propensity to block vents or otherwise manipulate the cigarette, increasing the number of puffs and the number of cigarettes smoked, puffing more frequently or with larger volumes and inhaling more deeply or holding smoke in the lungs longer. These usage patterns are consistent with the theory that low – "'tar"smokers seek to maintain a given nicotine level in the body, regardless of the cigarette. The patterns cited are instances which would tend to increase the "dosage" of nicotine to the smoker.'[197]

'… nicotine is the addictive agent in cigarettes'.[198]

'A short definition is that a cigarette supplies nicotine to the consumer in a palatable and convenient form.'[199]

'The cigarette's taste is a relatively unimportant benefit of smoking. Its taste is primarily a delivery vehicle[.]'[200]

'The paper *(by Benowitz N)* itself expresses what we in Biobehavioral have felt for quite some time. That is, smokers smoke differently than the FTC machine and may very well smoke to obtain a certain level of nicotine. in their bloodstream. If a given level of nicotine in the blood is the final goal of a smoker, one would predict that he would smoke an FFT [full flavor tar] and ULT [ultra low tar] cigarette differently.'[201]

'… was one of the first indications that smokers may in fact smoke to obtain a certain level of nicotine in their bloodstream'.[202]

'Defendants have long understood that cigarettes are addictive and that nicotine is the agent in cigarette smoke primarily responsible for addiction …'[203]

'Why do people smoke? … to relax; for the taste; to fill the time; something to do with my hands. […] But, for the most part, people continue to smoke because they find it too uncomfortable to quit.'[204]

'The amount of nicotine in the vapour phase can be modified by changing the acidity (pH) of the smoke. Hence it is readily feasible to have two cigarettes which deliver the same amount of nicotine (as measured on a Cambridge pad [the FTC method]) but which are easily differentiated on the sensory basis of impact since the acidity of the smoke (and hence amount of nicotine in the vapour phase) is different.'[205]

'Irrespective of the ethics involved, we should develop alternative designs (that do not invite obvious criticism) which will allow the smoker to obtain significant enhanced deliveries should he so wish … . Another area of importance is the exploitation of physical and chemical means to increase nicotine transfer, i.e. to increase the effective utilization of nicotine.'[206]

'Both Mr. Wrobleski *[Jacob, Medinger & Finnegan]* and Mr. Sirridge *[Shook, Hardy & Bacon]* warned, however, that there is very little literature favorable to the industry's position on addiction.'[207]

'"Addiction" has received little industry research attention. Nevertheless, many industry documents support the contention that there are types of persons whose psychological profile and smoking behavior is such that they have great difficulty in quitting. For example, documents describe a British American Tobacco Company sponsored conference in 1978, attended by PM and B&W representatives. One of the findings of the conference was: 'Serious smokers smoke to prevent withdrawal symptoms. Another study which Dr. Piehl (RJRT) cites recognizes "addictive" smokers: "People who find it unbearable to run out of cigarettes are described as using addictive-type smoking." The industry has also recognized that some smokers, especially smokers of high nicotine cigarettes "compensate" or regulate nicotine intake if it is lowered in individual cigarettes.'[208]

'… claims that cigarettes are addictive contradict common sense … An escalation of antismoking rhetoric … without medical or scientific foundation'.[209]

'After years of well-funded research, it has not been established that cigarette smoking produces a physical dependence to nicotine.'[210]

'Tobacco industry statements deal only sparsely with the issue of addiction. To the extent such statements exist they generally deny outright any addictive effect.'[211]

'Smoking cigarettes is not addictive because cigarettes are not like other addictive drugs, i.e., they are not illegal and are not necessarily linked to an anti-social lifestyle; smoking cigarettes is merely a pleasurable "habit" like playing tennis, jogging, eating chocolate, listening to rock music, etc.'[212]

'Clinically, cigarette smoking does not result in addiction-like behavior.'[213]

'The CNS effects obtained using the NC (nicotine citrate) cigarettes were approximately half the magnitude of those obtained with FB (free base nicotine) and unextracted cigarettes.'[214]

'I can't allow the claim that smoking is addictive to go unchallenged … . The majority of people who smoke make that decision, they can quit if they want to do it. It's a matter of willpower.'[215]

The 1990s

'It's not an addiction …'[216]

'Review the use of organic acids and nicotine salts in tobacco burning cigarettes, and recent attempts to develop an ultra low "tar" cigarette with enhanced nicotine yield.'[217]

'In my view, labeling tobacco use "addictive" is misleading and potentially harmful to the American public.'[218]

'We have shown that there are optimal cigarette nicotine deliveries for producing the most favorable physiological and behavioral responses.'[219]

'We are basically in the nicotine business. It is in the best long term interest for RJR to be able to control and effectively utilize every pound of nicotine we purchase. Effective control of nicotine in our products should equate to a significant product performance and cost advantage.'[220]

'Whilst the US Surgeon General has claimed that nicotine is addictive, he has also claimed that video games are addictive. This is a prime example of the misuse of the term "addiction" … [C]igarette smokers bear no resemblance to addicts … Smokers smoke because they enjoy smoking.'[221]

'Different people smoke for different reasons. But, the primary reason is to deliver nicotine into their bodies.' [222]

'Philip Morris has chosen to pursue a nicotine delivery device that, like RJR's Premier [previously marketed as a smokeless 'cigarette'], continues the cigarette tradition of sucking on a cylindrical mouthpiece to inhale flavorings and nicotine from a tobacco based product.'[223]

'Different people smoke cigarettes for different reasons. But, the primary reason is to deliver nicotine into their bodies. Nicotine is an alkaloid derived from the tobacco plant. It is a physiologically active nitrogen containing substance. Similar organic chemicals include nicotine, quinine, cocaine, atropine, and morphine. While each of these substances can be used to affect human physiology, nicotine has a particularly broad range of influence. During the smoking act, nicotine is inhaled into the lungs in smoke, enters the bloodstream and travels to the brain in about eight to ten seconds. The nicotine alters the state of the smoker by becoming a neurotransmitter and a stimulant. Nicotine mimics the body's most important neurotransmitter, acetylcholine (ACH), which controls heart rate and message sending within the brain. The nicotine is used to change psychological states leading to enhanced mental performance and relaxation. A little nicotine seems to stimulate, while a lot sedates a person. A smoker learns to control the delivery of nicotine through the smoking technique to create the desired mood state. In general, the smoker uses nicotine's control to moderate a mood, arousing attention in boring situations and calming anxiety in tense situations. Smoking enhances the smoker's mental performance and reduces anxiety in a sensorially pleasurable form.'[224]

'… a fast, highly pharmacologically effective and cheap "drug."'[225]

'This suggests that at the very least we should have contingency plans for a change in the predominant form of nicotine usage … . If these circuits do mediate nicotine intake and they could be blocked, then it is possible that cigarettes' appeal would decline'.[226]

'… on an "addiction scale," nicotine is less addictive than food'.[227]

'… those who term smoking an addiction do so for ideological, not scientific, reasons'.[228]

'… additional research on nicotine/acetaldehyde synergism may have shown that cigarettes were in fact addictive'.[229]

'Is nicotine addictive?' 'Absolutely not. Nicotine is first of all – I mean nicotine occurs naturally in cigarettes. Nicotine is also found in things as scary as potatoes.'[230]

'… [t]here is no chemical addiction' to nicotine'.[231]

'[D]oes the industry take the position that cigarettes are not addictive?' 'The industry does take that position.'[232]

'[d]o you – do you, in the industry, concede that nicotine is an addictive drug?' '[n]o we don't.'[233]

'No, nicotine is not addictive.'[234]

'REP. WYDEN: Let me ask you first, and I'd like to just go down the row, whether each of you believes that nicotine is not addictive. I've heard virtually all of you touch on it – yes or no, do you believe nicotine is not addictive?

WILLIAM I. CAMPBELL (Philip Morris): I believe that nicotine is not addictive, yes.

REP. WYDEN: Mr. Johnston …

JAMES JOHNSTON (RJR): Uh, Congressman, cigarettes and nicotine clearly do not meet the classic definition of addiction. There is no intoxication –

REP. WYDEN: We'll take that as a no. And again, time is short, if you can just, I think each of you believe nicotine is not addictive, I'd just like to have this for the record.

JOSEPH TADDEO (US Tobacco): 'I don't believe that nicotine or our products are addictive.'

ANDREW TISCH (P Lorillard): I believe that nicotine is not addictive.

EDWARD HORRIGAN (Liggett Group): I believe that nicotine is not addictive.

THOMAS SANDEFUR (Brown & Williamson): I believe that nicotine is not addictive.

DONALD JOHNSTON (American Tobacco Co.): And I too believe that nicotine is not addictive.'[235]

'The presence of nicotine, … does not make cigarettes a drug or smoking an addiction'.[236]

'Smokers are not drug addicts.'[237]

'Philip Morris does not believe cigarette smoking is addictive. People can and do quit all the time.'[238]

'To illustrate, a study was conducted on nicotine aerosols, where subjects inhaled the same amount of nicotine at pHs of 5.6, 7.5, and 11.0. It was found that higher peak concentrations of nicotine in blood were achieved at higher pHs. Since the amounts of inhaled nicotine were the same, the results indicate that the higher the pH, the more rapidly nicotine enters the bloodstream.'[239]

'As to the claim that smoking is addictive: this has been widely challenged by scientists working in the field.'[240]

(RJR) '… contests the consensus view of nicotine as addictive'.[241]

'Of course it's addictive. That's why you smoke the stuff.'[242]

'… neither cigarette smoking nor the nicotine delivered in cigarettes is addictive'.[243]

'In RJRT's opinion, cigarette smoking does not meet the classic definitions of "addiction," and the forty-five million Americans who smoke are not "addicts." To call nicotine "addictive" is to ignore significant differences between cigarettes and truly addictive drugs.'[244]

'Under scientifically verifiable criteria, nicotine and cigarette smoking are not addictive.'[245]

'… there is no accurate evidence establishing that any specific yield of nicotine causes "addiction."'[246]

'Nicotine has properties of a drug of abuse. It has properties of drug addiction … This [The results] was completely contradictory to the industry's position that nicotine is in cigarettes for taste. We know they [the rats] pressed the lever because of the drug effects on the animal's brain. We also know from studies that if the substance was cocaine or morphine or alcohol the rates would continue to press the lever. We found the same in nicotine.'[247]

'We have not concealed, we do not conceal and we will never conceal … we have no internal research which proves that smoking … is addictive'.[248]

'Those who term smoking an addiction do so for ideological – not scientific – reason.'[249]

'If [cigarettes] are behaviorally addictive or habit forming, they are much more like … . Gummi Bears, and I eat Gummi Bears, and I don't like it when I don't eat my Gummi Bears, but I'm certainly not addicted to them'.[250]

'We did decide that we needed a little more oomph, a little more pizzazz, if you will, in an ultra low tar cigarette. So we manipulated the blend to raise the nicotine level slightly ... . They didn't care what the nicotine level was. They just wanted a consumer acceptable product that was ultra low tar'.[251]

'We recognize that under common or popular definitions, cigarettes can understandably be viewed as "addictive." Many people find it exceedingly difficult to quit smoking. We recognize that cigarette smoking is a significant risk factor for lung cancer, emphysema and other diseases.'[252]

'On "addiction": Clearly cigarettes are "addictive" as most people understand the word.'[253]

'We make a product that is inherently risky. There is no safe cigarette. We know that. And we know that no other product or activity puts its users at greater risk of contracting lung cancer and other diseases. We also know that smoking is addictive, as that term is commonly understood today.'[254]

Into the twenty-first century

'*Well, what's your definition of addiction?* Well, my definition of addiction is a repetitive behavior that some people find difficult to quit. Sometimes that's associated with a psychoactive drug, which is the case of nicotine in a cigarette ...'[255]

'... cigarette smoking is addictive, as that term is most commonly used today'.[256]

'We agree with the overwhelming medical and scientific consensus that cigarette smoking is addictive.'[257]

'Public health authorities, e.g. the Institute of Medicine and the US Surgeon General, accept the role of nicotine as a primary determinant of "smoking addiction." Our core position is that smoking is a lot more than nicotine-taking, consisting of a complex set of interactive and interdependent behaviours.'[258]

'*At the present time*, based on our evaluation of the scientific/medical evidence, we do not believe that nicotine per se is addictive.' [emphasis in original][259]

'Cigarette smoking is addictive. It can be very difficult to quit but, if you are a smoker, this shouldn't stop you from trying to do so.'[260]

'...*nicotine is a* "significant contributor to addiction."'[261]

'Smoking is Addictive'[262]

'... agrees with the overwhelming medical scientific consensus that cigarette smoking is addictive'.[263]

'PM USA agrees with the overwhelming medical and scientific consensus that cigarette smoking is addictive. It can be very difficult to quit smoking, but this should not deter smokers who want to quit from trying to do so.'[264]

'Nicotine in tobacco products is addictive but is not considered a significant threat to health.'[265]

'Cigarette smoking can also be addictive.'[266]

'As part of the March 1997 settlement agreements, Liggett Group publicly acknowledged that cigarette smoking causes disease and is addictive.'[267]

Epilogue

'He who permits himself to tell a lie once, finds it much easier to do it a second and third time, till at length it becomes habitual'

Thomas Jefferson

Thus, even with as much as we have learned from the release of now nearly 70 million pages of previously secret tobacco industry documents we will never know the whole story because much of the evidence is beyond our reach in off shore laboratories.

> Ship all documents to Cologne ('a locale where we *{PM}* might do some of the things which we are reluctant to do in this *{USA}* country'[268]) ... . Keep in Cologne. OK to phone & telex (these will be destroyed). If *important* letters or *documents* have to be sent, please send to home – I will act on them and destroy.[269] *(emphasis in original)*

Or documents have been altered or destroyed,

> We do not foresee any difficulty in the event a decision is reached to remove certain reports from our Research files. Once it becomes necessary for successful defense of our present and future suits, we will promptly remove all such reports from our files ... . As an alternative to invalidation, we can have the authors rewrite the sections of the reports which appear objectionable.[270]

> I should advise you that I was requested by three of the largest Board members to prepare a Board paper, which could be used as the justification for the systematic destruction of pertinent documentation (from Infotab and the TDC). The aim of the document destruction exercise was to identify and remove all documents which could be viewed as 'problematic', damaging or useful to plaintiffs in any ongoing industry litigation. I have to admit that I undertook a complete document review and reduced the Infotab papers to only the bare statutory minimum ... . I should advise you that Authorized the destruction of close to a million individual pages in my seven years at TDC ...[271]

With this, the industry has spoken and now much of the truth is known – a truth that was intentionally hidden from view for over half a century. Federal District Court Judge Gladys Kessler summarized these revelations in her opinion (in which the industry was found guilty of violating the Racketeer Influenced and Corrupt Organizations Act – RICO):

> [O]ver the course of more than 50 years, Defendants lied, misrepresented, and deceived the American public, including smokers and the young people they avidly sought as 'replacement smokers', about the devastating health effects of smoking and environmental tobacco smoke, they suppressed research, they destroyed documents, they manipulated the use of nicotine so as to increase and perpetuate addiction, they distorted the truth about low tar and light cigarettes so as to discourage smokers from quitting, and they abused the legal system in order to achieve their goal – to make money with little, if any, regard for individual illness and suffering, soaring health costs, or the integrity of the legal system.[272]

> In short, defendants have marketed and sold their lethal product with zeal, with deception, with the single-minded focus on their financial success, and without regard for the human tragedy or social costs that success exacted.[273]

References

1. Wynder EL, and Graham E (1950). Tobacco Smoking as a Possible Etiologic Factor in Bronchiogenic Carcinoma: a Study of 684 Proven Cases. *JAMA* **143**:329–36.
2. Wynder EL, Graham EA, and Croninger AB (1953). Experimental Production of Carcinoma with Cigarette Tar. *Cancer Res* **13**:855–64.
3. Fields N and Chapman S (2003). Chasing Ernst Wynder: 40 years of Philip Morris' Efforts to Influence a Leading Scientist. *J. Epidemiology and Community Health* **57**:571–8.

4. http://www.tobacco.org/History/540104frank.html.

5. Teague C, and RJ Reynolds (1953). *Survey of Cancer Research with Emphasis upon Possible Carcinogens* from *Tobacco*, February 2.

6. *Advertisement for Parliament Cigarettes* (1953). American Tobacco Company, Bates 1002762253.

7. Quoted in Report of Special Master: *Findings of Fact, Conclusions of Law and Recommendations Regarding Non-Liggett Privilege Claims*, Minnesota Trial Court File Number C1-94-8565, 8 March 1998, quoting Pioneer Press, RJR, 24 October 1954.

8. Hill & Knowlton. Forwarding memorandum. Mid-1950s, http://www.tobacco.neu.edu/litigation/cases/mn_trial/TE18904.pdf.

9. Ibid.

10. Darkis F (1996). Untitled. Minutes of a meeting of Liggett scientists, 29 March 1954. In: Kluger R. *Ashes to Ashes*. New York:196.

11. Partridge EJ (Imperial Tobacco), Letter to Sir John Hawton, 9 March 1956.

12. TIRC Tobacco and Health Newsletter, 1957 US District Court for the District of Columbia, Civil Action No. 99-2496 (GK), USA *et al.* v. Philip Morris USA Inc. *et al.*, 9 September 2006, p. 263.

13. *RD 14 Smoke Group Programme for Coming 12–16 Week Period*, Southampton Research and Development Establishment [R&DE], British American Tobacco Company, Ltd, 1957.

14. Internal report, British Tobacco Research Council, Harrogate, England, dated 1 March 1957.

15. TIRC press release, 16 December 1957 US District Court for the District of Columbia, Civil Action No. 99-2496 (GK), USA *et al.* v. Philip Morris USA Inc. *et al.*, 9 September 2006, p. 261.

16. Report on Visit to USA and Canada by HR Bentley, DGI Felton and WW Reid of BAT, 17 April to 12 May 1958. Available at: http://www.tobacco.neu.edu/litigation/cases/mn_trial/TE11028.pdf.

17. Richards JP, President, Tobacco Institute, 30 June 1958 US District Court for the District of Columbia, Civil Action No. 99-2496 (GK), USA *et al.* v. Philip Morris USA Inc. *et al.*, 9 September 2006, p. 261–2.

18. Hilts PJ, *Smokescreen – The Truth Behind the Tobacco Industry Cover-Up*, 1996, Addison Wesley, p. 26 quoting CV Mace, memo to RN DuPuis, untitled, 24 July 1958.

19. Ibid.

20. Kloepfer W (VP Public Relations for the Tobacco Institute) to Clements E (President of the Tobacco Institute), ~1960 US District Court for the District of Columbia, Civil Action No. 99-2496 (GK), USA *et al.* v. Philip Morris USA Inc. *et al.*, 9 September 2006, p. 264.

21. Hilts PJ (1961). *Smokescreen – The Truth Behind the Tobacco Industry Cover-Up*, 1996, Addison Wesley, p. 25 quoting AD Little, Confidential Limited Memo, L&M – A Perspective Review, 15 March.

22. Wakeham H (1961). *Tobacco and Health R&D Approach*. November 15. Philip Morris. Available at: http://www.tobacco.neu.edu/litigation/cases/mn_trial/TE10300.pdf.

23. Rodgman A (1962). *A Critical and Objective Appraisal of The Smoking and Health Problem*. Available at: http://www.tobacco.neu.edu/litigation/cases/mn_trial/TE18187.pdf.

24. McCormick A (1962). *Smoking and Health: Policy on Research*, minutes of Southampton meeting. British American Tobacco Company.

25. Yeaman A (1963). *Implications of Battelle Hippo 1 & 11 and the Griffith Filter*, 17 July, Memo {1802.05}.

26. 1964 Report, Tobacco Institute, *Allen Outlines Some of Reasons Why Smoking-Health Theory is Disputed*, 11 October 1963 US District Court for the District of Columbia, Civil Action No. 99-2496 (GK), USA *et al.* v. Philip Morris USA Inc. *et al.*, 9 September 2006, p. 267.

27. Gray B, Chairman of the Board, RJR before the Committee on Interstate and Foreign Commerce, 25 June 1964 US District Court for the District of Columbia, Civil Action No. 99-2496 (GK), USA *et al.* v. Philip Morris USA Inc. *et al.*, 9 September 2006, p. 268.

28. Kornegay H, Chairman and President of the Tobacco Institute, 12 July 1964 US District Court for the District of Columbia, Civil Action No. 99-2496 (GK), USA *et al.* v. Philip Morris USA Inc. *et al.*, 9 September 2006, pp. 268–9.

29. Rodgman A (RJR), August 1964 US District Court for the District of Columbia, Civil Action No. 99-2496 (GK), USA *et al.* v. Philip Morris USA Inc. *et al.*, 9 September 2006, p. 280.

30. Rogers P and Todd G (1964). *Strictly Confidential, Reports on Policy Aspects of the Smoking and Health Situations in USA*, October.

31. Cullman H, board member Philip Morris. 1964. Cited in R Kluger, *Ashes to Ashes – America's Hundred-Year Cigarette War, the Public Health, and the Unabashed Triumph of Philip Morris*, Alfred A. Knopf, New York, 1996, p. 260.

32. Karnowski S, 'Gentlemen's Agreement' is one key to State's Tobacco Case, *AP/Minneapolis-St. Paul Star Tribune*, 23 February 1998; H. Wakeham, *Need for Biological Research by Philip Morris*, Research and Development, undated. Available at: http://www.tobacco.neu.edu/litigation/cases/mn_trial/TE2544.pdf.

33. Roe FJC and Pike MC. *Smoking and Lung Cancer*. Undated (mid 60s). British American Tobacco Company. Available at: http://www.tobacco.neu.edu/litigation/cases/mn_trial/TE11041.pdf.

34. Robb EW and Osdene TS, *Smoke Chemistry Control*, January 1964 to July 1965, Philip Morris Technical Report #239, 19 November 1965. Available at: http://legacy.library.ucsf.edu/tid/sbi54e00/pdf.

35. Luchsinger PC, Project Director (PM), *Project 6900 Semi-annual Report* (marked '(n)ot to be taken from this room', 1966 US District Court for the District of Columbia, Civil Action No. 99-2496 (GK), USA *et al.* v. Philip Morris USA Inc. *et al.*, 9 September 2006, p. 280.

36. Ibid.

37. Yeaman A (B&W) to McCormick AD (BATCo), February 1966 US District Court for the District of Columbia, Civil Action No. 99-2496 (GK), USA *et al.* v. Philip Morris USA Inc. *et al.*, 9 September 2006, pp.181–2.

38. Tobacco Institute public statement issued 21 October 1966 US District Court for the District of Columbia, Civil Action No. 99-2496 (GK), USA *et al.* v. Philip Morris USA Inc. *et al.*, 9 September 2006, p. 269.

39. B&W, *Smoking and Health Proposal*, US District Court for the District of Columbia, Civil Action No. 99-2496 (GK), USA *et al.* v. Philip Morris USA Inc. *et al.*, 9 September 2006, p. 301.

40. Kluger R, *Ashes to Ashes – America's Hundred-Year Cigarette War, the Public Health, and the Unabashed Triumph of Philip Morris*, Alfred A. Knopf, New York, 1996, p.325 quoting *Duns Review*, April 1968.

41. Kluger R, *Ashes to Ashes – America's Hundred-Year Cigarette War, the Public Health, and the Unabashed Triumph of Philip Morris*, Alfred A. Knopf, New York, 1996, p. 324 quoting C. Thompson, Memo to Kloepfer, 18 October 1968 [Cipollone 2725]; *Tobacco Institute Tobacco and Health Research Procedural Memo*, 1966 US District Court for the District of Columbia, Civil Action No. 99-2496 (GK), USA *et al.* v. Philip Morris USA Inc. *et al.*, 9 September 2006, p. 299.

42. Gilbert RS, Ruder & Finn Incorporated, for Philip Morris. Press release entitled: *Major tobacco company says that 'care, cooperation and confidence' will provide acceptable answers to smoking and health controversy.* 28 October 1968. Philip Morris. Bates range: 1005110104- 1005110108.

43. Kloepfer W, VP of Public Relations for the Tobacco Institute, 1968 US District Court for the District of Columbia, Civil Action No. 99-2496 (GK), USA *et al.* v. Philip Morris USA Inc. *et al.*, 9 September 2006, p. 331.

44. B&W, *How Eminent Men of Medicine and Science Challenged the Smoking-and-Health Theory During Recent Hearings in the US Congress*, 1969 US District Court for the District of Columbia, Civil Action No. 99-2496 (GK), USA *et al.* v. Philip Morris USA Inc. *et al.*, 9 September 2006, p. 301.

45. Ibid.

46. CTR press release, 3 February 1969 US District Court for the District of Columbia, Civil Action No. 99-2496 (GK), USA *et al.* v. Philip Morris USA Inc. *et al.*, 9 September 2006, p. 299.

47. Advertisement in the *New York Times* entitled, *'Why we're dropping the New York Times'*, 8 September 1969, American Tobacco Co. Bates range: ATX040303547-ATX040303550.

48. Gallaher Limited, Re, Auerbach/Hammond Beagle Experiment, 3 April 1970. Available at: http://www.tobacco.neu.edu/litigation/cases/mn_trial/TE21905.pdf.

49. Hargrove GC, Smoking and Health, 12 June 1970 [L&D BAT 9].

50. Sommers S, Scientific Director of CTR and Chairman of the SAB, *Smoking and Health: Many Unanswered Questions*, 7 September 1969 US District Court for the District of Columbia, Civil Action No. 99-2496 (GK), USA *et al.* v. Philip Morris USA Inc. *et al.*, 9 September 2006, p. 303.

51. Wakeham H to Cullman J. *'Best' Program for CTR*. 8 December 1970. Philip Morris. Available at: http://www.tobacco.neu.edu/litigation/cases/mn_trial/TE11586.pdf.

52. Cullman J, President of Philip Morris, 3 January 1971 US District Court for the District of Columbia, Civil Action No. 99-2496 (GK), USA *et al.* v. Philip Morris USA Inc. *et al.*, 9 September 2006, p. 304.

53. B&W, Presentation called *The Smoking /Health Controversy: A View from the Other Side*, 8 February 1971 {BW-W2-03113} {L&D BAT file 4}.

54. Short R, *A New Product*, BAT, 21 October 1971, http://www.tobacco.neu.edu/litigation/cases/mn_trial/TE10306.pdf.

55. Panzer F, *The Roper Proposal*, Memo to H. Kornegay, Tobacco Institute, 1 May 1972. Available at: http://www.tobaccofreedom.org/issues/documents/landman/holding/index.html.

56. Green SJ, *The Association of Smoking and Disease*, 26 July 1972 [L&D BAT 16].

57. Spears AW, Lorillard, 13 November 1973. Available at: http://www.tobacco.neu.edu/litigation/cases/mn_trial/TE14009.pdf.

58. Smith RE to Ave JR, Re: 1976 switching study, as found in Lorillard 1976 switching study summary. November 1976. Lorillard. Bates range: 03296484-03296544.

59. Ibid.

60. Nowland Organization Inc. *SHF Cigarette Marketplace Opportunities Search and Situation Analysis, II: Management Report*. Lorillard, December 1976. Available at: http://www.tobacco.neu.edu/litigation/cases/mn_trial/TE17994.pdf.

61. Ibid.

62. Ibid.

63. Millhiser, R, President of Philip Morris, 12 January 1978 US District Court for the District of Columbia, Civil Action No. 99-2496 (GK), USA *et al.* v. Philip Morris USA Inc. *et al.*, 9 September 2006, p. 311.

64. Conning DM, *The Concept of Less Hazardous Cigarettes*. 15 May 1978. Lorillard. Bates range: 01414847-01414853.

65. Ibid.

66. Facts About the Smoking Controversy, 1978. Philip Morris. Bates range: TIMN 0055129-TIMN0055135.

67 Oldman M, *Cigarette Smoking, Health, and Dissonance (Project Libra)*, BAT, 18 October 1979. Available at: http://www.tobacco.neu.edu/litigation/cases/mn_trial/TE11102.pdf.

68. Tobacco Institute, *Tobacco from Seed to Smoke Amid Controversy*, US District Court for the District of Columbia, Civil Action No. 99-2496 (GK), USA *et al.* v. Philip Morris USA Inc. *et al.*, 9 September 2006, p. 312.

69. Philip Morris Annual Report, 1979 US District Court for the District of Columbia, Civil Action No. 99-2496 (GK), USA *et al.* v. Philip Morris USA Inc. *et al.*, 9 September 2006, p. 315.

70. BATCo, 1980 US District Court for the District of Columbia, Civil Action No. 99-2496 (GK), USA *et al.* v. Philip Morris USA Inc. *et al.*, 9 September 2006, p. 290.

71. Green S, *Cigarette Smoking and Causal Relationships*, 1976, 27 October {2231.07}; Green S, Smoking, Associated Diseases and Causality, 1 January 1980.

72. BAT, *Secret – Appreciation*, 16 May 1980 [L&D RJR/BAT 8].

73. Sommers S, Scientific Director of CTR, testimony before US Congress, 1983 US District Court for the District of Columbia, Civil Action No. 99-2496 (GK), USA *et al.* v. Philip Morris USA Inc. *et al.*, 9 September 2006, p. 290.

74. Abrams T, Crist P, Kaczynski S, *et al.* for Jones, Day, Reavis & Pogue. Undated attorney work product. Brown & Williamson. Bates range: 681879254-681879715.

75. Ibid.

76. Ibid.

77. Dawson B, Tobacco Institute, 8 April 1987 US District Court for the District of Columbia, Civil Action No. 99-2496 (GK), USA *et al.* v. Philip Morris USA Inc. *et al.*, 9 September 2006, pp. 321–2.

78. Dawson B, Tobacco Institute, 11 January 1989 US District Court for the District of Columbia, Civil Action No. 99-2496 (GK), USA *et al.* v. Philip Morris USA Inc. *et al.*, 9September 2006, p. 322.

79. Tobacco Institute of Hong Kong Limited, Introducing the Tobacco Institute, March 1989 [C.7].

80. Advertisement for Now cigarettes, 1990. RJ Reynolds. Bates range: 509231506.

81. Spach JF, Response letter to principal of Willow Ridge School of Amherst, New York. 11 January 1990. RJ Reynolds.

82. Product Differentiation Group the Over-smoking Issue (tar to nicotine ratio). 1990. RJ Reynolds. Available at: http://www.tobacco.neu.edu/litigation/cases/mn_trial/TE13139.pdf.

83. Castanoso J, Man Who Once Helped Now Criticises Reynolds, *News and Record [Greensboro]*, 26–28 September 1992.

84. Philip Morris newspaper ad, 1994 US District Court for the District of Columbia, Civil Action No. 99-2496 (GK), USA *et al.* v. Philip Morris USA Inc. *et al.*, 9 September 2006, p. 325.

85. Sandefur T, CEO of B&W, 1994 US District Court for the District of Columbia, Civil Action No. 99-2496 (GK), USA *et al.* v. Philip Morris USA Inc. *et al.*, 9 September 2006, p. 324.

86. Broughton M, Chairman of BAT, 30 October 1996 US District Court for the District of Columbia, Civil Action No. 99-2496 (GK), USA *et al.* v. Philip Morris USA Inc. *et al.*, 9 September 2006, p. 325.

87. Tunistra T, *Speaking Up*. Tobacco Reporter. December 1997. British American Tobacco Company.

88. Shaffer D, *No Proof that Smoking Causes Disease, Tobacco Chief Says*, Pioneer Press, 3 March 1998 (Geoffery Bible, Chairman, Philip Morris, MN trial testimony).

89. Walker M, MN trial testimony, 1998.

90. Townsend D, Vice President of Product Development and Assessment, RJ Reynolds, MN trial testimony, 2 April 1998.

91. Townsend D, Vice President of Product Development and Assessment at RJ Reynolds Tobacco Co, Minneapolis-St Paul Star Tribune. 2 April 1998.

92. Philip Morris website, 13 October 1999 US District Court for the District of Columbia, Civil Action No. 99-2496 (GK), USA *et al.* v. Philip Morris USA Inc. *et al.*, 9 September 2006, pp. 326–7.

93. Derek I to Read G, BATCo Southampton, Bates 325153707, 2 May 2000.

94. Public apology by Philip Morris, 26 July 2001.

95. Schindler, A, RJR Chairman, January 2005 US District Court for the District of Columbia, Civil Action No. 99-2496 (GK), USA *et al.* v. Philip Morris USA Inc. *et al.*, 9 September 2006, p. 320.

96. Accessed 14 April 2009. Available at: http://www.philipmorrisusa.com/en/cms/Products/Cigarettes/Health_Issues/default.aspx.

97. Ibid.

98. Ibid.

99. Ibid.

100. Accessed 15 April 2009. Available at: http://www.rjrt.com/smoking/summaryCover.asp#PublicHealth.

101. Accessed 17 April 2009. Available at: http://www.bat.com/group/sites/UK__3MNFEN.nsf/vwPagesWebLive/DO52AMG6?opendocument&SKN=4.

102. Accessed 15 April 2009. Available at: http://www.bat.com/group/sites/uk__3mnfen.nsf/vwPagesWebLive/DO52AMG6?opendocument&SKN=1.

103. Accessed 15 April 2009. Available at: http://www.lorillard.com/index.php?id=32.

104. Accessed 15 April 2009. Available at: http://www.liggettvectorbrands.com/.

105. RDW, *Complexity of the PA 5A Machine and Variables Pool*. June 1959. British American Tobacco Company. Available at: http://www.tobacco.neu.edu/litigation/cases/mn_trial/TE10392.pdf.

106. Hurt RD and Robertson CR, Prying Open the Door to the Tobacco Industry's Secrets About Nicotine. *JAMA* 1998;280:1173–1181.

107. Ellis C, scientific advisor to BAT Board of Directors, 15 November 1961 US District Court for the District of Columbia, Civil Action No. 99-2496 (GK), USA *et al.* v. Philip Morris USA Inc. *et al.*, 9 September 2006, p. 386.

108. Project Ariel, BATCo, 3 January 1962 US District Court for the District of Columbia, Civil Action No. 99-2496 (GK), USA *et al.* v. Philip Morris USA Inc. *et al.*, 9 September 2006, p. 392.

109. McCormick A, *Smoking and Health: Policy on Research*, Minutes of Southampton Meeting, 1962 {1102.01}.

110. Ellis C, *The Effects of Smoking: Proposal for Further Research Contracts with Battelle*, BAT, 13 February 1962. Available at: http://www.tobacco.neu.edu/litigation/cases/mn_trial/TE11938.pdf.

111. Ibid.

112. General Counsel Addison Yeaman, Brown & Williamson, Memo dated: 17 July 1963.

113. Griffith RB, Letter to John Kirwan, B&W, 18 September 1963. Available at: http://www.tobacco.neu.edu/litigation/cases/mn_trial/TE10856.pdf.

114. Anderson HD. *Potassium Carbonate*, Memo to R. P. Dobson, BAT, 7 August 1964. Available at: http://www.tobacco.neu.edu/litigation/cases/mn_trial/TE10356.pdf.

115. Blackhurst JD, *Further Work on 'Extractable' Nicotine*. Report issued by I. W. Hughes, BAT, 30 September 1966. Available at: http://www.tobacco.neu.edu/litigation/cases/mn_trial/TE17825.pdf.

116. Green SJ (BATCo Chief Scientist) Memorandum to Hobson DSF (Deputy Chairman BATCo), 2 March 1967 US District Court for the District of Columbia, Civil Action No. 99-2496 (GK), USA *et al.* v. Philip Morris USA Inc. *et al.*, 9 September 2006, p. 396.

117. BAT, R&D Conference, Montreal, Proceedings, 24 October 1967 {1165.01}; BAT R&D Conference Montreal, 24–27 October 1967, Minutes written 8 November 1967. Available at: http://www.tobacco.neu.edu/litigation/cases/mn_trial/TE11332.pdf.

118. Nielson, ED (RJR), 16 November 1967 US District Court for the District of Columbia, Civil Action No. 99-2496 (GK), USA *et al.* v. Philip Morris USA Inc. *et al.*, 9 September 2006, p. 374.

119. Dunn WL Jr., *Jet's Money Offer*. Memo to Dr H. Wakeham, Philip Morris, 19 February 1969. Available at: http://www.tobacco.neu.edu/litigation/cases/mn_trial/TE10539.pdf.

120. Philip Morris Vice President for Research and Development, *Why One Smokes*, First Draft, Autumn, 1969. Available at: http://www.tobacco.neu.edu/litigation/cases/mn_trial/TE3681.pdf.

121. Johnson RR, *Comments on Nicotine*. B&W, 1971. Available at: http://www.tobacco.neu.edu/litigation/cases/mn_trial/TE13878.pdf.

122. Williams RL, *Development of a Cigarette with Increased Smoke pH*, Liggett, 16 December 1971. Available at: http://www.tobacco.neu.edu/litigation/cases/mn_trial/TE11903.pdf.

123. Teague, CE Jr., RJR Memorandum, 28 March 1972 US District Court for the District of Columbia, Civil Action No. 99-2496 (GK), USA *et al.* v. Philip Morris USA Inc. *et al.*, 9 September 2006, p. 375.

124. Teague CE Jr., *The Nature of the Tobacco Business and the Crucial Role of Nicotine Therein. Research Planning Memorandum*, RJR, 14 April 1972. Available at: http://www.tobacco.neu.edu/litigation/cases/mn_trial/TE12408.pdf.

125. Ibid.

126. Ibid.

127. Ibid.

128. Ibid.

129. Ibid.

130. Dunn WL Jr., *Motives and Incentives in Cigarette Smoking*. Philip Morris, 1972. Available at: http://www.tobacco.neu.edu/litigation/cases/mn_trial/TE18089.pdf.

131. Ibid.

132. Green SJ, BAT Group R&D Conference, October 1972 US District Court for the District of Columbia, Civil Action No. 99-2496 (GK), USA *et al.* v. Philip Morris USA Inc. *et al.*, 9 September 2006, p. 401.

133. B&W, Secondary Source Digest, ~1973. Available at: http://www.tobacco.neu.edu/litigation/cases/mn_trial/TE13809.pdf.

134. Pepples E (B&W Counsel), Memo to Blalock J, 14 February 1973.

135. B&W Confidential, 1973 US District Court for the District of Columbia, Civil Action No. 99-2496 (GK), USA et al. v. Philip Morris USA Inc. et al., 9 September 2006, p. 426.

136. Ibid.

137. Teague CE, Implications and Activities Arising from Correlation of Smoke pH with Nicotine Impact, Other Smoke Qualities, and Cigarette Sales. RJR, 1973. Available at: http://www.tobacco.neu.edu/litigation/cases/mn_trial/TE13155.pdf.

138. Ibid.

139. Colby FG, Cigarette Concept to Assure RJR a Larger Segment of the Youth Market, Memo to R. A. Blevins, Jr, RJR, 4 December 1973. Available at: http://www.tobacco.neu.edu/litigation/cases/mn_trial/TE12464.pdf.

140. Minutes B&W/BATCo conference, 1974 US District Court for the District of Columbia, Civil Action No. 99-2496 (GK), USA et al. v. Philip Morris USA Inc. et al., 9 September 2006, p. 428.

141. Raleigh Extra Milds Marketing Plan, January, 1974 US District Court for the District of Columbia, Civil Action No. 99-2496 (GK), USA et al. v. Philip Morris USA Inc. et al., 9 September 2006, p.428.

142. McCormick AD, Smoking and Health. BAT, 3 May 1974. Available at: http://www.tobacco.neu.edu/litigation/cases/mn_trial/TE10602.pdf.

143. Comer AK, BATCo Research Scientist, 1975 US District Court for the District of Columbia, Civil Action No. 99-2496 (GK), USA et al. v. Philip Morris USA Inc. et al., 9 September 2006, p. 403.

144. New Product Ideas Developed for B&W, August, 1975 US District Court for the District of Columbia, Civil Action No. 99-2496 (GK), USA et al. v. Philip Morris USA Inc. et al., 9 September 2006, p. 428.

145. Goodman B, Marlboro–Marlboro Lights Study Delivery Data. Report to L. F. Meyer, Philip Morris, 17 September 1975. Available at: http://www.tobacco.neu.edu/litigation/cases/mn_trial/TE11564.pdf.

146. Green SJ, The Product in the Early 1980s. BAT, 29 March 1976. Available at: http://www.tobacco.neu.edu/litigation/cases/mn_trial/TE11386.pdf.

147. Chen L, pH of Smoke: a Review. Lorillard, 12 July 1976. Available at: http://www.tobacco.neu.edu/litigation/cases/mn_trial/TE10110.pdf.

148. Ireland MS to Minnemeyer HJ (Lorillard), Research Proposal – Development of Assay for Free Nicotine, 16 July 1976 US District Court for the District of Columbia, Civil Action No. 99-2496 (GK), USA et al. v. Philip Morris USA Inc. et al., 9 September 2006, pp. 438–9.

149. Senkus M, RJR Director of Research, 4 August 1976 US District Court for the District of Columbia, Civil Action No. 99-2496 (GK), USA et al. v. Philip Morris USA Inc. et al., 9 September 2006, p. 378.

150. Ibid.

151. McKenzie JL, Product Characterization Definitions and Implications. Memo to AP Ritchy, RJR, 21 September 1976. Available at: http://www.tobacco.neu.edu/litigation/cases/mn_trial/TE12270.pdf.

152. Schachter S, Memorandum, 1March 1977 US District Court for the District of Columbia, Civil Action No. 99-2496 (GK), USA et al. v. Philip Morris USA Inc. et al., 9 September 2006, p. 362.

153. Hawkins, McCain & Blumenthal, Inc, Conference Report, 28 July 1977. Available at: http://www.tobacco.neu.edu/litigation/cases/mn_trial/TE13986.pdf.

154. Ibid.

155. Ibid.

156. Ibid.

157. Green SJ, Suggested Questions for CAC III. BAT, 26 August 1977. Available at: http://www.tobacco.neu.edu/litigation/cases/mn_trial/TE11390.pdf.

158. Dunn WL, (PM), Memorandum, 3 November 1977 US District Court for the District of Columbia, Civil Action No. 99-2496 (GK), USA et al. v. Philip Morris USA Inc. et al., 9 September 2006, p. 483.

159. Stungis GE, *B&W R&D Department, Long-Term Product Development Strategy*, 28 November 1977 US District Court for the District of Columbia, Civil Action No. 99-2496 (GK), USA *et al.* v. Philip Morris USA Inc. *et al.*, 9 September 2006, p. 430.

160. Osdene T, Memorandum, 29 November 1977 US District Court for the District of Columbia, Civil Action No. 99-2496 (GK), USA *et al.* v. Philip Morris USA Inc. *et al.*, 9 September 2006, p. 362.

161. Ibid.

162. Ibid.

163. Short PL, *Product and Process Innovation*, BATCo, 22 February 1978 US District Court for the District of Columbia, Civil Action No. 99-2496 (GK), USA *et al.* v. Philip Morris USA Inc. *et al.*, 9 September 2006, p. 406.

164. Ryan FJ, *Exit-Brand Cigarettes: A Study of Ex-Smokers*, March 1978 US District Court for the District of Columbia, Civil Action No. 99-2496 (GK), USA *et al.* v. Philip Morris USA Inc. *et al.*, 9 September 2006, p. 363.

165. Ibid.

166. Steele HD, *Future Consumer Reaction to Nicotine*. Memo to M. J. McCue, B&W, 24 August 1978. Available at: http://www.tobacco.neu.edu/litigation/cases/mn_trial/TE13677.pdf.

167. Ibid.

168. Todorovic D to PM President and CEO H Cullman, *The Slow Motion Self-Suicide of the Tobacco Industry*, 3 February 1979 US District Court for the District of Columbia, Civil Action No. 99-2496 (GK), USA *et al.* v. Philip Morris USA Inc. *et al.*, 9 September 2006, p.364.

169. Schori TR, *Free Nicotine: Its Implications on Smoking Impact*. 22 October 1979. Brown & Williamson. Bates range: 542001986-542001996.

170. BAT, *Key Areas for Product Innovation Over the Next 10 Years*, 28 August 1979. Available at: http://www.tobacco.neu.edu/litigation/cases/mn_trial/TE11283.pdf.

171. Ibid.

172. Green SJ, Transcript of Note By SJ Green, 1 January 1980 [Pollock 129].

173. Gregory CF, *Observations of Free Nicotine Changes in Tobacco Smoke/#528*. B&W, 4 January 1980. Available at: http://www.tobacco.neu.edu/litigation/cases/mn_trial/TE13182.pdf.

174. Smith RE, Memo to Ave JR, Flinn JG, and Spears AW, Lorillard, 13 February 1980. Available at: http://www.tobacco.neu.edu/litigation/cases/mn_trial/TE10170.pdf.

175. Dunn WL, *The Nicotine Receptor Program*. Memo to Seligman RB, Philip Morris, 21 March 1980. Available at: http://legacy.library.ucsf.edu/tid/vns87e00/pdf;jsessionid=4C93809168B3AFC2D0D895B FECB1EB13.

176. Ibid.

177. Ibid.

178. Ibid.

179. Dunn WL Jr., *High Nicotine, Low TPM Cigarettes*, Memo to Seligman RB, Philip Morris, 24 March 1980. Available at: http://www.tobacco.neu.edu/litigation/cases/mn_trial/TE10529.pdf.

180. Crellin RA, Ferris RP, Greig C, and Milner JK, *Brainstorming II: What Three Radical Changes Might, Through the Agency of R&D, Take Place in this Industry by the End of the Century?* BAT, 11 April 1980. Available at: http://www.tobacco.neu.edu/litigation/cases/mn_trial/TE11361.pdf.

181. Kidd TW, *BATCo Strictly Private and Confidential*, May 1980 US District Court for the District of Columbia, Civil Action No. 99-2496 (GK), USA *et al.* v. Philip Morris USA Inc. *et al.*, 9 September 2006, p. 412.

182. Osdene TS, *Evaluation of Major R&D Programs*. Letter to Seligman RB, Philip Morris, 12 August 1980. Available at: http://www.tobacco.neu.edu/litigation/cases/mn_trial/TE10255.pdf.

183. Knopick PC Memo to Kloepfer W, Tobacco Institute, 9 September 1980. Available at: http://tobacco. health.usyd.edu.au/site/gateway/docs/pdf2/pdf/TIMN0107822_7823.PDF.

184. Colby FG (RJR) *INFOTAB—EC Task Force.* [Memorandum to Witt SB], 1 April 1981. Available at: http://legacy.library.ucsf.edu/tid/nuu13a00.

185. Oldman M, *Products/Consumer Interaction: the Role of Human Smoking Studies in Subjective Testing, with Particular Reference to Machine vs. Human Smoking.* BAT, 19 May 1981. Available at: http://www.tobacco.neu.edu/litigation/cases/mn_trial/TE11357.pdf.

186. Spears A, Article presented to the 35th Tobacco Chemists Research Conference. 1981, Lorillard.

187. Mackin G, 4 December 1981 US District Court for the District of Columbia, Civil Action No. 99-2496 (GK), USA *et al.* v. Philip Morris USA Inc. *et al.*, 9 September 2006, p. 368.

188. Smoking Behavior and Attitudes, B&W market analysis, January 1982 US District Court for the District of Columbia, Civil Action No. 99-2496 (GK), USA *et al.* v. Philip Morris USA Inc. *et al.*, 9 September 2006, p. 433.

189. Ibid.

190. Horrigan E, RJR Chairman and CEO, Congressional Subcommittee hearings, 5–12 March 1982 US District Court for the District of Columbia, Civil Action No. 99-2496 (GK), USA *et al.* v. Philip Morris USA Inc. *et al.*, 9 September 2006, p.451.

191. Brooks GO, *Smoker Compensation Study.* Memo to William Telling, BAT, 7 April 1982. Available at: http://www.tobacco.neu.edu/litigation/cases/mn_trial/TE13668.pdf.

192. Ibid.

193. Smoker Personality Study, B&W, 1982 US District Court for the District of Columbia, Civil Action No. 99-2496 (GK), USA *et al.* v. Philip Morris USA Inc. *et al.*, 9 September 2006, p. 433.

194. Ibid.

195. Teague, CE to RJR R&D VP DiMarco R, 1 December 1982 US District Court for the District of Columbia, Civil Action No. 99-2496 (GK), USA *et al.* v. Philip Morris USA Inc. *et al.*, 9 September 2006, p. 380.

196. Mellman AJ, *Project Recommendations.* Memo to Blott RA, B&W, 25 March 1983. Available at: http://www.tobacco.neu.edu/litigation/cases/mn_trial/TE13344.pdf.

197. Smoker Compensation Review, RJR, 15 April 1983 US District Court for the District of Columbia, Civil Action No. 99-2496 (GK), USA *et al.* v. Philip Morris USA Inc. *et al.*, 9 September 2006, p. 381.

198. Bellman AJ, BATCo, Project Recommendations, 25 March 1983 US District Court for the District of Columbia, Civil Action No. 99-2496 (GK), USA *et al.* v. Philip Morris USA Inc. *et al.*, 9 September 2006, p. 415.

199. Roberts DL, Memo to Flavor and Biobehavioral Divisions Regarding Brainstorming Session, RJR, 13 October 1983. Available at: http://www.tobacco.neu.edu/litigation/cases/mn_trial/TE12743.pdf.

200. Ibid.

201. Robinson, J to Rodgman A (RJR), 1983 US District Court for the District of Columbia, Civil Action No. 99-2496 (GK), USA *et al.* v. Philip Morris USA Inc. *et al.*, 9 September 2006, pp. 381–2.

202. Ibid.

203. Farone, W, (PM) Testimony, 1984 US District Court for the District of Columbia, Civil Action No. 99-2496 (GK), USA *et al.* v. Philip Morris USA Inc. *et al.*, 9 September 2006, p. 369.

204. Philip Morris, internal presentation, 20 March 1984.

205. Proceedings of the Smoking Behavior-marketing Conference, July 9–12, 1984, Session I. To Blackman LCF and Heath AM, B&W, 30 July 1984. MN TE 13430.

206. R&D Views on Potential Marketing Opportunities. BAT, 9 December 1984. Available at: http://www.tobacco.neu.edu/litigation/cases/mn_trial/TE11275.pdf.

207. Report on Medical and Scientific Issues – Addiction, RJR, 3 June 1985 US District Court for the District of Columbia, Civil Action No. 99-2496 (GK), USA *et al.* v. Philip Morris USA Inc. *et al.*, 9 September 2006, pp. 382–3.

208. Smoking and Health Litigation, Tactical Proposals, RJR Memorandum from Jones Day lawyers, 10 August 1985 US District Court for the District of Columbia, Civil Action No. 99-2496 (GK), USA *et al.* v. Philip Morris USA Inc. *et al.*, 9 September 2006, p. 384.

209. The Tobacco Institute, Claims That Cigarettes are Addictive Contradict Common Sense, 16 May 1988. Available at: http://www.tobacco.neu.edu/litigation/cases/mn_trial/TE14384.pdf.

210. The Tobacco Institute, Claims That Cigarettes are Addictive Irresponsible and Scare Tactics, 16 May 1988 US District Court for the District of Columbia, Civil Action No. 99-2496 (GK), USA *et al.* v. Philip Morris USA Inc. *et al.*, 9 September 2006, p. 468.

211. Covington and Burling, summary by industry council, May 1988 US District Court for the District of Columbia, Civil Action No. 99-2496 (GK), USA *et al.* v. Philip Morris USA Inc. *et al.*, 9 September 2006, p. 446.

212. Ibid.

213. Raffle S, Tobacco Institute press release, 29 July 1988 US District Court for the District of Columbia, Civil Action No. 99-2496 (GK), USA *et al.* v. Philip Morris USA Inc. *et al.*, 9 September 2006, p. 468.

214. Gullota FP, Hayes CS, Martin BR, inter-office memorandum to Spielberg HL, *When Nicotine is Not Nicotine*, 2 August 1989. Available at: http://tobaccodocuments.org/product_design/26541.html.

215. Dawson B, VP Public Affairs, Tobacco Institute, *Good Morning America Interview*, 1989 US District Court for the District of Columbia, Civil Action No. 99-2496 (GK), USA *et al.* v. Philip Morris USA Inc. *et al.*, 9 September 2006, p. 469.

216. Dawson B, VP Public Affairs, Tobacco Institute, *Larry King Live Interview*, 1990 US District Court for the District of Columbia, Civil Action No. 99-2496 (GK), USA *et al.* v. Philip Morris USA Inc. *et al.*, 9 September 2006, p. 469.

217. Untitled report on Project GT. 1990, RJ Reynolds. Available at: http://www.tobacco.neu.edu/litigation/cases/mn_trial/TE13129.pdf.

218. Blau T, Tobacco Institute press release, 12 July 1990 US District Court for the District of Columbia, Civil Action No. 99-2496 (GK), USA *et al.* v. Philip Morris USA Inc. *et al.*, 9 September 2006, p. 470.

219. PM Memorandum from Gullotta F to Ellis C (R&D PM VP), *Raison d'etre*, 8 November 1990 US District Court for the District of Columbia, Civil Action No. 99-2496 (GK), USA *et al.* v. Philip Morris USA Inc. *et al.*, 9 September 2006, p. 370.

220. RJR R&D, *REST Program*, 3 May 1991, 1990 US District Court for the District of Columbia, Civil Action No. 99-2496 (GK), USA *et al.* v. Philip Morris USA Inc. *et al.*, 9 September 2006, p. 383.

221. BATCo, *Q&As*, 3 December 1990 US District Court for the District of Columbia, Civil Action No. 99-2496 (GK), USA *et al.* v. Philip Morris USA Inc. *et al.*, 9 September 2006, p. 457.

222. Reuter B, *TABLE*, Philip Morris, circa 1992. Available at: http://www.tobacco.neu.edu/litigation/cases/mn_trial/TE11559.pdf.

223. Ibid.

224. Reuter B, *TABLE*, Philip Morris, October 1992 US District Court for the District of Columbia, Civil Action No. 99-2496 (GK), USA *et al.* v. Philip Morris USA Inc. *et al.*, 9 September 2006, p. 373.

225. Greig C, BATCo Product Developer, Structured Creativity Group, 1992 US District Court for the District of Columbia, Civil Action No. 99-2496 (GK), USA *et al.* v. Philip Morris USA Inc. *et al.*, 9 September 2006, p. 420.

226. Levy, C, PM scientist, Memorandum to Campbell W, 2 October 1992 US District Court for the District of Columbia, Civil Action No. 99-2496 (GK), USA *et al.* v. Philip Morris USA Inc. *et al.*, 9 September 2006, p. 373.

227. *Arguments Against the EC Cigarette Warning Label 'Smoking Causes Addiction'*, RJR, 14 December 1992 US District Court for the District of Columbia, Civil Action No. 99-2496 (GK), USA *et al.* v. Philip Morris USA Inc. *et al.*, 9 September 2006, p. 452.

228. Philip Morris, Pamphlet, 1992 US District Court for the District of Columbia, Civil Action No. 99-2496 (GK), USA *et al.* v. Philip Morris USA Inc. *et al.*, 9 September 2006, p. 447.

229. Shook, Hardy & Bacon report, *Philip Morris Research on Nicotine Phamracology and Human Smoking Behavior*, 1994 US District Court for the District of Columbia, Civil Action No. 99-2496 (GK), USA *et al.* v. Philip Morris USA Inc. *et al.*, 9 September 2006, pp. 371–2.

230. Dawson B, VP Public Affairs, Tobacco Institute, *Crossfire Interview*, 10 March 1994 US District Court for the District of Columbia, Civil Action No. 99-2496 (GK), USA *et al.* v. Philip Morris USA Inc. *et al.*, 9 September 2006, p. 471.

231. Ibid p. 472.

232. Dawson B, VP Public Affairs, Tobacco Institute, *Face the Nation Interview*, 27 March 1994 US District Court for the District of Columbia, Civil Action No. 99-2496 (GK), USA *et al.* v. Philip Morris USA Inc. *et al.*, 9 September 2006, p. 472.

233. Dawson B, VP Public Affairs, Tobacco Institute, *MacNeil/Lehrer Newshour Interview*, 1 April 1994 US District Court for the District of Columbia, Civil Action No. 99-2496 (GK), USA *et al.* v. Philip Morris USA Inc. *et al.*, 9 September 2006, p. 472.

234. Dawson B, VP Public Affairs, Tobacco Institute, *Larry King Live Interview*, 13 April 1994 US District Court for the District of Columbia, Civil Action No. 99-2496 (GK), USA *et al.* v. Philip Morris USA Inc. *et al.*, 9 September 2006, p. 472.

235. The tobacco company executives who appeared before Henry Waxman's (D-CA) Subcommittee on Health and the Environment of the Committee on Energy and Commerce, House of Representatives, 103rd Congress, beginning 14 April 1994, were: William Campbell, CEO, Philip Morris; James Johnston, CEO, RJR Tobacco Co; Joseph Taddeo, President, U.S. Tobacco Co; Andrew Tisch, CEO, Lorillard Tobacc; Thomas Sandefur, CEO, Brown & Williamson Tobacco Co; Ed Horrigan, CEO, Liggett Group; Donald Johnston, CEO, American Tobacco Co.

236. Campbell WI, President and CEO of Philip Morris, House of Representatives Subcommittee on Health and the Environment, April 14, 1994 US District Court for the District of Columbia, Civil Action No. 99-2496 (GK), USA *et al.* v. Philip Morris USA Inc. *et al.*, 9 September 2006, pp. 447–8.

237. Ibid.

238. National Ad, Philip Morris, shortly after 14 April 1994 US District Court for the District of Columbia, Civil Action No. 99-2496 (GK), USA *et al.* v. Philip Morris USA Inc. *et al.*, 9 September 2006, p. 449.

239. *The Effects of Cigarette Smoke 'pH' on Nicotine Delivery and Subjective Evaluations.* Philip Morris, 24 June 1994. Available at: http://www.tobacco.neu.edu/litigation/cases/mn_trial/TE11752.pdf.

240. Boyse (Blackie) S, BATCo scientist, letter to The Daily Telegraph, 29 June 1994 US District Court for the District of Columbia, Civil Action No. 99-2496 (GK), USA *et al.* v. Philip Morris USA Inc. *et al.*, 9 September 2006, p. 457.

241. Robinson J, RJR scientist, New York Times, 2 August 1994 US District Court for the District of Columbia, Civil Action No. 99-2496 (GK), USA *et al.* v. Philip Morris USA Inc. *et al.*, 9 September 2006, p. 452.

242. Quoted (Johnson R, ex-Chief Executive of RJR) in the *Wall Street Journal*, 'Big Spender Finds a New Place to Spend', October 6, 1994, p1 quoted in Hilts PJ, *Smokescreen – The Truth Behind the Tobacco Industry Cover-Up*, 1996, Addison Wesley, p. 64.

243. Submission to NIDA's Drug Abuse Advisory Committee by Philip Morris and the American Tobacco Company, 2 August 1994 US District Court for the District of Columbia, Civil Action No. 99-2496 (GK), USA *et al.* v. Philip Morris USA Inc. *et al.*, 9 September 2006, p. 449.

244. Board of Directors of RJR Nabisco Holdings Corporation, 12 April 1995 US District Court for the District of Columbia, Civil Action No. 99-2496 (GK), USA *et al.* v. Philip Morris USA Inc. *et al.*, 9 September 2006, p. 454.

245. Joint submission – Philip Morris, B&W, BATCo, Lorillard, and the Tobacco Institute, 2 January 1996 US District Court for the District of Columbia, Civil Action No. 99-2496 (GK), USA *et al.* v. Philip Morris USA Inc. *et al.*, 9 September 2006, p. 454 & 460.

246. Board of Directors of RJR Nabisco Holdings Corporation, April 17, 1996 US District Court for the District of Columbia, Civil Action No. 99-2496 (GK), USA *et al.* v. Philip Morris USA Inc. *et al.*, 9 September 2006, p. 454.

247. Quoted on Channel 4, *Big Tobacco*, Dispatches, 31 October 1996 (referring to experiments conducted by Philip Morris researcher Victor DeNoble).

248. Stevenson T, BAT Denies Smoking Claims, *The Independent*, 31 October 1996, p. 20 – quoted from Martin Broughton, CEO BAT Industries and Director BATCo; also published in the Wall Street

Journal US District Court for the District of Columbia, Civil Action No. 99-2496 (GK), USA *et al.* v. Philip Morris USA Inc. *et al.*, 9 September 2006, p. 456.

249. Philip Morris, *Position Statement On A Wide Range of Issues*, believed to be 1996.

250. Morgan J, President and CEO Philip Morris, 12 May 1997 US District Court for the District of Columbia, Civil Action No. 99-2496 (GK), USA *et al.* v. Philip Morris USA Inc. *et al.*, 9 September 2006, p. 449.

251. Former RJ Reynolds manager of advanced product technologies, to the FDA, according to a transcript obtained by the 13 March 1998 *New York Times*. Available at: http://www.nty.com.

252. Parrish SC. (Sr. VP PM)*Unites [sic] States Hispanic Chamber of Commerce Kansas City, MO.*, 24 September 1998. Available at: http://legacy.library.ucsf.edu/tid/hql93c00.

253. Bible G. *To Everyone with Issues About Cigarette Companies and Philip Morris.* [Draft memorandum], 28 January 1999. Available at: http://legacy.library.ucsf.edu/tid/cxp80c00.

254. Greenberg D, Vice President Corporate Affairs, Strategy and Development, Philip Morris Management Corporation, *American Hospital Association*, 12 September 1999. Available at: http://legacy.library.ucsf.edu/tid/rwb45c00.

255. Szymanczyk M, President and CEO PM, 4 August 2000, Cited in: *Scientific Consensus—'Addiction'— Influence of Nicotine and Other Tobacco Smoke Constituents on Smoking Behavior as a Determinant of Smoke Exposure. DRAFT.* Available at: http://legacy.library.ucsf.edu/tid/cwp94c00.

256. Philip Morris website, October, 2000 US District Court for the District of Columbia, Civil Action No. 99-2496 (GK), USA *et al.* v. Philip Morris USA Inc. *et al.*, 9 September 2006, p. 477. Available at:.

257. Merlo E [Senior VP PM], *Letter to Tobacco Commission.* 14 February 2001, British American Tobacco. Available at: http://bat.library.ucsf.edu/tid/apu63a99.

258. Takada K, Materials for the Philip Morris Scientific Research Review Committee (SRRC) presentation on *Consensus – Addiction*, 24 April 2001. Available at: http://legacy.library.ucsf.edu/tid/qky31c00.

259. Anon, *PM WSA 20030000 Planning Meeting Presentation:Nnicotine Addiction Consensus*, 6 October 2003. Available at: http://legacy.library.ucsf.edu/tid/rci95a00.

260. Philip Morris International website, 2004.

261. Ivey S, former President and CEO of B&W and CEO of RJR & Reynolds American, 2004 US District Court for the District of Columbia, Civil Action No. 99-2496 (GK), USA *et al.* v. Philip Morris USA Inc. *et al.*, 9 September 2006, p. 476.

262. Liggett advertising and packaging, LeBow TT, February 7, 2005 US District Court for the District of Columbia, Civil Action No. 99-2496 (GK), USA *et al.* v. Philip Morris USA Inc. *et al.*, 9 September 2006, p. 478.

263. Philip Morris website, 2005 US District Court for the District of Columbia, Civil Action No. 99-2496 (GK), USA *et al.* v. Philip Morris USA Inc. *et al.*, 9 September 2006, p. 451.

264. Accessed 14 April 2009. Available at: http://www.philipmorrisusa.com/en/cms/Products/Cigarettes/Health_Issues/default.aspx.

265. Accessed 15 April 2009. Available at: http://www.rjrt.com/smoking/summaryCover.asp#PublicHealth.

266. Accessed 15 April 2009. Available at: http://www.lorillard.com/index.php?id=32.

267. Accessed 15 April 2009. Available at: http://www.liggettvectorbrands.com/.

268. Wakeham H to Goldsmith CH, Philip Morris, USA, Inter-Office Correspondence, 7 April 1970. Available at: http://legacy.library.ucsf.edu/tid/rzq24e00.

269. Osdene TS, Undated handwritten note. Available at: http://www.tobacco.neu.edu/litigation/cases/mn_trial/TE2501.pdf.

270. Senkus M, (research director RJR) to Crohn, M (Legal Department RJR). *Invalidation of some reports in the research department.* 1969. Trial exhibit 26216.

271. Tully R to Funck M (General Counsel Reemtsma), Bates 2070478713, 25 September 1998.

272. US District Court for the District of Columbia, Civil Action No. 99-2496 (GK), USA *et al.* v. Philip Morris USA Inc. *et al.*, 9 September 2006, pp.1500-01.

273. US District Court for the District of Columbia, Civil Action No. 99-2496 (GK), USA *et al.* v. Philip Morris USA Inc. *et al.*, 9 September 2006, p. 4.

Chapter 6

The changing cigarette: chemical studies and bioassays

Ilse Hoffmann and Dietrich Hoffmann

Introduction

In 1950, the first large-scale epidemiological studies on smoking and lung cancer (by Wynder and Graham in the United States and by Doll and Hill in the United Kingdom) strongly supported the concept of a dose response between the number of cigarettes smoked, and the risk for cancer of the lung (Doll and Hill 1950;Wynder and Graham 1950).

In 1953 the first successful induction of cancer in a laboratory animal with a tobacco product was reported, with the application of cigarette tar to mouse skin (Wynder *et al.* 1953). (Throughout this chapter, the term 'tar' is used as a descriptive noun only.) The particulate matter of cigarette smoke generated by an automatic smoking machine was suspended in acetone (1:1) and painted on to the shaven backs of mice three times weekly for up to 24 months. A clear dose response was observed between the amount of tar applied to the skin of mice and the percentage of animals in the test group bearing skin papillomas and carcinomas (Wynder *et al.* 1957). Since then, mouse skin has been widely used as the primary bioassay method for estimating the carcinogenic potency of tobacco tar and its fractions, as well as for particulate matters of other combustion products (Wynder and Hoffmann 1962, 1967; Hoffmann and Wynder 1977; National Cancer Institute 1977*a*, *b*, *c*, 1980; International Agency for Research on Cancer 1986*a*). Intratracheal instillation on rats of the polynuclear aromatic hydrocarbon (PAH)-containing neutral subfraction of cigarette tar led to squamous cell carcinoma of the trachea and lung (Davis *et al.* 1975). A cigarette tar suspension in acetone painted on to the inner ear of rabbits led to carcinoma, with metastasis in thoracic organs (Graham *et al.* 1957).

Dontenwill *et al.* (1973) developed a method whereby Syrian golden hamsters were placed, individually, into plastic tubes and exposed twice daily, 5 days a week, for up to 24 months to cigarette smoke diluted with air (1:15). The method led to lesions, primarily in the epithelial tissue of the outer larynx.Using an inbred strain of Syrian golden hamsters with increased suscep-tibility of the respiratory tract to carcinogens, long-term exposure to cigarette smoke produced a high tumour yield in the larynx (Bernfeld *et al.* 1974). A dose response was recorded between the amount of smoke exposure and the induction of benign and malignant tumours in the larynges of the hamsters.

In general, inhalation studies with tobacco smoke have not led to squamous cell carcinoma of the lung (Wynder and Hoffmann 1967; Mohr and Reznik 1978; International Agency for Research on Cancer 1986*a*, *b*). Dalbey *et al.*, from the National Laboratory in Oak Ridge, Tennessee, exposed female F344 rats to diluted smoke of up to seven cigarettes daily, five times a week for up to 2.5 years. A high percentage of the smoke-exposed rats developed hyperplasia and metaplasia in the epithelium of the nasal turbinates and in the larynx, and also some hyperplasia in the trachea. The sham-treated rats developed a small number of lesions in nasal and laryngeal epithelia, but none in the trachea. Ten tumours of the respiratory system were observed in 7 out of 80 smoke-exposed rats. These were: 1 adenocarcinoma, 1 squamous cell carcinoma in the nasal cavity, 5 adenomas of the lung, 2 alveologenic carcinomas, and 1 squamous cell carcinoma of the lung (Dalbey *et al.* 1980). In the control group of 93 sham-exposed rats, one developed an alveologenic carcinoma (Dalbey *et al.* 1980). In 1952, Essenberg reported that cigarette smoke induces an excessive number of pulmonary adenomas, whereas the sham-exposed mice, as well as the untreated mice, developed significantly lower rates of pulmonary tumours. In the following years, the Leuchtenbergers repeatedly confirmed the findings by Essenberg. They also demonstrated that even the gas phase, as such, increased the occurrence of pulmonary tumours in mice (Leuchtenberger *et al.* 1958; Leuchtenberger and Leuchtenberger 1970). Several additional studies demonstrated the induction of pulmonary tumours in several strains of mice exposed to diluted cigarette smoke (Mühlbock 1955;Wynder and Hoffmann 1967; Mohr and Reznik 1978; International Agency for Research on Cancer 1986*a*, *b*). Otto (1963) exposed mice to diluted cigarette smoke for 60 min daily, for up to 24 months. Of 30 exposed mice, 4 developed lung adenomas, and 1, an epidermoid carcinoma of the lung. In the untreated control group, 3 of 60 mice developed lung adenomas.

Identification of carcinogens and tumour promoters in tobacco smoke

Green and Rodgman estimated that there were about 4800 compounds in tobacco smoke. In addition, several additives out of a list of 599 compounds disclosed by tobacco companies (Doull *et al.* 1994) may be added to cigarette tobacco during the manufacturing process in the United States (Doull *et al.* 1994; Green and Rodgman 1996). Tables 6.1 and 6.2 list the major constituents of the vapour phase (Table 6.1) and the particulate phase (Table 6.2), and their concentrations in the mainstream smoke (MS) of non-filter cigarettes (Ishiguro and Sugawara 1980; Hoffmann and Hecht 1990). Agricultural chemicals and pesticides, as well as their specific thermic degradation products, are omitted from the two tables because of the many variations in the nature and amounts of these agents in tobacco from country to country, and from year to year (Wittekindt 1985). Table 6.3 lists the major toxic components in the MS of cigarettes (Hoffmann and Hoffmann 1995).

Development of highly sensitive analytical methods, as well as reproducible short-term and long-term assays, has led to the identification of 69 carcinogens in cigarette smoke (Table 6.4). Of these, 11 are known human carcinogens (Group I), 7 are probably carcinogenic in humans (Group 2A), and 49 of the animal carcinogens are possibly carcinogenic to humans (Group 2B). This classification of the carcinogens is according to the International Agency for Research on Cancer (IARC) (1983, 1984, 1986*b*, 1988, 1990, 1991, 1992, 1994*a*, *b*, *c*, *d*, 1995*a*, *b*, 1996, 1999*a*, *b*). Two suspected carcinogens have, so far, not been evaluated by the IARC.

Smoking conditions

In 1936, the American Tobacco Company began using standard machine-smoking conditions, which reflected, to some extent, the smoking habits of cigarette smokers at that time. The estimated sales-weighted average nicotine yields of the cigarettes smoked at that time were around 2.8 mg (Bradford *et al.* 1936). In 1969, in agreement with the United States tobacco industry, the Federal Trade Commission (FTC) adapted the standard method of 1936 with only slight modifications. Since then, machine-smoking conditions have been 1 puff/minute, with a volume of 35 ml drawn during 2 seconds, leaving a butt length of 23 mm for a non-filter (plain) cigarette and length of

Table 6.1 Major constituents of the vapour phase of the mainstream smoke of non-filter cigarettes

Compound[a]	Concentration/cigarette (% of total effluent)
Nitrogen	280–320 mg (56–64%)
Oxygen	50–70 mg (11–14%)
Carbon dioxide	45–65 mg (9–13%)
Carbon monoxide	14–23 mg (2.8–4.6%)
Water	7–12 mg (1.4–2.4%)
Argon	5 mg (1.0%)
Hydrogen	0.5–1.0 mg
Ammonia	10–130 μg
Nitrogen oxides (NO_x)	100–600 μg
Hydrogen cyanide	400–500 μg
Hydrogen sulfide	20–90 μg
Methane	1.0–2.0 mg
Other volatile alkanes (20)	1.0–1.6 mg[b]
Volatile alkenes (16)	0.4–0.5 mg
Isoprene	0.2–0.4 mg
Butadiene	25–40 μg
Acetylene	20–35 μg
Benzene	12–50 μg
Toluene	20–60 μg
Styrene	10 μg
Other volatile aromatic hydrocarbons (29)	15–30 μg
Formic acid	200–600 μg
Acetic acid	300–1700 μg
Propionic acid	100–300 μg
Methyl formate	20–30 μg
Other volatile acids (6)	5–10 μg
Formaldehyde	20–100 μg
Acetaldehyde	400–1400 μg
Acrolein	60–140 μg
Other volatile aldehydes (6)	80–140 μg
Acetone	100–650 μg
Other volatile ketones (3)	50–100 μg
Methanol	80–180 μg
Other volatile alcohols (7)	10–30 μg
Acetonitrile	100–150 μg
Other volatile nitriles (10)	50–80 μg[b]

(Continued)

Table 6.1 (continued) Major constituents of the vapour phase of the mainstream smoke of non-filter cigarettes

Compound[a]	Concentration/cigarette (% of total effluent)
Furan	20–40 µg
Other volatile furans (4)	45–125 µg[b]
Pyndine	20–200 µg
Picolines (3)	15–80 µg
3-Vinylpyridine	10–30 µg
Other volatile pyridines (25)	20–50 µg[b]
Pyrrole	0.1–10 µg
Pyrrolidine	10–18 µg
N-Methylpyrrolidine	2.0–3.0 µg
Volatile pyrazines (I8)	3.0–8.0 µg
Methylamine	4–10 µg
Other aliphatic amines (32)	3–10 µg

[a] Numbers in parentheses represent the individual compounds identified in a given group.
[b] Estimate.

Table 6.2 Major constituents of the particulate matter of the mainstream smoke of non-filter cigarettes

Compound[a]	µg/cigarette[b]
Nicotine	1000–3000
Nornicotine	50–150
Anatabine	5–15
Anabasine	5–12
Other tobacco alkaloids (17)	na
Bipyridyls (4)	10–30
n-Hentriacontane (n-$C_{31}H_{64}$)[c]	100
Total non-volatile hydrocarbons (45)[c]	300–400[c]
Naphthalene	2–4
Naphthalenes (23)	3–6[c]
Phenanthrenes (7)	0.2–0.4[c]
Anthracenes (5)	0.05–0.1[c]
Fluorenes (7)	0.6–1.0[c]
Pyrenes (6)	0.3–0.5[c]
Fluoranthenes (5)	0.3–0.45[c]
Carcinogenic polynuclear aromatic hydrocarbons (11)[b]	0.1–0.25
Phenol	80–160

Table 6.2 (continued) Major constituents of the particulate matter of the mainstream smoke of non-filter cigarettes

Compound[a]	µg/cigarette[b]
Other phenols (45)[c]	60–180[c]
Catechol	200–400
Other catechols (4)	100–200[c]
Other dihydroxybenzenes (10)	200–400[c]
Scopoletin	15–30
Other polyphenols (8)[c]	na
Cyclotenes (10)[c]	40–70[c]
Ouinones (7)	0.50
Solanesol	600–1000
Neophytadienes (4)	200–350
Limonene	30–60
Other terpenes (200–250)[c]	na
Palmitic acid	100–150
Stearic acid	50–75
Oleic acid	40–110
Linoleic acid	150–250
Linolenic acid	150–250
Lactic acid	60–80
Indole	10–15
Skatole	12–16
Other indoles (13)	na
Ouinolines (7)	2–4
Other aza-arenes (55)	na
Benzofurans (4)	200–300
Other O-heterocyclic compounds (42)	na
Stigmasterol	40–70
Sitosterol	30–40
Campesterol	20–30
Cholesterol	10–20
Aniline	0.36
Toluidines	0.23
Other aromatic amines (12)	0.25
Tobacco-specific N-nitrosamines (6)	0.34–2.7
Glycerol	120

[a] Numbers in parentheses represent individual compounds identified.
[b] For details, see Table 6.4.
[c] Estimate.
na, Not available.

Table 6.3 Major toxic agents in cigarette smoke[a] (from Hoffmann *et al.* 1998)

Agent	Concentration/ non-filter cigarette	Toxicity
Carbon monoxide	10–23 mg	Binds to hemoglobin, inhibits respiration
Ammonia	10–130 µg	Irritation of respiratory tact
Nitrogen oxide (NO_x)	100–600 µg	Inflammation of the lung
Hydrogen cyanide	400–500 µg	Highly ciliatoxic, inhibits lung clearance
Hydrogen sulfide	10–90 µg	Irritation of respiratory tract
Acrolein	60–140 µg	Ciliatoxic, inhibits lung clearance
Methanol	100–250 µg	Toxic upon inhalation and ingestion
Pyridine	16–40 µg	Irritates respiratory tract
Nicotine[b]	1.0–3.0 mg	Induces dependence, affects cardiovascular and endocrine systems
Phenol	80–160 µg	Tumour promoter in laboratory animals
Catechol	200–400 µg	Cocarcinogen in laboratory animals
Aniline	360–655 µg	Forms methemoglobin, and this affects respiration
Maleic hydrazide	1.16 µg	Mutagenic agent

[a] This is an incomplete list.
[b] Taxicity oral/rat, LD_{50} free nicotine 50 mg/kg, nicotine bitartrate 65 mg/kg.

Table 6.4 Carcinogens in cigarette smoke

Agent	Conc./non-filter cigarette	IARC evaluation of carcinogenicity		
		In lab animals	In humans	Group[a]
PAH				
Benz(*a*)anthracene	20–70 ng	Sufficient		2A
Benzo(*b*)fluoranthene	4–22 ng	Sufficient		2B
Benzo(*j*)fluoranthene	6–21 ng	Sufficient		2B
Benzo(*k*)fluafanthene	6–12 ng	Sufficient		2B
Benzo(*a*)pyrene	20–40 ng	Sufficient	Probable	2A
Dibenz(*a,h*)anthracene	4 ng	Sufficient		2A
Dibenzo(*a,l*)pyrene	1.7–3.2 ng	Sufficient		2B
Dibenzo(*a,e*)pyrene	Present	Sufficient		2B
Indeno (1,2,3-*cd*)pyrene	4–20 ng	Sufficient		2B
5-Methylchrysene	0.6 ng	Sufficient		2B
Heterocyclic compounds				
Quinoline[b]	1–2 ng			
Dibenz(*a,h*)acridine	0.1 ng	Sufficient		2B
Dibenz (*a,j*)acridine	3–10 ng	Sufficient		2B

Table 6.4 (continued) Carcinogens in cigarette smoke

Agent	Conc./non-filter cigarette	IARC evaluation of carcinogenicity		
		In lab animals	In humans	Group[a]
Dibenzo(c,g)carbazole	0.7 ng	Sufficient		2B
Benzo(b)furan	Present	Sufficient		2B
Furan	18–37 ng	Sufficient		2B
N-Nitrosamines				
N-Nitrosodimethylamine	2–180 ng	Sufficient		2A
N-Nitrosoethylmethylamine	3–13 ng	Sufficient		2B
N-Nitrosodiethylamine	ND–2.8 ng	Sufficient		2A
N-Nitroso-di-n-propylamine	ND–1.0 ng	Sufficient		2B
N-Nitroso-di-n-butylamine	ND–30 ng	Sufficient		2B
N-Nitrosopyrrolidine	3–110 ng	Sufficient		2B
N-Nitrosopiperidine	ND–9 ng	Sufficient		2B
N-Nitrosodiethanolamine	ND–68 ng	Sufficient		2B
N-Nitrosonornicotine	120–3700 ng	Sufficient		2B
4-(Methylnitrosamino)-1-(3-pyridyl)-1-butanone	80–770 ng	Sufficient		2B
Aromatic amines				
2-Toluidine	30–337 ng	Sufficient		2B
2,6-Dimethylaniline	4–50 µg	Sufficient		2B
2-Naphthylamine	1–334 ng	Sufficient	Sufficient	1
4-Aminobiphenyl	2–5.6 ng	Sufficient	Sufficient	1
N-Heterocyclic amines				
AaC	25–260 ng	Sufficient		2B
1Q	0.3 ng	Sufficient		2B
Trp-P-1	0.3–0.5 ng	Sufficient		2B
Trp-P-2	0.8–1.1 ng	Sufficient		2B
Glu-P-1	0.37–0.89 ng	Sufficient		2B
Glu-P-2	0.25–0.88 ng	Sufficient		2B
PhIP	11–23 ng	Sufficient	Possible	2A
Aldehydes				
Formaldehyde	70–100 µg	Sufficient	Limited	2A
Acetaldehyde	500–1400 µg	Sufficient	Insufficient	2B
Volatile hydrocarbons				
1,3-Butadiene	20–75 µg	Sufficient	Insufficient	2B
Isoprene	450–1000 µg	Sufficient		2B

(Continued)

Table 6.4 (continued) Carcinogens in cigarette smoke

Agent	Conc./non-filter cigarette	IARC evaluation of carcinogenicity		
		In lab animals	In humans	Group[a]
Benzene	20–70 µg	Sufficient	Sufficient	1
Styrene	10 µg	Limited		2B
Misc. organic compounds[c]				
Acetamide	38–56 µg	Sufficient		2B
Acrylamide	Present	Sufficient		2B
Acrylonitrile	3–15 µg	Sufficient	Limited	2A
Vinyl chloride	11–15 ng	Sufficient	Sufficient	1
DDT	800–1200 µg	Sufficient	Probable	2B
DDE	200–370 µg	Sufficient		2B
Catechol	100–360 µg	Sufficient		2B
Caffeic acid	<3 µg	Sufficient		2B
1,1-Dimethylhydrazine	Present	Sufficient		2B
Nitromethane	0.3–0.6 µg	Sufficient		2B
2-Nitropropane	0.7–1.2 µg	Sufficient		2B
Nitrobenzene	25 µg	Sufficient		2B
Ethyl carbamate	20–38 µg	Sufficient		2B
Ethylene oxide	7 µg	Sufficient	Sufficient	1
Propylene oxide	12–100 ng	Sufficient		2B
Methyleugenol	20 ng			
Inorganic compounds				
Hydrazine	24–43 ng	Sufficient	Inadequate	2B
Arsenic	40–120 µg	Inadequate	Sufficient	1
Beryllium	0.5 ng	Sufficient	Sufficient	1
Nickel	ND–600 ng	Sufficient	Sufficient	1
Chromium (only hexavalent)	4–70 ng	Sufficient	Sufficient	1
Cadmium	7–350 ng	Sufficient	Sufficient	1
Cobalt	0.13–0.2 ng	Sufficient	Inadequate	2B
Lead	34–85 ng	Sufficient	Inadequate	2B
Polonium-210	0.03–1.0 pCi	Sufficient	Sufficient	1

ND, not detected; PAH, polynuclear aromatic hydrocarbons; AaC, 2-amino-9*H*-pyrido[2,3-*b*]indole; 1Q,2-amino-3-methylimidazo[4,5-*b*]quinoline: Trp-P-1,3-amino-1,4-dimethyl-5*H*-pyrido[4,3-*b*|indole; Trp-2, 3-amino-1-methy1-5*H*-pyrido[4,3-*b*]indole;Glu-P-1, 2-amino-6-methyldipyridol[1,2-*a*: 3',2"-d]imidazole; Glu-P-2,2-aminodipyridol [1,2-*a*: 3',2"-*d*]imidazole; Phlp, 2-amino-1-methyl-6-phenylimidozo[4,5-*b*]pyridine.

[a] *IARC Monographs on the Evaluation of carcinogenic Risks.* Volume 1 and Supplements1–8, 1972–1999. (1) Human carcinogens; (2A) probably carcinogenic in humans; [2B] Possibly carcinogenic to humans; (3) not classifiable as to their carcinogenicity to humans.

[b] Unassigned carcinogenicity status by IARC at this time.

the filter plus overwrap, plus 3 mm for filter cigarettes (Pillsbury *et al.* 1969). In Canada and the United Kingdom, the standard smoking conditions of the International Standards Organization (ISO) have been accepted since 1991 (ISO 1991). In other European countries, the standard smoking conditions for cigarettes are those developed by CORESTA (Centre De Cooperation Pour Les Recherches Scientifiques Relative Au Tabac), which are similar to the FTC standard smoking conditions (CORESTA 1991). In Japan, the FTC standard smoking conditions are employed for machine smoking of cigarettes (Pillsbury *et al.* 1969). The FTC method defines tar as smoke particulates minus water and nicotine, whereas CORESTA defines tar as total particular minus water (Pillsbury *et al.* 1969; CORESTA 1991; ISO 1991). The standard conditions for machine smoking of tobacco products used by the different testing protocols are presented in Table 6.5. Using the FTC method, the sales-weighted average tar and nicotine yields of United States cigarettes decreased from about 37 mg and 2.7 mg, respectively, in 1954, to 12 mg and 0.85 mg in 1993 (Fig. 6.1).

More than 20 years ago, M. A. H. Russell in the United Kingdom and N. L. Benowitz in the United States reported that long-term smokers of cigarettes with lower nicotine yields took more than one puff per minute, drew puff volumes exceeding 35 ml, and inhaled the smoke more deeply than smokers of higher yield cigarettes (Russell 1976 1980; Benowitz *et al.* 1983).

Table 6.6 presents the smoking characteristics of 56 volunteer smokers who regularly consumed low-yield cigarettes (≤0.8 mg nicotine/cigarette according to the FTC machine-smoking method) and of 77 volunteer smokers regularly consuming medium-nicotine cigarettes (FTC, 0.9–1.2 mg nicotine/cigarette). These two ranges of nicotine yield constituted more than 73.4 per cent of all cigarettes smoked in the United States in 1993 (Federal Trade Commission 1995). The results of this study clearly indicate that the majority of smokers in the United States smoke their cigarettes much more intensely to satisfy their acquired need for nicotine. Comparing the yields of the same cigarettes smoked under FTC standard machine-smoking conditions with the smoke

Table 6.5 Standard conditions for machine smoking of tobacco products

Parameters	Tobacco product								
	Cigarettes		Bidis	Little cigars	Small cigars	Cigars	Premium	Pipes*	
	FTC	CORESTA	–	FTC	CORESTA	CORESTA	CORESTA	CORESTA	
Weight (g)	0.8–1.1	0.8–1.1	0.55–0.80	0.9–1.3	1.3–2.5	5–17	6–20		
Puff									
Frequency (s)	60.2	60.0	30.0	60.0	40.0	40.0	40.0	20.0	
Duration (s)	2.0	2.0	2.0	2.0	1.5	1.5	1.5	2.0	
Volume (ml)	35.0	35.0	35.0	35.0	40.0	40.0	40.0	50.0	
Butt length (mm)									
Non-filter	23.0	23.0	23.0	23.0	33.0	33.0	33.0		
Filtered	F and OW+ 3	F+8	F and OW + 3						

FTC Federal Trade Commission method; CORESTA, Centre De Cooperation Pour Les Recherches Scientifiques Relative Au Tabac Method; F, filter tip; OW, Overwarp.
* One gram of pipe tobacco smoked.
Sources: [a] Hoffmann *et al.* (1974); [b] International Committee for Cigar Smoking (1974); [c] Miller (1963).

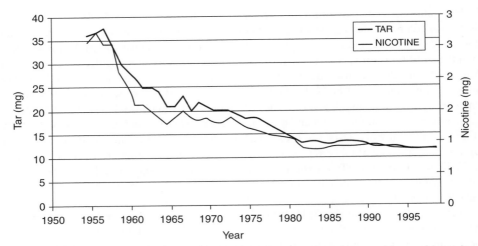

Figure 6.1 Sales-weighted tar and nicotine values for US cigarettes as measured by machine using the FTC method 1954–1998. Values before 1968 are estimated from available date (D. Hoffmann, personal communications).

inhaled by the consumers of cigarettes with low- and medium-nicotine content, reveals that smokers inhale 2.5 and 2.2 times more nicotine/cigarette, 2.6 and 1.9 times more tar, 1.8 and 1.5 times more carbon monoxide, 1.8 and 1.6 times more benzo(*a*)pyrene (BaP), and 1.7 and 1.7 times more 4-(methylnitrosamino)- 1-(3-pyridyl)-2-butanone (NNK) than is generated by the FTC machine-smoking method (Table 6.6, Djordjevic *et al.* 2000).

The discrepancy in exposure assessment between recent measurements and former interpretations of machine-smoking data has led to criticism of the FTC standard machine-smoking method for consumer guidance. The suggestion that there is a meaningful quantitative relationship between the FTC-measured yields and actual intake (by the cigarette smoker) is misleading (Benowitz 1996). In view of these concerns, it appears 'that the time has come for meaningful information on the yields of cigarettes' (Wilkenfeld *et al.* 2000*a*, *b*). The FTC agrees, in principle, that a better and more comprehensive test programme for cigarettes is needed (Peeler and Butters 2000).

Changes in cigarette smoke composition with various design changes

Filter tips

In 1959, Haag *et al.* reported the selective reduction of volatile smoke constituents by filtration through charcoal filter tips (Haag *et al.* 1959). Several of the compounds that are selectively removed from mainstream smoke (MS) in this fashion are major ciliatoxic agents, such as hydrogen cyanide, formaldehyde, acrolein, and acetaldehyde. Charcoal filters reduce the MS levels of these agents by up to 66 per cent (Kensler and Battista 1966; Battista 1976; Tiggelbeck 1976). However, for tar reduction, charcoal filters are less efficient than cellulose acetate filters. Several types of combination filters are in use. The early charcoal-activated dual and triple filter tips were cellulose acetate filters with embedded charcoal powder, or granulated charcoal sandwiched between cellulose acetate segments. These filters have been improved by innovative filter designs, incorporating cellulose acetate, charcoal, and cigarette filter paper (Shepherd 1994). However, in the United States, cigarettes with charcoal filters have accounted for only about 1 per cent of all

Table 6.6 A comparison of smoke data for two low-yield US filter cigarettes smoked according to the FTC method and by smokers (from Djordjevic *et al.* 2000)

Parameters	FTC machine smoking	Cigarette smokers	
		FTC 0.6–0.8 nicotine	FTC 0.9–1.2 nicotine
Puff			
Volume (ml)	35.0	48.6 (45.2–52.3)[a]	44.1 (40.8–46.8)[b]
Interval (s)	58.0	21.3(19.0–23.8)[a]	18.5(16.5–20.6)[b]
Duration (s)	2.0	1.5 (1.4–1.7)[a]	1.5 (1.4–1 6)[b]
Nicotine (mg/cigarette)	0.7 (0.6–0.8)	1.74(1.54–1.98)[c]	
	0.1 (1.09–1.13)		2.39 (2.20–2.60)[d]
Tar (mg/cigarette)	8.5 (7.7–9.5)	22.3(18.8–26.5)[e]	
	15.4 (14.2–14.9)		29.0 (25.8–32.5)[f]
CO (mg/cigarette)	9.7 (9.0–10.4)	17.3(15.0–20.1)[g]	
	14.6(14.2–14.9)		22.5 (20.3–25.0)[h]
BaP (ng/cigarette)	10(8.2–12.3)	17.9 (1 5.3–20.9)[i]	
	14(10.1–19.4)		21.4 (19.2–23.7)[j]
NNK (ng/cigarette)	112.9(96 6–113.0)	186.5(158.3–219.7)[i]	
	146.2(132.5–165.5)		250.9 (222.7–282.7)[j]

Test Groups: [a]56 smokers; [b]71 smokers; [c]3D smokers; [d]42 smokers; [e]18 smokers; [f]19 smokers; [g]15 smokers; [h]16 smokers; [i]6 smokers; [j]3 smokers.

BaP, benzo(a)pyrene; CO, carbon monoxide; NNK, 4-(methylnitrosamino)-1-(3-pyridyl)-2-butanone.

cigarette sales over the past 15 years. In most developed countries charcoal-filter cigarettes have had, at most, a few per cent of the open cigarette market. Exceptions are Japan, South Korea, Venezuela, and Hungary, where at least 90 per cent of the cigarettes have charcoal filter tips (John 1996; Fisher 2000).

Cellulose acetate filter cigarettes first became popular during the early 1950s in Switzerland and soon thereafter in Germany, then in the United States, later in the United Kingdom and Japan, and, finally, in France. In 1956, the market share of filter cigarettes in Switzerland, Germany, and the United States was 57.2 per cent, 16.7 per cent, and 29.6 per cent, respectively, with only a few per cent in Japan, England, and France. By 1965, the filter cigarette market share in these countries had risen to about 82 per cent (Switzerland), 80 per cent (Germany), 63 per cent (United States of America), 50 per cent (Japan), 52 per cent (England), and 21 per cent (France). At the present time, cellulose acetate filter cigarettes account for at least 95 per cent of the cigarette markets in all of the developed countries, except in France, where filter cigarettes remain at 85 per cent of all cigarette sales (Waltz and Häusermann 1963;Wynder and Hoffmann 1994; Hoffmann and Hoffmann 1997).

In the early 1960s, investigators found that cellulose acetate filter tips retained up to 80 per cent of the volatile phenols from the smoke. Reduction of the emissions of volatile phenols from cigarettes was desirable because their tumour-promoting activity had been demonstrated in carcinogenesis assays (Roe *et al.* 1959; Wynder and Hoffmann 1961; Hoffmann and Wynder 1971).When tested on a gram-for-gram basis, the tar from cellulose acetate-filtered smoke is somewhat more toxic, but less carcinogenic, than tars obtained from charcoal-filtered smoke, or from the smoke of non-filter cigarettes (Wynder and Mann 1957; Bock *et al.* 1962; Hoffmann and Wynder 1963; Spears 1963; National Cancer Institute 1977c). Cellulose acetate filter tips also selectively remove up to 75 per cent of the carcinogenic, volatile *N*-nitrosamines (VNAs) from the smoke; whereas charcoal filter tips are much less effective in removing VNA (Brunnemann *et al.* 1977). Exposure of Syrian golden hamsters to the diluted smoke from two different cellulose acetate filter cigarettes, twice daily for 5 days per week, over 60 weeks, elicited a significantly lower incidence of carcinoma of the larynx than exposure to the diluted smoke from the non-filter cigarette ($p < 0.01$). In contrast, the incidence rate of carcinoma of the larynx of hamsters exposed to diluted smoke from charcoal filter cigarettes did not differ significantly from that of larynx carcinoma in hamsters exposed to diluted smoke from the non-filter cigarette (Dontenwill *et al.* 1973).

Filter perforation allows air dilution of the smoke during puff drawing. The velocity of the airflow through the burning cones of cigarettes with perforated filters is slowed down. This is because the negative pressure generated by drawing a puff is reduced by drawing air through the filter perforations, and the pressure drop across the tobacco rod is reduced, thus slowing the flow of smoke through the rod. This results in less incomplete (more complete) combustion of the tobacco, and a higher retention of particulate matter by the cellulose acetate in the filter tip (Baker 1984; Durocher 1984; Norman *et al.* 1984; Hoffmann and Hoffmann 1997). Presently, more than 50 per cent of all cigarettes have perforated filter tips. Table 6.7 compares smoke yields of cigarettes without filter tips, cigarettes with cellulose acetate filter tips, and cigarettes with cellulose acetate filter tips that are perforated. The filling tobaccos of these experimental cigarettes were made of an identical blend. The conventional filter tip of cellulose acetate retains more tar, nicotine, and phenol but releases more CO and the ciliatoxic agents, hydrogen cyanide, acetaldehyde, and acrolein, into the smoke than does the cigarette with the perforated filter tip (National Cancer Institute 1976). In mouse skin assays, the tars from both types of filter cigarettes have

Table 6.7 Comparison of Experimental cigarettes (yield/Cigarette)[a,b] (from National Cancer Institute 1977c)

Smoke components	Unit of measurement	Non-filter cigarette	Cellulose acetate filter cigarette	Cellulose acetate filter w/perforation	Cellulose acetate filter w/perforation and highly porous paper
Carbon monoxide	ml	16.2	19.2	8.62	6.66
Hydrogen cyanide	µg	368	296	201	109
Nitrogen oxides—NO_x	µg	406	438	364	224
Formaldehyde	µg	36.0	20.9	31.7	21.4
Acetaldehyde	µg	1040	1290	608	550
Acrolein	µg	105	104	58.6	48.6
Tar	mg	27.0	14.7	19.2	19.5
Nicotine	mg	1.8	0.94	1.3I	1.5
Phenol	µg	161	61.7	122	129
Benz(a)anthracene	µg	40.6[1.40]	35.3 [2.25]	38.5 [1.88]	40.1 [1.91]
Benzo(a)pyrene	ng	29.9 [1.09]	19.6[1.25]	29.2 [1.13]	23.9 [1.14]

[a] The composition of the cigarette tobacco is identical in all four experimental cigarettes.
[b] Numbers in square brackets = µg/dry tar.

comparable tumourigenic activity. However, one needs to bear in mind: (1) that these comparative data are generated with tars obtained by the standardized machine-smoking method, with a 35-ml puff, taken once a minute over 2 s; (2) that more than 60 per cent of today's smokers in the United States and in many developed countries smoke cigarettes with nicotine yields of only 1.2 mg or less (according to FTC standards of smoking); and (3) that most of these smokers compensate for the low nicotine delivery.

Compensation and greater smoke intake is governed by the smokers' acquired need for nicotine and, in essence, negates the intended benefits of reducing smoke yields by technical means (Russell 1976, 1980; Schultz and Seehofer 1978;Moody 1980; Herning *et al.* 1981; Benowitz *et al.* 1983; Gritz *et al.* 1983; Nil *et al.* 1986; Benowitz and Henningfield 1994; Djordjevic *et al.* 1995, 2000).

Paper porosity

Since about 1960, higher cigarette paper porosity and treatment of paper with citrate has significantly contributed to the reduction of smoke yields of several smoke components. During and in between puff drawing, porous paper enhances the outward diffusion through the paper of hydrogen, NO, CO, CO_2, methane, ethane, and ethylene. On the other hand, it accelerates the diffusion of O_2 and N_2 into the tobacco column; this, in turn, causes more rapid smoldering during puff intervals (Hoffmann and Hoffmann 1997; Owens 1998). Porous cigarette paper causes a significant decrease of smoke yields of CO, hydrogen cyanide, nitrogen oxides, volatile aldehydes, yet it hardly changes the yields of tar, nicotine, benz(*a*)anthracene (BaA), and BaP. Importantly, the significant reduction of nitrogen oxides in the smoke of these cigarettes reduces the formation and, thus, significantly lowers the yields of volatile and tobaccospecific *N*-nitrosamines (TSNAs) (Brunnemann *et al.* 1994; Owens 1998).

Cigarette construction

Smoke yields of cigarettes are also dependent on physical parameters, such as length and circumference of the cigarette, and the width of the cut (number of cuts per inch) of the tobacco filler. Extending the cigarette length from 50 mm to 130 mm produces an increase in the level of oxygen in the mainstream smoke, while the absolute levels of hydrogen, carbon monoxide, methane, ethane, and ethylene decrease. The major reason for this lies in the diffusion of oxygen through the paper into the smoke stream (Terrell and Schmeltz 1970). This phenomenon is also reflected in an increased CO delivery with ascending number of puffs, because the available surface area of the paper diminishes as the cigarette is smoked.With increasing length of the cigarette, the overall yields of tar, nicotine, PAH, and other particulate components increase (DeBardeleben *et al.* 1978). A circumference of cigarettes smaller than the regular 24.8–25.5 mm, e.g. 23 mm or less, translates into less tobacco being burned but a greater volume of oxygen available during combustion. Thus, the smoke yields of tar, nicotine, and other particulate components are lowered (DeBardeleben *et al.* 1978; Lewis 1992; Brunnemann *et al.* 1994; Hoffmann and Hoffmann 1997). Cigarettes with a small circumference also have a lower ignition propensity toward inflammable materials than cigarettes that have a 24.8–25.5 mm circumference. In 1990, almost 5200 residents of the United States died in fires, an estimated 1200 of these deaths occurred in fires started by cigarettes (US Consumer Product Safety Commission 1993).

The number of cuts per inch (width of tobacco strands) applied to the filler tobacco of cigarettes has an impact on smoke yields and/or on the carcinogenicity of the tars. The first investigation on the importance of tobacco cuts per inch, with regard to smoke yields and tumourigenicity of the resulting tars, was published in 1965. It compared the smoke yields of tar and BaP when 8, 30, 50, and 60 cuts per inch of leaf were applied. Tar yields per cigarette decreased from 29.1 to

23.0 mg and BaP from 37 to 21 ng. The tumourigenicities of tars derived from cigarettes made with 8, 30, or 50 cuts per inch of tobacco declined from 27 per cent to 16 per cent and 13 per cent of tumourbearing mice. In a large-scale study of cigarettes filled with an identical blend, cut 20 and 60 times per inch, the smoke yields per cigarette of tar, nicotine, volatile aldehydes, BaA, and BaP were significantly reduced for the fine-cut tobacco. However, hydrogen cyanide was insignificantly increased. Gram-for-gram comparison of tumourigenicities of both tars on mouse skin revealed statistically insignificant differences (National Cancer Institute 1977a). As the large-scale bioassay was repeated twice, one has to conclude that in terms of mouse-skin carcinogenicity, activities of tars obtained from coarse-cut and fine-cut tobaccos are comparable.

Tobacco types

The botanical genus *Nicotiana* has two major subgenera: *N. rustica* and *N. tabacum*. *Nicotiana rustica* is grown primarily in Russia, the Ukraine, and other East European countries, including Georgia, Moldavia, and Poland. It is also grown in South America and, to a limited extent, in India. In the rest of the world, *N. tabacum* is grown as the major tobacco crop; it is classified into *flue-cured type* (often called bright, blond, or Virginia tobacco), *air-cured type* (often called burley tobacco; light air-cured tobacco grown in Kentucky, and dark air-cured type grown in parts of Tennessee and Kentucky, South America, Italy, and France), and *sun-cured* (often called oriental tobacco; primarily grown in Greece and Turkey). In addition, there are special classes of air-cured tobaccos for cigars, chewing tobacco, and snuff (Tso 1990).

Prior to the past two decades, flue-cured tobaccos were used exclusively for cigarettes in the United Kingdom and in Finland; they were also the predominate type used in Canada, Japan, China, and Australia. Air-cured tobaccos are preferred for cigarettes in France, southern Italy, some parts of Switzerland and Germany, and South America; cigarettes made exclusively from sun-cured tobaccos are popular in Greece and Turkey. In the rest of western Europe and in the United States, cigarettes contain blends of flue-cured and air-cured tobaccos as major components. Today, in many countries, such as the United Kingdom, France, and other developed nations, the US blended cigarette is gaining market share. In the United States, the composition of the cigarette blend has undergone gradual changes. In the 1960s and early 1970s, 45–50 per cent of the cigarette blend comprised flue-cured (Virginia) tobaccos; 35 per cent, air-cured (burley) tobaccos; and a few per cent were Maryland air-cured and oriental tobaccos. By 1980, the average blend was composed of 38 per cent flue-cured, 33 per cent air-cured, and a few per cent each of Maryland and oriental tobaccos. In the early 1990s, these proportions were about 35 per cent, 30 per cent, and, again, a few per cent of Maryland and oriental tobaccos (Spears and Jones 1981; Hoffmann and Hoffmann 1997). The blended cigarette is preferred in many countries, in part because each of the three major *N. tabacum* types adds a certain aroma to the smoke. Some isoprenoids, and a relatively high number of agents with carboxyl content, are associated with the aroma of flue-cured tobacco. Other isoprenoids, and especially the composition of the acidic fraction, are related to the special aroma of air-cured tobaccos (Roberts and Rowland 1962; Enzell 1976; Spears and Jones 1981; Tso 1990). 3-Methylbutanoic acid (isovaleric acid) is considered to impart the most important flavour characteristic to oriental tobacco (Stedman *et al.* 1963; Schumacher 1970).

However, in regard to the toxicity and carcinogenicity of tobacco and tobacco smoke, the difference in the nitrate content of the tobaccos is of primary significance. Flue-cured tobacco can contain up to 0.9 per cent of nitrate; yet, as it is used for regular cigarettes, it contains <0.5 per cent of NO_3. In oriental tobaccos one finds up to 0.6 per cent of NO_3, in air-cured tobaccos between 0.9 per cent and 5.0 per cent, but generally below 3 per cent in commercial cigarettes. The highest concentration of nitrate is present in the ribs, and the lowest concentration is in the laminae, especially in the laminae harvested from the top stalk positions of the tobacco plant (Neurath and Ehmke 1964; Tso *et al.* 1982).With the utilization of a greater proportion of air-cured tobacco in the American cigarette tobacco blend, the nitrate content of the blended US cigarette tobacco has risen from about 0.5 per cent in the 1950s to 1.2–1.5 per cent in the late 1980s (US DHHS 1989).

The concentrations of nitrogen oxides (NO_x) and methyl nitrite in smoke depend primarily on the nitrate concentrations in the tobacco, even though a portion of the nitrogen oxides is also formed during smoking from amino acids and certain proteins (Philippe and Hackney 1959; Sims *et al.* 1975; Norman *et al.* 1983). Cigarettes made with flue-cured tobaccos deliver up to 200 µg of NO_x, and 20 µg methyl nitrite in the smoke. Smoking US blended cigarettes produces up to 500 µg NO_2 and 200 µg methyl nitrite, and the smoke of air-cured tobacco cigarettes contains up to 700 µg NO_x and 400 µg methyl nitrite. The major source of nitrate is air-cured tobacco and, thus, the major source of NO_x in its smoke is nitrogen fertilizer (Sims *et al.* 1975). The stems of air-cured tobaccos are especially rich in nitrate (≤6.8 per cent). Consequently, stems, as components of expanded and reconstituted tobaccos, contribute in a major way to NO_x in the smoke (Brunnemann *et al.* 1983).

Freshly generated smoke, as it leaves the mouthpiece of a cigarette, contains NO_x virtually only in the form of nitric oxide (NO), and contains practically no nitrogen dioxide (NO_2). However, nitrogen dioxide is quickly formed upon aging of the smoke. It has been estimated that, within 500 seconds half of the NO in undiluted smoke is oxidized to NO_2 (Neurath 1972). Of major importance is the high reactivity of NO_x upon its formation in the burning cone and in the hot zones of a cigarette. The thermally activated nitrogen oxides serve as scavengers of C,H- radicals, whereby they inhibit the pyrosynthesis of carcinogenic polynuclear aromatic hydrocarbons. Table 6.8 presents data on the smoke yields of tar, nicotine, phenol, and BaP and the tumourigenicities of the tars on mouse skin (Wynder and Hoffmann 1963).

Freshly generated nitrogen oxides also react with secondary and tertiary amines to form volatile *N*-nitrosamines (VNAs) and several *N*-nitrosamines from amino acids, as well as from additives. The NO_x also form tobacco-specific *N*-nitrosamines (TSNAs) by *N*-nitrosation of nicotine and of the minor tobacco alkaloids (Brunnemann *et al.* 1977; Brunnemann and Hoffmann 1981; Tsuda and Kurashima 1991; Hoffmann *et al.* 1994). BaP declined while NNK increased in the smoke of

Table 6.8 Smoke yields and tumourigenicity of the tars from the four major *N.tabacum* varieties (from Wynder and Hoffmann 1963)

Factors	Flue-cured tobacco	Sun-cured tobacco	Air-cured tobacco	
			Kentucky[a]	Maryland
Yields/cigarette				
Tar (mg)	33.4	31.5	25.6	21.2
Nicotine (mg)	2.4	1.9	1.2	1.1
Phenol (µg)	95	I20	60	43
Benzo(a)pyrene(ng)	53(1.6)[b]	44 (1.4)[b]	24 (0.94)[b]	18 (0.85)[b]
Tumourigenicity[c]				
Percentage of mice with skin tumours	34	35	23	18

[a] Low-nicotine, air-cured tobacco (Kentucky).
[b] Number in parentheses: µg BaP/g dry tar.
[c] Bioassayed on a gram-for-gram basis of tar.

a leading US non-filter cigarette between 1974 and 1997. Both trends are correlated with the use of tobaccos with higher nitrate content. Recently, it was suggested (Peel *et al.* 1999) that the formation of tobacco-specific nitrosamines in flue-cured tobacco in the United States is, in part, due to the use of propane gas heaters in the curing process. Oxides of nitrogen generated during the burning of the liquid propane react with nicotine in the tobacco leaf to form TSNA. This change in the curing method, introduced in the mid-1960s, is a likely contributor to the increase of TSNA levels in cigarette tobacco. Other important factors are the proportionally greater use of air-cured tobacco and the use of reconstituted tobaccos in the cigarette tobacco blend (Neurath and Ehmke 1964; Brunnemann *et al.* 1983; Peel *et al.* 1999). Increased amounts of TSNAs in tobacco compound the carcinogenic potency of the resulting cigarette smoke (Hoffmann *et al.* 1994) and are considered to contribute to the rise of adenocarcinoma, which has become the dominant form of lung cancer in both male and female smokers during the past three decades (Vincent *et al.* 1977; Cox and Yesner 1979; El-Torkey *et al.* 1990; Devesa *et al.* 1991; Stellman *et al.* 1997). Increasing concentrations of nitrate in tobacco have also led to an increase in cigarette smoke of the human bladder carcinogens 2-naphthylamine and 4-aminobiphenyl, and of other aromatic amines (Patrianakos and Hoffmann 1979; Grimmer *et al.* 1995).

An important aspect relative to the toxicology of cigarette smoke is the correlation between the nitrate content of tobacco and the pH of cigarette smoke. Even though the different processes used to flue-cure and air-cure tobaccos have a significant impact on the smoke composition of the major types of tobacco, the role of nitrate is of major importance in determining the pH of the smoke. Whereas flue-cured tobacco and US cigarette tobacco blends deliver weakly acidic smoke (pH 5.8–6.3), the smoke of cigarettes made from air-cured tobacco delivers neutral to weakly alkaline smoke (pH 6.5–7.5). A major reason for the range of pH values encountered in the smoke of the two major tobacco types is the concentration of ammonia in the smoke, which is tied directly to the concentration of nitrate in the tobacco. When pH levels of the smoke rise above 6.0, the percentage of free, unprotonated nicotine increases to about 30 per cent at pH 7.4 and to about 60 per cent at pH 7.8 (Brunnemann and Hoffmann 1974). Protonated nicotine is only slowly absorbed in the oral cavity; yet, unprotonated nicotine, which is partially present in the vapour phase of the smoke, is quickly absorbed through the mucosal membranes of the mouth (Armitage and Turner 1970). The pH of cigar smoke rises with increasing puff numbers from pH 6.5 to 8.5; consequently, the rapid oral absorption of the free nicotine in the vapour phase gives a primary cigar smoker immediate nicotine stimulation so that he has no need for inhaling the smoke. Similarly, the smoker of black, air-cured cigarettes tends to inhale the smoke not at all, or only minimally (Armitage and Turner 1970; National Cancer Institute 1998).

In 1963, the first comparative study on the tumourigenicity on mouse skin of tars from the four major types of *N. tabacum* revealed the highest activity for tars from flue-cured and sun-cured tobaccos, and the lowest for the two varieties of air-cured tobaccos (Table 6.8; Wynder and Hoffmann 1963). The concentration of BaP, as an indicator of the concentrations of all carcinogenic PAHs, is correlated with the tumour initiation potential of the tars. Upon topical application to mouse skin and human epithelia, carcinogenic PAHs induce papilloma and carcinoma. In inhalation studies with Syrian golden hamsters, the smoke of a cigarette, made with a particular tobacco blend, was significantly more active in inducing carcinoma of the larynx than was the smoke of a cigarette with air-cured (black) tobacco (Dontenwill *et al.* 1973).

To verify whether a reduction of carcinogenic PAHs in the smoke due to the presence of high levels of nitrate in tobacco leads to reduced mouse skin tumourigenicity of the tar, sodium nitrate (8.3 per cent) was added to the standard tobacco blend. On a gram-for-gram basis, the tar from the cigarette with added nitrate (0.6 µg BaP/gram tar) induced skin tumours in only 2 of 50 mice, whereas the tar from the control cigarette (without the addition of nitrate; 1.05 µg BaP/gram tar) induced skin tumours in 25 of 100 mice (Hoffmann and Wynder 1967). In inhalation experiments with Syrian golden hamsters, smoke from the control cigarette plus 8.0 per cent of sodium nitrate induced laryngeal carcinomas in only 25 of 160 animals (15.6 per cent) compared to this type of neoplasm in 60 of 200 animals (30 per cent) in assays with the control cigarette (Dontenwill *et al.* 1973). Thus, all of these bioassays on the skin of mice and the inhalation studies with hamsters support the concept that increased nitrate content of the tobacco inhibits the pyrosynthesis of the carcinogenic PAHs and that the tars of these cigarettes, and their smoke as a whole, have a reduced potential for inducing benign and malignant tumours in epithelial tissues when compared to the tar or whole smoke of cigarettes with tobacco that is low in nitrate.

Reconstituted tobacco and expanded tobacco

In the early 1940s, the technology for making reconstituted tobacco (RT) was developed. Manufacturing RT enables the utilization of tobacco fines, ribs, and stems in cigarette tobacco blends (Halter and Ito 1979). Prior to this technology, tobacco fines and stems had been wasted. With the utilization of RT as part of the tobacco blend, less top-quality tobacco is needed, and thereby the cost of making cigarette has been reduced. Laboratory studies have shown that cigarettes made entirely of RT deliver a smoke with significantly reduced levels of tar, nicotine, volatile phenols, and carcinogenic PAHs.

The two major technologies for making RT for cigarettes are the slurry process and the paper process. Either process leads to RT with low density. The advantage of RT lies in the creation of a high degree of aeration of the tobacco, which enhances combustibility. Most of the tested tars from reconstituted tobaccos had significantly reduced carcinogenic activity on mouse skin (Wynder and Hoffmann 1965; National Cancer Institute 1977*a*). In inhalation assays with Syrian golden hamsters, diluted smoke from cigarettes made of reconstituted tobacco induced significantly fewer carcinomas in the larynx (19/160) than the diluted smoke from control cigarettes (60/200). The cigarette with RT gave, per cigarette, only 7 puffs and yielded 20.8 mg tar and 16 ng of BaP, compared to 10 puffs, 33.7 mg tar, and 35.4 ng BaP for the control cigarette (Dontenwill *et al.* 1973). This result supports the concept that, at least in the experimental setting, the carcinogenic PAHs, with BaP as a surrogate, are correlated with the induction of papilloma and carcinoma in epithelial tissues. The procarcinogenic TSNAs, on the other hand, are not activated by enzymes to their reactive species in epithelial tissues; thus, they induce few, if any, tumours in such tissues. Tobacco ribs and stems, the major components of RT, are richer in nitrate (and this applies especially to the ribs and stems of air-cured tobaccos) than the laminae of tobacco (Neurath and Ehmke 1964; Brunnemann *et al.* 1983; Brunnemann and Hoffmann 1991; Burton *et al.* 1992). Therefore, in general, the nitrate content of today's blended US cigarette, which may contain 20–30 per cent RT, is—at 1.2–1.5 per cent—much higher than the nitrate level in cigarettes during the 1950s and 1960s, when it was ≤0.5 per cent (Spears 1974; US DHHS 1989). Cigarettes with RT emit in their smoke significantly greater amounts of TSNAs than cigarettes of the past. These TSNAs include the adenocarcinoma-inducing NNK, which is metabolically activated to carcinogenic species in target tissues such as the lungs (Hoffmann *et al.* 1994). One major US cigarette manufacturer was awarded a patent in December of 1978 for developing a process that reduces more than 90 per cent of the nitrate content of the RT made from ribs and stems (Gellatly and Uhl 1978; Kite *et al.* 1978). It is unclear to what extent this patented method has been applied to RT manufacture for US commercial cigarettes.

There are at least three methods for expanding tobacco by freeze-drying (National Cancer Institute 1977*b*). As a result of freeze-drying, expanded tobacco has greater filling power than natural tobacco, meaning that less tobacco is needed to fill a cigarette. An 85-mm filter cigarette, filled entirely with expanded tobacco, requires 630 mg tobacco; while a regular non-filter control

Table 6.9 Smoke analyses of cigarettes made from puffed expanded, and freeze-dried tobacco and from a control cigarette (from National Cancer Institute 1980)

Smoke component	Puffed tobacco	Expanded tobacco	Freeze-dried tobacco	Expanded stems	Control
CO (mg)	9.33	11.8	12.3	23.1	18.0
Nitrogen oxides (μg)	247.0	293.0	235.0	349.0	269.0
HCN (μg)	199.0	287.0	234.0	248.0	413.0
Formaldehyde (μg)	20.7	21.7	33.4	58.0	31.7
Acetaldehyde (μg)	814.0	720.0	968.0	803.0	986.0
Acrolein (μg)	105.0	87.7	92.4	93.0	128.0
Tar (mg)	16	18	16	23	37
Nicotine (mg)	0.8	0.7	0.8	0.4	2.6
BaA(ng)	13.7	11.8	15.3	19.5	37.1
BaP(ng)	11.8	8.2	9.2	16.2	28.7

CO, carbon monoxide; HCN, hydrogen cyanide; BaA, benz(a)anthracene; BaP, benzo(a)pyrene.

cigarette of the same dimensions requires 920 mg tobacco. The tar yields in the smoke of both types of cigarettes amounted to 12.4 mg and 22.1 mg, respectively (National Cancer Institute 1977*b*, 1980). In 1982, incorporation of all possible modifications in the make-up of the cigarette required only 785 mg leaf tobacco; in contrast, in 1950, the blended US cigarette required 1230 mg leaf tobacco (Spears 1974). Table 6.9 presents analytical data for the smoke of experimental cigarettes filled with puffed tobacco, expanded or freeze-dried tobacco, and a control cigarette. Levels of most components measured in the smoke of cigarettes with puffed tobacco, expanded tobacco, or freeze-dried tobacco were reduced, compared with data for the control cigarette (National Cancer Institute 1977*b*, 1980).

The changes that have occurred between 1950 and 1995 in the make-up of US cigarettes, have significantly altered smoke composition. Table 6.10 compares data for individual components in the smoke of US blended cigarettes of the 1950s with corresponding data for the cigarette smoke composition profiles that have been established between 1988 and 1995. All of these cigarettes were smoked with the FTC method (Pillsbury *et al.* 1969).

Additives

Humectants

Humectants serve to retain moisture and plasticity in cigarette and pipe tobaccos. They prevent the drying of tobacco, which would lead to a harsh-tasting smoke; importantly, they also preserve those compounds that impart flavour to the smoke. Today, the principal humectants in cigarette tobacco are glycerol (propane-1,2,3-triol) and propylene glycol (PG; propane-1,2-diol); of lesser importance are diethylene glycol (2,2′-di[hydroxyethyl]ether) and sorbitol (Voges 1984). In the past, ethylene glycol (ethane-1,2-diol) has been used as a humectant for cigarette tobacco. However, because this compound leads to the formation of ethylene oxide, which is carcinogenic to both animals and humans, its use has been prohibited (IARC 1994*a*). In 1972, Binder and Lindner reported the presence of 20 μg ethylene oxide per cigarette in the smoke of the untreated tobacco of one cigarette brand (Binder and Lindner 1972). In this context, it is noteworthy that Törnqvist *et al.* (1986) found significant levels of the *N*-hydroxyethylvaline moiety of haemoglobin

Table 6.10 The changing cigarette: changes in the yields of selected toxic agents in the smoke of US cigarettes (FTC smoking conditions; Pillsbury *et al.* 1969)

Smoke component	Earlier cigarettes[a]		Current cigarettes[a]	
	Year	Concentration	Year	Concentration
Carbon monox ide (CO)	1953	33–38 mg (NF)	1994	11 mg (F)
Nitrogen oxides (HNO$_x$)	1965	330 μg (NF)	1994	500 μg (NF)
Benzene	1962	30 μg (NF)	1988	48 μg (NF)
	1962	25–30 μg (F)	1990	42 μg (F)
Acetaldehyde	1960	1000 μg (NF)	1992	400 μg (F)
NDMA	1976	43 ng (NF)	1989	65 ng (NF)
Tar	1953	38 mg (NF)	1994	12 mg (F)
Nicotine	1953	2.7 mg [NF)	1994	0.85 mg (F)
	1959	1.7mg (F)	1994	1.1 mg (F)
Phenol	1960	100 μg [NF)	1994	70 μg (NF)
	1960	46 μg (F)	1994	35 μg (F)
Catechol	1965	390 μg (NF)	1994	
	1976	790 μg (F)	1994	140 μg (F)
2-Naphthylamine	1968	22 ng (NF)	1985	35 ng (F)
BaP	1959	50 ng (NF)	1995	19ng (NF)
	1959	27 ng (F)	1995	8 ng (f)
NNN	1978	220 ng (NF)	1995	300 ng (NF)
	1978	240 ng (F)	1995	280 ng (F)
NNK	1978	110 ng (NF)	1995	190 ng (NF)
	1978	100 ng (F)	1995	144 ng (F)

[a]NF, non-filter; F, filter.
NDMA, *N*-nitrisodimethylamine; BaP, benzo(a)pyrene; NNN, *N*'-nitrosonornicotine; NNK, 4-(methylnitrosamino)-1-(3-pyridyl)-1 -butanone.

in the blood of smokers (ranging between 217 and 690 pmol/g Hb, averaging 389 ± 138 pmol/g); while levels in the blood of non-smokers ranged between 27 and 106 pmol/g Hb and averaged 58 ± 25 pmol/g Hb. The authors suggest that most of the ethylene oxide in the haemoglobin adduct is derived from endogenous oxidation of ethene in cigarette smoke (50–250 μg/cigarette).

Humectants may comprise up to 5 per cent of the weight of cigarette tobacco. In a 1964 study, 18 US cigarette tobacco blends that were analysed for humectants contained between 1.7 and 3.15 per cent of glycerol, which is, to some extent, decomposed to the ciliatoxic acrolein, and between 0.46 and 2.24 per cent of PG (Cundiff *et al.* 1964). The smoke of four American cigarettes contained between 0.34 and 0.96 mg/cigarette of PG (Lyerly 1967). However, PG may thermally degrade to yield propylene oxide. This would be of concern, because propylene oxide is regarded as possibly carcinogenic to humans (IARC 1994*b*). Four US cigarettes contained between 0.34 and 0.96 mg/cigarette (Lyerly 1967). In 1999, between 12 and 100 ng of propylene oxide were detected in the smoke of cigarettes filled with PG-treated tobacco. Several commercial samples of PG, used as a humectant for cigarette tobacco, already contained traces of propylene oxide (Kagan *et al.* 1999).

Flavour additives

Natural tobacco is composed of a wide spectrum of components that, upon heating, release agents that contribute to the flavour of the smoke. These include tobacco-specific terpenoids, pyrroles, and pyrazines, among others (Roberts and Rowland 1962; Gutcho 1972; Senkus 1976; Leffingwell 1987; Roberts 1988). The effective reduction of smoke yields by filter tips and by the incorporation of reconstituted tobacco also brought about a reduction of flavour components in the smoke. To counteract this loss of smoke flavour, the tobacco blends are treated with additives that are essentially precursors to smoke flavours. They include natural agents contributing to minty, spicy, woody, fruity, and flowery flavours. In some instances, such additives also include synthetic agents as flavour enhancers.While most of the flavour enhancers are chosen indiscriminately, it is realized that some of them may contribute to toxicity or carcinogenicity of cigarette smoke. A case in point was the cessation of the use of deer tongue extract which contained several per cent of the animal carcinogen coumarin (Voges 1984).

In 1993 and 1994, the tobacco industry convened an expert panel of toxicologists to screen agents that were in use, or considered for use, as tobacco additives. The panel established a list of 599 agents that were generally regarded as safe (GRAS), whereby the term 'safe' applied to each of the additives as such without consideration of the fate and reactivity of these agents during and after combustion (Doull *et al.* 1994). An exception was menthol, which was known to transfer into the smoke without yielding appreciable amounts of carcinogenic hydrocarbons (Jenkins *et al.* 1970). A recent toxicologic evaluation of flavour ingredients dealt with 170 such agents that are commonly used in the manufacture of American blended cigarettes, and examined their effects in four sub-chronic, nose-only smoke inhalation studies in rats compared to effects of the smoke of tobacco blends without additives. Control animals were exposed to filtered air (Gaworski *et al.* 1998). Smoke exposure was monitored with internal dose markers, including carboxyhaemoglobin, serum nicotine, and serum cotinine. The mainstream smoke (MS) of flavoured and non-flavoured cigarette types caused essentially the same responses in the respiratory tracts of the rats; specifically hyperplasia and metaplasia in the nose and larynx. As this study involved maximally 65 h of exposure (while induction of tumours would not be expected until animals reach half their life span), one cannot deduce with certainty that the addition of these flavouring agents to tobacco blends has no impact on the development of tumours.

New types of cigarettes

The tobacco companies have undertaken a substantial research effort to develop new types of nicotine delivery devices. These devices were intended to generate an aerosol with nicotine in the range of the levels present in conventional cigarettes but with very low emissions of tar and other toxic agents. Toward the end of the 1980s, the first prototype of these new types of cigarettes was on the test market, a product named 'Premier'. It was a cigarette that 'heats rather than burns tobacco' (R. J. Reynolds Tobacco Co. 1988; Borgerding *et al.* 1990*a*, *b*, 1997; DeBethizy *et al.* 1990). This 80-mm cigarette is comprised of three sections. The first 40-mm section of this cigarette is made with compressed charcoal, which is immediately linked to an inner aluminum tube containing tobacco, flavour additives, and glycerol. This tube is embedded in tobacco. Section 2 (~10 mm) is a cellulose acetate filter dusted with charcoal powder. The third section (~30 mm) is a cellulose acetate filter tip. Under FTC standard machine-smoking conditions, the 'Premier' delivers smoke containing 0.3 mg nicotine, 6.3 mg water, 4.6 mg glycerol, 0.4 mg propylene glycol, and 0.7 mg tar. Compared with the reference (conventional) cigarette, and disregarding nicotine, the majority of the known toxic and carcinogenic agents in the smoke are reduced by more than 90 per cent. Known exceptions are carbon monoxide (CO) (+3.5 per cent), ammonia (−5.6 per cent), formaldehyde (−35.3 per cent), resorcinol (−73.3 per cent), quinoline (−56.6 per cent), and acetamide (−18.2 per cent). This new type of cigarette did not gain consumer acceptance; possibly because of difficulty in igniting the 'Premier', the need for frequent puffing to ensure continuous burning, the lack of flavour, and the low nicotine delivery (0.3 mg/cigarette). Nicotine emission was below the level that would satisfy most smokers' acquired need for this agent, even with compensatory smoking.

In 1996, a modified 'Premier' came on the market. In the United States it is known as 'Eclipse', in Germany it is called 'HiQ', and in Sweden it goes by the name 'Inside'. The 'Eclipse' consists of four sections. Section 1, the heat source, is a specially prepared charcoal; section 2 consists of tobacco plus glycerol; section 3 contains finely shredded tobacco; and section 4 is a filter tip. Upon ignition, the special charcoal heats the air stream during puff drawing. The heated air-stream enters the tobacco sections and vapourizes glycerol, as well as the volatile and semi-volatile tobacco components, including nicotine. Under FTC smoking conditions, the 'Eclipse' delivers 8 mg CO (low-tar filter cigarette: 6–12 mg), 150 μg acetaldehyde (700 μg), 30 μg NO_x (200–300 μg), 180 μg hydrogen cyanide (300–400 μg), 5.1 mg tar (11–12 mg), and 0.2–0.4 mg nicotine (0.7–1.0 mg). The remainder of the smoke particulates consists of 33 per cent water, 47 per cent glycerol, and 17 per cent of various other compounds. The concentrations of the major carcinogens, such as BaP, 2-aminonaphthalene, 4-aminobiphenyl, and the TSNAs are lowered by 85–95 per cent (Rose and Levin 1996; Smith *et al.* 1996). Currently, the 'Eclipse' is being test marketed and it appears that response is somewhat more favorable than it was to its predecessor, the 'Premier'. The products labeled, 'Eclipse Full Flavour', 'Eclipse Mild', and 'Eclipse Menthol' produce FTC-standardized smoke yields of 0.2, 0.1, and 0.2 mg nicotine and of 3, 2, and 3 mg tar per cigarette. Regular cigarette smokers were asked to switch for 2 weeks to 'Eclipse'. There were four study groups, each composed of 26–30 volunteers, for a total of 109 smokers. Smoking of 'Eclipse' resulted in about a 30 per cent larger puff volume, about 50 per cent more puffs, which added up to a total puff volume per cigarette that was more than twice that of the total volume drawn from the control cigarettes (Stiles *et al.* 1999). These data suggest that the volunteers smoked 'Eclipse' more intensely than their non-filter cigarettes. This observation is also supported in the uptake of nicotine (Benowitz *et al.* 1997). The mutagenic activities of the urine of smokers of four types of 'Eclipse' were assayed on two bacterial strains and were reduced by 72–100 per cent, compared with the mutagenic activities of the urine of the same volunteers after smoking their regular cigarettes (Smith *et al.* 1996).

An Expert Committee from the Institute of Medicine of the National Academy of Sciences studied the scientific basis for a possible reduction of the 'harm' induced by 'Eclipse' relative to the 'harm' induced by smoking conventional cigarettes. On the basis of the available data, the committee came to the following conclusions: 'Eclipse' offers the committed smoker an option that is currently not available. 'Eclipse' does not add to the inherent biological activity of smoke from the range of cigarettes currently on the market. The elevated COHb levels should be regarded as a potential risk factor for cardiovascular diseases. The magnitude of this risk remains to be determined (Gardner 2000).

The high concentration of glycerol in the 'Eclipse' aerosol led to bioassays of glycerol in 2-week (1.0, 1.93, and 3.91 mg/l) and in 13-week (0.033, 0.167, and 0.662 mg/l) in 'nose only' inhalation studies with Sprague–Dawley rats, testing for toxicity and especially for irritating effects. The investigators detected metaplasia of the lining of the epiglottis (Gardner 2000). The 13-week inhalation studies with rats and hamsters had also resulted in some early histopathological changes in the upper respiratory tract in both laboratory animals. These observations signal the need for lifetime inhalation assays with the smoke of 'Eclipse' in rats, preferably Fisher 344 rats, or better yet, in Syrian golden hamsters, possibly with an inbred strain of hamsters susceptible to carcinogens in the respiratory tract (Bernfeld *et al.* 1974). Pauly *et al.*, from the Roswell Park Cancer Institute, Buffalo, New York, caution that harmful glass fibers have been found to migrate into the filter tip of the 'Eclipse' and may be inhaled during puffing (Pauly *et al.* 2000).

The Health Department of Massachusetts and the Society for Research on Nicotine and Tobacco disputed the claims made for 'Eclipse.' They requested that the FTC and the Food and Drug Administration (FDA) institute regulatory procedures to ensure that insufficiently documented health claims are not made for tobacco products. Declaring 'Eclipse' the 'next best choice,' or calling TSNA-reduced tobacco products 'safer tobacco' (Anonymous 2000; Society for Research on Nicotine and Tobacco 2000) is deceiving.

In 1998, Philip Morris USA released a new type of cigarette (EHC) that is heated electrically to release an aerosol. On the basis of chemical analyses and short-term bioassays, it has significantly lower toxicity and mutagenicity than the smoke of the Kentucky reference filter cigarette, 1R4F. The prototype, containing a tobacco filler wrapped in a tobacco mat, is kept in constant contact with eight electrical heater blades in a microprocessor-controlled lighter. This cigarette contains about half the amount of the tobacco of a conventional cigarette. Under FTC-standardized smoking conditions, the cigarette delivers, with an average of eight puffs, about 1 mg of nicotine, whereas all other smoke constituents analysed were significantly lower than those in the smoke of the low-yield Kentucky reference cigarette, 1R4F (Terpstra *et al.* 1998). However, formaldehyde yields were significantly higher in the smoke of the EHC and emissions of glycerol and 2-nitropropane were comparable to those recorded in the smoke of the 1R4F cigarette. Per gram of tar, the smoke of the EHC had significantly lower mutagenic activity than the smoke of the 1R4F reference cigarette in TA98 and TA100 tester strains with metabolic activation (Terpstra *et al.* 1998).

Observations on cigarette smokers

In mice, rats, and hamsters, NNK induces adenomas and adenocarcinomas (AC) in the peripheral lung. This effect is independent of route and form of application (Hoffmann *et al.* 1994). NNK is metabolically activated primarily to the unstable 4-(hydroxymethylnitrosamino)-1-(3-pyridyl)-1-butanone and to 4-(α-hydroxymethylene)- 1-(3-pyridyl)-1-butanol, which decomposes into methane diazohydroxide and 4-keto-4-(3-pyridyl)butane diazohydroxide, respectively. The diazohydroxides react with DNA bases to form 7-methyl guanine, O^6-methyl guanine, and O^4-methyl thymidine, respectively, and also form a pyridyloxobutyl adduct of presently unknown structure. Upon acid hydrolysis, this adduct releases 4-hydroxy-1-(3-pyridyl)-1-butanone. These adducts have been found in the lungs of mice and rats following treatment with NNK, and they have also been identified in human lungs. The origin of 7-methyl guanine in DNA from human lungs is unclear; conceivably, in addition to TSNA, nitroso compounds such as *N*-nitrosodimethylamine may also have been a source for this DNA methylation. However, it is clear that higher levels of 7-methyl guanine have been found in the lung of smokers than in the lung of non-smokers, thus strengthening the evidence that NNK is a major contributor to the methylation of the lung DNA of smokers (Hecht 1998).

PAHs induce squamous cell carcinoma of the lung in laboratory animals and in workers with exposures to aerosols that are high in PAH. NNK metabolites induce primarily AC of the lung in laboratory animals. Reactive PAH metabolites bind to DNA in epithelial tissues. In laboratory animals, metabolically activated forms of NNK react with the DNA of Clara cells in the peripheral lung (Belinsky *et al.* 1990) to form methylguanine and methylthymidine, as well as pyridyloxobutylated adducts. 7-Methylguanine has been found in smokers' lungs at higher levels than in the lungs of non-smokers. Additional support for the observation that adenocarcinoma of the lung, among cigarette smokers, has increased relative to squamous cell carcinoma during the past

25 years, and for the concept that the lung cancer risk of smokers of low-nicotine filter cigarettes is similar to that of smokers of non-filter cigarettes, comes from biochemical studies. In the mouse, the O^6-methylguanine pathway of metabolically activated NNK is clearly the major route for induction of lung tumours; this conclusion is consistent with the high percentage of GGT→GAT mutations in the K-*ras* oncogene induced by NNK (Singer and Essigmann 1991; Hecht 1998). A study from The Netherlands has shown that mutations on codon 12 of the K-*ras* oncogene are present in 24–50 per cent of human primary adenocarcinoma. These mutations occur more frequently in AC of the lung in smokers than in non-smokers. Twenty per cent of the mutations in codon 12 involve GGT→GAT conversions, which supports the concept that NNK plays a role in the induction of AC of the lung in smokers. Histochemical examination of human lung cancer showed cyclooxygenase (COX)-2 expression in 70 per cent of invasive carcinoma cases (Hida *et al.* 1998). COX-2 expression was also identified in adenocarcinoma of the lung in rats treated with NNK (El-Bayoumy *et al.* 1999). It is anticipated that future studies in molecular biology will fully elucidate the significance of TSNAs, especially of NNK, and of the carcinogenic PAHs in the induction of lung cancer in tobacco smokers.

Summary

Major modifications in the make-up of the commercial cigarette have been introduced between 1950 and 1975. Since then, there have been no substantive changes toward a further reduction of the toxic and carcinogenic potential of cigarette smoke, beyond reducing MS yields of tar, nicotine, and carbon monoxide. Some of these modifications have also resulted in diminished yields of several toxic and carcinogenic smoke constituents.

Cigarettes with charcoal filter tips deliver MS with significantly lower concentrations of the major ciliatoxic agents, such as hydrogen cyanide and volatile aldehydes. However, except in Japan, South Korea, Venezuela, and Hungary, cigarettes with charcoal filter tips account for less than 1 per cent (USA), and at most for a few per cent, of all cigarettes sold worldwide (Fisher 2000).

Cellulose acetate filters, with or without perforation, have the capacity for selective reduction of smoke yields of volatile *N*-nitrosamines and semi-volatile phenols. The latter are major tumour promoters in cigarette tar. In contrast to cigarettes manufactured in the 1950s, most of the cigarettes on the market today use a highly porous wrapper of paper treated with agents that enhance burning, thus contributing to the reduction of machine-measured yields of carbon monoxide, hydrogen cyanide, volatile aldehydes, volatile *N*-nitrosamines, PAH, and TSNA.

Reconstituted tobacco and expanded tobacco today amount to between 25 and 30 per cent of the cigarette tobacco blend. Reconstituted tobacco reduces the yields of smoke components such as tar and CO. The tar from cigarettes made entirely of reconstituted tobacco is less carcinogenic on mouse skin, and the smoke of these cigarettes reduces significantly the induction of carcinoma in the larynx of hamsters, compared to the smoke of reference cigarettes made of natural tobacco. Reconstituted tobaccos and expanded tobaccos have a significantly greater filling power than natural tobacco. An 85-mm filter cigarette that is filled entirely with expanded tobacco requires 363 mg tobacco while a regular filter-tipped cigarette requires 667 mg tobacco. The smoke of cigarettes made of expanded tobacco has significantly lower MS yields of tar, nicotine, CO, hydrogen cyanide, PAH, and TSNA. On the basis of weight-to-weight comparisons, the tar from these cigarettes is significantly less tumourigenic on mouse skin than the tar of a reference cigarette made of the corresponding natural tobacco.

Since 1959, each year the levels of tar, nicotine, and benzo(*a*)pyrene in the mainstream smoke of a leading US non-filter cigarette have been monitored. Beginning in 1977, the MS was also analysed for NNK and, in 1981, determinations of CO in the mainstream smoke were added. For all

Table 6.11 Tar, nicotine, CO, BaP, and NNK in the mainstream smoke of a leading US non-filter cigarette, 1959–1997[a]

Year	Tar (mg)	Nicotine (mg)	Carbon monoxide[b] (mg)	BaP (ng)	NNK[b] (ng)
1959	29.8	2.4		40	
1967	27.2	1.6		49	
1971	29.0	1.8		22	
1977	26.0	1.59		19	120
1981	24.3	1.52	16.7	19	130
1988	24	1.5	16	19	140
1991	25	1.7	16	18	190
1997	26	1.7	18	19	195

CO, carbon monoxide; NNK, 4-(methylnitrosamino)-1 -(3-pyridyl)-1 -butanone; BaP, benzo(a)pyrene.
[a] The analytical data were generated by smoking the leading US non-filter cigarette according to the FTC-mandated standard machine smoking method (Pillsbury et al. 1969).
[b] The open fields document the lack of analytical data for the years 1959,1967, 1971, and 1977 for CO and for 1959,1967, 1971 and 1977 for NNK.
From Wynder and Hoffmann (1960), Federal Trade Commission (1971, 1977, 1981, 1988, 1991, 1997), Hoffmann and Hoffmann (1997).

of these analyses, the MS was generated with the standardized machine smoking parameters that are mandated by the Federal Trade Commission. Table 6.11 documents the decline of tar levels, from 29.8 mg to 24.3 mg in the years between 1959 and 1984, while nicotine levels fell from 2.4 mg to 1.6 mg between 1959 and 1977. Since then, the smoke yields of tar and nicotine for this non-filter brand have not changed. Carbon monoxide has remained stable at 16–18 mg/cigarette since it was first reported in 1981. By 1997, it was clear that significant changes in the smoke yields of the major lung carcinogens BaP and NNK have occurred since 1977, in that BaP levels declined from 49 ng to 19 ng but NNK increased from 120 ng to 195 ng/non-filter cigarette.

It is important to note that we are lacking analytical data regarding the levels of these major carcinogens and toxins in the MS of leading cellulose acetate filter-tipped cigarettes with and without filter perforation, as well as in the MS of charcoal filter cigarettes. These cellulose acetate filter cigarettes were actually the ones dominating the US cigarette market as the use of cigarettes faded over the years and charcoal-filter cigarettes had only a modest market share. Most importantly, we are also lacking data on biological activities of the tars of leading brands of filter cigarettes produced since the 1960s, because tumourigenicity and carcinogenicity of tars have not been monitored on a regular basis. There is now also an urgent need for analytical profiles of the toxic and carcinogenic MS constituents that are generated under conditions reflecting the puff drawing profiles actually exhibited by humans who smoke these cigarettes with lower yields as per FTC measurements. Such analytical data would have to be established for major US cigarette brands manufactured since 1960. They would serve as the scientific basis in support of epidemiological observations regarding the risk of cancer of the lung and upper aerodigestive tract for smokers who have exclusively smoked filter-tipped brands, as compared to the risk for smokers who used non-filter cigarettes.

Changes in the agricultural, curing, and manufacturing processes of cigarettes have resulted in an increase in tobacco-specific nitrosamines in cigarette smoke that may have contributed to the increase in adenocarcinoma of the lung observed over the past several decades.

Conclusions

1. Major modifications in the make-up of the commercial cigarette were introduced between 1950 and 1975, but since that time there have been few substantive changes toward a further reduction of the toxic and carcinogenic potential of cigarette smoke.

2. A variety of changes in cigarette design and filtration have resulted in chemical changes in cigarette smoke, some of which have also demonstrated decreased toxicity in animal assays. Toxicity or carcinogenicity in animal assays has not been monitored to allow evaluation of changes over time that have occurred for cigarette smoke produced by commercial brands of cigarettes.

3. Changes in the agricultural, curing, and manufacturing processes of cigarettes have resulted in an increase over the past several decades in the amounts of tobacco-specific nitrosamines in cigarette smoke. These changes are considered to have contributed to the increase in adenocarcinoma of the lung observed over the past several decades.

4. On the basis of the standard machine-smoking method for cigarettes that has been mandated by the FTC, the sales-weighted average nicotine yields of US cigarettes decreased gradually from 2.7 mg/cigarette in 1953 to 0.85 mg by the mid-1990s. Today, the smoker of filter cigarettes will greatly increase his/her smoking intensity to satisfy an acquired need for nicotine. Thus, the inhaled smoke of one cigarette contains 2–3 times the amount of tar, nicotine, carbon monoxide, and 1.6–1.8 times the level of biomarkers for the major lung carcinogens BaP and NNK, compared to amounts in the smoke generated by the FTC method.

References

Anonymous (2000). Massachusetts disputes claims about Eclipse cigarettes. *Tobacco Reporter,* **127**(11):11–13.

Armitage, A.K. and Turner, D.H. (1970). Absorption of nicotine in cigarette and cigar smoke through the oral mucosa. *Nature (London),* **226**:1231–2.

Baker, R.R. (1984). The effect of ventilation on cigarette combustion mechanisms. *Recent Advances in Tobacco Science,* **10**:88–150.

Battista, S.P. (1976). Ciliatoxic components in cigarette smoke. In: E. L.Wynder, D. Hoffmann, and G. B. Gori (ed.) *Proceedings of the Third World Conference on Smoking and Health, New York, 2–5 June 1975. Vol. 1.Modifying the risk for the smoker.* US Department of Health, Education, and Welfare, Public Health Service, National Institutes of Health, National Cancer Institute.

Belinsky, S.A., Foley, J.F.,White, C.M., Anderson, M.W., and Maronpot, R. (1990). Dose–response relationship between O^6-methylguanine formation in Clara cells and induction of pulmonary neoplasia in the rat with 4-(methylnitrosamino)-1-(3-pyridyl)-1-butanone. *Cancer Research,* **50**(12):3772–80.

Benowitz, N.L. (1996). Biomarkers of cigarette smoking. *The FTC Cigarette Test Method for Determining Tar, Nicotine, and Carbon Monoxide Yields of U.S. Cigarettes. Report of the NCI Expert Committee.* Smoking and Tobacco Control Monograph No. 7. US Department of Health and Human services, National Institutes of Health, National Cancer Institute.

Benowitz, N.L. and Henningfield, J.E. (1994). Establishing a nicotine threshold for addiction. The implications for tobacco regulation. *New England Journal of Medicine,* **331**(2):123–5.

Benowitz, N.L., Hall, S.M., Herning, S.I., Jacob, P. III, Jones, R.T., and Osman, A.-L. (1983). Smokers of low yield cigarettes do not consume less nicotine during cigarette smoking. *New England Journal of Medicine,* **309**(3):139–42.

Benowitz, N.L., Jacob, P.J., Slade, J., and Yu, L. (1997). Nicotine content of the Eclipse nicotine delivery device. *American Journal of Public Health,* **87**(11):1865–6.

Bernfeld, P., Homberger, F., and Russfield, A.B. (1974). Strain differences in the response of inbred Syrian hamsters to cigarette smoke inhalation. *Journal of the National Cancer Institute*, **53**(4):1141–57.

Binder, H. and Lindner,W. (1972). Determination of ethylene oxide in the smoke of untreated cigarettes [in German]. *Fachliche Mitteilungen Austria Tabakwerke*, **13**:215–20.

Bock, F.G., Moore, G.E., Dowd, J.E. and Clark, P.C. (1962). Carcinogenic activity of cigarette smoke condensate. *Journal of the American Medical Association*, **181**:668–73.

Borgerding, M.F., Bodnar, J.A., Chung, H.L., Mangan, P.P., Morrison, C.C., Risner, C.H., *et al.* (1998). Chemical and biological studies of a new cigarette that primarily heats tobacco. Part 1. Chemical composition of mainstream smoke. *Food and Chemical Toxicology*, **36**(7):169–82.

Borgerding, M.F., Hicks, R.D., Bodnar, J.E., Riggs, D.M., Nanni, E.J., Fulp, G.W. Jr, *et al.* (1990*a*). Cigarette smoke composition. Part 1. Limitations of FTC method when applied to cigarettes that heat instead of burn tobacco. *Journal of the Association of Official Analytical Chemists*, **73**(4):605–9.

Borgerding, M.F., Milhous, L.A., Hicks, R.D., and Giles, J.A. (1990*b*). Cigarette smoke composition. Part 2.Method for determining major components in smoke of cigarettes that heat instead of burn tobacco. *Journal of the Association of Official Analytical Chemists*, **73**(4):610–15.

Bradford, J.A., Harlan,W.R., and Hanmer, H.R. (1936). Nature of cigarette smoke; technique of cigarette smoking. *Industrial Engineering and Chemistry*, **28**:836–9.

Brunnemann, K.D. and Hoffmann, D. (1974). Chemical studies on tobacco smoke. XXV. The pH of tobacco smoke. *Food and Cosmetics Toxicology*, **12**(1):115–24.

Brunnemann, K.D., Hoffmann, D. (1981). Chemical studies on tobacco smoke. LXIX. Assessment of the carcinogenic *N*-nitrosodiethanolamine in tobacco products and tobacco smoke. *Carcinogenesis*, **2**(11):1123–7.

Brunnemann, K.D. and Hoffmann, D. (1991). Analytical studies on *N*-nitrosamines in tobacco and tobacco smoke. *Recent Advances in Tobacco Science*, **17**:71–112.

Brunnemann, K.D., Yu, L., and Hoffmann, D. (1977). Chemical studies on tobacco smoke XVII. Assessment of carcinogenic volatile *N*-nitrosamines in mainstream and sidestream smoke from cigarettes. *Cancer Research*, **37**(9):3218–22.

Brunnemann, K.D., Masaryk, J., and Hoffmann, D. (1983). The role of tobacco stems in the formation of *N*-nitrosamines in tobacco and cigarette mainstream and sidestream smoke. *Journal of Agricultural and Food Chemistry*, **31**:1221–4.

Brunnemann, K.D., Hoffmann, D., Gairola, C.G., and Lee, B.C. (1994). Low ignition propensity cigarettes: smoke analysis for carcinogens and testing for mutagenic activity of the smoke particulate matter. *Food and Chemical Toxicology*, **32**(10):917–22.

Burton, H.R., Dye, N.K., and Bush, L.P. (1992). Distribution of tobacco constituents in tobacco leaf tissue. I. Tobacco-specific nitrosamines, nitrate, nitrite, and alkaloids. *Journal of Agricultural and Food Chemistry*, **40**:1050–5.

CORESTA (1991). Standard Smoking Methods 23: Determination of total and nicotine-free dry particulate matter using a routine analytical cigarette-smoking machine. Determination of total particulate matter and preparation for water and nicotine measurements. *CORESTA Information Bulletin*, **1991**–3:141–51.

Cox, J.D. and Yesner, R.A. (1979). Adenocarcinoma of the lung. Recent results from the Veterans Administration lung group. *American Review of Respiratory Disease*, **120**(5):1025–9.

Cundiff, R.H., Greene, G.H., and Laurene, A.H. (1964). Column elution of humectants from tobacco and determination by vapor chromatography. *Tobacco Science*, **8**:163–70.

Dalbey,W.E., Nettesheim, P., Griesemer, R., Caton, J.E., and Guerin, M.R. (1980). Chronic inhalation of cigarette smoke by F344 rats. *Journal of the National Cancer Institute*, **64**(2):383–90.

Davis, B.R., Whitehead, J.K., Gill, M.E., Lee, P.N., Butterworth, A.D., and Roe, F.J. (1975). Response of rat lung to tobacco smoke condensate or fractions derived from it ministered repeatedly by intratracheal installation. *British Journal of Cancer*, **31**(4):453–61.

DeBardeleben, M.Z., Claflin,W.E., and Gannon,W.F. (1978). Role of cigarette physical characteristics on smoke composition. *Recent Advances in Tobacco Science*, **4**:85–111.

DeBethizy, J.D., Borgerding, M.F., Doolittle, D.J., Robinson, J.H., McManus, K.T., Rahn, C.A., *et al.* (1990). Chemical and biological studies of a cigarette that heats rather than burns tobacco. *Journal of Clinical Pharmacology*, **30** (8): 755–63.

Devesa, S.S., Shaw, G.L., and Blot, W.J. (1991). Changing patterns of lung cancer incidence by histologic type. *Cancer Epidemiology Biomarkers and Prevention*, **1**(1): 29–34.

Djordjevic, M.V., Fan, J., Ferguson, S., and Hoffmann, D. (1995). Self-regulation of smoking intensity, smoke yields of low-nicotine, low 'tar' cigarettes. *Carcinogenesis*, **16**(9): 2015–21.

Djordjevic, M.V., Stellman, S.D., and Zang, E. (2000). Doses of nicotine and lung carcinogens delivered to cigarette smokers. *Journal of the National Cancer Institute*, **92**(2):106–11.

Doll, R. and Hill, A.B. (1950). Smoking and carcinoma of the lung. Preliminary report. *British Medical Journal*, **2**:739–48.

Dontenwill, W., Chevalier, H.J., Harke, H.-P., Lafrenz, U., Reckzeh, G., and Schneider, B. (1973). Investigations on the effects of chronic cigarette smoke inhalation in Syrian golden hamsters. *Journal of the National Cancer Institute*, **51**(6):1781–832.

Doull, J., Frawley, J.P., and George, W. (1994). List of ingredients added to tobacco in the manufacture of cigarettes by six major American cigarette companies. Covington and Burling, Washington, DC. [Reprinted: *Tobacco Journal International*, 196:32–9.]

Durocher, D.F. (1984). The choice of paper components for low-tar cigarettes. *Recent Advances in Tobacco Science*, **10**:52–71.

El-Bayoumy, K., Iatropoulos, M., Amin, S., Hoffmann, D., and Wynder, E.L. (1999). Increased expression of cyclooxygenase-2 in rat lung tumors induced by the tobacco-specific nitrosamine 4-(methylnitrosamine)-4-(3-pyridyl)-4-(3-pyridyl)-butanone: Impact of a high-fat diet. *Cancer Research*, **59**(7): 1400–3.

el-Torkey, M., el-Zeky, F., and Hall, J.C. (1990). Significant changes in the distribution of histologic types of lung cancer. A review of 4,928 cases. *Cancer*, **65**(10):2361–7.

Enzell, C. R. (1976). Terpenoid components of leaf and their relationship to smoking quality and aroma. *Recent Advances in Tobacco Science*, **2**:32–60.

Essenberg, J.M. (1952). Cigarette smoke and the incidence of primary neoplasm of the lung in the albino mouse. *Science*, **116**:561–2.

Federal Trade Commission (1971). *Report of 'Tar' and Nicotine Content of the Smoke of 121 Varieties of Cigarettes*. Federal Trade Commission, Washington, DC.

Federal Trade Commission (1977). *Report of 'Tar' and Nicotine Content of the Smoke of 166 Varieties of Cigarettes*. Federal Trade Commission, Washington, DC.

Federal Trade Commission (1981). *Report of 'Tar', Nicotine and Carbon Monoxide of the Smoke of 187 Varieties of Cigarettes*. Federal Trade Commission, Washington, DC.

Federal Trade Commission (1988). *Report of 'Tar', Nicotine and Carbon Monoxide of the Smoke of 272 Varieties of Domestic Cigarettes*. Federal Trade Commission, Washington, DC.

Federal Trade Commission (1991). *Tar, Nicotine, and Carbon Monoxide of the Smoke of 475 Varieties of Domestic Cigarettes*. Federal Trade Commission, Washington, DC.

Federal Trade Commission (1995). *Tar, Nicotine, and Carbon Monoxide of the Smoke of 1,107 Varieties of Domestic Cigarettes*. Federal Trade Commission, Washington, DC.

Federal Trade Commission (1997). *Tar, Nicotine, and Carbon Monoxide of the Smoke of 1,206 Varieties of Domestic Cigarettes*. Federal Trade Commission, Washington, DC.

Fisher, B. (2000). Filtering new technology. *Tobacco Reporter*, **127**(12):46–7.

Gardner, D.E. (ed.) (2000). A safer cigarette? *Inhalation Toxicology*, **12**(suppl. 5):1–58.

Gaworski, C.L., Dozier, M.M., Heck, J.D., Gerhard, J.M. Rajendran, N., David, R.M., *et al.* (1998). Toxicological evaluation of flavour ingredients added to cigarette tobacco: 13-week inhalation exposures in rats. *Inhalation Toxicology*, **10**:357–81.

Gellatly, G., and Uhl, R.G. (1978). Method for removal of potassium nitrate from tobacco extracts. US Patent 4,131,118, December 26, 1978.

Graham, E.A., Croninger, A.B., and Wynder, E.L. (1957). Experimental production of carcinoma with cigarette tar. IV. Successful experiments with rabbits. *Cancer Research*, 17:1058–66.

Green, C.R. and Rodgman, A. (1996). The Tobacco Chemists' Research Conference. A half-century of advances in analytical methodology of tobacco and its products. *Recent Advances in Tobacco Science*, 22:131–304.

Grimmer, G., Schneider, D., Naujack, K.-W., Dettbarn, G., and Jacob, J. (1995). Intercept-reactant method for the determination of aromatic amines in mainstream tobacco smoke. *Beitrage zur Tabakforschung International*, 16:141–56.

Gritz, E.R., Rose, J.E., and Jarvik, M.E. (1983). Regulation of tobacco smoke intake with paced cigarette presentation. *Pharmacology, Biochemistry, and Behavior*, 18:457–62.

Gutcho, S. (1972). *Tobacco flavoring substances and methods*. Noyes Data Corporation, Park Ridge, NJ.

Haag, H.B., Larson, P.S., and Finnegan, J.K. (1959). Effect of filtration on the chemical and irritating properties of cigarette smoke. *AMA Archives of Otolaryngology*, 69:261–5.

Halter, H.M. and Ito, T.I. (1979). Effect of reconstitution and expansion processes on smoke composition. *Recent Advances in Tobacco Science*, 4:113–32.

Hecht, S.S. (1998). Biochemistry, biology, and carcinogenicity of tobacco-specific *N*-nitrosamines. *Chemical Research in Toxicology*, 11(6):559–603.

Herning, R.I., Jones, R.T., Bachman, G., and Mines, A.H. (1981). Puff volume increases when low-nicotine cigarettes are smoked. *British Medical Journal (Clin Res Ed)*, 283(6285):187–9.

Hida, T., Yatabe, Y., Achiwa, H., Muramatsu, H., Kozaki, K-I., Makamura, S., *et al.* (1998). Increased expression of cyclooxygenase-2 occurs frequently in human lung cancers, especially in adenocarcinoma. *Cancer Research*, 58(17):3761–4.

Hoffmann, D. and Hecht, S.S. (1989). Advances in tobacco carcinogenesis. In: *Handbook of experimental pharmacology* (ed. C.S. Cooper and P.L. Grover). Springer Publications, New York.

Hoffmann, D. and Hoffmann, I. (1997). The changing cigarette, 1950–1995. *Journal of Toxicology and Environmental Health*, 50(4):307–64.

Hoffmann, D. and Wynder, E.L. (1963). Filtration of phenols from cigarette smoke. *Journal of the National Cancer Institute*, 30:67–84.

Hoffmann, D. and Wynder, E.L. (1967). The reduction in the tumorigenicity of cigarette smoke condensate by addition of sodium nitrate to tobacco. *Cancer Research*, 27(1):172–4.

Hoffmann, D. and Wynder, E.L. (1971). A study of tobacco carcinogenesis. XI. Tumor initiation, tumor acceleration, and tumor promoting activity of condensate fraction. *Cancer*, 27(4):848–64.

Hoffmann, D. and Wynder, E.L. (1977). Chemical analysis and carcinogenic bioassays of organic particulate pollutants. In: A. L. Stern (ed.), *Air pollution* pp. 361–455. Academic Press, New York.

Hoffmann, D., Sanghvi, L.D., and Wynder, E.L. (1974). Comparative chemical analysis of India bidi and American cigarette smoke. *International Journal of Cancer*, 14(1):49–53.

Hoffmann, D., Brunnemann, K.D., Prokopczyk, B., and Djordjevic, M.V. (1994). Tobacco-specific *N*-nitrosamines and *Areca*-derived *N*-nitrosamines. Chemistry, biochemistry, carcinogenicity, and relevance to humans. *Journal of Toxicology and Environmental Health*, 41(1):1–52.

Hoffmann, D., Hoffmann, I., and Wynder, E.L. (1998). The changing cigarette: 1950–1997: facts and expectations. In W. S. Rickert (ed.) *Report of Canada's Expert Committee on Cigarette Toxicity Reduction*. Health Canada, Toronto, Ontario, Canada.

International Agency for Research on Cancer (1982). Di(2-ethylhexyl)phthalate. *Some industrial chemicals and dyestuffs*. IARC Monographs on the Evaluation of Carcinogenic Risk of Chemicals to Humans 29, pp. 257–80. IARC, Lyon, France.

International Agency for Research on Cancer (1983). *Polynuclear aromatic compounds. Part 1. Chemical, environmental and experimental data*. IARC Monographs on the Evaluation of the Carcinogenic Risk of Chemicals to Humans 33. IARC, Lyon, France.

International Agency for Research on Cancer (1984). Coke production. *Polynuclear aromatic compounds, Part 3: Industrial exposure in aluminum production, coal gasification, coke production, and iron and steel founding.* IARC Monographs on the Evaluation of the Carcinogenic Risk of Chemicals to Humans 34, pp. 101–31. IARC, Lyon, France.

International Agency for Research on Cancer (1986*a*). *Tobacco smoking.* IARC Monographs on the Evaluation of Carcinogenic Risks to Humans 38. IARC, Lyon, France.

International Agency for Research on Cancer (1986*b*). Amino acid pyrolysis products in food. *Some naturally occurring and synthetic food components, furocoumarins, and ultraviolet radiation.* IARC Monographs on the Evaluation of Carcinogenic Risks to Humans 40, pp. 233–80. IARC, Lyon, France.

International Agency for Research on Cancer (1987). *Overall evaluation of carcinogenicity: An updating of IARC monographs 1 to 42.* IARC Monographs on the Evaluation of Carcinogenic Risks to Humans Suppl. 7. IARC, Lyon, France.

International Agency for Research on Cancer (1988). Radon. *Man-made mineral fibres and radon.* IARC Monographs on the Evaluation of Carcinogenic Risks to Humans 43, pp. 173–254. IARC, Lyon, France.

International Agency for Research on Cancer (1991). DDT and associated compounds. *Occupational exposures in insecticide application, and some pesticides.* IARC Monographs on the Evaluation of Carcinogenic Risks to Humans 53, pp. 179–249. IARC, Lyon, France.

International Agency for Research on Cancer (1992). 1,3-Butadiene. *Occupational exposures to mists and vapours from strong inorganic acids; and other industrial chemicals.* IARC Monographs on the Evaluation of Carcinogenic Risks to Humans 54, pp. 237–85. IARC, Lyon, France.

International Agency for Research on Cancer (1994*a*). Ethylene oxide. *Some industrial chemicals.* IARC Monographs on the Evaluation of Carcinogenic Risks to Humans 60, pp. 73–159. IARC, Lyon, France.

International Agency for Research on Cancer (1994*b*). Propylene oxide. *Some industrial chemicals.* IARC Monographs on the Evaluation of the Carcinogenic Risks of Chemicals to Humans 60, pp. 181–213. IARC, Lyon, France.

International Agency for Research on Cancer (1994*c*). Isoprene. *Some industrial chemicals.* IARC Monographs on the Evaluation of Carcinogenic Risks to Humans 60, pp. 215–32. IARC, Lyon, France.

International Agency for Research on Cancer (1994*d*). Styrene. *Some industrial chemicals.* IARC Monographs on the Evaluation of Carcinogenic Risks to Humans 60, pp. 233–320. IARC, Lyon, France.

International Agency for Research on Cancer (1994*e*) Acrylamide. *Some industrial chemicals.* IARC Monographs on the Evaluation of Carcinogenic Risks to Humans 60, pp. 389–433. IARC, Lyon, France.

International Agency for Research on Cancer (1995*a*). Furan. *Dry cleaning, some chlorinated solvents and other industrial chemicals.* IARC Monographs on the Evaluation of the Carcinogenic Risks to Humans 63, pp. 393–407. IARC, Lyon, France.

International Agency for Research on Cancer (1995*b*). Benzofuran. *Dry cleaning, some chlorinated solvents and other industrial chemicals.* IARC Monographs on the Evaluation of the Carcinogenic Risks to Humans 63, pp. 431–441. IARC, Lyon, France.

International Agency for Research on Cancer (1996). Nitrobenzene. *Printing processes and printing inks, carbon black and some nitro compounds.* IARC Monographs on the Evaluation of the Carcinogenic Risks to Humans 65, pp. 381–408. IARC, Lyon, France.

International Agency for Research on Cancer (1999*a*). 1,3-Butadiene. *Re-evaluation of some organic chemicals, hydrazine, and hydrogen peroxide.* IARC Monographs on the Evaluation of the Carcinogenic Risks to Humans 71, pp. 109–225. IARC, Lyon, France.

International Agency for Research on Cancer. (1999*b*). Acetaldehyde. *Re-evaluation of some organic chemicals, hydrazine, and hydrogen peroxide.* IARC Monographs on the Evaluation of the Carcinogenic Risks to Humans 71, pp. 319–44. IARC, Lyon, France.

International Agency for Research on Cancer (2000). Di(2-ethylhexyl)phthalate. *Some industrial chemicals.* IARC Monographs on the Evaluation of Carcinogenic Risk of Chemicals to Humans 77, pp. 41–148. IARC, Lyon, France.

International Committee for Cigar Smoking Study (1974). Machine smoking of cigars. *CORESTA Information Bulletin*, **1**:31–4.

International Standards Organization (1991). *Routine analytical cigarette smoking machine: Part I. Specifications and standard conditions*. ISO, Geneva, Switzerland.

Ishiguro, S. and Sugawara, S. (1980). The Chemistry of Tobacco Smoke [in Japanese; English translation 1981]. Central Institute, Japanese Tobacco Monopoly Corporation, Yokahama, Japan.

Jenkins, R.W.J., Neroman, P.H., and Charms, M.D. (1970). Cigarette smoke formation. II. Smoke distribution and mainstream pyrolytic composition of added 14C-menthol (U). *Beitrage zur Tabakforschung International*, **5**:299–301.

John, A.L. (1996). Japan. Always something new. *Tobacco International*, August, 30–5.

Kagan, M.R., Cunningham, J.A., and Hoffmann, D. (1999). Propylene glycol. A precursor of propylene oxide in cigarette smoke. *53rd Tobacco Science Research Conference*, Abstract Nos 41 and 42.

Kensler, C.J. and Battista, S.P. (1966). Chemical and physical factors affecting mammalian ciliary activity. *American Review of Respiratory Disease*, **93**(3):93–102.

Kite, G.F., Gellatly, G., and Uhl, R.G. (1978).Method for removal of potassium nitrate from tobacco extracts. US Patent 4,131,117, December 26.

Leffingwell, J.C. (ed.). (1987). Chemical and sensory aspects of tobacco flavor. *Recent Advances in Tobacco Science*, **14**:1–218.

Leuchtenberger, C. and Leuchtenberger, R. (1970). Effects of chronic inhalation of whole fresh cigarette smoke and of its gas phase on pulmonary tumorigenesis in Snell's mice. In: P. Nettesheim, M. G. Hanna Jr, and J.W. Deatherage Jr (eds) *Morphology of experimental respiratory carcinogenesis. Proceedings of a Biology Division, Oak Ridge National Laboratory, Conference, Gatlinburg, Tennesee, 13–16 May*, pp. 329–46. US Atomic Energy Commission, Washington, DC.

Leuchtenberger, C., Leuchtenberger, R., and Doolin, P.T. (1958). A correlated histological, cytological, and cytochemical study of tracheobronchial tree and lungs of mice exposed to cigarette smoke. *Cancer*, **11**:490–506.

Lewis, C.I. (1992). The effect of cigarette construction parameters on smoke generation and yield. *Recent Advances in Tobacco Science*, **16**:73–101.

Lyerly, L.A. (1967). Direct vapor chromatographic determination of menthol, propylene glycol, nicotine and triacetin in cigarette smoke. *Tobacco Science*, **11**:49–51.

Miller, J.E. (1963). Determination of the components of pipe tobacco smoke by means of a new pipe smoking machine. *Proceedings of the 3rd World Tobacco Congress, Salisbury, Rhodesia, CORESTA*, February, p. 11.

Mohr, U. and Reznik, G. (1978). Tobacco carcinogenesis. In C. C. Harris (ed.) *Pathogenesis and therapy of lung cancer*, pp. 263–361. Marcel Dekker, New York.

Moody, P.M. (1980). The relationships of qualified human smoking behavior and demographic variables. *Social Science and Medicine*, **14A**:49–54.

Mühlbock, O. (1958). Carcinogenicity of cigarette smoke in mice (Dutch). Nederlands Tijdschrift voor Geneeskunde, **99**:2276–8.

National Cancer Institute (1977*a*). *Tar and less hazardous cigarettes. First set of experimental cigarettes*. Smoking and Health Program. DHEW Publ. No. (NIH) 76–905.

National Cancer Institute (1977*b*). *Toward less hazardous cigarettes. Second set of experimental cigarettes*. Smoking and Health Program. DHEW Publ. No. (NIH) 76–111.

National Cancer Institute, Smoking and Health Program (1977*c*). *Toward less hazardous cigarettes. Third set of experimental cigarettes*. DHEW Publ. No. (NIH) 77–1280.

National Cancer Institute (1980). *Toward less hazardous cigarette. Fourth set of experimental cigarettes*. Smoking and Health Program. DHEW Publ. No. (NIH) 80.

National Cancer Institute (1998). Cigars: health effects and trends. In *Smoking and tobacco control monograph 9* (ed. D. M. Burns, D. Hoffmann, and K.M. Cummings). US DHHS, Public Health Service, NIH-NCI. NIH Publ. No. 98–1302, Bethesda, MD.

Neurath, G. (1972). Nitrosamine formation from precursors in tobacco smoke. In: P. Bogovski, R. Preussmann, and E. A.Walker (eds) *N-Nitroso compounds. Analysis and formation*. IARC Sci. Publ. 3, pp. 134–6. International Agency for Research on Cancer, Lyon, France.

Neurath, G. and Ehmke, H. (1964). Studies on the nitrate content of tobacco [in German]. *Beiträge zur Tabakforschung International*, **2**:333–44.

Nil, R., Buzzi, R., and Bättig, K. (1986). Effect of different cigarette smoke yields on puffing and inhalation. Is the measurement of inhalation volumes relevant for smoke absorption? *Pharmacology, Biochemistry, and Behavior*, **24**(3):587–95.

Norman,V., Ihrig, A.M., Larson, T.M., and Moss, B.L. (1983). The effect of nitrogenous blend components on NO/NO$_x$ and HCN levels in mainstream and sidestream smoke. *Beiträge zur Tabakforschung International*, **12**:55–62.

Norman,V., Ihrig, A.M., Shoffner, R.A., and Ireland, M.S. (1984). The effect of tip dilution on the filtration efficiency of upstream and downstream segments of cigarette filters. *Beiträge zur Tabakforschung International*, **12**:178–85.

Otto,H. (1963). Inhalation studies with mice exposed passively to cigarette smoke [in German]. *Frankfurter Zeitschrift für Pathologie*, **73**:10–23.

Owens,W.R., Jr. (1998). Effect of cigarette paper on smoke yield and composition. *Recent Advances in Tobacco Science*, **4**:3–24.

Patrianakos, C. and Hoffmann, D. (1979). Chemical studies on tobacco smoke. LXIV. On the analysis of aromatic amines in cigarette smoke. *Journal of Analytical Toxicology*, **3**:150–4.

Pauly, J.L., Lee, H.J., Hurley, E.L., Cummings, K.M., Lesser, J.D., and Streck, R.J. (1998). Glass fiber contamination of cigarette filters: an additional health risk to the smoker? *Cancer Epidemiology, Biomarkers and Prevention*, **7**(11):967–79.

Peel, D.M., Riddick, M.G., Edwards, M.E., Gentry, J.S., and Nestor, T.B. (1999). Formation of tobacco specific nitrosamines in flue-cured tobacco. Presented at the 53rd Tobacco Science Research Conference. Montreal, Quebec, Canada, 12–15 September.

Peeler, C.L. and Butters, G.R. (2000). Correspondence re: 'It's time for a change: cigarette smokers deserve meaningful information about their cigarettes'. *Journal of the National Cancer Institute*, **92**(10):842.

Philippe, R.J. and Hackney, E. (1959). The presence of nitrous oxide and methyl nitrite in cigarette smoke and tobacco pyrolysis gases. *Tobacco Science*, **3**:139–43.

Pillsbury, H.C., Bright, C.C., O'Connor, K.J., and Irish, F.W. (1969). Tar and nicotine in cigarette smoke. *Journal of the Association of Official Analytical Chemists*, **52**:458–62.

R. J. Reynolds Tobacco Company (1988). *New cigarette prototypes that heat instead of burn tobacco. Chemical and biological studies*. Reynolds Tobacco Co., Winston-Salem, NC.

Roberts, D.L. (1988). Natural tobacco flavor. *Recent Advances in Tobacco Science*, **14**:49–81.

Roberts,D.L. and Rowland, R.L. (1962). Macrocyclic diterpenes, α- and β-4,8,13-duvatriene-1,3-diol from tobacco. *Journal of Organic Chemistry*, **27**:3989–95.

Roe, J.F.C., Salaman, M.H. Cohen, J., and Burgan, J.C. (1959). Incomplete carcinogens in cigarette smoke condensate. Tumor promotion by phenolic fraction. *British Journal of Cancer*, **13**:623–33.

Rose, J.E. and Levin, E.D. (ed.) (1996). *Eclipse and the harm reduction strategy for smoking*. Conference, Duke University, Bryan Center, Durham, NC, 23 August.

Russell,M. A.H. (1976). Low-tar, medium nicotine cigarettes: A new approach to safer smoking. *British Medical Journal*, **6023**:1430–3.

Russell,M. A.H. (1980). The case for medium-nicotine, low-tar, low-carbon monoxide cigarettes. *Banbury Report 3*, pp. 297–310. Cold Spring Harbor, Cold Spring Harbor Laboratory, NY.

Schultz,W. and Seehofer, F. (1978). Smoking behavior in Germany. The analysis of cigarette butts. In: *Smoking behavior, physiological and psychological influences*, (ed. R.E. Thornton), pp. 259–76. Churchill Livingston, Edinburgh.

Schumacher, J.N. (1970). The isolation of 6-O-acetyl-2,3,4-tri-O-[(+)-3 methylvaleryl]-β-D-glucopyranose from tobacco. *Carbohydrate Research*, **13**:1–8.

Senkus, M. (ed.) (1976). Leaf composition and physical properties in relation to smoking quality and aroma. *Recent Advances in Tobacco Science,* **2**:1–135.

Shepherd, R.J.K. (1994). New charcoal filters. *Tobacco Reporter,* **121**(2):10–14.

Sims, J.L., Atkinson,W.D., and Benner, P. (1975). Nitrogen fertilization and genotype effects of selected constituents from all-burley cigarettes. *Tobacco Science,* **23**:11–13.

Singer, B. and Essigmann, J.M. (1991). Site-specific mutagenesis: Retrospective and prospective. *Carcinogenesis,* **12**(6):945–55.

Smith, C.J., McCarns, S.C., Davis, R.A., Livingston, S.D., Bombick, B.R., Avolos, J.T., *et al.* (1996). Human urine mutagenicity study comparing cigarettes which burn or primarily heat tobacco. *Mutation Research,* **361**(1):1–9.

Society for Research on Nicotine and Tobacco (2000). Policy committee urges regulation on Eclipse. *SRNT Newsletter,* **6**(2–3):21–2.

Spears, A.W. (1974). Effect of manufacturing variables in cigarette smoke composition. *CORESTA Bulletin* Montreux, Switzerland, Symp. p. 6.

Spears, A.W. (1963). Selective filtration of volatile phenolic compounds from cigarette smoke. *Tobacco Science,* **7**:76–80.

Spears, A.W. and Jones, S.T. (1981). Chemical and physical criteria for tobacco leaf of modern day cigarettes. *Recent Advances in Tobacco Science,* **7**:19–39.

Stedman, R.L., Burdick, D., and Schmeltz, I. (1963). Composition studies on tobacco. XVII. Steam-smoke, volatile acid fraction of cigarette. *Tobacco Science,* **7**:166–9.

Stellman, S.D., Muscat, J.E., Thompson, S., Hoffmann, D., and Wynder, E.L. (1997). Risk of squamous cell carcinoma and adenocarcinoma of the lung in relation to lifetime filter cigarette smoking. *Cancer,* **80**(3):362–8.

Stiles, M.F., Guy, T.D., Morgen,W.T., Edwards, D.W., Davis, R.W., and Robinson, J.H. (1999). Human smoking behavior study. ECLIPSE cigarette compared to usual brand. *Toxicologist,* **48**:119–20.

Terpstra, P.M., Renninghaus,W., and Solana, R.P. (1998). Evaluation of the electrically heated cigarette, *The Toxicologist. Toxicological Sciences,* **42**(1S):295; Abstract 1452.

Terrell, J.H. and Schmeltz, I. (1970). Alteration of cigarette smoke composition. II. Influence of cigarette design. *Tobacco Science,* **14**:82–5.

Tiggelbeck, D. (1976). Vapor phase modification. An under-utilized technology. *Proceedings of the 3rd World Conference on Smoking and Health.* Vol. 1, *Modifying the Risk for the Smoker.* DHEW Publ. No. (NIH) 76–1221, pp. 507–14.

Törnqvist, M., Osterman-Golkar, S., Kautiainen, A., Jensen, S., Farmer, P.B., and Ehrenberg, L. (1986). Tissue doses of ethylene oxide in cigarette smokers determined from adduct levels in hemoglobin. *Carcinogenesis,* **7**(9):1519–21.

Tso, T.C. (1990). *Production, physiology and biochemistry of tobacco Plant.* Ideals, Beltsville, MD.

Tso, T.C., Chaplin, J.P., Adams, J.D., and Hoffmann, D. (1982). Simple correlation and multiple regression among leaf and smoke characteristics of burley tobaccos. *Beiträge zur Tabakforschung International,* **11**:141–50.

Tsuda, M. and Kurashima, Y. (1991). Tobacco smoking, chewing and snuff dipping. Factors contributing to the endogenous formation of *N*-nitroso compounds. *Critical Reviews in Toxicology,* **21**(4): 243–53.

US Consumer Product Safety Commission (1993). *Practicability of developing a performance standard to reduce cigarette ignition propensity,* Vol. 1. USCPSC, Washington, DC.

US Department of Health and Human Services (1989). *Reducing the health consequences of smoking. 25 Years of progress.* A Report of the Surgeon General of the Public Health Service, Rockville, MD. DHHS Publ. No. (CDC) 89–8411.

Vincent, R.G., Pickren, J.W., Lane,W.W., Bross, I., Takita, H., Haten, L., *et al.* (1977). The changing histopathology of lung cancer. *Cancer,* **39**(4):1647–55.

Voges, E. (1984). *Tobacco encyclopedia.* Tobacco Journal International, Mainz, Germany.

Waltz, P. and Häusermann, M. (1963). Modern cigarettes and their effects on the smoking habits and on the composition of cigarette smoke [in German]. *Zeitschrift fur Präventivmedizin,* **8**:3–98.

Wilkenfeld, J., Henningfield, J., Slade, J., Burns, D., Pinney, J. (2000*a*). It's time for a change: cigarette smokers deserve meaningful information about their cigarettes. *Journal of the National Cancer Institute,* **92**(2):90–2.

Wilkenfeld, J., Henningfield, J., Slade, J., Burns, D., and Pinney, J. (2000*b*). Response to correspondence re: 'It's time for a change: cigarette smokers deserve meaningful information about their cigarettes'. *Journal of the National Cancer Institute,* **92**(2): 842–3.

Wittekindt,W. (1985). Changes in recommended plant protection agents for tobacco. *Tobacco Journal International,* **5**: 390–4.

Wynder, E.L. and Graham, E.A. (1950). Tobacco smoking as a possible etiologic factor in bronchiogenic carcinoma. A study of six hundred and eighty-four proved cases. *Journal of the American Medical Association,* **143**, 329–36 [reprinted in *Journal of the American Medical Association,* **253**(20): 2986–94].

Wynder, E.L., Graham, E.A., and Croninger, A.G. (1953). Experimental production of carcinoma with cigarette tar. *Cancer Research,* **13**: 855–64.

Wynder, E.L. and Hoffmann, D. (1960). Some practical aspects of the smoking—cancer problem. *New England Journal of Medicine,* **262**: 540–5.

Wynder, E.L. and Hoffmann, D. (1961). A study of tobacco carcinogenesis. VIII. The role of acidic fractions as promoters. *Cancer,* **14**: 1306–15.

Wynder, E.L. and Hoffmann, D. (1962). A study of air pollution carcinogenesis. III. Carcinogenic activity of gasoline engine exhaust. *Cancer,* **152**: 103–8.

Wynder, E.L. and Hoffmann, D. (1963). A contribution to experimental tobacco carcinogenesis [in German]. *Deut.Med.Wochenschr.,* **88**: 623–8.

Wynder, E.L. and Hoffmann, D. (1965). Reduction of tumorigenicity of tobacco smoke. An experimental approach. *Journal of the American Medical Association,* **192**: 85–94.

Wynder, E.L. and Hoffmann, D. (1967). *Tobacco and tobacco smoke. Studies in experimental carcinogenesis.* Academic Press, New York.

Wynder, E.L. and Hoffmann, D. (1994). Smoking and lung cancer: scientific challenges and opportunities. *Cancer Research,* **54**(20): 5284–95.

Wynder, E.L. and Mann, J. (1957). A study of tobacco carcinogenesis III. Filtered cigarettes. *Cancer,* **10**:1201–5.

Wynder, E.L., Kopf, P., and Ziegler, H. (1957). A study of tobacco carcinogenesis. II. Dose–response studies. *Cancer,* **10**:1193–200.

Chapter 7

Tobacco carcinogenesis: mechanisms and biomarkers

Stephen S. Hecht

Introduction

Why would anyone want to study mechanisms of tobacco carcinogenesis, when it is axiomatic that tobacco products cause about 3000 lung cancer deaths per day and 30% of all cancer mortality? By understanding mechanisms and developing relevant tobacco carcinogen biomarkers, we gain new insights for prevention of tobacco-induced cancer. Presently, we cannot predict which smoker will get cancer. If we could do that by identifying such susceptible individuals at a relatively young age, we could focus preventive efforts on those at high risk, arguably decreasing the huge toll of tobacco-related death.

The indisputable relationship between the world's most widespread exogenous chemical carcinogen exposure – tobacco smoke – and cancer, provides a framework for a better understanding of cancer mechanisms in general, particularly the interaction between carcinogen exposure and host factors, and for the development of novel preventive and therapeutic strategies. Furthermore, the biomarkers that are developed in this research can be applied in the approaching era of tobacco product regulation. In this chapter, mechanisms of tumour induction by tobacco carcinogens are discussed, and the status of tobacco carcinogen biomarkers is presented.

Overview of mechanisms of tumour induction by tobacco products

A conceptual model outlining mechanisms by which cigarette smoke causes cancer is shown in Fig. 7.1 [1, 2]. The major established pathway is summarized in the central track. Smokers inhale carcinogens which, either directly or after metabolism, covalently bind to DNA, forming 'DNA adducts'. DNA adducts are the hallmarks of chemical carcinogenesis because they can cause miscoding and permanent mutations. If these mutations occur in critical regions of important growth control genes such as oncogenes and tumour suppressor genes, the result can be loss of normal cellular growth control mechanisms, genomic instability, and cancer. A recent study validated this premise by finding multiple mutations in critical growth control genes in lung adenocarcinoma [3]. We will now consider each step of the conceptual model in more detail.

Most people begin smoking when they are teenagers. They become addicted to nicotine and cannot stop smoking in spite of their best intentions and efforts. Although many reports have described adverse cellular effects of nicotine, particularly with respect to uncontrolled growth, nicotine is not a carcinogen. However, it is accompanied in each puff of smoke by a complex mixture of carcinogens. As discussed in Chapter 6 of this book, there are over 60 carcinogens in cigarette smoke that have been evaluated by the International Agency for Research on Cancer (IARC) as having sufficient evidence for carcinogenicity. These carcinogens belong to a variety of chemical classes such as polycyclic aromatic hydrocarbons (PAH), typified by benzo[a]pyrene (BaP),

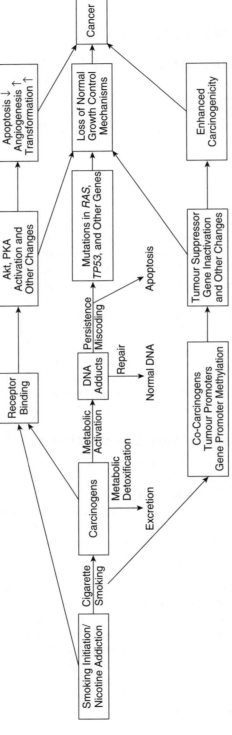

Figure 7.1 Conceptual model for understanding mechanisms of tobacco carciogenesis.

nitrosamines such as the tobacco-specific nitrosamines 4-(methylnitrosamino)-1-(3-pyridyl)-1-butanone (NNK) and *N*'-nitrosonornicotine (NNN), aromatic amines such as the well-known human bladder carcinogens 4-aminobiphenyl and 2-naphthylamine, aldehydes such as acetaldehyde and formaldehyde, volatile organic compounds such as benzene, 1,3-butadiene, and ethylene oxide, and other compounds including metals and the radioactive element [210]Po. Sixteen of these carcinogens, including BaP, NNK, NNN, 4-aminobiphenyl, 2-naphthylamine, formaldehyde, 1,3-butadiene, cadmium, and [210]Po are considered by IARC as carcinogenic to humans. There are also other carcinogens in cigarette smoke that have not been evaluated by IARC. Structures of tobacco smoke constituents and biomarkers discussed in this chapter are presented in Fig. 7.2.

Convincing studies demonstrate the uptake of these carcinogens by smokers, and confirm the expected higher levels of their metabolites in urine and blood of smokers than non-smokers. There are large differences in carcinogen exposure among people because of the number and types of cigarettes that they smoke and the ways in which they smoke them. These differences can be monitored in part by biomarkers of exposure such as those discussed in the section of this chapter on urinary metabolites as tobacco carcinogen biomakers. In one notable series of recent studies,

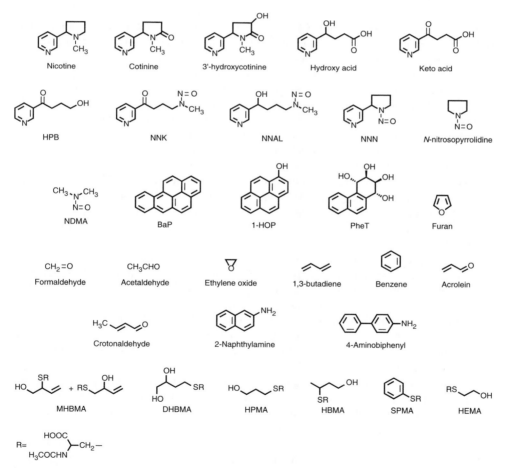

Figure 7.2 Structures of compounds discussed in this chapter.

polymorphisms in nicotinic receptor genes were associated with increased lung cancer risk due to increased uptake of nicotine and consequent increased exposure to carcinogens [4–7].

The body's response to cigarette smoke constituents is similar to its response to pharmaceutical agents and other 'foreign compounds'. Drug metabolizing enzymes, most frequently cytochrome P450s (P450s), convert these compounds to more water soluble forms facilitating excretion. But during this natural protective attempt, some reactive intermediates are formed. These intermediates are generally electrophilic (electron seeking, or bearing a partial or full positive charge). These electrophilic intermediates may react with water, generally resulting in detoxification, or may covalently bind to nucleophilic (electron rich) sites in DNA, forming DNA adducts [8, 9], which are absolutely critical in the carcinogenic process. Examples of DNA adduct formation from tobacco smoke carcinogens are given later in this chapter. P450s 1A1 and 1B1, repeatedly shown to be inducible by cigarette smoke via interactions of smoke compounds with the aryl hydrocarbon receptor [10,11], are particularly important in the metabolic activation of PAH, while P450 2A13 is critical for the metabolism of NNK [9,12]. The inducibility of certain P450s may be a critical aspect of cancer susceptibility in smokers. P450s 1A2, 2A6, 2E1, and 3A4 are also important in the metabolism of cigarette smoke carcinogens to DNA binding intermediates, and aldo-keto redcutase (AKR) enzymes, also induced by tobacco smoke [13], are involved in the metabolism of NNK and other tobacco smoke carcinogens. Competing with this process of 'metabolic activation' resulting in DNA binding is the intended metabolic detoxification, which leads to harmless excretion of carcinogen metabolites, and is also catalysed by P450s and a variety of other enzymes including glutathione-*S*-transferases, UDP-glucuronosyl transferases, and aryl-sulfatases [14,15]. The relative amounts of carcinogen metabolic activation and detoxification differ among individuals. It is widely hypothesized that this balance will affect cancer risk with those having higher activation and lower detoxification capacity being the most susceptible. This premise is supported in part by molecular epidemiologic studies of polymorphisms, or variants in more than 1% of the population, in the genes coding for these enzymes [16].

There is no reason to doubt that DNA adducts are critical in carcinogenesis. Many investigations demonstrate the presence of DNA adducts in human tissues, and some of these are summarized in the section of this chapter on carcinogen-DNA abducts as biomakers. There is massive evidence, particularly from studies which use relatively non-specific DNA adduct measurement methods, that DNA adduct levels in the lung and other tissues of smokers are higher than in non-smokers, and some epidemiologic data link these higher adduct levels to increased cancer risk [17, 18]. However, as also discussed later, there is much more limited evidence from studies using specific carcinogen-derived DNA adducts as biomarkers.

Cellular DNA repair systems can excise DNA adducts and restore normal DNA structure. These complex multiple systems include direct base repair by alkyltransferases, removal of DNA damage by base and nucleotide excision repair, mismatch repair, and double strand repair. If these DNA repair systems are unsuccessful in fixing the damage, then the DNA adducts can persist, increasing the probability of a permanent mutation. There are polymorphisms in genes coding for some DNA repair enzymes. If these variants lead to deficient DNA repair, the probability of cancer development can increase [19].

DNA adducts can cause miscoding during replication when DNA polymerase enzymes misread the DNA adduct and consequently insert the wrong base opposite to it. There is some specificity in the relationship between specific DNA adducts formed from cigarette smoke carcinogens and the types of mutations which they cause. G to T and G to A mutations have often been observed [1]. Extensive studies using state-of-the-art molecular biology techniques have characterized the mutations which occur because of specific carcinogen-DNA adducts [20]. As mentioned earlier, mutations have been reported in the *KRAS* oncogene in lung cancer and in the *p53* tumour suppressor gene in a variety of cigarette smoke-induced cancers [3, 21, 22]. The cancer causing role of these genes has been firmly established in animal studies [23, 24].

In addition to mutations, numerous cytogenetic changes are observed in lung cancer, and chromosome damage throughout the field of the aerodigestive tract is strongly associated with cigarette smoke exposure. Mutations resulting from DNA adducts can cause loss of normal cellular growth control functions, via a complex process of signal transduction pathways, ultimately resulting in genomic instability, cellular proliferation and cancer [3,25,26]. Apoptosis, or programmed cell death, is a protective process, and can remove cells which have DNA damage, thus serving as a counterbalance to these mutational events. The balance between apoptotic mechanisms and those suppressing apoptosis will have a major impact on tumour growth [26].

While the central track of Fig. 7.1 is the major pathway by which cigarette smoke carcinogens cause cancer, epigenetic mechanisms also contribute, as indicated in the top and bottom tracks [2, 27]. Nicotine, NNK, and NNN bind to nicotinic and other cellular receptors resulting in activation of Akt (also known as protein kinase B), protein kinase A, and other changes. This can cause decreased apoptosis, increased angiogenesis, and increased transformation [28, 29]. Although nicotine is not carcinogenic, it may enhance carcinogenicity in as yet undefined ways. Cigarette smoke activates the epidermal growth factor receptor and cyclooxygenase-2 [30], and contains well-established oxidants, co-carcinogens, tumour promoting fractions, and inflammatory agents. Many studies demonstrate the co-carcinogenic and cytotoxic effects of catechol, an important constituent of cigarette smoke. Another epigenetic pathway frequently observed in tobacco-induced cancers is enzymatic methylation of promoter regions of genes, resulting in gene silencing. When this occurs in tumour suppressor genes, the result can be unregulated proliferation [31]. Furthermore, inflammation due to smoking is associated with tumour promotion and cancer development.

Diverse tobacco carcinogens form DNA adducts

In this section, we focus on the formation of DNA adducts, which, as described earlier, are central to cancer causation in smokers. Many of the carcinogens in cigarette smoke require metabolic activation for DNA binding, but some can form adducts without metabolism. Figure 7.3 presents an overview of metabolism and DNA adduct formation from eight tobacco smoke constituents (clockwise from top left): BaP, NNK, N-nitrosodimethylamine (NDMA), NNN, acrolein, ethylene oxide, acetaldehyde, and 4-aminobiphenyl. There is evidence for DNA adduct formation from each of these carcinogens, based on studies of smokers' tissues or blood cells.

The major metabolic activation pathway of BaP leading to DNA adduct formation in human tissues is conversion to mutagenic 'bay region' diol epoxides. Competing with BaP metabolic activation reactions are detoxification reactions which produce phenols, dihydrodiols, and glutathione, glucuronide, and sulphate conjugates. Quinone metabolites are also commonly observed, and they result from initial 6-hydroxylation followed by further oxidation [32, 33].

The major metabolic activation pathways of NNK and its metabolite, 4-(methylnitrosamino)-1-(3-pyridyl)-1-butanol (NNAL), are hydroxylation of the carbons next to the N-nitroso group (α-hydroxylation) leading, via diazonium ions, to DNA adducts [34]. Glucuronidation of NNAL, at either the hydroxyl group or the nitrogen atom of the pyridine ring, and pyridine-N-oxidation of NNK and NNAL are detoxification pathways [34].

Metabolic activation of NDMA by α-hydroxylation leads to the unstable α-hydroxyNDMA. This metabolite spontaneously loses formaldehyde producing diazonium ions that react with DNA resulting in DNA adducts such as 7-methyldeoxyguanosine (7-methyl-dG) and O^6-methyl-dG. Denitrosation, which produces nitrite and methylamine, is a detoxification pathway [35].

α-Hydroxylation of NNN produces reactive diazonium ions and consequent DNA adducts. β-Hydroxylation of NNN, a minor metabolic pathway, and pyridine-N-oxidation, are

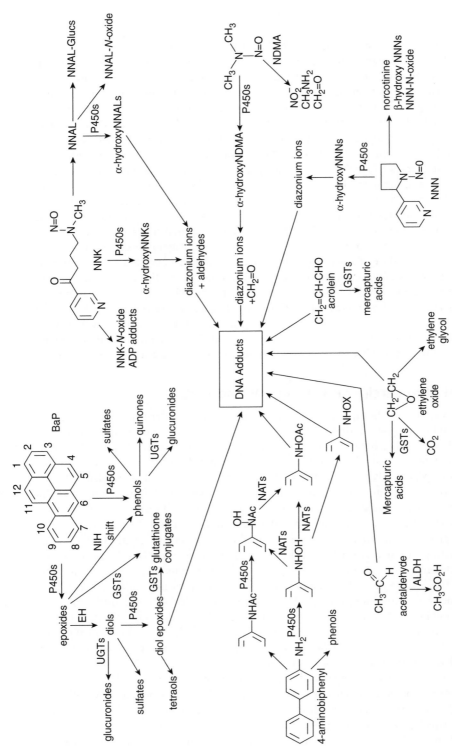

Figure 7.3 Overview of metabolism and DNA adduct formation from eight tobacco smoke constituents.

Sources: Adapted from references 1, 32, 34, 35, 37, 40.

Note

Abbreviations (in alphabetical order): 4-ABP = 4-aminobiphenyl; Ac = acetyl; ADP = adenosine diphosphate; ALDH = aldehyde dehydrogenase; B[a]P = benzo[a]pyrene; EH = epoxide hydrolase; Gluc = glucuronide; GSTs = glutathione S-transferases; NATs = N-acetyltransferases; NDMA = N-nitrosodimethylamine; NIH shift = phenomenon of epoxidation-induced intramolecular migration; NNAL = 4-(methylnitrosamino)-1-(3-pyridyl)-1-butanol; NNK = 4-(methylnitrosamino)-1-(3-pyridyl)-1-butanone; NNN = N'-nitrosonornicotine; NNN = N'-nitrosonornicotine; P450s = cytochrome P450 enzymes; UGTs = uridine-5'-diphosphate-glucuronosyl transferases detoxification reactions. NNN is also detoxified by denitrosation/oxidation yielding norcotinine, and by glucuronidation of the pyridine ring [34, 36].

Acrolein, ethylene oxide, and acetaldehyde all react directly with DNA to form well-characterized adducts [37–39]. There are competing metabolic detoxification pathways involving glutathione conjugation and, in the case of acetaldehyde, oxidation.

4-Aminobiphenyl is metabolically activated to reactive electrophiles by initial N-hydroxylation [40]. Conjugation of the resulting hydroxylamine with acetate or other groups such as sulphate ultimately results in the production of nitrenium ions which react with DNA producing adducts mainly at C-8 of dG. Other aromatic amines and heterocyclic aromatic amines are metabolically activated in similar ways. Acetylation of 4-aminobiphenyl can be a detoxification pathway if it is not followed by N-hydroxylation. Ring hydroxylation and conjugation of the phenolic metabolites results in detoxification [40].

The structures of DNA adducts of tobacco smoke carcinogens have been characterized in detail, and a complete accounting of these structures is beyond the scope of this chapter. Some of these adduct structures are illustrated in Fig. 7.4. The major DNA adduct formed from BaP (and several other PAH) results from trans-addition of BPDE to the N^2-position of dG [41]. Pyridyloxobutyl (POB)-DNA adducts of NNK and NNN are formed at the 7- and O^6-positions of dG, the O^2-position of thymidine, and the O^2-position of deoxycytidine [42]. Metabolic activation of NNK also results in the formation of 7-methyl-dG and O^6-methyl-dG, identical to the DNA adducts formed from NDMA (and other DNA methylating agents) [42]. Ethylating agents and ethylene oxide in cigarette smoke also alkylate dG [43, 44]. Acrolein and its homologue crotonaldehyde react with DNA to produce exocyclic $1,N^2$-dG adducts, while acetaldehyde forms a Schiff base adduct with the exocyclic (N^2) amino group of dG [38, 45]. There is evidence for the presence of all these DNA adducts in tissues or blood cells of smokers, but there are also many negative studies in which these specific adducts have been analysed for but not found [46, 47].

In summary, the major pathways of metabolic activation and detoxification of some of the most important carcinogens in cigarette smoke are well established. Reactive intermediates

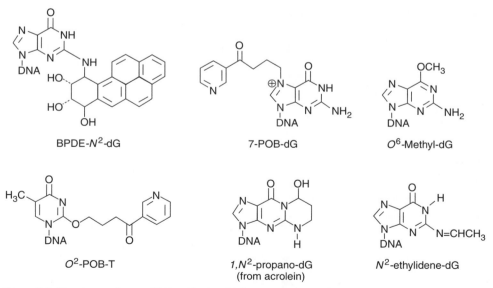

Figure 7.4 Structures of some DNA adducts of tobacco smoke carcinogens.

critical in forming DNA adducts include diol epoxides of PAH, diazonium ion products of nitrosamine α-hydroxylation, and nitrenium ions produced from esters of N-hydroxylated aromatic amines. Some other cigarette smoke compounds such as ethylene oxide, acrolein, and acetaldehyde react directly with DNA to form adducts. Glutathione and glucuronide conjugation are particularly important in the detoxification of cigarette smoke carcinogens.

Certain carcinogens are implicated in cancers caused by tobacco products

Data from product analyses, carcinogenicity studies, and biochemical and molecular biological investigations implicate certain carcinogens in specific types of tobacco-induced cancer, as summarized in Table 7.1. This represents a weight of the evidence approach. Proof of causation is difficult due to the complexity of tobacco smoke.

Substantial data support PAH and NNK as major causative agents for lung cancer. Many PAH are potent locally acting carcinogens, and tobacco smoke fractions enriched in these compounds cause lung tumours [48, 49]. PAH-DNA adducts have been detected in human lung, and the spectrum of mutations in the *p53* tumour suppressor gene isolated from lung tumours is similar to the spectrum of DNA damage produced in vitro by PAH diol epoxide metabolites and in cell culture by BaP (although a similar spectrum is produced by acrolein) [21, 46, 50, 51].

NNK is a potent lung carcinogen in rodents, inducing lung tumours systemically [34]. NNK is particularly strong in the rat, in which total doses as low as 6 mg/kg (and 1.8 mg/kg when considered as part of a dose-response trend) have induced lung tumours in significant numbers [52]. This compares to an estimated 1.1 mg/kg total dose of NNK in smokers [34]. DNA adducts of NNK and NNN are present in lung tissue from smokers [53–55], and metabolites of NNK are found in the urine and blood of smokers [56]. Other compounds that may

Table 7.1 Relationship of carcinogens to specific cancers

Cancer type	Likely carcinogen involvement[a]
Lung	PAH, NNK (major)
	1,3-butadiene, isoprene, ethylene oxide, ethyl carbamate, aldehydes, benzene, metals
Larynx	PAH
Nasal	NNK, NNN, other *N*-nitrosamines, aldehydes
Oral cavity	PAH, NNK, NNN
Oesophagus	NNN, other *N*-nitrosamines
Liver	NNK, other *N*-nitrosamines, furan
Pancreas	NNK, NNAL
Cervix	PAH, NNK
Bladder	4-aminobiphenyl, other aromatic amines
Leukaemia	benzene

Note

[a] Based on carcinogenicity studies in laboratory animals, biochemical evidence from human tissues and fluids, and epidemiological data, where available. NNAL, 4-(methylnitrosamino)-1-(3-pyridyl)-1-butanol; NNK, 4-(methylnitrosamino)-1-(3-pyridyl)-1-butanone; NNN, *N*'-nitrosonornicotine; PAH, polycyclic aromatic hydrocarbons. Adapted from US Surgeon General's Report 2010, in preparation.

contribute to lung cancer include 1,3-butadiene, ethylene oxide, aldehydes, benzene, metals, and oxidants but the collective evidence for each of these agents is not as convincing as for PAH and NNK [1, 57].

Cigarette smoke particulate phase causes tumours of the larynx in hamsters. This is most likely attributed to PAH [58], and is consistent with *p53* gene mutations identified in human larynx tumours [21]. *N*-Nitrosamines, as well as acetaldehyde and formaldehyde, cause nasal tumours in rodents and are the most likely causes of smoking associated nasal tumours [35] while, based on animal studies, PAH, NNK, and NNN are the most likely causes of oral cancer in smokers [59, 60]. *N*-Nitrosamines are the most effective oesophageal carcinogens known, and NNN, which causes oesophageal tumours in rats at relatively low doses, is the most prevalent of these carcinogens in cigarette smoke [60].

The nitrosamines NNK, NDMA, and *N*-nitrosopyrrolidine, as well as furan, are effective hepatocarcinogens in rats [35]. NNK and its metabolite NNAL are the only pancreatic carcinogens known to be present in tobacco products, and biochemical data from studies with human tissues provide some support for their role in smoking-related pancreatic cancer, although DNA adducts were not detected [61–63].

4-Aminobiphenyl and 2-naphthylamine are acknowledged human bladder carcinogens, and considerable data support their role, along with other aromatic amines, as causes of bladder cancer in smokers [64, 65]. Benzene is the most probable cause of leukaemia in smokers because it occurs in substantial quantities in cigarette smoke and is a known cause of acute myelogenous leukaemia in humans [66]. Formaldehyde is another potential cause of leukaemia in smokers [67].

Cigarette smoke causes oxidative damage, probably because it contains free radicals such as nitric oxide as well as mixtures of catechols, hydroquinones, semiquinones, and quinones which can induce redox cycling [1, 68]. Smokers have lower levels of ascorbic acid, higher levels of oxidized lipids, and sometimes higher levels of oxidized DNA bases such as 8-oxo-dG, than non-smokers but the role of oxidative damage as a cause of specific tobacco-induced cancers remains speculative [1, 69].

Some unanswered questions concerning mechanisms of tobacco carcinogenesis

There is no doubt that tobacco smoke carcinogens and their DNA adducts play a critical role in cancer induction by tobacco products. Mountains of bedrock evidence support this conclusion. But there are still some uncertainties. One involves dose. The strongest and well-established carcinogens – PAH, nitrosamines such as NNN and NNK, and aromatic amines – are present in cigarette smoke in relatively low quantities, typically 10–100 ng per cigarette while weaker carcinogens such as acetaldehyde are present in larger quantities of nearly 1 mg per cigarette. Which is more important – quantity or quality? A second question involves gas phase vs. particulate phase carcinogens. There is evidence in the literature that both are important, based on inhalation studies with rodents [70]. Which are more important in smokers – particulate phase carcinogens such as BaP, NNN, and NNK, or gas phase carcinogens such as benzene and 1,3-butadiene? One conclusion comes from a consideration of these complexities – it is very unlikely that one could design a safer combusted product by simply decreasing or eliminating one type of carcinogen.

It is also necessary to look beyond carcinogens and their genotoxic effects, and to consider more thoroughly the top and bottom tracks of Fig. 7.1. Prominent among these considerations is the role of tumour promotion and inflammation. We know from classic animal experiments – both inhalation and skin painting – that cigarette smoke and its condensate have tumour promoting activity, and there can be little doubt based on biomarker and other evidence that inflammation plays a significant role in the development of lung cancer and possibly other cancers by cigarette smoke [48, 71]. The reversibility of cancer risk upon smoking cessation, although slow, is completely consistent with what we know about tumour promotion and inflammation, yet overall our knowledge of these aspects of tobacco-induced cancer lags far behind our understanding of carcinogen induced events.

Furthermore, many recent studies demonstrate potentially damaging effects of nicotine and tobacco carcinogens, particularly NNK and NNN, that are apparently independent of their genotoxic effects and may contribute in important ways to cancer induction. These studies also raise some questions about the safety of nicotine replacement therapy.

Tobacco carcinogen biomarkers for investigating human carcinogen exposure and cancer susceptibility

Tobacco carcinogen biomarkers are quantifiable entities that can be *specifically* related to tobacco carcinogens. Specificity to a given carcinogen is critical because tobacco carcinogens vary widely in their potency and target organs. Lack of specificity can lead to misleading results and conclusions.

Considering the mechanistic framework outlined in Fig. 7.1, one could visualize various types of biomarkers. Currently, biomarkers of carcinogen/toxicant dose, reflecting the second box of the central track of Fig. 7.1, are by far the most extensively used and validated. The second most common are measurements of DNA adducts (or protein adducts as their surrogates), but few of these have both practical utility and validation with respect to tobacco carcinogen specificity.

The great advantage of tobacco carcinogen biomarkers is that their use bypasses many uncertainties in estimation of dose. The most commonly used estimation of dose is self-reported number of cigarettes per day, but this is really not a very good biomarker. It may not be reported accurately and it provides no information on the way in which the cigarettes were smoked, which is critical when one considers the common phenomenon of compensation. Brand information together with machine smoking measurements of specific components is another way of obtaining a measure of dose. However, machine smoking measurements are known to have limitations and the application of a given machine smoking protocol to a given smoker requires smoking topography measurements for that smoker. Estimation of tobacco carcinogen dose using biomarkers can be confounded to some extent by individual differences in metabolism, but studies of validated biomarkers have shown a significant relationship between biomarker levels and cigarettes per day. The variation in these studies result in part from the limitations of cigarettes per day as a biomarker. A stronger correlation between tobacco carcinogen biomarkers such as total NNAL and dose is observed when one compares the biomarker to total nicotine equivalents. Furthermore, some biomarkers have the unique attribute of being able to estimate dose plus metabolic activation in a given smoker, information that cannot be obtained in any other way.

The IARC monograph entitled 'Tobacco Smoking', published in 1986, contained no references describing tobacco carcinogen biomarkers [72]. There were over 350 citations on this topic in the 2004 IARC monograph entitled 'Tobacco Smoke and Involuntary Smoking', clearly demonstrating that this critical area of tobacco carcinogenesis has evolved remarkably in the past two to three decades [73]. Applications of tobacco carcinogen biomarkers include determining carcinogen dose in people who use tobacco products and in non-smokers exposed to secondhand smoke, identifying inter-individual differences in the uptake, metabolic activation, and detoxification of tobacco carcinogens, and ultimately predicting which tobacco user is susceptible to cancer. Tobacco carcinogen biomarkers will also be useful in regulation of tobacco products.

Validation

Validation of a tobacco carcinogen biomarker is accomplished in two steps. The first is analytical validation. The following questions must be answered affirmatively before the biomarker can be considered analytically validated:

a. Is the measurement chemically specific for the given substance? As an example, if one wishes to quantify the NNK metabolite NNAL in urine, it is necessary to demonstrate that the chromatographic peak being quantified does in fact represent NNAL and only NNAL. Co-eluting peaks, resulting from substances with similar polarity and structure, can confound specificity leading to incorrect results (values that are too high).

b. Is the measurement accurate? This is crucial, as conclusions regarding this biomarker will be drawn based on the numbers which are produced. Using the example of NNAL in urine, one could add increasing quantities of NNAL to urine samples from non-smokers, and carry out the anlaysis. The measured and added amounts should agree. A proper internal standard is critical for accuracy. The internal standard could be a closely related compound which is not found in the matrix being analysed, or if mass spectrometric detection methods are being used, it could be a stable isotope labelled version of the analyte.

c. Is the measurement reproducible? Intra-day and inter-day reproducibility can be established by splitting a sample into multiple aliquots and carrying out the analysis. Coefficients of variation should be relatively small. Analyte recovery, as determined by recovery of internal standard, will affect both accuracy and reproducibility and should be high enough such that analyte peak area is not compromised.

d. The method must be rugged, meaning that it should keep working in the hands of qualified analysts.

The second step is validation with respect to tobacco use. If the biomarker is not related to exposure via tobacco products, it may have limited utility in studies of tobacco and cancer. This is certainly true of biomarkers of carcinogen/toxicant dose and in most cases for carcinogen DNA or protein adducts. However, some biomarkers, such as those measuring oxidative damage to DNA or proteins, or those measuring inflammation, are not directly related to specific smoke constituents, but may still be useful. Validation with respect to tobacco use and exposure can be established using two main criteria. First, are levels of the biomarker higher in users than in non-users of tobacco (or in the case of secondhand smoke exposure, exposed vs. non-exposed)? Second, do levels of the biomarker decrease upon cessation of use or exposure? As a corollary, one would also expect a significant dose–response relationship between the biomarker and a questionnaire-based measure of dose such as cigarettes per day.

Types of tobacco carcinogen biomarkers

Examples of tobacco carcinogen biomarkers include tobacco carcinogens or their metabolites in urine, breath, blood, nails, and hair; tobacco carcinogen-DNA adducts; and tobacco carcinogen-protein adducts. Urinary metabolites, carcinogen-DNA adducts, and carcinogen-protein adducts will be discussed here.

Urinary metabolites

Probably the most practical and, to date, the most extensively applied tobacco carcinogen biomarkers are urinary metabolites of tobacco carcinogens [56]. Advantages include the ready availability of samples, and concentrations in urine that are easily quantifiable using modern analytical chemistry methods, most frequently liquid chromatography-tandem mass spectrometry (LC-MS/MS).

Metabolites of PAH and tobacco-specific nitrosamines, and mercapturic acids derived from benzene, acrolein, and 1,3-butadiene are commonly used urinary biomarkers. Among PAH metabolites, 1-hydroxypyrene (1-HOP) has been widely applied. 1-HOP is a metabolite of pyrene, a non-carcinogen but a component of all PAH mixtures. 1-HOP can be readily measured by HPLC with fluorescence detection and has been used in many studies to assess PAH uptake, which is frequently two to three times higher in smokers than in non-smokers [56, 74]. Our group has introduced r-1,t-2,3-c-4-tetrahydroxy-1,2,3,4-tetrahydrophenanthrene (PheT) as a biomarker of PAH uptake *plus* metabolic activation, as the metabolic pathway from phenanthrene, a non-carcinogenic PAH, to PheT is analogous to that involved in the metabolic activation of BaP to its ultimate carcinogenic diol epoxide metabolite illustrated in Fig. 7.3 [75, 76], but PheT is far more abundant in urine than BaP metabolites, thus facilitating measurement. PheT measurements will hopefully help to identify those smokers who are particularly able to catalyse this deleterious pathway.

Total NNAL, the sum of NNAL and its glucuronides, has emerged as a useful biomarker of NNK exposure [56, 77, 78]. The tobacco-specificity of NNK, and therefore total NNAL, is a key feature of this biomarker because studies in which it is applied are not confounded by other environmental or dietary exposures. Total NNAL has been used in numerous studies estimating uptake of the lung carcinogen NNK in smokers. In one example, smokers reduced their number of cigarettes smoked per day, but there was not a corresponding decrease in NNK uptake due to compensation [79, 80]. In another, NNK and PAH uptake, estimated by total NNAL and 1-HOP, respectively, were compared in smokers of regular, light, and ultra-light cigarettes, and found to be similar, consistent with epidemiologic studies which demonstrate no protection against lung cancer in smokers of light compared to regular cigarettes [81]. Other studies evaluated NNK uptake in smokers who switched from their current cigarette brand to products advertised as being less hazardous, but the results generally did not support these claims [82–84]. One of the most useful applications of total NNAL has been in studies of lung carcinogen uptake by non-smokers exposed to secondhand cigarette smoke [78]. The sensitivity and specificity of this biomarker are ideal for such studies, and it is the only tobacco carcinogen biomarker until now consistently elevated in non-smokers exposed to secondhand smoke. The only other biomarker demonstrated to be useful for such studies is cotinine (and other nicotine metabolites) but these are not carcinogen biomarkers. The results of these studies demonstrating NNK exposure throughout life in non-smokers exposed to secondhand smoke are summarized in Table 7.2 [85]. These results have had a significant impact on legislation prohibiting indoor smoking because non-smokers are highly adverse to the idea of having a lung carcinogen detected in their urine.

While total NNAL is a readily measured and established biomarker of uptake of the lung carcinogen NNK, it does not by itself provide any information on the extent of metabolic activation of NNK in a given smoker. Such information could be critical, as increased metabolic activation drives the central track of Fig. 7.1 towards a cancer endpoint. The urinary metabolites resulting from metabolic activation of NNK are 4-hydroxy-4-(3-pyridyl)butanoic acid (hydroxy acid) and 4-oxo-4-(3-pyridyl)butanoic acid (keto acid) (Fig. 7.2). As these two compounds are also minor metabolites of nicotine, their direct measurement in urine does not provide information about NNK metabolism because uptake of nicotine far exceeds that of NNK in smokers. However, they can be quantified in smokers who have used cigarettes to which [pyridine-D_4]NNK has been added. This approach is ethical because deuterium is non-radioactive and safe, and [pyridine-D_4] NNK can be added to low NNK cigarettes such that the total amount of NNK does not exceed that of the subjects' normal cigarette brand. Using this approach, it has been shown that hydroxy acid and keto acid, products of NNK metabolic activation, comprise about 80% of the NNK dose, and there is a 30-fold variation in NNK metabolic activation among smokers [86].

Table 7.2 Levels of total NNAL in the urine of non-smokers exposed to secondhand cigarette smoke

Exposed group	Type of exposure	Total NNAL (fmol/ml urine)	% of amount in smokers' urine[a]
Fetus	Transplacental	25 ± 29 (amniotic fluid)	1.3
Newborns	Transplacental	130 ± 150	6.5
Infants (<1 year old)	Air	83 ± 20	4.2
Elementary school children			
Minneapolis	Air	56 ± 76	2.8
Moldova	Air	90 ± 77	4.5
Women Living with smokers	Air	50 ± 68	2.5
Hospital workers	Air	59 ± 28	3.0
Casino patrons	Air	18 ± 15	0.9
Restaurant and bar workers	Air	33 ± 34	1.7

Note

[a] Based on 2 pmol/ml total NNAL in smokers. Adapted from SS Hecht, *Carcinogenesis* 23:907 (2002); SS Hecht *et al. CEBP* 15:988 (2006).

A series of urinary mercapturic acids, the normal degradation products of glutathione conjugates, have been investigated for estimating uptake of some of the volatile carcinogens and toxicants in cigarette smoke. Thus MHBMA (for monohydroxybutyl mercapturic acid) and DHBMA (for dihydroxybutyl mercapturic acid) are metabolites of 1,3-butadiene [87, 88]; HPMA (for 3-hydroxypropyl mercapturic acid) is a metabolite of acrolein [89]; HBMA (for 4-hydroxybut-2-yl mercapturic acid) is a metabolite of crotonaldehyde [90]; SPMA (for *S*-phenyl mercapturic acid) is a metabolite of benzene [91]; and HEMA (for 2-hydroxyethyl mercapturic acid) is a metabolite of ethylene oxide [92]. See Fig. 7.2 for structures of these metabolites.

These biomarkers represent some potentially important carcinogens and toxicants in cigarette smoke:1,3-butadiene, acrolein, crotonaldehyde, benzene, and ethylene oxide, found mainly in the gas phase of cigarette smoke (while PAH and NNK, represented by 1-HOP and total NNAL) are particulate phase constituents [93]. 1,3-Butadiene (20–40 μg per cigarette mainstream smoke), a potent multi-organ carcinogen in mice, with weaker activity in rats, is classified by IARC as 'carcinogenic to humans', Group 1 [94]. Acrolein (18–98 μg per cigarette) is highly cilia toxic and induces mutations in the *p53* gene similar to those caused by PAH diol epoxides and commonly found in lung tumours from smokers [57, 95]. Crotonaldehyde (15–20 μg per cigarette) is mutagenic in various systems and causes liver tumours in rats [96]. Benzene (12–50 μg per cigarette) is a known human leukemogen while ethylene oxide (7 μg per cigarette) is associated with lymphatic and haematopoietic cancers in humans and causes tumours at various sites in laboratory animals: both are IARC group 1 carcinogens [37, 66].

The relationship of these mercapturic acids, as well as total NNAL and 1-HOP, to cigarette smoking was evaluated in a study of 17 smokers who stopped smoking for 8 weeks. The results of this study are summarized in Table 7.3 and Fig. 7.5. Table 7.3 presents the baseline levels of each biomarker and the amounts detected at various intervals after stopping, while Fig. 7.5 illustrates these data as percentage decreases from baseline. The baseline data demonstrate that the levels of biomarkers could be split into three groups: low, medium, and high. Total NNAL, 1-HOP, and SPMA comprised the low group (1-3 nmol/24h), HEMA and MHBMA the medium group (60–100 nmol/24h), and DHBMA, HPMA, and HBMA the high group (1 000–10 000 nmol/24h).

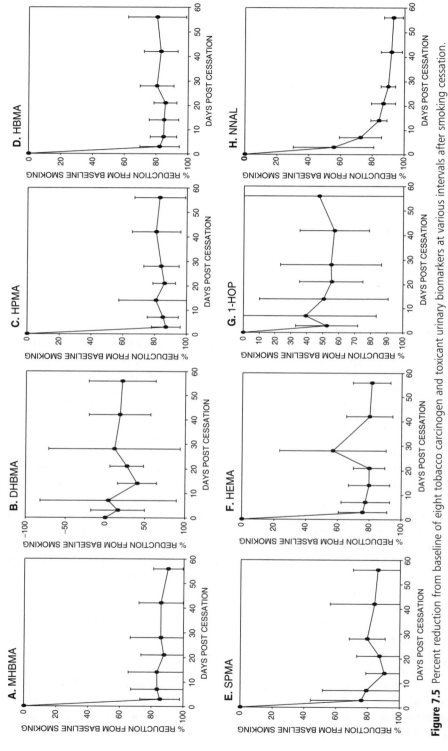

Figure 7.5 Percent reduction from baseline of eight tobacco carcinogen and toxicant urinary biomarkers at various intervals after smoking cessation.

Note

Values are means ± S.D. (N = 15) for which 2 subjects with highly variable data were omitted. Abbreviations: MHBMA, monohydroxybutyl mercapturic acid; DHBMA, dihydroxybutyl mercapturic acid; HPMA, 3-hydroxypropyl mercapturic acid; HBMA, 4-hydroxybut-2-yl mercapturic acid; SPMA, S-phenyl mercapturic acid; HEMA, 2-hydroxyethyl mercapturic acid; 1-HOP, 1-hydroxypyrene; NNAL, total NNAL, the sum of 4-(methylnitrosamino)-1-(3-pyridyl)-1-butanol and its glucuronides.

Table 7.3 Levels of biomarkers after smoking cessation

Mean ± S.D. (N = 17) amount (nmol/24h) at day

Biomarker	Baseline	3	7	14	21	28	42	56
MHBMA	66.1± 69.4	5.42 ± 4.35	6.12 ± 5.64	6.07 ± 5.10	4.67 ± 2.75	7.49 ± 13.81	5.08 ± 3.68	3.66 ± 2.41
DHBMA	1038 ± 514	875 ± 635	886± 558	622 ± 340	769 ± 316	791 ± 382	781 ± 269	662 ± 248
HPMA	10020 ± 5150	1336 ± 923	1362 ± 622	1626 ± 1587	1381 ± 653	1440 ± 741	1847 ± 1083	1500 ± 1005
HBMA	1965 ± 1001	265 ± 113	269 ± 95	270 ± 130	242 ± 83	331 ± 148	269 ± 118	273 ± 153
SPMA	3.20 ± 3.80	0.396 ± 0.345	0.276 ± 0.234	0.165 ± 0.136	0.203 ± 0.163	0.357 ± 0.249	0.254 ± 0.263	0.214 ± 0.214
HEMA	102 ± 47.1	24.0 ± 16.8	20.5 ± 11.3	21.2 ± 16.3	19.9 ± 15.0	38.8 ± 29.6	19.2 ± 18.1	19.2 ± 13.6
1-HOP	1.36 ± 0.776	0.826 ± 1.07	0.750 ± 0.545	1.06 ± 1.87	1.12 ± 1.81	0.783 ± 1.09	0.542 ± 0.224	1.09 ± 1.97
Total NNAL	2.70 ± 2.03	0.935 ± 0.496	0.761 ± 0.491	0.433 ± 0.321	0.343 ± 0.223	0.261 ± 0.175	0.199 ± 0.162	0.132 ± 0.113

The data in Table 7.3 and Fig. 7.5 demonstrate that, with the exception of DHBMA, levels of which did not change after cessation of smoking, all other biomarkers decreased significantly after three days of cessation ($P < 0.001$). The decreases in MHBMA, HPMA, HBMA, SPMA, and HEMA were rapid, nearly reaching their ultimate levels (81–91% reduction) after three days. The decrease in total NNAL was gradual, reaching 92% after 42 days, while reduction in 1-HOP was variable among subjects to about 50% of baseline. The results of this study clearly demonstrated that the tobacco smoke carcinogen/toxicant biomarkers MHBMA, HPMA, HBMA, SPMA, HEMA, 1-HOP, and NNAL are related to smoking and are good indicators of the impact of smoking on human exposure to 1,3-butadiene, acrolein, crotonaldehyde, benzene, ethylene oxide, PAH, and NNK.

Other studies of mercapturic acid biomarkers in smokers have reported results consistent with those illustrated in Fig. 7.5. Various methods including gas chromatography-mass spectrometry (GC-MS) [97,98], gas chromatography-tandem mass spectrometry (GC-MS/MS) [99, 100], and LC-MS/MS [87, 88,101–103] have been developed and applied for the quantitation of MHBMA and DHBMA in human urine after occupational exposure to 1,3-butadiene [88, 97–100, 102–106] and in smokers and non-smokers [87, 98, 101, 107]. Consistent with our results, most of these studies have shown that MHBMA is related to 1,3-butadiene exposure while DHBMA, which is present in far higher concentrations, is not related to exposure. Apparently there are significant sources of exposure to precursors of DHBMA other than metabolism of 1,3-butadiene. In one study of the effects of changes in smoking on 1,3-butadiene metabolites in urine, MHBMA levels decreased by 18% when smokers switched from cellulose acetate to charcoal filtered cigarettes [87], while a second study demonstrated a decrease of 50–80%, and also reported decreases of 90–95% when smokers stopped [107].

Analyses of HPMA and HBMA by LC-MS/MS have been reported [89, 90, 108]. The results shown in Fig. 7.5 are consistent with a previous study demonstrating that HPMA levels decreased significantly by 78% in smokers who abstained for four weeks [89]. In other studies, levels of HPMA were significantly higher in smokers than non-smokers in an investigation of 274 smokers and 100 non-smokers in Germany [91]. Levels of HPMA and HBMA decreased by 8% and 17%, respectively, when smokers switched from cellulose acetate to charcoal filter cigarettes [87], but in a second study HPMA decreased by 50–75% [107]. Small decreases in HPMA were observed in a study in which smokers switched from full-flavour to light or ultra-light cigarettes [109]. A significant 35% decrease in urinary HPMA was noted in smokers who switched to a second-generation electrically heated cigarette smoking system compared to those who continued smoking conventional cigarettes for 12 months [110].

SPMA has proven to be a useful and specific biomarker of benzene exposure [56, 111–115], with LC-MS/MS being used extensively for quantitation [87, 116–121]. Levels of SPMA are consistently higher in smokers than in non-smokers [56, 91, 120, 121]. Significant decreases in urinary SPMA were observed when smokers switched from conventional cellulose acetate to charcoal filter cigarettes [87, 107]. No or modest decreases in SPMA were observed in a study in which smokers switched from full-flavour to light or ultra-light cigarettes [109].

Variable amounts of HEMA were detected in workers exposed to ethylene oxide [122]. LC-MS/MS has been used to quantify HEMA in urine [92, 123], with higher levels found in smokers than in non-smokers.

In summary, urinary biomarkers of tobacco carcinogen exposure are readily measured and have been applied in many studies evaluating toxicant uptake by tobacco users. These biomarkers in particular are likely to play a major role in evaluating potential tobacco related harm in the coming era of tobacco product regulation.

Carcinogen-DNA adducts

Measurement of the carcinogen-DNA adducts such as those illustrated in Fig. 7.4 potentially can provide the most direct link between cellular exposure and cancer, as DNA adducts are critical in the carcinogenic process. But DNA adducts are challenging to quantify because their levels are extremely low, frequently ranging from 1 per 10^6 to 1 per 10^8 normal bases in humans [124], and the tissue or blood samples containing them are often available in only small quantities. In recent years, the sensitivity of mass spectrometers has improved dramatically, and the routine detection of amol levels of underivatized DNA adducts by conventional LC-MS/MS techniques is now feasible [125]. Although there are still relatively few examples of quantitation of specific DNA adducts in tissues of smokers using mass spectrometry, HPLC-fluorescence, HPLC with electrochemical detection, or post-labelling techniques, this literature is expanding rapidly and includes quantitation of DNA adducts of BaP, tobacco-specific nitrosamines [e.g. 4-hydroxy-1-(3-pyridyl)-1-butanone (HPB) releasing adducts of NNK or NNN], alkylating agents, aldehydes, and other lipid peroxidation products, and products of oxidative damage such as 8-oxo-dG [21, 38, 39, 45, 47, 55]. A much larger body of work has emerged from studies which have used the highly sensitive, but relatively non-specific ^{32}P-post-labelling and immunoassay methods for detection of DNA adducts. The advantages and disadvantages of ^{32}P-post-labelling and immunoassay have been discussed [50,126–128]. In summary, major advantages include high sensitivity allowing analysis of small amounts, generally micrograms, of DNA, relative simplicity of analysis, and no requirements for expensive equipment. Disadvantages include lack of chemical specificity, particularly in ^{32}P-post-labelling analyses, and difficulty in quantitation. Although the adducts detected using this method are often referred to in the literature as 'aromatic DNA adducts', there is strong evidence that they are not related to PAH [129]. The application of these methods to tissues obtained from smokers has been extensively reviewed [50]. Adduct levels are generally higher in lung tissues of smokers than non-smokers while studies using blood DNA have produced mixed results. Adducts have also been detected in many other tissues and fluids from smokers including larynx, oral and nasal mucosa, bladder, cervix, breast, pancreas, stomach, placenta, fetal tissue, cardiovascular tissues, sputum, and sperm. These studies have been comprehensively reviewed [50, 130]. A meta-analysis of the relationship of DNA adduct levels in smokers to cancer, as determined by ^{32}P-post-labelling, demonstrated a positive relationship in current-smokers [18, 131].

Still, these non-specific methods have severe problems and the quantitative measurement of DNA adducts by chemically specific methods in readily obtainable materials such as white blood cells, remains in relative infancy. Reliable validated methods exist only for BPDE and acetaldehyde-DNA adducts among those derived directly from tobacco carcinogens. 8-Oxo-dG, resulting from oxidative damage, has also been quantified in white blood cells, although there is some concern about artefact formation in this analysis.

Carcinogen-protein adducts

Carcinogen-haemoglobin (Hb) adducts levels have been used as surrogates for DNA adduct measurements [132, 133]. Serum albumin adducts could also be used in this way. Although these proteins are not considered as targets for carcinogenesis, all carcinogens that react with DNA will also react with protein to some extent. Advantages of Hb adducts as surrogates include the ready availability of relatively large amounts of Hb from blood and the relatively long lifetime of the erythrocyte in humans – 120 days – which provides an opportunity for adducts to accumulate. Studies on protein adducts in smokers have been comprehensively reviewed [50, 130].

Haemoglobin adducts of aromatic amines have emerged as a highly informative type of carcinogen biomarker, with levels which are consistently higher in smokers than in non-smokers, particularly for 3-aminobiphenyl and 4-aminobiphenyl-Hb adducts. Hb binds aromatic amines efficiently because haem accelerates the rate of nitrosoarene formation from the hydroxylamine, which is produced metabolically from the aromatic amine by P450 1A2 [134]. Binding of the nitrosoarene occurs at the β-93 cysteine residue of human Hb; the adduct is hydrolysed releasing the free amine which is quantified by GC-MS [134]. Adduct levels decrease upon smoking cessation and are related to numbers of cigarettes smoked per day [65,134,135]. Adducts which form with the amino terminal valine of Hb are also informative. Important examples include those derived from ethylene oxide, acrylonitrile, and acrylamide [136–138]. Ethylated N-terminal valine of Hb is also higher in smokers than in non-smokers [138].

A panel of biomarkers to assess tobacco carcinogen and toxicant uptake

On the basis of the studies described earlier, one can envision development of a standard panel of biomarkers which could be used to assess human uptake of tobacco smoke carcinogens and toxicants. This panel would include validated (analytically and with respect to smoking) tobacco carcinogen/toxicant biomarkers. The present members of the panel would be the following urinary biomarkers: nicotine equivalents (the sum of nicotine, nicotine-glucuronide, cotinine, cotinine-glucuronide, and trans-3'-hydroxycotinine and its glucuronides representing 75–90% of nicotine dose), total NNAL (representing NNK uptake), total NNN (representing NNN uptake), 1-HOP or PheT (representing PAH uptake), MHBMA, HPMA, HBMA, SPMA, and HEMA (representing uptake of 1,3-butadiene, acrolein, crotonaldehyde, benzene, and ethylene oxide), aminobiphenyl and other aromatic amine-Hb adducts (representing uptake of aromatic amines), and exhaled CO (representing CO exposure). Other biomarkers that could be included based on further validation studies are DNA adducts of acetaldehyde, formaldehyde, acrolein, and methylating or ethylating agents [39, 139, 140]; F_2-isoprostanes as biomarkers of oxidative damage [141]; and prostaglandin metabolites as biomarkers of inflammation [142]. These biomarkers not only include representatives of virtually all major toxicants and carcinogens in cigarette smoke but also cover the nine substances proposed by a WHO working group as targets for regulation under the Framework Convention on Tobacco Control: acrolein, acetaldehyde, formaldehyde, benzene, 1,3-butadiene, BaP, NNK, NNN, and CO [143]. As standard methods exist or are in development for all of these analytes, their application in regulation is feasible and can potentially bypass many of the vexing questions associated with machine measurements of smoke constituents. While some have argued that inter-individual differences in metabolism of these smoke constituents preclude their use in regulation [143], the data presented in this chapter clearly demonstrate that in most cases carcinogen/toxicant dose is the major factor in determining biomarker levels.

Tobacco carcinogen biomarkers: relationship to disease

Tobacco carcinogen biomarkers are validated with respect to exposure from tobacco products, as discussed earlier. But are these biomarkers also related to disease? This is a critical question if the ultimate goal of using biomarkers to predict susceptibility to tobacco-induced cancer is to be reached. Prior to 2008, there were no published studies attempting to relate specific tobacco carcinogen biomarkers to lung cancer, but three recently published studies on total NNAL changed this.

In one, a case-control study was nested in the National Cancer Institute's Prostate, Lung, Colorectum, and Ovarian (PLCO) Cancer Screening Trial, which began in 1993 and enlisted more than 77 000 subjects, of whom approximately 25 000 were current- or former-smokers [144]. Two hundred smokers of more than ten cigarettes per day who were free of cancer at baseline and contributed adequate serum samples to the repository upon enrollment were selected. One hundred of these individuals eventually presented with lung cancer, and 100 were cancer free at the cutoff date in 2007. The serum samples were analysed for total NNAL, PheT, and cotinine. Individual associations of age, smoking duration, and total NNAL with lung cancer risk were significant. After adjustment, total NNAL was the only biomarker significantly associated with risk (odds ratio 1.57 per unit standard deviation increase of 40 fmol/ml serum; 95% confidence interval, 1.08–2.28). Thus, the odds increase about 1.7 times from the 25th to the 75th percentiles of total NNAL in serum and about 4.2 times from the 5th to the 95th percentiles. These results suggest that, among long-term heavy smokers, total serum NNAL level is a major determinant of lung cancer risk conferred by cigarette smoking. The lack of a relationship with PheT may be due to confounding by exposures to phenanthrene in the diet or polluted air. The lack of a relationship to cotinine contrasts to a much larger study which demonstrated that cotinine levels were related to lung cancer, and may be due to the relatively small sample size [145].

A second study was carried out using a nested case control design in two Asian cohorts [146]. One was the Shanghai Cohort Study which consisted of 18 244 men enrolled from 1986–1989. The second was the Singapore Chinese Health Study which included 63 257 Chinese men and women enrolled in 1993–1998. The relationship between total NNAL in urine collected before diagnosis, and subsequent risk of lung cancer, was examined in 246 incident case of lung cancer and 245 matched controls who were current-smokers selected from these cohorts. Smokers who subsequently developed lung cancer had elevated levels of total NNAL in their urine at baseline relative to smokers who remained cancer free. Compared with the lowest tertile, relative risks of lung cancer for the 2nd and 3rd tertiles of total NNAL were 1.43 (95% confidence interval 0.86–2.37) and 2.11 (95% confidence interval 1.25–3.54), respectively (P for trend = 0.005) after adjustment for smoking intensity and duration, and urinary total cotinine levels. Smokers of more than 40 pack-years with high levels of total NNAL and total cotinine had more than ten times (95% confidence interval 4.98–23.02) the risk for lung cancer relative to smokers of less than 20 pack years with low levels of total NNAL and total cotinine. The finding of a joint effect of total NNAL and total cotinine in this study, as well as an independent effect of total cotinine, as compared to the PLCO study, may be due to the larger sample size. The results for total NNAL in this study were remarkably similar to those in the PLCO study. Collectively, these results provide powerful evidence linking the tobacco carcinogen biomarker total NNAL to lung cancer in smokers.

A third study focused on a locus at 15q24/15q25.1, which includes the nicotinic acetylcholine receptor A subunits 3 and 5 (CHRNA3, CHRNA5) genes, which were strongly associated with lung cancer susceptibility in three independent genome-wide association studies [4–6]. In this study, the relationship of variants in these genes to total NNAL and total nicotine equivalents in urine was examined [7]. A total of 819 smokers were studied. The results demonstrated that carriers of variants in these genes extracted a greater amount of nicotine per cigarette (P = 0.003) and had greater levels of total NNAL in their urine (P = 0.03) than non-carriers. Therefore, smokers with these variants are at higher risk for lung cancer because they extract more nicotine per cigarette and are therefore exposed to higher carcinogen levels, represented by total NNAL as a biomarker for NNK, than do smokers who do not carry these alleles.

Collectively, these data provide convincing evidence that total NNAL is a biomarker of lung cancer risk in smokers. This is completely consistent with the known lung carcinogenicity of NNK. The emergence of total NNAL as a biomarker of lung cancer risk is also undoubtedly related to the tobacco-specificity of NNK. Since there is no exposure to NNK, and therefore no total NNAL in serum or urine of non-exposed non-smokers, the baseline levels will be lower, thus providing more power and specificity to this biomarker.

Summary

Extensive research carried out over the past 50 years has brought forth a detailed understanding of mechanisms of tobacco carcinogenesis. Although there are still aspects of the overall mechanism which are unclear, the major pathway involving multiple tobacco smoke carcinogens and their DNA adducts, leading to mutations and malfunction of critical growth control genes, is now firmly established. A relatively complete picture of DNA adducts of tobacco smoke carcinogens has been developed in chemical and laboratory studies, although the identification and quantitation of specific DNA adducts in smokers has lagged behind. Tobacco carcinogen biomarkers, quantifiable metabolites or adducts directly related to carcinogen exposure, and in some cases to disease, have emerged as potentially powerful new entities which may find use in identifying individuals particularly predisposed to tobacco-induced cancer and in supporting the newly dawning era of tobacco product regulation. Thus, our improved understanding of tobacco carcinogenesis, representing a classic exposure-host interaction, promises to lead to new preventive and possibly therapeutic approaches to tobacco-induced cancer, which still causes approximately 30% of cancer death worldwide.

Acknowledgements

The author's research on mechanisms and prevention of tobacco-induced cancer is supported by grants CA-81301, 92025, and 102502 from the US National Cancer Institute, DA-13333 from the US National Institutes of Health, and RP-00-138 from the American Cancer Society.

References

1. Hecht, S.S. (1999). Tobacco smoke carcinogens and lung cancer. *J Natl Cancer Inst*, **91**:1194–1210.

2. Hecht, S.S. (2003). Tobacco carcinogens, their biomarkers, and tobacco-induced cancer. *Nature Rev Cancer*, **3**:733–744.

3. Ding, L., Getz, G., Wheeler, D.A., Mardis, E.R., McLellan, M.D., Cibulskis, K. *et al*. (2008). Somatic mutations affect key pathways in lung adenocarcinoma. *Nature*, **455**(7216):1069–1075.

4. Thorgeirsson, T.E., Geller, F., Sulem, P., Rafnar, T., Wiste, A., Magnusson, K.P. *et al*. (2008). A variant associated with nicotine dependence, lung cancer and peripheral arterial disease. *Nature*, **452**(7187): 638–642.

5. Hung, R.J., McKay, J.D., Gaborieau, V., Boffetta, P., Hashibe, M., Zaridze, D. *et al*. (2008). A susceptibility locus for lung cancer maps to nicotinic acetylcholine receptor subunit genes on 15q25. *Nature*, **452**(7187):633–637.

6. Amos, C.I., Wu, X., Broderick, P., Gorlov, I.P., Gu, J., Eisen, T. *et al*. (2008). Genome-wide association scan of tag SNPs identifies a susceptibility locus for lung cancer at 15q25.1. *Nat Genet*, **40**:616–622.

7. Le Marchand, L., Derby, K.S., Murphy, S.E., Hecht, S.S., Hatsukami, D., Carmella, S.G. *et al*. (2008). Smokers with the *CHRNA* lung cancer-associated variants are exposed to higher levels of nicotine equivalents and a carcinogenic tobacco-specific nitrosamine. *Cancer Res*, **68**(22):9137–9140.

8. Guengerich, F.P. (2001). Common and uncommon cytochrome P450 reactions related to metabolism and chemical toxicity. *Chem Res Toxicol*, **14**:611–650.

9. Jalas, J., Hecht, S.S., Murphy, S.E. (2005). Cytochrome P450 2A enzymes as catalysts of metabolism of 4-(methylnitrosamino)-1-(3-pyridyl)-1-butanone (NNK), a tobacco-specific carcinogen. *Chem Res Toxicol*, **18**:95–110.

10. Zhang, L., Lee, J.J., Tang, H., Fan, Y.-H., Xiao, L., Ren, H. *et al.* (2008). Impact of smoking cessation on global gene expression in the bronchial epithelium of chronic smokers. *Cancer Prev Res*, **1**:112–118.

11. Gümüs, Z.H., Du, B., Kacker, A., Boyle, J.O., Bocker, J.M., Mukherjee, P. *et al.* (2008). Effects of tobacco smoke on gene expression and cellular pathways in a cellular model of oral leukoplakia. *Cancer Prev Res*, **1**:100–111.

12. Nebert, D.W., Dalton, T.P., Okey, A.B., and Gonzalez, F.J. (2004). Role of aryl hydrocarbon receptor-mediated induction of the CYP1 enzymes in environmental toxicity and cancer. *J Biol Chem*, **279**(23):23847–23850.

13. Quinn, A.M., Harvey, R.G., and Penning, T.M. (2008). Oxidation of PAH *trans*-dihydrodiols by human aldo-keto reductase AKR1B10. *Chem Res Toxicol*, **21**:2207–2215.

14. Armstrong, R.N. (1997). Glutathione-S-transferases. In: F.P. Guengerich, editor. *Comprehensive Toxicology: Biotransformation*. New York: Elsevier Science, 307–327.

15. Burchell, B., McGurk, K., Brierley, C.H., and Clarke, D.J. (1997). UDP-Glucuronosyltransferases. In: Guengerich FP, editor. *Comprehensive Toxicology: Biotransformation*. New York: Elsevier Science, 401–436.

16. Vineis, P., Veglia, F., Benhamou, S., Butkiewicz, D., Cascorbi, I., Clapper, M.L. *et al.* (2003). CYP1A1 T3801 C polymorphism and lung cancer: a pooled analysis of 2451 cases and 3358 controls. *Int J Cancer*, **104**(5):650–657.

17. International Agency for Research on Cancer (2004). Tobacco Smoke and Involuntary Smoking. IARC Monographs on the Evaluation of Carcinogenic Risks to Humans. Lyon, FR: IARC, 1179–1187.

18. Veglia, F., Loft, S., Matullo, G., Peluso, M., Munnia, A., Perera, F., *et al.* (2008). DNA adducts and cancer risk in prospective studies: a pooled analysis and a meta-analysis. *Carcinogenesis*, **29**(5):932–936.

19. Liu, G., Zhou, W., and Christiani, D.C. (2005). Molecular epidemiology of non-small cell lung cancer. *Semin Respir Crit Care Med*, **26**(3):265–272.

20. Delaney, J.C. and Essigmann, J.M. (2008). Biological properties of single chemical-DNA adducts: a twenty year perspective. *Chem Res Toxicol*, **21**(1):232–252.

21. Pfeifer, G.P., Denissenko, M.F., Olivier, M., Tretyakova, N., Hecht, S.S., and Hainaut, P. (2002). Tobacco smoke carcinogens, DNA damage and p53 mutations in smoking-associated cancers. *Oncogene*, **21**:7435–7451.

22. Ahrendt, S.A., Decker, P.A., Alawi, E.A., Zhu Yr, Y.R., Sanchez-Cespedes, M., Yang, S.C. *et al.* (2001). Cigarette smoking is strongly associated with mutation of the K-ras gene in patients with primary adenocarcinoma of the lung. *Cancer*, **92**(6):1525–1530.

23. Johnson, L., Mercer, K., Greenbaum, D., Bronson, R.T., Crowley, D., Tuveson, D.A. *et al.* (2001). Somatic activation of the K-*ras* oncogene causes early onset lung cancer in mice. *Nature*, **410**(6832):1111–1116.

24. Lubet, R.A., Zhang, Z., Wiseman, R.W., and You, M. (2000). Use of p53 transgenic mice in the development of cancer models for multiple purposes. *Exp Lung Res*, **26**(8):581–593.

25. Sekido, Y., Fong, K.W., and Minna, J.D. (1998). Progress in understanding the molecular pathogenesis of human lung cancer. *Biochim Biophys Acta*, **1378**:F21–F59.

26. Bode, A.M. and Dong, Z. (2005). Signal transduction pathways in cancer development and as targets for cancer prevention. *Prog Nucleic Acid Res Mol Biol*, **79**:237–297.

27. Schuller, H.M. (2002). Mechanisms of smoking-related lung and pancreatic adenocarcinoma development. *Nat Rev Cancer*, **2**(6):455–463.

28. West, K.A., Brognard, J., Clark, A.S., Linnoila, I.R., Yang, X., Swain, S.M. *et al.* (2003). Rapid Akt activation by nicotine and a tobacco carcinogen modulates the phenotype of normal human airway epithelial cells. *J Clin Invest*, **111**(1):81–90.

29. Heeschen, C., Jang, J.J., Weis, M., Pathak, A., Kaji, S., Hu, R.S. *et al.* (2001). Nicotine stimulates angiogenesis and promotes tumor growth and atherosclerosis. *Nat Med*, **7**(7):833–839.

30. Moraitis, D., Du, B., De Lorenzo, M.S., Boyle, J.O., Weksler, B.B., Cohen, E.G. *et al.* (2005). Levels of cyclooxygenase-2 are increased in the oral mucosa of smokers: evidence for the role of epidermal growth factor receptor and its ligands. *Cancer Res*, **65**(2):664–670.

31. Belinsky, S.A. (2005). Silencing of genes by promoter hypermethylation: key event in rodent and human lung cancer. *Carcinogenesis*, **26**(9):1481–1487.

32. Cooper, C.S., Grover, P.L., and Sims, P. (1983). The metabolism and activation of benzo[*a*]pyrene. *Prog Drug Metab*, **7**:295–396.

33. Conney, A.H. (1982). Induction of microsomal enzymes by foreign chemicals and carcinogenesis by polycyclic aromatic hydrocarbons: G.H.A. Clowes Memorial Lecture. *Cancer Res*, **42**:4875–4917.

34. Hecht, S.S. (1998). Biochemistry, biology, and carcinogenicity of tobacco-specific *N*-nitrosamines. *Chem Res Toxicol*, **11**:559–603.

35. Preussmann, R. and Stewart, B.W. (1984). N-Nitroso Carcinogens. In: C.E. Searle, (ed.) Chemical Carcinogens, Second Edition, ACS Monograph 182. Washington, DC: American Chemical Society, 643–828.

36. Stepanov, I. and Hecht, S.S. (2005). Tobacco-specific nitrosamines and their *N*-glucuronides in the urine of smokers and smokeless tobacco users. *Cancer Epidemiol Biomarkers & Prev*, **14**:885–891.

37. International Agency for Research on Cancer (1994). Some Industrial Chemicals. IARC Monographs on the Evaluation of the Carcinogenic Risk of Chemicals to Humans. Lyon, FR: IARC, 73–159.

38. Zhang, S., Villalta, P.W., Wang, M., and Hecht, S.S. (2007). Detection and quantitation of acrolein-derived 1,N^2-propanodeoxyguanosine adducts in human lung by liquid chromatography-electrospray ionization-tandem mass spectrometry. *Chem Res Toxicol*, **20**:565–571.

39. Chen, L., Wang, M., Villalta, P.W., Luo, X., Feuer, R., Jensen, J. *et al.* (2007). Quantitation of an acetaldehyde adduct in human leukocyte DNA and the effect of smoking cessation. *Chem Res Toxicol*, **20**:108–113.

40. Kadlubar, F.F. and Beland, F.A. (1985). Chemical properties of ultimate carcinogenic metabolites of arylamines and arylamides. In: R.G. Harvey, (ed.) *Polycyclic Hydrocarbons and Carcinogenesis*. Washington, D.C.: American Chemical Society, 341–371.

41. Szeliga, J. and Dipple, A. (1998). DNA adduct formation by polycyclic aromatic hydrocarbon dihydrodiol epoxides. *Chem Res Toxicol*, **11**:1–11.

42. Hecht, S.S. (2008). Progress and challenges in selected areas of tobacco carcinogenesis. *Chem Res Toxicol*, **21**:160–171.

43. Zhao, C., Tyndyk, M., Eide, I., and Hemminki, K. (1999). Endogenous and background DNA adducts by methylating and 2- hydroxyethylating agents. *Mutat Res*, **424**(1–2):117–125.

44. Singh, R., Kaur, B., and Farmer, P.B. (2005). Detection of DNA damage derived from a direct acting ethylating agent present in cigarette smoke by use of liquid chromatography-tandem mass spectrometry. *Chem Res Toxicol*, **18**(2):249–256.

45. Zhang, S., Villalta, P.W., Wang, M., and Hecht, S.S. (2006). Analysis of crotonaldehyde- and acetaldehyde-derived 1,N^2-propanodeoxyguanosine adducts in DNA from human tissues using liquid chromatography-electrsopray ionization-tandem mass spectrometry. *Chem Res Toxicol*, **19**:1386–1392.

46. Boysen, G. and Hecht, S.S. (2003). Analysis of DNA and protein adducts of benzo[*a*]pyrene in human tissues using structure-specific methods. *Mutation Res*, **543**:17–30.

47. Beland, F.A., Churchwell, M.I., Von Tungeln, L.S., Chen, S., Fu, P.P., Culp, S.J. *et al.* (2005). High-performance liquid chromatography electrospray ionization tandem mass spectrometry for the detection and quantitation of benzo[a]pyrene-DNA adducts. *Chem Res Toxicol*, **18**(8):1306–1315.

48. Hoffmann, D., Schmeltz, I., Hecht, S.S., and Wynder, E.L. (1978). Tobacco carcinogenesis. In: H. Gelboin, P.O.P. Ts'o, (eds) *Polycyclic Hydrocarbons and Cancer*. New York: Academic Press, 85–117.

49. Deutsch-Wenzel, R., Brune, H., and Grimmer, G. (1983). Experimental studies in rat lungs on the carcinogenicity and dose–response relationships of eight frequently occurring environmental polycyclic aromatic hydrocarbons. *J Natl Cancer Inst*, **71**:539–544.

50. Phillips, D.H. (2002). Smoking-related DNA and protein adducts in human tissues. *Carcinogenesis*, **23**(12):1979–2004.

51. Liu, Z., Muehlbauer, K.R., Schmeiser, H.H., Hergenhahn, M., Belharazem, D., and Hollstein, M.C. (2005). p53 Mutations in benzo[*a*]pyrene-exposed human p53 knock-in murine fibroblasts correlate with p53 mutations in human lung tumors. *Cancer Res*, **65**(7):2583–2587.

52. Belinsky, S.A., Foley, J.F., White, C.M., Anderson, M.W., and Maronpot, R.R. (1990). Dose–response relationship between O6-methylguanine formation in Clara cells and induction of pulmonary neoplasia in the rat by 4-(methylnitrosamino)-1-(3-pyridyl)-1-butanone. *Cancer Res*, **50**:3772–3780.

53. Foiles, P.G., Akerkar, S.A., Carmella, S.G., Kagan, M., Stoner, G.D., Resau, J.H. *et al.* (1991). Mass spectrometric analysis of tobacco-specific nitrosamine-DNA adducts in smokers and nonsmokers. *Chem Res Toxicol*, **4**:364–368.

54. Schlöbe, D., Hölzle, D., Hatz, D., Von Meyer, L., Tricker, A.R., and Richter, E. (2008). 4-Hydroxy-1-(3-pyridyl)-1-butanone-releasing DNA adducts in lung, lower esophagus and cardia of sudden death victims. *Toxicology*, **245**(1–2):154–161.

55. Hölzle, D., Schlöbe, D., Tricker, A.R., and Richter, E. (2007). Mass spectrometric analysis of 4-hydroxy-1-(3-pyridyl)-1-butanone-releasing DNA adducts in human lung. *Toxicology*, **232**(3):277–285.

56. Hecht, S.S. (2002). Human urinary carcinogen metabolites: biomarkers for investigating tobacco and cancer. *Carcinogenesis*, **23**:907–922.

57. Feng, Z., Hu, W., Hu, Y., and Tang, M.S. (2006). Acrolein is a major cigarette-related lung cancer agent: Preferential binding at *p53* mutational hotspots and inhibition of DNA repair. *Proc Natl Acad Sci USA*, **103**(42):15404–15409.

58. International Agency for Research on Cancer (1986). Tobacco Smoking. IARC Monographs on the Evaluation of the Carcinogenic Risk of Chemicals to Humans. Lyon, FR: IARC, 37–385.

59. Hoffmann, D. and Hecht, S.S. (1990). Advances in tobacco carcinogenesis. In: C.S. Cooper, P.L. Grover, (eds) *Handbook of Experimental Pharmacology*. Heidelberg: Springer-Verlag, 63–102.

60. International Agency for Research on Cancer (2007). Smokeless tobacco and tobacco-specific nitrosamines. IARC Monographs on the Evaluation of Carcinogenic Risks to Humans, v. 89. Lyon, FR: IARC, 548–553.

61. Prokopczyk, B., Leder, G., Trushin, N., Cunningham, A.J., Akerkar, S., Pittman, B. *et al.* (2005). 4-Hydroxy-1-(3-pyridyl)-1-butanone, an indicator for 4-(methylnitrosamino)-1-(3-pyridyl)-1-butanone-induced DNA damage, is not detected in human pancreatic tissue. *Cancer Epidemiol Biomarkers Prev*, **14**(2):540–541.

62. Rivenson, A., Hoffmann, D., Prokopczyk, B., Amin, S., and Hecht, S.S. (1988). Induction of lung and exocrine pancreas tumors in F344 rats by tobacco-specific and *Areca*-derived N-nitrosamines. *Cancer Res*, **48**:6912–6917.

63. Prokopczyk, B., Hoffmann, D., Bologna, M., Cunningham, A.J., Trushin, N., Akerkar, S., *et al.* (2002). Identification of tobacco-derived compounds in human pancreatic juice. *Chem Res Toxicol*, **15**:677–685.

64. Skipper, P.L., Peng, X., SooHoo, C.K., and Tannenbaum, S.R. (1994). Protein adducts as biomarkers of human carcinogen exposure. *Drug Metab Rev*, **26**:111–124.

65. Castelao, J.E., Yuan, J.M., Skipper, P.L., Tannenbaum, S.R., Gago-Dominguez, M., Crowder, J.S. *et al.* (2001). Gender- and smoking-related bladder cancer risk. *J Natl Cancer Inst*, **93**(7):538–545.

66. International Agency for Research on Cancer (1982). Some Industrial Chemicals and Dyestuffs. IARC Monographs on the Evaluation of the Carcinogenic Risk of Chemicals to Humans. Lyon, FR: IARC, 93–148.

67. Zhang, L., Steinmaus, C., Eastmond, D.A., Xin, X.K., and Smith, M.T. (2008). Formaldehyde exposure and leukemia: a new meta-analysis and potential mechanisms. *Mutat Res* epub 15-July-2008.

68. Pryor, W.A., Stone, K., Zang, L.Y., and Bermudez, E. (1998). Fractionation of aqueous cigarette tar extracts: fractions that contain the tar radical cause DNA damage. *Chem Res Toxicol*, **11**:441–448.

69. Dietrich, M., Block, G., Hudes, M., Morrow, J.D., Norkus, E.P., Traber, M.G. *et al.* (2002). Antioxidant supplementation decreases lipid peroxidation biomarker F(2)- isoprostanes in plasma of smokers. *Cancer Epidemiol Biomarkers Prev*, **11**:7–13.

70. Hecht, S.S. (2005). Carcinogenicity studies of inhaled cigarette smoke in laboratory animals: old and new. *Carcinogenesis*, **26**:1488–1492.

71. Lee, J.M., Yanagawa, J., Peebles, K.A., Sharma, S., Mao, J.T., and Dubinett, S.M. (2008). Inflammation in lung carcinogenesis: new targets for lung cancer chemoprevention and treatment. *Crit Rev Oncol Hematol*, **66**(3):208–217.

72. International Agency for Research on Cancer (1986). Tobacco Smoking. IARC Monographs on the Evaluation of the Carcinogenic Risk of Chemicals to Humans. Lyon, FR: IARC, 37–375.

73. International Agency for Research on Cancer (2004). Tobacco Smoke and Involuntary Smoking. IARC Monographs on the Evaluation of Carcinogenic Risks to Humans. Lyon, FR: IARC, 1012–1065.

74. Jongeneelen, F.J. (2001). Benchmark guideline for urinary 1-hydroxypyrene as biomarker of occupational exposure to polycyclic aromatic hydrocarbons. *Ann Occup Hyg*, **45**:3–13.

75. Hecht, S.S., Carmella, S.G., Yoder, A., Chen, M., Li, Z., Le, C. *et al.* (2006). Comparison of polymorphisms in genes involved in polycyclic aromatic hydrocarbon metabolism with urinary phenanthrene metabolite ratios in smokers. *Cancer Epidemiol Biomarkers & Prev*, **15**:1805–1811.

76. Hecht, S.S., Chen, M., Yagi, H., Jerina, D.M., and Carmella, S.G. (2003). r-1,t-2,3,c-4-Tetrahydroxy-1,2,3,4-tetrahydrophenanthrene in human urine: a potential biomarker for assessing polycyclic aromatic hydrocarbon metabolic activation. *Cancer Epidemiol Biomarkers & Prev*, **12**:1501–1508.

77. Hatsukami, D.K., Benowitz, N.L., Rennard, S.I., Oncken, C., and Hecht, S.S. (2006). Biomarkers to assess the utility of potential reduced exposure tobacco products. *Nicotine and Tob Res*, **8**:600–622.

78. Hecht, S.S. (2003). Carcinogen derived biomarkers: applications in studies of human exposure to secondhand tobacco smoke. *Tob Control*, 13 (Suppl 1):i48–i56.

79. Hatsukami, D.K., Le, C.T., Zhang, Y., Joseph, A.M., Mooney, M.E., Carmella, S.G. *et al.* (2006). Toxicant exposure in cigarette reducers vs. light smokers. *Cancer Epidemiol Biomarkers & Prev*, **15**:2355–2358.

80. Hecht, S.S., Murphy, S.E., Carmella, S.G., Zimmerman, C.L., Losey, L., Kramarczuk, I. *et al.* (2004). Effects of reduced cigarette smoking on uptake of a tobacco-specific lung carcinogen. *J Natl Cancer Inst*, **96**:107–115.

81. Hecht, S.S., Murphy, S.E., Carmella, S.G., Li, S., Jensen, J., Le, C. *et al.* (2005). Similar uptake of lung carcinogens by smokers of regular, light, and ultra-light cigarettes. *Cancer Epidemiol Biomarkers & Prev*, **14**:693–698.

82. Mendoza-Baumgart, M.I., Hecht, S.S., Zhang, Y., Murphy, S.E., Le, C., Jensen, J., and Hatsukami, D.K. (2007). Pilot study on lower nitrosamine smokeless tobacco products compared to medicinal nicotine. *Nic Tob Res*, **9**:1309–1323.

83. Hatsukami, D.K., Ebbert, J.O., Anderson, A., Lin, H., Le, C., and Hecht, S.S. (2006). Smokeless tobacco brand switching: a means to reduce toxicant exposure? *Drug Alcohol Depend*, **87**:217–224.

84. Hatsukami, D.K., Lemmonds, C., Zhang, Y., Murphy, S.E., Le, C., Carmella, S.G. *et al.* (2004). Evaluation of carcinogen exposure in people who used 'reduced exposure' tobacco products. *J Natl Cancer Inst*, **96**:844–852.

85. Hecht, S.S., Carmella, S.G., Le, K., Murphy, S.E., Boettcher, A.J., Le, C., *et al.* (2006). 4-(Methylnitrosamino)-1-(3-pyridyl)-1-butanol and its glucuronides in the urine of infants exposed to environmental tobacco smoke. *Cancer Epidemiol Biomarkers & Prev*, **15**:988–992.

86. Stepanov, I., Upadhyaya, P., Feuer, R., Jensen, J., Hatsukami, D.K., and Hecht, S.S. (2008). Extensive metabolic activation of the tobacco-specific carcinogen 4-(methylnitrosamino)-1-(3-pyridyl)-1-butanone in smokers. *Cancer Epidemiol Biomarkers & Prev*, **17**:1764–1773.

87. Scherer, G., Urban, M., Engl, J., Hagedorn, H.W., and Riedel, K. (2006). Influence of smoking charcoal filter tipped cigarettes on various biomarkers of exposure. *Inhal Toxicol*, **18**(10):821–829.

88. Sapkota, A., Halden, R.U., Dominici, F., Groopman, J.D., and Buckley, T.J. (2006). Urinary biomarkers of 1,3-butadiene in environmental settings using liquid chromatography isotope dilution tandem mass spectrometry. *Chem Biol Interact*, **160**(1):70–79.

89. Carmella, S.G., Chen, M., Zhang, Y., Zhang, S., Hatsukami, D.K., and Hecht, S.S. (2007). Quantitation of acrolein-derived 3-hydroxypropylmercapturic acid in human urine by liquid chromatography-atmospheric pressure chemical ionization-tandem mass spectrometry: effects of cigarette smoking. *Chem Res Toxicol*, **20**:986–990.

90. Scherer, G., Urban, M., Hagedorn, H.W., Feng, S., Kinser, R.D., Sarkar, M. *et al.* (2007). Determination of two mercapturic acids related to crotonaldehyde in human urine: influence of smoking. *Hum Exp Toxicol*, **26**(1):37–47.

91. Scherer, G., Engl, J., Urban, M., Gilch, G., Janket, D., and Riedel, K. (2007). Relationship between machine-derived smoke yields and biomarkers in cigarette smokers in Germany. *Regul Toxicol Pharmacol*, **47**(2):171–183.

92. Calafat, A.M., Barr, D.B., Pirkle, J.L., and Ashley, D.L. (1999). Reference range concentrations of N-acetyl-S-(2-hydroxyethyl)-L-cysteine, a common metabolite of several volatile organic compounds, in the urine of adults in the United States. *J Expo Anal Environ Epidemiol*, **9**(4):336–342.

93. International Agency for Research on Cancer (2004). Tobacco Smoke and Involuntary Smoking. IARC Monographs on the Evaluation of Carcinogenic Risks to Humans. Lyon, FR: IARC, 33–1187.

94. International Agency for Research on Cancer (2008). 1,3-Butadiene, Ethylene Oxide and Vinyl Halides (Vinyl Fluoride, Vinyl Chloride, and Vinyl Bromide). IARC Monographs on the Evaluation of Carcinogenic Risks to Humans. Lyon, FR: IARC, 45–184.

95. Kensler, C.J. and Battista, S.P (1963). Components of cigarette smoke with ciliary-depressant activity. Their selective removal by filters containing activated charcoal granules. *N Engl J Med*, **269**:1161–1166.

96. International Agency for Research on Cancer (1995). Dry cleaning, some chlorinated solvents and other industrial chemicals. IARC Monographs on the Evaluation of Carcinogenic Risks to Humans. Lyon, FR: IARC, 373–391.

97. Bechtold, W.E., Strunk, M.R., Chang, I.Y., Ward, J.B. Jr., and Henderson, R.F. (1994). Species differences in urinary butadiene metabolites: comparisons of metabolite ratios between mice, rats, and humans. *Toxicol Appl Pharmacol*, **127**(1):44–49.

98. Fustinoni, S., Soleo, L., Warholm, M., Begemann, P., Rannug, A., Neumann, H.G. *et al.* (2002). Influence of metabolic genotypes on biomarkers of exposure to 1,3- butadiene in humans. *Cancer Epidemiol Biomarkers Prev*, **11**(10 Pt 1):1082–1090.

99. van Sittert, N.J., Megens, H.J., Watson, W.P., and Boogaard, P.J. (2000). Biomarkers of exposure to 1,3-butadiene as a basis for cancer risk assessment. *Toxicol Sci*, **56**(1):189–202.

100. Boogaard, P.J., van Sittert, N.J., and Megens, H.J. (2001). Urinary metabolites and haemoglobin adducts as biomarkers of exposure to 1,3-butadiene: a basis for 1,3-butadiene cancer risk assessment. *Chem Biol Interact*, **135–136**:695–701.

101. Urban, M., Gilch, G., Schepers, G., van Miert, E., and Scherer, G. (2003). Determination of the major mercapturic acids of 1,3-butadiene in human and rat urine using liquid chromatography with tandem mass spectrometry. *J Chromatogr B Analyt Technol Biomed Life Sci*, **796**(1):131–140.

102. Fustinoni, S., Perbellini, L., Soleo, L., Manno, M., and Foa, V. (2004). Biological monitoring in occupational exposure to low levels of 1,3-butadiene. *Toxicol Lett*, **149**(1–3):353–360.

103. McDonald, J.D., Bechtold, W.E., Krone, J.R., Blackwell, W.B., Kracko, D.A., and Henderson, R.F. (2004). Analysis of butadiene urinary metabolites by liquid chromatography-triple quadrupole mass spectrometry. *J Anal Toxicol*, **28**(3):168–173.

104. Albertini, R.J., Sram, R.J., Vacek, P.M., Lynch, J., Wright, M., Nicklas, J.A. *et al.* (2001). Biomarkers for assessing occupational exposures to 1,3-butadiene. *Chem Biol Interact*, **135–136**:429–453.

105. Hayes, R.B., Zhang, L., Yin, S., Swenberg, J.A., Xi, L., Wiencke, J. *et al.* (2000). Genotoxic markers among butadiene polymer workers in China. Carcinogenesis, **21**(1):55–62.

106. Albertini, R.J., Sram, R.J., Vacek, P.M., Lynch, J., Nicklas, J.A., van Sittert, N.J. *et al.* (2003). Biomarkers in Czech workers exposed to 1,3-butadiene: a transitional epidemiologic study. Res *Rep Health Eff Inst*, **116**:1–141.

107. Sarkar, M., Kapur, S., Frost-Pineda, K., Feng, S., Wang, J., Liang, Q. *et al.* (2008). Evaluation of biomarkers of exposure to selected cigarette smoke constituents in adult smokers switched to carbon-filtered cigarettes in short-term and long-term clinical studies. *Nicotine Tob Res*, **10**(12): 1761–1772.

108. Mascher, D.G., Mascher, H.J., Scherer, G., and Schmid, E.R. (2001). High-performance liquid chromatographic-tandem mass spectrometric determination of 3-hydroxypropylmercapturic acid in human urine. *J Chromatogr B Biomed Sci Appl*, **750**(1):163–169.

109. Mendes, P., Kapur, S., Wang, J., Feng, S., and Roethig, H. (2008). A randomized, controlled exposure study in adult smokers of full flavor Marlboro cigarettes switching to Marlboro Lights or Marlboro Ultra Lights cigarettes. *Regul Toxicol Pharmacol*, **51**(3):295–305.

110. Roethig, H.J., Feng, S., Liang, Q., Liu, J., Rees, W.A., and Zedler, B.K. (2008). A 12-month, randomized, controlled study to evaluate exposure and cardiovascular risk factors in adult smokers switching from conventional cigarettes to a second-generation electrically heated cigarette smoking system. *J Clin Pharmacol*, **48**(5):580–591.

111. Qu, Q., Melikian, A.A., Li, G., Shore, R., Chen, L., Cohen, B. et al. (2000). Validation of biomarkers in humans exposed to benzene: urine metabolites. *Am J Ind Med*, **37**(5):522–531.

112. Feng, S., Roethig, H.J., Liang, Q., Kinser, R., Jin, Y., Scherer, G. et al. (2006). Evaluation of urinary 1-hydroxypyrene, *S*-phenylmercapturic acid, *trans,trans*-muconic acid, 3-methyladenine, 3-ethyladenine, 8-hydroxy-2'-deoxyguanosine and thioethers as biomarkers of exposure to cigarette smoke. *Biomarkers*, **11**(1):28–52.

113. Kim, S., Vermeulen, R., Waidyanatha, S., Johnson, B.A., Lan, Q., Rothman, N. et al. (2006). Using urinary biomarkers to elucidate dose-related patterns of human benzene metabolism. *Carcinogenesis*, **27**(4):772–781.

114. Qu, Q., Cohen, B.S., Shore, R., Chen, L.C., Li, G., Jin, X. et al. (2003). Benzene exposure measurement in shoe and glue manufacturing: a study to validate biomarkers. *Appl Occup Environ Hyg*, **18**(12):988–998.

115. van Sittert, N.J., Boogaard, P.J., and Beulink, G.D. (1993). Application of the urinary *S*-phenylmercapturic acid test as a biomarker for low levels of exposure to benzene in industry. *Br J Ind Med*, **50**(5):460–469.

116. Barbieri, A., Sabatini, L., Accorsi, A., Roda, A., and Violante, F.S. (2004). Simultaneous determination of *t,t*-muconic, *S*-phenylmercapturic and *S*-benzylmercapturic acids in urine by a rapid and sensitive liquid chromatography/electrospray tandem mass spectrometry method. *Rapid Commun Mass Spectrom*, **18**(17):1983–1988.

117. Maestri, L., Negri, S., Ferrari, M., Ghittori, S., and Imbriani, M. (2005). Determination of urinary *S*-phenylmercapturic acid, a specific metabolite of benzene, by liquid chromatography/single quadrupole mass spectrometry. *Rapid Commun Mass Spectrom*, **19**(9):1139–1144.

118. Lin, L.C., Shih, J.F., Shih, T.S., Li, Y.J., and Liao, P.C. (2004). An electrospray ionization tandem mass spectrometry based system with an online dual-loop cleanup device for simultaneous quantitation of urinary benzene exposure biomarkers trans,trans-muconic acid and S-phenylmercapturic acid. *Rapid Commun Mass Spectrom*, **18**(22):2743–2752.

119. Lin, L.C., Tyan, Y.C., Shih, T.S., Chang, Y.C., and Liao, P.C. (2004). Development and validation of an isotope-dilution electrospray ionization tandem mass spectrometry method with an on-line sample clean-up device for the quantitative analysis of the benzene exposure biomarker S-phenylmercapturic acid in human urine. *Rapid Commun Mass Spectrom*, **18**(12):1310–1316.

120. Schettgen, T., Musiol, A., Alt, A., and Kraus, T. (2008). Fast determination of urinary S-phenylmercapturic acid (S-PMA) and S-benzylmercapturic acid (S-BMA) by column-switching liquid chromatography-tandem mass spectrometry. *J Chromatogr B Analyt Technol Biomed Life Sci*, **863**(2):283–292.

121. Sabatini, L., Barbieri, A., Indiveri, P., Mattioli, S., and Violante, F.S. (2008). Validation of an HPLC-MS/MS method for the simultaneous determination of phenylmercapturic acid, benzylmercapturic acid and o-methylbenzyl mercapturic acid in urine as biomarkers of exposure to benzene, toluene and xylenes. *J Chromatogr B Analyt Technol Biomed Life Sci*, **863**(1):115–122.

122. Popp, W., Vahrenholz, C., Przygoda, H., Brauksiepe, A., Goch, S., Muller, G. et al. (1994). DNA-protein cross-links and sister chromatid exchange frequencies in lymphocytes and hydroxyethyl mercapturic acid in urine of ethylene oxide-exposed hospital workers. *Int Arch Occup Environ Health*, **66**(5):325–332.

123. Barr, D.B. and Ashley, D.L. (1998). A rapid, sensitive method for the quantitation of N-acetyl-S-(2-hydroxyethyl)-L-cysteine in human urine using isotope-dilution HPLC-MS-MS. *J Anal Toxicol*, **22**(2):96–104.

124. De Bont, R. and van Larebeke, N. (2004). Endogenous DNA damage in humans: a review of quantitative data. *Mutagenesis*, **19**(3):169–185.

125. Singh, R. and Farmer, P.B. (2006). Liquid chromatography-electrospray ionization-mass spectrometry: the future of DNA adduct detection. *Carcinogenesis*, **27**(2):178–196.

126. Poirier, M.C., Santella, R.M., and Weston, A. (2000). Carcinogen macromolecular adducts and their measurement. *Carcinogenesis*, **21**(3):353–359.

127. Kriek, E., Rojas, M., Alexandrov, K., and Bartsch, H. (1998). Polycyclic aromatic hydrocarbon-DNA adducts in humans: relevance as biomarkers for exposure and cancer risk. *Mutat Res*, **400**:215–231.

128. Wild, C.P. and Pisani, P. (1998). Carcinogen DNA and protein adducts as biomarkers of human exposure in environmental cancer epidemiology. *Cancer Detection and Prevention*, **22**:273–283.

129. Arif, J.M., Dresler, C., Clapper, M.L., Gairola, C.G., Srinivasan, C., Lubet, R.A. *et al.* (2006). Lung DNA adducts detected in human smokers are unrelated to typical polyaromatic carcinogens. *Chem Res Toxicol*, **19**(2):295–299.

130. International Agency for Research on Cancer (2004). Tobacco Smoke and Involuntary Smoking. IARC Monographs on the Evaluation of Carcinogenic Risks to Humans. Lyon, FR: IARC, 35–102.

131. Veglia, F., Matullo, G., and Vineis, P. (2003). Bulky DNA adducts and risk of cancer: a meta-analysis. *Cancer Epidemiol Biomarkers & Prev*, **12**(2):157–160.

132. Golkar, S.O., Ehrenberg, L., Segerback, D., and Hallstrom, I. (1976). Evaluation of genetic risks of alkyating agents II. Haemoglobin as a dose monitor. *Mutat Res*, **34**:1–10.

133. Ehrenberg, L. and Osterman-Golkar, S. (1980). Alkylation of macromolecules for detecting mutagenic agents. *Teratogenesis Carcinog Mutagen*, **1**:105–127.

134. Skipper, P.L. and Tannenbaum, S.R. (1990). Protein adducts in the molecular dosimetry of chemical carcinogens. *Carcinogenesis*, **11**:507–518.

135. Maclure, M., Bryant, M.S., Skipper, P.L., and Tannenbaum, S.R. (1990). Decline of the hemoglobin adduct of 4-minobiphenyl during withdrawal from smoking. *Cancer Res*, **50**:181–184.

136. Bergmark, E. (1997). Hemoglobin adducts of acrylamide and acrylonitrile in laboratory workers, smokers and nonsmokers. *Chem Res Toxicol*, **10**:78–84.

137. Fennell, T.R., MacNeela, J.P., Morris, R.W., Watson, M., Thompson, C.L., and Bell, D.A. (2000). Hemoglobin adducts from acrylonitrile and ethylene oxide in cigarette smokers: effects of glutathione S-transferase T1-null and M1-null genotypes. *Cancer Epidemiol Biomarkers & Prev*, **9**(7):705–712.

138. Carmella, S.G., Chen, M., Villalta, P.W., Gurney, J.G., Hatsukami, D.K., and Hecht, S.S. (2002). Ethylation and methylation of hemoglobin in smokers and non-smokers. *Carcinogenesis*, **23**(11): 1903–1910.

139. Wang, M., Cheng, G., Villalta, P.W., and Hecht, S.S. (2007). Development of liquid chromatography electrospray ionization tandem mass spectrometry methods for analysis of DNA adducts of formaldehyde and their application to rats treated with *N*-nitrosodimethylamine or 4-(methylnitrosamino)-1-(3-pyridyl)-1-butanone. *Chem Res Toxicol*, **20**(8):1141–1148.

140. Chen, L., Wang, M., Villalta, P.W., and Hecht, S.S. (2007). Liquid chromatography-electrospray ionization tandem mass spectrometry analysis of 7-ethylguanine in human liver DNA. *Chem Res Toxicol*, **20**(10):1498–1502.

141. Morrow, J.D., Frei, B., Longmire, A.W., Gaziano, J.M., Lynch, S.M., Shyr, Y. *et al.* (1995). Increase in circulating products of lipid peroxidation (F2-isoprostanes) in smokers. *N Engl J Med*, **332**:1198–1203.

142. Murphey, L.J., Williams, M.K., Sanchez, S.C., Byrne, L.M., Csiki, I., Oates, J.A. *et al.* (2004). Quantification of the major urinary metabolite of PGE2 by a liquid chromatographic/mass spectrometric assay: determination of cyclooxygenase-specific PGE2 synthesis in healthy humans and those with lung cancer. *Anal Biochem*, **334**(2):266–275.

143. Burns, D.M., Dybing, E., Gray, N., Hecht, S., Anderson, C., Sanner, T. *et al.* (2008). Mandated lowering of toxicants in cigarette smoke: a description of the World Health Organization *TobReg proposal. Tob Control,* **17**(2):132–141.

144. Church, T.R., Anderson, K.E., Caporaso, N.E., Geisser, M.S., Le, C., Zhang, Y., *et al* . (2009). A prospectively measured serum biomarker for a tobacco-specific carcinogen and lung cancer in smokers. *Cancer Epidemiol, Biomarkers, & Prev***18**:260–266.

145. Boffetta, P., Clark, S., Shen, M., Gislefoss, R., Peto, R., and Andersen, A. (2006). Serum cotinine level as predictor of lung cancer risk. *Cancer Epidemiol Biomarkers Prev,* **15**(6):1184–1188.

146. Yuan, Y.-M., Koh, W.-P., Murphy, S.E., Fan, Y., Wang, R., Carmella, S.G. *et al.* (2009). Urinary levels of tobacco-specific nitrosamine metabolites in relation to lung cancer development in two prospective cohorts of cigarette smokers. *Cancer Res.,* **69**:2990–2995.

Chapter 8

Pharmacology of tobacco addiction

Jack E. Henningfield and Neal L. Benowitz

Since the 1980s, it has become recognized by clinicians, researchers, and public health experts that tobacco products are among the most addictive and deadly of all dependence-producing substances (Royal College of Physicians 2000; US DHHS 1988; WHO 2001). Nicotine meets all of the standard criteria for a dependence-producing drug and all types of tobacco products are capable of delivering dependence-producing levels of nicotine (Royal College of Physicians 2000; Royal Society of Canada 1989; US DHHS 1988). These conclusions are consistent with the neuropharmacology of nicotine (Henningfield, *et al.* 1996), with clinical studies of nicotine dependence and withdrawal (e.g., Hughes, *et al.* 1990; Henningfield, *et al.* 1995b), and with the epidemiology of tobacco use and dependence (Giovino, *et al.* 1995). In fact, if evaluated against the criteria used to determine the level of psychoactive scheduling set by the US Controlled Substance Act or the International Convention on Psychotropic Substances (described by McClain and Sapienza 1989 and McAllister 2003; Balster and Bigelow 2004), nicotine could be appropriately categorized as a controlled substance (Buchhalter, *et al.* 2008; Food and Drug Administration 1995, 1996). Regulation of tobacco products as controlled substances by the International Convention would probably be as unmanageable as regulation of alcoholic beverages by the Convention, whereas the World Health Organization's Framework Convention on Tobacco Products (FCTC) was developed with recognition that the addictive effects of nicotine must be addressed in tobacco control efforts (WHO 2009).

There are several reasons for the relatively recent widespread recognition of the dependence-producing effects of nicotine in tobacco as compared to the role of morphine in opium product use. For example, although the effects of nicotine on the nervous system have been investigated since the nineteenth century (e.g., Langely 1905), and the role of nicotine in tobacco since early in the twentieth century (e.g., Finnegan, *et al.* 1945; Johnston 1942), it was not until the 1980s that an overwhelming body of research established that nicotine itself met all criteria for a dependence-producing drug (National Institute on Drug Abuse 1984; US DHHS 1988).

Tobacco dependence and withdrawal were listed in the Diagnostic and Statistical Manual (DSM) of the American Psychiatric Association (APA) in its third edition in 1980. The International Classification of Diseases (ICD) of the World Health Organization (WHO) listed tobacco dependence and withdrawal in its tenth edition, in 1992. When the APA's DSM was revised in 1987, it replaced 'tobacco' with 'nicotine' as the identifying substance on the basis that evidence was sufficient to implicate nicotine as the primary determinant of dependence and withdrawal. In contrast, WHO (1992) continues to refer to the substance 'tobacco' as opposed to its drug, 'nicotine' just as it refers to the substance 'cannabinoids' as opposed to their drug, tetrahydrocannabinol. This is based on the reasoning that even though nicotine is the critical drug that defines the disorders, in practice, withdrawal signs from pure nicotine systems (e.g., nicotine gum and patches) are generally weak and the establishment of dependence on pure nicotine preparations is not a known public health problem.

Both the APA and WHO approaches have merit and scientific rationale. However, the WHO approach which emphasizes the importance of the tobacco vehicle is highly relevant to recent advances in the understanding of tobacco use that have begun to unravel the contributions of tobacco product ingredients and designs, which may be determinants of the risk, severity, and prevalence of nicotine addiction (FDA 1996; Henningfield, *et al.* 2004; Henningfield and Zeller 2006; WHO 2001, 2007). These issues will be addressed in the present analysis. Despite the many research questions that need to be explored to fully understand the mechanisms underlying dependence on tobacco and nicotine, there is a strong science foundation upon which to guide policy aimed at reducing the prevalence of tobacco use and eradicating tobacco caused diseases (WHO 2007; WHO TobReg 2004; US DHHS 2009).

Pharmacology of nicotine

Great advances have been made in understanding the pharmacology of nicotine as pertains to its addictiveness in recent years (Buchhalter, *et al.* 2008; US DHHS 2009). Nicotine is an alkaloid that is present in concentrations of about 1–3% in tobacco cultivated for commercial tobacco products (Browne 1990). The concept that the pharmacologic effects of tobacco primarily reflect the actions of nicotine has been widely accepted, at least since Lewin's analysis from the 1920s (translated into English in 1931 and reprinted in 1964) in which he concluded; 'The decisive factor in the effect of tobacco, desired or undesired, is nicotine…' For example, prominent effects of tobacco on muscle tone, heart rate, and blood pressure, as well as behavioural and mood altering effects, can be mimicked by administration of nicotine (Benowitz 1990; Henningfield, *et al.* 1996; Taylor 1996).

Nicotine is a potent and powerful agonist of several subpopulations of nicotinic receptors of the cholinergic nervous system (Buchhalter, *et al.* 2008; Henningfield, *et al.* 1996; Paterson and Nordberg 2000; Vidal 1996). Acute doses of 1 mg per 70 Kg accelerate heart rate and alter mood, although daily users are substantially less sensitive to such effects than non-users (Foulds, *et al.* 1997; Soria, *et al.* 1996; Taylor 1996; US DHHS 1988). The half-life of nicotine averages approximately two hours but is longer in persons in the presence of a genetic polymorphism of the liver enzyme CYP2A6, which is the primary metabolic pathway of nicotine (Benowitz, *et al.* 2002; Tyndale and Sellers 2001). The prevalence of CYP2A6 alleles that are associated with reduced enzymatic activity is higher in Asians than in Caucasians, and this difference may contribute to lower daily cigarette consumption and a lower risk of lung cancer in Asians compared to Caucasians. (Ahijevych 1999; Benowitz, *et al.* 2002; Haiman, *et al.* 2006; Tyndale and Sellers 2001). African Americans also have a higher prevalence of CYP2A6 gene variants associated with slow nicotine metabolism and also smoke fewer cigarettes per day in contrast to Caucasians, but for still unknown reasons have a higher risk of lung cancer compared to Caucasians (Mwenifumbo, *et al.* 2008; Perez-Stable, *et al.* 1998; Zhou Haiman *et al.* 2006). A primary nicotine metabolite, cotinine, has a 16–20 hour half-life and distribution in blood, urine, and saliva that makes it useful for studies of nicotine intake in the laboratory and at the population level (Benowitz 1996, 1999).

The peripheral nervous system actions of nicotine on ganglionic cholinergic receptors have been studied since the nineteenth century. Studies of nicotinic agonists and antagonists contributed to advances in methods, which formed the foundation for modern neuroscience research, including the use of selective agonists and antagonists to explore the mechanism of action of neurons and the concept of the 'receptive substance' as a mediator of effects (e.g., Langley 1905). The peripheral actions of nicotine include relaxation or stimulation of muscles, depending upon the dose and the muscle group, as well as a high dose 'paralysis', which can lead to respiratory depression and death; the latter is a mechanism exploited in the use of nicotine as a pesticide (Taylor 1996).

Central nervous system actions of nicotine are diverse (Buchhalter, *et al.* 2008; US DHHS 2009). The importance of variation in the structural and functional properties of nicotinic cholinergic receptors throughout the brain is an especially active area of neuropharmacological research. Identifying selective nicotinic agonists and antagonists could yield clinically important advances in medications for aiding smoking cessation as well as for treating disorders that appear to involve the various nicotinic receptor subpopulations, e.g., Parkinson's disease, Alzheimer's disease, attention deficit hyperactivity disorder, Tourette's syndrome, and various affective disorders (Balfour and Fagerstrom 1996; Levin, *et al.* 1996; Newhouse and Hughes 1991; Newhouse, *et al.* 1997; Paterson and Nordberg 2000; Santos, *et al.* 2002; Vidal 1996).

Abuse liability and physical dependence potential of tobacco products

All tobacco products are addictive with a high potential for abuse, physical dependence, and withdrawal (WHO 2006). This is because they contain and deliver behaviourally active amounts of nicotine to their users and do so in delivery systems which have often been highly engineered to enhance the addiction risk of the products (FDA 1995, 1996; WHO 2001, 2006, 2007; US DHHS 2009). Tobacco products without nicotine are not well accepted by chronic tobacco users (e.g., Finnegan, *et al.* 1945) and are not well accepted in the market place (FDA 1995, 1996). The abuse liability and physical dependence potential of nicotine have been well characterized and further exploration of the mechanism of these effects is an active are of research. In brief, nicotine produces dose-related psychoactive effects in humans that are identified as stimulant-like, and it elevates scores on standardized tests for liking and euphoria that are relied upon by WHO for assessing abuse potential (Henningfield, *et al.* 1995; Jones, *et al.* 1999; Royal College of Physicians 2000; US DHHS 1988). The subjective effects of nicotine are reduced by the centrally acting nicotinic cholinergic receptor blocker, mecamylamine (Rose, *et al.* 1989; Lundahl, *et al.* 2000), but not by the peripherally acting blocker, pentolinium (Stolerman, *et al.* 1973). Drug discrimination testing in animals has similarly revealed that nicotine is discriminated in a dose-related fashion and that these effects are blocked by centrally but not peripherally acting nicotinic cholinergic receptor blockers (Henningfield, *et al.* 1996; US DHHS 1988).

Nicotine can serve as a potent and powerful reinforcer for both humans and animals as demonstrated by intravenous self-administration studies (Corrigall 1999; Goldberg, *et al.* 1983; Goldberg and Henningfield 1988; Garrett, *et al.* 2004), patterns of self-administration are more similar to those of stimulants than of other drug classes (Griffiths, *et al.* 1980). However, the range of conditions under which it functions as a reinforcer is smaller than that under which cocaine serves as a reinforcer (US DHHS 1988).

Intravenous nicotine self-administration is reduced by centrally acting nicotinic cholinergic receptor blockers, but not by peripherally acting blockers (Corrigall 1999). Patterns of tobacco product self-administration are influenced by nicotine dose with manipulations of delivery resulting in changes in behaviour that tend to sustain similar levels of nicotine intake (Gritz 1980; Henningfield 1984; US DHHS 1988). Nicotine exposure results in a high degree of tolerance, which is mediated by several mechanisms, and which includes acute and long-term components (Perkins, *et al.* 1993; Perkins 2002; Swedberg, *et al.* 1990).

Tolerance

Tolerance to some effects may be related to the up-regulation of central nervous system nicotine receptors, but genetic factors also modulate nicotine effects including development of tolerance (Collins and Marks 1989). A practical consequence is that whereas first-time tobacco users often become profoundly sick and intoxicated, these effects generally dissipate within a few hours and are rarely experienced again due to a combination of learning to avoid overdosing, and tolerance (US DHHS 1988; Royal College of Physicians 2000). Laboratory studies of intravenous nicotine (Soria, *et al.* 1996) and nicotine gum administration (Heishman and Henningfield 2000) have demonstrated greater sensitivity to the mood-altering and behavioural effects of nicotine in subjects who do not use tobacco compared to tobacco users. The development of snuff products that are marketed as starter products in which the products delivered lower doses of nicotine more slowly than do the maintenance products takes advantage of the tolerance phenomenon and minimizes the likelihood that the initial users experience will be unpleasant (Connolly 1995; FDA 1995, 1996). With respect to cigarettes, because the nicotine dosing is puff by puff, with the physiologic response occurring quite quickly after each puff, this problem is less of a barrier to the acquisition of smoking than it is for the acquisition of snuff use (in which the dose is determined by the amount snuff put in the mouth) (Connolly 1995; Slade 1995).

Physical dependence and withdrawal

Tobacco withdrawal signs and symptoms, including changes in brain electrical activity, cognitive performance, anxiety, and response to stressful stimuli can be altered by administration of pure nicotine in a variety of forms (e.g., gum, patch, nasal delivery) (Heishman, *et al.* 1994; Hughes, Higgins and Hatsukami 1990; Pickworth, *et al.* 1995; Shiffman, *et al.* 1998). Humans report generally similar subjective effects from intravenous nicotine as from smoked tobacco (Henningfield, *et al.* 1985; Jones, *et al.* 1999). Tobacco craving is only partially relieved by pharmaceutical forms of nicotine, reflecting the facts that (1) cravings can be elicited by factors that are not mitigated by nicotine (e.g., the smell of smoke, the sight of other people smoking, and tobacco advertisements), and (2) tobacco smoke constituents other than nicotine (e.g., 'tar' and other smoke constituents) can reduce craving independently of nicotine (Butchsky, *et al.* 1995) and may have synergistic effects with nicotine in cigarettes to provide more effective nicotine relief than cigarette smoke-delivered nicotine (Rose, *et al.* 1993).

Rodent models of nicotine withdrawal have been developed and serve in the evaluation of medications for treating withdrawal (e.g., Malin, *et al.* 1992, 1998a, 1998b). The most useful is one in which the frequency of signs are observed and coded from a checklist which includes writhes and gasps, wet shakes and tremors, ptosis, bouts of teeth chattering and chewing, and miscellaneous less frequent signs such as foot licks, scratches, and yawns (Malin *et al.* 1992). Episodes of locomotor immobility lasting longer than a minute are also recorded. Another rodent model that might be of particular relevance to disruption of behavioural performance in humans is one in which acute nicotine abstinence disrupted food maintained learned behaviours (Carroll, *et al.* 1989).

Dose-related effects

As with many drugs, understanding the mechanisms of the effects of nicotine is complicated by the facts that total dose, rate of delivery, and amount of prior exposure are important determinants (Ernst, *et al.* 2001). For example, 1 mg nicotine delivered by smoke inhalation may produce cardiac acceleration and mood alteration, whereas the approximately 1 mg nicotine delivered per hour by transdermal nicotine patch produces no reliable change in mood or cardiovascular measure (Benowitz 1990; Pickworth, *et al.* 1994). Furthermore, observed effects involve a diverse array of mechanisms, which operate differentially at different dosages. For example, stimulation of nicotinic cholinergic receptors in the spinal cord may directly alter muscle tone, whereas heart rate acceleration and mood alteration appear to be primarily mediated by catecholamines release that is modulated by nicotine (e.g., release of norepinephrine and increased brain dopamine, respectively) (Benowitz 1990; Balfour and Fagerstrom 1996; Henningfield, Keenan and Clarke 1996).

Nicotine is rapidly and efficiently absorbed when inhaled into the lung (Benowitz 1990). It is also well absorbed though the skin, nasal passages, and the oral mucosa, although the speed of its absorption though the mucosa is directly related to the fraction of nicotine that is in a 'free-base' or unionized state, as opposed to that which is in the 'bound' or in the ionized state. The alkaloid nature of nicotine implies that the percentage of unionized nicotine molecules in tobacco material can be influenced by the pH of the product or its aqueous medium, with the concentration of free base nicotine increasing logarithmically as a function of increasing pH (Henningfield, Radzius and Cone 1995a). The pKa of nicotine is 8, and thus 50% of the nicotine is unionized and free to be rapidly absorbed at an aqueous pH of 8. The alkaline smoke typical of cigars (typically 7.0–8.5) enables efficient absorption of nicotine through the mouth without inhalation (Baker, *et al.* 2000; Henningfield, *et al.* 1999). The mildly acidic smoke of cigarettes (pH 5.5–6.5) produces less throat irritation and is easier to inhale than higher pH cigar smoke but no nicotine is absorbed in the mouth and smoke must be inhaled to absorb nicotine (Hoffman and Hoffman 1997). Since addictive drug effects are intensified by faster delivery (O'Brien 1996), the dual consequence of a potentially more addictive form of nicotine delivery and the well-documented greater lung toxicity due to the repetitive exposure of the lung to the smoke results (Hoffman and Hoffman 1997). Therefore, even though a cigar potentially delivers more nicotine and toxins, the risk of lung disease is less than that associated with cigarette smoking (Baker *et al.* 2000; National Cancer Institute 1998).

Smokeless tobacco products such as snuff, include 'starter' products (tobacco industry term) that are generally at pH levels of approximately 7.0, whereas products that experienced users tend to 'graduate' to (tobacco industry term) generally show an aqueous pH of 7.5–8.5) (Henningfield, Radzius and Cone 1995a). Snuff products with higher pH levels than products with similar nicotine content produce more rapidly rising and higher plasma nicotine levels as well as higher heart rates and stronger subjective effects (Fant, *et al.* 1999).

An additional consequence of smoke inhalation is the generation of arterial plasma nicotine spikes that can be up to ten times greater than simultaneously measured venous levels within the first minute following the smoking of a cigarette (Henningfield, *et al.* 1993). Similar effects occur with smoked cocaine and appear to contribute to its powerful reinforcing effects (Evans, *et al.* 1996). Consistent with these observations, tobacco products that deliver nicotine more rapidly are demonstrated to be of higher abuse liability in standard testing than pharmaceutical products, which deliver nicotine more slowly (Henningfield and Keenan 1993; Stitzer and DeWitt 1998). These observations are consistent with product design and ingredients: whereas, tobacco products are designed to maximize addictive potential, pharmaceutical products are designed and labelled to minimize the risk of addiction and abuse (Henningfield and Slade 1998; Slade and Henningfield 1998).

Cross population variation in nicotine metabolism

There is much individual variability in the CYP2A6 activity of human liver samples, and much variability in the rate of nicotine metabolism among individuals and populations. Studies of racial/ethnic differences have shown slower metabolism of nicotine and cotinine in Chinese Americans, and slower metabolism of cotinine in African Americans compared to American Caucasians and Hispanics (Benowitz, *et al.* 2002; Perez-Stable, *et al.* 1998). As mentioned previously the slower metabolism of nicotine and cotinine by Asians and African Americans can be explained by the high frequency of CYP2A6 gene alleles that are associated with diminished or absent enzyme activity (Haiman, *et al.* 2006; Nakajim, *et al.* 2006). Slower metabolism of nicotine among Asians may explain, at least in part, lower cigarette consumption among Asians compared to Caucasians (Benowitz, *et al.* 2002). African Americans also metabolize via the glucuronidation pathway more slowly than Caucasians, the genetic basis and biological consequences of which have not yet been determined (Benowitz, *et al.* 1999). Pregnancy is associated with a marked acceleration of nicotine and cotinine metabolism (Dempsey, *et al.* 2002). Thus the pregnant woman may require higher dose of nicotine medication to aid smoking cessation compared to the non-pregnant woman. Aging has been reported to be associated with slower metabolism of nicotine, as has the presence of kidney disease (Molander, *et al.* 2000, 2001). The importance of individual differences in nicotine metabolism in determining cigarette consumption and/or addiction risk is a subject of ongoing investigation.

Tobacco delivered nicotine

Nicotine is the critical and defining addictive drug in tobacco products, however, other ingredients and design features can contribute to the addictiveness of tobacco products (US DHHS 2009; WHO 2004, 2006, 2007). Tobacco products provide effective devices for storing nicotine and serving as vehicles for its delivery. Tobacco companies use a variety of techniques to control the nicotine dosing characteristics of cigarettes. The modern cigarette is elaborately designed, involving numerous patents for wrappers, manufacturing, filter systems, and processes for making 'tobacco' filler out of tobacco materials and other substances (Browne 1990; FDA 1995, 1996). The function of the cigarette has been described eloquently by senior Philip Morris researcher William Dunn, as reprinted in Hurt and Robertson (1998):

> The cigarette should be conceived not as a product but as a package. The product is nicotine. Think of the cigarette pack as a storage container for a day's supply of nicotine... Think of the cigarette as dispenser for dose unit of nicotine... Think of a puff of smoke as the vehicle of nicotine. Smoke is beyond question the most optimize vehicle of nicotine and the cigarette the most optimized dispenser of smoke.

Although both the tobacco industry and non-industry scientists and agencies have described cigarettes as nicotine delivery systems, not all of their effects are explained by nicotine delivery (e.g., Henningfield, *et al.* 2004; Hurt and Robertson 1998; FDA 1995, 1996; Slade, *et al.* 1995; US DHHS 2009; WHO 200, 2004, 2006, 2007). Most of the toxicity of the products is due to substances other than nicotine. Substances in tobacco smoke, in addition to nicotine, may also contribute to the development and maintenance of tobacco use (FDA 1995, 1996; Hurt and Robertson 1998; Slade, *et al.* 1995; WHO 2001).

Because the speed and nature of the absorption process is a strong determinant of the effects of nicotine, it is not surprising that the tobacco industry has focused much attention on tobacco product development and the control of nicotine dosing characteristics by means such as pH manipulation of tobacco and tobacco smoke (FDA 1995, 1996; Kessler, *et al.* 1996; Hurt and Robertson 1998; Slade, *et al.* 1995). For example, buffering compounds in smokeless tobacco products (FDA 1995, 1996; Tomar and Henningfield 1997) can alter the speed and amount of nicotine delivery of the products. Similarly menthol, and perhaps compounds such as levulinic acid (Bates, *et al.* 1999), may alter the effects of nicotine delivered by smoke by enabling smokers to inhale larger quantities of smoke by making the smoke feel less harsh and by reducing concerns about the smoke toxicity because of the perceived smoothness (Henningfield, *et al.* 2002). Product design and ingredients can also be employed to control the mean particle size to optimize the efficient inhalation of nicotine deep into the lungs where absorption is rapid and virtually complete (Royal College of Physicians 2000). Characteristics that contribute to larger amounts of smoke being more deeply absorbed into the lung could also contribute to more rapid absorption of nicotine as well as increasing the probability of diseases such as deep lung adenocarcinomas (Hoffman and Hoffman 1997; Thun and Burns 2001).

The idea that cigarette smoke is a chemical cocktail that produces effects beyond those produced by nicotine and/or which may modulate nicotine's effects has received increasing support since the 1990s. This has led to the conclusion that tobacco delivered nicotine is not only more toxic, but more addictive than pure nicotine forms (Henningfield *et al.* 2000; Royal College of Physicians 2000). Additionally, it appears that non-nicotine components of cigarette smoke inhibit monoamine oxidase which could contribute to an antidepressant effect of smoking (Lewis, *et al.* 2007; Volkow, *et al.* 1999). Acetaldehyde, a metabolite of alcohol, which contributes to its subjective effects, is present in cigarette smoke and can act synergistically with nicotine to produce stronger reinforcing effects than either nicotine or acetaldehyde alone (Bates, *et al.* 1999; FDA 1995, 1996). Research on this topic was conducted by the tobacco industry and modern cigarettes can be engineered to increase their delivery of acetaldehyde either by adding the substance or by including certain sugars, which yield acetaldehyde upon pyrolysis (Bates, *et al.* 1999; FDA 1995, 1996).

Nicotine toxicology

Although nicotine can be a lethal poison at very high dosages, relative to those typically delivered by use of tobacco or nicotine replacement medications, its toxicological effects in tobacco use are modest compared to the many carcinogens and other toxins present in tobacco products and the many more produced when tobacco products are burned (Benowitz 1998; Hoffman and Hoffman 1997). Nonetheless, nicotine delivered by tobacco products and medications is not entirely benign. Nicotine can produce a variety of potential adverse effects depending upon the dose and pattern of administration. 'For example, nicotine is a fetal neuroteratogen in rats and there is concern that nicotine from cigarette smoking during pregnancy might contribute to developmental and behavioral problems in children of mothers who smoke' (US DHHS 2001). At doses delivered by nicotine replacement medications, the risk of adverse effects from nicotine during pregnancy appears substantially lower than by smoking. But because the possibility of risks cannot be ruled out, it is generally recommended that a doctor be consulted concerning use of the medications during pregnancy (Windsor, *et al.* 2000). Similarly, nicotine is a possible contributor to coronary artery disease leading to labelling on nicotine medications advising persons with histories of heart disease to consult with a doctor before using the products.

Comparison across addictive drugs

As indicated by the foregoing discussion, nicotine delivered by tobacco meets criteria as a dependence producing drug. Moreover, there is sufficient epidemiological and clinical evidence for a systematic comparison of cigarettes to other addictive drugs. One such comparison was provided in a table (pp. 299–303) in the 1988 Surgeon General's Report (US DHHS 1988), and another by Henningfield, *et al.* (1995b), which was adapted for presentation in the report of the Royal College of Physicians (2000). The following comparison of drugs is based upon these prior analyses. Key findings were that the apparent severity of addictive effects of the various drugs depends upon the measure under consideration; no addictive drug exceeds all others on all points; nicotine delivered by tobacco is a highly addictive drug. Nonetheless, differences in specific features of addictive drugs and differences in consequences of their use have implications for regulatory approaches appropriate to each drug and for clinical approaches to treating individuals which are determined by the particular drug under consideration (Goldstein 1994).

Table 8.1 Ranking of nicotine in relation to other drugs in terms of addiction factors of concern (Royal College of Physicians 2000)

Dependence among users	nicotine>heroin>cocaine>alcohol>caffeine
Difficulty achieving abstinence	(alcohol=cocaine=heroin=nicotine)>caffeine
Tolerance	(alcohol=heroin=nicotine)>cocaine>caffeine
Physical withdrawal severity	alcohol>heroin>nicotine>cocaine>caffeine
Societal impact	serious effects due to secondary deaths (nicotine), accidents (alcohol) or crime (heroin, cocaine); no substantial impact for caffeine
Deaths	nicotine>alcohol>(cocaine=heroin)>caffeine
Importance in user's daily life	(alcohol=cocaine=heroin=nicotine)>caffeine
Intoxication	alcohol>(cocaine=heroin)>caffeine>nicotine
Animal self-administration	cocaine>heroin>(alcohol=nicotine)>caffeine
Liking by non-drug abusers	cocaine>(alcohol=caffeine=heroin=nicotine)
Prevalence	caffeine>nicotine>alcohol>(cocaine=heroin)

Incidence, prevalence, and risk of progression

Following initial use, development of dependence to nicotine is far more common than that to cocaine, heroin, or alcohol, and the rate of graduation from occasional use to addictive levels of intake is highest for nicotine (Anthony, *et al.* 1994; Giovino, *et al.* 1995). Depending upon the definition used for occasional use, between 33% and 50% escalate to become daily smokers in the United States (US DHHS 1994). In contrast, even when highly addictive dosage forms of cocaine (i.e., smokable 'crack' cocaine) are readily available in the United States, the risk of progression from any use to regular use is the exception and not the rule.

Remission and relapse

An evaluation of several data sets indicates that rates and patterns of relapse are similar for nicotine, heroin, and alcohol (e.g., Hunt and Matarazzo 1973; Maddux and Desmond 1986), and probably for cocaine (e.g., Wallace 1989). A closer analysis of relapse to cigarette smoking showed that in the context of a minimal treatment intervention approach, approximately 25% of persons relapsed within 2 days of their last cigarette and approximately 50% within 1 week (Kotke, *et al.* 1989), and that among people quitting on their own, two-thirds were smoking within 3 days of their scheduled quit date (Hughes, *et al.* 1992).

Reports of addictiveness by drug abusers

Two studies evaluated ratings across addictions by polydrug abusers. The first study found that when rating the degree of 'liking', tobacco, cocaine, and heroin were rated similarly and all were rated more highly than alcohol, and that tobacco was among the most highly rated drugs on a 'need' scale (Blumberg, *et al.* 1974). Another study found that compared to other substances, tobacco was associated with equal or greater levels of difficulty in quitting and urge to use, but its use was not as pleasurable (Kozlowski, *et al.* 1989).

Psychoactivity and euphoria

One correlate of addiction liability is that a drug produces pleasurable or euphoriant effects in standard tests of drug liking and morphine-benzedrine group scale (MBG) scores of the Addiction

Research Center Inventory (Fischman and Mello 1989; Jasinski 1979). Intravenous nicotine mimics mood-altering effects of tobacco and, when rapidly administered by intravenous injections in a similar manner as cocaine is often abuse, nicotine produces qualitatively similar effects as cocaine in poly drug abusers (Henningfield, *et al.* 1995b; Jones *et al.* 1999).

Reinforcing effects

As discussed earlier, nicotine serves as a reinforcer for a variety of species. Its reinforcing effects are related to the dose and are increased when sensory stimuli are associated with injections and by food deprivation (Corrigall 1999; USDHHS 1988).

Physical dependence

Among addictive drugs, the most severe withdrawal syndromes are those that occur following acute deprivation of extended administration of alcohol or short acting barbiturates; morphine-like opioids can also produce an overtly recognizable syndrome (O'Brien 1996). Deprivation after extended administration of cocaine and cannabis can also produce a diagnosable withdrawal syndrome; however, it is only since the mid-1980s that addiction experts have come to generally concur that these drugs can produce syndromes of withdrawal that can be distinguished from the lack of the effects of the drugs themselves; the role of the withdrawal syndromes in sustaining cocaine and cannabis use remains unclear (Gawin and Kleber 1986; O'Brien 1996). Acute deprivation from extended tobacco use produces a syndrome of withdrawal signs and symptoms that is intermediate between that of the opioids and cocaine in that it has been recognized for several decades, and is generally understood to serve as a barrier to even short-term efforts to achieve tobacco abstinence. Tobacco withdrawal can be occupationally and socially debilitating, but other than standing as a barrier to extended cessation, is not life-threatening in its own right (American Psychiatric Association 1996).

Tolerance

A high degree of tolerance develops to the acute effects of nicotine, and some degree of tolerance is gained during each day of smoking and lost during the approximately eight hours of tobacco deprivation during sleeping hours (Swedberg, *et al.* 1990). Tolerance to nicotine has been systematically explored for more than a century (e.g., Langley 1905). Its mechanisms are diverse and the time course of gain and loss of tolerance varies across responses under evaluation (Balfour and Fagerstrom 1996; Collins and Marks 1989; Perkins 2002; Royal College of Physicians 2000). Comparing drugs of abuse on measures of tolerance is complicated by the varying potential range of measures that can be considered, however, the general degree of tolerance that is produced by repeated nicotine exposure is comparable to that produced by other addictive drugs that produce high levels of tolerance such as the opioids.

Implications for treatment of tobacco dependence

Advances in the understanding of the neuropharmacology of nicotine and factors contributing to the addictiveness of tobacco products have had great implications for the use and development of treatment (Fant, *et al.* 2009; Henningfield, *et al.* 2009), Particular strides have been made in understanding the cognitive deficit and adverse mood effects which frequently accompany nicotine abstinence in dependent persons as well as the benefits of pharmacotherapy in providing relief of these symptoms (Fant, *et al.* 2009; Henningfield, *et al.* 2005, 2009). This includes understanding the cerebral correlates and potential mechanisms of such effects as revealed by brain imaging studies and other neuropsychopharmacology techniques (Henningfield, *et al.* 2009b; Stapleton, *et al.* 2005).

Although many people are able to quit smoking without formal intervention, this generally occurs only after many cessation attempts and after sufficient harm has been done to substantially increase the risks of premature mortality (Royal College of Physicians 2000; US DHHS 2000). For others, perhaps as a consequence of the pathological changes in brain structure and function produced by long-term nicotine exposure, achieving remission from dependence without treatment may be no more readily achievable than achieving remission from coronary artery disease or oral cancer without treatment. In fact, following surgery for coronary artery disease and lung cancer caused by smoking, many smokers resume smoking in face of the extraordinarily high risks (US DHHS 1988). The US Clinical Practice Guideline: Treating Tobacco Use and Dependence (Fiore, *et al.* 2000) and reports from the US Surgeon General (US DHHS 2000), and Royal College of Physicians (2000) describe behavioural and pharmacological treatment interventions that approximately double the chances of achieving cessation. These include intensive group behavioural counselling, other individualized behaviour therapies and several types of pharmacotherapy. Pharmacotherapies include different nicotine replacement medications (gum, patch, lozenge, oral inhaler, and nasal spray) and bupropion, as well as medications that have been demonstrated to be effective but have not been explicitly approved or marketed for smoking cessation (nortriptyline and clonidine). Many other substances have been used but show little evidence of efficacy (Fiore *et al.* 2000; Henningfield, *et al.* 1998; US DHHS 2000).

Acknowledgements

Preparation of this chapter was supported, in part, by a Robert Wood Johnson Foundation Innovators Combating Substance Abuse Award to Dr. Henningfield. Dr. Henningfield provides consulting services regarding treatments for tobacco dependence to GlaxoSmithKline Consumer Health Care through Pinney Associates, and also has a financial interest in a nicotine replacement product under development, and serves as an expert witness in litigation against the tobacco industry by the US Department of Justice and other plaintiffs. Dr. Benowitz work was supported, in part, by US Public Health Service Grants DA02277 and DA 12393.

References

Ahijevych, K. (1999). Nicotine metabolism variability and nicotine addiction. *Nicotine & Tobacco Research*, **1**, (Suppl.): S59–S62.

American Psychiatric Association. (1980). *Diagnostic and Statistical Manual of Mental Disorders* (Third edn). Washington, DC: American Psychiatric Association.

American Psychiatric Association. (1987). *Diagnostic and Statistical Manual of Mental Disorders* (Third revised edn). Washington, DC: American Psychiatric Association.

American Psychiatric Association. (1996). *Practice Guideline for the Treatment of Patients with Nicotine Dependence*. Washington, DC: American Psychiatric Association.

Anthony, J.C., Warner, L.A., and Kessler R.C. (1994). Comparative epidemiology of dependence on tobacco, alcohol, controlled substance, and inhalants: basic findings from the National Comorbidity Survey. *Experimental and Clinical Psychopharmacology*, **2**: 244–268.

Baker, F., Ainsworth, S.R., Dye, J.T., Crammer, C., Thun, M.J., Hoffmann, D. *et al.* (2000). Health risks associated with cigar smoking. *Journal of the American Medical Association*, **284**(6): 735–740.

Balfour, D.J. and Fagerstrom, K.O. (1996). Pharmacology of nicotine and its therapeutic use in smoking cessation and neurodegenerative disorders. *Pharmacology & Therapeutics*, **72**(1): 51–81.

Balster, R.L. and Bigelow, G.E. (2003). Guidelines and methodological reviews concerning drug abuse liability assessment. *Drug Alcohol Depend*, **70**: S13–40.

Bates, C., Connolly, G.N., and Jarvis, M. (1999). *Tobacco Additives: Cigarette Engineering and Nicotine Addiction*. London, UK: Action on Smoking and Health.

Benowitz, N.L. (1990). Pharmacokinetic considerations in understanding nicotine dependence. In: G. Bock and J. Marsh (eds), *The Biology of Nicotine Dependence*. (pp. 186–209). London, UK: John Wiley & Sons Ltd.

Benowitz, N.L. (1996). Biomarkers of cigarette smoking. In: National Institutes of Health, & National Cancer Institute *The FTC cigarette test method for determining tar, nicotine, and carbon monoxide yields of U.S. cigarettes: report of the NCI Expert Committee*. (pp. 93–111). Bethesda, MD: National Institutes of Health, & National Cancer Institute.

Benowitz, N.L. (ed) (1998). *Nicotine Safety and Toxicity*. Oxford: Oxford University Press.

Benowitz, N.L. (1999). Biomarkers of environmental tobacco smoke exposure. *Environmental Health Perspectives*, **107**(2): 349–355.

Benowitz, N.L., Perez-Stable, E.J., Herrera, B., and Jacob, P., III. (2002). Slower metabolism and reduced intake of nicotine from cigarette smoking in Chinese-Americans. *Journal of the National Cancer Institute*, **94**(2): 108–115.

Blumberg, H.H., Cohen, S.D., Dronfield, B.E., Mordecal, E.A., Roberts, J.C., and Hawks, D. (1974). British opiate users I. People approaching London drug treatment centers. *International Journal of Addiction*, **9**: 1–23.

Browne, C.L. (1990). *The Design of Cigarettes*. (Third edn). Charlotte, North Carolina: Filter Products Division Hoechst Celanese Corporation.

Buchhalter, A.R., Fant, R.V., and Henningfield, J.E. Nicotine. (2007). In: D.R. Sibley, I. Hanin, M. Kuhar, and P. Skolnick (eds) *Handbook of Contemporary Neuropharmacology, Volume 2, Substance Abuse and Addictive Disorders*. Hoboken, New Jersey: John Wiley & Sons, Inc., pp. 535–566.

Butschky, M.F., Bailey, D., Henningfield, J.E., and Pickworth, W.B. (1995). Smoking without nicotine delivery decreases withdrawal in 12-hour abstinent smokers. *Pharmacology Biochemistry and Behavior*, **50**(1): 91–96.

Carroll, M.E., Lac, S.T., Asencio, M., and Keenan, R.M. (1989). Nicotine dependence in rats. *Life Sciences*, **45**: 1381–1388.

Collins, A.C. and Marks, M.J. (1989). Chronic nicotine exposure and brain nicotinic receptors – influence of genetic factors. In: A. Nordberg, K. Fuxe, B. Holmstedt, and A. Sundwall (eds), *Progress in Brain Research*. Vol. 79.

Connolly, G.N. (1995). The marketing of nicotine addiction by one oral snuff manufacturer. *Tobacco Control*, **4**(1): 73–79.

Corrigall, W.A. (1999). Nicotine self-administration in animals as a dependence model. *Nicotine & Tobacco Research*, **1**: 11–20.

Ernst, M., Matochik, J.A., Heishman, S.J., Van Horn, J.D., Jons, P.H., Henningfield, J.E. *et al.* (2001). Effect of nicotine on brain activation during performance of a working memory task. *Proceedings of the National Academy of Sciences of the United States of America*, **98** (8): 4728–4733.

Evans, S.M., Cone, E.J., and Henningfield, J.E. (1996). Arterial and venous cocaine plasma concentrations in humans: relationships to route of administration, cardiovascular effects and subjective effects. *Journal of Pharmacology and Experimental Therapeutics*, **279**(3): 1345–1356.

Fant, R.V., Henningfield, J.E., Nelson, R., and Pickworth, W.B. (1999). Pharmacokinetics and pharmacodynamics of moist snuff in humans. *Tobacco Control*, **8**: 387–392.

Fant, R.F., Buchhalter, A.R., Buchman, A.C., and Henningfield, J.E. (2009). Pharmacotherapy for tobacco dependence. In: Henningfield, J.E., London, E.D., Pogun, S. (eds). *Nicotine Psychopharmacology. Handbook of Experimental Pharmacology 192*. Berlin Heidelberg: Springer-Verlag, pp. 487–510.

Finnegan, J.K., Larson, P.S., and Haag, H.B. (1945). The role of nicotine in the cigarette habit. *Science*, **102**, 94–96.

Fiore, M.C., Bailey, W.C., Cohen, S.J. *et al.* (2000). *Treating Tobacco Use and Dependence. Clinical Practice Guideline*. Rockville, MD: US Department of Health and Human Services. Public Health Service.

Fischman, M.W., and Mello, N.K. (eds.) (1989). *Testing for abuse liability of drugs in humans*. NIDA Research Monograph, No. 92. Washington., D.C., US Government. Printing Office, 73–100.

Food and Drug Administration. (1995). 21 CFR Part 801, *et al.* Regulations restricting the sale and distribution of cigarettes and smokeless tobacco products to protect children and adolescents; proposed rule analysis regarding FDA's jurisdiction over nicotine-containing cigarettes and smokeless tobacco products; notice. *Federal Register,* **60** (155): 41314–41792.

Food and Drug Administration. (1996). 21 CFR Part 801, *et al.* Regulations restricting the sale and distribution of cigarettes and smokeless tobacco to protect children and adolescents; final rule. *Federal Register,* **61** (168): 44396–45318.

Foulds, J., Stapleton, J., Bell, N., Swettenham, J., Jarvis, M.J., and Russell, M.A.H. (1997). Mood and physiological effects of subcutaneous nicotine in smokers and never-smokers. *Drug and Alcohol Dependence,* **44**: 105–115.

Garrett, B., Dwoskin, L., Bardo, M., and Henningfield, J.E. (2004). Behavioral pharmacology of nicotine reinforcement. In: P. Boyle, N. Gray, J. Henningfield, J. Seffrin, and W. Zatonski, *Tobacco and Public Health: Science and Policy.* Oxford: Oxford University Press, pp. 149–165.

Gawin, F.H. and Kleber, H.D. (1986). Abstinence symptomatology and psychiatric diagnosis in cocaine abusers, archives of general psychiatry. **43**: 107–113.

Giovino, G.A., Henningfield, J.E., Tomar, S.L., Escobedo, L.G., and Slade, J. (1995). Epidemiology of tobacco use and dependence. *Epidemiologic Reviews,* **17**(1): 48–65.

Goldberg, S.R., Spealman, R.D., Risner, M.E., and Henningfield, J.E. (1983). Control of behavior by intravenous nicotine injections in laboratory animals. *Pharmacology Biochemistry & Behavior,* **19**: 1011–1020.

Goldberg, S.R., & Henningfield, J.E. (1988). Reinforcing effects of nicotine in humans and experimental animals responding under intermittent schedules of IV drug injection. *Pharmacology Biochemistry & Behavior,* **30**: 227–234.

Goldstein, A. (1994). *Addiction: From Biology To Drug Policy.* New York: W.H. Freeman and Company.

Griffiths, R.R., Bigelow, G.E., & Henningfield, J.E. (1980). Similarities in animal and human drug-taking behavior. In: N.K. Mello (ed.), *Advances in Substance Abuse.* Greenwich, Connecticut: JAI Press, Inc., pp. 1–90.

Gritz, E.R. (1980). Smoking behavior and tobacco use. *Advances in Substance Abuse,* **1**: 91–158.

Haiman, C.A., Stram, D.O., Wilkens, L.R., Pike, M.C., Kolonel, L.N., Henderson, B.E. *et al.* (2006). Ethnic and racial differences in the smoking-related risk of lung cancer. *New England Journal of Medicine,* **354**(4): 333–342.

Heishman, S.J., Taylor, R.C., and Henningfield, J.E. (1994). Nicotine and smoking: a review of effects on human performance. *Experimental and Clinical Psychopharmacology,* **2** (4): 345–395.

Heishman, S.J. and Henningfield, J.E. (2000). Tolerance to repeated nicotine administration on performance, subjective, and physiological responses in nonsmokers. *Psychopharmacology,* **152**: 321–333.

Henningfield, J.E. (1984). Behavioral pharmacology of cigarette smoking. In: T. Thompson, P.B. Dews, and J. Barrett (eds), *Advances in Behavioral Pharmacology,* Vol. 4, (pp. 131–210). New York: Academic Press.

Henningfield, J.E., Miyasato, K., and Jasinski, D.R. (1985). Abuse liability and pharmacodynamic characteristics of intravenous and inhaled nicotine. *Journal of Pharmacology and Experimental Therapeutics,* **234** (1): 1–12.

Henningfield, J.E., and Keenan, R.M. (1993). Nicotine delivery kinetics and abuse liability. *Journal of Consulting and Clinical Psychology,* **61** (5): 1–8.

Henningfield, J.E., Stapleton, J.M., Benowitz, N.L., Grayson, R.G., and London, E.D. (1993). Higher levels of nicotine in arterial than in venous blood after cigarette smoking. *Drug and Alcohol Dependence,* **33**: 23–29.

Henningfield, J.E., Radzius, A., and Cone, E.J. (1995a). Estimation of available nicotine content of six smokeless tobacco products. *Tobacco Control,* **4** (1): 57–61.

Henningfield, J.E., Schuh, L.M., and Jarvik, M.E. (1995b). Pathophysiology of Tobacco Dependence. In: F.E. Bloom and D.J. Kupfer (eds), *Psychopharmacology: The Fourth Generation of Progress.* (pp. 1715–1729). New York: Raven Press, Ltd.

Henningfield, J.E., Keenan, R.M., and Clarke, P.B.S. (1996). Nicotine. In: C.R. Schuster and M. Kuhar (eds), *Pharmacological Aspects of Drug Dependence*. Berlin: Springer-Verlag, pp. 272–314.

Henningfield, J.E., Fant, R.V., and Gopalan, L. (1998). Non-nicotine medications for smoking cessation. *The Journal of Respiratory Diseases*, **19**(8): S33–S42.

Henningfield, J.E., and Slade, J. (1998). Tobacco-dependence medications: public health and regulatory issues. *Food and Drug Law Journal*, **53** (Suppl.): 75–114.

Henningfield, J.E., Fant, R.V., Radzius, A., and Frost, S. (1999). Nicotine concentration, smoke pH and whole tobacco aqueous pH of some cigar brands and types popular in the United States. *Nicotine & Tobacco Research*, **1**:163–168.

Henningfield, J.E., Fant, R.V., Shiffman, S., and Gitchell, J. (2000). Tobacco dependence: scientific and public health basis of treatment. *The Economics of Neuroscience*, **2**(1): 42–46.

Henningfield, J.E., Benowitz, N.L., Ahijevych, B., Garrett, G., Connolly, G., and Ferris Wayne, G. (2002). Developing leadership in reducing substance abuse. *Nicotine & Tobacco Research*, (in press).

Henningfield, J.E., Benowitz, N.L., Connolly, G.N., Davis, R.M., Myers, M.L., and Zeller, M. (2004). Reducing tobacco addiction through tobacco product regulation. *Tobacco Control*, **13**: 132–135.

Henningfield, J.E., Fant, R.V., Buchhalter, A.R., and Stitzer, M.L. (2005). Pharmacotherapy of nicotine dependence. *CA: A Cancer Journal for Clinicians*, **55**: 281–299.

Henningfield, J.E., and Zeller, M. (2006). Nicotine psychopharmacology research contributions to United States and global tobacco regulation: a look back and a look forward. *Psychopharmacology*, **184**: 286–291.

Henningfield, J.E., Shiffman, S., Ferguson, S.G., and Gritz, E.R. (2009a). Tobacco dependence and withdrawal: science base, challenges and opportunities for pharmacotherapy. *Pharmacology and Therapeutics*,

Henningfield, J.E., London, E.D., and Pogun, S. (eds) (2009b). *Nicotine Psychopharmacology. Handbook of Experimental Pharmacology 192*. Berlin Heidelberg: Springer-Verlag.

Hoffmann, D., & Hoffmann, I. (1997). The changing cigarette, 1950–1995. *Journal of Toxicology and Environmental Health*, **50**, 307–364.

Hughes, J.R., Higgins, S.T., and Hatsukami, D. (1990). Effects of abstinence from tobacco – a critical review. In: L.T. Kozlowski, H.M. Annis, H.D. Cappell, Fr. B. Glaser, M.S. Goodstadt, Y. Israel, H. Kalant, E. M. Sellers, and E.R. Vingilis (eds), *Research Advances in Alcohol and Drug Problems*. Plenum Publishing Corporation. pp. 317–398.

Hughes, J.R., Gulliver, S.B., Fenwick, J.W., Valliere, W.A., Cruser, K., Pepper, S. *et al.* (1992). Smoking cessation among self-quitters. *Health Psychology*, **11**: 331–334.

Hunt, W.A. and Matarazzo, J.D. (1973). Three years later: recent developments in the experimental modification of smoking behavior. *Journal of Abnormal Psychology*, **31**(2): 107–114.

Hurt, R.D. and Robertson, C.R. (1998). Prying open the door to the tobacco industry's secrets about nicotine: the Minnesota Tobacco Trial. *Journal of the American Medical Association*, **280**(13): 1173–1181.

Institutes of Medicine. (1997). *Dispelling the Myths about Addiction: Strategies to Increase Understanding and Strengthen Research*. Washington, D.C.: National Academy Press.

Jasinski, D.R. (1979). Assessment of the abuse potentiality of morphine-like drugs (methods used in man). *British Medical Journal*, **7**(Suppl.): 287S–290S.

Johnston, L.M. (1942). Tobacco smoking and nicotine. *Lancet*, **2**: 742.

Jones, H.E., Garrett, B.E., and Griffiths, R.R. (1999). Subjective and physiological effects of intravenous nicotine and cocaine in cigarette smoking and cocaine abusers. *Journal of Pharmacology and Experimental Therapeutics*, **288**(1): 188–197.

Kessler, D.A., Witt, A.M., Barnett, P.S., Zeller, M.R., Natanblut, S.L., Wilkenfeld, J.P. *et al.* (1996). The Food and Drug Administration's regulation of tobacco products. *New England Journal of Medicine*, **335**(13): 988–994.

Kotke, T.E., Breeke, M.L., Solberg, L.I., and Hughes, J.R. (1989). A randomized trail to increase smoking intervention by physicians, doctors helping smokers. Round 1. *Journal of American Medical Association*, **261**, 2101–2106.

Kozlowski, L.T., Wilkinson, D.A., Skinner, W., Kent, C., Franklin, T., and Pope, M. (1989). Measuring the heaviness of smoking: using self-reported time to the first cigarette of the day and number of cigarettes smoked per day. *British Journal of Addiction*, **84**(7): 791–799.

Langley, J.N. (1905). On the reaction of cells and of nerve-endings to certain poisons, chiefly as regards the reaction of striated muscle to nicotine and to curari. *Journal of Physiology (London)*, **33**: 374–413.

Levin, E.D., Wilson, W., Rose, J., and McEvoy. (1996). Nicotine-haloperidol interactions and cognitive performance in schizophrenics. *Neuropsychopharmacology*, **15** (5): 429–436.

Lewin, L. (1964). *Phantastica: Narcotic and Stimulating Drugs, Their Use and Abuse*. New York: E.P. Dutton and Company.

Lewis, A., Miller, J.H., and Lea, R.A. (2007). Monoamine oxidase and tobacco dependence. *Neurotoxicology*, **28**(1): 182–195.

Lundahl, L.H., Henningfield, J.E., and Lukas, S.E. (2000). Mecamylamine blockade of both positive and negative effects of IV nicotine in human volunteers. *Pharmacology Biochemistry and Behavior*, **66** (3): 637–643.

Maddux, J.F. and Desmond, D.P. (1986). Relapse and recovery in substance abuse careers. In: F.M. TiCms and C.G. Leukefeld (eds) *Relapse and recovery in drug abuse, NIDA research monograph* 72: 49–71. Bethesda, MD: US Department of Health and Human Services, Public Health Service, Alcohol, Drug Abuse, and Mental Health Administration, National Institute of Drug Abuse. DHHS Publication No. (ADM) 88–1473.

Malin, D.H., Lake, J.R., Newlin-Maultsby, P., Roberts, L.K., Lanier, J.G., Carter, V.A. *et al.* (1992). Rodent model of nicotine abstinence syndrome. *Pharmacology, Biochemistry & Behavior*, **43**: 779–784.

Malin, D.H., Lake, J.R., Shenoi, M., Upchurch, T.P., Johnson, S.C., Schweinle, W.E. *et al.* (1998a). The nitric oxide synthesis inhibitor nitro-L-arginine (L-NNA) attenuates nicotine abstinence syndrome in the rat. *Psychopharmacology*, **140**: 371–377.

Malin, D.H., Lake, J.R., Upchurch, T.P., Shenoi, M., Rajan, N., and Schweinle, W.E. (1998b). Nicotine abstinence syndrome precipitated by the competitive nicotinic antagonist dihydro-beta-erythroidine. *Pharmacology Biochemistry & Behavior*, **60**: 609–613.

McClain, H. and Sapienza, F. (1989). The role of abuse liability testing in drug procedures. In: M.W. Fischman, and N.K. Mello (eds), *Testing for Abuse Liability of Drugs in Humans. NIDA Research Monograph No.* 92, (pp.21–42). DHHS publication number (ADM) 89–1613. Rockville, MD: US Department of Health and Human Services.

Molander, L., Hansson, A. and Lunell, E. (2001). Pharmacokinetics of nicotine in health elderly people. *Clinical Pharmacology and Therapeutics*, **69**: 57–65.

Molander, L., Hansson, A., Lunell, E., Alainentalo, L., Hoffmann, M., and Larsson, R. (2001). Pharmacokinetics of nicotine in kidney failure. *Clinical Pharmacology and Therapeutics*, **68**: 250–260.

Mwenifumbo, J.C., Al Koudsi, N., Ho, M.K., Zhou, Q., Hoffmann, E.B., Sellers, E.M. *et al.* (2008). Novel and established CYP2A6 alleles impair in vivo nicotine metabolism in a population of Black African descent. *Human Mutation*, **29**(5): 679–688.

Nakajima, M., Fukami, T., Yamanaka, H., Higashi, E., Sakai, H., Yoshida, R. *et al.* (2006). Comprehensive evaluation of variability in nicotine metabolism and CYP2A6 polymorphic alleles in four ethnic populations. *Clinical Pharmacology Theraputics*, **80**(3): 282–297.

National Institute on Drug Abuse. (1984). *Drug Abuse and Drug Abuse Research, First Triennial Report to Congress*. Rockville, MD: National Institute on Drug Abuse.

National Cancer Institute. (1998). *Cigars: health effects and trends. Smoking and tobacco control monograph No. 9*. US Department of Health and Human Services, Public Health Service, National Institutes of Health National Cancer Institute.

Newhouse, P.A. and Hughes, J.R. (1991). The role of nicotine and nicotinic mechanisms in neuropsychiatric disease. *British Journal of Addiction*, **86**(5): 521–526.

Newhouse, P.A., Potter, A., and Levin, E.D. (1997). Nicotinic system involvement in Alzheimer's and Parkinson's – diseases – implications for therapeutics. *Nicotine and Neurodegenerative Diseases*, **11**(3): 206–228.

O'Brien, C.P. (1996). Drug addiction and drug abuse. In: J.G. Hardman, A.G. Gilman, and L.E. Limbird (eds), *Goodman & Gilman's The Pharmacological Basis of Therapeutics*. New York: McGraw-Hill, pp. 557–577.

Paterson, D. and Nordberg, A. (2000). Neuronal nicotinic receptors in the human brain. *Progress in Neurobiology*, **61**(1): 75–111.

Perkins, K.A., Grobe, J.E., Epstein, L.H., Caggiula, A.R., Stiller, R.L., and Jacob, R.G. (1993). Chronic and acute tolerance to subjective effects of nicotine. *Pharmacology Biochemistry and Behavior*, **45**: 375–381.

Perkins, K. (2002). Chronic tolerance to nicotine in humans and its relationship to tobacco dependence. *Nicotine and Tobacco Research*, **4**: 405–422.

Perez-Stable, E.J., Herrera, B., Jacob, P. III, and Benowitz, N.L. (1998). Nicotine metabolism and intake in black and white smokers. *Journal of the American Medical Association*, **280**: 152–156.

Pickworth, W.B., Bunker, E.B., and Henningfield, J.E. (1994). Transdermal nicotine: reduction of smoking with minimal abuse liability. *Psychopharmacology*, **115**: 9–14.

Pickworth, W.B., Heishman S.J., and Henningfield, J.E. (1995). Relationships between EEG and performance during nicotine withdrawal and administration. In: Domino, E.F. (ed.) *Brain Imaging of Nicotine and Tobacco Smoking*. Ann Arbor: NPP Books, pp. 275–287.

Rose, J.E., Sampson, A., Levin, E.D., and Henningfield, J.E. (1989). Mecamylamine increases nicotine preference and attenuates nicotine discrimination. *Pharmacology Biochemistry & Behavior*, **32**: 933–938.

Rose, J.E., Behm, F.M., and Levin, E.D. (1993). Role of nicotine dose and sensory cues in the regulation of smoke intake. *Pharmacology Biochemistry and Behavior*, **44**: 891–900.

Royal College of Physicians of London. (2000). *Nicotine addiction in Britain: a report of the Tobacco Advisory Group of the Royal College of Physicians*. London, U.K.: Royal College of Physicians.

Royal Society of Canada. (1989). *Tobacco Nicotine and Addiction: A Committee Report Prepared At the Request of the Royal Society of Canada*. Ottawa, Canada: Royal Society of Canada.

Santos, M.D., Alkondon, M., Pereira, E.F., Aracava, Y., Eisenberg, H.M., Maelicke, A. *et al.* (2002). The nicotinic allosteric potentiating ligand galantamine facilitates synaptic transmission in the mammalian central nervous system. *Molecular Pharmacology*, **61**(5): 1222–1234.

Shiffman, S., Mason, K.M., and Henningfield, J.E. (1998). Tobacco dependence treatments: review and prospectus. *Annual Review of Public Health*, **19**: 335–358.

Slade, J. (1995). Are tobacco product drugs? Evidence from US tobacco. *Tobacco Control*, **4**(1): 1–2.

Slade, J., Bero, L.A., Hanauer, P., Barnes, D.E., and Glantz, S.A. (1995). Nicotine and addiction. The Brown and Williamson documents. *Journal of the American Medical Association*, **274**(3): 225–233.

Slade, J. and Henningfield, J.E. (1998). Tobacco product regulation: context and issues. *Food and Drug Law Journal*, **53**(Suppl.): 43–74.

Soria, R., Stapleton, J.M., Gilson, S.F., Sampson-Cone, A., Henningfield, J.E., and London, E.D. (1996). Subjective and cardiovascular effects of intravenous nicotine in smokers and non-smokers. *Psychopharmacology (Berl)*, **128**(3): 221–226.

Spillane, J. and McAllister, W.B. (2003). Keeping the lid on: a centry of drug regulation and control. *Drug Alcohol Depend*, **70**: S5–12.

Stapleton, J.M., Gilson, S.F., Wong, D.F., Villemagne, V.L., Dannals, R.F., Grayson, R.F. *et al.* (2003). Intravenous nicotine reduces cerebral glucose metabolism: a preliminary study. *Neuropsychopharmacology*, **28**: 765–772.

Stitzer, M.L., and De Wit, H. (1998). Abuse liability of nicotine. In: N.L. Benowitz (ed.), *Nicotine Safety and Toxicity*. New York: Oxford University Press. pp.119–131.

Stolerman, I.P., Goldfarb, T., Fink, R., and Jarvik, M.E. (1973). Influencing cigarette smoking with nicotine antagonists. *Psychopharmacologia*, **28**: 217–259.

Swedberg, M.D.B., Henningfield, J.E., and Goldberg, S.R. (1990). Nicotine dependency: animal studies. In: S. Wonnacott, M.A.H. Russell, and I.P. Stolerman (eds), *Nicotine Psychopharmacology: Molecular, Cellular, and Behavioural Aspects*. Oxford University Press. pp. 38–76.

Taylor, P. (1996). Agents acting at the neuromuscular junction and autonomic ganglia. In: J.G. Hardman, L.E. Limbrid, P.B. Molinoff, R.W. Ruddon, and A.G. Gilman, T. (eds), *Goodman And Gilman's the Pharmacological Basis of Therapeutics*. New York: McGraw-Hill, pp.177–197.

Tomar, S.L. and Henningfield, J.E. (1997). Review of the evidence that pH is a determinant of nicotine dosage from oral use of smokeless tobacco. *Tobacco Control*, **6**: 219–225.

Thun, M.J. and Burns, D.M. (2001). Health impact of 'reduced yield' cigarettes: a critical assessment of the epidemiological evidence. *Tobacco Control*, **10**(Suppl 1): i4–i11.

Tyndale, R.F. and Sellers, E.M. (2001). Variable CYP2A6-mediated nicotine metabolism alters smoking behavior and risk. *Drug Metabolism and Disposition*, **29**(4 Pt 2): 548–552.

US Department of Health and Human Services. (1988). *The Health Consequences of Smoking: Nicotine Addiction, a Report of the Surgeon General*. Washington, D.C.: US Government Printing Office.

US Department of Health and Human Services. (1994). *Preventing tobacco use among young people. A report of the Surgeon General*. Washington, D.C.: US Government Printing Office.

US Department of Health and Human Services. (2000). *Reducing tobacco use. A report of the Surgeon General*. Washington, D.C.: US Government Printing Office.

US Department of Health and Human Services. (2001). *Women and Smoking: A Report of the Surgeon General*. Rockville, MD: US Department of Health and Human Services, Public Health Service, Office of the Surgeon General.

US Department of Health and Human Services (DHHS) (2009). How Tobacco Causes Disease – The Biology and Behavioral Basis for Tobacco-Attributable Disease: A Report of the Surgeon General. Washington, D.C.: US Government Printing Office.

Vidal, C. (1996). Nicotinic receptors in the brain. Molecular biology, function, and therapeutics. *Molecular Chemistry and Neuropathology*, **28**(1–3): 3–11.

Volkow, N.D., Fowler, J.S., Ding, Y.S., Wang, G.J., and Gatley, S.J. (1999). Imaging the neurochemistry of nicotine actions: studies with positron emission tomography. *Nicotine & Tobacco Research*, **1**(Suppl 2): S127–S132.

Wallace, B.C. (1989). Psychological and environmental determinants of relapse in crack cocaine smokers. *Journal of Substance Abuse Treatment*, **6**: 95–106.

Windsor, R., Oncken, C., Henningfield, J.E., Hartmann, K., and Edwards, N. (2000). Behavioral and pharmacological treatment methods for pregnant smokers: issues for clinical practice. *Journal of the American Medical Women's Association*, **55**(5): 304–310.

World Health Organization. (1992). *The ICD-10 Classification Of Mental And Behavioural Disorders: Clinical Description And Diagnostic Guidelines*. Geneva, Switzerland: World Health Organization.

World Health Organization. (2001). *Advancing Knowledge on Regulating Tobacco Products*. Geneva, Switzerland: World Health Organization.

World Health Organization Tobacco Regulation Study Group (2004). Study Group on Tobacco Product Regulation (TobReg) Recommendation: Guiding Principles for the Development of Tobacco Product Research and Testing Capacity and Proposed Protocols for the Initiation of Tobacco Product Testing. World Health Organization, Geneva, Switzerland.

World Health Organization (2006). *Tobacco: Deadly in Any Form or Disguise*, World No Tobacco Day Monograph, WHO, Geneva. (http://www.who.int/tobacco/communications/events/wntd/2006/Tfi_Rapport.pdf)

World Health Organization (2007). The Scientific Basis of Tobacco Product Regulation; Report of a WHO Study Group (TobReg). WHO Technical Report Series, No. 945, Geneva.

Chapter 9

Manipulating product design to reinforce tobacco addiction

Geoffrey Ferris Wayne and Carrie M. Carpenter

Introduction

Most tobacco-caused disease and premature death can be considered by-products of addiction, as addiction is what drives the extraordinarily high and persistent levels of exposure (Royal College of Physicians 2000; World Health Organization 2001, 2007; US DHHS 1988). Tobacco manufacturers have long been aware that nicotine is the central component of tobacco addiction, and that product sales, and ultimately profits, depend on creating and sustaining that addiction (Anderson and Read 1980; Teague 1972; Templeton 1984; Yearnan 1963). As observed by a researcher for Philip Morris (PM) in 1972: 'The cigarette should not be construed as a product but a package. The product is nicotine' (Dunn 1972a).

Beginning as early as the 1950s, and continuing to the present, tobacco industry documents highlight the importance of internal research seeking to determine optimum quantities and forms of delivered nicotine. The goal of these efforts was to ensure that smokers obtained sufficient nicotine to support dependence. Cigarettes were developed and marketed on the premise 'that the primary motivation for smoking is to obtain the pharmacological effect of nicotine' (Philip Morris 1969) and consequently, with the understanding that they 'must provide the appropriate levels of nicotine' (Brown & Williamson 1977).

However, the pharmacological addictiveness of a product is just one, albeit an important factor, in patterns of use on both individual and population levels. While the addictiveness of the product is a critical determinant of the risk of graduation from initiation of tobacco use to addiction, it does not drive initiation of use. Nor is initiation itself a sufficient condition for the development of addiction – many people try tobacco products and do not persist enough to develop pharmacological addiction. In fact, the effects of tobacco use are determined by a complex interaction of factors: sensory and physiological; social and personal; physical and behavioural (see Fig. 9.1. – taken from 1992 R.J. Reynolds document). Among the product factors that contribute to tobacco use and subsequent harm are those that encourage experimentation and initiation of use, reduce or mask negative product effects that would discourage further use and onset of addiction, and enable or assist frequency and ease of product use.

Cigarette manufacturers continually evaluate user response to products to inform increasingly sophisticated and highly targeted products matched to the needs and preferences of specific populations. New design technologies – ventilation, filters, processed tobaccos, flavours – have been developed and refined both in response to perceived health, social, and regulatory concerns, and with increased understanding of the interaction between product design and use. The result is a product which is wildly effective both at attracting and maintaining users despite overwhelming negative health outcomes and significant physical and social barriers to use.

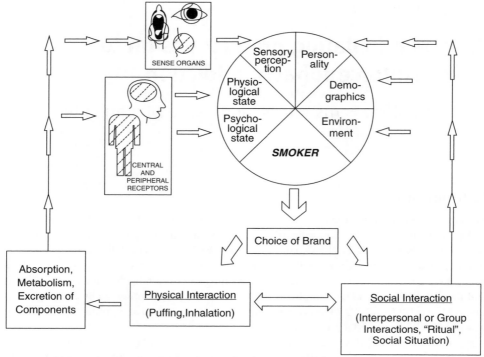

Figure 9.1 An illustration of the determinants of smoking satisfaction.

Source: Green *et al.* 1992.

Nicotine dosing

Cigarettes today are milder, less harsh, and more satisfying than their predecessors, enabling relatively easy inhalation of nicotine and other substances deep into the lung. Industry scientists optimized nicotine dosing, combining behavioural research and product technology to maximize nicotine effects, and, thus, improve commercial products and maintain smoking and addiction.

Smoke nicotine delivery

Smoke nicotine represents only a small fraction of the nicotine contained within the unburned cigarette, and all commercial cigarettes house sufficient nicotine to sustain dependence (Henningfield *et al.* 1998). The availability of nicotine from a single cigarette is highly variable and remains dependent on changes in human smoking patterns (Hammond *et al.* 2005; Kozlowski and O'Connor 2002). Indeed, compensatory behaviours (e.g. larger puff volume, more frequent puffs, vent blocking) have been demonstrated to increase the amount of nicotine delivered to as much as eight times the machine measured yield (Jarvis *et al.* 2001).

Nicotine in cigarette smoke is commonly measured using a smoking machine which draws smoke from the lit cigarette under a set of standard parameters (volume, puff duration, puff interval). While machine-based methods provide a means for quantifying relative product differences, they are generally recognized to be inadequate, and even deceptive with respect to their application to smokers (Hammond *et al.* 2006, 2007; National Cancer Institute 2001).

It is unknown whether an increase in machine-measured smoke nicotine yield is likely to reflect a real increase in the available dose. In one study, the Food and Drug Administration observed a trend of increasing smoke nicotine yield from 1982 to 1991, with the greatest increases in the lowest tar cigarettes (Kessler 1994). This trend strongly suggested that manufacturers had manipulated and controlled the levels of nicotine (Kessler *et al.* 1996). Similarly, in a recent analysis of machine-based nicotine yield data provided by manufacturers to the Massachusetts Department of Public Health, a small but statistically significant trend in increased smoke nicotine yield was observed from 1997 to 2005. The increasing trend was observed within all major market categories including full flavour, light, medium, and ultra light; mentholated, and non-mentholated; and within each major manufacturer, though at varying rates (Connolly *et al.* 2007).

In the latter study, Connolly *et al.* found that the increase in smoke nicotine yield reflected an underlying increase in nicotine concentration within commercial cigarettes, suggesting greater ease at obtaining nicotine dose within a given puff. This trend was further supported by the observed increase in per puff smoke nicotine yield. Increasing the availability of nicotine in cigarette tobacco means that cigarettes do not need to be smoked as intensively, or fewer cigarettes can be smoked to achieve the same daily level of nicotine intake. These findings illustrate how an apparent increase in smoke nicotine yield could in fact facilitate the ease with which a smoker obtains a given dose of nicotine, while supporting the same total nicotine dose.

Chemical form of nicotine

In cigarette smoke, nicotine may exist in either its protonated (bound) or unprotonated (free) forms, with the majority traditionally assumed to be protonated. A greater percentage of nicotine delivered in its unprotonated form, as determined by smoke basicity (often referred to as 'smoke pH'), may result in increased rates of absorption in the mouth and upper respiratory tract (increasing sensory impact through stimulation of receptors), as well as faster absorption from the lower respiratory tract to the brain (Henningfield *et al.* 2004; Hurt and Robertson 1998). These changes could alter the physiological response of smokers. Consequently, the chemical form of nicotine delivered by cigarettes has received increasing attention from public health researchers (Hurt and Robertson 1998; Kessler 1994).

Internal industry documents provide overwhelming evidence that manufacturers recognized and exploited differences in the chemical form of nicotine. For example, manufacturers monitored the free nicotine levels of competitor brands in the 1970s and found strong correlations between free nicotine delivery and market share (Leach and Shockley 1969; Teague 1973; Woods and Sheets 1975). Further, manufacturers identified free nicotine as a means to increase physiological satisfaction in lower nicotine products (Gregory 1980; Larson and Morgan 1976; Lorillard 1973; Schori 1979). As concluded by Philip Morris researchers in 1990, a low nicotine delivery cigarette with a higher proportion of free nicotine 'would be analytically similar to other cigarettes at comparable nicotine deliveries, but would be judged to have much more impact' (Gullotta *et al.* 1990c). Thus, manipulation of the form of nicotine was seen both as a means to maintain a competitive advantage across brand styles, and as a means to replace physiological impact among low nicotine cigarettes (Ferris Wayne *et al.* 2006; Hurt and Robertson 1998; Pankow 2001).

Pankow (2001) evaluated the considerable research conducted by tobacco manufacturers to describe patterns of deposition of nicotine related to differences in acid/base chemistry of smoke, noting the likely importance of 'smoke pH' and unprotonated ('free') nicotine in smoke delivery. This research led to independent confirmation of the utility of analytic techniques for assessment of the form of nicotine, demonstrating significant brand differences in free nicotine delivery (Pankow *et al.* 2003; Watson *et al.* 2004). One such finding was the conclusion that cigarettes marketed as lower in nicotine yield ('lights'and 'ultralights') had a greater percentage of free nicotine (Watson *et al.* 2004). Published reviews of the internal documents also demonstrate that even 'small' changes could significantly increase their ability to deliver an 'optimum' dose of nicotine and result in distinct differences readily recognizable among smokers (Ferris Wayne *et al.* 2006; Hurt and Robertson 1998; Pankow 2001). Further, industry scientists exhibited a clear understanding that free nicotine alters the rate of absorption and physiological impact among smokers (Hurt and Robertson 1998).

Tobacco as a vehicle for nicotine delivery

While nicotine is the primary active pharmacological agent, tobacco has been shown to be a particularly effective vehicle for delivery of nicotine (Food and Drug Administration 1995; Hurt and Robertson 1998; Slade *et al.* 1995; World Health Organization 2001). In fact, tobacco delivered nicotine is not only more toxic, but more addictive than nicotine in a pure form (e.g. nicotine replacement therapy) (Henningfield *et al.* 2000; Royal College of Physicians 2000). As noted by a Brown & Williamson scientist in 1990: 'Nicotine alone in smoke is not practical, nor are extreme tar/nicotine ratios, since nicotine is too irritating – other substances are required for sensoric reasons' (Baker 1990).

The importance of tobacco includes both those constituents in smoke that may interact with nicotine directly, as well as those which indirectly influence a smoker's perception and behaviours. For example, some tobacco smoke constituents may alter the site of absorption of nicotine, such as bronchodilators (e.g. cocoa, licorice) which allow deeper inhalation and subsequent deposition of constituents in more highly permeable areas of the respiratory tract. Likewise, product changes to alter or control particle size, or to provide particulate 'carriers' for vapour-phase smoke constituents, also could facilitate changes at the site of absorption (Ingebrethsen 1993). This would also include the use of acids or bases to alter the form of nicotine and basicity of smoke. Again, published tobacco document research describes a wide range of relevant findings (Ferris Wayne *et al.* 2006; Keithly *et al.* 2005; Pankow 2001).

Alternately, flavourants (e.g. menthol) and smoke 'smoothing' agents (e.g. sugars) may be used to mask or balance irritation and thereby facilitate nicotine dosing by offsetting the harshness of nicotine and removing natural physiological barriers (Burns 1992; National Cancer Institute 2001; Wayne and Connolly 2002; Wells 1995). Other approaches to reducing harshness would include the addition of a 'cooling' or anaesthetic compound (e.g. menthol, eugenol), altering smoke composition (such as the tar/nicotine ratio), or removing other tobacco constituents with irritant properties (Bates *et al.* 1999; Ferris Wayne and Connolly 2004; Hurt and Robertson 1998; Pankow 2001; Wayne *et al.* 2004). Reduced irritation may encourage or support increased frequency of use, and has been linked to increased rates of initiation and uptake of smoking among youth (Wayne and Connolly 2002).

Sensory factors and subjective response

Nicotine is an irritant, and reduction of harshness is a key component of tobacco product design. Yet the smoker also relies on sensory cues which affect smoking behaviour as well as reinforce the physiological impact of nicotine (Rose 2006). Sensory stimulus can elicit responses from the basic senses (sight, smell, touch, taste) as well as physiological responses from nerve systems such as the olfactory and trigeminal nerves (Carpenter *et al.* 2006; Rose 2006), and contribute to the overall subjective response apart from nicotine delivery. Cigarette manufacturers dedicated tremendous resources to investigation of perceived sensory stimulation in order to understand and maximize the role of sensory effects in the smoking experience. For example, industry researchers recognized that sensory properties were linked with smoking behaviour and puffing parameters produced by the smoker (British American Tobacco no date, 1983, 1994; Morgan *et al.* 1990). An undated R.J. Reynolds document summarized:

> The consumer may alter his smoking behavior based on sensory information so as to modify the sensory, chemical, and physiological properties of the smoke. This has implications for the physiological and psychological effects of smoking, since they may be affected by smoke dose and composition.

> (R.J. Reynolds, no date)

These findings are confirmed in the published literature. In a study comparing a high nicotine/high sensory cigarette, a low nicotine/low sensory cigarette, and a low nicotine/high sensory cigarette, subjects regulated their smoking behaviour according to sensory intensity rather than nicotine intake (Levin *et al.* 1993). In another study, pharmacological effects from denicotinized and regular cigarettes were compared (Pickworth *et al.* 1999). While subjects preferred the regular cigarettes, both types of cigarettes reduced subjective measures of craving and withdrawal.

Free nicotine was believed by manufacturers to be a critical sensory component (Brooks *et al.* 1974; Hirji and Wood 1973; Hurts and Robertson 1998; Maynor and Rosene 1981; Pankow 2001). Free nicotine provides a more immediate impact or 'kick' in the back of the mouth and throat, preceding the arrival of nicotine to the brain, with even a small amount of free nicotine discernible by the smoker (Hurts and Robertson 1998). As summarized in a 1976 memo: 'As the pH increases, the nicotine changes its chemical form so that it is more rapidly absorbed by the body and more quickly gives a "kick" to the smoker' (Mckenzie 1976). R.J. Reynolds funded studies in the late 1980s in an effort to understand trigeminal chemoreception in the nasal cavity, and concluded, 'Nicotine is the most effective trigeminal stimulus, and perhaps the most irritating' (Silver 1988).

While nicotine contributes to the sensory aspects of smoking, other physical and chemical properties of tobacco smoke also provide rewarding sensory stimulation to smokers. As described by Rose (2006), the smoking induced 'sensory package' influences smoking behaviour and dependence (Brauer *et al.* 2001; Carpenter *et al.* 2006; Rose 2006). A target of internal sensory research was the contribution of peripheral nerve responsivity to the total behavioural phenomenon (Philip Morris 1995; R.J. Reynolds 1987a). For example, a 1995 Philip Morris document described a series of research proposals identifying the sensory characteristics of nicotine and their relative contribution (alongside other stimuli) to smoker responses (Philip Morris 1995). Another related area of interest was the use of sensory stimulation to provide a bridge between product expectations and smoke delivery. As proposed by a Phillip Morris scientist: 'We might be able to produce the CNS effects of high delivery cigarettes by leading subjects to believe they [are] smoking high nicotine cigarettes when they [are] actually smoking low nicotine cigarettes. Experiments of this type might have important implications for the marketing of low delivery cigarettes' (Gullotta 1982).

Behavioural determinants of nicotine dosing

'Compensatory' smoking was recognized by the industry since the introduction of 'light'cigarettes more than thirty years ago (National Cancer Institute 2001). A Philip Morris memorandum observed in 1968 that 'since there is evidence that the smoker adapts his puff, it is reasonable to anticipate that he adapts to maintain a fairly constant daily dosage' (R.J. Reynolds 1997). Evidence to support this thesis was gathered in subsequent years by tobacco manufacturers (Dunn and Schori 1972c; Hurt and Robertson 1998; Phillip Morris 1974). Manufacturers acted to take advantage of compensatory behaviour that was driven by smoker's addiction to nicotine, and enhance it through cigarette designs that supported compensation. A 1977 British American Tobacco review observed:

> It is now possible to design cigarettes which would have the same smoking machine delivery but different deliveries to the compensating smoker. Broadly speaking, this could be achieved by developing cigarettes with a knowledge of the smoker's response to such factors as pressure drop, ventilation, irritation, impact, nicotine delivery, etc.

(Haslam 1977)

A 1984 British American Tobacco document lists as a 'high priority' the development of 'alternative designs (that do not invite obvious criticism) which will allow the smoker to obtain significant enhanced deliveries should he so wish' (British American Tobacco 1984b). The internal documents also indicate that other product design factors could be used to alter smoking behaviour. For example, smokers rate lower yield cigarettes as harder to draw because of the loss of sensory impact (Jeltema 1987), whereas the addition of an irritant makes it seem easier to puff (Walker *et al.* 1992). Internal studies investigated flavour discrimination of different compounds, with a particular goal of identifying olfactory responses with 'feel' (mild irritant) qualities. This work led to the development of specific additives aimed at enhancing both the flavour and physical 'feel' of tobacco smoke (Farnham 1995), as well as development of better puff profile characteristics (Jennings *et al.* 1991).

The internal application of behavioural research to nicotine dosing is illustrated in a model taken from a 1984 Brown & Williamson document [see Fig. 9.2, from Ayres and Greig 1984]. Researchers developed a methodology designed to measure the 'smoking dynamics' of a cigarette utilizing a reward for effort model, in which effort was the work done to obtain a volume of smoked and reward was the perceived delivery. This model was used to relate specific product changes to subjective product attributes affecting smoker response (Ayres and Greig 1984). Thus, behavioural determinants of smoke nicotine yield were incorporated alongside product characteristics to model expected delivery and to aid in development of new products.

Product modification

The conventional cigarette is relatively uniform, and many basic product differences are clearly defined by well-known market categories (e.g. length, circumference, 'menthol'). However, Connolly and others have demonstrated that additional product differences introduced by manufacturers may alter smoke chemistry, mechanisms of delivery, perception of smoke, bioavailability, and smoker behaviours (Carpenter *et al.* 2006; Cook *et al.* 2003; Ferris Wayne and Connolly 2004; Keithly *et al.* 2005; Wayne and Connolly 2002). For example, basicity of smoke ('smoke pH') may be controlled by tobacco processing and other changes, altering the route or speed of chemical uptake (Henningfield *et al.* 2004; Hurt and Robertson 1998). Likewise, new smoke compounds may be introduced or enhanced, including nicotine analogs and synergists, and bronchodilators (Bates *et al.* 1999; Wayne *et al.* 2004).

Tobacco manufacturers have successfully developed and utilized physical and chemical product design changes to control the quantity, form, and perception of nicotine dose. Methods included altering physical construction parameters, such as the tobacco, filter, ventilation, and paper; altering smoke chemistry, for example, by increasing 'smoke pH' through addition of ammonia or other bases; and introducing new smoke compounds to increase the potency of nicotine. Consequently these factors must be taken into account in assessment of nicotine dosing. Product features such as flavour and mildness play an important role in influencing acceptance, behaviour, and smoking effects. Marketing features (e.g. brand name, packaging, image, and advertising), though not discussed in the present chapter, warrant attention as well.

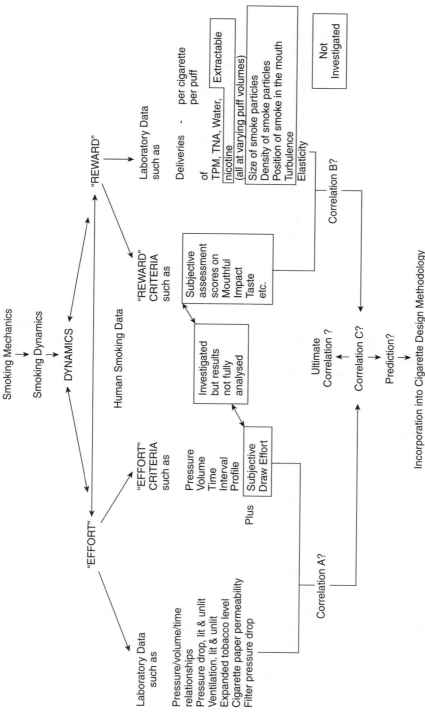

Figure 9.2 Internal BW model: 'An outline of those parameters thought to be involved in "effort" and "reward", and showing those experimentally accessible and examined.'

Source: Ayres and Greig 1984.

Physical construction parameters

Different tobacco types (e.g. flue-cured, Virginia, tobacco; air-cured, Burley, tobacco; sun-cured, Oriental tobacco) and leaves from different stalk positions affect the composition of cigarette smoke and the delivery of nicotine as well as sugars and other constituents to the smoker. For example, cigarettes that contain air-cured Burley tobacco (a major constituent of American blend cigarettes) produce greater smoke nicotine yields and a higher proportion of 'free' nicotine, whereas oriental Turkish-type cigarettes deliver substantially less nicotine, nearly all in the protonated or bound form (Bernasek *et al.* 1992). Consumption of some European cigarettes containing only Burley tobaccos can maintain blood nicotine levels with minimal smoke inhalation, similar to cigars.

In the 1980s, British American Tobacco and Brown & Williamson developed a tobacco referred to as 'Y-1' which was genetically engineered to have a nicotine content approximately twice the nicotine content of conventional tobacco. This nicotine-enhanced tobacco was blended with other tobaccos in order to alter nicotine to tar ratios in commercial cigarettes sold in the United States (Chakraborty 1985). Thus, differences in blend can produce significant variations in nicotine concentration in the tobacco rod, supporting differences in smoke composition and smoke yield. In Connolly *et al.* (2007), one of the design features that best defined smoke nicotine yield was concentration of nicotine in the tobacco rod, and significant increases over time were observed both in the concentration of (9%) and total nicotine (17%) in the tobacco rod, suggesting differences in blend.

Other physical characteristics such as length, circumference, porosity, ventilation, tobacco weight, and density combine to determine the basic machine-smoked yields of 'tar', nicotine, and other substances. The complex interaction among these different design features has been extensively studied within the tobacco industry in order to carefully control the resulting product delivery (Browne 1990).

Product design characteristics may affect the ability of the smoker to self-regulate dose, and are therefore introduced by the manufacturer and used by the smoker to control delivered smoke yields (Norman 1974, 1983). For example, an R.J. Reynolds review of 17 internal studies relating cigarette construction parameters to observed sensory properties, concluded that a number of cigarette design features play a significant role in determining how a cigarette is smoked – with key factors being air dilution, draw resistance, and filtration efficiency (Roberts 1985). A Lorillard presentation on development of 'low-yield' cigarettes describes the use of draw resistance as follows:

> ... the puff volume that the smoker extracts from a cigarette is a function of the resistance that he encounters in the cigarette unlike in the FTC smoking regime where the puff volume is constant regardless of draw resistance ... . If the object is to design a cigarette that has a very low FTC tar but that tastes like a 6 or 7 mg cigarette then the pressure drop distribution in the cigarette has to be manipulated in such a fashion that the smoker can draw larger than the standard FTC 35 cc 2 second puffs and still remain within his comfortable smoking effort range.
>
> (Norman 1983)

Specific product changes proposed include the use of ventilation, filtration, and tobacco rod density to alter draw resistance (Norman 1983; Thorne 1994); the introduction of channelled or other unique filter designs to enhance sensory properties such as sensations in the mouth referred to as 'mouthfull feeling' (Brown & Williamson 1983; Greig 1987; McMurtrie and Silberstein 1980); and the use of higher nicotine tobaccos, flavour additives, and alkaline additives to increase a range of sensory attributes (Shepperd 1993; Whitehead 1994).

Of all the design characteristics of cigarettes, filter ventilation may be the most important in determining machine-smoked yields (Djordjevic *et al.* 1995), as well as the most important determinant of the differences in machine-smoked yields and human smoking behaviour and smoke exposure. Filter ventilation dilutes mainstream smoke with air. Consequently, the rod characteristics become less important determinants of yield in the presence of filter ventilation (Schneider 1992). A recent study demonstrated that increases in filter ventilation increased the relative proportion of free-base nicotine in the mainstream smoke when measured in an unblocked machine-smoked condition (Watson *et al.* 2004). The practical importance of these results is that even without any compensatory smoking behaviour, a ventilated cigarette may deliver a greater proportion of total nicotine in free base on a puff-by-puff basis.

Product chemistry

Reconstituted tobacco is used at high levels in most American blend cigarettes, which are popular in many regions of the world (National Cancer Institute 1996). Reconstituted tobacco sheets are made from processing stems and other parts of the tobacco leaf that would otherwise go to waste. In the course of manufacturing reconstituted tobacco, numerous chemicals are added, including nicotine as the replacement for the amount lost in the manufacturing process (Browne 1990; National Cancer Institute 1996). Indeed, this also provides an effective means for manufacturers to control or even increase the amount of nicotine in the total blend (Minnemeyer 1977).

Ammonia compounds are a primary chemical component of many reconstituted tobaccos. The chemical impact of ammoniation is complex and appears to influence the form and delivery of nicotine in a variety of interconnected ways (see Fig. 9.3 from Brown & Williamson). The importance of ammoniation in the development of the characteristic flavour popularized by Marlboro has been widely publicized (Bates *et al.* 1999; Freedman 1995; Hurt and Robertson 1998). Ammoniated reconstituted tobacco has a characteristic mild sensory profile, and features a number of important compounds created through the reaction between ammonia and sugars (R.J. Reynolds 1980; Wells 1995). The addition of ammonia as a strong base leads to increased 'smoke pH', which then corresponds with increased levels of free nicotine in smoke (Hurt and

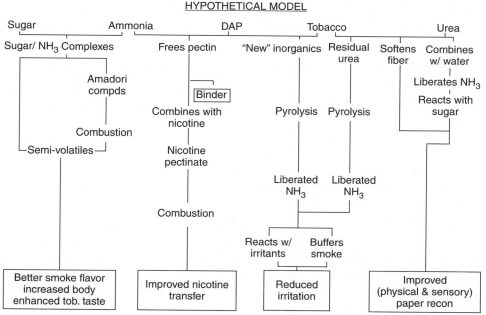

Figure 9.3 Industry model of the effects of ammonia on form and delivery of nicotine.
Source: Johnson 1989.

Robertson 1998). Thus, a 1982 position paper from R.J. Reynolds observed that '[a]mmonia in smoke is one of the major pH controlling components' and that '[s]tudies of the effect of ammonia on smoke composition showed… an increase in physiological satisfaction with increasing ammonia content' (Bernasek and Nystrom 1982).

Ammoniation also improves sheet tobacco strength and facilitates nicotine scavenging from the remaining cigarette tobacco, thus increasing the transfer efficiency of nicotine to smoke (British American Tobacco 1988; Wells 1995). Indeed, a recent review of the literature concluded that changes in nicotine kinetics (shorter $t_{1/2}$; higher C_{max}) due to ammoniation leads to higher concentrations of nicotine in the mainstream smoke rather than faster absorption of nicotine in the pulmonary tract (Willems *et al.* 2006).

Although ammoniation is the most commonly cited example of industry manipulation of smoke chemistry, the internal documents describe countless others. For example, sugars play a critical role in combination with ammonia in the formation of pyrazines and other compounds via reaction processes (Harllee and Leffingwell 1978; J.W. Swain and F.H. Crayton 1981; D.L. Wu and J.W. Swain 1983). Balancing the levels of sugars and nicotine may lower 'smoke pH' and reduce levels of free (unprotonated) nicotine, which also correspond with reduced harshness and impact (Bernasek *et al.* 1992; R.J. Reynolds 1992b; Smith 1992). Evaluation of smoke chemistry often focused on a combination of variables; sugars, for example, were combined with amino acid mixtures to alter smoke flavour (Crellin and Reihl 1984). A 1992 R.J. Reynolds document states: 'Based on initial testing it is highly likely that efforts in the area of sugar/nicotine balance will provide incremental improvements in the area of smoothness and harshness' (R.J. Reynolds 1992a). Industry scientists considered sugar/nicotine technology particularly important in the development of full flavour low tar products.

Other methods explored internally to alter the form of nicotine delivered included the use of base- or acid-coated filters. For example, researchers at R.J. Reynolds applied sodium hydroxide-coated filters to a cigarette yielding only 0.06 mg of nicotine, in order to heighten sensory impact (Shannon *et al.* 1992). Alternately, a filter coated with an acid (lactic, levulinic, citric) was used to reduce the impact of a high nicotine sheet, either by trapping the nicotine or changing the pH of the smoke so there is not as much nicotine in the vapour phase (Shannon *et al.* 1992). The researchers noted that,

> lactic and levulinic acids get into the smoke and they have a bigger smoothing effect than citric acid, which we are pretty sure does not get into the smoke. It does not smooth so much. In one case you have got both things going for you. You are restricting nicotine vapor plus you are dumping acids into the smoke. In the other case you are just absorbing nicotine vapor and you don't get as much of the nicotine.

> (Shannon *et al.* 1992)

Similarly, in a 1989 study titled 'When Nicotine is Not Nicotine', Philip Morris researchers observed that nicotine delivery of cigarettes that had been over sprayed with nicotine citrate were half as effective in nicotine transport and delivery when compared with those sprayed with nicotine as the base; the latter were perceived as having higher mouth/throat impact (Gullotta *et al.* 1989).

The ratio of nicotine versus other compounds delivered in smoke (e.g. nicotine/tar ratio) may also be a significant determinant of response. Philip Morris conducted multiple consumer research studies through the late 1970s to determine the acceptability of various nicotine to tar ratios, and found that consumers preferred nicotine to tar ratios that were higher than those that occur naturally in tobaccos (Dunn and Schori 1971, 1972b; Dunn *et al.* 1973, 1976; Houck *et al.* 1975, 1976). R.J. Reynolds pursued a project during this same time period 'to determine means to manipulate nicotine/tar ratio to provide a more satisfying smoke' (Henley 1977). Methods to increase the nicotine to tar ratios included blend modifications (i.e. the use of high nicotine tobaccos) the direct addition of nicotine to the blend, and addition of a 'nicotine salt complex… to increase the nicotine delivery' (R.J. Reynolds 1985, 1990a). A 1990 R.J. Reynolds document describing 'Project XB' observes that 'Nicotine is a key element in providing acceptable taste and satisfaction. Nicotine itself is harsh and irritating. High nicotine tobacco salts allow increase in smoke nicotine yields without corresponding increases in harshness attributes' (R.J. Reynolds 1990a).

New smoke compounds

Cigarette manufacturers may reinforce physiological effects of nicotine or otherwise influence response to nicotine through the introduction and use of compounds which interact with nicotine but do not directly alter its form or delivery. Manufacturers have acknowledged the use of hundreds of chemical additives in tobacco products (Leffingwell et al. 1972; Philip Morris 1994). Some of these additives may act synergistically with nicotine or demonstrate other reinforcing effects. Cocoa, for example, contains alkaloids, which themselves may have pharmacological effects when inhaled, or may modify the effects of nicotine. Pyridine is chemically a portion of the nicotine molecule, acting as a CNS depressant similar to nicotine, although it is less potent.

When burned, sugars also increase the smoke levels of acetaldehyde, another potential nicotine reinforcing agent. Recent studies demonstrate that acetaldehyde enhances behavioural and neuronal responses to nicotine in both adolescent and adult rats (Belluzzi et al. 2005; Cao et al. 2007). In the early 1980s, DeNoble and coworkers at Philip Morris studied the behavioural effects of nicotine and acetaldehyde in rats. The results of this research showed that the two compounds work synergistically, producing greater addictive effects. DeNoble claims that once this information was obtained, Philip Morris increased the level of acetaldehyde in Marlboro cigarettes by 40% between 1982 and 1992 through the addition of sugar (Bates et al. 1999).

Another area of research was the identification of analogs and synergists that could be used to imitate or alter response to nicotine. Industry research identified a number of analogs internally that could be used to imitate or enhance response to nicotine (Vagg and Chapman 2005; Wayne et al. 2004). R.J. Reynolds's analog research tested multiple potential nicotine analogs to compare with nicotine's effect on cholinergic receptor systems in the brain, cardiovascular activity and pharmacological potency, and cardiovascular and behavioural endpoints. In 1989, an R.J. Reynolds progress report indicated that 29 compounds competed for nicotine binding to receptors at physiologically relevant concentrations, based on relative potencies (Wayne et al. 2004).

Ferris Wayne and Connolly (2004) assessed the potential effects of menthol as an additive in cigarettes. Their findings linked menthol to a range of unique physiological and subjective effects in cigarettes including reduced harshness, increased nicotine-associated impact, greater ease of inhalation, and enhanced bioavailability of nicotine. Menthol has been shown to exhibit absorption-enhancing effects, as well as possible effects on drug metabolism that could alter the pharmacological action of other substances in tobacco smoke (Jori et al. 1969; Madyastha and Srivatsan 1988; Ferris Wayne and Connolly 2004).

Levulinic acid provides another example of the multiple influences that additives can demonstrate with respect to nicotine dose. R.J. Reynolds scientists generated considerable evidence that levulinic acid and nicotine levulinate decreased harshness and increased nicotine yield from tobacco smoke. Further, internal research demonstrated the capacity of levulinic acid to enhance the binding of nicotine in the brain, increasing its pharmacological effectiveness. The addition of levulinic acid also altered the composition of mainstream and sidestream smoke and introduced potentially toxic pyrolysis products to smoke. These combined effects could have significant implications for the increased addictiveness or toxicity of the cigarette and the progression of smoker behaviours including initiation and quitting. Measured increases in peak plasma nicotine levels among treated low-yield cigarettes confirm the importance of these internal findings in the assessment of brand deliveries (see Table 9.1 from Keithly 2005).

Product attractiveness

While tobacco users are primarily motivated by nicotine delivery, flavours and other physical design features elicit physiological as well as psychological responses which provide additional motivation for maintaining product use. The tobacco industry has been extraordinarily effective in its employment of product designs and marketing strategies to make tobacco products attractive, despite the fact that these products often produce noxious effects upon initial use, and despite the general knowledge that they are harmful. Much of the effort to make tobacco products attractive is targeted towards young people, but designs and marketing have also been targeted to adults and specific adult populations, with characteristics intended to appeal to these populations. These efforts contribute to the initiation of use, and along with addiction, play a role in persistence of use as well as relapse following the achievement of abstinence.

Table 9.1 Summary of effects of levulinic acid when used as an additive in cigarettes.

Potential effect	Measure used	Objective	Outcome
Sensory perception (Steele, 1989)	Subjective consumer panel testing of treated cigarettes	Offset harshness and irritation in development of low-yield cigarettes	"…physiological clues are being blocked, since people smoked the test cigarettes essentially the same as the control, even though more nicotine was obtained"
Smoke pH (Stewart & Lawrence, 1988)	Electrode-based measure of smoke pH of machine-smoked cigarettes	Offset harshness and irritation in development of low-yield cigarettes	Decreased smoke "pH" in Camel Light when used alone or added as nicotine levulinate
Nicotine delivery in smoke (Steele, 1989)	Puff profiles of smokers, followed by yield measures based on Human Mimic Smoking Machine	Increase smoke nicotine delivery of low-tar cigarettes relative to higher tar controls	Smoke nicotine delivery increased in a number of tested brands, including Camel Light, Vantage Ultra Light, and NOW
Plasma nicotine (Steele, 1989)	Plasma nicotine change from baseline measured comparing smokers of control and test cigarettes	Increase bioavailability of smoke nicotine in low-yield and low tar/nicotine cigarettes	Plasma nicotine for NOW about 6 ng/ml higher than the control (Winston King); for Winston Ultra Light, about 13 ng/ml higher than control
Tar/nicotine ratio (Steele, 1989)	Machine-measured smoke yields of tar and nicotine	Increase delivery of nicotine relative to tar in low-yield cigarettes	Levulinic acid alone had little effect: nicotine levulinate decreased tar and nicotine by half in Winston Ultra Light and NOW
Receptors in brain (Steele, 1989)	In vitro studies on binding of radiolabelled nicotine to pharmacological receptors in brain tissue	Determine whether levulinic acid affects nicotinic cholinergic receptors in the brain	Observed increased nicotine binding ranging from 20%–50%, with a mean value of around 30%; "…changes in receptor binding may lead to changes in physiological effects of nicotine…"

Note: Taken from Keithly et al. 2005, citing Stewart, C. A., & Lawrence, B. M. (1988). Effects of levulinic acid, tobacco essence and nicotine salts on smoke ph. August 8. R. J. Reynolds. Bates: 507862872–507862880. Available at: http://legacy.library.ucsf.edu/tid/zyk14d00, and Steele, R. (1989). Hrrc meeting. October 10. R.J. Reynolds. Bates: 507862810–507862812. Available at: http://legacy.library.ucsf.edu/tid/lyk14d00

Initiation and experimentation

The harsh and irritating character of nicotine and tobacco smoke provides a significant barrier to use. Younger and beginner smokers demonstrate a lower tolerance for irritation and an 'undeveloped' taste for tobacco smoke compared with regular smokers (Wayne and Connolly 2002); and youth who experience fewer adverse physiological effects from tobacco are more likely to progress to regular use (Robinson *et al.* 2007). Thus, development and promotion of products with minimal sensory and physiological impact is necessary to successfully capture young, new users. An analysis conducted by R.J. Reynolds in the 1980s concluded that for each cigarette brand that had achieved significant popularity among young and new smokers in the United States over the previous fifty years (including Pall Mall, Winston, Marlboro, and Newport), the most important design characteristic was its relative smoothness or mildness (Teague 1973).

Their conclusion is supported by independent analysis of the commercial market. According to Wayne and Connolly (2002), product changes applied to the US Camel brand in the early 1990s specifically targeting smoothness and mildness, and coordinated with the introduction of the Joe Camel 'Smooth Character' marketing campaign, corresponded not only to a five-fold increase in Camel US market share among youth, but to an increase in smoking initiation among youth overall during the same time period.

Internal industry research findings also indicate that masking tobacco with flavours more palatable to new users is a key strategy to support tobacco use among beginners (Wayne and Connolly 2002; Cummings *et al.* 2002). Examples include increased sweetness and higher levels of non-tobacco flavours, such as chocolate and vanillin. Among the flavours most successful in promoting early tobacco use is menthol. Menthol is particularly noted not only for its taste but for a physiological 'cooling' effect which masks the harshness as well as the taste of the tobacco. Hersey *et al.* (2006) found that menthol use among youth increased between 2000 and 2002, with highest use among younger, newer smokers, and suggested that menthol cigarettes may provide a 'starter product' for youth to begin smoking. Low-level menthol products were developed as part of a deliberate strategy by manufacturers to target youth smokers with reduced tobacco taste and harshness and without overwhelming or strong menthol flavour products (Kreslake *et al.* 2008b).

Targeted products and population differences

Product targeting efforts extend well beyond the acquisition of new smokers. A number of published studies have described the importance of additives and other product design characteristics in order to match preferences among specific populations of smokers (Keithly 2005; Carpenter 2005a, 2005b; Cook 2003; Connolly *et al.* 2000; Ferris Wayne and Connolly 2004; Wayne and Connolly 2002). In some cases the use of different product characteristics are more explicit – for example, longer and slimmer products. However, chocolate, licorice, and various sugars are used to modify the sensory properties of smoke without necessarily producing characteristic flavours that the smoker would recognize. For example, it is not evident that cigarette smokers characterize Marlboro branded cigarettes as 'chocolate' despite the fact that cocoa and chocolate are used in their manufacture. Although some brands are characterized and branded explicitly as 'menthol' cigarettes, it is acknowledged by manufacturers that menthol is present in many other cigarettes at reduced levels.

There is evidence in the internal documents that smokers develop a taste for specific flavours or characteristics of tobacco use other than nicotine, and come to associate use with these characteristics. For example, a 1991 PM document discusses the importance of the flavourant vanillin in the Japanese market. The researchers hypothesized that among smokers who have 'acquired the taste' for vanilla flavouring, it is both a preference and a barrier to exit, noting that switching data in Japan suggests that smokers switch readily between vanilla flavoured brands, but are reluctant to switch to non-vanilla flavoured brands (Philip Morris 1991). They also observe that vanilla increases mildness and smoothes harshness, and that some Japanese smokers link vanilla flavouring to perceived health benefits.

Menthol provides another example of this phenomenon. Although a primary advantage of menthol cigarettes for new or younger smokers is the masking of harshness and discomfort to facilitate use and allow a sufficient dose of nicotine, the wants of established menthol smokers incorporate a desire for menthol flavour. An internal R.J. Reynolds analysis summarizes the dilemma as follows: '[A]s smokers acclimate to menthol, their demand for menthol increases over time … Responsive brands whose strategy is to maximize franchise acceptance invariably increase menthol levels over time' (Lawson and Toben 1986). This process necessitated the eventual development of a two-pronged strategy of attracting new smokers with lower menthol content, while maintaining smokers with higher menthol content cigarettes (Kreslake 2008a).

Industry studies also suggest that certain sensory factors differ across ethnic groups. R.J. Reynolds highlighted ethnic differences in a report on sensorial differences among younger smokers suggesting that full flavour or taste as central brand features were not 'leverageable' among young adult white smokers, but were growing possibilities among young adult black smokers (R.J. Reynolds 1985). Another Brown & Williamson document describes a growing preference for 'strongly' flavoured cigarettes among black smokers indicating different sensory preferences from white smokers (Kapular & Associates 1984). These finding suggest that the role of flavours and other design features may differ depending on the user population.

Tobacco products in the commercial market

Both independent studies and internal industry research highlight the relevance of historical product differences. The evidence demonstrates the effectiveness of methods adopted by manufacturers to control nicotine dosing and target the needs of specific populations of smokers through commercial product development.

Commercial brand differences

Over the last several decades, manufacturers have significantly decreased tar and nicotine yields. Between 1954 and 1993, the average sales weighted 'tar' and nicotine yields of US cigarettes have declined from 38 and 2.7 to 12 and 0.9 mg, respectively (Hoffman *et al.* 1997). These changes have resulted from product design changes as discussed previously. Tar/nicotine ratios have also declined, resulting in more nicotine per unit of tar. In 1979, Brown & Williamson researchers found that the average nicotine to tar ratio for commercial brands had increased, and that the nicotine to tar ratio for low yield products was higher than for regular products (Esterle *et al.* 1979). Internal studies indicate that this decline was intentional and competition driven. R.J. Reynolds stated in 1990: 'PM [Philip Morris] has successfully raised the nicotine levels on all their products (across the line) by using high nicotine tobaccos. Thus, they already have a better T/N [tar/nicotine] ratio than their competitors. Adding nicotine could further improve that ratio' (R.J. Reynolds 1990c). R.J. Reynolds continued its own research into changing the nicotine to tar ratio throughout the 1990s, concentrating on development of an ultra low tar product that provided nicotine delivery similar to full-flavour products (Wilson 1991).

A published study (Wayne and Connolly 2002) on product changes in the Camel brand found an increased trend in nicotine levels between 1989 and 1994, while simultaneously tar/nicotine ratios were reduced. These changes corresponded with Camel's increase in popularity among youth smokers. Although increased nicotine delivery is typically associated with increased throat impact and irritation, product attribute measures for Camel brand styles between 1988 and 1991 demonstrate how increases in nicotine were offset by product changes targeting smoothness and harshness. The findings suggest that changes in tar/nicotine ratios may have offset the harshness commonly accompanying an increase in nicotine delivery, supporting increased intake of smoke nicotine particularly among new smokers unaccustomed to nicotine.

R.J. Reynolds researchers discussed differences among their products and those of competitor Philip Morris. They observed that Marlboro has less smoke nicotine than Winston, but a higher level of weaker bases, such as pyrazines. These weaker bases accounted for the slightly higher 'smoke pH' of Marlboro – and equivalent levels of volatile or 'free' nicotine – despite the fact that nicotine was not as high. One difference that the researchers noted with respect to Philip Morris products was that following the initial production of reaction products (via ammoniation), their products remained extremely consistent over time. By contrast, the process used by R.J. Reynolds 'did not quench that reaction and that product continued to change over time' (Shannon *et al.* 1992).

Ferris Wayne *et al.* (2006) observed consistent relationships among brands for internal 'smoke pH' and free nicotine measurements, supporting the utility of these measures in brand comparisons. For example, during the period 1965–1980, Marlboro exhibited consistently higher 'smoke pH' values relative to Winston, regardless of testing method or manufacturer; after 1980, both brands gave similar 'smoke pH' values. Similarly, 'low yield' brands such as Merit and Barclay exhibited higher values relative to 'regular' brands. Consistent patterns of relative brand differences such as these explain the long-term use of 'smoke pH' measurements by the tobacco industry, and contrasts with public claims by the industry that little or no variation in 'smoke pH' exists among brands (Philip Morris Inc. *et al.* 1997, 1998). Internal results obtained for 'low yield' brands are also consistent with the view that such brands may compensate for reduced total nicotine delivery by maintaining a certain level of free-base nicotine delivery.

Product targeting

There is no single approach to tailoring tobacco products to all populations. For example, initiation can be fostered by marketing strategies and development or promotion of products that enhance product attractiveness without necessarily altering the pharmacological addictiveness or abuse liability of the product. Some product factors affecting attractiveness may seem obvious, such as tobacco products that are branded and manufactured with candy-like flavourings. Other factors are more insidious, such as the use of menthol and other ingredients to mask throat irritation, smooth the smoke, and produce sensory effects specific to the target market, for example, 12–16 year olds. Filters can be used to make cigarettes more attractive in several ways such as by making it possible to smoke without putting tobacco in the mouth, by making the smoke cooler and easier to inhale, and by reinforcing the deception that such cigarettes are less harmful. Taken together, these factors may be considered to contribute to the appeal of the product and, hence, promote the initiation of use and development of addiction.

In recent years, a number of heavily flavoured tobacco products (including cigarettes, smokeless, bidis, and waterpipes) have been introduced commercially in the United States and elsewhere, many of which are marketed as extensions of popular commercial brands, particularly brands favoured by youth. None of these flavoured brands have achieved significant market penetration, and it has been speculated in the literature that these products are intended primarily to increase experimentation and 'someday smoking' among youth and newer users (Carpenter *et al.* 2005b; Connolly 2004; Lewis and Wackowski 2006). Thus, in contrast to mild products which are intended to enable and foster repeated product use, these new products appear designed to provide a bridge between never-users and initial use and perhaps cultivate niche (but potentially financially lucrative) markets for the manufacturers of such products.

Indeed, a recent survey of college students found that flavoured cigarettes elicited higher positive expectancies than non-flavoured counterparts across all groups, including non-smokers, and supported a greater 'intention to try' among experimenters (Ashare *et al.* 2007). Data from two national surveys of youth smokers which report experimentation with flavoured products suggested highest rates of use among those under 25 years of age (Giovino *et al.* 2005); and a 2008 study concluded that uniquely flavoured cigarette brands were most attractive to the youngest smokers, aged 17–19 (Klein *et al.* 2008).

Internal industry studies of differences in taste and flavour preferences by age confirm that younger smokers are more open to unique and exotic flavours (Carpenter *et al.* 2005b). The internal research suggests that young and novice smokers may also be especially vulnerable to product benefits related to flavoured cigarettes (Kapular & Associates 1984). For example, in 1992, Philip Morris tested several flavours among young adult smokers and identified a number of possible consumer benefits including increased social acceptance via pleasant aroma and aftertaste, increased excitement (e.g. sharing flavours), smoking enjoyment, and a 'high-curiosity to try factor' (Philip Morris 1992).

Other examples highlight the importance of product design matched to preferences of the target population. A distinguishing characteristic of brands more popular among youth than adults in the United States today is their smoothness and mildness as compared with competitive products (Kreslake *et al.* 2008a). On the other hand, industry research identified expectations of heightened menthol delivery among a subset of primarily male, black smokers in the United States. These expectations were successfully matched to a set of products with menthol levels exceeding those of products developed and targeted to new smokers and women (Kreslake *et al.* 2008a).

Likewise, a study by Carpenter *et al.* (2005a) found that manufacturers used a variety of product parameters including physical features such as longer length and reduced circumference as well as additives and tobacco blends to meet female-targeted product preferences. Such design features conveyed perceptions of reduced risk, less strength, and lower delivery, thereby targeting needs (i.e. health, weight loss, reduced taste) previously identified among women smokers. These physical design changes heightened product appeal among women and, over time, resulted in the introduction of a number of commercial female brands (e.g. Virginia Slims, Misty, More).

Conclusions

The historical evidence with respect to manipulation of nicotine is overwhelming. Tobacco manufacturers began programmes for manipulation of nicotine more than fifty years ago and refined these efforts over decades, altering product characteristics in order to sustain addictive levels of nicotine delivery despite reduced machine measured levels of tar and nicotine delivery.

In the August 2006 decision of a suit between the US federal government and major US cigarette manufacturers, federal Judge Gladys Kessler concluded that tobacco manufacturers:

'… designed their cigarettes to precisely control nicotine delivery levels and provide doses of nicotine sufficient to create and sustain addiction.' [p. 515]

'… extensively studied smoking intake and inhalation, compensation, addiction physiology, smoker psychology, the pharmacological aspects of nicotine, the effects of nicotine on brain waves, and related subjects.' [p. 515]

'… intentionally developed and marketed cigarettes which, in actuality, delivered higher levels of nicotine than those measured by the FTC method.' [p. 516]

There is no evidence to suggest that this historical pattern of nicotine manipulation has changed. Numerous product adjustments are used to optimize both levels of nicotine as well as effects. Manufacturers have concealed much of their nicotine-related research, and have continuously and vigorously denied their efforts to control nicotine levels and delivery. Nonetheless, the modern cigarette reflects many decades of sophisticated internal research on nicotine dosing, incorporating sensory, behavioural, psychological, and social factors alongside a highly engineered chemical delivery system designed to increase ease of use, enhance the physiological effects of smoking, and most effectively match the needs of smokers.

Product design and ingredients facilitate tobacco addiction through diverse addiction potentiating mechanisms. In addition to designs and ingredients that enhance nicotine self-administration and absorption (e.g. filter tip ventilation, menthol, and levulinic acid), ingredients may have their own direct pharmacologic effects that potentiate those of nicotine (e.g. acetaldehyde), ingredients may increase the free base fraction of nicotine (e.g. ammonia and urea-based compounds), and still other designs may increase the attractiveness of the product through the illusion of reduced harmfulness and even candy-like flavourings. These observations are also consistent with the conclusion that tobacco products in general, and cigarettes in particular, though addictive by nature, carry enhanced addiction risk through modern designs that were intended to achieve this effect (Henningfield *et al.* 2004 US FDA 1995, 1996; World Health Organization 2007).

The results of the few laboratory studies conducted with bidis and clove cigarettes – highly flavoured and unique tobacco products – indicate that in spite of large differences in the availability of nicotine in these products, experienced smokers will extract quantities of nicotine similar to those extracted when smoking their usual brand of cigarettes. However, to the extent that cigarette designs make addictive levels of nicotine delivery easier to achieve, such designs may facilitate the path to addiction for youth or new smokers, and enable smokers to sustain their addiction in the face of smoking restrictions, increased prices, or other obstacles.

The evidence supports the need for regulatory oversight of both nicotine and tobacco as its delivery mechanism. Cigarette manufacturers have dedicated extensive resources to careful investigation of nicotine manipulation in order to understand and optimize the role of nicotine in the smoking experience. Regulation of tobacco products is needed to assess product changes that are used to reinforce or contribute to tobacco dependence. Assessment should include not only levels of nicotine in smoke, but also factors known to influence dose and effects. Among these are the form of delivery of nicotine, the role of 'impact' or other sensory cues, and physical or chemical design differences (e.g. ventilation) likely to influence puffing and inhalation behaviour.

Acknowledgments

The present chapter is based on a chapter published previously in the volume Nicotine Psychopharmacology (2008) in the *Handbook of Experimental Pharmacology* book series. Research was conducted at the Harvard School of Public Health and funded through National Cancer Institute Grant R01 CA87477-08.

References

Anderson, I.G.M. and Read, G.A. (1980). Method for nicotine and cotinine in blood and urine. Report No. Rd.1737c. 21 May. Bates: 650032386-650032428. Available at: http://tobaccodocuments.org/bw/18184.html

Ashare, R.L., Hawk, L.W. Jr, Cummings, K.M., O'Connor, R.J., Fix, B.V., and Schmidt, W.C. (2007). Smoking expectancies for flavored and non-flavored cigarettes among college students. *Addict Behav*. June; **32**(6): 1252–61.

Ayres, C.I. and Greig, C.C. (1984). Smoking dynamics: exploratory studies. 22 June. Brown & Williamson. Bates: 650371156-650371229. Available at: http://tobaccodocuments.org/product_design/79706.html

Baker, R.R. (1990). Chemosensory research. 28 February. British American Tobacco. Bates: 400854060-400854066. Available at: http://tobaccodocuments.org/ness/21044.html

Barton, H.C. (2000). Marketing committee. British American Tobacco. Bates: 325051442-1444. Available at: http://legacy.library.ucsf.edu/tid/dbk50a99

Bates, C., Jarvis, M., and Connolly, G. (1999). *Tobacco additives: cigarette engineering and nicotine addiction*. London: Action on Smoking and Health.

Belluzzi, J.D., Wang, R., and Leslie, F.M. (2005). Acetaldehyde enhances acquisition of nicotine self-administration in adolescent rats. *Neuropsychopharmacology*, **30**: 705–12.

Bernasek, E. and Nystrom, C.W. (1982). Ammonia. 09 August. R.J. Reynolds. Bates: 504438506-504438512. Available at: http://tobaccodocuments.org/rjr/504438506-8512.html

Bernasek, P.F., Furin, O.P., and Shelar, G.R. (1992). Sugar/Nicotine Study. 29 July. R.J. Reynolds. Bates: 510697389-510697410. Available at: http://tobaccodocuments.org/product_design/510697389-7410.html

Brauer, L.H., Behm, F.M., Lane, J.D., Westman, E.C., Perkins, C., and Rose, J.E. (2001). Individual differences in smoking reward from de-nicotinized cigarettes. *Nicotine & Tobacco Research*, **3**: 101–9.

British American Tobacco. (Undated). Smoking behavior study – German Marlboro Lights consumers. Bates: 400474215-400474232. Available at: http://bat.library.ucsf.edu/tid/zga72a99

British American Tobacco. (1983). Comments of Brown & Williamson Tobacco Corporation on the Federal Trade Commission's proposal to modify the official cigarette testing methodology. Bates: 400800808-400801051. Available at: http://bat.library.ucsf.edu/tid/jjn42a99

British American Tobacco. (1984a). Nicotine Conference: Southampton 6–8 June. Summary. 06 June. Bates: 101234971-101235018 Exhibit 10. http://tobaccodocuments.org/product_design/HmNcBAT19840606.Sm.html

British American Tobacco. (1984b). R&D Views on Potential Marketing Opportunities. 12 September. Bates: 109869437-109869440 Exhibit 11. Available at: http://tobaccodocuments.org/youth/PdToBAT19840912.Rm.html

British American Tobacco. (1988). Nicotine scavenging-A consequence of ammonia-release taste modifier No. 7. Available at: http://tobaccodocuments.org/product_design/402363924-3962.html

British American Tobacco. (1994). Proceedings of chemosensory meeting held in Southampton 8-10 931100. Bates: 570354096-570354354. Available at: http://legacy.library.ucsf.edu/tid/yzc51f00

Brooks, G.O., Cousins, A.R., and Crellin, R.A. (1974). Puff by puff impact – extractable nicotine studies on Hallmark cigarettes from Australia report No. Rd. 1108-R. 21 May. Brown & Williamson. Bates: 650318361-650318421. Available at: http://tobaccodocuments.org/bw/70032.html

Brown & Williamson. (1977). Long-term product development strategy. 28 November. Bates:501011512-501011515. Available at: http://tobaccodocuments.org/bw/90839.html

Brown & Williamson. (1983). Directed flows of smoke. 17 February. Bates: 509001468-509001475. Available at: http://tobaccodocuments.org/product_design/1334.html

Browne, C.L. (1990). *The design of cigarettes*, 3rd edn. Charlotte, NC, C Filter Products Division, Hoechst Celanese Corporation.

Burns, D.M. (1992). Assessing changes in topography (inhalation profile) and biological effects of tobacco smoke in humans. Available at: http://tobaccodocuments.org/product_design/87795497-5520.html

Cao, J., Belluzzi, J.D., Loughlin, S.E., Keyler, D.E., Pentel, P.R., and Leslie, F.M. (2007). Acetaldehyde, a major constituent of tobacco smoke, enhances behavioral, endocrine, and neuronal responses to nicotine in adolescent and adult rats. *Neuropsychopharmacology*, **32**: 2025–35.

Carpenter, C.M., Ferris Wayne, G., and Connolly, G.N. (2005a). Designing cigarettes for women: new findings from the tobacco industry documents. *Addiction*, **100**: 837–51.

Carpenter, C., Ferris Wayne, G., Connolly, G.N., Pauly, J., and Koh, H. (2005b). New cigarette brands with flavors that appeal to youth. *Health Affairs*, **24**(6): 1601–10.

Carpenter, C.M., Ferris Wayne, G., and Connolly, G.N. (2006). The role of sensory perception in the development and targeting of tobacco products. *Addiction*, **102**: 136–47.

Chakraborty, B.B. (1985). Subject: Status of High Nicotine Tobacco Evaluation/377. 16 July. Brown & Williamson. Bates: 510003880-510003882Exhibit13. Available at: http://tobaccodocuments.org/youth/CgNcBWC19850416.Me.html

Connolly, G.N., Wayne, G.D., Lymperis, D., and Doherty, M. (2000). How cigarette additives are used to mask environmental tobacco smoke. *Tobacco Control*, **9**: 283–91.

Connolly, G.N. (2004). Sweet and spicy flavours: new brands for minorities and youth. *Tobacco Control*, **13**(3): 211–12.

Connolly, G.N., Alpert, H.A., Ferris Wayne, G., and Koh, H. (2007). Trends in smoke nicotine yield and relationship to design characteristics among popular US cigarette brands, 1997–2005. *Tobacco Control*, October; **16**(5): e5.

Cook, B.L., Wayne, G.F., Keithly, L., and Connolly, G. (2003). One size does not fit all: how the tobacco industry has altered cigarette design to target consumer groups with specific psychological and psychosocial needs. *Addiction*, **98**: 1547–61.

Crellin, R. and Reihl, T. (1984). Project SHIP. 2 May. Brown & Williamson. Bates: 621062393-621062413. Available at: http://tobaccodocuments.org/product_design/1462302.html

Cummings, K.M., Morley, C.P., Horan, J.K., Steger, C., and Leavell, N.R. (2002). Marketing to America's youth: evidence from corporate documents. *Tobacco Control*, **11**(90001): i5–17.

Djordjevic, M.V., Fan, J., Ferguson, S., and Hoffmann, D. (1995). Self-regulation of smoking intensity. Smoke yields of the low-nicotine, low-'tar' cigarettes. *Carcinogenesis*, **16**: 2015–21.

Dunn, W.L. and Schori, T.R. (1971). 1600 – Consumer psychology tar, nicotine, and smoking behavior. November. Philip Morris. Bates: 1000350158-1000350188. Available at: http://tobaccodocuments.org/pm/1000350158-0188.html

Dunn, W.L. (1972a). Motives and incentives in cigarette smoking. (est.). Philip Morris. Bates: 1001541594/1596. Available at: http://legacy.library.ucsf.edu/tid/vkb97e00

Dunn, W.L. and Schori, T.R. (1972b). Smoking and low delivery cigarettes. 23 June. Philip Morris. Bates:1000351570-1000351595. Available at: http://tobaccodocuments.org/pm/1000351570-1595.html

Dunn, W.L. and Schori, T.R. (1972c). Tar, nicotine, and cigarette consumption. Jan. Philip Morris. Bates:1003285403-1003285416. Available at: http://tobaccodocuments.org/landman/1003285403-5416.html

Dunn, W.L., Jones, B.W., and Schori, T.R. (1973). Project 1600 – smoker psychology smoking and low delivery cigarettes – II (Tnt-3). October. Philip Morris. Bates: 1000048633-1000048654. Available at: http://tobaccodocuments.org/pm/1000048633-8654.html

Dunn, W.L. Houck, W., Jones, B.W., and Meyer, L.F. (1976). 1600 – Smoker psychology low delivery cigarettes and increased nicotine/tar ratios, III (Pol-1606). (est.) Philip Morris. Bates: 2024545758-2024545773. Available at: http://tobaccodocuments.org/pm/2024545758-5773.html

Esterle, J.G., Honeycutt, R.H., and Nall, J.F. (1979). Tar/nicotine ratios and nicotine transfer efficiencies of B&W and competition brands. 20 September. Brown & Williamson. Bates: 505003431-505003438. Available at: http://tobaccodocuments.org/bw/94764.html

Farnham, F. (1995). List of additives in the manufacture of tobacco products and their substitutes. Philip Morris. Bates No. 2050755566-5578. Available at: http://tobaccodocuments.org/product_design/2050755566-5578.html

Ferris Wayne, G. and Connolly, G.N. (2004). Application, function, and effects of menthol in cigarettes: a survey of tobacco industry documents. *Nicotine & Tobacco Research*, **6**(Suppl 1): S43–54.

Ferris Wayne, G., Connolly, G.N., and Henningfield, J.E. (2006). Brand differences of free-base nicotine delivery in cigarette smoke: the view of the tobacco industry documents. *Tobacco Control*, **15**: 189–98.

Freedman, A.M., and Wall Street Journal. (1995). Impact booster: tobacco firm shows how ammonia spurs delivery of nicotine. 18 October. Brown & Williamson. Bates No. 450180185/0188. Available at: http://legacy.library.ucsf.edu/tid/bsv01f00

Giovino, G.A., Yang, J., Tworek, C., Cummings, K.M., O'Connor, R.J., Donohue, K. *et al.*(2005). Use of flavored cigarettes among older adolescent and adult smokers: United States. Presentation at the National Conference on Tobacco or Health. Chicago, Illinois. 6 May 2005.

Green, C.R., Benezet, H.J., and Guess, H.E. (1992). Tobacco technology training program. R.J. Reynolds. 13 July. R.J. Reynolds. Bates No. 511291871/2200. Available at: http://tobaccodocuments.org/rjr/511291871-2200.html

Gregory, C F. (1980). Observation of free nicotine changes in tobacco smoke/#528. 04 January. Brown & Williamson. Bates: 510000667. Available at: http://tobaccodocuments.org/product_design/3355.html

Greig, C.A. (1987). Review of filters which generate smoke swirl, and their sensory properties. 23 March. British American Tobacco. Bates: 570365201-570365258. Available at: http://tobaccodocuments.org/product_design/954800.html

Gullotta, F. (1982). Electrophysiological Studies – 1982 Annual Report. Philip Morris. Bates: 028814487-4523. Available at: http://tobaccodocuments.org/youth/NcSrPMI19820705.An.html

Gullotta, F.P., Hayes, C.S., and Martin, B.R. (1989). When nicotine is not nicotine. 02 August. Philip Morris. Bates: 2029082240-2029082244. Available at: http://tobaccodocuments.org/pm/2029082240-2244.html

Gullotta, F.P., Hayes, C.S., and Martin, B.R. (1990). Subject: the electrophysiological and subjective consequences of tobacco filler Ph modifications: a proposal. 14 December. Philip Morris. Bates: 2023107993-7994. Available at: http://tobaccodocuments.org/product_design/2023107993-7994.html

Hammond, D., Fong, G.T., Cummings, K.M., and Hyland, A. (2005). Smoking topography, brand switching, and nicotine delivery: results from an in vivo study. *Cancer Epidemiology Biomarkers & Prevention*, 14: 1370–5.

Hammond, D., Fong, G.T., Cummings, K.M., O'Connor, R.J., Giovino, G.A., and McNeill, A. (2006). Cigarette yields and human exposure: a comparison of alternative testing regimens. *Cancer Epidemiology Biomarkers & Prevention*, 15: 1495–501.

Hammond, D., Wiebel, F., Kozlowski, L.T., Borland, R., Cummings, K.M., O'Connor, R.J., *et al.* (2007). Revising the machine smoking regime for cigarette emissions: implications for tobacco control policy. *Tobacco Control*, 16(1): 8–14.

Harllee, G.C. and Leffingwell, J.C. (1978). Composition of casing material: cocoa, its constituents, and their organoleptic properties. Brown & Williamson. Bates No. 566613142/3177. Available at: http://legacy.library.ucsf.edu/tid/wfk51f00

Haslam, F. [Re:] Compensation. 21 September 1977. British American Tobacco. Bates: 100236543Exhibit1048. Available at: http://tobaccodocuments.org/product_design/CnTuBAT19770921.Me.html

Henley, W.M. (1977). Project 1250: methods of controlling tar, nicotine and satisfaction. 19 May. RJ Reynolds, Bates: 504476706. Available at: http://tobaccodocuments.org/rjr/504476706-6706_D1.html

Henningfield, J.E., Benowitz, N.L., Connolly, G.N., Davis, R.M., Gray, N., Myers, M.L. *et al.* (2004). Reducing tobacco addiction through tobacco product regulation. *Tobacco Control*, 13: 132–5.

Henningfield, J., Pankow, J., and Garrett, B. (2004). Ammonia and other chemical base tobacco additives and cigarette nicotine delivery: issues and research needs. *Nicotine & Tobacco Research*, 6: 199–205.

Henningfield, J.E., Benowitz, N.L., Slade, J., Houston, T.P., Davis, R.M., and Deitchman, S.D. (1998). Reducing the addictiveness of cigarettes. *Tobacco Control*, 7: 281–93.

Henningfield, J.E., Fant, R. V., Shiffman, S., and Gitchell, J. (2000). Tobacco dependence: Scientific and public health basis of treatment. *The Economics of Neuroscience*, 2: 42–46.

Hersey, J.C., Ng, S.W., Nonnemaker, J.M., Mowery, P., Thomas, K.Y., Vilsaint, M.C. *et al.* (2006). Are menthol cigarettes a starter product for youth? *Nicotine and Tobacco Research*, 8(3): 403–13.

Hirji, T. and Wood, D.J. (1973). Impact: its relationship with extractable nicotine and with other cigarette variables (Report No. Rd. 1052-R). 29 Oct. Brown & Williamson. BatesL 650318009. Available at: http://tobaccodocuments.org/product_design/70021.html

Hoffman, D., Djordievic, M.V., and Hoffman, I. (1997). The changing cigarette. *Preventive Medicine*, 26: 427–34.

Houck, W.G., Jones, B., Martin, P., and Meyer, L.F. (1975). 1600 – Smoker psychology low delivery cigarettes and increased nicotine/tar ratios, a replication. October. Philip Morris. Bates: 1003288950-1003288967. Available at: http://tobaccodocuments.org/pm/1003288950-8967.html

Houck, W.G., Jones, B.W., and Meyer, L. 1600 – Smoker psychology low delivery cigarettes and increased nicotine/tar ratios, III. 1976 (est.). Bates: 1003288934-1003288949. Available at: http://tobaccodocuments.org/pm/1003288934-8949.html

Hurt, R.D. and Robertson, C.R. (1998). Prying open the door to the tobacco industry's secrets about nicotine: the Minnesota Tobacco Trial. *JAMA*, **280**: 1173–81.

Ingebrethsen, B.J. (1993). The physical properties of mainstream cigarette smoke and their relationship to deposition in the respiratory tract. 10 February. RJ Reynolds. Bates: 512293419 -3456. Available at: http://tobaccodocuments.org/product_design/512293419-3456.html

Jarvis, M.J., Boreham, R., Primatesta, P., Feyerabend, C., and Bryant, A. (2001). Nicotine yield from machine-smoked cigarettes and nicotine intakes in smokers: evidence from a representative population survey. *Journal of the National Cancer Institute*, **93**: 134–8.

Jeltema, M. (1987). Subject: ease of draw. 23 April. Philip Morris. Bates: 2022195514- 2022195518. Available at: http://tobaccodocuments.org/product_design/2022195514-5518.html

Jennings, R.A., Morgan, W.T., and Walker, J.C. (1991). Title: effect of a chemical stimulant on the perception of draw: a pilot study. 08 February. RJ Reynolds. Bates: 508258180-508258191. Available at: http://tobaccodocuments.org/product_design/508258180-8191.html

Johnson, R.R. (1989). Ammonia technology conference minutes. 12 June. Brown & Williamson. Bates: 620941483. Available at: http://tobaccodocuments.org/product_design/1097876.html

Jori, A., Bianchetti, A., and Prestini, P.E. (1969). Effect of essential oils on drug metabolism. *Biochemical Pharmacology*, **18**: 2081–5.

Kapular & Associates. (1984). Smokers reaction to a flavored cigarette concept – a qualitative study. January. Brown & Williamson. Bates No. 679235846-679235893. Available at: http:// tobaccodocuments.org/product_design/11924518.html

Keithly, L., Ferris Wayne, G., Cullen, D.M., and Connolly, G.N. (2005). Industry research on the use and effects of levulinic acid: a case study in cigarette additives. *Nicotine Tobacco Research*, **7**: 761–71.

Kessler, D.A. (1994). Statement. In: Regulation of tobacco products. Part 1. Hearing before the Subcommittee on Health and the Environment of the Committee on Energy and Commerce, House of Representatives. Washington, D.C.: Government Printing Office, 143–4. (Serial no 103-149).

Kessler, D.A., Witt, A.M., Barnett, P.S., Zeller, M.R., Natanblut, S.L., Wilkenfeld, J.P., *et al.* (1996). The Food and Drug Administration's Regulation of Tobacco Products. *New England Journal Medicine*, **335**: 988–94.

Klein, S.M., Giovino, G.A., Barker, D.C., Tworek, C., Cummings, K.M., and O'Connor, R.J. (2008). Use of flavored cigarettes among older adolescent and adult smokers: United States, 2004–2005. *Nicotine & Tobacco Research*, **10**(7): 1209–14.

Kozlowski, L.T., and O'Connor, R.J. (2002). Cigarette filter ventilation is a defective design because of misleading taste, bigger puffs, and blocked vents. *Tobacco Control*, **11**: i40–50.

Kreslake, J.M., Ferris Wayne, G., Alpert, H.R., Koh, H.K., and Connolly, G.N. (2008a). Tobacco industry control of menthol in cigarettes and targeting of adolescents and young adults. *American Journal of Public Health*, **98**(9): 1685–92.

Kreslake, J., Ferris Wayne, G., and Connolly, G.N. (2008b). The menthol smoker: tobacco industry research on consumer sensory perception of menthol cigarettes and its role in smoking behavior. *Nicotine and Tobacco Research*, **10**(4): 705–15.

Larson, T.M. and Morgan, J.P. (1976). Application of free nicotine to cigarette tobacco and the delivery of that nicotine in the cigarette smoke. 08 June. Lorillard. Bates: 87231657-87231667. Available at: http://tobaccodocuments.org/lor/87231657-1667.html

Lawson, J.L. and Toben, T.P. (1986). 'New Business Research and Development Report. Low Level Menthol Opportunity Analysis.' R.J. Reynolds. 24 November. Bates: 505930469-505930487. Available at: http://tobaccodocuments.org/rjr/505930469-0487.html

Leach, J. and Shockley, L. (1969). The aqueous extract Ph and extractable nicotine studies of major cigarette brands from Brown & Williamson and some domestic competitive companies. Report No. 69-19. Project No. 313. 13 June. Brown & Williamson. Bates: 598001443-598001467. Available at: http://tobaccodocuments.org/bw/971434.html

Leffingwell, J.C., Young, H.J., and Bernasek. E. (1972). *Tobacco flavoring for smoking products*. Winston-Salem, NC: RJ Reynolds.

Levin, E.D., Behm, F., Carnahan, E., LeClair, R., Shipley, R., and Rose, J.E. (1993). Clinical trials using ascorbic acid aerosol to aid smoking cessation. *Drug and Alcohol Dependence*, **33**: 211–23.

Lewis, M.J. and Wackowski, O. (2006). Dealing with an innovative industry: a look at flavored cigarettes promoted by mainstream brands. *Am J Public Health*, February, **96**(2): 244–51.

Lorillard (1973). Research 1-3-5 Year Projection of Major Projects. 02 November. Bates: 83250679-83250693. Available at: http://tobaccodocuments.org/lor/83250679-0693.html

Madyastha, K.M. and Srivatsan, V. (1988). Studies on the metabolism of l-menthol in rats. *Drug Metabolism and Disposition*, **16**: 765–72.

Maynor, B.W. and Rosene, C.J. (1981). A comparison of the extractable nicotine content of smoke from Barclay and Cambridge cigarettes. 20 January. Brown & Williamson. Bates: 680600845-680600853. Available at: http://tobaccodocuments.org/bw/329242.html

Mckenzie, J.L. (1976). Product characterization definitions and implications. 21 September. RJ Reynolds. Bates: 509195711-509195714. Available at: http://tobaccodocuments.org/rjr/509195711-5714.html

McMurtrie, A. and Silberstein, D.A. (1980). Further Investigation of Barclay Mainstream Turbulence. 02 December. Brown & Williamson. Bates: 650521259-650521262. Available at: http://tobaccodocuments.org/product_design/53691.html

Minnemeyer, H.J. (1977). Present status of the nicotine enrichment project. 13 April. Lorillard. Bates: 00044787-00044799. Available at: http://tobaccodocuments.org/lor/00044787-4799.html

Morgan, W.T., Villegas, E.H., Davis, C.C., Stevenson, M.D., and Hege, K.A. (1990). NPT menthol human smoking behavior basic learning study. RJ Reynolds. Bates: 508025121-508025162. Available at: http://tobaccodocuments.org/product_design/508025121-5162.html

National Cancer Institute (1996). *The FTC Cigarette Test Method for Determining Tar, Nicotine, and Carbon Monoxide Yields of U.S. Cigarettes. Report of the NCI Expert Committee.* Smoking and Tobacco Control Monograph No. 7. Bethesda, MD: US Department of Health and Human Services, Public Health Service, National Institutes of Health. NIH Publication No. 96-4028, August.

National Cancer Institute (2001). *Risks Associated with Smoking Cigarettes with Low Tar Machine-Measured Yields of Tar and Nicotine.* Smoking and Tobacco Control Monograph No. 13. Bethesda, MD: US Department of Health and Human Services, Public Health Service, National Institutes of Health. NIH Publication No. 02-5047, October.

Norman, V. (1974). The effect of perforated tipping paper on the yield of various smoke components. *Beitr Tabakforsch*, **7**: 282–7.

Norman, V. (1983). Puffing effort and smoke yield. Lorillard. Bates: 87633182-3199. Available at: http://tobaccodocuments.org/lor/87633182-3199.html

Pankow, J.F. (2001). A consideration of the role of gas/particle partitioning in the deposition of nicotine and other tobacco smoke compounds in the respiratory tract. *Chemical Research in Toxicology*, **14**: 1465–81.

Pankow, J.F., Takavoli, A.D., Luo, W., and Isabelle, L.M. (2003). Percent free-base nicotine in the tobacco smoke particulate matter of selected commercial and reference cigarettes. *Chemical Research & Toxicology*, **16**: 1014–18.

Philip Morris (1969). Why One Smokes. Bates: 1003287836-1003287848 Exhibit 3. Available at: http://tobaccodocuments.org/youth/NcSrPMI19690000.An.html

Philip Morris (1974). Europe. 32. Human Smoking Habits. June. Bates: 1001812883- 1001812903. Available at: http://tobaccodocuments.org/pm/1001812883-2903.html

Philip Morris (1991). Qualitative Research on Menthol/Nonmenthol Smokers. 26 September. Bates: 2057096413-2057096532. Available at: http://tobaccodocuments.org/ahf/2057096413-6532.html

Philip Morris (1992). New flavors qualitative research insights 921000. October. Bates No. 2023163698-2023163710. Available at: http://legacy.library.ucsf.edu/tid/wzj48e00

Philip Morris (1994). Ingredients added to tobacco in the manufacture of cigarettes by the six major American cigarette companies. Bates No. 202301127411322. Available at: http://legacy.library.ucsf.edu/tid/pqy74e00

Philip Morris (1995). Sensory research activities nicotine sensory research. Bates: 2063127630-2063127632. Available at: http://tobaccodocuments.org/product_design/2063127630-7632.html

Philip Morris Inc. *et al.* (1997). Submission Before the Massachusetts Department of Public Health Regarding Proposed Refinements in Sampling and Testing Procedures Set Forth in 105 CMR 660.500 and Certain Other Matters. 8 April.

Philip Morris Inc. *et al.* (1998). Comments before the Massachusetts Department of Public Health on proposed amendments to regulations entitled cigarette and smokeless tobacco products: Reports of added constituents and nicotine ratings. 2 October.

Pickworth, W.B., Fant, R.V., Nelson, R.A., Rohrer, M.S., and Henningfield, J.E. (1999). Pharmacodynamic effects of new de-nicotinized cigarettes. *Nicotine & Tobacco Research*, 1: 357–64.

Reynolds, R.J. (Undated). Psychophysics of tobacco use. Bates: 501542595. Available at: http://tobaccodocuments.org/product_design/501542595-2595.html

Reynolds, R.J. (1979). Response surface methodology (RSM). Bates: 512327145-7148. Available at: http://tobaccodocuments.org/product_design/512327145-7148.html

Reynolds, R.J. (1980). Technology: ammoniation. Available at: http://tobaccodocuments.org/rjr/509018864-8865A.html

Reynolds, R.J. (1985). Now-type cigarettes with increased nicotine. 09 October. Bates: 509108038-509108040. Available at: http://tobaccodocuments.org/rjr/509108038-8040.html

Reynolds, R.J. (1986). Support Brand R&D. R.J. Reynolds. 12 December. Bates: 515395107-515395119. Available at: http://tobaccodocuments.org/product_design/515395107-5119.html

Reynolds, R.J. (1987a). Taste & olfaction. Bates: 509859364-509859400. Retrieved from: http://tobaccodocuments.org/rjr/509859364-9400.html

Reynolds, R.J. (1987b). 988-90 (880000-900000) Strategic plan. action programs. 15 August. Bates: 511266804-511266819. Available at: http://tobaccodocuments.org/product_design/511266804-6819.html

Reynolds, R.J. (1989). Inrc. Nicotine related research areas: nicotine optimization. Bates: 507028876. Available at: http://tobaccodocuments.org/rjr/507028876-8876.html

Reynolds, R.J. (1990a). Project Xb. Bates: 511282950-511282968. Available at: http://tobaccodocuments.org/women/511282950-2968.html

Reynolds, R.J. (1990b). Mission statement. Investigate the pharmacological effects of nicotine and other tobacco constituents to support the development and marketing of superior products. Bates: 509787523-509787549. Available at: http://tobaccodocuments.org/rjr/509787523-7549.html

Reynolds, R.J. (1990c). There are several reasons why Philip Morris would find it strategically advantageous to master nicotine manuipulation in cigarettes. 15 November. Bates: 509348227-509348229. Available at: http://tobaccodocuments.org/rjr/509348227-8229.html

Reynolds, R.J. (1991). Nicotine Rsm review II – FFLT Smokers. 16 December. Bates: 510961381-510961445. Available at: http://tobaccodocuments.org/product_design/510961381-1445.html

Reynolds, R.J. (1992a). Sugar nicotine balance. Bates: 512802860-512802862. Available at: http://tobaccodocuments.org/rjr/512802860-2862.html

Reynolds, R.J. (1992b). Status update of sugar/nicotine balance technology assessment. March. Bates: 512842551-512842552. Available at: http://tobaccodocuments.org/rjr/512842551-2552.html

Reynolds, R.J. (1994). Acceptance & strength perceptions by nicotine level. 8 April. Bates: 514314536-514314565. Available at: http://tobaccodocuments.org/product_design/514314536-4565.html

Reynolds, R.J. (1997). Table of contents. I. Additives. 31 January. Bates: 521097968-521097974. Available at: http://tobaccodocuments.org/rjr/521097968-7974.html

Roberts, D.L. (1985). The effects of construction parameters on cigarette sensory properties. 9 September. R.J. Reynolds. Bates: 512134464-512134492. Available at: http://tobaccodocuments.org/product_design/512134464-4492.html

Robinson, J.D., Cinciripini, P.M., Tiffany, S.T., Carter, B.L., Lam, C.Y., & Wetter, D.W. (2007). Gender differences in affective response to acute nicotine administration and deprivation. *Addictive Behaviors*, **32**(3): 543–61.

Rose, J.E. (2006). Nicotine and nonnicotine factors in cigarette addiction. *Psychopharmacology*, **184**: 274–85.

Royal College of Physicians of London. (2000). Nicotine addiction in Britain: a report of the Tobacco Advisory Group of the Royal College of Physicians. London, UK: Royal College of Physicians.

Schneider, W. (1992). Elasticity of cigarettes. 9 September. Brown & Williamson. Bates: 575251611-43. Available at: http://tobaccodocuments.org/bw/956817.html

Schori, T.R. (1979). Free nicotine: its implications on smoke impact. 22 October. Brown & Williamson. Available at: http://tobaccodocuments.org/product_design/166104.html

Slade, J., Bero, L.A., Hanauer, P., Barnes, D.E. and.Glantz, S.A. (1995). Nicotine and addiction. The Brown and Williamson documents. *JAMA*, **274**: 225–33.

Shannon, M.D., Dube, M.F., Walker, J.R., Reynolds, J., Smith, K., Norman, A.B., *et al.* (1992). We are looking at smoothness from a different perspective. R.J. Reynolds. Bates: 508408649-508408770. Available at: http://tobaccodocuments.org/rjr/508408649-8770.html

Shepperd, C. (1993). The sensory enhancement of the intial puffs of low tar products using an alkaline additive. 16 December. British American Tobacco. Bates: 570267693-570267726. Available at: http://tobaccodocuments.org/product_design/951740.html

Silver, W. (1988). Physiology of trigeminal chemoreceptors in the nasal cavity. R.J. Reynolds. Bates No. 506797834-506797868. Available at: http://tobaccodocuments.org/product_design/506797834-7868.html

Smith, K. (1992). Technology assessment status update. 29 May. R.J. Reynolds. Bates: 512775555-512775597. Available at: http://tobaccodocuments.org/product_design/512775555-5597_D1.html

Swain, J.W. and Crayton, F.H. (1981). *US Patent No. 4,286,606*. Washington, D.C: US Patent and Trademark Office.

Teague, C.E. Jr. (1972). Research planning memorandum on the nature of the tobacco business and the crucial role of nicotine therein. 14 April. Bates: 500915630-500915638. Available at: http://tobaccodocuments.org/rjr/500915630-5638.html

Teague, C.E. (1973). Implications and activities arising from correlation of smoke Ph with nicotine impact, other smoke qualities, and cigarette sales. 23 July. R.J. Reynolds. Bates: 501136994-501137023. Available at: http://tobaccodocuments.org/rjr/501136994-7023.html

Templeton, W.W. (1984). Receptors for nicotine in the central nervous system: I Radioligand Binding Studies Report No. Rd.1960 Restricted. 22 March. Brown & Williamson. Bates: 650000996-650001034. Available at: http://tobaccodocuments.org/bw/17198.html

Thorne, N. (1994). The role of smoking behaviour in sensory evaluation Paper 4. British American Tobacco. Bates: 505303409-505303427. Available at: http://tobaccodocuments.org/product_design/944668.html

US Department of Health and Human Services (1988). The health consequences of smoking: nicotine addiction. Department of Health and Human Services, Public Health Service, Centers for Disease Control and Prevention, Center for Health Promotion and Education, Office on Smoking and Health, Rockville, MD.

US Food and Drug Administration. (1995). 21 CFR Part 801, *et al.* Regulations restricting the sale and distribution of cigarettes and smokeless tobacco products to protect children and adolescents; proposed rule analysis regarding FDA's jurisdiction over nicotine-containing cigarettes and smokeless tobacco products; notice. *Federal Register*, **60**: 41314–792.

US Food and Drug Administration. (1996). 21 CFR Part 801, *et al.* Regulations restricting the sale and distribution of cigarettes and smokeless tobacco to protect children and adolescents; final rule. *Federal Register*. **61**: 44396–5318.

Vagg, R. and Chapman, S. (2005). Nicotine analogues: a review of tobacco industry research interests. *Addiction*, **100**: 701–12.

Walker, J.R., Jennings, R., and Reynolds, J. (1992). Subject: perception of draw (Integrating Lab and Consumer Data). 21 February. R.J. Reynolds. Bates: 513325096-513325098. Available at: http://tobaccodocuments.org/product_design/513325096-5098.html

Watson, C.H., Trommel, J.S., and Ashley, D.L. (2004). Solid-phase microextraction-based approach to determine free-base nicotine in trapped mainstream cigarette smoke total particulate matter. *Journal of Agricultural and Food Chemistry*, **52**: 7240–5.

Wayne, G.F. and Connolly, G.N. (2002). How cigarette design can affect youth initiation into smoking: Camel cigarettes 1983–93. *Tobacco Control*, **11**: i32–9.

Wayne, G.F., Connolly, G.N., and Henningfield, J.E. (2004). Assessing internal tobacco industry knowledge of the neurobiology of tobacco dependence. *Nicotine Tobacco Research*, **6**: 927–40.

Wells, J.K., III. (1995). Subject: Technology Handbook. 22 August. Brown & Williamson. Bates: 505500002. Available at: http://tobaccodocuments.org/product_design/945335.html

Whitehead, P. (1994). Visual and sensory cues in the control of smoking behaviour P Whitehead Paper 5. British American Tobacco. Bates: 505303428-505303444. Available at: http://tobaccodocuments.org/product_design/944669.html

Willems, E.W., Rambali, B., Vleeming, W., Opperhuizen, A., and van Amsterdam, J.G. (2006). Significance of ammonium compounds on nicotine exposure to cigarette smokers. *Food and Chemical Toxicology*, **44**: 678–88.

Wilson, D.J. Project Xb. (1991). Product Development – Phase 1. 06 August. R.J. Reynolds. Bates: 509308455-509308459. Available at: http://tobaccodocuments.org/rjr/509308455-8459.html

World Health Organization. (2001). Advancing knowledge on regulating tobacco products. Geneva, Switzerland: World Health Organization.

World Health Organization. (2007). Tobacco free Initiative. The scientific basis of tobacco product regulation. Available at: http\://www.who.int/tobacco/global_interaction/tobreg/tsr/en/index.html

Woods, J.D. and Sheets, S.H. (1975). Updated review and analyses of 1974 (740000) Competitive Brand Data. 15 January. R.J. Reynolds. Bates: 500615944-500615960. Available at: http://tobaccodocuments.org/rjr/500615944-5960.html

Wu, D.L. and Swain, J.W. (1983). *US Patent 4,379,464*. Washington, D.C.: US Patent and Trademark Office.

Yearnan, A. (1963). Implications of Battelle Hippo I & II and the Griffith Filter. 17 July. Bates No: 1802.05. Available at: http://legacy.library.ucsf.edu/tid/xrc72d00

Chapter 10

Nicotine content in tobacco and tobacco smoke

Mirjana V. Djordjevic

Introduction

Since the 1968 article by Stedman (1968), the number of identified tobacco and tobacco smoke components has increased several fold, to 8 089 and 7 357, respectively (Rodgman and Perfetti 2009). However, regardless of the complexity of tobacco and tobacco smoke chemical composition and cross reactivity among different constituents, tobacco use initiation and maintenance is primarily due to psychopharmacological effects of nicotine (Henningfield *et al.* 2006). Nicotine is a tobacco alkaloid, a basic substance which contains a cyclic nitrogenous nucleus. In *Nicotiana* plants most alkaloids are 3-pyridyl derivatives.[1] In cured leaf of Maryland Robinson Medium Broadleaf, 24-pyridine derivatives were identified including nicotine, nornicotine, anabasine, oxynicotine, myosmine, 3-acetylpyridine, 2,3′-dipyridyl, nicotinamide, anatabine, nicotinic acid, and unidentified pyridine alkaloids of derivatives thereof (Tso 1990). Nicotine is the principal alkaloid in commercial tobaccos (this was confirmed in 34 out of 65 *Nicotiana* species); nornicotine appears to be the main alkaloid in 19 out of 65 species rather than nicotine; and anabasine is the third most important. In addition to the above-mentioned principal and minor alkaloids, the presence of many trace amounts of new alkaloids or their derivatives were frequently reported including, for example, 2.4′-dipyridyl, 4,4′-dipyridyl, *N*′-formylanabasine, *N*′-formylanatabine, *N*′-acetylanatabine, *N*′-hexanoyl-nornicotine, *N*′-octanoyl-nornicotine, 1′-(6-hydroxyoctanoyl) nornicotine, and 1′-(7-hydroxyoctanoyl) nornicotine. The latter were reported in flue-cured tobacco leaves (Djordjevic *et al.*, 1990a).

Commercial tobacco, or *Nicotiana tabacum* (*N. tabacum*), is one of the more than 64 established species in the genus *Nicotiana*. Among those species, 45 are indigenous to North or South America and 15 to Australia. Of the many American species, *N. tabacum* is the only one grown commercially in the United States at present (Tso 1990). In Russia and some of the Asiatic countries, *N. rustica* also is grown more or less extensively, though chiefly for local consumption. All 64 of the *Nicotiana* species tested by Sisson and Severson (1990) contained a measurable alkaloid fraction (at least 10 µg/g). There was a wide range in total-alkaloid levels with a 400-fold difference among field grown species.

Tobacco types, leaf position on the plant, agricultural practices, fertilizer treatment, and degree of ripening, and curing technologies are among some prominent factors which determine the levels of alkaloids in *Nicotiana* plants. In fact, every step in tobacco production that affects plant metabolism will influence the level of alkaloid content to a certain degree (Tso 1990).

---

[1] Indole alkaloids, such as harmane and norharmane, were also reported to be present in tobacco but in minute quantities.

The Maryland and Turkish types of tobacco are generally low in nicotine, the flue-cured, burley, Cuban, and Connecticut cigar wrapper are medium, and the Pennsylvania, dark fire-cured, and especially *N. rustica* are high in nicotine content (Djordjevic *et al.*, 1989, 1991; Idris *et al.*, 1991). Under favourable conditions (e.g., fertile soils under irrigation over period of years), *N. rustica* consistently produced more nicotine than *N. tabacum* (Bhide *et al.* 1987; Sisson and Severson 1990). From a random examination of 152 cultivated varieties of *N. tabacum*, a range of alkaloid variation between 0.17% and 4.93% was found (Tso 1990).

Tobacco leaves have the highest content of nicotine, roots have less, and stalks have the least. Alkaloid level increases as plants mature, especially during the period after topping (Burton *et al.* 1983, 1989b, 1994; DeRoton *et al.*, 2005; Djordjevic *et al.* 1989; Peele *et al.*, 1995; Walton *et al.*, 1995). Marked increase of nicotine was generally achieved with the increased rate of nitrogen fertilization (Chamberlain and Chortyk 1992). In lamina of air-cured and flue-cured tobacco, nicotine content increased from 41.82 to 65.77 mg/g tobacco and 30.66 to 33.51 mg, respectively, when nitrogen was applied from 0–300 lbs/acre; in midribs of air-cured and flue-cured tobacco, nicotine content increased from 2.74 to 6.5 mg/g tobacco and 6.46 to 6.78 mg, respectively.

Nicotine content in cured tobacco

Nicotine content varies considerably in different tobacco types (e.g., sun-cured oriental, flue-cured Virginia, air-cured burley, and air-cured dark tobacco; Table 10.1). Oriental tobacco commonly used for manufacturing cigarettes in the former USSR contained 1.8–12.6 mg nicotine per gram of dry tobacco (Djordjevic *et al.*, 1991). Nicotine content in flue-cured laminae from the third priming (leaves from upper stalk position) of NC alkaloid isolines (Virginia bright tobacco) contained 6.52–60.4 mg nicotine per gram of dry tobacco (Djordjevic *et al.*, 1989). Burley tobacco lamina contained 35.6–47.73 mg nicotine per gram dry tobacco (Burton *et al.*, 1989a; MacKown *et al.*, 1988). Nornicotine and anatabine concentrations also show wide range of concentrations in different tobacco types. The concentrations of nicotine, nornicotine, and anatabine in Burley midribs were significantly lower than in laminae: 5.5–19.48 mg, 0.33–0.51 mg, and 0.15–0.45 mg, respectively. As reported by MacKown *et al.* (1988), reconstituted tobacco sheets contained 5.1 mg nicotine per gram, 0.2 mg of nornicotine and 0.1 mg anatabine.

Tobacco leaves harvested from the bottom of Virginia tobacco plant contained the lowest amount of nicotine whereas the leaves from the top contained the highest amount (37.37 mg/g dry tobacco and 60.4 mg/g, respectively) (Djordjevic *et al.* 1989). The concentration of alkaloids was reported to be the lowest at the base and the tip of the leaf and greatest at the periphery of the leaf and decreased towards the tip of the leaf. Thus nicotine content in the lamina of a dark air-cured tobacco (Ky 171) varies from 33.06 to 76.10 mg per gram; nornicotine from 0.37–0.76 mg; and anatabine from 0.41 to 0.82 g (Burton *et al.*, 1992).

Nicotine and secondary amine alkaloids, such as nornicotine, anatabine, and anabasine, give rise to tobacco-specific *N*-nitrosamines (TSNA; Fig. 10.1) during all stages of tobacco production,

Table 10.1 Alkaloid content in lamina of different tobacco types[a]

Alkaloid (mg/g dry weight)	Oriental tobacco	Virginia tobacco	Burley tobacco
Nicotine	1.80–12.6	6.52–60.4	35.6–47.73
Nornicotine	0.05–1.32	0.14–6.47	0.9–2.09
Anatabine	0.02–1.60	0.14–2.17	0.9–2.31

Note

[a] Djordjevic *et al.* (1991); Djordjevic *et al.* (1989); Burton *et al.* (1989a); MacKown *et al.* (1988).

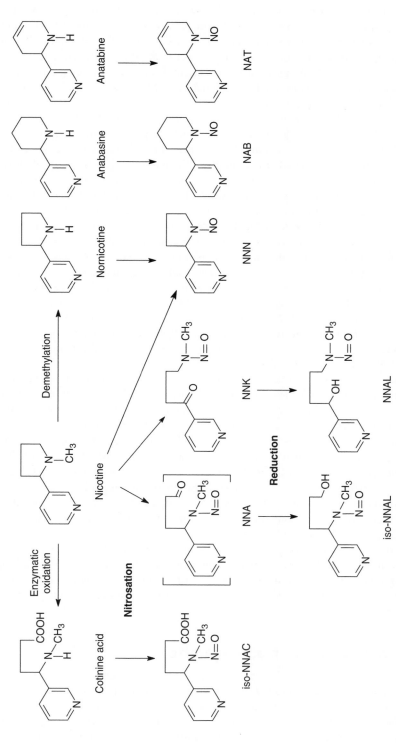

Figure 10.1 Formation of tobacco-specific N'-nitrosamines (*) (Hoffmann et al., 1995).

Note

(*) iso-NNAC, 4-(methylnitrosoamino)-4-(3-pyridyl)butyric acid; iso-NNAL, 4-(methylnitrosoamino)-4-(3-pyridyl)-1-butanol; NAB, N'-nitrosoanabasine; NAT, N'-nitrosoanatabine; NNA, 4-(methylnitrosoamino)-4-(3-pyridyl)butanal; NNAL, 4-(methylnitrosoamino)-1-(3-pyridyl)-1-butanol; NNK, 4-(methylnitrosoamino)-1-(3-pyridyl)-1-butanone; NNN, N'-nitrosonornicotine (Note: NNA is a very reactive aldehyde and has therefore never been quantified in tobacco or tobacco smoke).

from growing in the field to curing, processing, and storage, as well as during product manufacturing and puffing of combustible products (Hoffmann *et al.* 1994). TSNA are present in both smoked and non-smoked tobacco products and their concentrations vary dramatically from one product type to another, from one brand of product to another, and from one country to another (IARC 2004, 2007). Upon the evaluation of scientific evidence regarding carcinogenic risks to humans and mechanistic pathways, International Agency for Research on Cancer (IARC) designated nicotine-derived 4-(methylnitrosoamino)-1-(3-pyridyl)-1-butanone (NNK) and N'-nitrosonornicotine (NNN) as *carcinogenic to humans (Group 1)* (IARC 2007).

During the past two decades, the existence of available technologiesto control the formation of carcinogenic TSNA from their precursors in tobacco, primarily curing practices, has been well documented (O'Connor *et al.*, 2008). The availability of these technologies is of critical importance for the implementation of regulation of tobacco products as relates to mandated lowering of toxicants such as NNN and NNK in cigarette smoke (Burns *et al.*, 2008). Genetically, flue-cured and dark tobaccos have fairly low levels of nornicotine and the trait is stable while burley tobaccos have higher levels and tend to be highly variable. Nornicotine accumulation in burley tobacco is of concern because burley is one of the major constituents of American blend cigarettes (Adam *et al.*, 2006) and nornicotine is the major precursor of carcinogenic NNN both in tobacco and tobacco smoke (Hoffmann *et al.*, 2001; Moldoveanu and Borgerding 2008). As a result of screening burley lines, low convertor varieties (plants which convert or demethylate nicotine to nornicotine) have been released and this greatly reduced the level of nornicotine and hence NNN in the national burley crop (Jack *et al.*, 2007; Siminszky *et al.*, 2007). In addition to TSNA formation during tobacco curing, manufacturing, aging, and pyrolysis, some NNN formation may occur endogenously, both in animals and humans, from nornicotine and nitrosating agents (Carmella *et al.*, 1997; Stepanov *et al.*, 2009).

Similarly to reduction of NNN, NNK, and nornicotine, new technologies and approaches should be utilized to reduce nicotine levels in tobacco in order to curb the addiction to tobacco products (Benowitz and Henningfield 1994; Henningfield *et al.*, 1998; Benowitz *et al.*, 2007, 2009). To that end, several cigarette brands with low content of nicotine in tobacco were introduced in the market during the past two decades. These were: Next (Philip Morris USA) containing 0.03 mg nicotine per gram of dry tobacco (tobacco blend was de-nicotinized by supercritical fluid extraction method) (Djordjevic *et al.*, 1990), three versions of Quest (Vector Tobacco Inc.) containing 0.6, 0.3, and <0.05 mg nicotine, respectively (cigarette blend was made using genetically modified tobacco) (Chen *et al.*, 2008; Strasser *et al.*, 2006, 2007), and three versions of Marlboro Ultra Smooth (Philip Morris USA) containing 0.42–0.56 mg nicotine per cigarette in the mainstream smoke (Laugesen and Fowles 2006; Rees *et al.*, 2007).

Given a wide range of nicotine content in various tobacco types or leaves harvested from different plant positions, including the country of origin and variability from year-to-year crops due to climate conditions and agricultural practices, manufacturers have unparallel opportunity to manipulate nicotine content in cigarettes as well as delivery to the smoker by chiefly blending different tobaccos.

Nicotine content in factory-made cigarettes

Until the recent two decades, only flue-cured tobaccos were used in cigarettes in the United Kingdom, and Finland, and they were the predominant type used in Canada, Japan, China, Australia, and New Zealand. Air-cured tobaccos were preferred in France, southern Italy, some parts of Switzerland, Germany, and South America; cigarettes made exclusively from sun-dried tobaccos are popular in Greece and Turkey. In the rest of Western Europe and in the

United States, cigarettes contain blends of flue-cured and air-cured tobaccos as major components (Hoffmann *et al.*, 2001). Today, in many countries all over the world, including United Kingdom and France, the American blend cigarettes are gaining market shares. The 2R4F Kentucky reference cigarette, designed for research purposes and modelled to represent the typical American blend cigarette, contains 32.5% Virginia flue-cured tobacco, 20% Burley air-cured tobacco, 1.06 Maryland tobacco, 11.1% Oriental sun-cured tobacco, 27.2% reconstituted tobacco sheets, 2.8% glycerol, and 5.3% invert sugar (Adam *et al.*, 2006)

Nicotine content in cigarette filler

Nicotine content in tobacco from cigarettes sold worldwide shows a wide variation (IARC 2004). Counts and co-authors reported on the nicotine content in the tobacco filler of 48 Philip Morris (USA) and Philip Morris International commercial filtered cigarettes from numerous international market regions (Counts *et al.*, 2005). The majority contained blends of bright flue-cured (Virginia), burley air-cured, and sun-cured oriental tobaccos, with inclusions of expanded tobaccos, processed tobacco, or processed stems. Four cigarettes contained primarily bright tobaccos. Nine brands contained carbon (also known as 'charcoal') in their filter construction.

The nicotine concentrations in Philip Morris' sample of international brands ranged from 13.79 to 23.18 mg per gram of dry tobacco and those of ammonia from 0.16 to 3.51 mg/g. Data presented in Table 10.2 show that cigarettes ranked as very low yield ($\leq$ 4.9 mg tar/cigarette), low yield (5-9.9 mg tar), and moderate yield (10–14.9 mg tar), based on 'tar' and nicotine yields determined by the Federal Trade Commission (FTC)/ISO machine-smoking method (IARC 1986), contained similar amounts of nicotine and ammonia in tobacco filler. It was observed that very low-yield cigarettes, both American- and Virginia-blend, tend to contain somewhat higher amounts of nicotine and ammonia in tobacco filler. The latter suggests that even smokers of very low-yield cigarettes can obtain high nicotine dose by adjusting puffing intensity or exercising other compensatory smoking behaviours. As for cigarette brands with charcoal in the filter tip, there is no apparent difference in nicotine content in tobacco filler compared to American blend cigarettes which are manufactured with filter tips made exclusively of cellulose acetate fibres.

Table 10.2 Content of nicotine and ammonia in tobacco filler of cigarettes (mg/g dry tobacco) with different smoke yields as determined by standard FTC/ISO machine-smoking method (Counts *et al.* 2005)

	Moderate[a] 10–14.9 mg FTC tar	Low[a] 5–9.9 mg FTC tar	Very low[a] $\leq$4.9 mg FTC tar
American-blend cigarettes ($n = 44$)			
Nicotine	13.70–20.12	13.79–19.48	16.26–23.18
Ammonia	0.85–3.32	0.84–3.51	1.27–3.28
Virginia-blend cigarettes ($n - 4$)			
Nicotine	16.91–17.11	15.36	18.64
Ammonia	0.18–0.45	0.46	0.24
Charcoal-filter cigarettes ($n = 9$)			
Nicotine	15.8–18.82	14.42–19.17	20.24
Ammonia	1.17–2.83	0.84–3.25	1.54

Note

[a] IARC 1986.

Cigarette characteristics that influence nicotine delivery to the smoker, particularly nicotine and ammonium content in tobacco filler and human smoking topography, deserve special attention because nicotine induces and maintains addiction that promotes long-term chronic exposure to chemical toxicants with known harmful health effects including cancer, cardiovascular, and pulmonary diseases (IARC 2004, 2007; US DHHS 2004).

Kozlowski and co-authors reported on the nicotine content in 92 brands of cigarettes (32 American, 23 Canadian, and 37 British) (Kozlowski et al., 1998). The total nicotine content of tobacco averaged 10.2 mg/g tobacco (7.2–13.4 range) in the United States, 13.5 mg (8.0–18.3 range) in Canada, and 12.5 mg (9–17.5 range) in the United Kingdom. It is apparent, from the data presented in Table 10.3 that there are no differences in the nicotine content of tobacco, regardless of the type of cigarettes defined by the FTC/ISO machine-smoking method.

Stepanov and co-authors compared nicotine content in tobacco from cigarettes produced in the United States, Moldavia, and foreign cigarettes commercialized in Moldavia (Stepanov et al., 2002). They reported similar levels of nicotine in domestic Moldavian cigarettes (9.6–19.6 mg nicotine per gram wet weight), imported brands (13.5–15.1 mg), and cigarettes consumed in the United States (17.6–19.5 mg).

In summary, similar nicotine content in the filler of cigarettes with a wide range of FTC/ISO machine smoke yields, as shown by Djordjevic et al. (1990b), Kozlowski et al. (1998), and Counts et al. (2005), clearly show that the elasticity was built into the design of the cigarette so that smokers can extract as much nicotine as they need by changing puffing topography.

Nicotine content in cigarette smoke (standard machine-smoking methods)

Almost all parameters involved in cigarette design will change nicotine delivery. However, eight technologies in the design of 'less hazardous' cigarettes were classified by cigarette manufacturers as significant. These include: the tobacco blend, the filter tip, filter tip additives, reconstituted tobacco sheet, paper additives, air dilution via paper porosity, expanded tobacco, air dilution via filter-tip perforation (Hoffmann et al., 2001; Green et al., 2007a). For example, depending on the ratio of expanded tobacco in cigarette blend, nicotine can range from 1.01 mg/cigarette (100% expanded tobacco) to 2.01 mg/cigarette (no expanded tobacco) (Green et al., 2007b). The incorporation of a substitute for some or all of the tobacco in the cigarette filler was also considered important in manipulating smoke chemistry including nicotine yield (Green et al., 2007a). The application of additives (e.g., ammonia or ammonia-derived agents) play an important role in nicotine bioavailability as well as physiological and addictive effects (Henningfield et al., 2004).

Table 10.3 Content of nicotine in tobacco filler of cigarettes (mg/g tobacco) with different smoke yields as determined by standard FTC/ISO machine-smoking method (Kozlowski et al., 1998)

Country	High[a] >15 mg tar	Moderate[a] 10–14.9 mg tar	Low[a] 5–9.9 mg tar	Very low[a] ≤4.9 mg FTC tar
United States, n = 32	9.5–13.4	8.9–11.4	7.2–11.5	8.7–10.9
Canada, n = 23	8.0–15.4	11.6–18.3	11.9–16.7	11.2–14.4
United Kingdom, n = 37	NR[b]	9.0–17.5	9.9–14.3	10.7–15.7

Note
[a] IARC 1986.
[b] NR, not reported.

Ammonium concentrations in 10 cigarettes brands range from 0.07 to 0.49 g/100g of tobacco (Geiss and Kotzias 2003). However, ammonia in the gas phase is the key factor that impacts nicotine bioavailability not the soluble ammonia in the tobacco. Nicotine manipulation using the free base form of nicotine has been studied independently (Pankow et al., 2003a, 2003b; Watson et al., 2004; Chen and Pankow 2009; Ashley et al., 2009). The effect of tobacco blend additives on the retention of nicotine in the human respiratory tract was also described in the literature (Armitage et al., 2004; Pankow 2001).

Traditionally, smoke yields of 'tar', nicotine, and carbon monoxide (TNCO) were determined by machine-smoking method that was adopted by the FTC in 1967 and was based on the protocol developed by the American Tobacco Company in the 1930s (Bradford et al., 1936; Pillsbury 1996). Internationally, this method is also known as the International Standards Organization (ISO) method. The TNCO is measured in the mainstream smoke (MS) obtained when cigarettes are smoked by machine with a puff volume of 35 cm^3, puffs are taken once every 60 seconds and the duration of the puff is 2 seconds. Cigarettes are smoked to a prescribed final butt length and are inserted in the Cambridge filter holder without blocking of ventilation holes in the cigarette filter. The Cambridge filter pad used in the FTC/ISO method provides greater than 99% trapping efficiency for MS nicotine from cigarettes, including those with widely different soluble ammonia levels in the filler and MS smoke ammonia yields (Callicutt et al., 2006). Based on the FTC report, per cigarette tar and nicotine delivery in US cigarettes, weighed by sales, declined from 21.6 mg and 1.35 mg, respectively, in 1967 to 12.0 mg and 0.88 mg, respectively, in 1998 (FTC 2000).

Calafat and co-authors conducted a survey of TNCO deliveries from 77 cigarette brands, purchased in 35 countries from the six WHO regions, using the FTC/ISO machine-smoking methods (Calafat et al. 2004). Mainstream smoke nicotine deliveries varied from 0.5–1.6 mg per cigarette. Analysis of the smoke deliveries suggested that cigarettes from the Eastern Mediterranean, Southeast Asia, and Western Pacific WHO regions tended to have higher tar, nicotine, and CO smoke deliveries than brands from the European, American, or African WHO regions surveyed.

The FTC/ISO yields of nicotine in 25 commercial UK cigarettes made from bright tobaccos ranged from 0.11–0.94 mg/cigarette (Gregg et al. 2004). These data reflect the compliance with the directive of the European Parliament which mandated that 'from January 1, 2004, the yields of cigarettes released for free circulation, marketed or manufactured in the Member states shall not be greater than 10 mg per cigarette for tar, 1 mg per cigarette for nicotine, 10 mg per cigarette for carbon monoxide.' (Official Journal of the European Communities 2001).

International comparison of the ranges of mainstream smoke nicotine yields showed a wide variation (0.1–2.7 mg/cigarette) with the highest emissions measured in cigarettes from France, Thailand, United Kingdom, and the United States (IARC 2004). On the basis of scientific evidence accumulated over the past several decades, the consensus is that FTC/ISO per cigarette smoke yields do not provide valid estimates of human exposure or of relative human exposure when smoking different brands of cigarettes (Burns et al., 2008; Harris 2001; National Cancer Institute 2001; Stratton et al., 2001). Machine-smoking regimens other than FTC/ISO regimen have also been examined, particularly ones with more intense puffing parameters and ventilation holes in cigarette filters partially or completely blocked during smoking. The examples include those developed by the US State of Massachusetts and the Canadian Government. The Massachusetts method prescribes drawing 45-cm^3 puffs once every 30 seconds, the duration of the puff is 2 seconds, and 50% of filter ventilation holes are blocked during smoking; the Health Canada Method prescribes drawing 55-cm^3 puffs once every 30 seconds, the duration of the puff is 2 seconds, and 100% of filter ventilation holes are blocked during smoking (Borgerding and Klus 2005; Hammond et al., 2006). These two regimens generally produce higher yields per cigarette (Table 10.4; Counts et al., 2005) and reduce differences between brands in the yields.

Table 10.4 Nicotine yields (mg/cigarette) in the mainstream smoke of Philip Morris cigarettes ($n = 48$), sold internationally, generated under different smoking conditions (Counts *et al.* 2008)

Method	Moderate[a] 10–14.9 mg FTC tar	Low[a] 5–9.9 mg FTC tar	Very low[a] ≤4.9 mg FTC tar
FTC	0.67–1.04	0.44–0.77	0.10–0.46
Massachusetts	1.65–2.17	1.07–1.70	0.51–1.20
Health Canada	1.48–2.56	1.43–2.17	1.07–1.85

Note

[a] IARC 1986

Nevertheless, these regimens continue to maintain a ranking of brands, based on 'tar' and nicotine yield per cigarette, and the rankings by yield per cigarette using these more intense regimens also do not provide valid estimates of human exposure, or of the relative exposure, experienced by smokers when they smoke different brands of cigarettes (Burns *et al.*, 2008; Laugesen and Fowles 2006). The alternative smoking regimens, introduced in the state of Massachusetts and Canada, have not been evaluated against human smoking behaviour and biomeasures of exposure. Hammond and co-investigators compared the emissions of nicotine in cigarette smoke generated by ISO, Massachusetts, Health Canada, Compensatory, and Human Mimic methods (Hammond *et al.*, 2006) and concluded that none of the existing smoking regimens adequately represents human smoking behaviour nor do they generate yields associated with human measures of nicotine uptake.

Normalization of the machine-generated yields per mg nicotine, or per mg tar, does not eliminate the variation in the values measured by the different smoking regimens. For example, the differences in the yields of nine smoke toxicants per mg nicotine (e.g., NNK, NNN, acetaldehyde, acrolein, form aldehyde, benzene, benzo(a)pyrene, 1,3-butadiuene, carbon monoxide), as recommended for regulation by the WHO Study Group on Tobacco Regulation (WHO, 2008), obtained with these different regimens likely reflect differences in temperature of combustion, rates of air flow at the point of combustion, and other factors that result from the differences in puff profiles used (Burns *et al.*, 2008). The fate of nicotine in a burning full flavour cigarettes is affected by the manner in which cigarette is smoked. The greater percentage of labelled nicotine in the tobacco column remains intact during the smoking process as smoking intensity increases (Yu *et al.*, 2006). As smoking regimen intensity increased, the amount of nicotine pyrolisis and oxidation products detected in sidestream smoke decreased, while marginal increases in these compounds were observed in mainstream smoke and in the cigarette butt.

Connolly and co-authors undertook the study to find out whether nicotine yields in the smoke of cigarettes sold in the United States, as measured by Massachusetts machine-smoking method, would show an overall increase over time or an increasing trend limited to any particular market category (e.g., full flavour vs. light, medium/mild or ultra light; mentholated vs. non-mentholated), manufacturer, or brand family or brand style, and whether nicotine yields in smoke would be associated with measurable trends in cigarette design (Connolly *et al.*, 2007). They reported a statistically significant trend in increased nicotine yield of 0.019 (1.1%) mg/cig/year over the period of 1997–2005, and 0.029 (1.6%) mg/cig/year over the period 1998–2005. The increasing trend was observed in all major market categories. Nicotine yield in smoke was positively associated with nicotine concentration in the tobacco and number of puffs per cigarette, both of which showed increasing trends during the study period. Although nicotine yield in smoke (mean mg/cig) based on Massachusetts smoking regimen appears to be slightly higher in mentholated vs.

non-mentholated brands (1.71–1.95 vs. 1.62–1.91) (Connolly *et al.*, 2007), the sales-weighted average nicotine per cigarette is significantly higher in mentholated cigarettes (Farrelly *et al.*, 2007).

O'Connor and co-investigators examined data from two cross-sectional surveys to find out whether observed decreases in cigarette use over time among smokers in the United States were followed by reduction of their nicotine uptake (O'Connor *et al.*, 2006). The findings of this study suggest that cigarettes per day (CPD) may represent a proxy for exposure to nicotine on the population level since the decline in serum cotinine (a metabolite of nicotine) levels observed among smokers closely paralleled the decline in self-reported CPD.

Nicotine in cigarette smoke (machine-smoking mimicking human patterns)

A single machine testing regimen produces a single set of toxicant yields. In contrast to the machine, individual smokers vary puffing patterns (e.g., drawing larger puffs more frequently, blocking filter ventilation holes, and smoking to a certain butt length) with which they smoke different cigarettes of the same brand, and cigarette design changes can lead smokers to systematically change how they puff cigarettes. Thus even more intense Massachusetts and Health Canada machine-smoking regimens have a potential to mislead smokers when smoke yields are expressed on per cigarette basis. As noted earlier, machine measured yields should not be used to support claims of reduced exposure or risk (Burns *et al.*, 2008; Djordjevic *et al.*, 2000; Harris 2001; Hammond *et al.*, 2006; NCI 2001).

Compared with the FTC/ISO protocol values, 56 smokers of low- and 77 smokers of medium-yield brands took in statistically significantly larger puffs (48.6 and 44.1 mL, respectively) at statistically significantly shorter intervals (21.3 and 18.5 seconds, respectively) (Djordjevic *et al.* 2000). Thus, they received, respectively, 2.5 and 2.2 times more nicotine and 2.6 and 1.9 times more 'tar' than FTC-derived amounts as well as about two-fold higher levels of nicotine-derived carcinogen NNK. Smokers of low-yield cigarettes received 1.74 mg (1.54–1.98) nicotine from their cigarette whereas smokers of medium-yield cigarettes received 2.39 mg (2.2–2.6) nicotine. Delivery of NNK among smokers of low-yield cigarettes was 112.9 ng (158.3–219.7) per cigarette and of medium-yield cigarettes 250.9 ng (222.7–282.7) per cigarette. Although there was a slight difference in 'at the mouth' delivery of smoke toxicants, as shown by Djordjevic *et al.* (2000), the exposure, as measured by urinary biomarkers revealed similar uptake of nicotine and lung carcinogen NNK by smokers of regular, light, and ultra light cigarettes (Hecht *et al.*, 2005).

Levels of urinary metabolites expressed per unit of delivered parent compounds, measured in the mainstream smoke generated by mimicking human smoking patterns, decreased with increased smoke emissions (Melikian *et al.* 2007a). In smokers of low-, medium-, and high-yield cigarettes, the respective cotinine (ng/mg creatinine)-to-nicotine (mg/day) ratios were 89.4, 77.8, and 57.1 (low vs. high; $P = 0.06$); the 4-(methylnitrosoamino)-1-(3-pyridil)-1-butanol (NNAL) (pmol/mg creatinine)-to-NNK (ng/day) ratios were 0.81, 055, and 0.57 (low vs. high; $P = 0.05$). Similarly, means of cotinine per unit of delivered nicotine in smokers who consumed < 20 cigarettes per day was 3.5-fold higher than in those who smoked >20 cigarettes per day. Likewise, a negative correlation was observed between cotinine–nicotine ratios and delivered doses of nicotine in subgroups of smokers who used the identical brand of cigarette, namely filter tip-ventilated Marlboro ($r = -0.59$), which is popular brand among European Americans, and Newport ($r = -0.37$), a menthol-flavoured cigarette without filter tip vents that is preferred by African Americans. Thus, intensity of the exposure significantly affects the levels of urinary biomarkers of exposure and this inverse relationship phenomenon should be considered and further explored.

Melikian and co-workers also reported on gender differences in delivered nicotine dosages as a result of specific puffing behaviours (Melikian *et al.*, 2007b). The geometric means of emissions of nicotine from cigarettes were 1.92 mg/cigarette (95% CI = 1.8–2.05) for women vs. 2.2 (95% CI = 2.04–2.37 for men ($p = 0.005$). Similarly, cigarettes smoked by women yielded 139.5 ng/cigarette of carcinogenic NNK (95% CI = 128.8–151.0), compared with 170.3 ng/cigarette (95% CI = 156.3–185.6) for men ($p = 0.0007$). The gender differences with regard to cigarette smoke yields of toxicants were more profound in European Americans than in African Americans. On average, African American men's smoking behaviour produced the highest emissions of select toxicants from cigarettes, and European American female smokers had the lowest exposure to nicotine and carcinogens.

Nicotine content in other combustible tobacco products

Roll-your own cigarettes

Although factory-made (FM) cigarettes dominate the world market, the use of roll-your-own (RYO) cigarettes has increased substantially in Thailand (58%), New Zealand (32%), the United Kingdom (28.4%), Australia (24.2%), Malaysia (17%), Canada (17.1%), the United States (6.7%), and some European countries such as Norway (15.5%) (Laugesen 2003; Wangan and Biørn 2002; Young *et al.*, 2006, 2008). Most RYO smokers choose to make their own cigarettes because they are less expensive than FM products or because they perceive RYO as less harmful. The increase of cigarette prices also leads to increases in sales of cigarettes with high tar and nicotine FTC/ISO yields (Farrelly *et al.*, 2007). According to Young and co-authors, the use of RYO cigarettes was associated with having lower annual income, male sex, younger average age, higher level of nicotine addiction, and more positive perception of tobacco use (Young *et al.*, 2006). RYO cigarette contain less tobacco compared to factory-made (FM) brands (Laugesen *et al.*, 2009). Yet, RYO smoking is associated with increased smoke exposure per cigarette (smoke volume: 952 mL smoke vs. 743 ml for FM cigarettes, $p = 0.025$; puff number 16.9 vs. 13.6, $p = 0.035$).

The smoke nicotine yields reported for the five brands of fine-cut tobaccos used for making RYO cigarettes were 1.5–1.8 mg per units based on the FTC/ISO machine-smoking method whereas the nicotine delivery from 35 commercial factory-made cigarettes was lower 0.09–1.4 mg/cigarette (Kaiserman and Rickert 1992a). In addition, the levels of a lung carcinogen benzo[a]pyrene (BaP) in the smoke of RYO cigarettes were 22.9–26,3 ng/unit compared to 3.36–28.39 ng/cigarette in commercial cigarettes. In a subsequent study, Kaiserman and Rickert examined the importance of the cigarette tube in the delivery of smoke toxicants from RYO cigarettes. Results showed that 'tar' and nicotine yields were related to the type of tube but generally not related to the various tobacco types (Kaiserman and Rickert 1992b). Appel *et al.* (1990) compared BaP levels in mainstream smoke from cigars, RYO, and pipe tobacco. Combustion of all products produced similar levels of BaP- averaging 45 ng/g of tobacco combusted. The mainstream smoke of three brands of hand-rolled cigarettes from Thailand delivered 1.1–5.5 mg nicotine per cigarette (Mitacek *et al.*, 1991).

To date, there are no available data on nicotine in mainstream smoke of RYO delivered either by more intense machine-smoking or mimicking human smoking topography.

Cigars

There are many types of cigars in the international markets. In North America and in many parts of Europe, there are at lest four types of cigars, namely little cigars, small cigars (also called cigarillos), regular cigars, and premium cigars. In 1997 in the United States, the leading brands of little, large, and premium cigars (ranging in length from 7.3 to 17.6 cm and in weight from 1.24 to 8.1 g) were analysed and the levels of nicotine and selected carcinogens (e.g., B[a]P, NNN, and NNK) were reported in the mainstream smoke (Djordjevic *et al.* 1997). The nicotine yields in mainstream smoke of little, large, and premium cigars, as measured by standard International Committee for Cigar Smoke Study method (puffs of 20 cm^3 taken every 40 seconds, duration of puffs 1.5 second; butt length 33 mm), were 1.5, 1.4, and 3.4 mg per unit, respectively (Hoffmann and Hoffmann, 1998). The levels of nicotine and NNK in the smoke of premium cigars were higher by three and 17 times, respectively, than in cigarette smoke of best selling cigarettes on the US market. When little filter-tipped cigars were machine smoked in a manner that mimicked human smoking behaviour, the emissions of nicotine and TSNA were higher than those measured by standard method. Thai cigars deliver 7.95–11.4 mg nicotine in mainstream smoke per piece (Mitacek *et al.*, 1991).

Seventeen brands of cigars ranging in weight from 0.53 to 21.5 g showed considerable variation in the total nicotine content of the tobacco, 5.9–335.2 mg per cigar (Henningfield *et al.*, 1999). The aqueous pH of cigar tobacco ranged from 5.7 to 7.8. The smoke pH values of the smallest cigars were generally acidic, changed little across the puffs and more closely resembled the profiles previously reported for tobacco of typical commercial cigarettes. The smoke pH of smaller cigars and cigarillos only became acidic after the first third of the rod had been smoked and remained acidic thereafter. The smoke pH of larger cigars was acidic during the smoking of the first third of the rod and became quite alkaline during the smoking of the last third. This phenomenon needs to be taken into consideration when evaluation the bio-availability and addictive potential of cigars.

In the study of 30 smokers of pipes or cigars only, 28 cigarette smokers only, and 30 non-smokers male subjects matched for age, urinary cotinine and 1-hydroxypyrene (a biological marker of exposure to carcinogenic polycyclic aromatic hydrocarbons -PAH) levels were found to be higher in cigarette smokers than in pipe or cigar smokers and higher in the later than in non-smokers (Funk-Brentano *et al.*, 2006). In multivariate analysis, cigarette smoking was the only independent predictor of CYP1A2 activity ($p < 0.0001$) and of 1-hydroxypyrene excretion in urine ($p = 0.0012$). In this study, pipe or cigar smoking was associated with lower exposure to products of tobacco metabolism than cigarette smoking and to an absence of CYP 1A2 induction. However, inhalation behaviour, rather than the type of tobacco smoked, may be the key factor linked to the extent of tobacco toxicants exposure and CYP 1A2 induction. It has been suggested that switching from smoking cigarettes to cigars, or smoking both products intermittently, may increase the exposure of smokers to toxic and carcinogenic agents (Henningfield *et al.*, 1999). In contrast with 'only cigar smokers' who relatively seldom inhale smoke into the lung, former cigarette smokers, and concurrent cigar and cigarette smokers have a tendency to maintain their cigarette smoke inhalation pattern when they smoke cigars thus inhaling larger quantities of smoke toxicants including nicotine.

Bidis (hand-rolled Indian cigarettes) and chutta (hand-made Indian cigar)

A chutta is a type of a small hand-made cigar consumed in India, without a wrapper and a single tobacco leaf as a binder and usually weighing 1–7.5 g (Malik and Behera 1985; Pakhale and Maru 1998). It consists of air-cured and fermented tobacco folded into a dried tobacco leaf. Chuttas are usually without a filter and characterized by being open-ended. They are frequently associated with the remarkable habit of 'reverse' smoking, during which the burning end is held inside the mouth (the reverse smoker inhales both the mainstream and sidestream smoke). The nicotine content in chutta tobacco is comparable with that of bidi tobacco (30.84 mg/g vs. 35.2 mg/g). However, the nicotine level in mainstream smoke from chutta is higher (6.98 mg/piece) than that from bidis (1.87 mg/piece). The nicotine content in sidestream smoke of chutta was 2.07 mg/

product. The highest amounts of TSNA in tobacco products, besides most snuff, were measured in chutta tobacco (Malik and Behera 1985).

The construction and appearance of bidi cigarettes differ markedly from commercial cigarettes. Bidis are manufactured primarily in India and consist of about 150–500 mg of pulverized (or flakes) sun-dried locally grown tobacco (*N. tabacum*) wrapped in a dried leaf of temburni (*Diospyros melanoxylon*) or tendi (*Diospyrosebenum*) (Pakhale and Maru 1998; Richter and Watson 2008).

As reported by Malson and co-authors, the concentration of nicotine in the tobacco of 12 bidi cigarettes (mean value: 21.2 mg/g; range:15.7–27 mg/g) was significantly higher than that in the tobacco from commercial filter-tipped cigarettes (16.3 mg/g) and unfiltered cigarettes (13.5 mg/g) (Malson *et al.*, 2001). The amount of nicotine par bidi was on average 4.7 mg (range: 3.3–12.4 mg). In 10 smokers who switched to Irie bidi, strawberry-flavoured, cigarettes, plasma nicotine levels increased above the levels recorded when they smoked regular filter tipped cigarettes (26 ng/mL vs. 18.5 ng/mL) (Malson *et al.* 2002).

The amount of nicotine and nornicotine in Indian bidi tobacco was higher than that in Indian filter-tipped cigarettes (35.2 and 3.4 mg/g, respectively vs. 14.2 and 1.56 mg/g, respectively). Curiously, the mainstream smoke of Indian bidis delivered less nicotine than Indian cigarettes (1.87 mg vs. 2.58 mg/cigarette) (Pakhale and Maru 1998; Pakhale *et al.*, 2009).

A survey of the nicotine levels in mainstream smoke from 21 brands of bidi cigarettes, both filtered and unfiltered, was conducted using a variation of the FTC standardized cigarette machine-smoking method (Watson *et al.*, 2003). The primary difference between this method and the FTC method was a reduction of the 60-second puff interval to 15 seconds. The shorter puff interval was required to prevent the bidi cigarettes from self-extinguishing and may represent a closer approximation to human usage. In this study, bidi cigarettes delivered 2.7 ± 0.4 mg nicotine/unit in mainstream smoke. Unlike cigarettes, the filtered and unfiltered bidis delivered comparable smoke yields (2.82 ± 0.23 mg/bidi and 2.57 ± 0.22, respectively). When commercial cigarettes were machine-smoked using the same modified FTC method, nicotine deliveries were from 1.94 mg/cigarette (filtered brands) to 2.87 mg/cigarette (unfiltered brands).

The levels of TSNA in the tobacco filler and mainstream smoke from 14 bidi cigarette brands were reported by Wu *et al.*, (2004). In the bidi tobacco filler, the NNK amounts ranged from 0.09 to 0.85 µg/g tobacco and NNN from 0.15 to 1.44 µg/g. These amounts are similar to those reported for typical American blended cigarette (Hoffmann and Hoffmann 1997). The levels of NNK in mainstream smoke from bidis ranged from 2.13–25.9 ng/cigarette, and those of NNN from 8.5.6 to 62.3 ng/cigarette (Wu *et al.*, 2004).

Clove (kreteks) cigarettes

Clove cigarettes are produced in Indonesia and exported throughout the world. They are composed of a mixture of tobacco (60–80%) and ground clove buds (20–40%), available with or without filters, and are usually machine rolled in white, brown, or black paper. These cigarettes have a distinctive aroma because of the cloves. Eugenol, an analgesic, is naturally occurring in cloves and is present in milligram quantities in the clove cigarette filler (Stanfill *et al.*, 2006). Like menthol, eugenol diminishes the harshness of the tobacco smoke. The reported FTC/ISO nicotine yield in mainstream smoke of clove cigarette was reported to be 2.0 mg per unit (Malson *et al.*, 2003).

Waterpipe tobacco smoking

The waterpipe (WP), also known as shiha, hookah, narghile, goza, and hubble bubble, has long been used for tobacco consumption in the middle East, India, and parts of Asia, and more recently has been introduced into the smokeless tobacco market in western nations. Using WP is often associated with Indian Subcontinent and Southwest Asia. It is particularly popular among young adults and teens in Southwest Asia. For example, in Syria, 45% of college students at Aleppo University report ever use (Maziak *et al.*, 2004, 2005); in Israel, 22% of 12–18 year olds reported that they use WP to smoke tobacco every weekend (Varsano *et al.* 2003); in Lebanon, 23–30% of Beirut university students reported weekly use (Tamim *et al.*, 2003); and 25.6% of 11–17 year olds in Beirut reported past 30 day use (Tamim *et al.*, 2007). Current use was also reported among 29–34% adolescents in Estonia and Latvia. In the United States, 9.5–20.3% college students used WP during the past 30 days (Eissenberg *et al.*, 2008; Primack *et al.*, 2008, 2009; Smith *et al.*, 2006).

Waterpipe smoking is so different from cigarette smoking that data on smoke composition and toxicity cannot be extrapolated from one to the other. Neergard and co-authors reviewed six studies to estimate daily nicotine exposure among adult WP users (Neergaard *et al.* 2007). These studies measured the nicotine or cotinine levels associated with WP smoking in four countries (Lebanon, Jordan, Kuwait, and India). Four of these studies directly measured nicotine or cotinine levels in human subjects. The remaining two studies used smoking machines to measure nicotine yield in smoke condensate generated by WP. In Lebanon, Shihadeh (2003) designed a first-generation smoking machine to determine the chemical profile of the WP mainstream smoke. Ten grams of tobacco smoked per session (100 puffs at 3 seconds/puff, 300 mL/puff, 30 seconds between puffs) generated 2.25 mg nicotine. Two years later, Shihadeh and Saleh (2005) reported a delivery of 2.94 mg nicotine per session under different machine-smoking conditions (171 puffs at 2.6 seconds/puff, 530 mL/puff, 2.8 puffs/min). The latter study reported high deliveries of CO (143 mg vs.1–22 mg per single cigarette), carcinogeic PAH (phenanthrene: 0.748 µg vs. 0.2–04; fluoranthene: 0.221 µg vs. 0.009–0.099; chrysene: 0.112 vs. 0.004–0.041). The source of high emissions of CO and PAH is a burning charcoal which is normally placed atop the tobacco to smoke the narghile WP (Monzer *et al.* 2008).

Urinary cotinine values reported among WP users ranged from 0.184 µg/mL (at least 3 WP per week; $n = 14$ male users) to 6.08 µg/mL (at least 1 WP per day/$n = 15$ male users and 1 female) (Neergaard *et al.*, 2007). To put this in prospective, cotinine values reported for users of other tobacco products were: cigarette smokers: 1.28 µg/mL ($n = 12$; urine taken from an 8-h collection in people who smoked from 15–40 cigarettes per day; cigar smokers 0.67 µg/mL($n = 8$), traditional pipe smokers: 1.36 µg/mL ($n = 5$); and users of smokeless tobacco: 0.92 µg/mL ($n = 9$) (Jacob III *et al.* 1999).

Potential reduced-exposure products PREPs

Since the late 1980s there has been a proliferation of new potential reduced-exposure products (PREPs), promoted by industry with the implicit or explicit claims of reduced harm (Stratton *et al.* 2001; Hatsukami *et al.* 2002, 2005). These include, (a) modified tobacco products such as several denicotinized brands and reduced TSNA emission cigarettes, (b) chewing gum impregnated with tobacco, (c) smokeless tobacco products with reduced nitrosamine levels, and (d) cigarette-like products (carbon-heated 'smoking' devices).

Two prototypes of the new carbon-filtered Marlboro UltraSmooth (MUS), marketed as PREPs, were investigated using both standard (FTC/ISO) and intensive (Health Canada) machine methods to measure gas/vapour and particulate phase smoke constituents (Rees *et al.* 2007). FTC nicotine yields in mainstream smoke of two MUS varieties containing 180 mg and 120 mg carbon were 0.53 and 0.42 mg per cigarette, respectively, compared to Marlboro ultra light brand which delivered 0.56 mg nicotine per cigarette. Under more intense puffing conditions nicotine emissions were 1.5, 1.32 and 1.6 mg per cigarette. The latter data suggest that MUS, although designed to reduce yields of select toxicants, primarily volatile organic compounds, preserved nicotine addiction and consumer appeal potential. Thus, claims made by the manufacturer for reduced harm status of MUS depend heavily on standard machine smoke yields but not on clinical and long-term health outcome data. In June 2008, after three years of test marketing, Philip Morris pulled MUS off the market because it drew a little attention from consumers.

Two versions of reduced-nicotine cigarette Quest delivered 0.53 and 0.032 mg nicotine per cigarette under standard FTC machine-smoking method (Chen *et al.* 2008). Historical research on low nicotine cigarettes demonstrated that smokers compensated for lower nicotine delivery by increasing their puffing behaviour to extract more nicotine (National Cancer Institute 2001). In a study by Strasser and co-workers, among 50 smokers of 0.6, 0.3, and 0.05 mg nicotine Quest cigarettes, total puff volume was greatest for the 0.05 mg nicotine cigarette and CO boost was moderately greater after smoking the 0.3 and 0.05 mg cigarettes compared to the 0.6 mg nicotine cigarette suggesting that this product can potentially be a harm-increasing product (Strasser *et al.*, 2007). Other study using research cigarettes with progressively reduced nicotine content (0.6–10.1 mg nicotine per gram tobacco; 0.1–0.8 mg in smoke per cigarette) showed that intake of nicotine declined progressively, with little evidence of compensation (Benowitz *et al.*, 2007). The Ames test revealed that cigarette smoke condensates (CSC) from the nicotine-free and low-nicotine Quest cigarettes had a similar mutagenic potency as regular cigarettes (Chen *et al.* 2008). Authors concluded that this finding, and the findings of other toxicological assays carried out in this study, are not consistent with a perception that low-nicotine or nicotine-free cigarettes may have less toxicity in human cells. Nicotine, as it exists in CSC, attenuates cytotoxicity possibly in part through inhibition of apoptotic pathways.

Smokers who switched to Advance, a cigarette with purportedly reduced levels of toxicants, got exposed to significantly higher levels of nicotine, than when they smoked their own brand (23.3 ng/ml vs. 18.6 ng/mL $p < 0.05$ (Breland *et al.*, 2002).However, smokers who switched to Advance were exposed to lower concentrations of CO and TSNA as determined by urinary biomarkers (Breland *et al.*, 2003).

In 1997, R.J. Reynolds Tobacco Co. introduced Eclipse, a nicotine delivery device purported to deliver lower levels of smoke toxicants than conventional cigarettes. Eclipse uses a carbon fuel element to vaporize nicotine in the rod; the user then inhales the nicotine vapour. Venous plasma nicotine boost among 10 smokers was significantly lower 2 minutes after they smoked Eclipse as compared with their own brand (10.7 ng/mL vs. 16.4 ng/mL) (Lee *et al.*, 2004). Nevertheless, Eclipse exposes the user to significant quantities of nicotine, CO (7.3 ppm vs 4.2 ppm from conventional cigarette), and possibly other harmful components of tobacco smoke.

Nicotine in smokeless tobacco products

While cigarette sales in the United States declined 18% from 21 billion packs in 2000 to 17.4 billion pack in 2007, during the same time period sales of other products, such as moist snuff, increased by 1.10 billion cigarette pack equivalents (Connolly and Alpert 2008). In the United States, most common smokeless tobacco (ST) products are chewing tobacco (loose leaf, plug, and twist), moist snuff, and dry snuff. Many other forms of smokeless tobacco that are used globally are described in the IARC Monograph Vol. 89 (2007). All smokeless tobacco products contain nicotine and other tobacco alkaloids that are inherent to tobacco leaf.

The Massachusetts Department of Public Health (MDPH) promulgated regulations in 1996 that required cigarette and smokeless tobacco manufacturers to file annual reports on nicotine yield by brand (IARC 2004). The Table 10.5 presents the mean values of total nicotine, pH, and unprotonated (free) for each type of smokeless tobacco products sold in the United States.

Table 10.5 Ranges of pH and nicotine concentrations in smokeless tobacco sold in Massachusetts (USA) in 2003 (IARC 2004).

Constituent	Chewing tobacco ($n = 74$) Mean (range)	Dry snuff ($n = 33$) Mean (range)	Moist snuff ($n = 106$) Mean (range)
Moisture (%)	22.8 (14.57–28.57)	8.2 (5.38–23.9)	52.6 (21.58–55.77)
Nicotine (%, dry wt)	1.22 (0.45–4.65)	1.82 (1.14–2.69)	2.58 (0.49–3.70)
Nicotine (mg/g product)	9.9 (3.41–39.74)	16.8 (10.48–24.84)	12.6 (4.7–24.29)
pH	5.82 (5.07–6.91)	6.36 (5.50–7.61)	7.43 (5.41–8.38)
Unprotonated (free) nicotine (mg/g product)	0.11 (0.02–1.77)	0.71 (0.05–3.12)	3.52 (0.03–8.57)

On average, moist snuff contained the highest levels of total and free nicotine (2.58% dry weight and 3.52 mg/g product, respectively) followed by dry snuff (1.82 % and 0.71 mg/g, respectively) and chewing tobacco (1.22% and 0.11 mg/g, respectively). The analysis of MDPH database revealed the following: (a) free nicotine levels vary widely between brands and are controlled by manufacturer primarily by pH, consistent with well-known graduation strategy; (b) high market share products have high and/or increasing free nicotine; (c) increasing numbers of sub-brands with designs to enhance or ease the delivery of nicotine; (d) combination of above factors, price discounts, clean indoor air policies, and other marketing strategies are most likely responsible for increasing moist snuff sales (Alpert *et al.*, 2008).

Free nicotine concept and biological applications were discussed in a greater detail in peer reviewed literature (Ashley *et al.*, 2009; Ayo-Yusuf *et al.*, 2004; Djordjevic *et al.*, 1995; Fant *et al.*, 1999; Henningfield *et al.* 1995; Hoffmann *et al.*, 1995; Idris *et al.* 1991, 1998) as well as in the IARC Monograph (2007). In the countries such as South Africa, because of the high pH (up to10.1) of popular commercial and traditional smokeless tobacco, calculated percentage of free-base nicotine was reported at 99.1% (total nicotine, up to 29.29 mg/gram dry tobacco) (Ayo-Yusuf *et al.*, 2004). In Sudan, snuff, locally known as *toombak*, was introduced approximately 400 years ago (Idris *et al.* 1998) Tobacco used for manufacture of *toombak*, is of the species *Nicotiana rustica*, and the fermented ground powder is mixed with an aqueous solution of sodium bicarbonate. The resultant product is moist, with a strong aroma, highly addictive and its use is widespread particularly among males. Its pH is 8–11, moisture content ranges from 6 to 60%, and nicotine content from 8 to 102 mg/g dry weight (Idris *et al.* 1991).

McNeill and co-authors analysed 11 smokeless products most popular in the United Kingdom including Gutkha and Zarda varieties that have an origin in India and 4 products purchased outside the United Kingdom (McNeill *et al.* 2006). United Kingdom purchased products contained a very wide concentrations of nicotine (3.1 mg/g to 83.5 mg/g). Products purchased outside of United Kingdom included snus from Sweden (15.2 mg nicotine), Baba 120 from India (55 mg nicotine), and Copenhagen from the United States (9.2 mg nicotine). Some of the products purchased in the United Kingdom contained a very high pH (up to 9.94) resulting in a very high concentration of free nicotine (98.75%). Smokeless tobacco products available to consumers in India have pH ranging from 5.21 to 10.1 and contain 0.7–10.16 mg nicotine per gram of the product (Gupta 2004).

The most recent analysis of new smokeless tobacco products marketed as potential reduced-exposure products (PREPs) on the US market, namely Philip Morris' Taboka and Marlboro Snus, R.J. Reynolds' Camel Snus, and US Tobacco's Skoal Dry, revealed a very wide range of pH as well as total and free nicotine content: 6.47–7.75; 11.3–28.8 mg/g dry weight and 0.35–9.16 mg/g, respectively (Stepanov *et al.* 2008). These products are available in a variety of flavours including 'original', 'green', 'rich', 'mild', 'spice', 'mint', 'frost', 'regular', 'cinnamon', and 'menthol. The highest pH and both total and free nicotine were measured in Camel Snus and the lowest in Skoal Dry. The nornicotine content ranged from 0.31 to 1.04 mg. The comparison of contents of new PREPs and traditional forms of smokeless tobacco such as Copenhagen, Skoal, and Kodiak (17.7–26.7 mg of total nicotine and 4.88–12.1 mg of free nicotine) show that PREPs have a high nicotine content; thus a propensity to initiate and sustain addiction among users.

The conclusions of the IARC Monograph on smokeless tobacco (2007) and Scientific Committee on Emerging and Newly Identified Health Risks (SCENIHR) opinion on Health Effects of Smokeless Tobacco (2008) can be summarized as follows: (a) all forms of ST are potentially addictive, (b) all forms of ST are carcinogenic, (c) probable reproductive health effects, (d) probable risk factor for myocardial infarction, (e) limited and inconsistent evidence for ST as effective smoking cessation aid, and (f) inconsistent association in patterns of smoking and ST use across countries.

Summary

The data presented in this chapter show clearly that all tobaccos used for factory- and hand-made products (e.g., Oriental, Virginia, burley, reconstituted tobacco sheets) contain nicotine and many other alkaloids. The concentrations of nicotine vary dramatically across different types of tobacco and greatly depend on genetic potential, agricultural practices including fertilization and plant density in the field, curing and processing methods, leaf position on the plant, storage practices, country of origin, and production year. The content of nicotine in tobacco products, both smoked and smokeless, largely depend on blending strategies, namely the types of tobaccos and their proportion in the blend, product design features as well as additives that are employed to enhance nicotine bioavailability and appeal to the user. It is evident that all tobacco products contain enough nicotine to induce and sustain tobacco dependence. However, human exposure to nicotine does not depend solely on its content in the tobacco product and products design characteristics, but also on the way each individual is using the product such as puffing intensity and filter vents blocking among smokers and frequency and the duration of dipping among smokeless tobacco users.

References

Adam, T., Mitschke, S., Streibel, T., Baker, R.R., and Zimmermann, R. (2006) Puff-by-puff resolved characterization of cigarette mainstream smoke by single photon ionization (SPI)-time-of-flight mass spectrometry (TOFMS): comparison of the 2R4F research cigarette and pure Burley, Virginia, Oriental and Maryland tobacco cigarettes. *Anal Chimica Acta*, 572:219–229.

Alpert, H.R., Koh, H., and Connolly, G.N. (2008) Free nicotine content and strategic marketing of moist snuff tobacco products in the United States: 2000–2006. *Tob Control*, 18:332–338.

Appel, B.R., Guirguis, G., Kim, I.S., Garbin, O., Fracchia, M., Flessel, C.P. *et al.* (1990) Benzene, benzo(a)pyrene, and lead in smoke from tobacco products other than cigarettes. *Am J Public Health*, 80:560–564.

Armitage, A.K., Dixon, M., Fros, B.E., Mariner, D.C., and Sinclair, N.M. (2004) The effect of tobacco blend additives on the retention of nicotine and solanesol in the human respiratory tract and on subsequent plasma nicotine concentrations during cigarette smoking. *Chem Res Toxicol*, 17(4):537–544.

Ashley, D.L., Pankow, J.F., Tavakoli, A.D., and Watson, C.H. (2009) Approaches, challenges, and experience in assessing free nicotine. *Handb Exp Pharmacology*, 192:437–456.

Ayo-Yusuf, O.A., Swart, T.J., and Pickworth, W.B. (2004) Nicotine delivery capabilities of smokeless tobacco products and implications for control of tobacco dependence in South Africa. *Tob Control*, 13:186–189.

Benowitz, N.L. and Henningfield, J.E. (1994) Establishing a nicotine threshold for addiction. The implication of tobacco regulation. *New England J Med*, **331**:123–125.

Benowitz, N.L., Hall, S.M., Stewart, S., Wilson, M., Dempsay, D., and Jacob, P. III (2007) Nicotine and carcinogen exposure with smoking of progressively reduced nicotine content cigarette. *Cancer Epi Biomark Prev*, **16**:2479–2485.

Benowitz, N.L., Dains, K.M., Hall, S.M., Stewart, S., Wilson, M., Dempsey, D. *et al.* (2009) Progressive commercial cigarette yield reduction: biochemical exposure and behavioral assessment. *Cancer Epi Biomark Prev*, **18**(3):876–883.

Bhide, S.V., Nair, J., Maru, G.B., Nair, U.J., Kameshwar Rao, B.V., Chakraborty, M.K. *et al.* (1987) Tobacco-specific N-nitrosamines (TNSA) in green mature and processed tobacco leaves from India. *Beitr Tabakforsch*, **14**:29–32.

Bradford, J.A., Harlan, W.R., and Hanmer, H.R. (1936) Nature of cigarette smoke: technic of experimental smoking. *Industrial Engineering Chem*, **29**:836–839.

Breland, A.B., Evans, S.E., Buchhalter, A.R., and Eissenberg, T. (2002) Acute effects of Advance™: a potential reduced exposure product for smokers. *Tob Control*, **11**:376–378.

Breland, A.B., Acosta, M.C., and Eissenberg, T. (2008) Tobacco-specific nitrosamines and potential reduced exposure products for smokers: a preliminary evaluation of Advance ™. *Tob Control*, **12**:317–321.

Borgerding, M., Klus, H. (2005) Analysis of complex mixtures – cigarette smoke. *Experimental Toxicologic Pathology*, **57**:43–73.

Burns, D.M., Dybing, E., Gray, N., Hecht, S., Anderson, C., Sanner, T. *et al.* (2008) Mandated lowering of toxicants in cigarette smoke: a description of the World Health Organization TobReg proposal. *Tob Control*, **17**:132–141.

Burton, H.R., Bush, L.P., and Hamilton, J.L. (1983) Effect of curing on the chemical composition of burley tobacco. *Recent Adv Tob Sci*, **9**:91–153.

Burton, H.R., Bush, L.P., Djordjevic, M.V. (1989a) Influence of temperature and humidity on the accumulation of tobacco-specific nitrosamines in stored burley tobacco. *J Agric Food Chem*, **37**:1372–1377.

Burton, H.R., Childs, G.H. Jr, Andersen, R.A., and Fleming, P.D. (1989b) Changes in chemical composition of burley tobacco during senescence and curing. 3. Tobacco-specific nitrosamines. *J Agric Food Chem*, **37**:426–430.

Burton, H.R., Dye, N.K., and Bush, L.P. (1992) Distribution of tobacco constituents in tobacco leaf tissue. 1. Tobacco-specific nitrosamines, nitrate, nitrite and alkaloids. *J Agric Food Chem*, **40**:1050–1055.

Burton, H.R., Dye, N.K., and Bush, L.P. (1994) Relationship between tobacco-specific nitrosamines and nitrite from different air cured tobacco varieties. *J Agric Food Chem*, **42**:2007–2011.

Calafat, A.M., Polzin, G.M., Saylor, J., Richter, P., Ashley, D.L., and Watson, C.H. (2004) Determination of tar, nicotine, and carbon monoxide yields in the mainstream smoke of selected international cigarettes. *Tob Control*, **13**:45–51.

Callicutt, C.H., Cox, R.H., Farthing, D., Hsu, F.S., Johnson, L., Laffoon, S. *et al.* (2006) The ability of the FTC method to quantify nicotine as a function of ammonia in mainstream smoke. *Beitr Tabakforsch*, **22**(2):71–78.

Carmella, S.G., Borukhova, A., Desai, D., and Hecht, S.S. (1997) Evidence for endogenous formation of tobacco-specific nitrosamines in rats treated with tobacco alkaloids and sodium nitrate. *Carcinogenesis*, **18**(3):587–592.

Chamberlain, W.J. and Chortyk, O.T. (1992) Effects of curing and fertilization on nitrosamine formation in bright and burley tobacco. Chemical composition of nonsmoking tobacco products. *Beitr Tabakforsch*, **15**:87–92.

Chen, J., Higby, R., Tian, D., Tan, D., Johnson, M.D., Xiao, Y. *et al.* (2008) Toxicological analysis of low-nicotine and nicotine free-cigarettes. *Toxicology*, **249**:194–203.

Chen, C. and Pankow, J.F. (2009) Gas/particle partitioning of two acid-base active compounds in mainstream tobacco smoke: nicotine and ammonia. *J Agric Food Cgem*, **57**(7):2678–2690.

Connolly, G.N., Alpert, H.R., Wayne, G.F., and Koh, H. (2007) Trends in nicotine yield in smoke and its relationship with design characteristics among popular US cigarette brands, 1997–2005. *Tob Control*, **16**:e5,1–8.

Connolly, G.N. and Alpert, H.R. (2008) Trends in the use of cigarettes and other tobacco products, 2000–2007. *JAMA*, **299**:2629–2630.

Counts, M.E., Morton, M.J., Lafoon, S.W., Cox, R.H., and Lipowicz, P.J. (2005) Smoke composition and potential relationship for international commercial cigarettes smoked with three machine-smoking conditions. *Regulatory Toxicol Pharmacol*, **41**:185–227.

DeRoton, C., Wiernik, A., Wahlberg, I., and Vidal B (2005) Factors influencing the formation of tobacco-specific nitrosamines in french air-cured tobaccos in trials and at the farm level. *Beitr Tabakforsch*, **21**:305–320.

Djordjevic, M.V., Gay, S.L., Bush, L.P., and Chaplin, J.F. (1989) Tobacco-specific nitrosamine accumulation and distribution in flue-cured tobacco isolines. *J Agric Food Chem*, **37**:752–756.

Djordjevic, M.V., Bush, L.P., Gay, S.L., and Burton, H.R. (1990a) Accumulation and distribution of acylated nornicotine derivatives in flue-cured tobacco alkaloid isolines. *J Agric Food Chem*, **38**:347–350.

Djordjevic, M.V., Sigountos, C.W., Brunnemann, K.D., and Hoffmann, D. (1990b) Tobacco-specific nitrosamine delivery in the mainstream smoke of high– and low–yield cigarettes smoked with varying puff volume. In: CORESTA Information Bulletin. Symposium 1990, Oct. 7–11 Hellas, p. 209.

Djordjevic, M.V., Sigountos, C.W., Hoffmann, D., Brunnemann, K.D., Kagan, M., Bush, L.P. *et al.* (1991) Assessment of major carcinogens and alkaloids in the tobacco and mainstream smoke of USSR cigarettes. *Int J Cancer*, **47**:348–351.

Djordjevic, M.V., Hoffmann, D., Glynn, T., Connolly, G.N. (1995) US commercial brands of moist snuff, 1994. I. Assessment of nicotine, moisture, and pH. *Tob Control*, **4**:62–66.

Djordjevic, M.V., Eixarch, L., and Hoffmann, D. (1997) Self-administered and effective dose of cigar smoke constituents. The 51st Tobacco Chemists' Research Conference, Abstr. # 9, Winston-Salem, NC, September 14–17.

Djordjevic, M.V., Stellman, S.D., and Zang, E. (2000) Dosages of nicotine and lung carcinogens delivered to cigarette smokers. *J Natl Cancer Inst*, **92**:106–111.

Eissenberg, T., Ward, K.D., Smith-Simone, S., and Maziak, W. (2008) Waterpipe tobacco smoking on a US College campus: prevalence and correlates. *J Adolesc Health*, **42**(5):526–529.

Fant, R.V., Henningfield, J.E., Nelson, R.A., and Pickworth, W.B. (1999) Pharmacokinetcs and pharmcodynamics of moist snuff in humans. *Tob Control*, **8**:387–392.

Farrelly, M.C., Loomis, B.R., and Mann, N.H. (2007) Do increases in cigarette prices lead to increases in sales of cigarettes with hightar and nicotine yields? *Nicotine Tob Res*, **9**(10):1015–1020.

FTC, Federal Trade Commission (2000) 'Tar', nicotine, and carbon monoxide of the smoke of 1294 varieties of domestic cigarettes for the year 1998. Federal Trade Commission Report p. 9.

Funk-Brentano, C., Raphaël, M., Lafontaine, M., Arnould, J.-P., Verstuyft, C., Lebot, M. *et al.* (2006) Effects of type of smoking (pipe, cigars or cigarettes) on biological indices of tobacco exposure and toxicity. *Lung Cancer*, **54**:11–18.

Geiss, O. and Kotzais, D. (2003) Determination of ammonium, urea, and chlorinated pesticides in cigarette tobacco. *Fresenius Env. Bull*, **12**(12):1562–1565 PSP 1018–4619.

Green, C.R., Schumacher, J.N., Lloyd, R.A., and Rodgman, A. (2007a) Comparison of the composition of tobacco smoke and the smokes from various tobacco substitutes. *Beitrage Tabakforsch*, **22**(4): 258–289.

Green, C.R., Scumacher, J.N., and Rodgman, A. (2007b) The expansion of tobacco and its effect on cigarette mainstream smoke properties. *Beitrage Tabakforsch*, **22**(5):317–345.

Greg, E., Hill, C., Hollywood, M., Kearney, M., McAdam, K., Mclaughlin, D. *et al.* (2004) The UK smoke constituents testing study. Summary of results and comparison with other studies. *Beitr Tabakforsch*, **21**:117–138.

Gupta, P. (2004) *Laboratory Testing of Smokeless Tobacco Products. Final Report to the India Office of the WHO* (allotment No. SE IND TOB 001.RB.02). New Delhi.

Hammond, D., Fong, G.T., Cummings, K.M., O'Connor, R.J., Giovino, G.A., and McNeill, A. (2006) Cigarette yields and human exposure: a comparison of alternative testing regimens. *Cancer Epidemiol Biomarkers Prev*, **15**(8):1495–1501.

Harris, J.E. (2001) Smoke yields of tobacco-specific nitrosamines in relation to FTC tar level and cigarette manufacturer: analysis of the Massachusetts Benchmark Study. *Public Health Reports*, **116**:336–343.

Hatsukami, D.K., Slade, J., Benowitz, N.L., Giovino, G.A., Gritz, E.R., Leischow, S. *et al.* (2002) Reducing tobacco harm: research challenges and issues. *Nicotine Tob Res*, (Suppl 2):S89–S101.

Hatsukami, D.K., Giovino, G.A., Eissenberg, T., Clark, P.I., Lawrence, D., and Leischow, S. (2005) Methods to asses potential reduced exposure products. *Nicotine Tob Res*, **7**:827–844.

Hecht, S.S., Murphy, S.E., Carmella, S.G., Li, S., Jensen, J., Le, C. *et al.* (2005) Similar uptake of lung carcinogens by smokers of regular, light, and ultralight cigarettes. *Cancer Epidemiol Biomar Prev*, **14**:693–698.

Henningfield, J.E., Radzius, A., and Cone, E.J. (1995) Estimation of available nicotine content in six smokeless tobacco products. *Tob Control*, **4**:57–61.

Henningfield, J.E., Benowitz, N.L., Slade, J., Houston, T.P., Davis, R.M., and Deitchman, S.D. (1998) Reducing the addictiveness of cigarettes. *Tob Control*, **7**:281–293.

Henningfield, J.E., Fant, R.V., Radzius, A., and Frost, S. (1999) Nicotine concentrations, smoke pH and whole tobacco aqueous pH of some cigar brands and types popular in the United States. *Nicotine Tob Res*, **1**:163–168.

Henningfield, J.E., Pankow, J., and Garrett, B. (2004) Ammonia and other chemical base tobacco additives and cigarette nicotine delivery: issues and research needs. *Nicotine Tob Res*, **6**:199–205.

Henningfield, J.E., Stolerman, I.P., Miczek, K.A. (2006) Nicotine psychopharmacology research: advancing science, public health, and global policy. *Psychopharmacology*, **184**:263–265.

Hoffmann, D., Brunnemann, K.D., Prokopczyk, B., and Djordjevic, M.V. (1994) Tobacco-specific N-nitrosamines: chemistry, biochemistry, carcinogenicity, and relevance to humans. *J Toxicol Env Health*, **41**:1–52.

Hoffmann, D., Djordjevic, M.V., Fan, J., Zang, E., Glynn, T., and Connolly, G.N. (1995) Five leading US commercial brands in moist snuff in 1994: Assessment of carcinogenic N-nitrosamines. *J Natl Cancer Inst*, **87**:1862–1869.

Hoffmann, D. and Hoffmann, I. (1997) The changing cigarette, 1950–1995. *J Toxicol Environ Health*, **50**:307–364.

Hoffmann, D. and Hoffmann, I. (1998) Chemistry and Toxicology. In: *Smoking and Tobacco Control Monograph No. 9*. Cigars. Health Effects and Trends. Washington, DC, USA: US Department of Health and Human Services, Public Health Service, National Institutes of Health, National Cancer Institute.

Hoffmann, D., Hoffmann, I., and El-Bayoumy, K. (2001) The less harmful cigarette: A controversial Issue. A tribute to Ernst L. Wynder. *Chem Res Toxicol*, **14**:767–790.

Idris, A.M., Nair, J., Oshima, H., Friesen, M., Bronet, I., Faustman, E.M. *et al.* (1991) Unusually high levels of carcinogenic tobacco-specific nitrosamines in Sudan snuff *(toombak)*. *Carcinogenesis*, **12**:1115–1118.

Idris, A.M., Ibrahim, S.O., Vasstrand, E.N., Johannessen, A.C., Lillehaug, J.R., Magnusson, B. *et al.* (1998) The Swedish snus and the Sudanese toombak: are they different? *Oral Oncol*, **34**:558–566.

IARC, International Agency for Research on Cancer (1986) Tobacco Smoking. In: *IARC Monographs on the Evaluation of the Carcinogenic Risk of Chemicals to Humans*. Vol. 38, p. 61. IARC, Lyon, France.

IARC, International Agency for Research on Cancer (2004) Tobacco Smoke and Involuntary Smoking. In: *IARC Monographs on the Evaluation of the Carcinogenic Risk of Chemicals to Humans*. Vol. 83, IARC, Lyon, France.

IARC, International Agency for Research on Cancer (2007) Smokeless Tobacco and Some Tobacco-specific N-nitrosamines In: *IARC Monographs on the Evaluation of the Carcinogenic Risk of Chemicals to Humans*. Vol. 89, IARC, Lyon, France.

Jack, A., Fennin, N., and Bush, L.P. (2007) Implications of reducing nornicotine accumulation in burley tobacco. *Recent Adv Tob Sci*, **33**:39–92.

Jacob, III P., Yu, L., Shulgin, A.T., and Benowitz, N.L. (1999) Minor tobacco alkaloids as biomarkers for tobacco use: comparison of users of cigarettes, smokeless tobacco, cigars and pipes. *Am J Pub Health*, **89**:731–736.

Kaiserman, M.J. and Rickert, W.S. (1992a) Carcinogens in tobacco smoke: benzo[a]pyrene from Canadian cigarettes and cigarette tobacco. *Am J Pub Health*, **82**:1023–1026.

Kaiserman, M.J. and Rickert, W.S. (1992b) Handmade cigarettes: it's the tube that counts. *Am J Pub Health*, **82**:107–109.

Kozlowski, L.T., Mehta, N.Y., Sweeney, C.T., Schwartz, S.S., Vogler, G.P., Jarvis, M.J. *et al.* (1998) Filter ventilation and nicotine content of tobacco of cigarettes from Canada, the United Kingdom, and the United States. *Tob Control*, **7**:369–375.

Laugesen, M. (2003) Tobacco Manufacturers' returns for calendar year 2002. Report to the Ministry of Health, New Zealand, Health New Zealand.

Laugesen, M. and Fowles, J. (2006) Marlboro UltraSmooth: a potentially reduced exposure cigarette? *Tob Control*, **15**:430–435.

Laugesen, M., Epton, M., Frampton, C.M.A., Glower, M., and Lea, R.A. (2009) Hand-rolled cigarette smoking patterns compared with factory-made cigarette smoking in New Zealand men. *BMC Public health*, **9**(194):1–6.

Lee, E.M., Malson, J.L., Moolchan, E.T., and Pickworth, W.B. (2004) Quantitative comparison between a nicotine delivery device (Eclipse) and conventional cigarette smoking. *Nicotine Tob Res*, **6**:95–102.

MacKown, C.T., Douglas, B., Djordjevic, M.V., and Bush, L.P. (1988) Tobacco-specific nitrosamines: formation during processing of midvein and lamina fines. *J Agric Food Chem*, **36**:1031–1035.

McNeill, A., Bedi, R., Islam, S., Alkhatib, M.N., and West, R. (2006) Levels of toxins in oral tobacco products in the UK. *Tob Control*, **15**:64–67.

Malik, S.K. and Behera, D. (1985) Chemistry of tobacco and tobacco smoke in chutta – a home made cigar; a preliminary study. *Int J Clin Pharmacol Ther Toxicol*, **23**(11):604–605.

Malson, J.L., Sims, K., Murty, R., and Pickworth, W.B. (2001) Comparison of the nicotine content of tobacco used in bidis and conventional cigarettes. *Tob Control*, **10**:181–183.

Malson, J.L., Lee, E.M., Moolchan, E.T., and Pickworth, W.B. (2002) Nicotine delivery from smoking bidis and additive-free cigarette. *Nicotin Tob Res*, **4**:485–490.

Malson, J.L., Lee, E.M., Murty, R., Moolchan, E.T., and Pickworth, W.B. (2003) Clove cigarette smoking: biochemical, physiological, and subjective effects. *Pharmacol Biochem Behavior*, **74**:739–745.

Maziak, W., Ward, K.D., Afifi Soweid, R.A., and Eissenberg, T. (2004) Tobacco smoking using a waterpipe: a re-emerging strain in a global epidemic. *Tob Control*, **13**:327–333.

Maziak, W., Eissenberg, T., and Ward, K.D. (2005) Patterns of waterpipe use and dependence: implications for intervention development. *Pharmacol Biochem Behavior*, **80**:173–179.

Melikian, A.A., Djordjevic, M.V., Chen, S., Richie, J.P. Jr, and Stellman, S.D. (2007a) Impact of delivered dosage of cigarette smoke toxins on the levels of urinary biomarkers of exposure. *Cancer Epi Biomarkers Prev*, **16**:1408–1415.

Melikian, A.A., Djordjevic, M.V., Hosey, J., Zhang, J., Chen, S., Zang, E. *et al.* (2007b) Gender differences relative to smoking behavior and emission of toxins from mainstream cigarette smoke. *Nicotine Tob Res*, **9**(3):377–387.

Mitacek, E.J., Brunnemann, K.D., Polednak, A.P., Hoffmann, D., and Suttajit, M. (1991) Composition of popular tobacco products in Thailand and its relevance to disease prevention. *Prev Med*, **20**:764–773.

Moldoveanu, S.C., Borgerding, M. (2008) Formation of tobacco specific nitrosamines in mainstream cigarette smoke; Part 1, FTC smoking. *Beitrage Tabakforsch*, **23**(1):19–31.

Monzer, B., Sepetdjian, E., Saliba, N., and Shihadeh, A. (2008) Charcoal emissions as a source of CO and carcinogenic PAH in mainstream narghile WP smoke. *Food Chem Toxicol*, **46**(9):2992–2995.

National Cancer Institute (2001) Risk associated with smoking cigarettes with low machine-measured yields of tar and nicotine. In: *Smoking and Tobacco Control Monograph No.13.* Washington, DC, USA: US Department of Health and Human Services, Public Health Service, National Institutes of Health, National Cancer Institute.

Neergaard, J., Singh, P., Job, J., and Montgomery, S. (2007) Waterpipe smoking and nicotine exposure: E review of the current evidence. *Nicotine Tob Res,* 9:987–994.

O'Connor, R.J., Giovino, G.A., Kozlowski, L.T., Shiffman, S., Hyland, A., Bernert, J.T. *et al.* (2006) Changes in nicotine intake and cigarette use over time in two nationally representative cross-sectional samples of smokers. *Am J Epidemiol,* 164:750–759.

O'Connor, R.J. and Hurley, P.J. (2008) Existing technologies to reduce specific toxicant emissions in cigarette smoke. *Tob Control Suppl,* 1:i39–48.

Official Journal of European Communities (2001) Directive 2001/37/EC of the European Parliament and of the Council of 5 June.

Pakhale, S.S. and Maru, G.B. (1998) Distribution of major and minor alkaloids in tobacco, mainstream, and sidestream smoke of popular Indian smoking products. *Food Chem Toxicol,* 36:1131–1138.

Pakhale, S.S., Jayant, K., and Bhide, S.V. (1989) Total particulate matter and nicotine in Indian bidis and cigarettes: a comparative study of standard machine estimates and exposure levels in smokers in Bombay. *Indian J Cancer,* 26(4):227–232.

Pankow, J.F. (2001) A consideration of the role of gas/particle partitioning in the deposition of nicotine and other tobacco smoke compounds in the respiratory tract. *Perspective. Chem Res Toxicol,* 14(11):1465–1481.

Pankow, J.F., Barsanti, K.C., and Peyton, D.H. (2003a) Fraction of free-base nicotine in fresh smoke particulate matter from the Eclipse 'cigarette' by ^{1}H NMR spectroscopy. *Chem Res Toxicol,* 16: 1014–1018.

Pankow, J.F., Tavakoli, A.D., Luo, W., and Isabelle, L.M. (2003b) Percent free base nicotine in the tobacco smoke particulate matter of selected commercial and reference cigarettes. *Chem Res Toxicol,* 16:23–27.

Peele, D.M., Danehower, D.A., and Goins, G.D. (1995) Chemical and biochemical changes during flue curing. *Recent Adv Tob Sci,* 21:81–133.

Pillsbury, H.C. (1996) Review of the Federal Trade Commission Method for determining cigarette tar and nicotine yield. In: *The FTC Cigarette Test Method for Determining Tar, Nicotine, and Carbon Monoxide Yields of US Cigarettes.* Report of the NCI Expert Committee. Smoking and Tobacco Control Monograph No.7, Bethesda (MD): US Department of Health and Human Services. National Institutes of Health, National Cancer Institute, NIH Publication No. 96-4028.

Primack, B.A., Sidani, J., Agarwal, A.A., Shadel, W.G., Donny, E.C., and Eissenberg, T.E. (2008) Prevalence and associations with waterpipe tobacco smoking among US university students. *Ann Behav Med,* 36(1):81–86.

Primack, B.A., Walsh, M., Bryce, C., and Eissenberg, T. (2009) Water-pipe tobacco smoking among middle and high school students in Arizona. *Pwediatrics,* 123(2):e282–288.

Rees, V.W., Wayne, J.F., Thomas, B.F., and Connolly, G.N. (2007) Physical design analysis and mainstream smoke constituent yields of new potential reduced exposure product, Marlboro UltraSmooth. *Nicotine Tob Res,* 9(11):1197–1206.

Richter, P. and Watson, C. (2008) Chemistry and Toxicology. In: P.C. Gupta and S. Asma (eds), *Bidi Smoking and Public Health.* New Delhi: Ministry of Health and Family Welfare. Government of India.

Rodgman, A. and Perfetti, T.A. (2009) The chemical components of tobacco and tobacco smoke. CRS Press, Taylor & Francis Group, LLC.

SCENIHR, Scientific Committee on Emerging and Newly Identified Health Risks (2008) Opinion on Health Effects of Smokeless Tobacco. Opinion adopted by SCENIHR at the 22nd plenary on 6 February. Available at: http://ec.europa.eu/health/ph_risk/committees/04_scenihr/scenihr_cons_06_en.htm

Shihadeh, A. (2003) Investigation of mainstream aerosol of the argileh waterpipe. *Food Chem Toxicol*, **41**:143–152.

Shihadeh, A. and Saleh, R. (2005) Polycyclic aromatic hydrocarbons, carbon monoxide, 'tar', and nicotine in the mainstream smoke aerosol of the narghile water pipe. *Food Chem Toxicol*, **43**:655–661.

Siminszky, B., Gavilano, L.B., and Chakrabarti, M. (2007) Evolution of nicotine N-demethylaze genes and their use in reducing nornicotine levels in tobacco. *Recent Adv Tob Sci*, **33**:27–38.

Sisson, V.A. and Severson, R.F. (1990) Alkaloid composition of the *Nicotiana* species. *Beitr Takforsch*, **14**:327–340.

Smith *et al.* (2006)

Stanfill, S.B., Brown, C.R., Yan, X., Watson, C.H., and Ashley, D.L. (2006) Quantification of flavor-related compounds in the unburned contents of bidi and clove cigarettes. *J Agric Food Chem*, **54**:8580–8588.

Stedman, R.L. (1968) The chemical composition of tobacco and tobacco smoke. *Chem Rev*, **68**:153–207.

Stepanov, I., Carmella, S.G., Hecht, S.S., and Duca, G. (2002) Analysis of tobacco-specific nitrosamines in Moldovan cigarette tobacco. *J Agric Food Chem*, **50**:2793–2797.

Stepanov, I., Jensen, J., Hatsukami, D., and Hecht, S.S. (2008) New and traditional smokeless tobacco: comparison of toxicant and carcinogen levels. *Nicotine Tob Res*, **10**(12):1773–1782.

Stepanov, I., Carmella, S.G., Han, S., Pinto, A., Strasser, A., Lerman, C. *et al.* (2009) Evidence for endogenous formation of *N'*-nitrosonornicotine in some long-term nicotine patch users. *Nicotine Tob Res*, **11**(1):99–105.

Strasser, A.A., Lerman, C., and Capella, J.N. (2006) Lower nicotine cigarettes may not lower harm. *LDI Issue brief*, **12**(2):1–4.

Strasser, A.A., Lerman, C., Sanborn, P.M., Pickworth, W.B., and Feldman, E.A. (2007) New lower nicotine cigarettes can produce compensatory smoking and increased carbon monoxide exposure. *Drug Alcohol Depend*, **86**:294–300.

Stratton, K., Shetty, P., Wallace, R., and Bondurant, S. (2001) Clearing the smoke. Assessing the science base for tobacco harm reduction. Washington DC, USA: National Academy Press.

Tamim, H., Terro, A., Kassem, H., Ghazi, A., Khamis, T.A., Hay, M.M. *et al.* (2003) Tobacco use by university students, Lebanon 2001. *Addictions*, **98**(7):933–939.

Tamim *et al.* (2007)

Tso, T.C. (1990) Organic metabolism- alkaloids. In: T.C.Tso (ed.) *Production, Physiology and Biochemistry of Tobacco Plant*. IDEALS, Inc., Beltsville, MD, pp 427–486.

US DHHS (Department of Health and Human Services) (2004). *The Health Consequences of Smoking: A Report of the Surgeon General*. Atlanta, GA: US Department of Health and Human Services, Centers for Disease Control and Prevention, National Center for Chronic Disease Prevention and Health Promotion, Office on Smoking and Health.

Varsano, S., Ganz, I., Eldor, N., and Garenkin, M. (2003) [Water-pipe tobacco smoking among school children in Israel: frequencies, habits, and attitudes]. *Harefuah*, **142**(11):736–741.

Walton, L.R., Burton, H.R., and Swetnam, L.D. (1995) Effect of mechanization on the physical appearance and chemical composition of burley tobacco. *Recent Adv Tob Sci*, **21**:3–38.

Wangan, K.R. and Biørn, E. (2001) Prevalence and substitution effects in tobacco consumption: a discrete choice analysis of panel data. No. 312. Statistics Norway, Research Department.

Watson, C.H., Polzin, G.M., Calafat, A.M., and Ashley, D.L. (2003) Determination of tar, nicotine, and carbonmonoxide yields in the smoke of bidi cigarettes. *Nicotine Tob Res*, **5**:747–753.

Watson, C.H., Trommel, J.S., and Ashley, D.L. (2004) Solid-phase microextraction-based approach to determine free-base nicotine in trapped mainstream cigarette smoke total particulate matter. *J Agric Food Chem*, **52**:7240–7245.

Wu, W., Song, S., Ashley, D.L., and Watson, C.H. (2004) Assessment of tobacco-specific nitrosamines in the tobacco and mainstream smoke of Bidi cigarettes. *Carcinogenesis*, **25**(2):283–287.

WHO, World Health Organization (2008) Mandated lowering of toxicants in cigarette smoke: tobacco-specific nitrosamines and selected other constituents. *Technical Report Series*, **951**:45–260.

Young, D., Borland, R., Hammond, D., Cummings, K.M., Devlin, E., Yong, H.-H. *et al.* (2006) Prevalence and attributes of roll-your-own smokers in the International Tobacco Control (ITC) four country survey. *Tob Control*, **15**(Suppl III): iii76–iii82.

Young, D., Yong, H.-H., Borland, R., Ross, H., Sirirassamee, B., Kin, F. *et al.* (2008) Prevalence and correlates of roll-your-own smoking in Thailand and Malaysia: Findings of the ITC-South East Asia survey. *Nicotine Tob Res*, **10**:907–915.

Yu, J., Taylor, L.T., Aref, S., Bodnar, J.A., and Borgerding. M.F. (2006) Influence of puffing parameters and filter vent blocking condition on nicotine fate in a burning cigarette. Part 1. Full flavor cigarette. *Beitr Takforsch*, **144**:185–195.

Chapter 11

Tobacco smoking and tobacco-related harm in the European Union with special attention to the new EU member states

Witold A. Zatoński and Marta Mańczuk

Introduction

Smoking tobacco is a major cause of mortality from chronic diseases in most countries, in particular in young adulthood (35–44 years) and middle age (45–64 years).[1] It has been estimated that in the year 2000 tobacco caused 13% of deaths in men and 4% in women worldwide (Ezzati *et al.* 2004). These estimates reflect gender differences that are linked to the pattern of smoking in previous decades. Europe has experienced some of the highest rates of smoking in both men and women, and the epidemic of tobacco-related mortality has been one of the most important public health events in the region in the second half of the twentieth century (WHO 2007).

This chapter assesses the role of tobacco smoking as a cause of premature mortality in Europe, and its contribution to the health gap between the EU10[2] and EU15[3] countries, using several complementary approaches. It reviews the history of tobacco smoking in the EU10 countries, and analyses the patterns of tobacco smoking. Since lung cancer is the cause of death most strongly associated with tobacco smoking, the chapter also analyses temporal trends in lung cancer mortality in Europe. Finally, it estimates the mortality attributable to tobacco smoking in the EU countries.

History of tobacco smoking

Before World War II (WWII), tobacco consumption in central and eastern European (CEE) countries was lower than in most western European countries (Forey *et al.* 2002). At that time, tobacco was mostly consumed by men as hand-rolled cigarettes. After WWII, tobacco products consisted nearly exclusively of factory-made cigarettes, whose production was standardized across the entire Soviet block. Cigarette production became a priority, cigarette prices were low,

---

[1] For calculations of tobacco-attributable mortality, analysis was undertaken for the population aged 35 years and over.

[2] EU10: Bulgaria, Czech Republic, Estonia, Hungary, Latvia, Lithuania, Poland, Romania, Slovakia, and Slovenia – European Union new member states in May 2004 (excluding Malta and Cyprus, which also joined the EU at the time), and next in January 2007 (Bulgaria, Romania).

[3] EU15: Austria, Belgium, Denmark, Finland, France, Germany, Greece, Ireland, Italy, Luxembourg, Netherlands, Portugal, Spain, Sweden, and United Kingdom – European Union member states before enlargement in May 2004, also 'the old EU' or 'countries of the old EU'.

and the product itself was widely available. This situation hardly changed until the end of the 1980s. Until the 1990s, information on the frequency of smoking and tobacco consumption in the CEE countries was fragmentary (Forey *et al.* 2002).

Before the 1990s scientific knowledge on the health effects of smoking did not reach the CEE countries. As a consequence, awareness of the harm done by tobacco was low prior to the political changes in 1990s (Zatoński & Przewoźniak 1992) and the CEE countries were at the top of the list of world cigarette consumers from the early 1960s until the end of the twentieth century (Shafey *et al.* 2003). An unusual aspect was that smoking was more common among the better educated and better-off people, both men and women (Zatoński & Przewoźniak 1992; Zatoński 2004). The rapid rise in tobacco consumption in the CEE countries after WWII was followed by an increase in the incidence of, and mortality from, tobacco-related diseases (Peto *et al.* 2004).

The socioeconomic transformation in the 1990s quickly restored a normal cigarette market. The tobacco industry was among the first to undergo privatization and cigarette manufacturers were almost completely taken over by trans-national companies (Gilmore & McKee 2004). A structured market was soon established. Constant availability was ensured while prices were kept at a very low level. In the early 1990s, the price of a pack of cigarettes in Poland was, on average, lower than the price of a loaf of bread (Zatoński 2004). Cigarettes also became the most heavily advertised product; for example, in the late 1990s, the industry was spending US$100 million per year on tobacco advertisements in Poland (Zatoński 2004).

After the political changes, health advocacy movements began their struggle in the CEE countries to avert the tobacco-related health consequences. In Poland, the health advocates (mostly medical professionals), collaborated with members of the parliament (many of whom were also medical professionals) to prepare a comprehensive tobacco control legislation, during a five-year confrontation with the international tobacco companies (Zatoński & Przewoźniak 1999; Zatoński 2004). They finally succeeded in 1995 in having a first law on tobacco control, which was extended in 1999 and 2003. According to WHO, it was one of the most comprehensive tobacco laws of its time in the world (WHO 2004). Provisions included a total ban on advertising and promotion; the allocation of 0.5% of tobacco excise tax to tobacco control activities; a ban on sponsorship of political parties by tobacco companies; a smoking ban in health care establishments, schools, other educational facilities, sport facilities and workplaces; a ban on selling tobacco products to minors under 18 years, ban on selling tobacco products by vending machines, and in small packs or individual units; a ban on producing and selling smokeless tobacco; health warnings on cigarette packs (30% of front and back of cigarette pack, at the time the biggest health warnings in the world); a gradual reduction of tar and nicotine levels; and the free provision of treatment for smoking dependence (Zatoński 2003a). After 1990, tobacco consumption in Poland began to decrease for the first time (Zatoński 2003b; Zatoński 2004).

Similar developments took place in the 1990s in Czech Republic, Slovakia, and Slovenia, while in the remaining CEE countries, and notably in the former USSR countries, the situation remained different, in some of former Soviet Union countries tobacco products consumption and smoking prevalence is increasing still today (Bobak *et al.*, 2006), in the other the 1990s were a period of stagnation with no significant changes in tobacco consumption (Zatoński 2004; WHO 2007).

Characteristics of tobacco products

The kind of tobacco used before 1990 for making cigarettes was usually domestic black shag, and most cigarettes were made with low amounts of additives. Cigarettes seldom had filters and had a high content of nicotine and tar (Zatoński & Przewoźniak 1992). Fragmentary data from Hungary show that the tar level in cigarettes sold in the 1970s often exceeded 30 mg per cigarette (Forey *et al.* 2002). In Poland, where systematic studies on harmful substances in cigarettes were conducted since the beginning of the 1980s, the average content of tar varied in the 1980s from about 21 to 24 mg per cigarette, and average nicotine content reached 2 mg per cigarette (Fig. 11.1). During the 1980s, the tar and nicotine levels in cigarettes sold in eastern Europe were about 1.5 to 2 times higher than in western Europe (Forey *et al.* 2002). After 1990, international companies successively took over the entire industry and cigarettes were manufactured in central

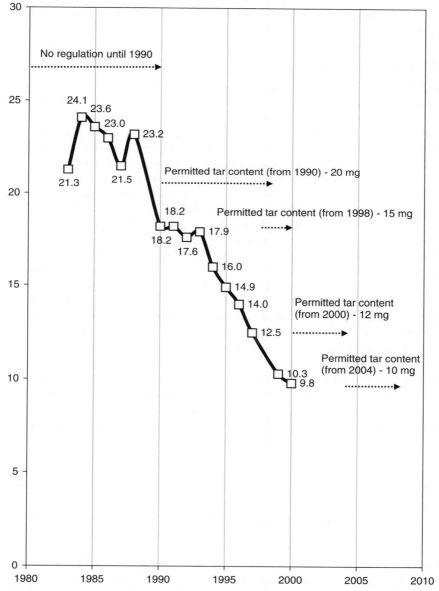

Figure 11.1 Mean tar content (mg/cigarette) in cigarettes sold in Poland (1983–2000) in relation to permitted norms.

Source: Chemical studies conducted in Polish and foreign laboratories and coordinated by the Cancer Center and Institute of Oncology in Warsaw.

and eastern Europe according to international standards (Gilmore & McKee 2004). Most ciga-rettes are manufactured from light tobacco and the proportion of filter cigarettes which were equipped with acetate or charcoal filters rose to 90% (Zatoński 2004). The toxic properties of cigarettes, 'power' additives and taste enhancers are now similar to those used in western Europe. As an effect of the new tobacco control regulations and the European Union requirements, the national norms for permitted levels of tar, nicotine, and carbon monoxide were introduced in the accession countries. In Poland, this policy was enforced for the first time in 1990, and then con-tinuously implemented, and average tar content was reduced from about 23 mg in 1988 to about 10 mg per cigarette in 2000 (Fig. 11.1).

Smoking prevalence

Although there are many data sources on tobacco exposure in Europe, international comparisons are not straightforward, especially in central and eastern Europe. For the EU10 countries, his-torical data on cigarette sale and consumption are very difficult to collect reliably and compare internationally for a number of reasons. Before WWII, tobacco use in the region was mostly limited to hand-rolled cigarettes and the market of manufactured cigarettes was small. Between WWII and the beginning of the 1990s, consumption of manufactured cigarettes has grown dramatically, reaching worldwide levels in such countries as Poland, Hungary, and Bulgaria (Forey et al. 2002). However, filter cigarettes were not produced until the end of the 1950s. The tobacco industry, including its databases, was controlled by the state government and the major-ity of tobacco products were produced from black or brown tobacco for the domestic or Soviet Union market. Data on cigarette consumption per adult were first published at the beginning of the 1960s (Zatoński & Przewoźniak 1992). After the 1990s, the state monopoly of the tobacco industry in the CEE countries was passed to the hands of transnational tobacco companies that totally changed the structure of the tobacco market (see previous section) and limited access to information on cigarette sale and consumption (Gilmore & McKee 2004). In addition, central Europe became a transfer path for cigarette smuggling from eastern to western Europe (ASPECT 2004). Furthermore, international comparisons of cigarette sales and consumption became dif-ficult due to changes in the political map of Europe (new states) and due to subsequent changes in country populations.

Therefore, data on smoking prevalence seem now to be a better source for tobacco use estimates than cigarette sale or consumption. However, due to the methodological differences in country-specific surveys (see www.hem.waw.pl); these data should be critically evaluated and carefully used. In general, they are collected in the CEE countries since the beginning of the 1980s, the earliest in Poland (since 1974). In certain countries, studies on smoking behaviours were conducted in dif-ferent periods and based on different research design, sometimes as separate tobacco use surveys, sometimes within health status and behaviours studies. Although all studies were based on national random samples, these samples represented different age categories and knowledge on sampling methods and selected social strata is general. In central and eastern Europe, face-to-face interview or mail surveys were more often used and population data were taken from national population registers. In western European countries, telephone surveys were also carried out and samples were based in a few countries on data from census studies. Therefore, CEE studies were smaller and precise cross-sectional statistical analysis was more difficult. Due to different study designs, response rates in particular studies varied from 55% to 100%. Finally, studies also differ in the definition of smoking categories or in the focus on specific behaviours (e.g., daily smoking).

To overcome methodological differences, comparative analysis of smoking prevalence was limited to adults aged 20 to 64 years. The analysis was based on well-documented data taken from the most recent nation-wide randomized surveys of the adult population. It was decided to focus on current smoking that was defined in all studies in similar terms (smoking at least one cigarette a day). Data on prevalence of current smoking was adjusted for world standard population and its presentation included the same gender and age groups (see www.hem.waw.pl).

The prevalence of current smoking in men aged 20–64 years is higher in the EU10 countries (42.7%) than in the EU15 countries (35.5%) (Fig. 11.2a). Among the EU10 countries, Slovenia has a lower (30.1%), Czech Republic has a similar (35.4%), and Romania (37.6%) and Slovakia (39.2%) have a slightly higher prevalence than the average of the EU15 countries. In Latvia and Bulgaria, smoking prevalence exceeds 50%, while in Estonia, Poland, Lithuania, and Hungary it ranges from 40% to 50%. The highest rates in the EU10 countries are comparable to those in Greece (51%) and Portugal (47.2%), but are still much lower than those observed in Russia (66.2%) where they reach the highest level in Europe. These patterns characterize both young-adult (20–44 years) and middle-aged (45–64 years) male population.

In contrast to men, there are no major differences in women's smoking between the EU10 and the EU15 countries (Fig. 11.2b). The average prevalence of current smoking in women aged 20–64 years is slightly higher in the EU15 (27.4%) than in the EU10 countries (24.8%). The differences in smoking prevalence between countries are larger in the EU10 than in the EU15 countries: Bulgaria has the highest prevalence in Europe (32.5%), while Romania (12.5%) and Lithuania (13.2%) have the lowest. In addition to Bulgaria, smoking prevalence in adult women exceeds 30% in Hungary and Poland, as well as in Portugal, Greece, and the Netherlands. In young-adult women (20–44 years), average smoking prevalence is higher in the EU15 countries (31.2%) than in the EU10 countries (26.3%); in Greece, Portugal, and Bulgaria, the prevalence exceeds 40%. In middle-aged women (45–64 years), smoking prevalence in the EU10 countries (22%) is similar to that in the EU15 countries (21%), and Poland is the leading country in this age group (30.8%).

A gap in smoking prevalence among men between the EU15 and EU10 countries remains present, despite a sharp decline in smoking rates in some EU10 countries, notably Poland and Czech Republic (Fig. 11.3). However, in the Baltic States and Bulgaria, the prevalence of smoking in men has not decreased since the 1990s. Unfortunately, reliable long-term data on smoking habits are not available in many EU10 countries. For example, in the absence of historical data from Hungary, it is difficult to understand how male smoking prevalence in that country (currently in the middle of the distribution) can match lung cancer mortality (the highest ever recorded in Europe), and why smoking prevalence is now at such a low level in Romanian women. In general, patterns of smoking prevalence in women are not so homogenous by age as in men, reflecting large inter-country differences in cohort effects (Figs 11.3a and 11.3b).

Lung cancer mortality

Because 80–90% of lung cancer in European populations is attributable to smoking, lung cancer mortality rates provide a convenient indicator of temporal trends in the cumulative health effects from past smoking (Didkowska *et al.* 2005). Analysing trends in lung cancer in age groups, starting from young adults (20–44 years), and middle-aged persons (45–64 years) to the population after the age of 65 years, can relatively quickly document changes in tobacco exposure (and health consequences of tobacco use).

Standardized lung cancer mortality rates for the years 1968–2002 were calculated for the two European regions, EU15 and EU10, in the following age groups: 20–44, 45–64, 65+, and 20+ years, separately for men and women (Figs 11.4 and 11.5).

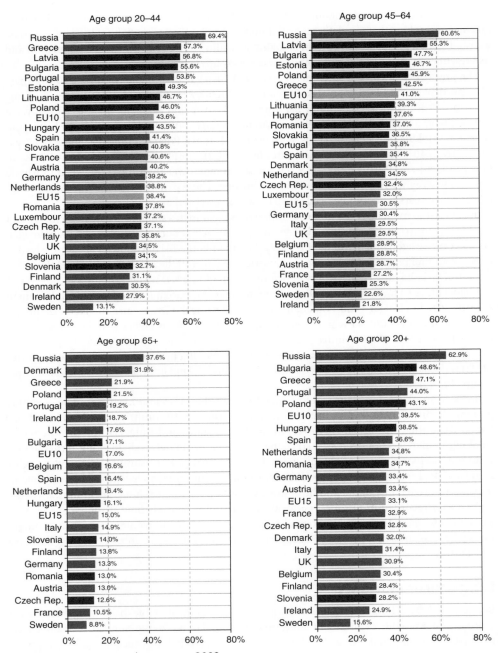

Figure 11.2a Current smokers, men – 2002.

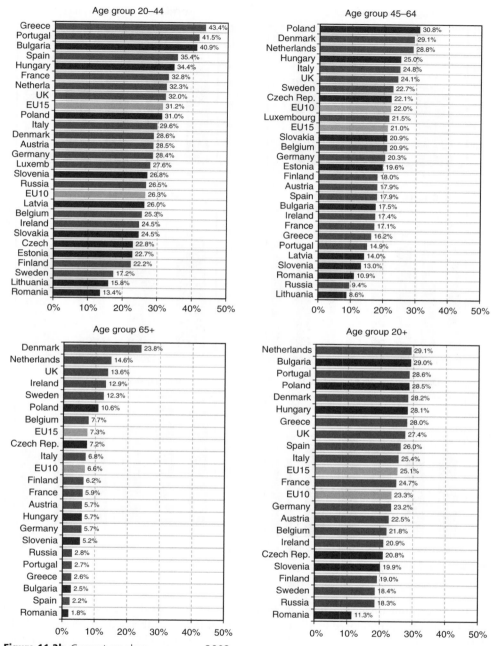

Figure 11.2b Current smokers, women – 2002.

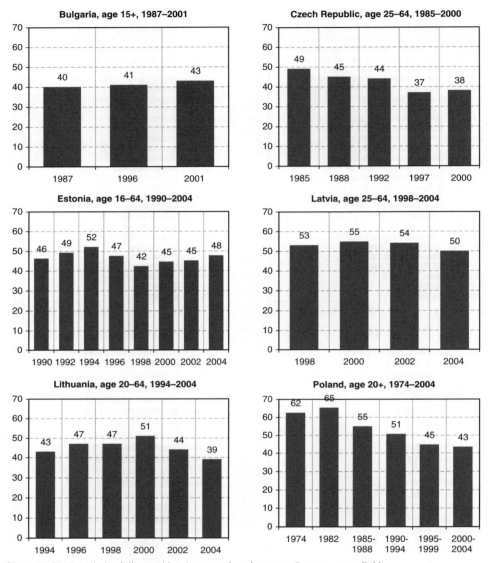

Figure 11.3a Trends in daily smoking in central and eastern Europe, men (%)*

* Data based on original age-specific study samples.

Lung cancer time trends in young-adult men in the EU10 showed a strong increase until the early 1980s, a less pronounced increase until a peak in 1994, and then a decline (Fig. 11.4). In 1994, rates in the EU10 countries (7.2/100 000 p-y) were twice as high as in the EU15 countries (3.6/100 000 p-y). Since the early 1990s, mortality also declined in the EU15 countries, but less so than in the EU10 countries, and by the year 2002, the rate ratio between the EU10 (4.7/100 000 p-y) and the EU15 countries (2.7/100 000 p-y), was reduced to 1.7.

In middle-aged men, lung cancer mortality increased dramatically in the EU10 until 1991 (177/100 000 p-y), after which it began to fall appreciably (Fig. 11.4). In the EU15 countries, lung cancer mortality showed a slight increase until 1985 (116/100 000 p-y), after which it started to

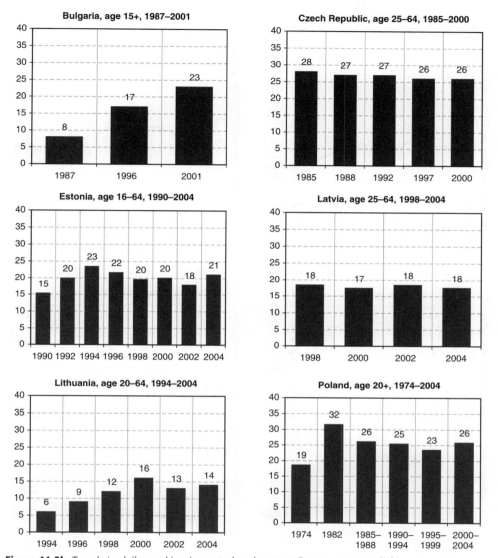

Figure 11.3b Trends in daily smoking in central and eastern Europe, women (%)*

* Data based on original age-specific study samples.

decrease. In the year 2002, the rate ratio between the EU10 (149/100 000 p-y) and the EU15 countries (85/100 000 p-y) was 1.8. Lung cancer mortality has increased among men in the EU10
countries until the recent years, when the increase ceased. In the EU15 countries, rates increased
until 1988, but then started to decrease. As a consequence, mortality in EU10 countries in the
group 65+ years was initially lower than in the EU15 countries, but, in 1995, the rates in the two
regions crossed, and during the last decade they were higher in the EU10 than in the EU15. In the
year 2002, the rate ratio between EU10 (409/100 000 p-y) and EU15 countries (351/100 000 p-y)
was 1.2. When country-specific rates are considered, Hungarian men had the highest mortality
both in young adulthood and middle age.

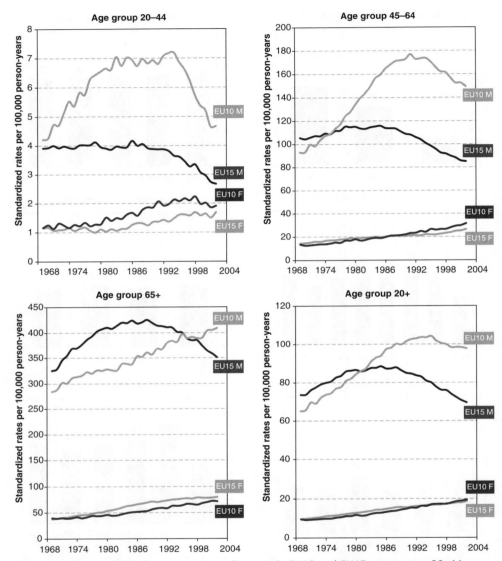

Figure 11.4 Time trends in lung cancer mortality rates in EU10 and EU15, age groups 20–44, 45–64, 65+, 20+

In women, time trends of lung cancer showed similar patterns in the EU10 and the EU15 countries in all age groups (Fig. 11.4). Among young adults, stagnation was apparent in recent years in both regions. No significant gap in lung cancer mortality was observed in women between the EU10 and the EU15 countries. As in men, mortality among young-adult and middle-aged women was higher in Hungary than in any other European country.

Tobacco-attributable mortality

The proportion of deaths attributable to tobacco smoking was calculated by deriving for each country the prevalence of smokers (in the past) that would have produced the observed mortality

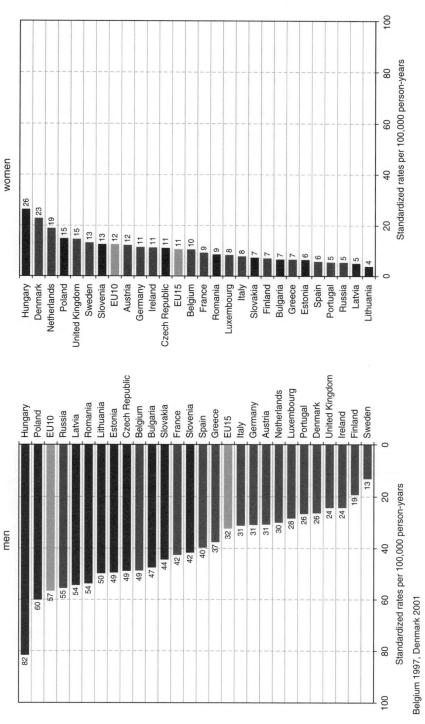

Belgium 1997, Denmark 2001

Figure 11.5 Lung cancer mortality 20–64 years – 2002.

rates of lung cancer in that country, and by using this prevalence to calculate the burden of other tobacco-related causes of death (Peto *et al.* 2004; Table 2).

Among men, 41% of adult (35–64 years) deaths in the EU10 countries were attributable to tobacco smoking compared with 33% in the EU15 countries. The figures for women were 17% in the EU10 countries and 14% in the EU15 countries. In both men and women and in both groups of countries, the proportion of tobacco-attributable mortality was higher in middle age (45–65 years) than in young adulthood (35–44 years). For example, among men in the EU10 countries, 20% of young-adult deaths and 45% of middle-age deaths were attributable to tobacco smoking.

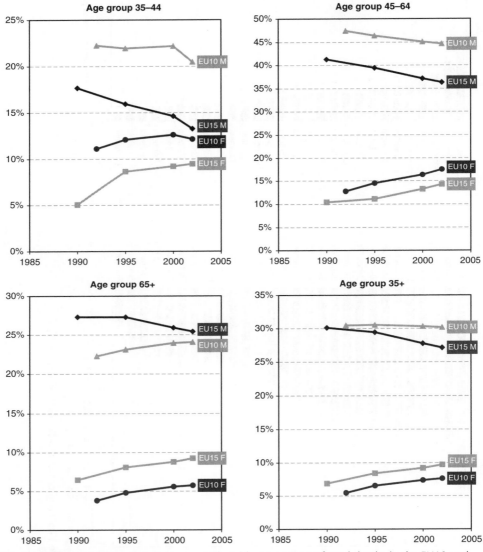

Figure 11.6 Temporal trends in tobacco-attributable percentage of total deaths in the EU10 and EU15 countries.

No difference in the proportion of deaths attributable to tobacco between the EU10 and the EU15 countries was observed among men after 65 years of age, while the tobacco-attributable fraction in elderly women was higher in the EU15 than in the EU10 countries.

Among men aged 45–64 years, 39% of tobacco-attributable deaths in the EU10 countries resulted from cancer and 46% from cardiovascular diseases, while in the EU15 countries, 52% of tobacco-attributable deaths were from cancer and 30% were from cardiovascular diseases. The same pattern (a larger contribution of cardiovascular deaths in the EU10 countries and of cancer deaths in the EU15 countries) was observed among women (EU10 countries: 40% and 49%; EU15 countries: 49% and 27%, respectively).

In country-specific analyses, it is apparent that tobacco-attributable mortality among middle-aged men is larger in many EU10 countries than in EU15 countries, with the notable exception of Slovenia, where tobacco-attributable mortality is lower than the EU15 average (Fig. 11.7a). Among men aged 35–44 years, Latvia, Hungary, Romania, and Bulgaria show the highest tobacco-attributable mortality, but no clear difference is seen between the remaining EU10 countries and the EU15 (the proportion is notably low in Czech Republic). Among middle-aged women, the tobacco-attributable mortality is higher in Hungary than in any other European country, followed by Denmark, the Netherlands, and the United Kingdom, while in young-adult women the effects of the tobacco epidemic among women is strong in Hungary, and starting to appear in France, Poland, and Slovakia (Fig. 11.7b). Tobacco-attributable mortality is very low among women from several EU15 countries (notably Portugal and, in women aged 45–64 years, Spain) and from some EU10 countries, notably Lithuania.

Between the early 1990s and 2002, a clear decrease in tobacco-attributable mortality was apparent among young-adult and middle-aged men in the EU15 countries, while among women, an increase was apparent in both age groups. In the EU10 countries, tobacco-attributable mortality among men decreased in both the young and the middle-age groups. Among women, a decrease in tobacco-attributable mortality was apparent only in recent years in the young-adult age group, while there was a clear increase in the middle-age group.

Nineteen per cent of the male mortality differences[4] in the age group 35–44 years between the EU10 and the EU15 was caused by tobacco, and 53% in the age group 45–64 years. Among women, 15% of the mortality difference in the age group 35–44 years was a result of tobacco consumption, and 21% in the age group 45–64 years.

The present analysis has clearly identified tobacco as the major determinant of the health gap between the EU10 and EU15 countries. Over half of the excess mortality among middle-aged men in the EU10 countries might have been avoided if the tobacco consumption of these men had been the same as that of their equivalents in the EU15. The contribution of tobacco to the excess mortality in young adults seems less important than in middle-age adults. While this is a reassuring result, suggesting that tobacco-related health disparities between the two regions of Europe are reducing, caution should be applied in its interpretation, because the global picture of the health effects of tobacco is not fully apparent until middle age. As expected, the role of tobacco in shaping mortality differences between the EU10 and EU15 countries in women is less prominent than men: nevertheless, about one fourth of the excess mortality among middle-aged women in EU10 countries can be attributed to their higher tobacco consumption.

Tobacco-attributable mortality is decreasing among middle-aged men in both EU15 and EU10 countries. Among women, the trends are less favourable, with the possible exception of mortality

---

[4] These values were calculated as $(TM_{10} - TM_{15}) / (M_{10} - M_{15})$, where TM is the tobacco-attributable mortality rate and M is total mortality rate (the subscripts 10 and 15 refer to the two groups of countries).

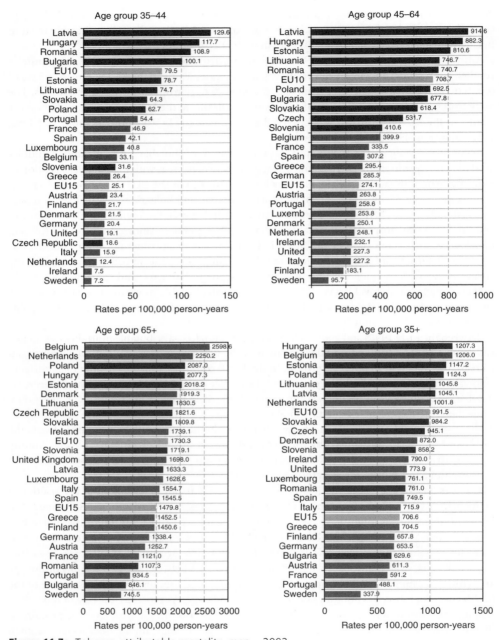

Figure 11.7a Tobacco-attributable mortality, men – 2002.

in the age group 35–44 years in the EU10 countries. Despite these encouraging results, however, the gap in tobacco-attributable middle-age mortality between EU10 and EU15 countries remains alarming, and the effect of the tobacco-epidemic in central and eastern European countries will greatly affect the mortality patterns in this region for the following decades. It is worth noting, however, that in some EU10 countries, the policies and programmes implemented to

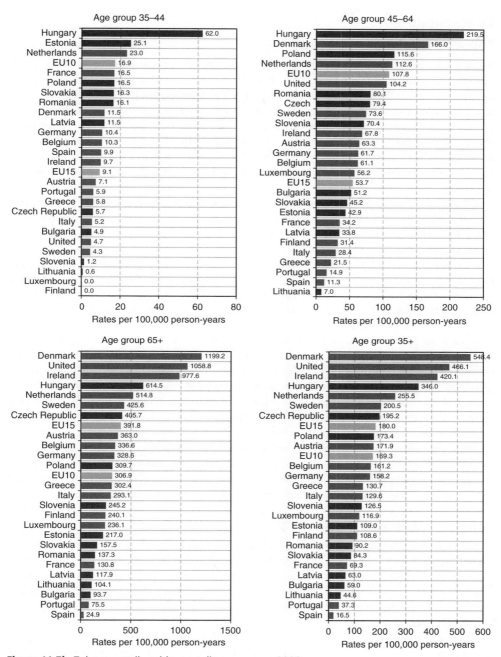

Figure 11.7b Tobacco-attributable mortality, women – 2002.

reduce tobacco consumption, in particular among men, have already produced notable results on tobacco-attributable mortality. For example, tobacco-attributable lung cancer mortality rates among men aged 35–44 years are 2.0/100 000 p-y in Czech Republic and 5.1/100 000 p-y in Slovenia, compared with an average of 4.4/100 000 p-y in the EU15 countries, and of 9.5/100 000 p-y in the EU10 countries.

Conclusions

Tobacco smoking

Among men, smoking prevalence has tended to reduce in many countries of central and eastern Europe over recent years (Fig. 11.3). There has been a constant declining trend in all age groups in Czech Republic, Poland, and Slovenia, although data from Slovenia are based on only a few time points. Male smoking also seems to have declined in Slovakia and Romania, but these observations are not consistent with other data sources or are based on regional surveys. In the Baltic States, there are no consistent changes in male smoking during the whole period of observation, although smoking prevalence has reduced in Lithuania and grown in Estonia over the last few years. In Bulgaria, there has been a slight but consistent increase in male smoking since the end of the 1980s.

Although the gap in male smoking has reduced between the EU10 and the EU15 over the past 20 years, recent survey data still show a higher prevalence of current smoking in the new members of the European Union, with Latvian and Bulgarian men aged 20–64 years having the highest smoking rates (>50%) in Europe (except for Russia).

In women, the patterns of current smoking in the EU10 countries are different to those of men. In contrast to men, time trends in smoking differ by age groups and the average level of female smoking is still lower in the newer than in the older EU member states (Fig. 11.3). In addition, the differences in smoking rates of women are larger than of men. On the one hand, there are countries with very low (Romania and Lithuania have the lowest level of female smoking in Europe) or moderately low (Estonia, Latvia, Slovenia, Czech Republic, Slovakia) smoking rates when compared with other European countries. On the other hand, Bulgaria, Hungary, and Poland have one of the highest smoking prevalence rates in European women, especially in the young-adult and middle-aged populations. Unfortunately, besides Slovenia, Czech Republic, and Poland (only in the youngest adult women), smoking prevalence has not tended to decrease, but, on the contrary, it has even increased in recent years. In Bulgaria, this increasing trend has been observed for many years. In middle-age groups, where the level of smoking is still increasing in many CEE countries, this phenomenon seems to be linked with a birth cohort effect. In young-adult women, the increase in smoking rates is associated with sharp changes in experimentation with smoking that took place in the 1990s, when cigarettes were massively advertised in women's magazines and weekly smoking rates even doubled among young girls (Woynarowska 2002).

Tobacco-attributable mortality

The most important result of the analysis is that tobacco smoking is the single greatest contributor to the gap in premature mortality between the EU10 and EU15 countries, especially in men. Although the difference has narrowed since the political changes and developments of tobacco control policy in central and eastern Europe, premature mortality from tobacco-related causes remains higher in men in most EU10 countries than in the EU15 countries.

The heterogeneity between the EU10 countries in the importance of tobacco as the cause of premature mortality is an additional important result. Countries such as Slovenia and Czech Republic have reduced their rates of tobacco-related mortality to well within the range of the EU15 countries. However, Hungary and the Baltic States (as well as the Russian Federation, which was not systematically included in our analysis) experience very high rates among men.

Among women, differences in tobacco-related premature mortality between the EU10 and EU15 countries are less important, since the epidemic of smoking has not yet reached its maturity (see the above paragraph on tobacco smoking). However, this pattern does not concern all countries and all age groups. Hungarian women lead in lung cancer mortality (all age groups) in

Europe, having almost twice as high lung cancer mortality rates than the second leading European country (Netherlands) in the young adult population (20–44 years). The situation in tobacco-attributable mortality in the EU10 countries could even worsen in the future, since the prevalence of female smoking has not decreased in many CEE countries and smoking prevalence among girls has tended to increase in recent years.

Tobacco control policy

The collapse of the economic and political system at the end of the 1980s had two consequences for tobacco control. On one hand, it caused a rapid privatization of the tobacco industry in the region and the restoration of a structured tobacco market. Eastern Europe became one of the leading markets for transnational tobacco companies. Cigarette prices remained low, and teenagers were exposed to aggressive tobacco advertisements. On the other hand, democracy allowed the establishment of a health advocacy movement that was based on medical and scientific societies which helped parliaments to prepare and introduce comprehensive tobacco control legislation in the CEE countries. According to the resolution of the UICC International Conference 'Tobacco Free New Europe' that was held in November 1990 in Kazimierz, Poland, most eastern European countries started to work on the development of future comprehensive tobacco control strategies (Zatoński 2003c). Today, all EU10 countries have tobacco control legislation and strategies and have ratified the WHO Framework Convention on Tobacco Control (with the exception of the Czech Republic), although there are still gaps and challenges for the future (WHO 2004). In some CEE countries, comprehensive tobacco control policies were developed according to the best WHO standards and practices. In the 1990s, Poland's legislation was evaluated by international public health experts (and the tobacco industry as well!) as a strong policy measure that can diminish cigarette consumption on a national scale[5] (WHO 2004; Zatoński 2003c). Poland was one the first countries in the world where the total ban of tobacco advertising, promotion and sponsorship, including political parties, has been enforced. During discussions on the new EU Directive on enlarged health warnings on cigarette packs, policy makers gave an example of best practice from the Polish cigarette market. Membership of the CEE countries in the European Union was another milestone in the development of tobacco control policy and programmes. Today, enlarged health warnings are on all cigarette packs sold in CEE markets, and the content of tar, nicotine, and carbon monoxide is consistent with EU requirements. Since 1995 Poland has introduced ban on smoking in public places (at the time one of the first bans on smoking in public places in Europe), but with possibility of rooms for smokers. It is a very well implemented ban with the exception of hospitality industry. The ban is not effectively introduced only in 15% of the hospitality industry, mainly in discotheques and pubs. After the year 2000, already as members of the EU, following the example of Ireland, Norway, Italy, and other western European countries, Lithuania, Slovenia, and Estonia have enforced a ban on smoking in public places, including bars and pubs. In recent years (2008–2009) Poland have prepared and discussed legislative regulations in their parliaments for total ban on smoking in public places (Zatoński 2003a). Romania introduced pictorial health warnings on cigarette packs as the second country in Europe.

However, there are also big challenges that have to be confronted to help new members of the European Union to achieve worldwide standards in tobacco control. Probably the most important issue that has to be discussed within the family of European Union countries is the price and

---

[5] In fact, cigarette sale declined in Poland about 20–25% in the past 15 years, although industry predicted 10% increase on the sale market.

tax policy for tobacco products, including cigarette smuggling and tobacco subsidies for eastern European farmers. Despite attempts for harmonization of this policy made by the European Commission, prices for tobacco products remain at a low level in the eastern part of the European Union. Big differences in cigarette prices between the EU10 and EU15 countries (and within the EU10 countries), lead to cigarette smuggling and losses in government revenue from tobacco taxes. The chance to effectively intervene in the smoking behaviours of teenagers and economically disadvantaged people[6] through sharp increases in cigarette prices is passing by. CEE countries should also focus more on effective enforcement of existing strategies and action plans and take combined actions aimed to both prevent smoking initiation and to help smokers to quit. The Great Smokeout in Poland or smoking cessation programmes for medical doctors in the Czech Republic are good examples of the best practice in the EU10 countries (WHO 2007). Unfortunately, the participation of non-government organizations and local communities in tobacco control is still limited in central and eastern Europe. In general, they have to apply for government or European Union support and, in many cases, are too weak to separately contribute to these programmes.

Summary

Tobacco smoking is the single greatest contributor to the gap in premature mortality between eastern (EU10) and western (EU15) part of European Union, especially in the population of men. In some EU10 countries, the huge efforts made to reduce tobacco consumption have already produced notable results on tobacco-attributable mortality. The strong temporal decrease in tobacco-attributable mortality among young men is particularly encouraging. The gap in tobacco-attributable premature mortality between EU10 and EU15 countries remains impressive, and the effect of the tobacco-epidemic in central and eastern European countries will greatly affect the mortality patterns in this region for the next decades.

European Union has been faced with the necessity of closing the gap in tobacco control between eastern and western part of the community. There exist science and evidence-based premises that it can be done through:

1. creating progressive tax and price policy for tobacco products according to best standards in the EU

2. changing the attitude towards tobacco smoking through health information, public awareness campaigns, and counter-tobacco advertising

3. increasing relevant funding for effective tobacco control policy, programmes, and research, and ensuring support for tobacco control civil society movement

4. involving and educating health professionals, especially medical doctors, in smoking cessation treatment, and building capacity for developing smoking cessation programmes and services

5. introducing pictorial health warnings on cigarette packs

6. enforcing a complete ban of smoking in public places and worksites.

Acknowledgements

We would like to acknowledge all HEM – Closing the Gap project team members for their contribution to this chapter on all levels (collecting and submitting data, analysing the data, preparing

---

[6] Unemployed people are smokers two times more often than well-educated employees in CEE countries.

figures, writing paragraphs, and proofreading the final text). Especially we would like to thank to one of the HEM project Principal Co-Investigators Paolo Boffetta, who actively participated in the tobacco analysis in the project. Furthermore we would like to thank to Urszula Sulkowska, Krzysztof Przewoźniak, and Jakub Łobaszewski, who partly conducted the analysis and inspired creating the tables and figures (full list of the project team members with their affiliations is available on the project's website: www.hem.waw.pl).

References

Balabanova, D., Bobak, M., and McKee, M. (1998). Patterns of smoking in Bulgaria. *Tob Control*, 7(4): 383–5.

Bobak, M., Gilmore, A., McKee, M., Rose, R., and Marmot, M. (2006). Changes in smoking prevalence in Russia, 1996–2004. *Tob Contr*, **15**:131–15.

Didkowska, J., Mańczuk, M., McNeill, A., Powles, J., and Zatoński, W. (2005). Lung cancer mortality at ages 35–54 in the European Union: ecological study of evolving tobacco epidemics. *BMJ*, **331**(7510): 189–91.

Differences in worldwide tobacco use by gender: findings from the Global Youth Tobacco Survey (2003). *J Sch Health*, **73**(6):207–15.

Ezzati, M., Hoorn, S.V., Rodgers, A., Lopez, A.D., Mathers, C.D., and Murray, C.J. (2003). Comparative risk assessment collaborating group. Estimates of global and regional potential health gains from reducing multiple major risk factors. *Lancet*, **362**(9380):271–80.

Ezzati, M., Lopez, A.D. (2004). Smoking and oral tobacco use. In: M. Ezzati, A.D. Lopez, A. Rodgers, and C.J.L. Murray (eds), *Comparative quantification of health risks. Global and regional burden of disease attributable to selected major risk factors*. Vol. 1, p. 883–957. Geneva: World Health Organization.

Forey, B., Hamling, J., Lee, P., and Wald, N. (2002). *International Smoking Statistics. A collection of historical data from 30 economically developed countries*. 2nd edn. Oxford: The Wolfson Institute of Preventive Medicine.

Gilmore, A., Pomerleau, J., McKee, M., Rose, R., Haerpfer, C.W., Rotman, D. *et al.* (2004). Prevalence of smoking in 8 countries of the former Soviet Union: results from the living conditions, lifestyles and health study. *Am J Public Health*, **94**(12):2177–87.

Gilmore, A.B. and McKee, M. (2004). Tobacco and transition: an overview of industry investments, impact and influence in the former Soviet Union. *Tob Control*, **13**(2):136–42.

Jha, P., Peto, R., Zatoński, W., Boreham, J., Jarvis, M.J., and Lopez, A.D. (2006). Social inequalities in male mortality, and in male mortality from smoking: indirect estimation from national death rates in England and Wales, Poland, and North America. *Lancet*, **368**(9533):367–70.

Peto, R., Lopez, A.D., Boreham, J., and Thun, M. (2004). *Mortality from Smoking in Developed Countries 1950–2000*. 2nd edn. Imperial Cancer Research Fund and the World Organization. Oxford University Press.

Shafey, O., Dolwick, S., Guindon, G.E. (eds) (2003). *Tobacco Control Country Profiles*. 2nd edn. Atlanta, GA: American Cancer Society.

Sovinová, H., Csémy, L., Procházka, B., and Kottnauerová, S. (2008). Smoking-attributable mortality in the Czech Republic. *J Public Health*, **16**(1):37–42.

Strong, K., Guthold, R., Yang, J., Lee, D., Petit, P., and Fitzpatrick, C. (2008). Tobacco use in the European region. *Eur J Cancer Prev*, **17**(2):162–8.

The ASPECT Consortium. (2004). *Tobacco or Health in the European Union. Past, present and future*. Luxembourg: Office for Official Publications of the European Communities.

West R., Zatoński, W., Przewoźniak, K., and Jarvis, M.J. (2007). Can we trust national smoking prevalence figures? Discrepancies between biochemically assessed and self-reported smoking rates in three countries. *Cancer Epidemiol Biomarkers Prev*, **16**(4):820–2.

World Health Organization (2007). *The European Tobacco Control Report.* Copenhagen, Denmark: WHO., pp. 184–7

World Health Organization (2004). *Tools for advancing tobacco control in the 21st century. Tobacco control legislation: an introductory guide.* Geneva: WHO; pp. 184–7.

World Health Organization, Research for International Tobacco Control (2008). WHO Report on the Global Tobacco Epidemic, The MPOWER package. Geneva: World Health Organization.

Woynarowska, B. and Mazur, J. (2002). *Zachowania zdrowotne, zdrowie i postrzeganie szkoły przez młodzie ż w Polsce w 2002 r. Raport techniczny z bada ń.* [Health Behaviours, Health and Perception of School by Youth in Poland in 2002. A Technical Research Report]. Warsaw: Warsaw University and Institute of Mother and Child; 2002.

Zatoński W. (2003a). *A Nation's Recovery. Case Study of Poland's Experience in Tobacco Control.* Warsaw: Health Promotion Foundation; Available at: http://www.hem.home.pl/index.php?idm=58,59&cmd=1s

Zatoński W. (2003b). Decreasing smoking in Poland: the importance of a comprehensive governmental policy. *J Clin Psychiatry Monograph,* **18**(1):74–82.

Zatoński W. (2003c). Democracy and health: tobacco control in Poland. In: de Beyer J, Waverley Bridgen L, editors. *Tobacco Control Policy, Strategies, Successes, and Setbacks.* World Bank and Research for International Tobacco Control (RITC); pp. 97–120.

Zatoński W. (2003d). *Lung cancer trends in selected European Countries: What we can learn from the Swedish Experience with oral tobacco (snuff). ENSP Status Report on Oral Tobacco.* Brussel: European Network for Smoking Prevention; pp. 37–54.

Zatoński W. (2004). Tobacco smoking in central European Countries: Poland. In: P. Boyle, N. Gray, J. Henningfield, J. Seffrin, W. Zatoński (eds), *Tobacco and Public Health: Science and Policy,* pp. 235–52. Oxford University Press.

Zatoński, W.A., Mańczuk, M., Powles, J., and Negri, E. (2007). Convergence of male and female lung cancer mortality at younger ages in the European Union and Russia. *Eur J Public Health,* **17**(5):450–4.

Zatoński, W., Przewoźniak, K. (eds) (1992). *Zdrowotne nast ępstwa palenia tytoniu w Polsce* [Health Consequences of Tobacco Smoking in Poland]. Warsaw: Ariel Publishing Co.

Zatoński, W., Przewoźniak, K. (eds) (1999). *Palenie tytoniu w Polsce: Postawy, nast ępstwa zdrowotne i profilaktyka.* [Tobacco Smoking in Poland: Behaviors, Health Consequences, and Prevention]. 2nd edn. Warsaw: Cancer Center and Institute.

Chapter 12

The epidemic in India

Prakash C. Gupta and Cecily S. Ray

The introduction of tobacco

The story of tobacco in India began with royalty, but soon spread to the masses, despite health concerns. During the late sixteenth century, Portuguese traders introduced tobacco to the Bijapur kingdom (now Karnataka) ruled by Adil Shah. After a visit to Bijapur in around 1604–1605, Assad Beg, the Ambassador of the Mughal Emperor, Akbar, in Delhi, brought him back tobacco and jewel-encrusted European-style pipes. The appreciation at court was marred only by the Emperor's physicians who forbade him to inhale the smoke, since tobacco was an unknown substance. A compromise was reached wherein the smoke was to be first passed through water for purification, resulting in the invention of the hookah.

Hookah smoking became popular in parts of India where a strong Mughal influence prevailed; it was especially favoured among the aristocratic and elite classes despite health concerns. Ornately crafted in engraved silver, brass, or other precious materials and decorated with enamel or jewels, the hookah became a status symbol. Paintings of the Mughal period show both men and women smoking hookahs. The lower classes began to make them out of common woods and coconut shells and as the hookah was often shared, hookah smoking became associated with social acceptance, brotherhood, and equality. A common expression for social boycott in North India is to stop sharing the hookah and water from the village well.

In 1617, Emperor Jehangir, Akbar' son, decided that tobacco use produced adverse physical and mental effects on his subjects and tried to stop its use by declaring that any user would have his lips slit, but the practice continued nevertheless (Bhonsle et al. 1992).

Well before the introduction of tobacco smoking in India, the inhalation and smoking of aromatic herbs was practised as a form of therapy. When tobacco smoking was introduced, it was assigned medicinal qualities – as a calmative, relaxant, and stimulant. Aromatic substances were often added to tobacco smoked through hookah. A conical clay pipe, known as a *chilum*, traditionally used for smoking narcotics, began to be used for tobacco smoking as well (Bhonsle et al. 1992). Tobacco was often used to stave off hunger during travel and sustain long hours of work (Sanghvi 1992).

Evolution of tobacco use

Smoking

Tobacco began to be smoked in many ways, besides in the hookah and the chilum. The *hookli* is a European-style pipe with a clay bowl and stem (sometimes of wood) about 7–10 cm long, commonly used in western India for smoking sun-dried tobacco. The habit of smoking a rolled tobacco leaf, tied with a thread, known as a *chutta*, was documented as early as 1670 on the east coast of India, where women commonly smoke them in reverse, that is, with the glowing end inside the mouth. The *dhumti*, a large, cone-shaped roll of tobacco in a jack-fruit leaf

(*Artocarpus integrefolia L.*), is mainly used in the Konkan region, including Goa, and it, too, is often smoked in reverse by women. Reverse smoking is supposed to be convenient while doing household work and tending to children. It also generates extreme heat in the mouth, thought to be good for toothache, and the smoke is believed to mask halitosis. Girls learn to imitate the habit when asked by their mothers to light up for them. Some men practice reverse smoking too. The most popular smoking product in India today is the *bidi*, first documented in 1711 and mainly smoked by men (Bhonsle *et al.* 1992; Sanghvi 1992).

Smokeless tobacco

In addition to smoking, tobacco began to be used in a wide variety of ways in India. It found its way into betel quid (*paan*) at the Mughal court, where it was served from ornate boxes. Betel quid consists of a leaf of the *Piper betle* vine smeared with slaked lime (aqueous calcium hydroxide paste), pieces of the nut of the *Areca catechu* palm and, frequently, spices. The practice of chewing betel quid had reached South Asia by the first century or earlier, through contacts with the South Pacific Islands (Gode 1961). Chewing tobacco in betel quid soon became the most popular form of smokeless tobacco use.

Other smokeless tobacco preparations containing areca nut and slaked lime were developed. *Mainpuri* tobacco, popular in Uttar Pradesh, contains tobacco with slaked lime, finely cut areca nut, camphor, and cloves. *Mawa*, a relatively new preparation containing thin shavings of areca nut with some tobacco and slaked lime, is popular in Gujarat among youth. *Gutka*, a dry preparation containing areca nut, slaked lime, catechu, flavourings, powdered tobacco, and other additives, originally available custom-mixed from pan vendors, later began to be industrially manufactured and sold in tins and later, also in convenient sachets. Gutka, like mawa, contains both tobacco and areca nut, making it is highly addictive. The same mixture without tobacco is called *pan masala*. Offering pan masala to others is advertised as an act of hospitality, brotherhood, and equality, just like the traditional offering of betel quid to guests. Gutka and pan masala have been widely advertised since 1975 and have become very popular especially among youth (Jaiswal 2009). Since the enforcement of bans on the advertisement of tobacco products, pan masala advertisements are considered surrogate for gutka ads by tobacco control advocates.

Various combinations of tobacco, spices, molasses, and lime were developed for use in betel quid or separately. Raw tobacco is sold as bundles of long strands in Kerala. *Hogesoppu* is a leaf tobacco used by women in Karnataka. *Kaddipudi* are cheap 'powdered sticks' of raw tobacco used in Karnataka. Bricks and blocks of powdered tobacco mixed with jaggery (solid molasses) are also used. *Gundi* and *kadapan* are mixtures of coarsely powdered, cured tobacco, coriander seeds, other spices and aromatic, resinous oils, used in Gujarat, Orissa and West Bengal. *Kiwam*, used mainly in north India, is a thick paste of boiled tobacco mixed with powdered spices like saffron, cardamom, aniseed and musk, also available as granules or pellets. *Pattiwala* is sun-dried, flaked tobacco, used with or without lime, mainly in north India. North Indian tobacco and slaked lime preparations include *zarda*, coarsely cut tobacco, boiled till dry with slaked lime, with added colouring and flavouring agents, often expensive ones like saffron and cardamom. Zarda is sold in small sachets and tins, used by itself or in betel quid. *Khaini*, a mixture of sun-dried tobacco and slaked lime, is placed in the mandibular or labial groove and sucked slowly for 10–15 minutes, occasionally over night.

The nasal use of dry snuff, introduced by the Europeans and once fairly common, has all but died out. Snuff-like preparations became especially popular with women due to the misconception that they were good for teeth and gums (Bhonsle *et al.* 1992). *Masheri* or *mishri*, is a powdered black-roasted tobacco preparation used mainly in Goa and Maharashtra; *bajjar* is a dry snuff commonly used in Gujarat; *gudhaku* is a moist form of powdered tobacco and molasses from eastern India; tobacco toothpaste, also called 'creamy snuff', advertised as antibacterial, became popular in western parts of India; and, tobacco water, that is, water through which tobacco smoke has been passed, is sold for gargling in Manipur and Mizoram, where it is called hidakphu or tuibur, respectively.

With globalization, Swedish *snus* was launched in India in 2001 in pouch form in large cities of India under a brand name, 'Click', and marketed for a few years.

Tobacco production

From its earliest days in India, tobacco has played an important role in international trade and economic growth. Indeed, tobacco cultivation was inherited from the colonial period. During the seventeenth century, the Portuguese traders imported tobacco for sale in India, using the income to buy Indian cotton textiles for Portugal. After displacing the Portuguese in India, the British imported American tobacco to India to finance foreign trade. This lasted until the American Revolution in 1776, after which the East India Company began growing tobacco as a cash crop. The area under tobacco cultivation tripled during 1891–1921 (Sanghvi 1992).

Bidi making began as a small-scale activity in rural areas. Different kinds of leaves were tried as wrappers until the early 1890s when leaves of the tendu tree, also called temburni (*Diospyros melanoxylon*), growing mainly in the forests of Madhya Pradesh, were found to be the best suited. The oldest bidi manufacturing firm was established around 1887 and by 1930 the bidi industry had spread across the country. Some of the firms became very large, although the process of manufacturing by hand-rolling has remained the same (Chauhan 2001). Bidi manufacture, by far the most labour intensive of all tobacco industries, enjoys government protection, as bidis are made mostly at home by women.

The first Indian cigarette factory was established in 1906, by the Imperial Tobacco Company that was to become the Indian Tobacco Company (ITC), partly owned by British American Tobacco (Bhonsle 1992). From 1920 onwards, the growing urban market for cigarettes grew with the urban populace. Several smaller Indian cigarette companies also emerged. Later, in 1968, Philip Morris Inc entered India as the holding company of the pre-existing Godfrey Phillips India Ltd.

In 1938, the British Raj in India established a cigarette tobacco research station at Guntur, Andhra Pradesh, from where scientific inputs began to be provided for tobacco production. After independence in 1947, the Indian Government continued this practice through the Central Tobacco Research Institute at Rajahmundry, Andhra Pradesh (Chari and Rao 1992). Tobacco is currently a highly subsidised sector: farmers receive subsidies on water, electricity, and fertilizers as well as price support.

Independent India's tobacco production grew with the population from 1949 to 1997 as shown in Fig. 12.1. India currently produces over half a million kilos (680 million kg as of 2004–2005) of tobacco (Tobacco Board – About us, 2008). India is currently the world's third largest tobacco producer after China and Brazil, but produces only about 3.3% of the world's Flue Cured Virginia (FCV) (240 million kgs), according to the Tobacco Board (2002). India consumes about four-fifths of its total tobacco production. A small portion of tobacco used in India is imported.

Less than one-fifth of tobacco consumed in India is in the form of cigarettes (19%), more than half as bidis (about 54%), and the remaining 27% mostly as smokeless forms of tobacco (Panchamukhi *et al.* 2008).

Revenue and foreign exchange from tobacco

Tobacco produced in India contributes about Rs.82 billion or 12% of total excise revenue. State taxes on cigarettes bring in revenue equivalent to more than 10% of total excise collections from cigarettes (TIC 2003).

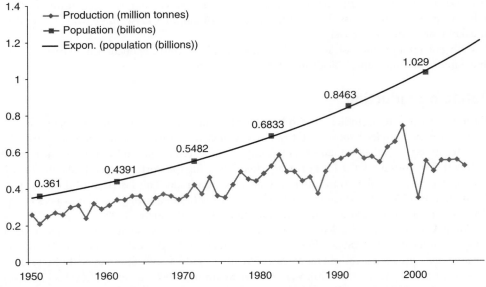

Figure 12.1 Tobacco Production* & Population Growth** in India, Year 1950–2006.

* Moon-Stone Group, 2000, FAOSTAT, 1999–2007.

** National Census figures: 1951–1991, Visaria, 2002; Census 2001: New Delhi: Office of the Registrar General & Census Commissioner, India; 2007.

Exported Indian tobacco earns about Rs.9.3 billion or 4% of agri-export revenue as foreign exchange earnings. The Tobacco Board has a vision for India to grab 5% of world market and earning Rs.50 billion (TIC 2003).

India exports about one-fifth of its tobacco production. Of the exported tobacco, 85% is in the unmanufactured form. In 2007–2008 India exported nearly 175 thousand metric tons of unmanufactured tobacco and 31 thousand metric tons of tobacco products. At least 70% of the exported tobacco, especially unmanufactured cigarette tobacco, is sent to western and eastern Europe, especially Belgium and Russia. Exports have shown a generally upward trend since 1988–1989 (Fig. 12.2).

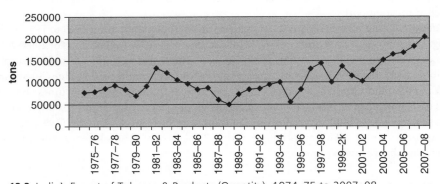

Figure 12.2 India's Export of Tobacco & Products (Quantity), 1974–75 to 2007–08.

Data source: Tobacco Board, 2008.
http://tobaccoboard.com/images/stats/1256207931exports1974-75.htm
Exports have shown a generally upward trend since 1988–89.

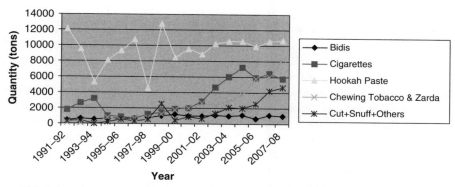

Figure 12.3 Tobacco Exports from India, Productwise, 1991–92 to 2007–08.

Data sources: Panchamukhi *et al.* 2008 and Tobacco Board, Exports Data: 2004 to 2008.
The increase in exports since 2001-02 is mainly due to smokeless tobacco.

The government sets targets for tobacco exports; some years these include specific product-wise targets. In 2003–2004, 2004–2005, 2005–2006, and 2006–2007, product-wise targets were exceeded in quantity and value. One-quarter of unmanufactured tobacco is exported to South and Southeast Asia; one half is sent to Europe and the rest elsewhere (Tobacco Board, Statistics 2008). Figure 12.3 shows the break-up of the tobacco exports quantity-wise by type.

Due to a depressed international market and a fall in domestic prices, the Indian Tobacco Board declared a crop holiday for the growing season of 1999–2000 in Andhra Pradesh and a cap on production in Karnataka. This was with the influence of the growers of Andhra Pradesh, who were left with most of their stocks from the previous year after the auctions were over (Menon and Sharma 2000).

The Tobacco Board of India views growing global demand for tobacco as an opportunity for export both in leaf form as well as products, which would translate into foreign exchange and employment. Projected growth in domestic consumption is also expected to lead to greater revenue (Hindu Business Line 2000)

Tobacco use

About 470 M (metric) tons of tobacco are consumed in India yearly. During 1950–1955, the annual per capita adult consumption of tobacco in India was around 900 g, which declined to 700 g by the late 1980s, small values compared to developed country standards. Consumption of tobacco was said to be increasing around 3% per year by Price Waterhouse Coopers in 2000. Until the end of the 1940s, tobacco was used mostly for hookah smoking and for chewing. Thereafter, bidi and cigarette smoking increased tremendously with bidis becoming the predominant tobacco habit (Sanghvi 1992). In recent years India has been witnessing a resurgence of smokeless tobacco consumption in industrially manufactured forms, especially among the young. By far most tobacco products consumed are produced in the country.

Prevalence in the general population

The most recent national measures of tobacco use prevalence come from the third round of the National Family Health Survey, conducted in 2005-6 (IIPS and ORC Macro, 2007), in which it was found that 57% of men and 10.9% of women aged 15–49 years were users of tobacco in some form. There was considerable variation in prevalence across the country (for men ranging from a low of 28% in Goa to a high of 83% in Mizoram and for women from a low of 1% in Punjab and Himachal Pradesh to a high of 61% in Mizoram). There was a preference for smokeless tobacco: 38.1% of men; 9.9% of women were smokeless tobacco users, while 33.3% of men and 1.6% of women were smokers. A considerable proportion of men (14.4%) were both smokeless tobacco users and smokers.

The most accurate information on tobacco use prevalence comes from house-to-house surveys carried out in individual areas. In these studies, conducted over a 40-year time span in different parts of India, the percentage using tobacco among men (>15 years age) ranged from 19% to 86% and among women from 7% to 77% (Table 12.1). Overall, tobacco use prevalence was higher in rural areas. Gender-wise, chewing habits were practised about equally by men and women, while most smokers were men. The prevalence of chewing in men varied from 11% to 55% and in women from 10% to 39%. Smoking prevalence varied from 8% to 77% in men and 2% to 12% in women with some exceptions.

In a few regional pockets where certain indigenous forms of smoking have been practised, women may smoke at equal or higher rates compared to men (Table 12.1). In one study in rural Srikakulam, Andhra Pradesh, 'reverse' chutta smoking was practised by 59% of women and 35% of men. In rural Darbhanga, Bihar, smoking was practised by nearly 11.4% of men and 21.8% of women – mainly hookah smokers (Mehta *et al.* 1971). Also, in an area of Orissa 85% of women smoked chuttas, compared to 30% of men (Jindal and Malik 1989). Among school personnel in rural and urban Bihar, 47.4% of men and 31% of women reported smoking (Sinha *et al.* 2002).

In some parts of Gujarat, like Bhavnagar and Ahmedabad, chewing of a new product called *mawa* became very popular among young men during the 1980s and 1990s. During a survey carried out in 1993–1994 in Bhavnagar, the prevalence of mawa use was 19%, whereas in 1969 it was around 4.7% (Gupta 2000; Mehta *et al.* 1971; Sinor *et al.* 1992). Another relatively new industrially manufactured tobacco and areca nut product, *gutka*, has become very popular, not only in Gujarat (Gupta 1999), but also in all of India.

Overall, tobacco use in India is inversely related to educational level. Using cross-sectional survey data from Mumbai, cigarettes smoking appears to increase with education (Gupta 1996), However, after controlling for age, cigarette smoking prevalence shows an inverse relationship with education, although with a small incline. In Mumbai, cigarette smoking is most common among professionals and traders, while bidis smoking is most common among unskilled workers and the unemployed (Sorensen *et al.* 2005). In Delhi, nearly a third of highly educated men in Delhi and Chandigarh reported smoking, mainly cigarettes (Bhattacharjee *et al.* 1994; Sarkar *et al.* 1990).

Prevalence among youth

While smoking continues be a threat, an easily observable trend among youth in India today is an increasing use of smokeless tobacco. One-third to one-half of children under the age of ten years in rural areas of different states experiment with smoking or smokeless tobacco in some form (Kapoor *et al.* 1995; Krishnamurthy *et al.* 1997; Vaidya *et al.* 1992). Despite Punjab's tradition of low tobacco use, Punjabi youth today are falling prey to gutka, as shown in a recent survey of rural school-going teenagers in five villages, where two-thirds regularly used it (Kaur and Singh 2002). The popularization of gutka in urban and rural areas of Gujarat, urban Bihar and Maharashtra has also been documented (Gupta and Ray 2002). In recent surveys conducted in secondary schools in Mumbai, about one-fifth of boys in the eighth, ninth, and tenth standards (aged about 13–15 years) were using gutka. In a municipal school, 9% of girls in ninth standard used gutka and in a private one, 5% of girls in seventh, eighth, and ninth standards used it. Surveys of street boys in Mumbai have shown that most start chewing gutka and smoking bidis by the age of eight years.

Table 12.1 Tobacco use prevalence among adults from population-based studies in rural and urban India

Area	Population Type	Reference	Sample size	% Tobacco users		
				Men	**Women**	**Overall**
National						
NFHS-3	15–48 yrs	IIPS & ORC Macro, 2007	198,754	57.0	10.8	--
Rural						
Maharashtra & Karnataka	Village	Khanolkar (1959)	9,996	84	a	a
Uttar Pradesh	Village	Khanolkar (1959)	12,637	82	a	a
Andhra Pradesh	Village	Khanolkar (1959)	7,249	86	a	a
Mainpuri, Uttar Pradesh	Village	Wahi (1968)	34,997	82	21	57
Bhavnagar, Gujarat	Village	Mehta et al. (1969)	10,071	71	15	44
Ernakulam, Kerala	Village	Mehta et al. (1969)	10,287	81	39	59
Srikakulam, Andhra Pradesh	Village	Mehta et al. (1969)	10,169	81	67	74
Singbhum, Bihar	Village	Mehta et al. (1969)	10,048	81	33	56
Darbhanga, Bihar	Village	Mehta et al. (1969)	10,340	78	51	64
Pune, Maharashtra	Village	Mehta et al. (1972)	101,761	62	49	64
Punjab	Village	Mohan et al. (1986)	24 villages	19	Very small	b
Goa	Village	Vaidya et al. (1992)	29,713	33	20	27
Bihar schools 60 rural 40 urban	School personnel	Sinha et al. (2002)	637 Smokeless: Smoking:	78 59 47	77 53 31	77 57 43
Urban						
Bombay	Police-men	Mehta et al. (1961)	4,734	76.5	a	a
Ahmedabad	Mill workers	Malaowalla et al. (1976)	57,518	b	b	85 (mostly men)
Mumbai	Lower SES group	Gupta (1996)	99,598	69	57.5	b
Delhi	All SES groups	Narayan et al. (1996)	13,558	45 c	7 c	b
Delhi	Mid-high SES group	Bhattacharjee et al. (1994)	508	31 c	a	a

a Women were not interviewed in these areas.

b Not reported.

c Only Smoking habits were assessed. SES = Socio-Economic Status.

Table 12.2 Tobacco use prevalence among adolescent students in the Global Youth Tobacco Survey – India, 2006.

Area	Age group	Reference	Sample size	% Tobacco Users		
				Males	Females	Overall
GYTS, 2006	13–15 yrs	Sinha et al., 2007	12,086	17.3	9.7	14.1

Two complete rounds of the Global Youth Tobacco Survey (GYTS) on school-going adolescents (grades 8–10 corresponding to ages 13–15 years) have been completed in India so far. In the round for 2006 (Table 12.2), current use of any form of tobacco by students (defined as use within the last 30 days) was overall 14.1% (95% CI: 11.9–16.7). This varied region-wise from 8% in the West (and 8.2% South) to 30.3% in the East and was greater than 20% in three regions. Cigarette smoking was 4.2% overall (1.8% females, 5.9% males) and varied from 0.7% in the West to 18.2% in the Northeast (Sinha *et al.* 2007). In the earlier round for 2003, with a much larger sample, the statewise prevalence of any current tobacco use ranged from 3.3% in Goa to 62.8% in Nagaland (Reddy and Gupta 2004). The GYTS results show that tobacco use among adolescent students is quite high. The use varies by state and region, the use of non-cigarette tobacco products is widespread and the prevalence is higher in males. Students reported smoking bidis, using smokeless tobacco products like gutka and khaini as well as pan masala.

In both rounds of the GYTS, over two-thirds of children who currently smoked cigarettes reported wanting to quit and many had made unsuccessful attempts (Reddy and Gupta 2004; Sinha *et al.* 2008). Nationwide in 2003, about half reported having been taught in school about the dangers of tobacco. This varied from 2.7% in Bihar to 75.5% in Punjab (Reddy and Gupta 2004).

Among college students in Maharashtra state, at least one-fifth reported using some form of tobacco. Cigarette smoking was reported by 10.6%, tobacco chewing by 6.7%, pan masala by 9.9%, and gutka by 9.6% – many had more than one habit. Awareness of the ill-effects of tobacco was generally low, especially for smokeless products (Hans 1998). A high prevalence (20–80%) has been observed among medical and dental students, raising a concern that in future they may not provide appropriate professional advice to tobacco users.

A survey of 1 587 male college students (aged 16–23 years) undertaken in 1998 in Karnataka revealed that 45% had ever tried tobacco products: 36.1% had tried cigarettes, 18.3% gutka, 9.9% bidis, 6.4% pan with tobacco, and 5.1% khaini (Nichter *et al.* 2004). The most popular products were cigarettes and 8.6% were daily users. Gutka was the next popular, but only 23 (1.4%) were daily users. The survey was conducted in 11 colleges in Mangalore (7) and surrounding towns (4). Daily smokers were 3.6 times more likely to have urban origin than be from villages.

Reasons for tobacco use

There are a wide variety of reasons why people use tobacco. Among lower socio-economic strata, people often use it to suppress hunger. In rural areas, people believe that tobacco has medicinal properties to cure or palliate common discomforts, like toothache, headache, and stomachache. Children copy the behaviour of their parents and other elders. People are largely unaware of the dangers posed by tobacco. Young working boys start smoking because they see others smoking and local shopkeepers give bidis to young boys to attract them for work. Labourers use smoking as a pretext to take a break from work.

The most common reason among children of the urban poor is their film hero who smokes. In higher socio-economic classes, children may smoke due to peer pressure, as a status symbol, family influence, and advertising. Advertisements on television, although banned on government channels, continue to be broadcast on cable and satellite channels. These, as well as ads on public buses and in print media influence tobacco use especially gutka, among children. Fun and enjoyment are among the most common reasons given by school and college students for using various addictive substances. The easy availability and low cost of most tobacco products are also important factors.

In the study among college students in Karnataka, smoking cigarettes was a way to relieve boredom, get a kick, relax, forget problems, get respect, etc. Smoking was also a response to how and when film heroes smoked (Nichter *et al.* 2004).

Burden due to tobacco

Premature mortality

Tobacco users experience a significantly higher mortality compared to nonusers, as shown by three cohort studies in different parts of India. Using conservative estimates (relative risk 1.4 for men and 1.3 for women) and prevalence of tobacco use (60% in men and 15% in women), it was estimated that about 630 000 deaths, that is, 12.6% of overall deaths, were attributable to tobacco use in 1986 (Gupta 1989). A later study by the Indian Council for Medical Research (ICMR) estimated that in 1996 the total number of tobacco-related deaths was 800 000 (Ministry of Health and Family Welfare 2001).

The most recent national case-control study providing information on number of tobacco-related deaths in adults aged 20 years and above, predicted that 930 000 deaths would be caused in 2010 due to smoking in India, that is, 10.5% of total adult deaths $\geq$ 20 years of age (8 846 000 deaths). Among men, smoking attributable deaths represented 16.7% of deaths. Significantly, among persons aged 30-69 years, men who smoked had a 2.3 fold higher risk (99%CI: 2.1-2.6) of dying of tuberculosis than nonsmokers. For women smokers the risk ratio was 3.0 (99%CI: 2.4-3.9) for dying of tuberculosis (Jha *et al.* 2008).

Disease risks

Tobacco use in India contributes to high incidence rates and numbers of cases of certain cancers (especially those of the head and neck and lung), lung diseases and cardiovascular disease. In various studies, the relative risks of cancers of the different sites of the upper alimentary and respiratory tracts have varied from 2.5–6.2 in chewers and 2.2–11.8 in smokers and 6.2–31.7 in those who both chew and smoke. The relative risk for smokers developing myocardial infarction and coronary artery disease (CAD) have varied from 2 to 3 fold. A four-fold prevalence of chronic obstructive lung disease (COLD) was found in smokers (Notani *et al.* 1989). An Expert Committee constituted by the ICMR used conservative risk estimates to calculate the number of avoidable cases of the three major disease groups due to tobacco use in 1999 (GOI 2001). This was updated for the year 2001–2002 as follows (Reddy and Gupta 2004):

* Incident tobacco-related cancers amounted to at least 200 000 cases.
* Prevalent CAD cases attributable to smoking amounted to 4.6 million.
* Prevalent cases of COLD attributable to smoking amounted to 40.7 million.

Financial costs

In the ICMR study on costs of tobacco-related diseases, the direct (medical and non medical, like travel and lodging) and indirect costs, like loss of income due to absenteeism during treatment and premature death were assessed. Cost information was collected on a cohort of 195 cancer patients for three years from 1990 and one year on 500 patients of CAD, 423 of COLD, and 28 patients of both CAD and COLD. The average cost per cancer patient, projected to the rates of 2001–2002, amounted to Indian Rupees (INR) 382 000, with direct costs amounting to 13% of total cost. The average yearly per capita costs in 1999 terms for CAD and COLD respectively amounted to INR 30 310 and INR 25 478 (USD 645 and USD 542), with direct costs accounting for 55% and 17%, respectively.

The cost of the tobacco-related cases of the three major diseases amounted to at least:

+ Total cost of Cancers: INR 65.04 billion (USD 1.4 billion)
+ Total cost of CAD: INR 139.7 billion (USD 3.0 billion)
+ Total cost of COLD: INR 103.57 billion (USD 2.2 billion)
+ Total cost of the three diseases: INR 308.33 billion (USD 6.6 billion).

These totals were updated to 2001–2002 using current prices and incomes in order to estimate the income and production losses, assuming that the other aspects remained unchanged – that is, assuming no acceleration in the burden of diseases or the cost of management of the disease. This conservative estimate of the social cost of tobacco use in India exceeded the total medical and public health outlay of the Central and State Governments (by around 5%) (Reddy and Gupta 2004).

For the sake of comparison, in 2000–2001, total excise revenues from tobacco corresponded to around INR 81.8 billion or USD 1.7 billion, and the nationwide annual consumer expenditure (in 1999–2000 – latest available data) on all tobacco products was INR 237 billion or around USD 5.0 billion (Panchamukhi et al. 2008). Clearly the economic benefit of tobacco to the country is unable to outweigh the costs accrued due to the diseases it causes.

Interventions
Primary prevention of tobacco-related diseases

Attempts have been made by NGOs to conduct educational campaigns through various media. In Mumbai, the Preventive Oncology Department of the Tata Memorial Centre, a cancer diagnosis and treatment centre, organized an anti-tobacco campaign in July–August, 2002, through college students volunteering in the National Social Service Scheme. After being informed of the harmful effects of tobacco use, the students developed street plays on the topic. They performed these plays in schools and public places.

In Delhi, a controlled anti-tobacco intervention among adolescent students of 30 schools (Project MYTRI – Mobilizing Youth for Tobacco Related Initiatives in India) was conducted to raise their awareness and involve them in activities like peer interaction within and between schools, family discussions, a signature campaign in the community, and an appeal to the Prime Minister. The post-test showed that students in the intervention group were significantly less likely than controls to have been offered, received, experimented with, or have intentions to use tobacco (Reddy et al. 2002).

Efforts in persuading illiterate villagers to stop or reduce their tobacco use have been attempted in rural areas. A large, controlled, educational intervention trial in tobacco users with ten years of annual follow-ups was conducted during 1967–1988 in three areas of India. Personal communication with visual aids after oral examination addressed factors for decision-making on tobacco use. Messages through personal communication were reinforced by documentaries, slides, posters, exhibitions, folk-dramas, radio messages, and newspaper articles (Gupta et al. 1986). The educational intervention was helpful in reducing tobacco use and in significantly increasing quit

Box 12.1 Performance of the first 13 Tobacco Cessation Centres (Dec. 2003 to Nov. 2004)

- 12 813 patients attended the centres: 11 918 males (93%) and 895 females (7%)
- Quit rates at 4 weeks were about 10% with about half (52%) having disappeared from follow-up by that time
- About one-fifth had been referred from other departments with co-morbidities
- Outreach by the TCCs into the surrounding communities, including corporations, resulting in increased attendance at the centres
- About 29% received pharmacotherapy
- Quit rates for patients given behavioural counselling alone or using pharmacotherapy also were both about 10%
- Rates of reduction in tobacco use were 26.1% for pharmacotherapy users and 18.4% of those receiving counselling alone
- Follow-up of patients was carried out through telephone calls, post cards, and fellow TCC subjects, but still around half (51.8%) of patients were lost to follow-up by 4 weeks (56.3% of patients treated by counselling only and 40.7% of patients treated with pharmacotherapy and counselling pharma).

Source: WHO-India 2004.

rates in two areas assessed after five and ten years of follow-up (9% and 14.3% in Ernakulam and 17% and 18.4% in Srikakulam) (Gupta *et al.* 1992).

In another intervention study conducted in Karnataka, after a five-year interval, quit rates in men and women respectively were 26.5% and 36.7% (Anantha *et al.* 1995).

The Government of India and the World Health Organization in India (WHO-India) have been collaborating on awareness campaigns, World No Tobacco Day events and setting up of tobacco cessation clinics (Kaur 2009). In 2002 they jointly set up 13 cessation clinics (Box 12.1), mostly in major cities of the country and mainly in tertiary care health institutions (cancer treatment centres, psychiatric centres, medical colleges, and NGOs) (WHO-India TFI 2008). In 2005, five additional centres were set up in five different states. The training programme was organized by the Bangalore tobacco cessation centre, that is part of the National Institute of Mental Health and Neuro-Sciences (NIMHANS).

In 2008, Pfizer, a US pharmaceutical multinational, began setting up 600 specialized smoking cessation clinics called Champix Clinics, where smokers who want to quit will be offered a three month treatment with Champix for Rs.9500 (≈ USD 195). This treatment is targeted at the affluent (Shrivastava 2008).

Government programmes

In addition to conducting an awareness campaign on tobacco use, the Central Government has been gearing up a new vertical programme: the National Tobacco Control Programme, under the Eleventh Plan Period (2007–2012), also in collaboration with the World Health Organization. So far this programme has been in the pilot phase, working in 9 states (18 districts) (Kaur 2009). When completely set up, its main components will include:

- A National Regulatory Authority (NRA)

- State Tobacco Control Cells
- District Tobacco Control Programmes
- Anti-tobacco Public Awareness Campaigns
- Establishment of tobacco testing labs.

Legislation

It is well known that raising the price of items like alcohol and tobacco decreases their consumption. Over 80% of total tobacco excise revenue in India comes from cigarettes. From early 1990s, bidis have begun to be taxed, albeit at very low level. Many smokeless tobacco products, which are becoming increasingly popular, are taxed at a low level but evasion is rampant. There is a great scope to control tobacco use through higher taxation.

As a result of a case filed in the Rajasthan High Court by a manufacturer of tobacco tooth powder against an amendment to the Drugs and Cosmetics Act, 1940, prohibiting tobacco in dental care products, the Central Committee on Food Standards recommended a ban on smokeless tobacco products. This has not been implemented but several states took the step of banning the sale, manufacture, and storage of gutka under Prevention of Food Adulteration Act as gutka is classified as a food product. Opposition from the producers resulted in a Supreme Court order stating that States cannot permanently ban tobacco products; only the Central Government can.

After years of groundwork, a comprehensive tobacco control law, reflecting the articles of the Framework Convention on Tobacco Control, began to go into force on 25 February 2004: The Cigarettes and Other Tobacco Products (Prohibition of Advertisement and Regulation of Trade and Commerce, Production, Supply and Distribution) Act, 2003. This Act of Parliament had received the assent of the President on 18 May 2003. It was meant to supersede a previous Act of 1975 that related solely to cigarettes. The new Act was framed so that its provisions would come into force by notification by the Central Government in the Official Gazette, which could be on different dates. Thus the first provisions to go into force included the prohibition of smoking in public places, a ban on advertising of tobacco products, except at points of sale, and of sale to minors. In addition, this notification granted power to the Central Government to make rules by notification in the Official Gazette, to carry out the provisions of the Act. On 16 November 2008 another Gazette notification was made for the provisions on health warnings to come into force on 1 December 2007. There have been various limitations to the effectiveness of this law for tobacco control: (1) The exclusion of points of sale from the prohibition on adverting, which led to a profusion of signboards with colourful cigarette logos and key words, like light, mild, and low; (2) Hurdles in implementing the bans on smoking in public places and sale to minors, including authorizing, sensitizing, and training enforcing personnel; (3) Protests to the government and in courts by tobacco industry representatives against newer rules limiting advertising at point of sale, prohibiting smoking, and pack placement in films and specifying health warnings. NGOs are working to overcome some of the problems, such as that of sensitizing and training government personnel in the states to implement the ban on smoking in public places and this has borne fruit. In places such as Rajasthan, Chandigarh, Maharashtra, and NGOs are trying to intervene where the law is tied up in courts.

Summary and conclusions

With an initial introduction into Indian royal courts by the Portuguese, tobacco use spread quickly throughout society, taking on many indigenously developed forms to suit local tastes.

The British colonizers promoted tobacco as a cash crop and as an industry. The independent Indian Government continued to support tobacco as a revenue earner and employment generator. Among the middle classes, smoking is not socially accepted for women and adolescents but smokeless tobacco is more widely accepted. The poor and uneducated have little awareness of health effects of tobacco, especially smokeless tobacco. Tobacco use, especially smoking, is more prevalent among men than women, except in some small regions. The youth have shown eagerness to experiment with new tobacco products like mawa and gutka along side more traditional products. Young children are prone to take up tobacco use, especially in rural areas and among the urban poor. Intervention studies have demonstrated that it is possible to reduce tobacco use through education but this needs to be done nationally. National legislative action to combat tobacco menace is now conforming to the Framework Convention for Tobacco Control, although implementation is taking time due to constraints in identifying, sensitizing, and training enforcement personnel, and interference from the tobacco industry. New plans and budgets have incorporated elements dedicated to tobacco control.

References

Anantha, N., Nandakumar, A., Vishwanath, N., Venkatesh, T., Pallad, Y.G., Manjunath, P. *et al.* (1995). Efficacy of an anti-tobacco community education program in India. *Cancer Causes and Control*, **6**: 119–29.

Bhattacharjee, J., Sharma, R.S., and Verghese, T. (1994). Tobacco smoking in a defined community of Delhi. *Indian Journal of Public Health*, **38**:22–6.

Bhonsle, R.B., Murti, P.R., and Gupta, P.C. (1992). Tobacco habits in India. In: P.C. Gupta, J.E. Hamner III, and P.R. Murti (eds) *Control of tobacco-related cancers and other diseases*, pp. 25–46. International Symposium, 1990. Oxford University Press, Bombay.

Census of India (2001). New Delhi: Office of the Registrar General & Census Commissioner, Government of India; 2007. Available from: http://www.censusindia.gov.in/Census_Data_2001/National_Summary/National_Summary_DataPage.aspx (Accessed 20th October, 2008).

Chari, M.S. and Rao, B.V.K. (1992). Role of tobacco in the national economy: past and present. In: P.C. Gupta, J.E. Hamner III, and P.R. Murti (eds) *Control of Tobacco-Related Cancers and Other Diseases*, pp. 57–76. International Symposium, 1990. Oxford University Press, Bombay.

Chauhan, Y. (2001). *History and struggles of Beedi workers in India*. All India Trade Union Congress, New Delhi.

Food and Agriculture Organization. Major Food and Agricultural Commodities and Producers. Data extracted from the FAOSTAT database. Rome, 2003. http://www.fao.org/es/ess/top/commodity.jsp?commodity=27&lang=EN (Accessed 2 July 2003).

Gode, P.K. (1961). Studies in Indian Cultural History. *Indological Series 9, Institute Publication, No. 189.* Hoshiarpur: Vishveshvaranand Vedic Research Institute. Vol. I, pp. 111–90.

Gupta, P.C. (1989). An assessment of excess mortality caused by tobacco usage in India. In: L.D. Sanghvi and P.P. Notani (eds) *Tobacco and Health: The Indian Scene*, pp. 57–62. Proceedings of the UICC workshop, 'Tobacco or Health', April 15–16, 1987, Tata Memorial Centre, Bombay.

Gupta, P.C. (1996). Survey of sociodemographic characteristics of tobacco use among 99,598 individuals in Bombay, India using handheld computers. *Tobacco Control*, **5**:114–20.

Gupta, P.C. (1999). Mouth cancer in India: a new epidemic? *Journal of Indian Medical Association*, **97**: 370–3.

Gupta, P.C. (2000). Oral cancer and tobacco use in India: a new epidemic. In: *Tobacco the Growing Epidemic* – Proceedings of the 10th World Conference on Tobacco or Health, 24–28 August 1997, pp. 20–21. Beijing, China.

Gupta, P.C. and Mehta, H.C. (2000). A cohort study of all-cause mortality among tobacco users in Mumbai, India. *Bulletin of the World Health Organization*, **78**:877–83.

Gupta, P.C., Mehta, F.S., Pindborg, J.J., Aghi, M. B., Bhonsle, R.B., Daftary, D.K. *et al.* (1986). Intervention study for primary prevention of oral cancer among 36 000 Indian tobacco users. *Lancet*, **i**:1235–9.

Gupta, P.C., Mehta, F.S., Pindborg, J.J., Bhonsle, R.B., Murti, P.R., Daftary, D.K. *et al.* (1992). Primary prevention trial of oral cancer in India: a 10-year follow-up study. *Journal of Oral Pathology and Medicine*, **21**:433–9.

Gupta, P.C. and Ray, C. (2002). Tobacco and youth in the South East Asian region. *The Indian Journal of Cancer*, **39**:5–35.

Gupta, P.C., Pednekar, M.S., Parkin, D.M., and Sankaranarayanan, R. (2005). Tobacco associated mortality in Mumbai (Bombay) India. Results of the Bombay Cohort Study. *Int. J. Epidemiol.*, **34**: 395–402. Available from: http://ije.oxfordjournals.org/cgi/content/full/34/6/1395

Hans, G. (1998). *Prevention of Cancer in Youth with Particular Reference to Intake of Paan Masala and Gutkha*, NSS Unit, TISS, Mumbai, India.

Indian tobacco industry must go global *Hindu Business Line* (2000). 16 February, Internet edition. Available at: http://www.thehindubusinessline.com/2000/02/16/stories/141644b7.htm

International Institute for Population Sciences (IIPS) and ORC Macro International, *National Family Health Survey (NFHS-3), 2005–06: India* (Volume II) (2007). pp. 426-429. IIPS, Mumbai. Available from:http://www.nfhsindia.org/NFHS-3%20Data/VOL-1/Chapter%2013%20-%20Morbidity%20and%20Health%20Care%20(475K).pdf

Jaiswal, A. (2009) Tobacco consumption: gutka leads over cigarette. Chandigarh: *The Tribune*. 18 January. Available at: http://www.tribuneindia.com/2009/20090118/cth1.htm (Accessed 3 April 2009).

Jha, P., Jacob, B., Gajalakshmi, V., Gupta, P.C., Dhingra, N., Kumar, R. *et al.* (2008). A nationally representative case-control study of smoking and death in India. *New England Journal of Medicine*, **358**:1137–47.

Jindal, S.K., and Malik, S.K. (1989). Tobacco smoking and non-neoplastic respiratory disease. In: L.D. Sanghvi and P.P. Notani (eds) *Tobacco and Health: The Indian Scene*, pp. 30–6. Proceedings of the UICC workshop, 'Tobacco or Health', 15–16 April 1987, Tata Memorial Centre, Bombay.

John, R.M. (2006). Household's tobacco consumption decisions: evidence from India. *Journal of South Asian Development*, **1**:119–47.

Kapoor, S.K., Anand, K., and Kumar, G. (July–August 1995). Prevalence of tobacco use among school and college going adolescents of Haryana. *Indian Journal of Paediatrics*, **62**:461–6.

Kaur J. (2009). National Tobacco Control Programme. Ministry of Health and Family Welfare, Government of India. Powerpoint presentation for the Second National Capacity Building Workshop for NGO personnel organised by HRIDAY-SHAN on behalf of AFTC at PHD House, New Delhi (2–3 February 2009). Available at: http://www.hriday-shan.org/NCB%20Workshop2/Presentations/Day1/Government%20of%20India's%20Tobacco%20Control%20Initiatives%20and%20National%20Tobacco%20Control%20Program/Government%20of%20India's%20Tobacco%20Control%20Initiatives%20and%20National%20Tobacco%20Control%20Program.ppt (Accessed 3 April 2009).

Kaur, S. and Singh, S. (2002). Cause for concern in Punjab villages. High levels of Gutkha intake among students. *Lifeline*, January, **7**:3–4.

Khanolkar, V.R. (1959). Oral Cancer in India. *Union International Contra Cancrum Acta*, **15**:68–77.

Krishnamurthy, S., Ramaswamy, R., Trivedi, U., and Zachariah, V. (October 1997). Tobacco use in Rural Indian Children. *Indian Journal of Paediatrics*, **34**:923–27.

Malaowalla, A.M., Silverman, S., Mani, N.J., Bilimoria, K.F., and Smith, L.W. (1976). Oral cancer in 57,518 industrial workers of Gujarat, India. A prevalence and follow-up survey. *Cancer*, **37**:1882–6.

Mehta, F.S., Gupta, P.C., Daftary, D.K., Pindborg, J.J., and Choksi, S.K. (1972). An epidemiologic study of oral cancer and precancerous conditions among 101,761 villagers in Maharashtra, India. *International Journal of Cancer*, **10**:134–41.

Mehta, F.S., Pindborg, J.J., Gupta, P.C., and Daftary, D.K. (1969). Epidemiologic and histologic study of oral cancer and leukoplakia among 50,915 villagers in India. *Cancer*, **24**:832–49.

Mehta, F.S., Pindborg, J.J., Hamner, J.E., Gupta, P.C., Daftary, D.K., Sahiar, B.E. *et al.* (1971). Report on investigations of oral cancer and precancerous conditions in Indian rural populations, 1966–1969. Munksgaard, Copenhagen.

Mehta, F.S., Sanjana, M.K., Shroff, B.C., and Doctor, R.H. (1961). Incidence of leukoplakia among 'Pan' (betel leaf) chewers and bidi smokers: a study of a sample survey. *Indian Journal of Medical Research*, **49**:393–9.

Menon, P. and Sharma, R. (2000). A crop holiday for tobacco. *Frontline*, 13–26 May; **17**(10): Available at: http://www.flonnet.com/fl1710/17100940.htm

Ministry of Health and Family Welfare (2001). Report of the expert committee on the economics of tobacco use. Department of Health, Ministry of Health and Family Welfare, Government of India, New Delhi, pp. 9–19; 39–45; 50; 89; 152 (unpublished).

Mohan, D., Sundaram, K.R., and Sharma, H.K. (May 1986). A study of drug abuse in rural areas of Punjab (India). *Drug and Alcohol Dependence*, **17**:57–66.

Moon-Stone Group (2000). *Tobacco, all-India area, production and yield of tobacco.* Hyderabad: Moonstone Group. Available at: http://www.indiancommodity.com/statistic/tobaco.htm (Accessed 16 August 2002).

Narayan, K.M.V., Chadha, S.L., Hanson, R.L., Tandon, R., Shekhawat, S., Fernandes, and R.J., Gopinath N. (Jun 1996). Prevalence and patterns of smoking in Delhi: cross sectional study. *British Medical Journal*, **312**:1576–9.

Nichter, M., Nichter, M., and Van Sickle, D. (2004). Popular perceptions of tobacco products and patterns of use among male college students in India. *Social Science and Medicine* 2004, **59**:415–31.

Notani, P.N., Jayant, K., and Sanghvi, L.D. (1989). Assessment of morbidity and mortality due to tobacco usage in India. In: L.D. Sanghvi and P.P. Notani (eds) *Tobacco and Health: The Indian Scene*, pp. 63–78. Proceedings of the UICC workshop, 'Tobacco or Health', 15–16 April 1987. Tata Memorial Centre, Bombay.

Panchamukhi, P.R., Woolery, T., and Nayantara, S.N. (2008). Economics of bidis in India. In: P. Gupta and S. Asma (eds) *Bidi Smoking and Public Health.*, Ministry of Health and Family Welfare, Government of India, New Delhi,. pp. 167-195. Available from: http://www.whoindia.org/LinkFiles/Tobacco_Free_Initiative_bidi_and_public_health.pdf

Price Waterhouse Coopers (2000). Selangaor Darul Ehsani: British American Tobacco, Malaysia. Available at: Batmalaysia.com-Corporateinformation-investorRelations-The TobaccoIndustry-India Final Report.pdf (Accessed 16 August 2002).

Reddy, K.S. and Gupta, P.C. (eds). (2004). *Report on Tobacco Control in India*. Ministry of Health and Family Welfare, Government of India, New Delhi, pp. 129–38. Available at: http://www.whoindia.org/SCN/Tobacco/Report/TCI-Report.htm (Accessed 14 November 2008).

Reddy, K.S., Arora , M., Perry, C.L., Nair, B., Kohli , A., Lytle, L.A., *et al.* (2002). Tobacco and alcohol use outcomes of a school-based intervention in New Delhi. *Am J Health Behav.* May-Jun, **26**(3):173–81.

Sanghvi, L.D. (1992). Challenges in tobacco control in India: a historical perspective. In: P.C. Gupta, J.E. Hamner III, and P.R. Murti (eds) *Control of Tobacco-Related Cancers and other Diseases.* International Symposium, 1990, pp. 47–55. Oxford University Press, Bombay.

Sarkar, D., Dhand, R., Malhotra, A., Malhotra, S., and Sharma, B.K. (January to March 1990). Perceptions and attitude towards tobacco smoking among doctors in Chandigarh. *Indian Journal of Chest Diseases and Allied Sciences*, **32**:1–9.

Shrivastava B. (2008). Dilemma over anti-smoking drug. New Delhi: OneWorld South Asia. 29 Apr. Available at: http://southasia.oneworld.net/Article/dilemma-over-anti-smoking-drug (Accessed 8 December 2008).

Sinha, D.N., Gupta, P.C., Pednekar, M.S., Jones, J.T., and Warren, C.V. (2002). Tobacco use among school personnel in Bihar, India. *Tobacco Control*, **11**:82–85.

Sinha, D.N., Gupta, P.C., and Gangadharan, P. (2007). Tobacco Use among students and school personnel in India. *Asian Pacific Journal of Cancer Prevention*, **8**:417–21.

Sinha, D.N., Gupta, P.C., Reddy, K.S., Prasad, V.M., Rahman, K., Warren, C.W. *et al.* (2008). Linking Global Youth Tobacco Survey 2003 and 2006 data to tobacco control policy in India. *The Journal of School Health* 2008, **78**:368–73.

Sinor, P.N., Murti, P.R., Bhonsle, R.B., and Gupta, P.C. (1992). Mawa chewing and oral submucous fibrosis in Bhavnagar, Gujarat, India. In: P.C. Gupta, J.E. Hamner III, and P.R. Murti (eds) *Control of Tobacco-Related Cancers And Other Diseases*, International Symposium, 1990, pp. 107–12. Oxford University Press, Bombay.

Sorensen, G., Gupta, P.C., and Pednekar, M.S. (2005). Social disparities in tobacco use in Mumbai, India: the roles of occupation, education, and gender. *American Journal of Public Health*, **95**:1003–8.

TIC Economic Bureau. (2003) National symposium on tobacco to focus on future challenges news. Navi Mumbai (Belapur): The Information Company Pvt Ltd (TIC); 22 January. Available at: http://www.domain-b.com/economy/trade/20030122_symposium.html (Accessed 22 October 2008).

Tobacco Board (2008) About us. Available at: http://www.indiantobacco.com/aboutus.php (Accessed 14 November 2008).

Tobacco Board (2008) Statistics. Exports of tobacco and tobacco products since 1974–75. Guntur, AP: Tobacco Board. Ministry of Commerce, Government of India. Available at: http://www.indiantobacco.com/reports.php; http://tobaccoboard.com/images/stats/1256207931exports1974–75.htm (Accessed 14 November 2008).

Tobacco Board (2008) Statistics. Exports data. Guntur, AP: Tobacco Board. Ministry of Commerce, Government of India. Available at: http://tobaccoboard.com/component/option,com_tobstats/Itemid,182/cat,Exports%20data/lang,english/ (Accessed 11 December 2008).

Vaidya, S.G., Vaidya, N.S., and Naik, U.D. (1992). Epidemiology of tobacco habits in Goa, India. In: P.C. Gupta, J.E. Hamner III, and P.R. Murti (eds) *Control of Tobacco-Related Cancers and Other Diseases*, International Symposium, 1990, pp. 315–22. Oxford University Press, Bombay.

Visaria, P. (2002). Population policy in India, performance and challenges. *The National Medical Journal of India*, 15, Suppl.1:6–18.

Wahi, P.N. (1968). Epidemiology of oral and oropharyngeal cancer. *Bulletin of the World Health Organization*, 38:495–521.

WHO-India Core Program Clusters, Non-communicable Diseases and Mental Health, Tobacco Free Initiative, Tobacco Cessation Clinics. (2008). Available at: http://www.whoindia.org/EN/Section20/Section25_952.htm (Accessed 8 December 2008).

WHO-India. (2004). Draft Compiled Report on TCCs in India December 2003 to November 2004 (Unpublished).

Chapter 13

Tobacco—the growing epidemic*

Richard Peto, Zheng-Ming Chen, and Jillian Boreham

The largest study ever undertaken to examine the health effects of tobacco finds that there are already a million deaths a year from smoking in China, and it predicts large increases in mortality over the next few decades. This pattern is likely to be repeated in other developing countries.

CHINA, WITH 20% of the world's population, produces and consumes about 30% of the world's cigarettes. The first nationwide study of the effects of smoking in any developing country now shows that China already suffers almost a million deaths a year from tobacco [1,2] (the full reports are freely available at *http://www.bmj.com*). This is more than in any other country, and the hazards are expected to increase substantially over the next few decades as a delayed effect of the recent rise in cigarette use. To monitor the current and future hazards of tobacco use, the Chinese study consisted of two parts: one retrospective [1] and one prospective [2]. The retrospective study, which assessed current mortality from tobacco use in China, was of a new design (see legend to Figure 13.1) and involved analysis of one million deaths. The prospective study (the early results from which confirm the retrospective results) began by interviewing a quarter of a million adults and will continue for decades, monitoring the long-term growth of the epidemic.

Apart from HIV/AIDS, tobacco is the only major cause of death that is increasing rapidly[3]. Worldwide, smoking caused about 3 million deaths in 1990, out of a total of 30 million adult deaths from all causes, and it will cause about 10 million in 2030, out of a total of about 60 million [4,5]. Most of this projected increase in tobacco deaths will take place in Asia, Africa and South America. Until recently, such projections had to be based chiefly on extrapolation from studies in developed countries such as Britain or the United States [6,7]. But, most of the world's one billion smokers live in developing countries, where the effects of smoking could well be different, so local studies are urgently needed.

This new Chinese evidence needs to be seen in the context of Western epidemiological evidence, which demonstrates the peculiarly long delay between cause and full effect. In countries such as Britain and the United States, most of those who now smoke cigarettes began to do so in early adult life, and recent UK/US prospective studies show that about half of all persistent smokers are eventually killed by their habit [6,7]. Fifty percent of these tobacco deaths occur in middle age (here defined as 35–69 years), and half in old age [4]. But only those who have smoked cigarettes since early adulthood are at particularly high risk in middle and old age, so earlier UK/US prospective studies—conducted after the rise in cigarette use but only halfway through the increase in mortality—misleadingly suggested that the risks of tobacco use were lower [8]. The need for prolonged smoking before the full risks become evident means that if a country experiences a

* This chapter was originally published in *Nature Medicine* journal (Peto *et al.*, Tobacco—the growing epidemic, *Nature Medicine* 1999; **5**: 15–17) and is reproduced with the kind permission of the authors and Nature Publishing Group.

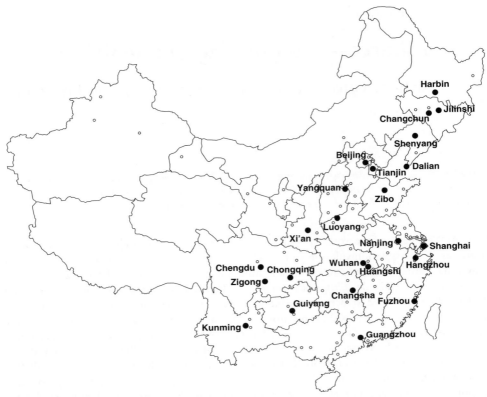

Figure 13.1 For the one million people who died between 1986 and 1988 in 24 cities (filled circles on map) and in various rural areas of China (open circles), the disease that caused death was determined and the family was interviewed to discover what the deceased person had smoked. The smoking habits of 0.7 million Chinese adults who had died of neoplastic, respiratory or vascular causes were compared with the habits of the 'reference group' of 0.2 million adults who had died of other causes. The threefold excess of lung cancer deaths among smokers could then be inferred from the excess, in comparison with the reference group, of smokers in the lung cancer death category. (Similarly, the excesses of various other diseases among smokers could be calculated.) In each city the local relative risk, the local prevalence of smoking and the local lung cancer rate (standardized for age by averaging the seven death rates at ages 35–9, 40–4 ... 65–9) could then be combined to calculate the absolute lung cancer rates among smokers and non-smokers separately (see Fig.13.2).

This figure was reproduced from ref. 1 with permission from the *Br. Med. J.*

nationwide surge in cigarette use by young adults then this will cause a large increase in tobacco deaths about a half-century later. Until then, however, there may be several decades during which cigarette consumption is high but mortality from tobacco is still relatively low.

In developed countries, cigarette smoking became popular during the first half of the twentieth century, so the main increase in tobacco deaths has been seen during the second half of this century. For example, mean US cigarette consumption per adult in 1910, 1930 and 1950 was 1, 4 and 10 a day, respectively, after which it remained fairly constant for a few decades. Therefore, the proportion of all US deaths at ages 35–69 attributed to tobacco rose from 12% in 1950 to 33% in 1990 [4].

In many developing countries, cigarette smoking became widespread only during the last 30 years, so the main consequences of this will emerge next century. For example, the US pattern of an increase in cigarette smoking between 1910 and 1950 has been repeated 40 years later in China. Mean cigarette consumption per Chinese man in 1952, 1972 and 1992 was 1, 4 and 10 per day, respectively, after which it seems to have leveled off [1]. Both the retrospective study and the early results from the prospective study in China indicate that in 1990 tobacco caused about 12% of adult male deaths, and by 2030 it will probably be a cause of about one third of them. About two thirds of young Chinese men become cigarette smokers in early adult life, and in China, as in America, about half of those who do so will eventually be killed by their habit. Thus, about one third of all young Chinese men will eventually, in middle or old age, be killed by tobacco. As about 10 million a year reach manhood in China, the annual number of tobacco deaths will rise from almost 1 million now to about 3 million in the middle of the next century. Hence, there will be a total of about 100 million deaths caused by tobacco in China during the first half of the next century.

But even if the overall 50% hazard is about the same in China as elsewhere, these new studies show that the chief diseases by which tobacco causes death are very different in China (and, within China, between one city and another). In the United States, for example, tobacco causes far more deaths from heart attacks than from emphysema, whereas in China the opposite is true. Of Chinese tobacco deaths, almost half involve emphysema, and the proportions involving tuberculosis, esophageal cancer, stomach cancer and liver cancer are each about as large (5–8%) as the proportions involving heart disease or stroke.

Lung cancer, which was the first major disease to be reliably linked to smoking in Western studies, is also an important hazard for Chinese smokers, but, unexpectedly, there is a tenfold variation from one Chinese city to another in the magnitude of this hazard (see Fig. 13.2). In each city, the lung cancer rate is about three times as great among smokers as among non-smokers, but there is a tenfold variation in the non-smoker lung cancer rates, which in some cities, perhaps chiefly because of domestic heating and cooking fumes, are ten times greater than the rates among US non-smokers. There was even wider variation between one city and another in the non-smoker emphysema death rates, which in some cities were almost 100 times greater than those in US non-smokers.

From a public health perspective, the main finding of the Chinese study is the alarming overall risk of death, which can be stated in various ways: tobacco will eventually kill one third of all young men in China; it will kill half of all persistent cigarette smokers; there will be one million tobacco deaths a year in China during the first decade of the next century, 2 million a year by 2025, 3 million a year by mid-century, and a total of 100 million during the first 50 years of the next century. In comparison, most of the intriguing little details of how tobacco kills are of less immediate importance.

The chief exception, however, concerns women. The bad news is that if women smoke like men they die like men; their overall risks are about the same. But the good news is that on the whole Chinese women don't smoke like men; unexpectedly (and unexplainedly), the proportion of women who became smokers before the age of 25 has decreased enormously over the past few decades. If this low uptake rate of smoking by young women continues then, although the proportion of deaths attributed to smoking in 1990 and in 2030 will increase from 12% to about 33% for Chinese men, it will decrease from 3% to 1% for Chinese women. Tobacco would then be responsible for most of the difference in life expectancy between men and women in China.

The only hope of substantially limiting worldwide tobacco deaths in the first half of the next century is for many of the adults who now smoke to stop doing so, because discouraging young people from starting will take half a century to produce its main health benefits. Western studies

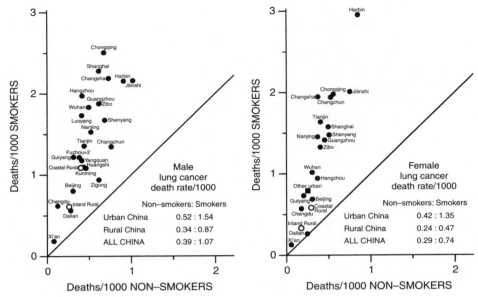

Figure 13.2 Death rates at ages 35–69 from lung cancer in various parts of China: smokers versus nonsmokers (1986–1988). The lung cancer rates show wide variation, with extremely high rates in some cities among non-smokers and, particularly, among smokers. In comparison, the nationwide US lung cancer death rates in 1990, similarly standardized for age, were 1.4 per 1,000 men and 0.6 per 1,000 women, and were 0.1 per 1,000 male or female US non-smokers.

This figure was reproduced from ref. 1 with permission from the *Br. Med. J.*

show that, even in middle age, cessation of smoking is remarkably effective, removing most of the 50% risk of death from tobacco if smoking persists. Stopping at earlier ages is even more effective [6]. Britain, which is now experiencing the most rapid decrease in the world in premature deaths from tobacco, shows that large improvements are possible: over the past 30 years, UK cigarette sales have halved, as have UK tobacco deaths in middle age [3]. At present, however, such changes are chiefly limited to educated Western smokers; Chinese smokers, for example, rarely stop until

Tobacco control in China: economically favourable options for central government

♦ Big tax increases will make some smokers stop, preventing many future deaths, but will still increase total government income from tobacco.

♦ Big packet health warnings in Chinese, stating that tax has been paid in China, will help some smokers to stop and will help the government prevent smuggling.

♦ Absolute ban on all types of tobacco advertising or promotion will help prevent women from ever starting and will help keep out foreign tobacco companies.

On present smoking patterns, where 2/3 of the young men in China start smoking, and few smokers quit the habit, there will be about 100 million tobacco deaths in China over the next 50 years, **unless** there is widespread cessation of smoking.

they are too ill to continue. So, the worldwide network of epidemiological studies of tobacco deaths in developing countries—such as India, Mexico, Cuba, Egypt and South Africa—that are being modeled on these Chinese studies, is likely to document a growing epidemic in these nations over the next few decades.

Acknowledgment

We thank the Chinese principal investigators [1,2] and our funding organizations.

References

1. Liu, B.Q. *et al.* (1998). Emerging tobacco hazards in China: 1. Retrospective proportional mortality study of one million deaths. *Br.Med. J*, **317**:1411–1422.

2. Niu, S.R. *et al.* (1998). Emerging tobacco hazards in China: 2. Early mortality results from a prospective study. *Br.Med. J*, **317**:1423–1424.

3. Ad Hoc Committee on Health Research (1996). Investing in health research and development. The World Health Organization, Geneva, Switzerland.

4. Peto, R., Lopez, A.D., Boreham, J., Thun, M., and Heath, C. Jr. (1994). Mortality from smoking in developed countries 1950–2000: Indirect estimates from national vital statistics. Oxford University Press.

5 Murray, C.J.L. and Lopez, A.D. (eds) (1996). In *The global burden of disease*. Harvard School of Public Health, Boston, Massachusetts.

6. Doll, R., Peto, R., Wheatley, K., Gray, R., and Sutherland, I. (1994). Mortality in relation to smoking: 40 years' observations on male British doctors. *Br.Med. J*, **309**:901–911.

7. Thun, M.J. *et al.* (1997). Alcohol consumption and mortality among middle-aged and elderly U.S. adults. *N. Engl. J. Med*, **337**:1705–1714.

8. U.S. Department of Health & Human Services (1989). Reducing the health consequences of smoking: 25 years of progress. A Report of the Surgeon General. U.S. Department of Health & Human Services, Public Health Service, Centers for Disease Control, Center for Chronic Disease Prevention and Health Promotion, Office on Smoking and Health. DHHS Publication No. (CDC) 89–8411.

Chapter 14

Tobacco control in the Republic of South Korea, an Asian example

Jae-Gahb Park, Ji Won Park, Hong-Gwan Seo, Jin Soo Lee, Il Soon Kim, Yong-Ik Kim, Jong-Koo Lee, and Dae-Kyu Oh

Introduction

There has been a huge recognition on harmfulness of smoking in the Republic of South Korea in a relatively short period of time. Adult male smoking rates rapidly fell over the past 7 years, from 67.6% to 43.4%. Along with government and nongovernmental organizations (NGOs), the National Cancer Center (NCC) in Korea also contributed to this trend by promoting anti-smoking activities.

It is well known that smoking damages nearly every organ in the human body and it is linked to an increased risk of at least 15 different human cancers, most notably the lung, larynx, oral cavity, pharynx, oesophagus, and bladder cancers[1]. About 4 000 different toxic chemicals have been found in cigarette smoke and 62 of them are known carcinogens in humans[2]. In 2006 alone, smoking-related deaths exceeded 5.1 millions worldwide and it is estimated that if the smoking pattern continues at its present rate, about 450 million people will die of the variety of diseases caused by smoking in the first half of this century[3, 4]. Anti-smoking movements can be initiated by educating the population about the harmful effects of smoking on health and also about the socioeconomic impact on society. However, what is deemed to be more important is to ensure that the general population and the policy makers are aware of the entire situation related to the tobacco issues and to persuade them to participate in the measures to avert this public health threat.

Over the past quarter of the century, smoking rates in adult males continued to fall in many high-resource countries of Europe, North America, and Australia. In those countries, active anti-smoking efforts had been made to reduce tobacco consumption through a variety of means including public health education, banning advertising and promotion, increasing prices of tobacco products, restricting access of minors to tobacco products, and bans on smoking in public places, bars, and restaurants[5].

Republic of South Korea has been one of the countries with a high prevalence of smoking among adult males. The population is about 50 million, or 0.75% of the world's population. Korean cancer cases make up 1% of the world's cancer cases, and also the number of Korean smokers was 1% of the world's smokers for a long time. Every year more than 5 million people die due to smoking-related disease in the world, of them approximately 1%, about 50 000 people, are Koreans. That means that approximately one in five Korean people eventually die due to smoking-related disease. It is also estimated that tobacco smoking would incur social and economic costs worth over US$10 billion per year. The smoking rate of adult males peaked at 79.3%

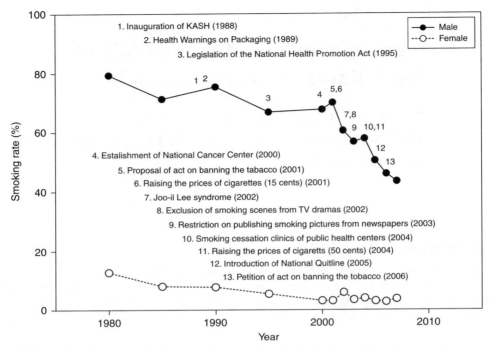

Figure 14.1 Adult smoking prevalence and anti-smoking events in Korea.

in the 1980s and it has been on a steady decline reaching 67.6% in 2000[6]. However, it has rapidly fallen to 43.4% over recent 7 years (Fig. 14.1).

We may not exactly identify the cause of this decline in smoking prevalence, but we may be able to list several factors that might have contributed to the reduction in the smoking rates. In this chapter we will discuss the role of Korean government, NGOs, as well as NCC in Korea, whose mission was to prevent cancer, decrease cancer mortality, and improve the quality of life of Korean cancer patients, together with the other anti-smoking movements. In order to protect people from cancer, it was thought that the most effective cancer prevention strategy is to protect them from tobacco exposure and that Cancer Centers and Cancer Institutes should set an example of how to deal with major carcinogenic threats like tobacco smoking.

Korean Association of Smoking & Health (KASH): beginning of anti-smoking activities

The anti-smoking movement in the Republic of South Korea began with the launch of KASH in 1988. KASH led a nationwide anti-smoking campaign and conducted seminars publicizing the hazard of smoking, widely distributed relevant reports to the public and undertook a boycott smoking campaign. Since 1988, KASH has conducted an annual or biannual survey to examine the smoking rate in collaboration with Ministry of Health, Welfare, Gender Equality and Family.

The first warnings on cigarette packages began in 1976 at the urging of the World Health Organization. The warning stated: 'Do not smoke too much for your health.' In 1989, the warning was significantly strengthened by KASH. The changed warning was 'Smoking may cause lung cancer and it is especially dangerous for teenagers and pregnant women.'

Interventions of Korean government

Other Interventions at the government level began in 1995 with the legislation of the National Health Promotion Act. This landmark law in the history of Korean anti-tobacco activities introduced regulations on smoke-free areas, bringing fundamental changes to the public awareness of the hazardous effects of secondhand smoke. The Health Promotion Act mandates not only the regulation of tobacco use but also the levying of a health enhancement tax on cigarettes, which can be used for the anti-smoking movement and health enhancement programmes. The budget for smoking cessation projects increased as much as 46 times from US$670 000 in 1998 to US$31 million in 2007. According to The Health Promotion Act, public facilities are required to designate non-smoking and smoking zones as follows: office buildings, performance halls, hotels, sports facilities, general restaurants, public buildings and etc. Since 2003, anti-smoking zones that considered completely non-smoking facilities are as follows: kindergarten, school buildings, hospitals, nursery facilities, etc.

Role of the National Cancer Center in the anti-smoking movement

Non-smoking campaign at the NCC

Since the opening of the NCC on 13 March 2000, several anti-smoking policies have been introduced. Accompanying the proclamation of non-smoking within the NCC compound, all the staff members pledged to abstain from smoking when they first become employed and are required to adhere to their commitment, trying to set a good example for creating a smoke-free workplace. NCC started a series of symposia to summarize the dangers and risks of smoking, to give anti-smoking expert educational directions for anti-smoking activities and to provide support for quitting nicotine addiction, these were held once or twice each year[7]. A NCC non-smoking declaration ceremony was held in December 2002 to demonstrate the commitment of the NCC in setting an example of anti-smoking activity[8].

Proposal for raising the cigarette price

Since 1994, the Republic of South Korea has increased cigarette prices seven times but only by a small percentage so that the price has stayed relatively low. In fact, it is only 20–30% of the absolute price of cigarettes in Western countries. Even with income level and purchasing power considered, it remains at 50–70% level. Also a health promotion tax in the tobacco tax was less than 0.2 cents in the Republic of South Korea.

As a means to reduce cigarettes consumption in Korea, NCC proposed to President Kim DJ in 2001 and Rho MH in 2003 to increase the cigarette price. The Ministry of Health, Welfare, Gender Equality and Family raised the tobacco price by 15 cents per pack in 2001. The Korean government hiked cigarette prices again by 50 cents (about 29%) in December 2004, which is notable in that the purpose of this measure was to reduce tobacco consumption for the first time, unlike previous attempts just to increase tax revenues. As a result, the adult male smoking rate dropped by 7.5 percentage points from 57.8% in September 2004 to 50.3% a year after. Price elasticity of cigarette demand was −0.39 in adult males and −1.15 to −1.56 in youth. Efforts are under way to increase the tobacco price by another 50 cents (about 22%).

Proposal for prohibiting scenes showing smoking on mass media

To prevent youths and adolescents from imitating the unhealthy habits of dignitaries and famous actors and actresses in TV dramas or in newspaper photographs, NCC proposed to prohibit smoking scenes or photos in two major broadcasting companies (Korea Broadcasting System, Seoul Broadcasting System) and twelve newspaper companies in 2002 and 2003, respectively. The restriction decision was made by broadcasting companies in December 2002 and twelve newspaper companies announced it on 5 May 2003, which carries a special meaning since May 5 is designated as Children's day in the Republic of South Korea. Munhwa Broadcasting Corporation also joined this restriction campaign and announced that they will not show smoking scenes on news and drama series in 2004. Since then, smoking scenes have been remarkably reduced in major mass media.

Anti-smoking campaigns in the social community and the army

The NCC proposed that the Presidents of nine universities should implement an admission policy that gives advantage to non-smoking candidates in 2002. Konkuk University was poised to be the first school in the nation to adopt this policy to give special advantage to the non-smoking students seeking admission in 2007 in cases where their admission evaluation scores tied with smokers. NCC also received letters from two major trade unions and six medical associations with written signatures of officers of each organization seeking to actually ban tobacco.

South Korean men have a compulsory military service of two years. Because of the high prevalence of smoking among males in the military, an anti-smoking campaign during military service is expected to have the greatest impact in decreasing the rate of male smoking. As the anti-smoking campaign progressed, the Minister of National Defence and also the Commissioner General of the National Police Agency agreed to stop selling duty-free cigarettes to the military personnel from 2009 and the police from 2008 by the request of NCC[9].

Proposal for designating non-smoking areas at the public places

Since 1995, non-smoking areas have been designated in large buildings, theaters, stores, hospitals, schools, private tutoring institutes, social welfare facilities, as well as on public transportation and its related facilities. To establish perhaps the most important milestone of the national non-smoking campaign in the Republic of South Korea, the designation of portion of the National Assembly Building as a non-smoking area was initiated in 2003 by the plea from the NCC. On January 2004, a ceremony was held to hang a signboard for the non-smoking section at the National Assembly Building.

Promotion of a legislative petition for prohibiting the manufacture and sales of tobacco products

J-G Park (president of NCC, from 13 March 2000 to 12 March 2006) proposed to prohibit the sale of cigarettes in Korea to President DJ Kim at the opening ceremony of NCC on 20 June 2001. On 22 February 2006, J-G Park and 157 dignitaries representing various sectors in Korean Society filed a petition requesting a law that would ban the manufacture, sales, exportation, and importation of tobacco, as well as the possession of cigarettes for selling purposes, to be applied within ten years. A survey conducted by Gallup showed that 61% of men and 77.0% of women were in favour of the legislation, which means that 69% of the total population are in favour of banning tobacco manufacture and sales in the Republic of South Korea. The approval rates for the legislation were lower among the current-smokers, both male and female, as anticipated, and also for men in their twenties and women with no exposure to anti-smoking campaign message. Even so, 51% of current-smokers favoured the legislation[10].

This effort has received wholehearted support from the international community. The Asian National Cancer Center Alliance (ANCCA), the organization of NCCs in Asian countries also resolved to ban the manufacture and sales of tobacco products eventually. Further, a meeting of National Cancer Institute Directors (organized at the International Agency for Research on Cancer [IARC] in October 2005) adopted the Lyons Declaration which resolved to support every initiative to reduce the consumption of tobacco products in their countries, and ultimately to reach a complete ban on tobacco products[11].

Anti-smoking activities in Korea

Joo-il Lee syndrome

Amidst the successful anti-smoking campaign in the Republic of South Korea, we acknowledge a famous comedian, Joo-il Lee, who passed away in 2002 at the NCC after losing his battle against lung cancer. The 'emperor of comedy' spearheaded an anti-smoking campaign after he was at the NCC hospital in October 2001 with lung cancer, caused by decades of heavy smoking. The television images of the bedridden and emaciated comedian, with oxygen tubes coming out of his nostrils shocked many. 'Please quit smoking', he appealed in a TV interview. 'Or you may end up like me.' Partly because of Lee, anti-smoking sentiment has increased in the Republic of South Korea since early 2002. His struggle against lung cancer has prompted many smokers to quit the chronic habit of smoking. The media called it 'Joo-il Lee syndrome.' No official statistics are available on how many smokers have joined the big tide of the stop-smoking drive. However, if sales figures of products that help mitigate nicotine withdrawal symptoms are anything to go by, the number of smokers attempting to quit had doubled in 2002 compared to 2001.

Anti-smoking education

In Korea, quit smoking education was initiated in 1998 by the KASH. In 1999, KASH started a 'quit smoking model schools' programme in the Republic of South Korea. The Korean National Tuberculosis Association also conducted smoking prevention classes, touring 400 schools nationwide every year since 2001. Health centers nationwide dispatch speakers on smoking prevention to schools for health education. These health-care teachers take the leadership roles in anti-smoking education[12]. Also, one of the authors, J-G Park, gave over 500 anti-smoking lectures in local communities, as well as in the private sectors during the past seven years.

Anti-smoking campaigns

Inspired by the effects of non-smoking campaigns on TV, which have been available since 2000, the health authorities began using a wide variety of media in 2005 such as internet, subway signboard, nursery tale books, posters, and leaflets. Such diversification also took place in defined target groups ranging from children to teens, college students to soldiers and women, so as to develop anti-tobacco messages specific to each group. In particular, the TV advertisements presented in 2005 were enthusiastically supported by teens and young adults, helping establish anti-tobacco activities as a social trend.

Smoking cessation clinic and Quitline

Smoking cessation counselling in health centre and treatment services have been established since 2005 at no cost to smokers who want to quit, regardless of their gender, age, and income level, at 246 public health centres throughout the country. These public health activities began in 2004, when the health authorities launched the pilot trial of smoking cessation clinics at ten public health centres from October through December 2004. Among 719 people who used these services for more than four weeks, 61% reported that they stayed smoke-free for the entire four weeks. On the basis of these results, the public health authorities expanded these services to public health centres nationwide in 2005, where more than 200 000 smokers benefited from free counselling and treatment services (nicotine replacement therapy, prescription of Bupropion, etc.) in only half a year. Quitline, a toll-free counselling service, was introduced in selected areas in 2005. It will be expanded nationwide to reach out to the smokers who find it difficult to visit smoking cessation clinics in public health centres as well as to inform non-smokers of health hazards of smoking cigarettes for the purpose of prevention[13]. From April 2006 to January 2008, the Quitline helped 5 663 persons with smoking cessation.

Through these various initiatives and efforts smoking prevalence in the Republic of South Korea has continuously fallen. It is hoped that this declining tendency will last and the act on banning the manufacture and sale of tobacco products will be promulgated in the near future in Korea. Also, it is hoped to move towards a tobacco-free world by joining the international network, Tobacco Free World Alliance (ToFWA, http://www.tofwa.org), for banning tobacco manufacture and sales.

References

1. International Agency for Research on Cancer IARC monographs on the evaluation of the carcinogenic risk to chemicals to humans. Vol 83. (2004). *Tobacco smoking and involuntary smoking*. Lyons, IARC Press.

2. Hoffmann, D. and Hoffmann, I. (2001). The changing cigarette – chemical studies and bioassays. In: D. Shopland, D. Burns, and N. Benowitz (eds) *Risks Associated With Smoking Cigarettes With Low-Machine Measured Yields of Tar and Nicotine Smoking and Tobacco Control Monograph*, pp 159–184. No 13. Bethesda, MD, US Department of Health and Human Services, National Institutes of Health, National Cancer Institute, NIH Publication.

3. Keeler, T.E., Hu, T.W., Barnett, P.G., and Manning, W.G. (1993). Taxation, regulation, and addiction: a demand function for cigarettes based on time-series evidence. *J Health Econ*, **12**:1–18.

4. World Health Organization (2002). *The World Health Report 2002: Reducing risks, promoting healthy life*. Geneva, World Health Organization.

5. Shafey, O., Dolwick, S., and Guindon, G.E. (2003). Tobacco control: country profiles. Atlanta, American Cancer Society. World Health Organization, and International Union Against Cancer.

6. Korean Association of Smoking and Health: Report on smoking prevalence in Korea. Available at: http://www.kash.or.kr (accessed on 2 January 2008).

7. National Cancer Center Korea: NCC anti-smoking symposium. Available at: http://www.ncc.re.kr (accessed on 2 February 2007).

8. Boyle, P., Ariyaratne, M., Bartelink, H., Baselga, J., Berns, A., Brawley, O.W. *et al*. (2005). Curbing tobacco's toll starts with the professionals: world no tobacco day. *Lancet*, **365**:1990–2.

9. Park, J.G. (2006). Anti-smoking activities of National Cancer Center: UICC World Cancer Congress 2006. Washington DC, In: Education/Abstract Book, pp 160–1.

10. Park, J.G., Park, J.W., Kim, D.W., Seo, H.G., Nam, B.H., Lee, J.S. *et al*. (2008). Factors influencing attitudes to legislation banning the manufacture and sale of tobacco products. *Tob Control*, **17**:142–3.

11. International Agency for Research on Cancer: Lyon declaration. Lyon. Available at: http://www.tofwa.org (accessed on 23 December 2007).

12. Korean Association of Smoking and Health (2004). Tobacco control policy and anti-smoking activities in Korea: The 7th Asia Pacific Conference on Tobacco or Health. Gyeongju, Korean Association of Smoking and Health, p 22.

13. Myung, S.K., Seo, H.G., Park, J.G., Bae, W.K., Lee, Y.J., and Kim, Y. (2008). Effectiveness of proactive Quitline service at 30 days and predictors of successful smoking cessation: Findings from a preliminary study of Quitline service for smoking cessation in Korea. *J Korean Med Sci*, **23**:888–94.

Chapter 15

The hazards of smoking and the benefits of stopping: cancer mortality and overall mortality*

This *Handbook* is concerned with the health benefits of smoking cessation and, in particular, with the full eventual effects of cessation on life expectancy. It is chiefly concerned not with how to achieve cessation, but merely with the health benefits that smokers can expect if they do stop—and stay stopped—in comparison with the hazards that they would face if they were to continue. In general, for smokers who stop before middle age the resulting difference in life expectancy is about 10 years. This conclusion comes chiefly from studies of males in populations where the full hazards of smoking are already apparent, but it is likely to apply approximately equally to females and to populations where the hazards are not yet fully apparent, as young smokers in those populations will eventually experience substantial hazards if they continue.

Different sections of the main report deal separately (citing full references) with the eventual effects of smoking, and of smoking cessation, on particular conditions such as cancers of the lung, mouth, pharynx, larynx, oesophagus, stomach, liver, pancreas, kidney, bladder or cervix, heart disease, stroke, other vascular diseases and chronic obstructive lung disease. This Introductory section, however, stands back from such detail and summarises the eventual effects of smoking, and the eventual effects of smoking cessation, on overall mortality and on lung cancer mortality (or on the total cancer mortality attributed to smoking, most of which involves lung cancer). As long as due allowance is made for the remarkably long delay between cause and full effect, reliable quantitative conclusions emerge about the hazards that will eventually be faced by those in their 20s, 30s, or 40s who have been habitual cigarette smokers since early adult life if they continue to smoke and, correspondingly, about the eventual benefits for such persistent smokers of stopping permanently.

Smoking is extraordinarily destructive (Table 15.1). Cigarette smoking is common in many populations, and where the habit has been widespread among young adults for many decades, about half of all persistent cigarette smokers are eventually killed by it, unless they stop. Bidi smoking ('bidis' consist of a small amount of tobacco wrapped in the leaf of another plant), which is common in parts of Asia, probably causes similar risks (Gajalakshmi *et al.*, 2003). Cigarette smoking causes relatively few deaths before about 35 years of age, but it causes many deaths in middle age (here defined as 35–69 years) and at older ages. Although some of those killed by tobacco in middle age might have died soon anyway, many could have lived on for another 10, 20, 30, or more good years. Those who stop smoking in early middle age, however (before they have incurable lung cancer or some other fatal disease), avoid most of their risk of being killed by tobacco, and stopping before middle age is even more effective, gaining on average about an extra 10 years of life.

---

* Reproduced, with permission, from pp. 15–27 of IARC Handbooks of Cancer Prevention, Volume 11, *Reversal of Risk after Quitting Smoking*, IARC, Lyon, 2007, with updated figures supplied in 2009 by Richard Peto.

Table 15.1 Main findings for the individual who becomes a habitual cigarette smoker in adolescence or early adult life

The risk is big

- About half are eventually killed by smoking, if they continue.
  [Among persistent cigarette smokers, male or female, the overall relative risk of death is greater than 2 throughout middle age and well into old age. Thus, among smokers of a given age more than half of those who die in the near future would not have done so at never smoker death rates.]
- On average, smokers lose about 10 years of life.
  [This average combines a zero loss for those not killed by tobacco, and an average loss of much more than 10 years for those who are killed by it.]

Those killed in middle age (35–69 years of age) can lose many years of life

- Some of those killed in middle age might have died soon anyway, but others might have lived on for another 10, 20, 30, or more good years.
- On average, those killed in middle age lose about 20 years of never smoker life expectancy.

Stopping smoking works

- Even in early middle age, those who stop (before they have incurable lung cancer or some other fatal disease) avoid most of their risk of being killed by tobacco.
- Stopping before middle age works even better.
- Those who have habitually smoked cigarettes since early adult life but stop at 60, 50, 40, or 30 years of age gain, respectively, about 3, 6, 9, or almost the full 10 years of life expectancy, in comparison with those who continue to smoke.

Main reference: Doll *et al.* (2004)

Effects of cessation on lung cancer mortality and on all-cause mortality in Europe and North America

Lung cancer is one of the main diseases caused by smoking. Even though it accounts for less than half of all smoking-attributed mortality, when the lung cancer death rates among persistent cigarette smokers, former smokers and never smokers are compared, the relative risks are so extreme that the long-term hazards of smoking and benefits of stopping can be seen particularly clearly. Figures 15.1–15.3 compare, for men in Western Europe, Eastern Europe and North America, the lung cancer rates in continuing smokers, never smokers, and former smokers who stopped at about 30, 40, or even 50 years of age (although the risks among continuing smokers are slightly under-estimated in the North American study–see Figure 15.3). In each population the hazards of persistent cigarette smoking are substantial, and in each population the former smokers still have some excess risk many years after stopping. There is, however, a large absolute difference between the eventual risks in those who stop at about 30 to 50 years of age and in those who continue smoking. This is true for lung cancer, and it is also true for overall mortality (see below)—indeed, during the first decade or two after stopping smoking, the absolute mortality difference may well be much greater for other diseases than for lung cancer.

British males born in the 20th century were the first large population in which many began to smoke substantial numbers of cigarettes in early adult life, and continued to do so. The lifelong effects of persistent cigarette smoking, and the corresponding benefits of stopping, can therefore be illustrated by the experience of male British doctors born during the first few decades of the 20th century (1900–1930) and followed prospectively throughout the last half of it (1951–2001). Their smoking habits were ascertained in 1951 and every few years thereafter, and their mortality was monitored reliably. Figure 15.4 compares cigarette smokers with never smokers, showing the

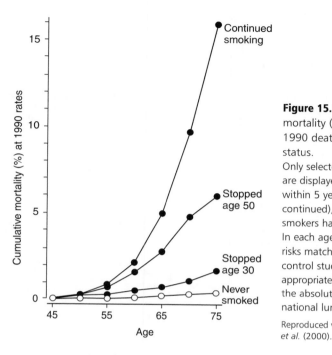

Figure 15.1 Lung cancer mortality (%) in UK males at 1990 death rates by smoking status.

Only selected smoking categories are displayed (never, stopped within 5 years of stated age, continued), and almost all smokers had used cigarettes. In each age range the relative risks match those in a case-control study of smoking, and an appropriately weighted average of the absolute risks matches the national lung cancer death rate.

Reproduced with permission from Peto *et al.* (2000).

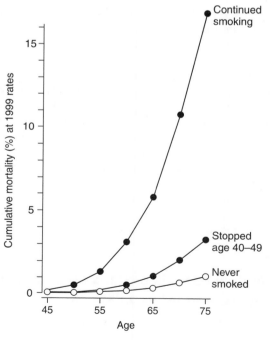

Figure 15.2 Lung cancer mortality in Polish males at 1999 death rates by smoking status.

Only selected smoking categories are displayed (never, stopped within 5 years of stated age, continued), and almost all smokers had used cigarettes. In each age range the relative risks match those in a case-control study of smoking, and an appropriately weighted average of the absolute risks matches the national lung cancer death rate.

Reproduced with permission from Brennan *et al.* (2006).

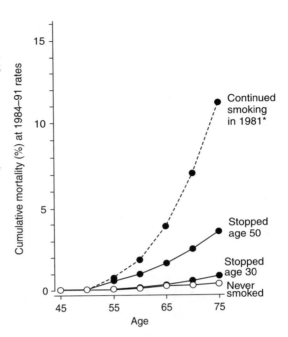

Figure 15.3 Lung cancer mortality in US males, 1984–91, by smoking status in 1981: ACS CPS–II prospective study. Only selected smoking categories are displayed (never, stopped within 5 years of stated age, continued), and almost all smokers had used cigarettes. From the American Cancer Society (ACS) CPS-II 10-year prospective study of one million adults, omitting the earlier years (1981–83). *Re-survey of a sub-sample suggested that about half of those who were continuing to smoke in 1981 stopped during the 1980's but that few who had stopped by 1981 would restart.

Data provided in 2006 by M. Thun, personal communication.

10-year decrease in life expectancy. During middle age (35–69) 19% of the never smokers and 42% of the cigarette smokers died (i.e. the respective probabilities of survival were 81% and 58%), and much of this absolute difference of 23% in mortality was actually caused by smoking. For, it mainly involved differences in the numbers dying from diseases that can be caused by smoking (lung cancer, heart disease, chronic lung disease, etc.); most of the participants had much the same profession (as all were male doctors who had been on the UK Medical Register in 1951); and there were no material differences between smokers, former smokers and never smokers in mean alcohol consumption or obesity.

Figure 15.5 shows, however, that those who stopped at around 40 (35–44) years of age lost only about 1 year of life expectancy instead of 10 years, even though they had already smoked cigarettes for a mean of some 20 years before stopping. On average, the life expectancy gained by stopping at about 60, 50, 40, or 30 years of age, in comparison with those who continued, was, respectively, about 3, 6, 9, or almost the full 10 years in this study. Other studies indicate that those who smoke until 30 years of age and then stop do have a small but significant excess risk of lung cancer in old age (Figures 15.1–15.3), but agree that cessation avoids most of the excess mortality among continuing smokers.

The study of mortality in relation to smoking among British doctors assessed the effects of men who had not yet developed a life-threatening disease stopping before middle age or during middle age, but other studies have shown that even after the onset of disease cessation may well remain important (Table 15.2).

Under-estimation of eventual hazards of smoking and benefits of stopping in many studies of other populations

Cigarette consumption was low worldwide in 1900, but among men in many developed countries such as the United Kingdom or United States it increased substantially during the first few

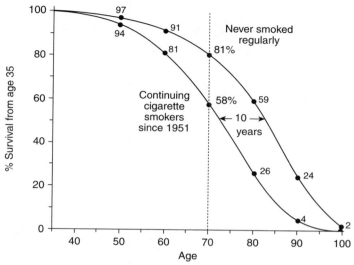

Figure 15.4 Survival from age 35: continuing cigarette smokers vs never smokers.
50-year prospective follow-up (1951–2001) of mortality in relation to smoking among male British doctors born 1900–1930. Men were asked in 1951, and again every few years until 2001, what they smoked. Few never smokers or ex-smokers became smokers, but many smokers became ex-smokers. Analyses are by habit last reported. Among men born 1900–1930, the continuing smokers (and ex-smokers) would on average have started at about 18 years of age, and smoked about 20 cigarettes per day.

Reproduced with permission from Doll *et al*. (2004).

decades of the 20th century (IARC, 2004). In recent decades it has also increased substantially among women in many developed countries and among men in many developing countries, including China. When in a particular population there is an upsurge of cigarette smoking among young adults, it may be about 30 or 40 years before the main upsurge of tobacco deaths in middle age is seen, and then another 20 years before the main upsurge of tobacco deaths in old age.

The United Kingdom was the first major country in the world to experience a large increase in lung cancer from cigarette smoking. Even in Britain, however, it is only among men born early in the 20th century, many of whom started in youth the habit of smoking substantial numbers of cigarettes, that we can assess directly the full hazards of continuing to do so throughout adult life, and, correspondingly, the full long-term benefits of stopping at various ages. That is why the results for such men (Figures 15.4 and 15.5) are particularly relevant to predicting the future worldwide health effects of current smoking patterns, and the eventual importance of cessation, particularly before middle age. For, even in populations where there is not yet a high death rate from smoking (because relatively few who are now in middle or old age have been habitual cigarette smokers throughout adult life), many of those who start smoking cigarettes nowadays do so in adolescence or early adult life, as did many of the British doctors described in Figures 15.4 and 15.5, so the young smokers in those populations will eventually also face substantial risks in middle and old age if they continue to smoke, and have much to gain from prompt cessation.

Many previous epidemiological studies of smoking and disease took place in populations where the middle-aged or, particularly, the older smokers had not at the time of the study been smoking substantial numbers of cigarettes throughout adult life, and where the national lung cancer rates in middle or old age were still relatively low, or rising steeply. This is true for many previous

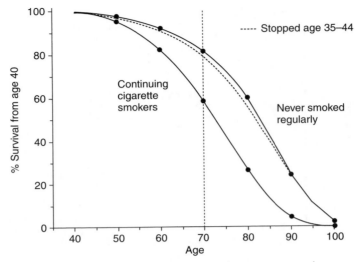

Figure 15.5 Survival from age 40: continuing cigarette smokers vs never smokers vs smokers who stopped at about age 40.

50-year prospective follow-up (1951–2001) of mortality in relation to smoking among male British doctors born 1900–1930. Men were asked in 1951, and again every few years until 2001, what they smoked. Few never smokers or ex-smokers became smokers, but many smokers became ex-smokers. Analyses are by habit last reported. Among men born 1900–1930, the continuing smokers (and ex-smokers) would on average have started at about 18 years of age, and smoked about 20 cigarettes per day.

Dotted line corresponds to the survival of those stopping smoking.

Reproduced with permission from Doll *et al.* (2004).

studies of men and may well be true for all previous studies of women. The risks found by comparing the smokers and the former smokers (or never smokers) in those studies may therefore greatly underestimate the risks that the younger cigarette smokers of today will eventually face if they continue. Hence, in those previous studies the apparent absolute benefits after 20, 30 or more years of cessation are likely to be substantially less than the absolute benefits that the younger cigarette smokers of today could gain from cessation (in comparison with the risks they would otherwise face if they were to continue).

In many studies the proportional excess mortality in middle and old age from smoking is greater among male than among female smokers, but this may be chiefly because they smoked

Table 15.2 Effects of cessation at different ages

Time of stopping smoking	Effect on later risk of death from smoking
Before middle age, e.g. at about age 20–30	Avoids nearly all of the future mortality from tobacco in middle and old age
During middle age, e.g. at about 40–50, but before major disease onset	Avoids much hazard over the next few decades, but some hazard remains
After the onset of life-threatening disease	Rapid benefit (particularly for vascular mortality), unless the existing disease causes death

Main reference: IARC Handbooks of Cancer Prevention, Volume 11, *Reversal of Risk after Quitting Smoking*, IARC, Lyon, 2007.

cigarettes more intensively when young than the female smokers did. If, however, smoking cigarettes throughout adult life eventually produces about as great a proportional increase in female as in male overall death rates, then in terms of years of life expectancy lost or gained the eventual hazards of persistent cigarette smoking (and the corresponding benefits of cessation) may well be about as great for women as for men.

Likewise, among men in developing countries such as China, the hazards that younger cigarette smokers will eventually face in middle and old age may well be substantially greater than the risks now seen among Chinese smokers in middle and old age (Peto *et al.*, 1999). Indeed, for any cigarette smoker, male or female, in any part of the world who started smoking substantial numbers of cigarettes when young and has continued doing so, the eventual hazards may well be similar: about half will be killed by their habit unless they stop, and cessation before age 40 (or, better, before age 30) would avoid most of that risk. In any population in the world, therefore, the prevalence of cigarette (or bidi) smoking among young adults can be used as a proxy to predict the eventual future impact of smoking on mortality in that population several decades hence if those who now smoke continue to do so, and to predict the corresponding importance for those who now smoke of prompt cessation.

Contrasting national trends in tobacco-attributed mortality at ages 35–69

In many countries the trends in cigarette smoking and, more recently, in cessation have been so extreme that they have dominated the recent national trends in cancer mortality and in overall mortality, at least among middle-aged men. The United Kingdom, Poland and the USA offer three contrasting examples of this (Figures 15.6–15.11).

In the United Kingdom (Figures 15.6 and 15.7), cigarette smoking became widespread during the first few decades of the 20th century among men, and around the middle of the century among women. By the 1960s the male death rates attributed to tobacco in the United Kingdom were among the worst in the world, with smoking causing more than half of the cancer mortality and almost half of the overall mortality among men in middle age, and the death rates from smoking among women were rising. Over the past few decades, however, there has been widespread cessation, a substantial decrease in the male death rates and, more recently, some decrease in the female death rates from smoking in the UK. Had UK female smokers all continued smoking, there could well have been a substantial rise in the UK female death rates from smoking in recent decades instead of the moderate decrease actually seen.

In Poland (Figures 15.8 and 15.9), the main increase in cigarette smoking took place around the middle of the century among males, and was followed by a large increase in tobacco-attributed mortality during the second half of the century (to levels comparable with those seen earlier in the UK). However, a decrease in smoking during the 1990s has been associated with the start of a decrease in this mortality. Women have thus far been less severely affected than men in Poland, although young Polish women who smoke will also face substantial hazards if they do not stop.

In the USA (Figures 15.10 and 15.11), a rapid increase in tobacco-attributed mortality among males was still in progress when it was halted (before the cancer or overall death rates from smoking were as high as they had been in the United Kingdom, and would become in Poland) by a substantial decrease in cigarette consumption over the past few decades. Since 1970 male lung cancer mortality in early middle age has fallen substantially, and male lung cancer mortality at later ages is beginning to do likewise. The death rate from smoking among women in the USA was still very low in 1950, but it rose rapidly and by the 1990s the female death rates attributed to

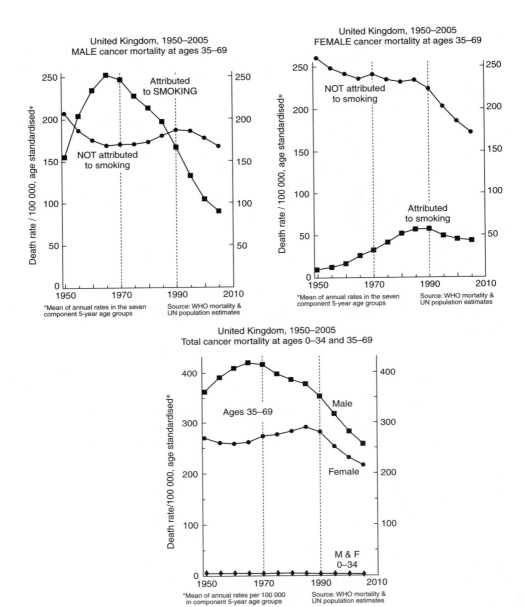

Figure 15.6 United Kingdom, 1950–2005. Total annual cancer mortality rates at ages 0–34 and 35–69 years, with the total male and total female rates at ages 35–69 years subdivided into the parts attributed, and not attributed, to smoking.

Rates are calculated from WHO mortality data and UN population estimates, and are standardised to a uniform age distribution (so the standardised rate for a 35-year age range is the mean of the 7 rates in the component 5-year age ranges). In the absence of other causes of death, an annual rate of death of R per 100 000 would correspond to a 35-year probability of death of 1-exp(−35R/100 000). Thus, a rate of 300 would correspond to a probability of 10%.

The mortality attributed to smoking is estimated indirectly from the national mortality statistics (using the absolute lung cancer rate as a guide to the fraction of the deaths from other causes, or groups of causes, attributable to smoking).

Source: WHO mortality & UN population estimates

UNITED KINGDOM: 1950–2006 MALES

**Population risk of a 35-year-old dying at ages 35–69
from smoking (shaded) or from any cause (shaded and white)**

*eg, at year 2006 male death rates, out of 100 men aged 35, 21 would
die before age 70 (with 5 of these deaths attributed to smoking)

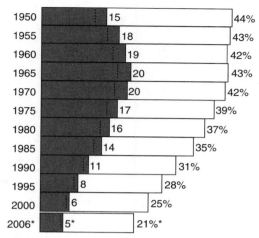

Year	Smoking	Total
1950	15	44%
1955	18	43%
1960	19	42%
1965	20	43%
1970	20	42%
1975	17	39%
1980	16	37%
1985	14	35%
1990	11	31%
1995	8	28%
2000	6	25%
2006*	5*	21%*

Note: Most of those killed by smoking would otherwise have survived beyond age 70,
but a minority (shaded area to right of dotted line) would died by 70 anyway

UNITED KINGDOM: 1950–2006 FEMALES

**Population risk of a 35-year-old dying at ages 35–69
from smoking (shaded) or from any cause (shaded and white)**

*eg, at year 2006 female death rates, out of 100 women aged 35, 14 would
die before age 70 (with 3 of these deaths attributed to smoking)

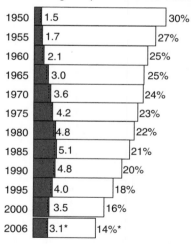

Year	Smoking	Total
1950	1.5	30%
1955	1.7	27%
1960	2.1	25%
1965	3.0	25%
1970	3.6	24%
1975	4.2	23%
1980	4.8	22%
1985	5.1	21%
1990	4.8	20%
1995	4.0	18%
2000	3.5	16%
2006	3.1*	14%*

Note: Most of those killed by smoking would otherwise have survived beyond age 70,
but a minority (shaded area to right of dotted line) would died by 70 anyway

Figure 15.7 United Kingdom, 1950–2006. Probabilities of death at ages 0–34 and 35–69 at the
death rates of particular calendar years, with the male and female probabilities of death from
smoking at ages 35–69 shaded.

Rates are calculated from WHO mortality data and UN population estimates, and are standardised to a
uniform age distribution (so the standardised rate for a 35-year age range is the mean of the 7 rates in
the component 5-year age ranges).

The mortality attributed to smoking is estimated indirectly from the national mortality statistics (using the
absolute lung cancer rate as a guide to the fraction of the deaths from other causes, or groups of causes,
attributable to smoking).

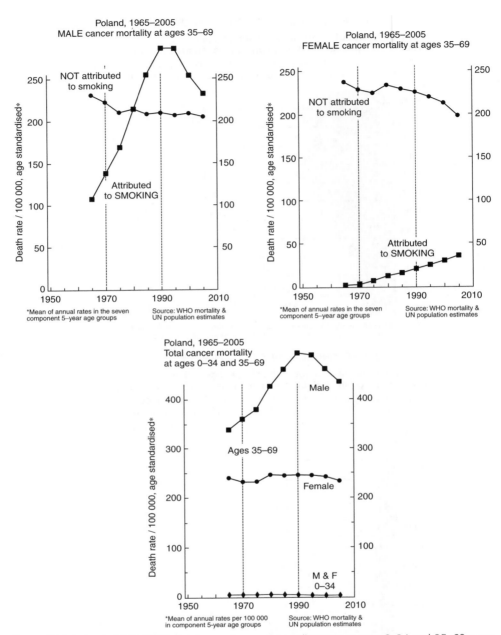

Figure 15.8 Poland, 1965–2005. Total annual cancer mortality rates at ages 0–34 and 35–69 years, with the total male and total female rates at ages 35–69 years subdivided into the parts attributed, and not attributed, to smoking.

Rates are calculated from WHO mortality data and UN population estimates, and are standardised to a uniform age distribution (so the standardised rate for a 35-year age range is the mean of the 7 rates in the component 5-year age ranges). In the absence of other causes of death, an annual rate of death of R per 100 000 would correspond to a 35-year probability of death of 1-exp (−35R/100 000). Thus, a rate of 300 would correspond to a probability of 10%.

The mortality attributed to smoking is estimated indirectly from the national mortality statistics (using the absolute lung cancer rate as a guide to the fraction of the deaths from other causes, or groups of causes, attributable to smoking).

Source: WHO mortality & UN population estimates

Poland: 1955–2006 MALES

Population risk of a 35-year-old dying at ages 35–69 from smoking (shaded) or from any cause (shaded and white)

*eg, at year 2006 male death rates, out of 100 men aged 35, 39 would die before age 70 (with 14 of these deaths attributed to smoking)

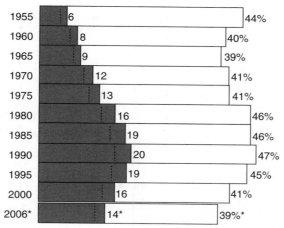

Note: Most of those killed by smoking would otherwise have survived beyond age 70, but a minority (shaded area to right of dotted line) would died by 70 anyway

Poland: 1955–2006 FEMALES

Population risk of a 35-year-old dying at ages 35–69 from smoking (shaded) or from any cause (shaded and white)

*eg, at year 2006 female death rates, out of 100 women aged 35, 17 would die before age 70 (with 3 of these deaths attributed to smoking)

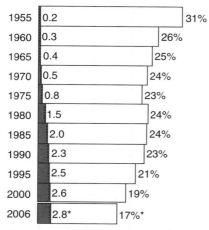

Note: Most of those killed by smoking would otherwise have survived beyond age 70, but a minority (shaded area to right of dotted line) would died by 70 anyway

Figure 15.9 Poland, 1955–2006. Probabilities of death at ages 0–34 and 35–69 at the death rates of particular calendar years, with the male and female probabilities of death from smoking at ages 35–69 shaded.

Rates are calculated from WHO mortality data and UN population estimates, and are standardised to a uniform age distribution (so the standardised rate for a 35-year age range is the mean of the 7 rates in the component 5-year age ranges).

The mortality attributed to smoking is estimated indirectly from the national mortality statistics (using the absolute lung cancer rate as a guide to the fraction of the deaths from other causes, or groups of causes, attributable to smoking).

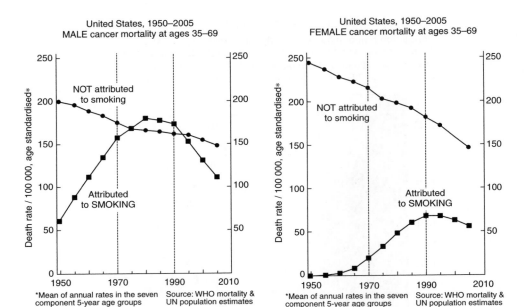

United States, 1950–2005
MALE cancer mortality at ages 35–69

NOT attributed
to smoking

Attributed
to SMOKING

Death rate / 100 000, age standardised*

*Mean of annual rates in the seven
component 5-year age groups

Source: WHO mortality &
UN population estimates

United States, 1950–2005
FEMALE cancer mortality at ages 35–69

NOT attributed
to smoking

Attributed
to SMOKING

Death rate / 100 000, age standardised*

*Mean of annual rates in the seven
component 5-year age groups

Source: WHO mortality &
UN population estimates

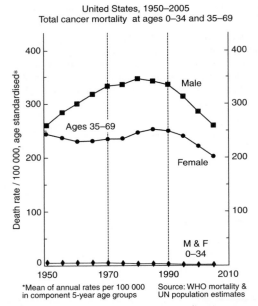

United States, 1950–2005
Total cancer mortality at ages 0–34 and 35–69

Death rate / 100 000, age standardised*

Male

Ages 35–69

Female

M & F
0–34

*Mean of annual rates per 100 000
in component 5-year age groups

Source: WHO mortality &
UN population estimates

Figure 15.10 USA, 1950–2005. Total annual cancer mortality rates at ages 0–34 and 35–69 years,
with the total male and total female rates at ages 35–69 years subdivided into the parts attributed,
and not attributed, to smoking.

Rates are calculated from WHO mortality data and UN population estimates, and are standardised to a
uniform age distribution (so the standardised rate for a 35-year age range is the mean of the 7 rates in
the component 5-year age ranges). In the absence of other causes of death, an annual rate of death of R
per 100 000 would correspond to a 35-year probability of death of 1-exp (-35R/100 000). Thus, a rate of
300 would correspond to a probability of 10%.

The mortality attributed to smoking is estimated indirectly from the national mortality statistics (using the
absolute lung cancer rate as a guide to the fraction of the deaths from other causes, or groups of causes,
attributable to smoking).

Source: WHO mortality & UN population estimates

Population risk of a 35-year-old dying at ages 35–69 from smoking (shaded) or from any cause (shaded and white)

*eg, at year 2005 male death rates, out of 100 men aged 35, 26 would die before age 70 (with 7 of these deaths attributed to smoking)

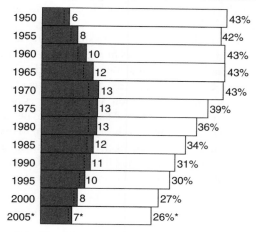

Year	Smoking	Any cause
1950	6	43%
1955	8	42%
1960	10	43%
1965	12	43%
1970	13	43%
1975	13	39%
1980	13	36%
1985	12	34%
1990	11	31%
1995	10	30%
2000	8	27%
2005*	7*	26%*

Note: Most of those killed by smoking would otherwise have survived beyond age 70, but a minority (shaded area to right of dotted line) would died by 70 anyway

UNITED STATES: 1950–2005 FEMALES

Population risk of a 35-year-old dying at ages 35–69 from smoking (shaded) or from any cause (shaded and white)

*eg, at year 2005 male death rates, out of 100 men aged 35, 17 would die before age 70 (with 5 of these deaths attributed to smoking)

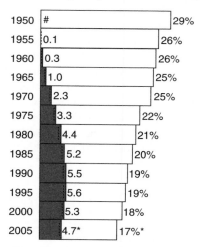

Year	Smoking	Any cause
1950	#	29%
1955	0.1	26%
1960	0.3	26%
1965	1.0	25%
1970	2.3	25%
1975	3.3	22%
1980	4.4	21%
1985	5.2	20%
1990	5.5	19%
1995	5.6	19%
2000	5.3	18%
2005	4.7*	17%*

Note: Most of those killed by smoking would otherwise have survived beyond age 70, but a minority (shaded area to right of dotted line) would died by 70 anyway

Figure 15.11 USA, 1950–2005. Probabilities of death at ages 0–34 and 35–69 at the death rates of particular calendar years, with the male and female probabilities of death from smoking at ages 35–69 shaded.

Rates are calculated from WHO mortality data and UN population estimates, and are standardised to a uniform age distribution (so the standardised rate for a 35-year age range is the mean of the 7 rates in the component 5-year age ranges).

The mortality attributed to smoking is estimated indirectly from the national mortality statistics (using the absolute lung cancer rate as a guide to the fraction of the deaths from other causes, or groups of causes, attributable to smoking).

smoking in the USA were among the worst in the world, although (as in men in the USA) the rise was eventually halted by a decrease in cigarette consumption. Again, had US female smokers all continued smoking, there could well have been a substantial rise in recent decades in the US female death rates from smoking.

The methods used in these three populations to estimate smoking attributed mortality, past and present, are indirect, so the absolute death rates in Figures 15.6–15.11 are somewhat uncertain (although they cannot be greatly in error for smoking-attributed cancer mortality, as most of this involves lung cancer), and some of the recent changes in the overall mortality attributed to smoking may be due to factors other than cessation, such as changes in other causes of vascular disease, or in its treatment. Nevertheless, the overall patterns should be reasonably trustworthy, confirming the enormous potential relevance of smoking cessation to overall mortality rates in such countries, and the practicability of substantial changes accumulating over a period of several years. This is true both in populations where smoking is already a major cause of death and in populations where it is not, but where it could become so if current smoking patterns persist.

Worldwide trends

Worldwide, about 100 million people a year reach adult life. Based on present smoking patterns about 50% of the young men and 10% of the young women will start to smoke, and most will continue. Of those who continue to smoke cigarettes or bidis, whether in Asia, America, Africa or Europe, about half will eventually be killed by their habit (unless they die before middle age of something else). Hence, if more than 20 million of these 30 million new smokers a year continue smoking cigarettes, and do not stop, and half of those who do so are killed by it, then eventually more than 10 million people per year will be killed by tobacco.

Based on current smoking patterns, worldwide annual mortality from tobacco is likely to rise to about 10 million per year (i.e. 100 million per decade) by around the year 2030 (Peto *et al*, 1994, 2001), and will rise somewhat further in later decades. Tobacco is therefore expected to cause about 150 million deaths in the first quarter of the twenty-first century and 300 million in the second quarter. Predictions for the third and, particularly, the fourth quarter of the century are inevitably more speculative. However, if over the next few decades about 30% of the young adults become persistent cigarette or bidi smokers and about half who do are eventually killed by it, then about 10–15% of adult mortality in the second half of the century will be due to tobacco smoking (probably implying more than 500 million deaths due to tobacco in the second half of the century; Table 15.3).

Table 15.3 Projected numbers of deaths from tobacco during the 21st century, if current smoking patterns persist

Period (years)	Tobacco deaths (millions)
2000–2024	~150
2025–2049	~300
2050–2099	>500
Total, 21st century	~1000
20th century, for comparison	~100

Source: Peto & Lopez (2001)

The number of tobacco deaths predicted to occur before 2050 cannot be greatly reduced unless a substantial proportion of the adults who have already been smoking for some time give up the habit. A decrease over the next decade or two in the proportion of children who become smokers will not have its main effects on mortality until the middle and second half of the century. The effects of adult smokers quitting on deaths before 2050 and of young people not starting to smoke on deaths after 2050 will probably be approximately as follows:

♦ *Quitting:* If many of the adults who now smoke were to give up over the next decade or two, thus halving global cigarette consumption per adult by the 2020s, this would prevent about one-third of tobacco-related deaths in the 2020s and would almost halve tobacco-related deaths thereafter. Such changes could avoid about 20 or 30 million tobacco-related deaths in the first quarter of the century and could avoid 100 million in the second quarter.

♦ *Not starting:* If, by progressive reduction over the next decade or two in the global uptake rate of smoking by young people, the proportion of young adults who become smokers were to be halved by the 2020s, this would avoid hundreds of millions of deaths from tobacco after 2050. It would, however, avoid almost none of the 150 million deaths from tobacco in the first quarter of the century, and would probably avoid 'only' about 10 or 20 million of the 300 million deaths from tobacco in the second quarter of the century.

Thus, using widely practicable ways of helping large numbers of young people not to become smokers could avoid hundreds of millions of tobacco-related deaths in the middle and second half of the twenty-first century, but not before. In contrast, widely practicable ways of helping large numbers of adult smokers to quit (preferably before middle age, but also in middle age) might avoid one or two hundred million tobacco-related deaths in the first half of this century. Large numbers of deaths during the second half of the century could also be avoided if many of those who, despite warnings, still start to smoke in future years could be helped to stop before they are killed by the habit. Such calculations suggest that the effect of quitting could be more rapidly apparent on a population scale than the effects of not starting to smoke. Both, however, are of great importance.

References

Brennan, P., Crispo, A., Zaridze, D., *et al.* (2006). High cumulative risk of lung cancer death among smokers and nonsmokers in Central and Eastern Europe. *Am J Epidemiol*, **164**(12):1233–1241.

Doll, R., Peto, R., Wheatley, K. *et al.* (1994). Mortality in relation to smoking: 40 years' observations on male British doctors. *BMJ*, **309**(6959):901–911.

Doll, R., Peto, R., Boreham, J. *et al.* (2004). Mortality in relation to smoking: 50 years' observations on male British doctors. *BMJ*, **328**(7455):1519–1527.

Gajalakshmi, V., Hung, R.J., Mathew, A., *et al.* (2003). Tobacco smoking and chewing, alcohol drinking and lung cancer risk among men in southern India. *Int J Cancer*, **107**(3):441–447.

IARC (2004). IARC Monographs on the Evaluation of Carcinogenic Risks to Humans, Vol. 83, Tobacco Smoke and Involuntary Smoking. Lyon, IARC Press.

Peto, R., Lopez, A.D., Boreham, J. *et al.* (1992). Mortality from tobacco in developed countries: indirect estimation from national vital statistics. *Lancet*, **339**(8804):1268–1278.

Peto, R., Lopez, A.D., Boreham, J. *et al.* (1994). *Mortality from Smoking in Developed Countries 1950–2000: Indirect Estimates from National Vital Statistics.* Oxford, Oxford University Press.

Peto, R., Lopez, A.D., Boreham, J. *et al.* (1996). Mortality from smoking worldwide. *Br Med Bull*, **52**(1):12–21.

Peto, R., Chen, Z.M., Borehamm, J. (1999). Tobacco–the growing epidemic. *Nat Med*, **5**(1):15–17.

Peto, R., Darby, S., Deo, H. *et al.* (2000). Smoking, smoking cessation, and lung cancer in the UK since 1950: combination of national statistics with two case-control studies. *BMJ*, **321**(7257):323–329.

Peto, R. and Lopez, A.D. (2001). Future worldwide health effects of current smoking patterns. In C.E. Koop, C. Pearson, M.R. Schwarz, (eds) *Critical issues in Global Health*, pp. 154–161. New York, Jossey-Bass.

Website

Deaths from smoking http://www.deathsfromsmoking.net

Chapter 16

Passive smoking and health

Jonathan M. Samet

Overview

Evidence on the many adverse health effects of tobacco smoking, both active and passive, and of using smokeless tobacco has been central in driving initiatives to control tobacco use. In some countries, the evidence on passive smoking has had particularly powerful consequences in shaping public policy in recent decades, as strategies have been implemented to protect non-smokers from involuntarily inhaling tobacco smoke in public places, workplaces, and their homes. Over the last decade, and particularly the past five years, progress has been rapid as a number of countries, such as Ireland, Scotland, Uruguay, and Italy have implemented strong smoke-free measures that cover workplaces and public places.

This chapter provides an overview and introduction to the now-vast data on the adverse health consequences of passive smoking, covering the risks to passive smokers, including the fetus, infants and children, and adults. Since the 1980s, the evidence has been periodically examined and synthesized in various governmental reports, which should be used by those seeking comprehensive summaries to supplement this chapter. Notable reports over the last decade include those prepared by the Environmental Protection Agency of the state of California in the United States (Cal/EPA) (California Environmental Protection Agency et al. 2005), the United Kingdom's Scientific Committee on Tobacco (Scientific Committee on Tobacco Health and HSMO 1998), the World Health Organization (WHO) (World Health Organization 1999), the International Agency for Research on Cancer (IARC) (International Agency for Research on Cancer 2004) and the US Surgeon General (US Department of Health and Human Services 2006). Samet and colleagues (2009b) have also recently and comprehensively reviewed the literature.

Although there were writings on the dangers to health of tobacco use centuries ago, the body of evidence that constitutes the foundation of our present understanding of tobacco as a cause of disease dates to approximately the mid-twentieth century. Even earlier, case reports and case series had called attention to the likely role of smoking and chewing tobacco as a cause of cancer. The rise of diseases that had once been uncommon, such as lung cancer and coronary heart disease, was noticed early in the twentieth century and motivated clinical and pathological studies to determine if the increases were 'real' or an artefact of changing methods of detection. By mid-century, there was no doubt that the increases were real and the focus of research shifted to the causes of the new epidemics of 'chronic diseases', such as lung cancer and coronary heart disease.

The epidemiological studies that were implemented to find the causes of these new epidemics quickly linked active cigarette smoking to cancers of the lung and other organs, coronary heart disease, and 'emphysema and chronic bronchitis', now termed chronic obstructive pulmonary disease (COPD). The studies were observational, that is comparing risks of disease in those who smoked with those who did not, and were primarily of the cohort (following smokers and non-smokers and measuring the rate at which disease develops in the two groups) and case-control designs (comparing rates of smoking in persons with the disease under study and in controls who are similar but do not have the disease). Surveys, or cross-sectional studies, were also carried out, particularly to compare rates of lung disease in smokers and non-smokers. These same designs were subsequently used to investigate the risks of passive smoking.

By the 1960s, there was strong evidence that active smoking was a powerful cause of disease. For example, the risk of lung cancer in men who smoked was increased ten-fold or more compared to men who had never smoked, and the risk increased with the number of cigarettes smoked and the duration of smoking (US Department of Health Education and Welfare 1964). These initial observations quickly sparked complementary laboratory studies on the mechanisms by which tobacco smoking causes disease. The multidisciplinary approach to research on tobacco has been key in linking active and passive smoking to various diseases; the observational evidence has been supported with an understanding of the mechanisms by which smoking causes disease. By 1953, for example, Wynder and colleagues (1953) had shown that painting the skin of mice with the condensate of cigarette smoke caused skin tumours. In combination with the emerging epidemiologic evidence on smoking and lung cancer, this observation was sufficiently powerful to be followed by the US tobacco industry's dramatic response of establishing the Tobacco Industry Research Committee, later to become the Tobacco Research Council, and to initiate a campaign to discredit the emerging scientific evidence on the danger of smoking (Brandt 2007). This same tactic has since been used by the tobacco industry to maintain controversy around the emerging evidence on passive smoking (Michaels 2008).

By the late 1950s and early 1960s, the mounting evidence on active smoking received formal review and evaluation by government committees, leading to definitive conclusions on causation in the early 1960s. In the United Kingdom, the 1962 report of the Royal College of Physicians (Royal College of Physicians of London 1962) concluded that smoking was a cause of lung cancer and bronchitis and a contributing factor to coronary heart disease. In the United States, the 1964 report of the Advisory Committee to the Surgeon General concluded that smoking was a cause of lung cancer in men and of chronic bronchitis (US Department of Health Education and Welfare 1964). This conclusion was based on a systematic and comprehensive evaluation of evidence and application of criteria for judgement as to the causality of association. The criteria included the association's consistency, strength, specificity, temporal relationship, and coherence. By law, a US Surgeon General's report was subsequently required annually and new conclusions have been reached periodically with regard to the diseases caused by smoking. The Royal College of Physicians has also continued to release periodic reports, as have other organizations. These reports and other expert syntheses of the evidence have proved effective for translating the findings on smoking, both active and passive, and disease into policy.

The issue of passive smoking and health has a briefer history. Some of the first epidemiological studies on secondhand smoke (SHS) or environmental tobacco smoke (ETS) and health were reported in the late 1960s (Cameron 1967; Colley and Holland 1967; Cameron et al. 1969). Prior to that point, there had been scattered case reports; the Nazi government had campaigned against smoking in public, and one German physician, Fritz Lickint, used the term 'passive smoking' in his 1939 book on smoking (Proctor 1995). In the 1960s, the initial investigations focused on parental smoking and lower respiratory illnesses in infants; studies of lung function and respiratory symptoms in children soon followed (US Department of Health and Human Services 1986; Samet et al. 2009b). The 1971 report of the US Surgeon General raised concern about possible adverse effects of passive smoking (US Department of Health Education and Welfare 1971).

The first major studies on passive smoking and lung cancer in non-smokers were reported in 1981, a cohort study in Japan and a case-control study in Athens (Hirayama 1981a, 1981b; Trichopoulos et al. 1981) and by 1986 the evidence supported the conclusion that passive smoking was a cause of lung cancer in non-smokers, a conclusion reached by the IARC, the US Surgeon General, and the

US National Research Council (International Agency for Research on Cancer 1986; US Department of Health and Human Services 1986). The evidence on child health and passive smoking was also reviewed in 1986 by the US Surgeon General and the US National Research Council. A now-substantial body of evidence has continued to identify new diseases and other adverse effects of passive smoking, including increased risk for coronary heart disease (Table 16.1) (California Environmental Protection Agency and Office of Environmental Health Hazard Assessment 1997; Scientific Committee on Tobacco Health and HSMO 1998; World Health Organization 1999; US Department of Health and Human Services 2006; Samet *et al.* 2009b).

Table 16.1 Adverse effects from exposure to tobacco smoke

Health effect	SGR 1984	SGR 1986	EPA 1992	Cal/EPA 1997	UK 1998	WHO 1999	IARC 2004	Cal/EPA[a] 2005	SGR 2006
Increased prevalence of chronic respiratory symptoms	Yes/a	Yes/a	Yes/c	Yes/c	Yes/c	Yes/c		Yes/c	Yes/c
Decrement in pulmonary function	Yes/a	Yes/a	Yes/a	Yes/a		Yes/c		Yes/a	Yes/c
Increased occurrence of acute respiratory illnesses	Yes/a	Yes/a	Yes/a	Yes/c		Yes/c		Yes/c	Yes/c
Increased occurrence of middle-ear disease		Yes/a	Yes/c	Yes/c	Yes/c	Yes/c		Yes/c	Yes/c
Increased severity of asthma episodes and symptoms			Yes/c	Yes/c		Yes/c		Yes/c	Yes/c
Risk factor for new asthma			Yes/a	Yes/c				Yes/c	Yes/c
Risk factor for SIDS				Yes/c	Yes/a	Yes/c		Yes/c	Yes/c
Risk factor for lung cancer in adults		Yes/c	Yes/c	Yes/c	Yes/c		Yes/c	Yes/c	Yes/c
Risk factor for breast cancer for younger, primarily postmenopausal women								Yes/c	
Risk factor for nasal sinus cancer								Yes/c	
Risk factor for heart disease in adults			Yes/c	Yes/c				Yes/c	Yes/c

Source: Samet *et al.* 2009b.

Note

Yes/a = association; Yes/c = cause.

SGR 1984: US Department of Health and Human Services (1984); SGR 1986: US Department of Health and Human Services (1986); EPA 1992: US Environmental Protection Agency (1992); Cal/EPA 1997: California Environmental Protection Agency and Office of Environmental Health Hazard Assessment (1997); UK 1998: Scientific Committee on Tobacco and Health and HSMO (1998); WHO 1999: World Health Organization (1999); IARC 2004: International Agency for Research on Cancer (2004); Cal/EPA 2005: California Environmental Protection Agency and Air Resources Board (2005); SGR 2006: US Department of Health and Human Services (2006).

[a] Only effects causally associated with SHS exposure are included.

This evidence and the associated causal conclusion have been the primary impetus for smoke-free policies worldwide. Beginning several decades ago, many countries began to pass bans on smoking in public places and workplaces. Smoking was banned on almost all airplane flights. Now, many countries have passed legislation making all public and workplaces smoke-free and the Framework Convention on Tobacco Control (FCTC) mandates smoke-free environments (World Health Organization 2003).

Toxicology of tobacco smoke

Tobacco smoke is generated by the burning of a complex organic material, tobacco, along with the various additives and paper, at a high temperature, reaching about a thousand degrees centigrade in the burning coal of the cigarette (US Department of Health Education and Welfare 1964). The resulting smoke, comprising numerous gases and also particles, includes myriad toxic components that can cause injury through inflammation and irritation, asphyxiation, carcinogenesis, and other mechanisms. Some examples are carbon monoxide, cyanide, radioactive polonium, benzo-(a)-pyrene, oxides of nitrogen, acrolein, benzene, and particles. Active smokers inhale mainstream smoke (MS), the smoke drawn directly through the end of the cigarette. Passive smokers inhale smoke that is now generally referred to as SHS or ETS, comprising a mixture of mostly sidestream smoke (SS) given off by the smouldering cigarette and some exhaled MS. The term SHS is currently preferred because ETS originated with the tobacco industry. Sidestream smoke is generated at lower temperatures than MS, and consequently concentrations of many toxic compounds are greater in SS than MS. However, SS is rapidly diluted following its generation as it disperses into the air. Concentrations of tobacco smoke components in SHS are far below the levels of MS inhaled by the active smoker, but there are qualitative similarities between SHS and MS (US Department of Health and Human Services 1986; International Agency for Research on Cancer 2004).

Both active and passive smokers absorb tobacco smoke components through the lung's airways and alveoli and many of these components, such as the gas carbon monoxide, then enter into the circulation and are distributed systemically. There is also uptake of such components as benzo-(a)-pyrene directly into the cells that line the upper airway and the lung's airways. Some of the carcinogens undergo metabolic transformation into their active forms and evidence now indicates that metabolism-determining genes may affect susceptibility to tobacco smoke (Hecht *et al.* 2007). The genitourinary system is exposed to toxins in tobacco smoke through the excretion of compounds in the urine, including carcinogens. The gastrointestinal tract is exposed through direct deposition of smoke in the upper airway and the clearance of smoke-containing mucus from the trachea through the glottis into the oesophagus. Not surprisingly, tobacco smoking has proved to be a multisystem cause of disease.

There is a substantial scientific literature on the mechanisms by which tobacco smoking causes disease. This body of research includes characterization of many components in smoke, some having well-established toxicity, such as nicotine, hydrogen cyanide, benzo(a)-pyrene, carbon monoxide, and nitrogen oxides. The toxicity of smoke has been studied by exposing animals to tobacco smoke and smoke condensate, in cellular and other laboratory systems for evaluating toxicity, and by assessing smokers for evidence of injury by tobacco smoke, using biomarkers such as tissue changes and levels of damaging enzymes and cytokines. The data from these studies amply document the powerful toxicity of tobacco smoke. The mechanisms of disease causation by tobacco smoke include changes in the genetic material of cells that leads to malignancy; inflammatory injury to the cells lining the surfaces, such as the lung's airways where smoke deposits, and to more distant sites, such as the blood vessels, that are affected by circulating tobacco smoke components; impairment of the body's defence mechanisms; and specific effects reflecting pharmacologic consequences of specific components, for example, nicotine, and reduction of oxygen-carrying capacity from carbon monoxide in tobacco smoke.

Exposure to secondhand smoke

Concentrations of secondhand smoke

Tobacco smoke is a complex mixture of gases and particles that contains myriad chemical species (US Department of Health Education and Welfare *et al.* 1979; US Department of Health and Human Services 1984; Jenkins *et al.* 2000; International Agency for Research on Cancer 2004). Not surprisingly, tobacco smoking in indoor environments increases levels of respirable particles, nicotine, polycyclic aromatic hydrocarbons, carbon monoxide (CO), acrolein, nitrogen dioxide (NO_2), and many other substances. Figure 16.1 from the 2006 Surgeon General's report summarizes major studies on nicotine concentrations in homes, offices, other workplaces, and restaurants where smoking is permitted (US Department of Health and Human Services 2006). The extent of the increase in concentrations of these markers varies with the number of smokers, the intensity of smoking, the rate of exchange between the indoor air space and with the outdoor air, and the use of air-cleaning devices. Ott (Ott 1999) has used mass balance models to characterize factors influencing concentrations of tobacco smoke indoors. Using information on the source

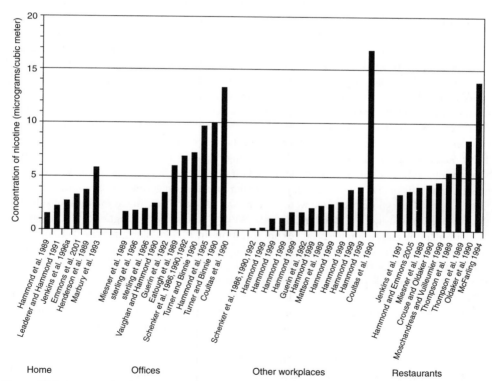

Figure 16.1 Average nicotine concentrations in homes, offices, other workplaces, and restaurants where smoking is permitted.

Source: US Department of Health and Human Services 2006.

strength (i.e., the generation of emissions by cigarettes) and on the air exchange rate, researchers can apply mass balance models to predict tobacco smoke concentrations. Such models can be used to estimate exposures and to project the consequences of control measures (Repace *et al.* 2007).

Several components of cigarette smoke have been measured in indoor environments as markers of the contribution of tobacco combustion to indoor air pollution. Particles, a non-specific marker, have been measured because both SS and MS contain high concentrations of particles in the respirable size range (National Research Council and Committee on Passive Smoking 1986; US Department of Health and Human Services 1986). Other, more specific markers have also been measured, including nicotine, solanesol, and ultraviolet light (UV) absorption of particulate matter (Jenkins *et al.* 2000; US Department of Health and Human Services 2006). Nicotine in SHS can be readily measured with passive diffusion badges (Jenkins *et al.* 2000; US Department of Health and Human Services 2006). Studies of levels of SHS components have been conducted largely in public buildings; fewer studies have been conducted in homes and offices (US Department of Health and Human Services 2006; Wipfli *et al.* 2008).

The contribution of various environments to personal exposure to tobacco smoke varies with the time-activity pattern, namely the distribution of time spent in different locations. Time-activity patterns may heavily influence lung airway exposures in particular environments for certain groups of individuals. For example, exposure in the home predominates for infants who do not attend day care (Harlos *et al.* 1987). For adults residing with non-smokers, the workplace may be the principal location where exposure takes place.

The contribution of smoking in the home to indoor air pollution has been demonstrated by studies using personal monitoring and monitoring of homes for respirable particles. In one of the early studies, Spengler *et al.* (1981) monitored homes in six US cities for respirable particle concentrations over several years and found that a smoker of one pack of cigarettes daily contributed about 20 $\mu g/m^3$ to 24-hour indoor particle concentrations. Because cigarettes are not smoked uniformly over the day, higher peak concentrations must occur when cigarettes are actually smoked and also when the non-smoker is in close proximity to the smoker. Spengler *et al.* (1985) measured the personal exposures to respirable particles sustained by non-smoking adults in two rural Tennessee communities. The mean 24-hour exposures were substantially higher for those exposed to smoke at home: 64 $\mu g/m^3$ for those exposed versus 36 $\mu g/m^3$ for those not exposed. These measurements indicate the strength of burning cigarettes as a source of indoor air pollution.

In several studies, homes have been monitored for nicotine, which is a vapour-phase constituent of SHS. In a study of SHS exposure of day-care children, average nicotine concentration during the time that the SHS-exposed children were at home was 3.7 $\mu g/m^3$; during home without smoking, the average was 0.3 $\mu g/m^3$ (Henderson *et al.* 1989). Coultas and colleagues (1990) measured 24-hour nicotine and respirable particle concentrations in 10 homes on alternate days for a week and then on five more days during alternate weeks. The mean levels of nicotine were comparable to those in the study of Henderson *et al.* (1989), but some 24-hour values were as high as 20 $\mu g/m^3$. Nicotine and respirable particle concentrations varied widely in the homes.

The total exposure assessment methodology (TEAM) study, conducted by the US Environmental Protection Agency, provided extensive data on concentrations of 20 volatile organic compounds in a sample of homes in several communities (Wallace and Pellizzari 1987). Indoor monitoring showed increased concentrations of benzene, xylenes, ethylbenzene, and styrene in homes with smokers compared to homes without smokers (Wipfli *et al.* 2008).

Extensive information is available on levels of SHS components in public buildings and workplaces of various types (US Department of Health and Human Services 2006) (Fig. 16.1). Monitoring in locations where smoking may be intense, such as bars and restaurants, has generally shown elevations of particles and other markers of smoke pollution where smoking takes place (National Research Council and Committee on Passive Smoking 1986; US Department of Health and Human Services 2006). For example, Repace and Lowrey (1980) in a 1980 study used a portable piezobalance to sample aerosols in restaurants, bars, and other locations. This study provided early documentation of the strength of smoking as a source of particles. In the places sampled, respirable particle levels ranged up to 700 μg/m^3, and the levels varied with the intensity of smoking. More recently, a number of studies have used portable particle monitors to measure short-term concentrations of respirable particles in bars, casinos, and other hospitality settings (Repace 2004; Jones *et al.* 2006; Repace *et al.* 2006; Hyland *et al.* 2008). The findings similarly show that very high levels of particles may occur. Similar data have now been reported for the office environment (National Cancer Institute 1999; Jenkins *et al.* 2000; US Department of Health and Human Services 2006). More recent studies indicate low concentrations in many workplace settings, reflecting declining smoking prevalence in recent years and changing practices of smoking in the workplace. Using passive nicotine samplers, studies showed that worksite smoking restriction or prohibition policies can sharply reduce SHS exposure (US Department of Health and Human Services 2006).

Transportation environments may also be polluted by cigarette smoking. Contamination of air in trains, buses, automobiles, airplanes, and submarines has been documented (National Research Council and Committee on Airliner Cabin Environment Safety Committee 1986; US Department of Health and Human Services 1986). A National Research Council report (National Research Council and Committee on Airliner Cabin Environment Safety Committee 1986) on air quality in airliners summarized studies for tobacco smoke pollutants in commercial aircraft. In one study, during a single flight, the NO$_2$ concentration varied with the number of passengers with a lighted cigarette. In another study, respirable particles in the smoking section were measured at concentrations five or more times higher than in the non-smoking section. Peaks as high as 1000 μg/m^3 were measured in the smoking section. Mattson and colleagues (1989) used personal exposure monitors to assess nicotine exposures of passengers and flight attendants. All persons were exposed to nicotine, even if seated in the non-smoking portion of the cabin. Exposures were much greater in the smoking than in the non-smoking section and were also greater in aircraft with recirculated air. Fortunately, with the banning of tobacco-smoking on all domestic flights in 1987 and on all flights into and out of the United States in 1999, the issue has for the most part been resolved, as reflected in the National Research Council's 2002 updated report (National Research Council *et al.* 2002). Most recently, several studies have addressed the impact of smoking on air quality in motor vehicle (Edwards *et al.* 2006; Rees and Connolly 2006). Rees and Connolly conducted driving experiments under different smoking and ventilation conditions, and monitored the level of respirable suspended particles ≤2.5 microns in aerodynamic diameter (PM$_{2.5}$) and carbon monoxide using a personal aerosol monitor. Over a 5-minute mean smoking phase PM$_{2.5}$ concentration increased over ten-fold under closed-ventilation condition and over two-fold under open-ventilation condition (Rees and Connolly 2006). In a pilot study in New Zealand, researchers found that mean PM$_{2.5}$ concentration in a car with three cigarettes smoked and extinguished consecutively did not return to baseline level until almost 40 minutes after the last cigarette with windows closed (Edwards *et al.* 2006).

Health effects of passive smoking

Overview

Evidence on the health risks of passive smoking comes from epidemiologic studies, which have directly assessed the associations of measures of SHS exposure with disease outcomes. Judgements about the causality of associations between SHS exposure and health outcomes are based not only on this epidemiologic evidence, but also on the extensive evidence derived from epidemiologic and toxicologic investigation on the health consequences of active smoking. To date, the evidence has supported causal conclusions on a range of acute and chronic adverse effects in children and adults (Table 16.1). This chapter provides an overview of the now extensive data on adverse health effects of passive smoking on women and children, drawing on various synthesis reports and other reviews (US Department of Health and Human Services 2006; Samet *et al.* 2009b). The evidence is reviewed separately for adults and children.

In interpreting this evidence, a principal competing explanation to causality for associations between SHS exposure and disease risk is confounding; that is, the association between SHS exposure and disease risk reflects the action of another factor, besides SHS exposure, which is correlated with SHS exposure and also a risk factor for the health outcome of concern. Critics of the evidence, largely affiliated with the tobacco industry, have repeatedly raised concerns about confounding, citing such factors as diet for lung cancer and socioeconomic status for respiratory illnesses in children. The various syntheses of evidence have given close attention to the issue of confounding and have concluded that confounding alone cannot explain the observed findings. This repeated emphasis on confounding was one component of the industry's strategy to maintain controversy about the scientific evidence on passive smoking, and was also figured permanently in litigations (Francis *et al.* 2006).

Concerns related to misclassification of active smoking status and also to the extent of exposure to SHS have also been raised. Misclassification of active smoking status has been offered as one potential explanation for the association of lung cancer with SHS exposure, particularly as assessed by the smoking status of the spouse (Lee 1986, 1988). Since smokers tend to marry smokers, any misreporting of active smoking status would tend to introduce a positive association of lung cancer risk with spouse smoking, given the much higher risk for lung cancer in active smokers compared with never smokers. The potential for this source of bias to explain the observed association of spouse smoking with lung cancer risk in never smokers has been examined quantitatively and set aside by, for example, the US Environmental Protection Agency in its 1992 risk assessment (US Environmental Protection Agency 1992) and Hackshaw *et al.* (1997) in their meta-analysis. Exposure to SHS is inevitably assessed with some misclassification with the extent of error depending on the exposure setting. In general, random misclassification is anticipated, which tends to reduce the strength of association. Thus, estimates of risk of exposure to SHS may tend to be underestimates.

Adverse effects of secondhand smoke exposure on children

Overview

The evidence on passive smoking and children was most recently reviewed by the US Surgeon General and the Cal/EPA (California Environmental Protection Agency *et al.* 2005; US Department of Health and Human Services 2006); the conclusions were even stronger than those of prior reviewing groups on the effects of passive smoking on children (Table 16.1). Exposure to SHS has been classified as a cause of slightly reduced birth weight, lower respiratory illnesses, chronic respiratory symptoms, middle ear disease, and reduced lung function growth. Maternal smoking was characterized as a major cause of sudden infant death syndrome (SIDS) by WHO in its 1999 consultation (World Health Organization 1999), and more recently postnatal exposure to SHS has been classified as a cause of SIDS as well (California Environmental Protection Agency *et al.* 2005; US Department of Health and Human Services 2006). The specific adverse effects are considered briefly below.

Fetal effects

Researchers have demonstrated that active smoking by mothers during pregnancy results in a variety of adverse health effects in children, postulated to result predominantly from transplacental exposure of the fetus to tobacco smoke components and from reduced oxygen delivery (US Department of Health and Human Services 2001). Maternal smoking during pregnancy reduces birth weight (US Department of Health and Human Services 2001) and causes increased risk for SIDS. Secondhand smoke exposure of non-smoking mothers is associated with reduced birth weight as well, although the extent of the reduction is far less than that for active maternal smoking during pregnancy. In a meta-analysis, the summary estimate of the reduction of birth weight associated with paternal smoking was only 28 g (Windham *et al.* 1999), compared with about 200 g for maternal smoking.

Health effects on the child postnatally, resulting from either SHS exposure to the fetus or to the newborn child, include SIDS, and adverse effects on neuropsychologic development and physical growth. A number of components of SHS may produce these effects, including nicotine and carbon monoxide. Possible longer term health effects of fetal SHS exposure include increased risk for childhood cancers of the brain, leukaemia, and lymphomas, among others. A meta-analysis of the evidence on childhood cancer through the time of the 1999 WHO consultation, subsequently reported elsewhere, did not show a significant association of SHS exposure with overall risk for childhood cancer or for leukaemia (Boffetta *et al.* 2000). The evidence available to date has been considered insufficient to reach any conclusion with regard to causality (US Department of Health and Human Services 2006; Samet *et al.* 2009b).

Perinatal health effects

These health effects include reduced fetal growth, growth retardation, and congenital abnormalities. In most studies, paternal smoking status has been used as the exposure measure to assess the association between SHS exposure and these nonfatal perinatal health effects. Low birth weight was first reported in 1957 to be associated with maternal smoking (Simpson 1957), and maternal cigarette smoking during pregnancy is considered to be causally associated with low birth weight (US Department of Health and Human Services 1989). Recent studies report lower birth weight for infants of non-smoking women passively exposed to tobacco smoke during pregnancy (Martin and Bracken 1986; Rubin *et al.* 1986).

Other nonfatal perinatal health effects possibly associated with SHS exposure are growth retardation and congenital malformations, and a few studies assessed fatal perinatal health effects. Martin and Bracken (1986) demonstrated a strong association with growth retardation in their 1986 study, and several more recent studies provide support (Zhang *et al.* 1992; Roquer *et al.* 1995). The few studies conducted to assess the association between paternal smoking and congenital malformations (Seidman *et al.* 1990; Savitz *et al.* 1991; Zhang *et al.* 1992) have demonstrated risks ranging from 1.2 to 2.6 for those exposed compared with those nonexposed. These studies are too limited to support any conclusions.

Postnatal health effects

Secondhand smoke exposure due to maternal or paternal smoking may lead to postnatal health effects, including increased risk for SIDS, reduced physical development, decrements in cognition and behaviour, and increased risk for childhood cancers. For cognition and behaviour, evidence is limited and is not considered in this review. There is more extensive information available on maternal smoking during pregnancy and subsequent neurocognitive development (US Department of Health and Human Services 2001).

SIDS

SIDS refers to the unexpected death of a seemingly healthy infant while asleep. Although maternal smoking during pregnancy has been causally associated with SIDS, these studies measured maternal smoking after pregnancy, along with paternal smoking and household smoking generally. In the WHO consultation, the evidence on passive smoking (i.e., post-birth) and SIDS was considered to be inconclusive, although there was some indication of increased risk (World Health Organization 1999). Subsequent studies have led to far stronger conclusions on SHS and SIDS (Table 16.1). A number of studies of paternal smoking showed increased risk, thus documenting that exposure to SHS after birth was sufficient to cause SIDS (US Department of Health and Human Services 2006).

Cancers

Secondhand smoke exposure has been evaluated as a risk factor for the major childhood cancers. The evidence is limited and does not yet support conclusions about the causal nature of the observed associations. In the meta-analysis conducted for the WHO consultation (Boffetta *et al.* 2000), the pooled estimate of the relative risk for any childhood cancer associated with maternal smoking was 1.11 (95% confidence interval (CI):1.00, 1.23) and that for leukaemia was 1.14 (95% CI: 0.97, 1.33). Subsequent reports remain mixed (Samet *et al.* 2009b).

Lower respiratory tract illnesses in childhood

Lower respiratory tract illnesses are extremely common during childhood. Studies of involuntary smoking and lower respiratory illnesses in childhood, including the more severe episodes of bronchitis and pneumonia, provided some of the earliest evidence on adverse effects of SHS (Colley *et al.* 1974; Harlap and Davies 1974). Presumably, this association represents an increase in the frequency or in the severity of illnesses that are infectious in aetiology and not a direct response of the lung to the toxic components of SHS. Effects of exposure to tobacco smoke *in utero* on the airways may also play a role in the effect of postnatal exposure on risk for lower respiratory illnesses. Infants of mothers who smoke during pregnancy have evidence of damage to their airways during gestation on lung function testing shortly after birth, and this damage may increase the likelihood of having a more severe infection (US Department of Health and Human Services 2006). The evidence indicates that the airways of the exposed infants are functionally narrowed and have a higher degree of non-specific responsiveness.

Investigations conducted throughout the world have demonstrated an increased risk of lower respiratory tract illness in infants with parents who smoked (Strachan and Cook 1997; US Department of Health and Human Services 2006). These studies indicate a significantly increased frequency of bronchitis and pneumonia during the first year of life of children with parents who smoked. Strachan and Cook (1997) reported a quantitative review of this information that was updated in the 2006 Surgeon General's report (US Department of Health and Human Services 2006). Overall, the approximate increase in illness risk was 50% if either parent smoked, with odds ratios for maternal smoking somewhat higher. Although the health outcome measures varied somewhat among the studies, the relative risks associated with involuntary smoking were similar, and dose–response relations with extent of parental smoking were demonstrable. Although most of the studies have shown that maternal smoking rather than paternal smoking underlies the increased risk of parental smoking, studies from China and elsewhere show that paternal smoking alone can increase incidence of lower respiratory illness (Chen *et al.* 1986; Strachan and Cook 1997; US Department of Health and Human Services 2006). In these studies, an effect of passive smoking has not been readily identified after the first year of life. During the first year of life, the strength of its effect may reflect higher exposures consequent to the time-activity patterns of young infants, which place them in proximity to cigarettes smoked by their mothers, as well as the particular susceptibility of infants.

Respiratory symptoms and illness in children

Data from numerous surveys demonstrate a greater frequency of the most common respiratory symptoms: cough, phlegm, and wheeze in the children of smokers (Table 16.2) (US Department of Health and Human Services 1986; Cook and Strachan 1997; US Department of Health and Human Services 2006). In these studies, the subjects have generally been schoolchildren, and the effects of parental smoking have been examined. Thus, the less prominent effects of passive smoking, in comparison with the studies of lower respiratory illness in infants, may reflect lower exposures to SHS by older children who spend less time with their parents. The 2006 Surgeon General's report (US Department of Health and Human Services 2006) offers a quantitative summary of the relevant studies (Table 16.2), including 58 with data on wheeze, 44 on chronic cough, 12 on chronic phlegm, and 6 on breathlessness. Overall, this synthesis indicates increased risk for respiratory symptoms for children whose parents smoke (US Department of Health and Human Services 2006). There was even increased risk for breathlessness (OR = 1.31, 95% CI: 1.14, 1.50). Having both parents smoke was associated with the highest levels of risk.

Childhood asthma

Exposure to SHS might cause asthma as a long-term consequence of the increased occurrence of lower respiratory infection in early childhood or through other pathophysiologic mechanisms, including inflammation of the respiratory epithelium (Samet *et al.* 1983; US Department of Health and Human Services 2006). The effect of SHS may also reflect, in part, the consequences of *in utero* exposure. Assessment of airways responsiveness shortly after birth has shown that infants whose mothers smoke during pregnancy have increased airways responsiveness, a characteristic of asthma, compared with those whose mothers do not smoke (Young *et al.* 1991). Maternal smoking during pregnancy also reduces ventilatory function measured shortly after birth (Hanrahan *et al.* 1992). These observations suggest that *in utero* exposures from maternal smoking may affect lung development and may increase risk for asthma and also for more severe lower respiratory illnesses, as reviewed above.

While the underlying mechanisms remain to be better characterized, the epidemiologic evidence linking SHS exposure and childhood asthma is mounting (California Environmental Protection Agency *et al.* 2005; US Department of Health and Human Services 2006). Quantitative syntheses show a significant excess of prevalent childhood asthma if both parents smoke or the mother smokes (Table 16.2). Evidence also indicates that involuntary smoking worsens the status of those with asthma. For example, Murray and Morrison (1986, 1988) evaluated asthmatic children followed in a clinic in Canada. Level of lung function, symptom frequency, and responsiveness to inhaled histamines were adversely affected by maternal smoking. Population studies have also shown increased airways responsiveness for SHS-exposed children with asthma (O'Connor *et al.* 1987; Martinez *et al.* 1988). The increased level of airway responsiveness associated with SHS exposure would be expected to increase the clinical severity of asthma. In this regard, exposure to smoking in the home has been shown to increase the number of emergency room visits made by asthmatic children (Burnett *et al.* 1997). Asthmatic children with mothers who smoked are more likely to use asthma medications (Weitzman *et al.* 1990), a finding that confirms the clinically significant effects of SHS on children with asthma. Guidelines for the management of asthma urge cessation of smoking by parents of young children with asthma in the household (National Heart Lung and Blood Institute and National Asthma Education and Prevention Program 2007).

Table 16.2 Summary of pooled random effects odds ratios with 95% confidence intervals

Symptom	Number of studies	Odds ratios (95% confidence interval)				
		Either parent smokes	One parent smokes	Both parents smoke	Only mother smokes	Only father smokes
Asthma	31[a]	1.23 (1.14–1.33)				
	7		1.01 (0.84–1.22)			
	10			1.42 (1.30–1.56)		
	21				1.33 (1.24–1.43)	
	12					1.07 (0.97–1.18)
Wheeze[b]	45[a,c]	1.26 (1.20–1.33)				
	13		1.18 (1.10–1.26)			
	14			1.41 (1.23–1.63)		
	27[d]				1.28 (1.21–1.35)	
	14					1.13 (1.08–1.20)
Cough	39	1.35 (1.27–1.43)				
	18		1.27 (1.14–1.41)			
	18			1.64 (1.48–1.81)		
	16[d]				1.34 (1.17–1.54)	
	10					1.22 (1.12–1.32)
Phlegm[e]	10	1.35 (1.30–1.41)				
	7		1.24 (1.10–1.39)			
	6			1.42 (1.19–1.70)		
Breathlessness[e]	6	1.31 (1.14–1.50)				

Source: (US Department of Health and Human Services 2006).

Note
[a] Two age groups from Moyes et al. 1995 were included as separate studies.
[b] Excluded the European Communities Study, in which pooled odds ratio was 1.20.
[c] Agabiti et al. 1999 included as two separate studies.
[d] Bracback et al. 1995 included as three separate studies.
[e] Data for phlegm and breathlessness restricted as several comparisons were based on fewer than five studies.

The 2006 report of the US Surgeon General (US Department of Health and Human Services 2006) found the evidence on SHS and incident asthma to be suggestive of a causal association but not conclusive. The relevant evidence comes largely from cohort studies and relatively few have been conducted. Investigations on incident asthma are further complicated by the non-specificity of asthma phenotypes across infancy and childhood (US Department of Health and Human Services 2006).

Lung growth and development

During childhood, measures of lung function increase, more or less parallel to the increase in height. On the basis of the primarily cross-sectional data available at the time, the 1984 report of the Surgeon General (US Department of Health and Human Services 1984) concluded that the children of parents who smoked in comparison with those of non-smokers had small reductions of lung function, but the long-term consequences of these changes were regarded as unknown. On the basis of further longitudinal evidence, the 1986 report (US Department of Health and Human Services 1986) concluded that involuntary smoking reduces the rate of lung function growth during childhood. Evidence from cohort studies has continued to accumulate (California Environmental Protection Agency *et al.* 2005; US Department of Health and Human Services 2006). The difficulty of separating effects of *in utero* exposure from those of childhood SHS exposure because most mothers who smoke while pregnant continue to do so after the birth of their children needs consideration in interpreting these studies. Cross-sectionally, children whose parents smoke have about a 5% reduction in measures of the functioning of the lung's small airways (US Department of Health and Human Services 2006).

Secondhand smoke and middle-ear disease in children

Numerous studies have addressed SHS exposure and middle-ear disease (US Department of Health and Human Services 2006). Positive associations between SHS and otitis media have been consistently demonstrated in studies of the prospective cohort design, but not as consistently in case-control studies. This difference in findings may reflect the focus of the cohort studies on the first two years of life, the peak age of risk for middle-ear disease. The case-control studies, however, have been directed at older children who are not at lower risk for otitis media. Exposure to SHS has been most consistently associated with recurrent otitis media and not with incident or single episodes of otitis media. In their 1997 meta-analysis, Cook and Strachan (1997a) found a pooled odds ratio of 1.48 (95% CI: 1.08, 2.04) for recurrent otitis media if either parent smoked, 1.38 (95% CI: 1.23, 1.55) for middle-ear effusions, and 1.21 (95% CI: 0.95, 1.53) for outpatient or inpatient care for chronic otitis media or 'glue ear'. Similar estimates were reported in the updated analysis in the 2006 Surgeon General's report (Fig. 16.2) (US Department of Health and Human Services 2006). The US Surgeon General's Office and the Cal/EPA (California Environmental Protection Agency *et al.* 2005; US Department of Health and Human Services 2006) reviewed the literature on SHS and otitis media most recently and concluded that there is a causal association between SHS exposure and otitis media in children.

Health effects of involuntary smoking on adults

Lung cancer

In 1981, reports published from Japan (Hirayama 1981a) and from Greece (Trichopoulos *et al.* 1981) indicated increased lung cancer risk in non-smoking women married to cigarette smokers. Subsequently, this still-controversial association has been examined in many investigations

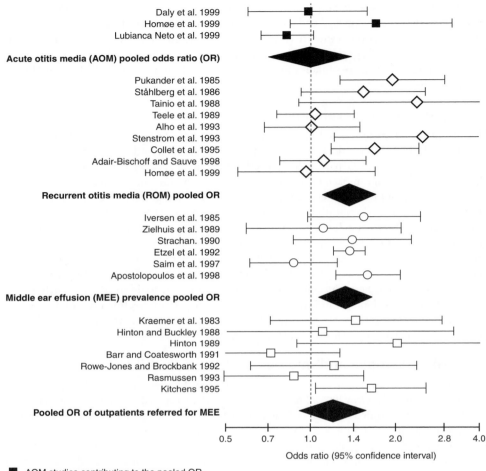

Figure 16.2 Odds ratios for the effect of smoking by either parent on middle-ear disease in children.

Source: (US Department of Health and Human Services 2006).

conducted in the United States and other countries around the world, including a substantial number of studies in Asia. The association of involuntary smoking with lung cancer derives biologic plausibility from the presence of carcinogens in SS and the lack of a documented threshold dose for respiratory carcinogenesis in active smokers (US Department of Health and Human Services 1982; International Agency for Research on Cancer 1986). Moreover, genotoxic activity, the ability to damage DNA, has been demonstrated for many components of SHS (Claxton *et al.* 1989; Lofroth 1989; Weiss *et al.* 1989). Experimental exposure of non-smokers to SHS leads to their excreting 4-(methylnitrosamino)-1-(3-pyridyl)-1-butanol (NNAL), a tobacco-specific carcinogen, in their urine. Non-smokers exposed to SHS in their homes also excrete higher levels of this carcinogen (Anderson *et al.* 2001). Non-smokers, including children, exposed to SHS also have increased concentrations of adducts of tobacco-related carcinogens, that is detectable binding of the carcinogens to DNA of white blood cells, for example (Maclure *et al.* 1989; Crawford *et al.* 1994).

The first major epidemiological studies on SHS and lung cancer were reported in 1981. The early report by Hirayama (1981a) was based on a prospective cohort study of 91 540 non-smoking women in Japan. Standardized mortality ratios for lung cancer increased significantly with the amount smoked by the husbands. The findings could not be explained by confounding factors and were unchanged when follow-up of the study group was extended (Hirayama 1984). On the basis of the same cohort, Hirayama also reported significantly increased risk for non-smoking men married to wives who smoked 1–19 cigarettes and 20 or more cigarettes daily (Hirayama 1984). In 1981, Trichopoulos *et al.* (1981) also reported increased lung cancer risk in non-smoking women married to cigarette smokers. These investigators conducted a case-control study in Athens, Greece, which included cases with a diagnosis other than for orthopaedic disorders. The positive findings reported in 1981 were unchanged with subsequent expansion of the study population (Trichopoulos *et al.* 1983). By 1986, the evidence had mounted, and the three synthesis reports published in that year concluded that SHS was a cause of lung cancer (International Agency for Research on Cancer 1986; National Research Council and Committee on Passive Smoking 1986; US Department of Health and Human Services 1986).

In 1992, the US Environmental Protection Agency (US Environmental Protection Agency 1992) published its risk assessment of SHS as a carcinogen. The Agency's evaluation drew on the toxicologic evidence on SHS and the extensive literature on active smoking. A meta-analysis of the 31 studies published to that time was central to the decision to classify SHS as a class A carcinogen, that is, a known human carcinogen. The meta-analysis considered the data from the epidemiologic studies by tiers of study quality and location and used an adjustment method for misclassification of smokers as never-smokers. Overall, the analysis found a significantly increased risk of lung cancer in never-smoking women married to smoking men; for the studies conducted in the United States, the estimated relative risk was 1.19 (90% CI: 1.04, 1.35).

The meta-analysis included pooled estimates by geographic region. The data from China and Hong Kong were notable for not showing the increased risk associated with passive smoking that was found in other regions (US Environmental Protection Agency 1992). The epidemiologic characteristics of lung cancer in women in this region of the world have been distinct with a relatively high proportion of lung cancers in non-smoking women. Explanations for this pattern have centred on exposures to cooking fumes and indoor air pollution from coal-fuelled space heating (Samet *et al.* 2009a).

A 1997 meta-analysis by Hackshaw and colleagues (1997) included 37 published studies. The excess risk of lung cancer for smokers married to non-smokers was estimated as 24% (95% CI: 13%, 36%). Adjustment for potential bias, including misclassification of some smokers as never smokers, and confounding by diet did not alter the estimate. More recently, the IARC (International Agency for Research on Cancer 2004) reviewed more than 50 studies, finding a similar increase in risk. Stayner *et al.* (2007) reported an analysis on workplace exposure, also finding an increased risk.

Secondhand smoke and coronary heart disease (CHD)

Causal associations between active smoking and fatal and nonfatal CHD outcomes have long been demonstrated (US Department of Health and Human Services 2004). The risk of CHD in active smokers increases with the amount and duration of cigarette smoking and decreases relatively quickly with cessation. Active cigarette smoking is considered to (1) increase the risk of cardiovascular disease by promoting atherosclerosis; (2) increase the tendency to thrombosis;

(3) cause spasm of the coronary arteries; (4) increase the likelihood of cardiac arrhythmias; and (5) decrease the oxygen-carrying capacity of the blood (US Department of Health and Human Services 2004). Barnoya and Glantz (2005) summarized the pathophysiologic mechanisms by which passive smoking might increase the risk of heart disease, giving emphasis to the same mechanisms considered to be relevant to active smoking. It is biologically plausible that passive smoking could also be associated with increased risk for CHD through these same mechanisms, although the lower exposures to smoke components of the passive smoker have raised questions regarding the relevance of the mechanisms cited for active smoking. Several experimental studies have shown that exposure to SHS may affect platelets and endothelial cell functioning (US Department of Health and Human Services 2006). Studies of human volunteers show that even brief exposures to SHS adversely affect measures of endothelial cell functioning (Celermajer *et al.* 1996; Sumida *et al.* 1998; Otsuka *et al.* 2001). Complementary evidence is available from research on other inhaled pollutants. A substantial body of evidence links particulate air pollution, which has many properties comparable to the particles in SHS, to adverse cardiovascular effects (Brook *et al.* 2004; Pope and Dockery 2006).

Epidemiologic data first raised concern that passive smoking may increase risk for CHD with the 1985 report of Garland *et al.* (1985), based on a cohort study in southern California. There are now more than 20 studies on the association between SHS and cardiovascular disease (US Department of Health and Human Services 2006). These studies assessed both fatal and nonfatal cardiovascular heart disease outcomes, and most used self-administered questionnaires to assess SHS exposure. They cover a wide range of populations, both geographically and racially. While many of the studies were conducted within the United States, studies were also conducted in Europe (Scotland, Italy, and the United Kingdom), Asia (Japan and China), South America (Argentina), and the South Pacific (Australia and New Zealand). The majority of the studies measured the effect of SHS exposure due to spousal smoking; however, some studies also assessed exposures from smoking by other household members or occurring at work or in transit. Several studies included measurement of SHS exposure biomarkers (Whincup *et al.* 2004; Venn and Britton 2007).

While the risk estimates for the association of SHS with CHD outcomes vary in these studies, they range from null to modest, but statistically significant increases in risk, with the risk estimates for fatal outcomes generally higher. In their 1997 meta-analysis, Law and Hackshaw (1997) estimated the excess risk from SHS exposure as 30% (95% CI: 22%, 38%) at age 65 years. The findings were similar in a meta-analysis of 18 studies reported by He and colleagues (1999). The overall increase in risk associated with passive exposure was 25% and the risk increased with duration and level of smoking. Based on 16 studies, the pooled estimate in the 2006 Surgeon General's Report was 1.27 (95% CI: 1.19, 1.36) (US Department of Health and Human Services 2006). A number of groups have concluded that SHS exposure causes CHD (Table 16.1).

Additional, powerful evidence reflecting a causal role for SHS and CHD comes from studies of morbidity and mortality after the implementation of smoking bans (Samet 2006). The first such study was carried out in Helena, Montana; the authors tracked hospital admissions across a time period when a ban was implemented and then ended (Sargent *et al.* 2004). The ban was followed by a surprisingly large reduction in the number of admissions, about 40%. Similar reports have followed from other locations including not only the United States (Bartecchi *et al.* 2006; Juster *et al.* 2007), but also Italy (Cesaroni *et al.* 2008) and Scotland (Pell *et al.* 2008). The report from Scotland estimated the decrease for both smokers and non-smokers with the finding that the bulk of the reduction was among non-smokers (Pell *et al.* 2008). Richiardi *et al.* (2008) used a modelling approach to estimate that bans should reduce rates of acute myocardial infarction by 5–15%. Further reports can be anticipated as additional national bans are implemented.

The American Heart Association's Council on Cardiopulmonary and Critical Care concluded that SHS both increases the risk of heart disease and is 'a major preventable cause of cardiovascular disease and death' (Taylor *et al.* 1992). This conclusion was echoed in 1998 by the Scientific Committee on Tobacco and Health in the United Kingdom (Scientific Committee on Tobacco Health and HSMO 1998). The Cal/EPA (California Environmental Protection Agency *et al.* 2005) recently concluded that there is an overall excess risk of 20–50% for CHD due to exposure from SHS. The Centers for Disease Control and Prevention (CDC) estimated 46 000 annual deaths due to CHD from 2000–2004 among non-smokers exposed to SHS (2008). A much smaller body of evidence on SHS and stroke has not yet been found sufficient to reach a causal conclusion (US Department of Health and Human Services 2006).

Respiratory symptoms and illnesses in adults

This topic was most recently reviewed in the 2006 report of the Surgeon General (US Department of Health and Human Services 2006). Largely cross-sectional investigations provide the available information on the association between respiratory symptoms in non-smokers and involuntary exposure to tobacco smoke. These studies have primarily considered exposure outside the home. Among the 13 epidemiologic studies that were reviewed in the 2006 Surgeon General's report, only a few were longitudinal in their design (Schwartz and Zeger 1990; Robbins *et al.* 1993; Jaakkola *et al.* 1996). Consistent evidence of an effect of SHS exposure on acute respiratory symptoms in adults has been found (US Department of Health and Human Services 2006). However, the evidence of an effect of SHS on chronic respiratory symptoms has been less consistent (US Department of Health and Human Services 2006). Overall, symptoms of chronic cough and dyspnea have been more consistently associated with exposure to SHS than have chronic phlegm and wheeze (US Department of Health and Human Services 2006).

Active smoking is causally associated with increased risk for pneumonia and influenza (US Department of Health and Human Services 2004). Several studies suggest that exposure to SHS may also cause acute respiratory morbidity. Analysis of National Health Interview Survey data showed that being married to a pack-a-day smoker increases respiratory restricted days by about 20% for a non-smoking spouse (Ostro 1989). A study of determinants of daily respiratory symptoms in Los Angeles student nurses found a significantly increased risk of an episode of phlegm associated with having a smoking roommate, after controlling for personal smoking (Schwartz and Zeger 1990).

A number of studies have addressed chronic respiratory symptoms (US Department of Health and Human Services 2006). For example, Leuenberger *et al.* (1994) describe associations between passive exposures to tobacco smoke, at home and in the workplace, and respiratory symptoms in 4 197 randomly selected never-smoking adults in the Swiss Study on Air Pollution and Lung Diseases in Adults, a multicenter study in eight areas of the country. Exposed subjects were those who reported any exposure during the past 12 months; exposed persons were then asked about workplace exposure and also about the number of smokers and the duration of exposure at home and work together. Involuntary smoke exposure was associated with asthma, dyspnea, bronchitis and chronic bronchitis symptoms, and allergic rhinitis. The increments in risk were substantial, ranging from approximately 40% to 80% for the different respiratory outcome measures. Dose–response relationships were found with the quantitative indicators of exposure. For several of the outcome measures, the dose–response relationships tended to be steeper for those who also reported workplace exposure. In a cross-sectional study of 1 954 women, Baker and Henderson (1999) found a significant association (OR = 1.73; 95% CI: 1.05, 2.85) of wheeze in non-smoking mothers living with a smoking partner. No association was found in fathers.

Acute effects of SHS exposure have also been documented. Studies of bar workers, before and after implementation of smoking bans, have shown reduction of respiratory symptoms on a short-term basis. In a 1998 report, Eisner *et al.* (1998) described the respiratory benefits for bar workers of the California smoking ban. At baseline before the ban, 74% had respiratory symptoms; after the ban, the majority of those with symptoms were no longer symptomatic. In studies of the smoking bans in Ireland (Goodman *et al.* 2007) and Scotland (Menzies *et al.* 2006), reduced symptoms were shown in bar workers after the bans.

Asthma could be plausibly worsened by SHS, which contains irritant gases as well as respirable particles. The relevant evidence comes from a small set of experimental studies and diverse epidemiological studies. The experimental evidence primarily comes from studies that assessed acute responses of asthmatics who were exposed to SHS in a chamber. This experimental approach cannot be readily controlled because of the impossibility of blinding subjects to SHS. However, suggestibility does not appear to underlie physiological responses of asthmatics to SHS (Urch *et al.* 1988). Of the three studies involving exposure of unselected asthmatics to SHS, only one showed a definite adverse effect (Shephard *et al.* 1979; Dahms *et al.* 1981; Hargreave *et al.* 1981; Murray and Morrison 1986; Qin *et al.* 1991). Stankus *et al.* (1988) recruited 21 asthmatics who reported exacerbation with exposure to SHS. With challenge in an exposure chamber at concentrations much greater than that typically encountered in indoor environments, seven subjects experienced a more than 20% decline in FEV_1.

Several epidemiologic studies have investigated the roles of SHS exposure in the onset of asthma and in exacerbating asthma in adults. Mannino *et al.* (1997), using data from the 1991 National Health Interview Survey found that lifetime non-smokers exposed to SHS had a 44% increased risk of exacerbated chronic respiratory conditions, compared to unexposed non-smokers, after adjusting for potential confounders. In a small case-control study, Tarlo *et al.* (2000) found that asthma patients with an exacerbation were more likely to have been exposed to SHS than asthma patients without an exacerbation. In a cohort study of lifetime non-smoking asthma patients in India by Jindal *et al.* (1994), SHS exposure was found to increase the risk of acute episodes and impaired lung function. Ostro *et al.* (1994) also found an increased risk of shortness of breath, cough, and restricted activity among asthmatics exposed to SHS compared to unexposed asthmatics. Sippel *et al.* (1999) found a significant increase in the use of hospital services, such as urgent care and emergency room visits, among asthma patients exposed to SHS compared to those who were unexposed. In a prospective cohort study of adult non-smokers admitted to the hospital for asthma, Eisner *et al.* (2005) found a significant association between the severity of asthma symptoms and SHS exposure after controlling for potential confounders.

As for cardiovascular disease, the implementation of smoking bans provides an opportunity to assess the consequences of SHS exposure for persons with asthma. In a study published in 2006, Menzies *et al.* (2006) reported findings of a beneficial health effect of the smoking ban in Scotland on the health of bar workers. The investigators measured FEV_1 level in nonasthmatic and asthmatic non-smoking bar workers before and after the ban was implemented. They found that the FEV_1 level increased after the ban was implemented. They also found a decrease in the prevalence of respiratory symptoms among non-smoking bar workers. The bar workers with asthma experienced a reduction in the level of exhaled nitrous oxide and an improvement on a respiratory health quality-of-life scale.

In 1999 review, Weiss *et al.* (1999) identified two prospective cohort studies and a population-based case-control study that found a significant association between SHS exposure and the onset of asthma in adults. They concluded that because the evidence is scant and has potential problems in study design, 'a definitive conclusion cannot be made at this time'. Subsequently, a population-based case-control study by Jaakkola *et al.* (2003) investigated the association between SHS exposure and the onset of adult asthma in the Pirkanmaa district of Finland. They recruited all incident cases of asthma in the district and selected population-based controls. There were 239 lifetime non-smoking cases and a comparison group of 487 lifetime non-smoking controls. They found a two-fold increased risk of asthma among those exposed to SHS in the home and the workplace compared with those who were unexposed.

The 2006 Surgeon General's report (US Department of Health and Human Services 2006) considered the relevant evidence on SHS and causation and exacerbation of asthma in adults. For both, the evidence was found to be 'suggestive, but not sufficient' for causation.

Lung function in adults

With regard to involuntary smoking and lung function in adults, exposure to SHS has been associated in cross-sectional investigations with reduction of the FEF_{25-75}. In one of the first studies to address this consequence of exposures to SHS, White and Froeb (1980) compared spirometric test results in middle-aged non-smokers with at least 20 years of involuntary smoking in the workplace to the results in an unexposed control group of non-smokers. The mean FEF_{25-75} of the exposed group was significantly reduced, by 15% of predicted value in women and by 13% in men. This investigation was intensely criticized, largely by tobacco industry-related scientists, when published with regard to the spirometric test procedures, the determination and classification of exposures, and the handling of former smokers in the analyses. An investigation in France examined the effect of marriage to a smoker in over 7 800 adults in seven cities (Kauffmann et al. 1983). The study included 849 male and 826 female non-smokers exposed to tobacco smoke by their spouses' smoking. At age above 40 years, the FEF_{25-75} was reduced in non-smoking men and women with a smoking spouse. The investigators interpreted this finding as representing a cumulative adverse effect of marriage to a smoker. In a subsequent report, the original findings in the French women were confirmed, but a parallel analysis in a large population of US women did not show effects of involuntary smoking on lung function (Spengler and Ferris 1985).

The results of an investigation of 163 non-smoking women in the Netherlands also suggested adverse effects of tobacco smoke exposure in the home on lung function (Brunekreef et al. 1985; Remijn et al. 1985). Cross-sectional analysis of spirometric data collected in 1982 demonstrated adverse effects of tobacco smoke exposure in the home, but in a sample of the women, domestic exposure to tobacco smoke was not associated with longitudinal decline of lung function during the period 1965–1982.

Svendsen et al. (1987) assessed the effects of spouse smoking on 1 400 non-smoking male participants in the Multiple Risk Factor Intervention Trial (MRFIT). The participants, aged 35–57 years at enrolment, were at high risk for mortality from coronary artery disease. At baseline, the maximum FEV_1 was approximately 3% lower for the men married to a smoker.

Masi et al. (1988) evaluated lung function of 293 young adults, using spirometry and measurement of the diffusing capacity and lung volumes. The results varied with gender. In men, reduction of the maximal midexpiratory flow rate was associated with maternal smoking and exposure to SHS during childhood. In women, reduction of the diffusing capacity was associated with exposure to SHS at work.

In the study of a general population sample in western Scotland, non-smokers living with another household member who was a smoker had significantly reduced lung function in comparison to unexposed non-smokers (Hole et al. 1989); the reduction of FEV_1 associated with involuntary smoking was about 5%. Secondhand smokers with higher exposure had greater reduction of the FEV_1.

Masjedi et al. (1990) investigated the effects of exposure to SHS on lung function of 288 non-smoking volunteers living in Tehran. Ventilatory function was reduced significantly for men exposed at work, although an additional effect of exposure at home was not found. Secondhand smoke exposure at home and at work did not reduce the lung function of the female subjects.

In a meta-analysis of 15 cross-sectional studies, Carey *et al.* found a mean deficit of 1.7% in FEV_1 level due to SHS exposure (Carey *et al.* 1999). They also conducted a separate cross-sectional investigation of 1 623 adults in Britain and found similar results, with a stronger effect in men than in women. Subsequently, Chen *et al.* found an inverse dose–response relationship between SHS and FEV_1 level in 301 adults in Scotland for exposure to SHS at work (Chen *et al.* 2001).

In a study of young Canadian adults, Jaakkola *et al.* (1995) did not find effects of home and workplace exposures on eight-year change in lung function. In persons less than 26 years of age at enrolment, workplace SHS exposure was associated with greater decline. In another cohort study of 1 391 lifetime non-smokers and former smokers in California, Abbey *et al.* found a decrease in the ratio of FEV_1 to FVC in both women exposed at home and men exposed at work (Abbey *et al.* 1998). However, the results were not statistically significant.

Using NHANES III data, Eisner (2002) conducted a cross-sectional study to investigate the association between level of SHS exposure and pulmonary function in 10 581 non-smoking adults and 440 non-smoking adults with asthma. He found that FVC and FEV_1 levels were significantly lower in adult females with the highest concentration of serum cotinine levels compared to adult females with lower serum cotinine levels. He did not find a significant association in adult males.

Several investigators have reported associations of involuntary smoking with COPD in non-smokers. In the Japanese cohort study, a nonsignificant trend of increasing mortality from chronic bronchitis and emphysema with increasing passive exposure of non-smoking women was reported (Hirayama 1984). Kalandidi *et al.* (1987) conducted a case-control study of involuntary smoking and COPD; the cases were non-smoking women with obstruction and reduction of the FEV_1 by at least 20%. Smoking by the husband was associated with a doubling of risk. Dayal *et al.* (1994) conducted a case-control study of self-reported obstructive lung disease in 219 never-smoking residents of Philadelphia. Household SHS exposure from one or more packs per day was associated with a doubling of risk. In a prospective cohort study of 3 914 non-smoking Adventists, SHS exposure was associated with report of symptoms considered to be reflective of 'airway obstructive disease' (Robbins *et al.* 1993). An association of SHS exposure with COPD seems biologically implausible, however, since only a minority of active smokers develop this disease, and adverse effects of involuntary smoking on lung function in adults have not been observed consistently (US Department of Health and Human Services 1984). The autopsy study of Trichopoulos *et al.* (1992) did show, however, that airways of non-smokers can be affected by SHS.

The 2006 report of the Surgeon General states that the evidence is suggestive but not sufficient to infer a causal association for the effects of SHS exposure on lung function in adults (US Department of Health and Human Services 2006). However, further research is warranted because of widespread exposure in workplaces and homes.

Odour and irritation

Tobacco smoke contains numerous irritants, including particulate matter and gases (US Department of Health and Human Services 1986). Both questionnaire surveys and laboratory studies involving exposure to SHS have shown annoyance and irritation of the eyes and upper and lower airways from involuntary smoking. Consequently, SHS has long been regarded as a cause of irritation (US Department of Health and Human Services 1986; US Department of Health and Human Services 2006). The odour and irritation associated with SHS merit special consideration because a high proportion of non-smokers are annoyed by exposure to SHS, and control of concentrations in indoor air poses difficult problems in the management of heating, ventilating, and air-conditioning systems.

Conclusion

In about three decades, we have progressed from the first studies on passive smoking and health to definitive evidence that passive smoking causes disease. The evidence includes not only epidemiological studies, but studies with biomarkers documenting that tobacco smoke inhaled by non-smokers delivers doses of toxic components and metabolites to target organs. There are also animal studies and extensive data on patterns of exposure. The strength of the evidence and its public health implications have been a strong force for motivating tobacco control policy.

References

(2008). 'Smoking-attributable mortality, years of potential life lost, and productivity losses – United States, 2000–2004.' *MMWR Morb Mortal Wkly Rep*, **57**(45): 1226–8.

Abbey, D.E., Burchette, R.J. *et al.* (1998). 'Long-term particulate and other air pollutants and lung function in nonsmokers.' *American Journal of Respiratory and Critical Care Medicine*, **158**(1): 289–98.

Anderson, K.E., Carmella, S.G. *et al.* (2001). 'Metabolites of a tobacco-specific lung carcinogen in nonsmoking women exposed to environmental tobacco smoke.' *Journal of the National Cancer Institute*, **93**(5): 378–81.

Baker, D. and Henderson J. (1999). 'Differences between infants and adults in the social aetiology of wheeze. The ALSPAC Study Team. Avon Longitudinal Study of Pregnancy and Childhood.' *Journal of Epidemiology and Community Health*, **53**(10): 636–42.

Barnoya, J. and Glantz S.A. (2005). 'Cardiovascular effects of secondhand smoke: nearly as large as smoking.' *Circulation*, **111**(20): 2684–98.

Bartecchi, C., Alsever, R.N. *et al.* (2006). 'Reduction in the incidence of acute myocardial infarction associated with a citywide smoking ordinance.' *Circulation*, **114**(14): 1490–6.

Boffetta, P., Tredaniel, J. *et al.* (2000). 'Risk of childhood cancer and adult lung cancer after childhood exposure to passive smoke: A meta-analysis.' *Environmental Health Perspectives*, **108**(1): 73–82.

Brandt, A.M. (2007). *The Cigarette Century: The Rise, Fall, and Deadly Persistence of the Product That Defined America*. New York, Basic Books.

Brook, R.D., Franklin, B. *et al.* (2004). 'Air pollution and cardiovascular disease: a statement for healthcare professionals from the Expert Panel on Population and Prevention Science of the American Heart Association.' *Circulation*, **109**(21): 2655–71.

Brunekreef, B., Fischer, P. *et al.* (1985). 'Indoor air pollution and its effect on pulmonary function of adult nonsmoking women. III. Passive smoking and pulmonary function.' *International Journal of Epidemiology*, **14**: 227–30.

Burnett, R.T., Cakmak, S. *et al.* (1997). 'The role of particulate size and chemistry in the association between summertime ambient air pollution and hospitalization for cardiorespiratory diseases.' *Environmental Health Perspectives*, **105**(6): 614–20.

California Environmental Protection Agency and Office of Environmental Health Hazard Assessment (1997). Health Effects of Exposure to Environmental Tobacco Smoke, California Environmental Protection Agency.

California Environmental Protection Agency, Office of Environmental Health Hazard Assessment, *et al.* (2005). Proposed identification of environmental tobacco smoke as a toxic air contaminant Sacramento, CA California Environmental Protection Agency.

Cameron, P. (1967). 'The presence of pets and smoking as correlates of perceived disease.' *Journal of Allergy*, **67**(1): 12–15.

Cameron, P., Kostin, J.S. *et al.* (1969). 'The health of smokers' and nonsmokers' children.' *Journal of Allergy*, **43**(6): 336–41.

Carey, I.M., Cook, D.G. *et al.* (1999). 'The effects of environmental tobacco smoke exposure on lung function in a longitudinal study of British adults.' *Epidemiology*, **10**(3): 319–26.

Celermajer, D.S., Adams, M.R. *et al.* (1996). 'Passive smoking and impaired endothelium-dependent arterial dilatation in healthy young adults.' *New England Journal of Medicine*, **334**(3): 150–4.

Cesaroni, G., Forastiere, F. *et al.* (2008). 'Effect of the Italian smoking ban on population rates of acute coronary events.' *Circulation*, **117**(9): 1183–8.

Chen, R., Tunstall-Pedoe, H. *et al.* (2001). 'Environmental tobacco smoke and lung function in employees who never smoked: the Scottish MONICA study.' *Occupational and Environmental Medicine*, **58**(9): 563–8.

Chen, Y., Li, W. *et al.* (1986). 'Influence of passive smoking on admissions for respiratory illness in early childhood.' *British Medical Journal*, **293**: 303–06.

Claxton, L.D., Morin, R.S. *et al.* (1989). 'A genotoxic assessment of environmental tobacco smoke using bacterial bioassays.' *Mutation Research*, **222**(2): 81–99.

Colley, J.R. and Holland, W.W. (1967). 'Social and environmental factors in respiratory disease. A preliminary report.' *Archives of Environmental Health*, **67**(1): 157–61.

Colley, J.R., Holland, W.W. *et al.* (1974). 'Influence of passive smoking and parental phlegm on pneumonia and bronchitis in early childhood.' *Lancet*, **2**(7888): 1031–4.

Cook, D.G. and Strachan, D.P. (1997). 'Health effects of passive smoking. 3. Parental smoking and prevalence of respiratory symptoms and asthma in school age children.' *Thorax*, **52**(12): 1081–94.

Coultas, D.B., Samet, J.M. *et al.* (1990). 'Variability of measures of exposure to environmental tobacco smoke in the home.' *American Review of Respiratory Disease*, **142**: 602–06.

Crawford, F.G., Mayer, J. *et al.* (1994). 'Biomarkers of environmental tobacco smoke in preschool children and their mothers.' *Journal of the National Cancer Institute*, **86**(18): 1398–402.

Dahms, T.E., Bolin, J.F.*et al.* (1981). 'Passive smoking: effects on bronchial asthma.' *Chest*, **80**(5): 530–4.

Dayal, H.H., Khuder, S. *et al.* (1994). 'Passive smoking in obstructive respiratory disease in an industrialized urban population.' *Environmental Research*, **65**(2): 161–71.

Edwards, R., Wilson, N. *et al.* (2006). 'Highly hazardous air quality associated with smoking in cars: New Zealand pilot study.' *The New Zealand Medical Journal*, **119**(1244): U2294.

Eisner, M.D. (2002). 'Environmental tobacco smoke exposure and pulmonary function among adults in NHANES III: impact on the general population and adults with current asthma.' *Environmental Health Perspectives*, **110**(8): 765–70.

Eisner, M.D., Klein, J. *et al.* (2005). 'Directly measured second hand smoke exposure and asthma health outcomes.' *Thorax*, **60**(10): 814–21.

Eisner, M.D., Smith, A.K. *et al.* (1998). 'Bartenders' respiratory health after establishment of smoke-free bars and taverns.' *Journal of the American Medical Association*, **280**(22): 1909–14.

Francis, J.A., Shea, A.K. *et al.* (2006). 'Challenging the epidemiologic evidence on passive smoking: tactics of tobacco industry expert witnesses.' *Tobacco Control*, 15 Suppl 4: iv68–iv76.

Garland, C., Barret-Connor, E. *et al.* (1985). 'Effects of passive smoking on ischemic heart disease mortality of nonsmokers: a prospective study.' *American Journal of Epidemiology*, **121**(5): 645–50.

Goodman, P., Agnew, M. *et al.* (2007). 'Effects of the Irish smoking ban on respiratory health of bar workers and air quality in Dublin pubs.' *American Journal of Respiratory and Critical Care Medicine*, **175**(8): 840–5.

Hackshaw, A.K., Law, M.R. *et al.* (1997). 'The accumulated evidence on lung cancer and environmental tobacco smoke.' *British Medical Journal*, **315**(7114): 980–8.

Hanrahan, J.P., Tager, I.B. *et al.* (1992). 'The effect of maternal smoking during pregnancy on early infant lung function.' *American Review of Respiratory Disease*, **145**: 1129–35.

Hargreave, F.E., Ryan, G. *et al.* (1981). 'Bronchial responsiveness to histamine or methacholine in asthma: measurement and clinical significance.' *Journal of Allergy and Clinical Immunology*, **68**: 347–55.

Harlap, S. and Davies, A.M. (1974). 'Infant admissions to hospital and maternal smoking.' *Lancet*, **1**: 529–32.

Harlos, D.P., Marbury, M. *et al.* (1987). 'Relating indoor NO 2 levels to infant personal exposures.' *Atmospheric Environment*, **21**(2): 369–78.

He, J., Vupputuri, S. *et al.* (1999). 'Passive smoking and the risk of coronary heart disease – a meta-analysis of epidemiologic studies.' *New England Journal of Medicine*, **340**(12): 920–6.

Hecht, S.S., Samet, J.M. *et al.* (2007). Cigarette smoking. *Environmental and Occupational Medicine*, 4th edn. Philadelphia, Wolters Kluwer/Lippincott Williams & Wilkins: 1521–51.

Henderson, F.W., Reid, H.F. *et al.* (1989). 'Home air nicotine levels and urinary cotinine excretion in preschool children.' *American Review of Respiratory Disease*, 140(1): 197–201.

Hirayama, T. (1981a). 'Non-smoking wives of heavy smokers have a higher risk of lung cancer: a study from Japan.' *Br Med J (Clin Res Ed)*, 282(6259): 183–5.

Hirayama, T. (1981b). 'Passive smoking and lung cancer.' *British Medical Journal*, 282: 1393–4.

Hirayama, T. (1984). 'Cancer mortality in nonsmoking women with smoking husbands based on a large-scale cohort study in Japan.' *Preventive Medicine*, 13(6): 680–90.

Hole, D.J., Gillis, C.R. *et al.* (1989). 'Passive smoking and cardiorespiratory health in a general population in the west of Scotland.' *British Medical Journal*, 299(6696): 423–7.

Hyland, A., M. Travers, J. *et al.* (2008). 'A 32-country comparison of tobacco smoke derived particle levels in indoor public places.' *Tobacco Control*, 17(3): 159–65.

International Agency for Research on Cancer (1986). IARC Monographs on the Evaluation of the Carcinogenic Risk of Chemicals to Humans: Tobacco Smoking. Lyon, France, World Health Organization, IARC.

International Agency for Research on Cancer (2004). Tobacco smoke and involuntary smoking. IARC monograph 83. Lyon, France, International Agency for Research on Cancer.

Jaakkola, M.S., Jaakkola, J.J. *et al.* (1996). 'Effect of passive smoking on the development of respiratory symptoms in young adults: an 8-year longitudinal study.' *Journal of Clinical Epidemiology*, 49(5): 581–6.

Jaakkola, M.S., Jaakkola, J.J.K. *et al.* (1995). 'Passive smoking and evolution of lung function in young adults. An eight-year longitudinal study.' *Journal of Clinical Epidemiology*, 48: 317–27.

Jaakkola, M.S., Piipari, R. *et al.* (2003). 'Environmental tobacco smoke and adult-onset asthma: a population-based incident case-control study.' *American Journal of Public Health*, 93(12): 2055–60.

Jenkins, R.A., Guerin, M.R. *et al.* (2000). The Chemistry of Environmental Tobacco Smoke: Composition and Measurement (2nd edn). Boca Raton, Lewis Publishers.

Jindal, S.K., Gupta, D.*et al.* (1994). 'Indices of morbidity and control of asthma in adult patients exposed to environmental tobacco smoke.' *Chest*, 106: 746–9.

Jones, S.C., Travers, M.J. *et al.* (2006). 'Secondhand smoke and indoor public spaces in Paducah, Kentucky.' *The Journal of the Kentucky Medical Association*, 104(7): 281–8.

Juster, H.R., Loomis, B.R. *et al.* (2007). 'Declines in hospital admissions for acute myocardial infarction in New York state after implementation of a comprehensive smoking ban.' *American Journal of Public Health*, 97(11): 2035–9.

Kalandidi, A., Trichopoulos, D. *et al.* (1987). 'Passive smoking and chronic obstructive lung disease.' *Lancet*, 2(8571): 1325–6.

Kauffmann, F., Tessier, J.F. *et al.* (1983). 'Adult passive smoking in the home environment: a risk factor for chronic airflow limitation.' *American Journal of Epidemiology*, 117(3): 269–80.

Law, M.R. and Hackshaw, A.K. (1997). 'A meta-analysis of cigarette smoking, bone mineral density and risk of hip fracture: recognition of a major effect.' *British Medical Journal*, 315(7112): 841–6.

Lee, P.N. (1986). 'Misclassification as a factor in passive smoking risk [letter].' *Lancet*, 86(8511): 867.

Lee, P.N. (1988). *Misclassification of Smoking Habits and Passive Smoking*. Berlin, Springer Verlag.

Leuenberger, P., Schwartz, J. *et al.* (1994). 'Passive smoking exposure in adults and chronic respiratory symptoms (SAPALDIA Study).' *American Journal of Respiratory and Critical Care Medicine*, 150(5 Pt 1): 1222–8.

Lofroth, G. (1989). 'Environmental tobacco smoke: overview of chemical composition and genotoxic components.' *Mutation Research*, 222(2): 73–80.

Maclure, M., Katz, R.B. *et al.* (1989). 'Elevated blood levels of carcinogens in passive smokers.' *American Journal of Public Health*, 89(10): 1381–4.

Mannino, D.M., Siegel, M. *et al.* (1997). 'Environmental tobacco smoke exposure in the home and worksite and health effects in adults: results from the 1991 National Health Interview Survey.' *Tobacco Control*, 6(4): 296–305.

Martin, T.R. and Bracken, M.B. (1986). 'Association of low birth weight with passive smoke exposure in pregnancy.' *American Journal of Epidemiology*, **124**(4): 633–42.

Martinez, F.D., Antognoni, G. *et al.* (1988). 'Parental smoking enhances bronchial responsiveness in nine-year-old children.' *American Review of Respiratory Disease*, **138**: 518–523.

Masi, M.A., Hanley, J.A. *et al.* (1988). 'Environmental exposure to tobacco smoke and lung function in young adults.' *American Review of Respiratory Disease*, **138**(2): 296–9.

Masjedi, M.R., Kazemi, H. *et al.* (1990). 'Effects of passive smoking on the pulmonary function of adults.' *Thorax*, **45**(1): 27–31.

Mattson, M.E., Boyd, G. *et al.* (1989). 'Passive smoking on commercial airline flights.' *Journal of the American Medical Association*, **261**: 867–72.

Menzies, D., Nair, A. *et al.* (2006). 'Respiratory symptoms, pulmonary function, and markers of inflammation among bar workers before and after a legislative ban on smoking in public places.' *Journal of the American Medical Association*, **296**(14): 1742–8.

Michaels, D. (2008). *Doubt is their Product: How Industry's Assault on Science Threatens Your Health.* New York, NY, Oxford University Press.

Murray, A.B. and Morrison, B.J. (1986). 'The effect of cigarette smoke from the mother on bronchial responsiveness and severity of symptoms in children with asthma.' *Journal of Allergy and Clinical Immunology*, **77**(4): 575–81.

Murray, A.B. and Morrison, B.J. (1988). 'Passive smoking and the seasonal difference of severity of asthma in children.' *Chest*, **88**(4): 701–08.

National Cancer Institute (1999). Health effects of exposure to environmental tobacco smoke. The report of the California Environmental Protection Agency. Monograph 10. [NIH Pub. No. 99–4645]. Bethesda, MD US Department of Health and Human Services, National Institutes of Health, National Cancer Institute.

National Heart Lung and Blood Institute and National Asthma Education and Prevention Program (2007). Expert Panel Report 3: Guidelines for the Diagnosis and Management of Asthma. Bethesda, MD, US Department of Health and Human Services; National Institutes of Health.

National Research Council, Committee on Air Quality in Passenger Cabins of Commercial Aircraft, *et al.* (2002). *The Airliner Cabin Environment and the Health of Passengers and Crew.* Washington, D.C., National Academy Press.

National Research Council and Committee on Airliner Cabin Environment Safety Committee (1986). *The Airliner Cabin Environment: Air Quality and Safety.* Washington, D.C., National Academy Press.

National Research Council and Committee on Passive Smoking (1986). *Environmental Tobacco Smoke: Measuring Exposures and Assessing Health Effects.* Washington, D.C., National Academy Press.

O'Connor, G.T., Weiss, S.T. *et al.* (1987). 'The effect of passive smoking on pulmonary function and nonspecific bronchial responsiveness in a population-based sample of children and young adults.' *American Review of Respiratory Disease*, **135**: 800–04.

Ostro, B.D. (1989). 'Estimating the risks of smoking, air pollution, and passive smoke on acute respiratory conditions.' *Risk Analysis*, **9**(2): 189–96.

Ostro, B.D., Lipsett, M.J. *et al.* (1994). 'Indoor air pollution and asthma. Results from a panel study.' *American Journal of Respiratory and Critical Care Medicine*, **149**: 1400–06.

Otsuka, R., Watanabe, H. *et al.* (2001). 'Acute effects of passive smoking on the coronary circulation in healthy young adults.' *Journal of the American Medical Association*, **286**(4): 436–41.

Ott, W.R. (1999). 'Mathematical models for predicting indoor air quality from smoking activity.' *Environmental Health Perspectives*, **107**(Suppl 2): 375–81.

Pell, J.P., Haw, S. *et al.* (2008). 'Smoke-free legislation and hospitalizations for acute coronary syndrome.' *New England Journal of Medicine*, **359**(5): 482–91.

Pope, C.A., III and Dockery, D.W. (2006). 'Health effects of fine particulate air pollution: lines that connect.' *Journal of the Air and Waste Management Association*, **56**(6): 709–42.

Proctor, R.N. (1995). *Cancer Wars. How Politics Shapes What We Know and Don't Know About Cancer.* New York, Basic Books.

Qin, D.X., Li, J.Y. *et al.* (1991). 'Sputum occult blood screening for lung cancer. Stage II screening of 14,431 subjects.' *Cancer,* **67**(7): 1960–3.

Rees, V.W. and Connolly, G.N. (2006). 'Measuring air quality to protect children from secondhand smoke in cars.' *American Journal of Preventive Medicine,* **31**(5): 363–8.

Remijn, B., Fischer, P. *et al.* (1985). 'Indoor air pollution and its effect on pulmonary function of adult nonsmoking women. I. Exposure estimates for nitrogen dioxide and passive smoking.' *International Journal of Epidemiology,* **14**: 215–20.

Repace, J. (2004). 'Respirable particles and carcinogens in the air of delaware hospitality venues before and after a smoking ban.' *Journal of Occupational and Environmental Medicine,* **46**(9): 887–905.

Repace, J.L., Hyde, J.N. *et al.* (2006). 'Air pollution in Boston bars before and after a smoking ban.' *BMC Public Health,* **6**: 266.

Repace, J.L. and Lowrey, A.H. (1980). 'Indoor air pollution, tobacco smoke, and public health.' *Science,* **208**: 464–72.

Repace, J.L., Ott, W.R. *et al.* (2007). Exposure to secondhand smoke. *Exposure Analysis.* Boca Raton, FL, CRC Press-Taylor & Francis Group: 201–35.

Richiardi, L., Vizzini, L. *et al.* (2009). 'Cardiovascular benefits of smoking regulations: The effect of decreased exposure to passive smoking.' *Preventive Medicine,* **48**(2): 167–72.

Robbins, A.S., Abbey, D.E. *et al.* (1993). 'Passive smoking and chronic respiratory disease symptoms in non-smoking adults.' *International Journal of Epidemiology,* **22**(5): 809–17.

Roquer, J.M., Figueras, J. *et al.* (1995). 'Influence on fetal growth of exposure to tobacco smoke during pregnancy.' *Acta Paediatrica,* **84**: 118–21.

Royal College of Physicians of London (1962). Smoking and Health. Summary of a report of the Royal College of Physicians of London on smoking in relation to cancer of the lung and other diseases. London, Pitman Medical Publishing Co., LTD: S2–70.

Rubin, D.H., Krasilnikoff, P.A. *et al.* (1986). 'Effect of passive smoking on birth-weight.' *Lancet,* **2**(8504): 415–17.

Samet, J.M. (2006). 'Smoking bans prevent heart attacks.' *Circulation,* **114**(14): 1450–1.

Samet, J.M., Avila-Tang, E. *et al.* (2009a). 'Lung cancer in never smokers: clinical epidemiology and environmental risk factors.' *Clinical Cancer Research,* **15**(18): 5626–45.

Samet, J.M., Neta, G.I. *et al.* (2009b). Secondhand smoke. *Environmental Toxicants: Human Exposures and Their Health Effects,* 3rd Edition. M. Lippmann. Hoboken, N.J., John Wiley & Sons, Inc.: 709–61.

Samet, J.M., Tager, I.B. *et al.* (1983). 'The relationship between respiratory illness in childhood and chronic airflow obstruction in adulthood.' *American Review of Respiratory Disease,* **127**: 508–23.

Sargent, R.P., Shepard, R.M. *et al.* (2004). 'Reduced incidence of admissions for myocardial infarction associated with public smoking ban: before and after study.' *British Medical Journal,* **328**(7446): 977–80.

Savitz, D.A., Schwingl, P.J. *et al.* (1991). 'Influence of paternal age, smoking, and alcohol consumption on congenital anomalies.' *Teratology,* **44**(4): 429–40.

Schwartz, J. and Zeger, S. (1990). 'Passive smoking, air pollution, and acute respiratory symptoms in a diary study of student nurses.' *American Review of Respiratory Disease,* **141**(1): 62–7.

Scientific Committee on Tobacco Health and HSMO (1998). Report of the Scientific Committee on Tobacco and Health, The Stationary Office.

Seidman, D.S., Ever-Hadani, P. *et al.* (1990). 'Effect of maternal smoking and age on congenital anomalies.' *Obstetrics & Gynecology,* **76**(6): 1046–50.

Shephard, R.J., Collins, R. *et al.* (1979). '"Passive" exposure of asthmatic subjects to cigarette smoke.' *Environmental Research,* **20**(2): 392–402.

Simpson, W.J. (1957). 'A preliminary report on cigarette smoking and the incidence of prematurity.' *American Journal of Obstetrics and Gynecology,* **73**(4): 808–15.

Sippel, J., Pedula, K. *et al.* (1999). 'Associations of smoking with hospital based care and quality of life in patients with obstructive airway disease.' *Chest*, **115**: 691–6.

Spengler, J.D., Dockery, D.W. *et al.* (1981). 'Long-term measurements of respirable sulfates and particles inside and outside homes.' *Atmospheric Environment*, **15**: 23–30.

Spengler, J.D. and Ferris, B.G. Jr. (1985). 'Harvard air pollution health study in six cities in the USA.' *The Tokai Journal of Experimental and Clinical Medicine*, **10**(4): 263–86.

Spengler, J.D., Treitman, R.D. *et al.* (1985). 'Personal exposures to respirable particulates and implications for air pollution epidemiology.' *Environmental Science and Technology*, **19**: 700–07.

Stankus, R.P., Menan, P.K. *et al.* (1988). 'Cigarette smoke-sensitive asthma: challenge studies.' *Journal of Allergy and Clinical Immunology*, **82**(3 Pt 1): 331–8.

Stayner, L., Bena, J. *et al.* (2007). 'Lung cancer risk and workplace exposure to environmental tobacco smoke.' *American Journal of Public Health*, **97**(3): 545–51.

Strachan, D.P. and D.G. Cook (1997). 'Health effects of passive smoking. 1. Parental smoking and lower respiratory illness in infancy and early childhood.' *Thorax*, **52**(10): 905–14.

Sumida, H., Watanabe, H. *et al.* (1998). 'Does passive smoking impair endothelium-dependent coronary artery dilation in women?' *Journal of the American College of Cardiology*, **31**(4): 811–5.

Svendsen, K.H., Kuller, L.H. *et al.* (1987). 'Effects of passive smoking in the multiple risk factor intervention trial.' *American Journal of Epidemiology*, **126**(5): 783–95.

Tarlo, S.M., Broder, I. *et al.* (2000). 'A case-control study of the role of cold symptoms and other historical triggering factors in asthma exacerbations.' *Canadian Respiratory Journal*, **7**(1): 42–8.

Taylor, A.E., Johnson, D.C. *et al.* (1992). 'Environmental tobacco smoke and cardiovascular disease: a position paper from the council on cardiopulmonary and critical care, American Heart Association.' *Circulation*, **86**(2): 1–4.

Trichopoulos, D., Kalandidi, A. *et al.* (1983). 'Lung cancer and passive smoking: conclusion of Greek study.' *Lancet*, **2**: 677–8.

Trichopoulos, D., Kalandidi, A. *et al.* (1981). 'Lung cancer and passive smoking.' *International Journal of Cancer*, **27**(1): 1–4.

Trichopoulos, D., Mollo, F. *et al.* (1992). 'Active and passive smoking and pathological indicators of lung cancer risk in an autopsy study.' *Journal of the American Medical Association*, **268**(13): 1697–701.

US Department of Health and Human Services (1982). The health consequences of smoking: Cancer. A report of the Surgeon General. Washington, D.C., US Department of Health and Human Services, Public Health Service, Office on Smoking and Health.

US Department of Health and Human Services (1984). The health consequences of smoking: chronic obstructive lung disease. A report of the Surgeon General. Washington, D.C., US Department of Health and Human Services, Public Health Service, Office on Smoking and Health.

US Department of Health and Human Services (1986). *The Health Consequences of Involuntary Smoking. A Report of the Surgeon General*. Washington, D.C., US Department of Health and Human Services, Public Health Service, Office on Smoking and Health.

US Department of Health and Human Services (1989). *Reducing the Health Consequences of Smoking: 25 Years of Progress. A Report of the Surgeon General*. Washington, D.C., US Department of Health and Human Services, Public Health Service, Office on Smoking and Health.

US Department of Health and Human Services (2001). *Women and Smoking. A Report of the Surgeon General*. Rockville, MD, US Department of Health and Human Services, Centers for Disease Control and Prevention, National Center for Chronic Disease Prevention and Health Promotion, Office on Smoking and Health.

US Department of Health and Human Services (2004). *The Health Consequences of Smoking. A Report of the Surgeon General*. Atlanta, GA, US Department of Health and Human Services, Centers for Disease Control and Prevention, National Center for Chronic Disease Prevention and Health Promotion, Office on Smoking and Health.

US Department of Health and Human Services (2006). *The Health Consequences of Involuntary Exposure to Tobacco Smoke. A Report of the Surgeon General*. Atlanta, GA, US Department of Health and Human Services, Centers for Disease Control and Prevention, Coordinating Center for Health Promotion, National Center for Chronic Disease Prevention and Health Promotion, Office on Smoking and Health.

US Department of Health Education and Welfare (1964). *Smoking and Health. Report of the Advisory Committee to the Surgeon General*. Washington, DC, US Government Printing Office.

US Department of Health Education and Welfare (1971). *The health consequences of smoking. A report of the Surgeon General*: 1971. [None Specified]. Washington, DC, US Government Printing Office.

US Department of Health Education and Welfare, US Environmental Protection Agency, *et al.* (1979). Changes in Cigarette Smoking and Current Smoking Practices Among Adults: United States, 1978. Washington, D.C., US Government Printing Office.

US Environmental Protection Agency (1992). *Respiratory Health Effects of Passive Smoking: Lung Cancer and Other Disorders*. Washington, D.C., US Government Printing Office.

Urch, R.B., Silverman, F. *et al.* (1988). 'Does suggestibility modify acute reactions to passive cigarette smoke exposure?' *Environmental Research*, **47**(1): 34–47.

Venn, A. and Britton, J. (2007). 'Exposure to secondhand smoke and biomarkers of cardiovascular disease risk in never-smoking adults.' *Circulation*, **115**(8): 990–5.

Wallace, L.A. and Pellizzari, E.D. (1987). 'Personal air exposures and breath concentrations of benzene and other volatile hydrocarbons for smokers and nonsmokers.' *Toxicology Letters*, **35**(1): 113–16.

Weiss, B., McClellan, R.O. *et al.* (1989). Behavior as an endpoint for inhaled toxicants. *Concepts in Inhalation Toxicology*. New York, Hemisphere Publishing: 475–93.

Weiss, S.T., Utell, M.J. *et al.* (1999). 'Environmental tobacco smoke exposure and asthma in adults.' *Environmental Health Perspective*, **107** Suppl 6: 891–5.

Weitzman, M., Gortmaker, S. *et al.* (1990). 'Maternal smoking and childhood asthma.' *Pediatrics*, **85**(4): 505–11.

Whincup, P.H., Gilg, J.A. *et al.* (2004). 'Passive smoking and risk of coronary heart disease and stroke: prospective study with cotinine measurement.' *British Medical Journal*, **329**(7459): 200–05.

White, J.R. and Froeb, H.F. (1980). 'Small-airways dysfunction in nonsmokers chronically exposed to tobacco smoke.' *New England Journal of Medicine*, **302**(13): 720–3.

Windham, G.C., Eaton, A. *et al.* (1999). 'Evidence for an association between environmental tobacco smoke exposure and birthweight: a meta-analysis and new data.' *Paediatric and Perinatal Epidemiology*, **13**(1): 35–7.

Wipfli, H., Avila-Tang, E. *et al.* (2008). 'Secondhand smoke exposure among women and children: evidence from 31 countries.' *American Journal of Public Health*, **98**(4): 672–9.

World Health Organization (1999). International Consultation on Environmental Tobacco Smoke (ETS) and Child Health. Consultation Report. Geneva, World Health Organization.

World Health Organization (2003). WHO Framework Convention on Tobacco Control. Geneva.

Wynder, E.L., Graham, E.A. *et al.* (1953). 'Experimental production of carcinoma with cigarette tar.' *Cancer Research*, **13**: 855–64.

Young, S., Le Souef, P.N. *et al.* (1991). 'The influence of a family history of asthma and parental smoking on airway responsiveness in early infancy.' *New England Journal of Medicine*, **324**(17): 1168–73.

Zhang, J., Savitz, D.A. *et al.* (1992). 'A case-control study of paternal smoking and birth defects.' *International Journal of Epidemiology*, **21**(2): 273–8.

Chapter 17

Adolescent smoking

John P. Pierce, Janet M. Distefan, and David Hill

Introduction

It is over 40 years since the public health community came to the consensus that smoking tobacco, particularly cigarettes, caused lung cancer. Despite widespread dissemination of the likely health consequences, cigarette smoking is still a prevalent behaviour in all developed countries and is a rapidly increasing behaviour in developing countries. There is an extensive literature on quitting studies indicating that, for many smokers, successful quitting is one of the hardest lifestyle changes to achieve. Given this, many argue that the majority of the emphasis should be on preventing initiation of smoking in the first place. This chapter focuses on influences encouraging young people to become smokers.

Trends in who initiates smoking

Cigarette smoking can be considered the epidemic of the twentieth century. In 1900, cigarette smoking was rare, with total cigarette sales at 54 cigarettes per person in the United States. Over the next half century, the prevalence of smoking rose rapidly, with sales peaking in 1963 at 4 345 cigarettes per person (FTC 2000). The peak of cigarette smoking for men was seen in those who were born between 1915 and 1930, of whom 70% were addicted. Importantly, all of the men in this highest smoking prevalence cohort were over 20 years of age when the first evidence was published in scientific journals demonstrating that smoking caused lung cancer in men. The highest prevalence of cigarette smoking for women was observed in those who were born between 1935 and 1950, of whom 45% were addicted (Burns *et al.* 1997). Importantly, cigarette smoking among women was a very rare event prior to 1925 at the start of the first cigarette advertising campaign that specifically targeted women (Pierce and Gilpin 1995). Notably, women in the highest prevalence birth cohorts were all exposed to cigarette advertising targeted to them throughout their teenage years.

In all of these early birth cohorts, the vast majority of people who started to smoke did so between the ages of 14 and 25 years, with the peak starting ages being 18–24 years (Lee *et al.* 1993). However, throughout the latter half of the twentieth century, this uptake pattern changed dramatically. At the end of the twentieth century, the vast majority of those who started smoking regularly were between the ages of 14 and 19 years, with the peak starting age group being 14 and 17 years. Among both genders, the initiation rates among 18–21- and 22–24-year-olds have continuously declined since the public health consensus that smoking caused disease in 1964 (Gilpin *et al.* 1994).

A study of trends across birth cohorts in the proportion of adolescents who started smoking as 14–17-year-olds adds further evidence implicating cigarette advertising and promotions as a major factor in adolescent smoking (Table 17.1). The incidence of initiation in 14–17-year-old males increased considerably during both World Wars I and II, by 71 and 62%, respectively,

Table 17.1 Events associated with marked change in incidence of initiation among 14–17-year-old adolescents

Historical event	Period	Targeted audience	% Change in incidence of Initiation
World war I	1916–18	Males	71%
Lucky Strike campaign	1925–30	Females	280%
World war II	1941–45	Males	62%
Virginia Slims campaign	1967–73	Females	41%

Source: Pierce and Gilpin (1995).

when cigarettes became viewed as important in helping soldiers be better fighters by 'soothing the nerves' and were freely distributed to the armed forces (Pierce and Gilpin 1995). As noted above, 14–17-year-old females did not smoke before the first 'Reach for a Lucky instead of a sweet' advertisements in 1925. During the period 1925–30, initiation rates of 14–17-year-old females increased dramatically by 280% (Pierce *et al.* 1994). Thereafter, the rates progressively increased with each birth cohort through 1950. In 1967, the tobacco industry launched a series of cigarettes with advertising campaigns announcing that they were specifically designed for women, the most well known of which was the Virginia Slims cigarette. Coincident with the starting of these campaigns, the uptake of smoking among girls, particularly those who would not proceed to higher education, jumped dramatically by 41% for the period 1967–73 (Pierce *et al.* 1994).

In 1971, Congress enacted a ban on all broadcast advertising of cigarettes in the United States. Shortly thereafter, the initiation rate in all 14–17-year-olds started a 12-year decline (CDCP 1998). The tobacco industry's reaction to this decline in adolescent smoking was to progressively increase tobacco advertising and promotional expenditures. By the mid-1980s, the decline in adolescent smoking was halted. Thereafter, the tobacco industry increased its advertising and promotional expenditures almost exponentially. This was associated with a rapid increase in the uptake of smoking through 1996 that was confined almost completely to the 14–17-year-old age group.

This volatility in trends in the uptake of smoking among adolescents demonstrates that it is possible to rapidly impact the rate of smoking initiation. The question is what would be the impact of this on population prevalence? Obviously, smoking prevalence cannot be maintained if there is no initiation to replace those who successfully quit or who die. The rapidity of the effect on prevalence of smoking in the population can be seen from the experience of United States physicians. At the time of the consensus that smoking caused lung cancer, approximately half the physicians and medical students smoked. However, the report appeared to have a huge effect on medical students; by the early 1980s, only 2% of students in US medical schools in the United States were smoking (Pierce and Gilpin 1994). On the other hand, successful quitting among physicians increased only slowly, in a pattern very similar to other highly educated people in the society. However, within 20 years, the rapid and sustained decline in smoking initiation led to a 6% prevalence of smoking among US physicians (USDHHS 1989).

Studying trends in smoking uptake also provides valuable information on the likely impact of different health promotion messages aimed at discouraging adolescents from smoking. Between 1950 and 1964, there was a barrage of news media coverage on the health consequences of smoking that was associated with many smokers quitting (Pierce and Gilpin 2001). However, there was no discernable effect on initiation rates of people aged 14–24 years. However, after the public health consensus that smoking caused disease in 1964, there has been a continual decline in the proportion of neversmoking adults (aged 18–24 years) who initiated smoking. This effect of the dissemination of the health consequences of smoking in reducing the incidence of initiation in young adults has been replicated in many countries. This declining pattern was not observed among 14–17-year-old adolescents in the United States or anywhere else.

What is the process by which someone becomes a smoker?

Longitudinal studies of adolescents in the late 1980s and 1990s have shown that, at the end of elementary school, children are generally committed never smokers, that is, they do not envisage that there is any way that they will become a smoker. However, for many this certainty does not last, and they eventually become unwilling to rule out smoking in all situations, which we have defined as becoming susceptible to smoking. Susceptible smokers indicate that their decision depends on the particular situation they are in and many would describe themselves as curious about smoking. A series of studies have demonstrated that susceptible never smokers are at twice the risk of smoking of committed never smokers (Pierce *et al.* 1996; Unger *et al.* 1997; Jackson 1998).

Many studies have shown that the more experience a person has with smoking, the greater the likelihood they will be a continuing smoker. Indeed, each increase in the level of experience increases the probability of future smoking.However, this probability decreases with time since the last smoking experience.What people expect they will do in the future is also important. If an adolescent is certain that they will not try a cigarette again, then their risk level is reduced (Choi *et al.* 2001). These variables can be put together to create a continuum for assessing the probability of future smoking for any individual at any point in time.

We use three age-specific indices to identify where a community or population is on this uptake continuum. The first is the proportion of the group who are committed never smokers. In the United States, the main movement out of the committed neversmoking group occurs between the ages of 10 and 14 years. The second marker is the proportion of adolescents who have experimented with smoking, even a few puffs. The modal age of experimentation in the United States is between 12 and 14 years. There is thought to be an important age window for completing experimentation during the teenage years that influences the probability of later daily smoking. The marker used to indicate completion of the experimentation phase is having smoked at least 100 cigarettes in one's lifetime, which is the accepted definition of an adult smoker in the United States. It has been estimated that 50% of adolescents who reach at least 100 cigarettes will still be smoking at age 35 years (Pierce and Gilpin 1996). Interestingly, previously secret tobacco industry documents obtained through the US lawsuits have indicated that the tobacco industry felt that brand loyalty occurred generally after smoking as little as 200 cigarettes of the same brand. Despite this research and concerns relating to recall bias, the traditional measure of adolescent smoking is a period prevalence measure, the proportion who have smoked in the previous 30 days.

How strong is genetics in determining who will become a smoker?

In 1958, the famous statistician, Sir Ronald Fisher, argued that it was possible that people who were genetically at risk to develop cancer were the same people who were genetically at risk to start smoking (Fisher 1958). Given the overwhelming evidence supporting a causal association between smoking and lung cancer, this argument was not at all persuasive in the public policy debate of the time. However, it did raise the issue that there is probably a genetic component to smoking initiation. There has now been considerable research on identical twins, some who have been raised apart. These studies allow the separation of the social environmental influences from genetic influences, and have generally found that there is an important genetic influence on who becomes a smoker. However, the genetic influence is not related to the development of a susceptibility to smoking. Instead, people respond differently to exposure to nicotine, with some appearing to be genetically predisposed to become dependent. In a series of different studies, it appears that a relatively constant 30–50% of experimenters go on to become addicted smokers. As there is a lot of research in this area at the present time, we can expect the knowledge base in this area to expand rapidly in the next decade.

How do friends who smoke affect initiation?

One of the most consistent findings in research on adolescent smoking is that nonsmokers who have friends who smoke soon become smokers themselves (USDHHS 1994). Indeed, the majority of early smoking experiences occur in social settings with cigarettes obtained from a friend, often in the company of a best friend (Bauman *et al.* 1984).

Peer groups are particularly important in the early adolescent years (Steinberg 2002). At the start of adolescence, there is a sharp increase in the amount of time spent with peers, most often without adult supervision. Brown (1990) noted that adolescents in schools quickly start to identify with one of a series of large, reputation-based collectives of similarly stereotyped individuals, even if they don't spend much time with them. In the United States, commonly used labels for these different collectives include 'jocks', 'brains', 'druggies', 'populars', 'nerds', etc. Identifying with one of these collectives locates the teen within the school social structure. To identify with a particular collective, an adolescent will often need to follow the dress code of the collective and to adhere to lifestyle and behaviour preferences of the collective, which includes choice of friends (Brown *et al.* 1993). These collectives serve as the reference group for the adolescent and a source of identity. Adolescents judge one another on the basis of the company they keep, the clothes they wear, the music they listen to, the language that they use, and the places in which they 'hang out'. It is the desire/need of the adolescent to be seen to belong to one of these collectives that provides the 'peer pressure' on adolescents. This is particularly strong in the middle school years, where, typically, the number of peer collectives is limited. It isn't until high school that the collectives become more differentiated and permeable, and thus there is less pressure to conform.

Clearly, if a middle school adolescent is seeking to identify with a collective that has smoking as a condoned lifestyle, then the likelihood of the adolescent starting to smoke will increase significantly. Adolescents do choose the collective they wish to identify with, thus they can influence the type of 'peer pressure' to which they will be subject. However, in the recent studies of the progress toward smoking by committed never smokers, the influence of peers has been somewhat muted (Pierce *et al.* 1998, 2002). This suggests that adolescents who have been influenced to become curious about smoking may seek out peers or friends who smoke as a way of obtaining the first cigarette.

What is the role of parents as an influence on initiation?

Numerous studies have demonstrated that parents and parenting practices are one of the major influences on how an adolescent adjusts in society (Steinberg 2002). A series of studies have identified high levels of responsiveness (good bidirectional communication and support) and demandingness (setting limits and ceding independence with evidence of responsibility) as the most important factors in appropriate adolescent socialization (Baumrind 1978). Contrary to some people's belief, adolescents generally share the value system of their parents. Thus, parenting which comprises high levels of both responsiveness and demandingness, which is considered recommended parenting, can influence adolescent behavior in many ways, including which 'collective' the adolescent associates with at school.

When parents value not smoking, recommended parenting can be expected to be associated with a much lower level of adolescent smoking. This appears to be the situation in most of the United States in the early twenty-first century, and many studies indicate that recommended parenting practices are associated with a halving of the use of nonsanctioned substances, including cigarettes (Mounts and Steinberg 1995; Jackson *et al.* 1994, 1998; Pierce *et al.* 2002). One way this appears to be achieved is by reducing the probability that the adolescent has best friends who smoke (Pierce *et al.* 2002).

Measures of the importance of not smoking in the parental value system include whether or not the parents smoke themselves, their attitudes and behaviour toward other smokers, whether they have a smoke-free home, and the adolescent's expectations of how parents will respond to him or her smoking. Within the tobacco control literature, the measure of parental influence most emphasized has been parental smoking behaviour.While many studies have shown that parental smoking increases the probability of adolescent smoking, there is a growing literature on studies that do not report such an association. Differences in effect would be expected between adolescents who interpret parent smoking as evidence of the difficulty of overcoming a nicotine addiction compared to those who interpret it as evidence that smoking has some real advantages (such as weight or stress control).

How can advertising and promotions entice adolescents to start smoking?

Advertising and promotions have the goal of building sales and profits for a company. A tobacco company's sales can be increased if current smokers change brands, however, the future of the industry requires a continuing supply of new smokers. Over the past century, every time a tobacco company advertising campaign was acclaimed as innovative and successful, adolescent smoking increased (Pierce *et al.* 1994, 1996).

Ray (1982) uses a farming analogy to explain the different tasks of advertising and promotion. The farmer must invest in seeds, plant them, and nurture them before he can reap a crop and sell it to make a profit. To be successful, the farmer needs to balance the amount of sowing and nurturing that he does with the amount of reaping that can be done. Advertising and publicity, as well as some promotional efforts, aim at building the product franchise. Therefore, they can be considered to be in the 'sowing' category. The goals of these types of communication for the tobacco industry are to build awareness of the brand, to increase the proportion of the population who see a benefit to smoking, and to have a positive (or not so negative) feeling toward smoking. Image marketing attempts to associate values with the product (i.e. the cigarette) that the target group would like to have, nearly always through visual imagery. Thus, by buying Marlboro cigarettes, adolescents present a symbol to others that they have reached independence. The initial goal is to build curiosity to try smoking (equivalent to susceptibility to smoking).

Once people are susceptible to smoking, converting them to smoking a particular brand is the goal of 'reaping' activities. The first goal of the tobacco industry is to ensure that cigarettes are fairly easily accessible and at a low cost to the person who is susceptible to smoking. Pricing, package design, and promotions (such as two-for-one and free gift with purchase) are activities that can be described as in the 'reaping' category. One of the secret industry documents outlined a 'reaping' strategy that had as its goal getting the young person to smoke 200 cigarettes, claimed as sufficient to achieve brand loyalty in a new smoker (Young and Rubicam 1990).

The tobacco industry documents outline that they evaluate their advertising campaigns using the standard 'hierarchy of effects' approach. This approach assumes that the adolescent initially needs to be exposed to the message, with the goal of saturation exposure. The 'hierarchy of effects' model of advertising takes account of the fact that not everyone who sees an advertising message will be receptive to it. An individual's level of receptivity to an advertising campaign can be measured.We classify people who label an ad as one of their favourites as moderately receptive. Companies that have been successful in branding their product with an image that resonates with the target audience frequently use brand-extenders such as tee-shirts or tote bags. The person who is willing to wear the image of the product on a piece of clothing, for example, is classified as highly receptive to the marketing campaign.

Using the hierarchy of effects approach to evaluating tobacco advertising, there is very strong evidence that vast majority of adolescents are not only exposed to cigarette advertising but are well aware of the images of the advertised cigarette brands. The vast majority of adolescents understand that cigarette advertising promotes one of the following benefits of smoking: smoking is enjoyable; it helps people relax; it helps people feel comfortable in social situations; it helps people stay thin; it helps people with stress; helps them overcome boredom; and, the 'in-crowd' are smokers. Further, the majority of United States adolescents (even as young as 12–14 years) have a favourite cigarette advertisement. Around 30% of 15–17-year-old adolescents are willing to wear a tee-shirt displaying the brand image used to advertise a cigarette. These results place cigarettes at the top of the products that have good advertising penetration with adolescents.

There are now four separate longitudinal studies in the United States (Pierce *et al.* 1998, 2002; Biener and Siegel 2000; Sargent *et al.* 2000) that have shown that the more receptive an adolescent is to cigarette advertising and promotions (using the above hierarchy of effects) the higher the probability that they will experiment with smoking and become dependent on it. The most recent of these studies indicates that receptivity to tobacco industry advertising can undermine the effectiveness of good parenting in protecting adolescents from starting to smoke (Pierce *et al*).

Public health approaches to reduce smoking initiation

In the United States and in many other countries, there is strong public support for using the public sector to discourage adolescents from starting to smoke. Four of the major approaches used are: the conduct of counter-advertising campaigns, increases in cigarette price through increases in state excise taxes on cigarettes, and increasing enforcement of regulations and laws forbidding merchants to sell cigarettes to minors and school programmes.

Can a mass media campaign lead to a reduction in initiation rates?

The first population-based antismoking mass media campaign occurred in the late 1960s and was associated with a marked decline in the per capita consumption of cigarettes (Warner 1977). During the 1980s the Office on Smoking and Health in the United States ran a sporadic national mass media programme through public service announcements (Pierce *et al.* 1992) and many of these productions targeted adolescent smoking. The first statewide antismoking mass media campaigns started in Australia in 1983 using health consequences messages in paid media. These were demonstrated to effectively reduce adult-smoking prevalence (Dwyer *et al.* 1986; Pierce *et al.* 1990). While adolescents were a target of some of the early campaigns, effective changes in adolescent smoking behaviour were not demonstrated.

Clear evidence that mass media antismoking campaigns could affect youth smoking was demonstrated with the Florida Tobacco Control Program (Bauer *et al.* 2000). The Florida 'Truth' campaign sought to engage youth in a movement that included questioning tobacco industry public messages. This programme achieved extremely high awareness among 12–17-year-olds (92%). More than 10 000 youth signed up for an action program. Over 2 years, this programme achieved dramatic changes in youth smoking across all levels of the smoking uptake continuum in both middle and high schools. The level of committed never smokers increased from 67% to 76% in middle schools. The level of experimentation decreased by 25% and the prevalence of current smokers dropped by more than one-third in middle school and by 18% in high school. These changes are unprecedented, and this programme is the model for the American Legacy National antismoking programme that began in the United States in 1999 with money supplied by the tobacco industry in their legal settlement agreement with the Attorneys General of the various states.

What is the effect of price on initiation?

Econometric studies abound demonstrating that smoking behaviour is heavily influenced by cigarette price, as predicted by standard economic theory. The price elasticity of demand is the phrase used to describe the estimated impact of a change in price on subsequent consumption. Most studies estimate that a 10% increase in price will reduce overall per capita consumption among the overall population by between 2% and 5%. Several studies of adolescents suggest that they are more than twice and possibly three times as responsive to price changes than are adults, as would be expected from their lower level of disposable income (Chaloupka and Grossman 1996; Lewit et al. 1997). Further, as expected, the effect of price in reducing adolescent smoking is mainly seen on those who purchase cigarettes. As discussed earlier, initial experimentation usually involves cigarettes supplied from social sources and evidence supports the hypothesis that price changes will have a considerably lower impact on the proportion of adolescents who experiment than on subsequent purchasing behaviour (Gruber 2000; Tauras et al. 2000; Emery et al. 2001).

It is important to remember that the public health approach is limited to setting the excise tax, while the tobacco industry sets the price as part of their marketing strategy. Indeed, a major component of the advertising and promotional budget is the use of retail value added items that can selectively reduce the actual price that an individual pays for cigarettes. Many of these promotions are focused on the small convenience store, the source of cigarettes for the majority of adolescent smokers and potential smokers.

Does accessibility of cigarettes matter?

During the twentieth century world wars, cigarettes became perceived as essential to the United States war effort and were provided to all soldiers both in their ration packs and on street corners by the Red Cross. This made access to cigarettes relatively easy for 14–17-year-old males. As presented earlier in Table 18.1, these two periods were associated with rapid increases in the initiation of smoking by these adolescents.

In the last 20 years, public policy on reducing teens' access to cigarettes has focused on effectively barring sales of cigarettes to minors. Limiting the ability of minors to purchase cigarettes or other tobacco products is a seemingly practical and politically popular measure (in the United States) aimed at curbing teen smoking, by making it difficult for adolescents to purchase cigarettes. Whether this strategy actually limits teens' access to cigarettes is controversial. Several studies have shown that such laws have minimal impact on teen perceptions that cigarettes are accessible to them or on teen smoking (Chaloupka and Grossman 1996; Rigotti et al. 1997). However, there may be a threshold effect. Analyses of the impact of California's strong enforcement of laws banning tobacco sales to minors have demonstrated a major reduction in the perceived accessibility of cigarettes and that, for the first time, perceived ease of access of cigarettes predicts later smoking behaviour (Gilpin et al. 2001).

What influence do schools have on initiation?

School smoking prevention efforts have the potential to influence adolescent smoking in several ways. A study from Australia indicates that many adolescents start smoking regularly at school

(Hill and Borland 1991). The implementation and enforcement of smoke-free school policies limits the opportunity for teens to smoke. Further, the existence and enforcement of these policies promote norms against smoking as an acceptable behaviour for everyone, including teachers, who are important role models for adolescents. Finally, antismoking curricula can provide vital information on the health dangers and the addictive nature of cigarettes.

For decades, schools have played a central role in educational efforts aimed at smoking prevention (USDHHS 1989, 1994; Hansen 1992; Glynn 1993). It is recognized that such programs have the best chance of success in the setting of comprehensive community-based tobacco control programs (Glynn 1993). If tobacco policies are not consistently enforced in schools, they can convey a mixed message to students (Bowen *et al.* 1995). However, Pentz *et al.* (1989) showed that, when consistently enforced and coupled with cessation education, school-smoking policies are associated with decreased smoking prevalence among adolescents.

By the time adolescents have reached high school, students routinely have had smoking prevention education classes that discuss the health dangers of smoking. The level of smoking experience of the adolescent is associated with how effective they perceive these classes to be. In California, a majority of adolescents who have smoked do not credit the classes with influencing their peers against smoking (Gilpin *et al.* 2001). Therefore, such classes likely have minimal personal impact as well.

Compliance with smoke-free school policies is associated with decreased levels of exposure to smoking at school, including teachers' smoking and increased levels of students who think that the classes on the health effects of smoking are effective. General acceptance of school smoking bans for everyone at school may be a factor in reducing adolescent smoking.

References

Bauer, U.E., Johnson, T.M., Hopkins, R.S., and Brooks, R.G. (2000). Changes in youth cigarette use and intentions following implementation of a tobacco control program: Findings from the Florida Youth Tobacco Survey, 1998–2000. *JAMA*, **284**:723–8.

Bauman, K.E., Fisher, L.A., Bryan, E.S., and Chenoweth, R.L. (1984). Antecedents, subjective expected utility and behavior: A panel study of adolescent cigarette smoking. *Addictive Behaviors*, **9**:121–36.

Baumrind, D. (1978). Parental disciplinary patterns and social competence in children. *Youth and Society*, **9**:239–75.

Biener, L. and Siegel, M. (2000). Tobacco marketing and adolescent smoking: More support for a causal inference. *American Journal of Public Health*, **90**:407–11.

Brown, B. (1990). Peer groups. In: S. Feldman and G. (ed.) Elliott *At the threshold: the developing adolescent*, pp. 171–96. Harvard University Press, Cambridge, MA.

Brown, B.B., Mounts, N., Lamborn, S.D., and Steinberg, L. (1993). Parenting practices and peer group affiliation in adolescence. *Child Development*, **64**:467–82.

Bowen, D.J., Kinne, S., and Orlandi, M. (1995). School policy in COMMIT: A promising strategy to reduce smoking by youth. *Journal of School Health*, **65**:140–4.

Burns, D., Garfinkel, L., and Samet, J.M. (1997). Introduction, summary, and conclusions. In: *Smoking and tobacco control, Monograph 8*. National Cancer Institute, pp. 1–11.

Centers for Disease Control and Prevention (CDCP) (1998). Incidence of initiation of cigarette smoking—United States, 1965–1996. *MMWR*, **47**:837–40.

Chaloupka, F. and Grossman, M. Price (1996). *Tobacco control policies and youth smoking*. National Bureau of Economic Research, Cambridge, MA.

Choi, W.S., Gilpin, E.A., Farkas, A.J., and Pierce, J.P. (2001). Determining the probability of future smoking among adolescents. *Addiction*, **96**:313–23.

Dwyer, T, Pierce, J.P., Hannam, C.D., and Burke, N. (1986). Evaluation of the Sydney 'Quit For Life' Anti-Smoking Campaign. Part II. Changes in smoking prevalence. *Medical Journal of Australia*, **144**:344–7.

Emery, S., White, M.M., and Pierce J.P. (2001). Does cigarette price influence adolescent experimentation? *Journal of Health Economics*, **20**:261–70.

Fisher, R.A. (1958). Cancer and smoking. *Nature*, **182**:596.

FTC (US Federal Trade Commission) (2000). Cigarette Report for 2000. Issued 2002. (http://www.ftc.gov/bcp/menu-tobac.htm). Accessed July 20, 2002.

Gilpin, E.A., Lee, L., Evans, N., and Pierce, J. (1994). Smoking initiation rates in adults and minors: United States, 1944–1988. *American Journal of Epidemiology*, **140**:535–43.

Gilpin, E.A., Emery, S.L., Farkas, A.J., Distefan, J.M., White, M.M., and Pierce, J.P. (2001). *The California tobacco control program: A decade of progress, 1989–1999.* University of California, San Diego, La Jolla, CA.

Glynn, Thomas, J. (1993). Improving the health of U.S. children: The need for early interventions in tobacco use. *Preventative Medicine*, **22**:513–9.

Gruber, J. (2000). Youth smoking in the US: Prices and policies. National Bureau of Economic Research Working Paper, No. 7506.

Hansen,W.B. (1992). School-based substance abuse prevention: A review of the state of the art in curriculum, 1980–1990. *Health Education Research.*, **7**:403–30.

Hill, D. and Borland, R. (1991). Adults' accounts of onset of regular smoking: Influences of school, work, and other settings. *Public Health Reports*, **106**:181–5.

Jackson, C., Henriksen, L., and Foshee, V.A. (1998). The Authoritative Parenting Index: Predicting health risk behaviors among children and adolescents. *Health Education and Behavior*, **25**:319–37.

Jackson, C., Bee-Gates, D.J., and Henriksen, L. (1994). Authoritative parenting, child competencies, and initiation of cigarette smoking. *Health Education Quarterly*, **21**:103–16.

Jackson, C. (1998). Cognitive susceptibility to smoking and initiation of smoking during childhood: A longitudinal study. *Preventive Medicine*, **27**:129–34.

Lee, L.L., Gilpin, E.A., and Pierce, J.P. (1993). Changes in the patterns of initiation of cigarette smoking in the United States: 1950, 1965, and1 980. *Cancer Epidemiol. Biomarkers Prev.*, **2**:593–7.

Lewit, E.M., Hyland, A., *et al.* (1997). Price, public policy, and smoking in young people. *Tob Control*, (Suppl 2):S17–24.

Mounts, N.S. and Steinberg, L.D. (1995). An ecological analysis of peer influence on adolescent grade point average and drug use. *Developmental Psychology*, **31**:915–22.

Pentz, M.A., Brannon, B.R., Charlin, V.L., Barrett, E.J., MacKinnon, D.P., and Flay, B.R. (1989). The power of policy: The relationship of smoking policy to adolescent smoking. *American Journal of Public Health*, **79**:857–62.

Pierce, J.P., Macaskill, P., and Hill, D. (1990). Long term effectiveness of Mass Media Led Anti-Smoking Campaigns in Australia. *American Journal of Public Health*, **80**(5):565–9.

Pierce, J.P., Anderson, M., Romano, R.M., Meissner, H.I., and Odenkirchen, J.C. (1992). Promoting smoking cessation in the United States: Effect of public service announcements of the Cancer Information Service Telephone Line. *Journal of the National Cancer Institute*, **84**(9):677–83.

Pierce, J.P., Lee, L., and Gilpin, E.A. (1994). Smoking initiation by adolescent girls, 1944 through 1988 in association with targeted advertising. *JAMA*, **271**:608–11.

Pierce, J.P. and Gilpin, E.A. (1994). Trends in physicians' smoking behavior and patterns of advice to quit. In: *Tobacco and the clinician: Interventions for medical and dental practice, smoking and tobacco control, Monograph No. 5.* National Institutes of Health, National Cancer Institute, pp. 12–23.

Pierce, J.P. and Gilpin, E.A. (1995). A historical analysis of tobacco marketing and the uptake of smoking by youth in the United States: 1890–1977. *Health Psychology*, **14**:500–8.

Pierce, J.P., Choi,W.S., Gilpin, E.A., Farkas, A.J., and Merritt, R.K. (1996). Validation of susceptibility as a predictor of which adolescents take up smoking in the U.S. *Health Psychology*, **15L**:355–61.

Pierce, J.P, and Gilpin, E. (1996). How long will today's new adolescent smokers be addicted to cigarettes? *American Journal of Public Health*, **86**:253–6.

Pierce, J.P., Choi,W., Gilpin, E.A., Farkas, A.J., and Berry C.C. (1998). Tobacco industry promotion of cigarettes and adolescent smoking. *JAMA*, **279**:511–15.

Pierce, J.P. and Gilpin, E.A. (2001). News media coverage of smoking and health is associated with changes in population rates of smoking cessation but not initiation. *Tobacco Control*, **10**:145–53.

Pierce, J.P., Distefan, J.M., Jackson, C., White, M.M, and Gilpin, E.A. (2002). Does tobacco marketing undermine the influence of recommended parenting in discouraging adolescents from smoking? *American Journal of Preventive Medicine*, **23**:73–81.

Ray, M.L. (1982). *Advertising and communication management*. Prentice Hall, Englewood Cliffs, NJ.

Rigotti, N.A., DiFranza, J.R., Chang, Y., Tisdale, T., Kemp, B., and Singer, D. (1997). The effect of enforcing tobacco sales laws on adolescents' access to tobacco and smoking behavior. *New England Journal of Medicine*, **337**:1044–51.

Sargent, J.D., Dalton, M., Beach, M., Bernhardt, A., Heatherton, T., and Stevens, M. (2000). Effect of cigarette promotions on smoking uptake among adolescents. *Preventive Medicine*, **30**:320–7.

Steinberg, L. (2002). *Adolescence*. (6th edn) McGraw-Hill, New York.

Tauras, J.A., Johnston, L.D., and O'Malley, P.M. (2000). An analysis of teenage smoking initiation: the effects of government intervention. Impact Teen/YES! Research Paper No. 2.

Unger, J.B., Johnson, C.A., Stoddard, J.L., Nezami, E., and Chou, C.P. (1997). Identification of adolescents at risk for smoking initiation: Validation of a measure of susceptibility. *Addictive Behaviors*, **22**:81–91.

US Department of Health and Human Services (1989). Reducing the health consequences of smoking: 25 years of progress. A report of the surgeon general. USDHHS, Centers for Disease Control and Prevention, National Center for Chronic Disease Prevention and Health Promotion, Office on Smoking and Health, Atlanta, GA. DHHS Pub. No. (CDC) 89-8411.

US Department of Health and Human Services (1994). Preventing tobacco use among young people: A report of the surgeon general. USDHHS, Centers for Disease Control and Prevention, National Center for Chronic Disease Prevention and Health Promotion, Office on Smoking and Health, Atlanta GA.

Warner, K.E. (1977). The effects of the anti-smoking campaign on cigarette consumption. *American Journal of Public Health*, **67**:645–50.

Young and Rubicam (1990). Mangini Document No. RJR472678.

Chapter 18

Tobacco and women

Amanda Amos and Judith Mackay

The epidemic
The global picture

Smoking is still seen mainly as a male problem, since in most countries smoking prevalence is lower among women than men. Yet, it is currently estimated that there are already about 250 million women in the world who are daily smokers, and in addition, there are others who chew tobacco (Ezzati *et al.* 2004). Approximately 22% of women in high-income countries and 9% of women in low- and middle-income countries smoke, but because most women live in low- and middle-income countries, there are numerically more women smokers in these countries. Unless effective, comprehensive, and sustained initiatives are implemented to reduce smoking uptake among young women and increase cessation rates among women, the global prevalence of female smoking could rise to 20% by 2025 (Brundtland 2001). This would mean that by 2025 there could be 532 million women smokers. Even if prevalence levels do not rise, the number of women who smoke will increase because the population of women in the developing world is predicted to rise from the current 2.5 billion to 3.5 billion by 2025 (Ezzati and Lopez 2003). Thus, while the epidemic of tobacco use among men is in slow decline, the epidemic among women will not reach its peak until well into the twenty-first century. This will have enormous consequences not only for women's health and economic wellbeing but that of their families.

The prevalence of smoking and smoking-related diseases in countries across the world varies markedly by gender and socioeconomic status. Women have traditionally started smoking later and consumed fewer cigarettes than men. Thus the patterning of smoking among and between women and men differs according to the stage of the smoking epidemic which countries inhabit (Fig. 18.1).

The differences in smoking rates between girls and boys around the world are not as large as one might expect. In one in seven countries covered by the Global Youth Tobacco Survey (GYTS), more girls than boys smoke cigarettes (Warren *et al.* 2008). The overwhelming majority of female smokers become addicted to tobacco before reaching adulthood (Fig. 18.2).

The factors that increase the risk of girls smoking are broadly similar to those of boys: tobacco industry promotion, especially that which targets girls and women; easy access to tobacco products; low prices and greater purchasing power of girls; peer pressure; tobacco use and approval by peers, parents, and siblings; and the misperception that smoking enhances social popularity. However there is also evidence that there are important gender differences in relation to the role and meaning of smoking in young people's lives (Amos and Bostock 2007).

In cultures where women are subjected to unrealistic images of slimness, girls and young women may initiate smoking and continue to smoke in the mistaken belief that smoking keeps them thin. In fact, cigarette smoking is not associated with a lower body mass index (BMI) in young women. Smoking prevention and cessation programmes designed for girls and young women would benefit from the inclusion of support related to body image.

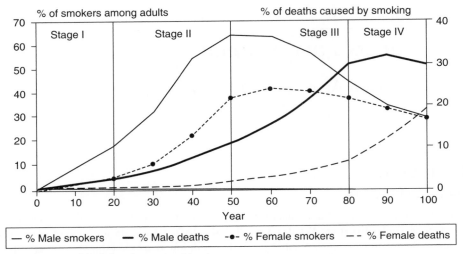

Figure 18.1 A model of the cigarette epidemic.

Source: From Lopez AD, Collishaw NE, Piha T (1994) A descriptive model of the cigarette epidemic in developed countries. Tobacco Control, 3, 242–7 with permission

High-income countries

Currently, about 22% of women aged 15 years and above in high-income countries smoke cigarettes, almost 80 million women. In the earlier decades of the smoking epidemic in high-income countries, smokers were much more likely to be male than female. In the past four decades, however, the pattern in many of these countries has changed dramatically. Drawing on a widely used four stage model of the global smoking epidemic (Fig. 18.1), some countries in Southern Europe

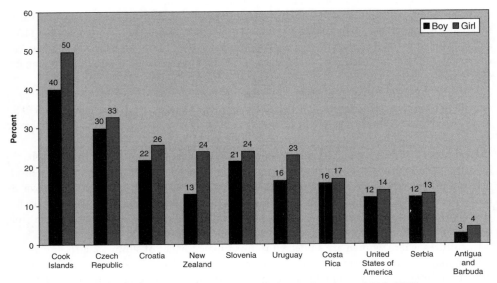

Figure 18.2 GYTS surveyed countries where girls smoke more than boys, 2000–2007.

Source: Warren *et al.* (2008).

(e.g. Portugal) and some high-income countries in Asia and the Western pacific (e.g. Japan) can be located currently at stage 2 with smoking rates peaking at between 50% and 80% among men while the trend among women is rising. Stage 3 countries have a longer history of widespread smoking and include many Southern, Central, and Eastern European countries (e.g. Italy, Spain, Greece). In these countries prevalence rates among men are decreasing but cigarette smoking is either still increasing among women or has not shown any decline. Women's smoking rates typically peak at 35–45%.

Stage 4 countries have the longest history of cigarette smoking (e.g. the USA, UK, Canada, Australia, Finland, Germany) and in these countries cigarette smoking is declining among both women and men (Cavelaars *et al.* 2000; Huisman *et al.* 2005; WHO Europe 2007). However the gap in smoking between women and men in these countries has also greatly decreased. Indeed, in Sweden smoking rates in women are now higher than in men. This has been due to a combination of a narrowing in the gap between uptake rates of smoking in girls and boys (Fig. 18.3), and relatively lower cessation rates in cigarette smoking women compared to men. The Health Behaviour in School-Aged Children Survey (HBSC), which includes 39 countries in Europe and N. America, found that in nearly half the countries weekly smoking rates among 15-year-old girls were higher than those among boys (Currie *et al.* 2008). In addition smoking in these countries has now become highly concentrated among the poorer and more disadvantaged sections of the population. This reflects relatively lower uptake rates and higher quit rates in more affluent groups. In these countries smoking is therefore an increasingly important cause of inequalities in health.

The following are the reasons why some young women initiate smoking

♦ Global trends in women's emancipation

♦ Concern with weight, body image and fashion

♦ Cigarette marketing campaigns targeting women

♦ Positive images of smoking in movies, magazines, and youth culture

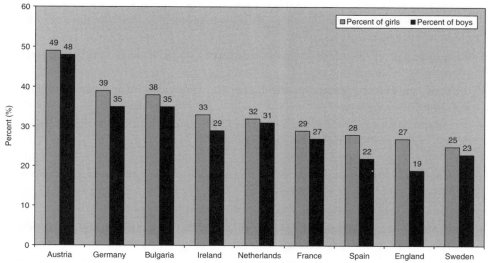

Figure 18.3 Tobacco use initiation: percentage of 15-year-old females who report smoking initiation at age 13 or younger, Europe 2006.

Source: Currie *et al.* (2008).

♦ Improved economic conditions

♦ Drug-positive subcultures

Source: International Network of Women Against Tobacco (2005)

Another cause for concern in high income countries is that the speed of transition from one stage of the epidemic to the next seems to be getting faster, in part due to tobacco companies targeting of young women in countries undergoing rapid social and economic change. In Lithuania, for example, smoking among women doubled over a five-year period in the 1990s and increased by five-fold among the youngest groups (Amos and Haglund 2000). In Sweden, one of Lithuania's neighbours, where women started to smoke in large numbers in the 1950s, it took almost 20 years for the female prevalence to double. Between 1993 and 1997, rates of smoking among 12–25-year-old young women in former East Germany nearly doubled from 27% to 47%. In contrast rates among young men showed a less steep increase from 38% to 45%, and there was little change in smoking rates among the same age group in former West Germany (Corrao *et al.* 2000).

Low- and middle-income countries

Most women live in low- and middle-income countries, where currently only between 2% and 10% smoke cigarettes, although in some regions, such as South Asia, women more commonly chew tobacco. Therefore most of these countries are at stage 1 or stage 2 of the epidemic, with much higher rates of smoking in men compared to women. Typically rates of smoking are highest among well-educated, affluent, urban young women. Although smoking prevalence among women in these countries is generally lower than in high-income countries, this is no cause for complacency as it does not reflect health awareness, but rather social and religious traditions and women's low economic resources. Also in many low- and middle-income countries, such as China, there is evidence that the age of first smoking is becoming younger. The numbers of women smokers in low- and middle-income countries will inevitably increase because:

♦ the female population in low and middle-income countries is predicted to rise from the current 2.5 billion to 3.5 billion by 2025, so even if the prevalence remains low, the absolute numbers of smokers will increase

♦ the spending power of girls and women is increasing so that cigarettes are becoming more affordable

♦ the social and cultural constraints which previously prevented many women smoking are weakening in some places

♦ the tobacco companies are targeting women with well-funded, alluring marketing campaigns, linking smoking with emancipation and glamour

♦ many gender specialists, women's organizations, women's magazines, models, film and pop stars, and other female role models have not yet acted on the basis that smoking is a women's issue, or their need to take an appropriate role

♦ women-specific health promotion and quitting programmes are rare

♦ governments in low- and middle-income countries may be less aware of the harmfulness of tobacco use and are preoccupied with other health issues; where they are concerned with smoking, they focus on the higher levels of male smoking. In fact, no low- and middle-income country is addressing the emerging female epidemic to the extent the problem warrants.

Regional cameos

Africa

Data are now available for most African countries (Shafey *et al.* 2009). Smoking rates vary, but overall it is estimated that about 10% of African women smoke. This ranges from less than 2% in Nigeria, Ivory Coast, and Zimbabwe to 8% in South Africa. Studies from the few countries where more than one survey has been undertaken show a rising trend, especially in urban areas (Elegbeleye *et al.* 1976). Smoking patterns and trends may also differ considerably by ethnic group. For example, in South Africa 59% of coloured women smoked in 1995 compared to 10% of black women and 7% of Indians (WHO 1997). Rates of smoking have declined among white South African women but are increasing among black women.

Americas

Rates of smoking in women vary considerably between the 36 countries. In the United States and Canada rates among women peaked at over 30% and are now declining. In contrast low rates of female smoking are reported in Caribbean countries. Prevalence in women varies from 6% in Paraguay to 27% in Venezuela (Mackay and Eriksen 2002; Shafey *et al.* 2009). Rates of female smoking can vary considerably by ethnic group. While in the United States smoking rates among white women have been consistently higher than those among Black women, a study in Trinidad and Tobago found that there was a higher prevalence among women of European origin (14%) than among women of African (7%) or Indian origin (8%).

South East Asia

The prevalence of cigarette smoking is generally very low among women. Only 3% of women smoke manufactured cigarettes but in several countries other forms of tobacco use by women have been integrated into cultural practices for several decades. In several areas of India, for example, 50% to 60% of women chew tobacco, and rural women smoke the kretek, dhumti, khi yo, ya muan, chilum, and water pipe, and 'reverse smoke' bidis and chutta, with the lighted end inside the mouth (Aghi *et al.* 1988). Very high rates of tobacco smoking are found in women in Nepal.

Western Pacific

Although the overall smoking rate across these 31 countries is estimated to be less than 10%, there are wide variations. For example, in some parts of Papua New Guinea 80% of women smoke, and rates are also high among women in the Pacific Islands (Tuomilehto *et al.* 1986). Less than 4% of women in China smoke (Shafey *et al.* 2009) and 3% in Hong Kong, Malaysia, and Thailand (Shafey *et al.* 2009). Tobacco chewing is uncommon. China deserves special mention because of its size. The prevalence of smoking remains high among older women in cities such as Beijing and Tianjin. Although a substantial minority of women born before 1940 became smokers by age 25, only about 2% of those born since 1950 have done so. In two large nationwide surveys the prevalence of smoking among women aged 15–24 was 0.5% both in 1984 and in 1996 (Chinese Academy of Preventive Medicine 1999). However, it is still possible that the number of young women becoming smokers will increase. Surveys have reported 10% of young women smoking in selected small areas in China (Liu *et al.* 1998).

Eastern Mediterranean

Smoking by women in these countries is often considered vulgar, improper, even immoral. Only 2% of Egyptian women smoke compared with 35% of men (Shafey *et al.* 2009).

In the Gulf region, about 8% of women smoke in contrast to 33% of men. The highest reported female smoking prevalence is 57% in Lebanon (Shafey *et al.* 2009). However surveys may significantly underestimate smoking prevalence among women in these countries as, due to religious and cultural reasons, women may be reluctant to admit to their smoking.

Europe

Prevalence rates in some countries in Central and Eastern Europe (Czech Republic, Hungary, Poland, and Bulgaria) are now similar to those in Western Europe, around 20% to 30% and are increasing. In countries such as Russia, where it has been less acceptable for women to smoke in public places, the rates are generally lower, around 10–15%. However, this may be changing as in Russia smoking prevalence in women doubled from 6.9% to 14.8% between 1992 and 2003 (Perlman *et al.* 2007).

Health effects of tobacco use

Active tobacco use

Because the health effects of smoking only become fully evident 40–50 years after the widespread uptake of smoking (Fig. 18.1), we have yet to see the full global impact of smoking on women's health. This also means that most of what is known about the health effects of smoking has come from studies of cigarette smoking in high-income countries which have tended to focus more on men than women. However, it is now clear that women around the world who smoke, as with male smokers, have markedly increased risks of many cancers, particularly lung cancer, heart disease, stroke, emphysema, and other fatal diseases (see Chapter 15 in this volume). Indeed there is now evidence that the health effects of smoking for women may be even more serious than those for men as there are additional sex specific effects, for example, on the reproductive system (WHO 2007). Smoking currently kills around a million women in the world each year and this number is increasing rapidly (Ezzati and Lopez 2003). Between 1950 and 2000, around 10 million women died from tobacco use. It is estimated that over the next 30 years, tobacco-attributable deaths among women will more than double (Jacobs 2001).

In countries which have the longest history of widespread female smoking, such as United States, Canada and United Kingdom, smoking is now the single most important preventable cause of premature death in women, accounting for around 20% of deaths (Ezzati and Lopez 2003). It is also a major cause of inequalities in health among women (USSG 2001, Department of Health 2002; NICE 2008). In the United States, as in the United Kingdom and Japan, lung cancer has overtaken breast cancer as the leading cause of cancer deaths in women. Death rates from lung cancer among white women in the United States increased by 600% between 1950 and 2000 (USSG 2001). In 1950 lung cancer accounted for only 3% of all female cancer deaths, whereas in 2000 it accounted for an estimated 25%. WHO has identified the epidemic in lung cancer among women as most worrying health trend in Europe (WHO 1999). The number of women developing lung cancer in Europe doubled during the last half of the twentieth century. In high-income countries cardiovascular diseases are the major cause of death among women. As in men, women who smoke have a greater risk of developing these diseases. Nor are the serious effects confined to older women. The relative risk for coronary heart disease associated with smoking is higher among younger than older women (Ernster 2001).

In most low- and middle-income countries the impact of smoking on women's health is currently much lower than in many high-income countries because they are at an earlier stage of the epidemic. For example, in China, the risks for those who smoke have been found to be much the same for women and men, but because smoking has been low among women, only 2.7% of the deaths of women aged 35–69 are attributed to smoking compared with 13.0% of those of men (Liu *et al.* 1998). Also the impact on women's health can vary depending on the type of tobacco use in these countries. For example, in India where betel quid chewing is common among women, oral cancer is more common among women than breast cancer (Jacobs 2001). Female smokers in India die an average of 8 years earlier than their non-smoking peers (Jha *et al.* 2008).

In addition to the health risks that women share with men, women face particular problems linked to tobacco use (USSG 2001; BMA 2004; Ernster 2001; Jacobs 2001; WHO 2007). These include:

♦ Cancer: female-specific cancers, such as breast cancer and cancer of the cervix.

♦ Coronary heart disease: increased risk with use of oral contraceptives.

♦ Menstruation: irregular cycles, higher incidence of painful cramps (dysmenorrhea).

♦ Menopause: women who smoke tend to enter menopause at age 49 – 1–2 years before non-smokers. This places them at a greater risk for heart disease and osteoporosis, including hip fractures (SG), as well as an increased incidence of hot flushes.

♦ Pregnancy: smoking in pregnancy causes increased risks of spontaneous abortion (miscarriage), ectopic pregnancy, low birth weight, higher perinatal mortality, long-term effects on growth/development of the child. Many of these problems affect not only the health of the foetus, but also the health of the mother. For example, a miscarriage with bleeding is dangerous for the mother, especially in poor countries where health facilities are inadequate or non-existent.

♦ Infertility: smoking is also linked to infertility and delays in conceiving.

However, many women are unaware of these risks, even in countries such as the United States. For example, a US study found a serious lack of knowledge among women regarding gender-specific health risks of smoking (Roth and Taylor 2001). The study surveyed female hospital employees, who represented a wide span of age, socioeconomic and educational backgrounds, as to their awareness of reproductive health risks associated with smoking. While nearly all were aware of increased complications in pregnancy (91%), only a minority new of the increased risk of miscarriage (39%), and even fewer knew of the increased risk of ectopic pregnancy (27%), cervical cancer (24%), and infertility (22%).

Secondhand smoke

Secondhand smoke (SHS), environmental tobacco smoke (ETS) or passive smoking, has a negative impact on women's general and reproductive health, causing many illnesses, including lung cancer and heart disease (USSG 2001, Samet and Yang 2001; Amos *et al.* 2008). As with active smoking, SHS exposure is linked with sex-specific effects including cervical cancer (Amos *et al.* 2008). Few countries have sex disaggregated estimates of death due to SHS, but in Scotland (a stage 4 country) it is estimated that 75% of deaths from non-smokers are in women (Hole 2005). As the majority of smokers in the world are men, women are at particular risk from SHS at home. Surveys from high-income countries show that smoking in the home is more common in low socioeconomic households (Borland *et al.* 2006; Amos *et al.* 2008). As the majority of people who work outside the home in the world are also male, women working in these workplace settings may also be exposed to passive smoking.

Women's own smoking may impact on the health of her family. As well as women's smoking during pregnancy having an impact on the health of the foetus, smoking by the father (or other close adult) can cause complications during pregnancy, such as low birth weight. Smoking, especially by the mother or father, around a baby or child also increases the risk of childhood chest infections and worsening of asthma, and can have long-term effects on growth/development (BMA 2004; Muller 2007; Amos *et al.* 2008). Children of smokers are also more likely to become smokers themselves. Women continue to undertake most domestic and child care responsibilities in the home and therefore mothers who smoke may be a more important source of SHS exposure for their children than fathers who smoke (Amos *et al.* 2008). However, many mothers, particularly those living in disadvantaged circumstances, face social, physical and economic barriers that make it difficult for them to reduce SHS exposure in the home (Amos *et al.* 2008).

Economic impact of tobacco use on women

Tobacco use results in a net loss of US$200 billion per year to the global economy, with half of these losses occurring in low-income countries. There are immeasurable personal, social, and economic costs to women, particularly those living in poverty, in low-income countries and in rural settings. Women tend to have fewer resources than men and are more likely to be poor lone parents. More than 70% of the estimated 1.3 billion people living in poverty are women (Hunter 2001). There are also considerable impacts of the cost of smoking on other aspects of the family budget such as expenditure on diet.

Smoking and socioeconomic status

Recent international comparisons of the variation in cigarette smoking by educational level (a proxy indicator of socioeconomic status) show that in mature smoking economies (i.e. stage 4 countries) higher smoking prevalence is associated with lower educational attainment (Bostock 2003; Huisman *et al.* 2005). In these countries, over the past few decades, relatively higher uptake rates and lower quit rates among lower socioeconomic groups have resulted in smoking becoming overwhelmingly associated with social and material disadvantage, with rates highest in areas of low income and multiple deprivation. In the United Kingdom, for example, a study found that the odds of smoking for women who left full-time education at the minimum age were over three times higher than those who stayed beyond 21, and their odds of quitting were more than halved (Graham *et al.* 2006). Similarly in the United States, smoking prevalence is nearly three times higher among women with 9–11 years of education (30.9%) than among women with 16 or more years of education (10.6%) (USSG 2001). In the United States, Canada, New Zealand, and Australia the highest female smoking rates are found among native and aboriginal populations, which characteristically experience high levels of disadvantage and deprivation (Corrao *et al.* 2000; Greaves *et al.* 2006). In these countries, therefore, smoking is both a direct and indirect cause of inequalities in women's health and their wider social and economic wellbeing. Directly, it impacts on women's health and consequently their economic productivity and prosperity. Indirectly, expenditure on tobacco means less resources are available for other essential household requirements.

Purchasing cigarettes

The economic impact of purchasing cigarettes can have a considerable effect on personal and family income. This may be more serious for women, given their initial lower earning power. In particular it will hit poor women the hardest irrespective of whether cigarettes are purchased by men and/or women in a family (Greaves *et al.* 2006). Women who smoke a pack of 20 cigarettes daily in Hong Kong spend approximately US$1 500 per annum on the habit. In China, research carried out in the outskirts of Shanghai showed that farmers spend more on cigarettes and wine than on grains, pork, and fruits. Another study on 2 716 households in Minhang District showed that smokers spent an average of 60% of their personal income and 17% of household income on

Box 18.1 A pack of Marlboro is equal to ...

% of Daily Income:
66.3% – China
62.5% – Moldova
62% – Pakistan
60% – Papua New Guinea (BAT's Benson and Hedges)
56% – Ghana
56% – Bangladesh (15% of average income of the wealthiest 5% of the population)
30% – Romania
28% – Bulgaria
14% – France
6% – United States (using Marlboro price in Oregon)

Source: Global Partnerships (2001).

cigarettes (Gong *et al.* 1995). In Bangladesh smoking is twice as high among the poor as the wealthy (Efroymson *et al.* 2001). Male smokers on average spend more than twice as much on cigarettes as per capita expenditure on clothing housing, health, and education combined. An estimated 10.5 million Bangladeshis who are currently malnourished could have an adequate diet if money spent on tobacco was spent on food instead. In Vietnam, a survey showed that the average smoker spends as much on cigarettes in one month as spent on health care in one year, or which could have bought 169 kilos of rice, more than enough to feed one person for one year (Thuy 1998). The impact on diet is not only restricted to developing countries. In the United Kingdom, for example, family diet has been shown to be adversely affected among smokers on low income (Jarvis 1997) (Box 18.1).

Health costs

By 2025 the transmission of the tobacco epidemic from rich to poor countries will be well advanced, with 85% of the world's smokers living in developing countries (Ezzati and Lopez 2003). Health care facilities will be hopelessly inadequate to cope with this epidemic, especially among women. Also, as smokers (in addition to earlier death) have significantly higher rates of illness, they incur higher health care costs and also loss of income. This will impact particularly on women as they usually have to care for family smokers when they are ill. Structural adjustment and the global financial crisis have severely increased health costs for women and children.

Tobacco taxation

> The Parties recognize that price and tax measures are an effective and important means of reducing tobacco consumption by various segments of the population...
>
> WHO Framework Convention on Tobacco Control, Article 6 [9]

Despite the addictive components of tobacco, there is strong global evidence that smokers' demand for tobacco is strongly affected by price. Higher taxes reduce cigarette consumption (USDHHS 1998; WHO 2008), as illustrated in Fig. 18.4 for South Africa, and postpone initiation of smoking (Lewit *et al.* 1997). For example, tax increases in Canada between 1982 and 1993 led to a steep increase in the real price of cigarettes and consumption fell considerably. When tax was reduced in an attempt to counter smuggling consumption rose sharply again until a subsequent

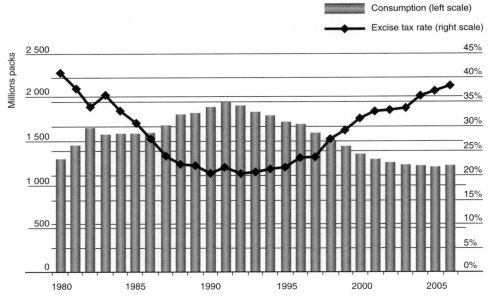

Figure 18.4 Relationship between cigarette consumption and excise tax rate in South Africa.

Source: van walbeek C. Tobacco excise taxation in South Africa: tools for advancing tobacco control in the 21st century success stories and lessons learned, Geneva, World Health Organization, 2003. Additional information obtained from personal communication with C. van Walbeek (http://www,introint/tobacco/training/success_stories/en/best_practices_south-africa_taxation.pdf. accessed 6 December 2007).

tax increase in 1995, when consumption levelled off (World Bank 1999). Increases in the price of tobacco appears to have a disproportionately greater impact on low- and middle-income countries than in high-income countries, and among lower socioeconomic groups in high-income countries (Townsend *et al.* 1994).

In addition, tax revenues go up as cigarette taxes go up, as demonstrated in South Africa (Fig. 18.5).

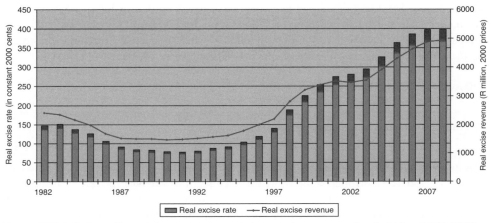

Figure 18.5 Inflation adjusted cigarette taxes and cigarette tax revenue, South Africa, 1982–2008.

Source: Reproduced with permission from The Tobacco Atlas, 3rd edition. Published by American Cancer Society, 2009.

There has been very little economic research on gender sensitivity to price in low- and middle-income countries. Research from high-income countries is somewhat conflicting (Jacobs 2001). In the United States, for example, it has been found that men, particularly young men, are most sensitive to price (Lewit *et al.* 1981; Lewit and Coate 1982). While most British research has concluded that women are more price sensitive than men. Price was found to have a significant effect on the prevalence of smoking in women in the lowest socioeconomic groups where prevalence is highest. However the number of cigarettes smoked by women on low income seemed not to vary with price changes in the expected way. It has been suggested that while they may respond more than other groups to price increases by quitting, those who continue to smoke, will smoke cheaper, smaller, hand rolled, or smuggled cigarettes rather than reduce the number of cigarettes smoked (Jacobs 2001; Wiltshire *et al.* 2001).

Thus, despite their overall positive effects, policies to increase tobacco taxation can be seen as regressive, penalizing female smokers within the very poorest groups of society which are least able to find a way out of addiction. Therefore non-price measures in conjunction with price measures may be more effective in helping women to quit (Jacobs 2001). In addition, interventions and public policies relevant to smoking should take account of the needs of the poorest female smokers. For example, a proportion of tobacco tax revenues could be hypothecated to address both the dimensions of disadvantage that bind women to smoking as well as providing specifically targeted smoking interventions (Marsh 1997; Graham 1998; Gaunt-Richardson *et al.* 1999, INWAT Europe 2000).

In China, it is estimated that a 10% increase in cigarette price would reduce consumption by 5% and raise enough revenue to cover basic health needs of 33 million rural residents (Hu and Mao 2002).

Smoking cessation

Our understanding of smoking cessation among women is mainly drawn from research carried out in countries with the longest history of smoking, in particular the United States and United Kingdom. In these countries the decline in cigarette smoking has been faster in men than women. This may in part be due to some men changing from smoking cigarettes to cigar and/or pipes. However, several studies have suggested that women may indeed find it more difficult to quit smoking than men, and that as well as similarities, there may be important differences between men and women as to the reasons why they smoke which have implications for policy and practice.

The reasons why women seem to find it more difficult to quit than men are not well understood (Hunter 2001). It is likely to be due to a combination of biological, psychological, and social factors. There is increasing evidence that while most smokers are addicted to nicotine, factors other than nicotine may be more important in reinforcing smoking among women than men. For example, a meta-analysis of cessation studies using nicotine patches found that women had lower quit rates compared to men (Perkins and Scott 2008). Women who used the English NHS Stop Smoking services were also slightly less likely to be quit at four weeks than men (NHSIC 2008). Similarly, studies of self-quitters have found that women were less likely to quit initially or to remain abstinent at follow-up. British data show that women feel more dependent on their smoking than men despite having lower levels of consumption (Goddard 2008).

Social and environmental factors are believed to be a more important influence on the smoking behaviour of women than men. For example, British and Canadian qualitative sociological research has shown how the social circumstances of disadvantage play an important part in reinforcing smoking among women (Graham 1993; Greaves 1996). This research illustrates how smoking is one mechanism which women use to cope with living and caring in disadvantaged circumstances. That is, smoking may constitute an important source of pleasure and satisfaction for women in caring roles by helping them to deal with frustration, stress, boredom, and material insecurity. This research has made important inroads into our understanding of the difficulties of quitting for low-income mothers and to the development of new approaches to tackle this issue (Gaunt-Richardson *et al.* 1999).

Thus while in many high-income countries men and women smokers show similar levels of motivation to quit, many women appear to face additional barriers to quitting, particularly those living in disadvantaged circumstances such as low income and lone mothers (Graham *et al.* 2006). It is becoming more widely accepted therefore that tailored approaches to cessation are needed which address the particular personal, social, and cultural factors that make it difficult for women to quit successfully (Gaunt-Richardson *et al.* 1999; INWAT Europe 2000; Samet and Yoon 2001; Bostock 2003). These programmes and services need to be accessible to women throughout the life course and should be integrated into high quality and affordable health services. However, the true potential of such programmes will only be fully realized when the wider social and economic factors that bind women to smoking, their life circumstances, are also addressed by action at national and international levels (Greaves *et al.* 2006; Graham *et al.* 2006).

The tobacco industry

A review of the marketing of tobacco to women concluded that 'selling tobacco products to women currently represents the single largest product marketing opportunity in the world' (Kaufman and Nichter 2001). And it is clear from tobacco companies' own internal documents and proclamations that they are seizing this opportunity with gusto by manipulating various aspects of the marketing mix (product, price, packaging, and promotion) to make their products more appealing and accessible to girls and women around the world. While tobacco companies have only started marketing tobacco relatively recently to women in low- and middle-income countries, they can draw on over eighty years experience of successful marketing to women in countries such as the United States and United Kingdom (Amos 1996; Joossens and Sasco 1999; Amos and Haglund 2000; Kaufman and Nichter 2001; USSG 2001; Tinkler 2006).

High-income countries

The development of cheap mass produced cigarettes at the end of the nineteenth century greatly affected tobacco consumption. However, although cigarette smoking became increasingly popular among men, smoking was seen by many as a dirty habit that corrupted both men and women. The tobacco companies responded by employing new modern marketing methods to help spread their message (Amos and Haglund 2000). Although women often featured in promotional materials their role was to entice male rather than female customers. There is little evidence that tobacco companies directly targeted women to any significant extent at this time or attempted to challenge the dominant social stigma attached to female smoking.

World War I was a watershed in both the emancipation of women and the spread of smoking among women. During the war many women not only took on traditionally 'male' occupations but also started to wear trousers, play sports, cut their hair short, and smoke. Subsequently attitudes towards women smoking began to change, and more women started to use the cigarette as a weapon in challenging traditional ideas about female behaviour. The cigarette became a symbol of new roles and expectations of women's behaviour. But its questionable whether smoking would have become as popular among women as it did if tobacco companies had not seized on this opportunity in the 1920s and 1930s to exploit ideas of liberation, power, and other important values for women to recruit them to the cigarette market. Smoking was repositioned as being respectable, sociable, fashionable, stylish, feminine, and an aid to slimming.

The Lucky Strike campaign 'Reach for Lucky instead of a Sweet' of 1925 was one of the first media campaigns targeted at women. The message was highly effective and made Lucky Strike the best selling brand. Another important element in the marketing campaign was to challenge the social taboo against women smoking in public. In 1929 there was the much publicized event in the Easter Sunday Parade in New York where Great American Tobacco hired several young women to smoke their 'torches of freedom' (Lucky Strikes) as they marched down Fifth Avenue protesting against women's inequality. This event generated widespread newspaper coverage and provoked a national debate. Tobacco companies also needed to ensure that women felt confident about smoking in public. While to some extent they tackled this by using images of women smoking in cigarette advertisements, they also ensured that Hollywood stars were well supplied with cigarettes and often paid them to give endorsements in advertisements (Lum *et al.* 2008). Philip Morris even went so far as to organize a lecture tour in the United States giving women lessons in cigarette smoking. Within 20 years of starting to target women, over half the young women (20–24 years) in Britain, for example, had become smokers.

Since starting to target women in North America and Northern Europe in the 1920s and 1930s the tobacco industry has become more sophisticated in its marketing strategies, developing a diverse range of messages, products, and brands to appeal to different segments of the female market (Anderson *et al.* 2005; Toll and Ling 2005). Such marketing messages, and the way that they have been reflected in and reinforced by the mass media such as films and magazine, has led to the cultural meaning of women's smoking changing from being a symbol of being *bought* by men (prostitute), to being *like* men (lesbian/mannish), to being able to *attract* men (glamorous/heterosexual) (Greaves 1996). To this could also be added its symbolic value of freedom, that is, being *equal* to men (feminism) and to being your *own woman* (emancipation).

The tobacco companies have also used other elements of the marketing mix to target women. One of the most important strategies has been the production of cigarette brands and versions of current brands, notably low tar brands, to appeal to women, particularly young women. In recent years, for example, there has been the launch of the new brand Camel No9 in the United States with advertisements including slogans such as 'light and luscious' and colours such as hot pink, with imagery suggestive of luxury perfumes such as Channel No 5 (Simpson 2007).

New markets

In the latter decades of the twentieth century up to today, tobacco companies have been seizing the opportunities presented by often very rapid cultural, economic, social, and political change to promote the 'liberating' symbolic value of smoking to women (Amos and Haglund 2000). For example, in Spain after the fall of the Franco regime, ads for Kim in the 1980s promoted the slogan 'Asi, como soy' (It's so me) and in the 1990s West ads in Spain showed women in traditionally male occupations such as fighter pilots. Some of the most blatant targeting of young women has occurred in the former socialist countries of Central and Eastern Europe, which are now exposed to the commercial forces of 'free' markets and often have few restrictions on tobacco advertising. Here cigarettes have been promoted as a potent symbol of Western freedom, as in Czech Republic 'West – the taste of now'. Young women are encouraged to join men in their 'western' male leisure pursuits. In Germany in the 1990s young women became a prime target for cigarette ads, many of which promoted smoking as synonymous with western images of modern emancipated womanhood (Poetschke-Langer and Schunk 2001). Cigarette advertisements were among the first to appear on the Berlin Wall with slogans such as 'Test the West'. It is therefore not surprising that between 1993 and 1997, rates of smoking among young women in former East Germany nearly doubled from 27% to 47%. In addition, the desire to quit among 12–25-year-old smokers declined from two-thirds to less than half over this period (Corrao *et al.* 2000). In Russia between 1992 and 2003 smoking prevalence in women doubled from 6.9% to 14.8%, with the increase being greatest among least educated women (Perlman *et al.* 2007). During this period Russia was undergoing transition to a market economy which included a massive increase in marketing by tobacco companies, in particular targeting women and young people.

The marketing of cigarettes as both a passport to and symbol of emancipation, independence, and success is not restricted to countries in the West. A 1990 editorial in Tobacco Reporter noted the growth opportunities represented by women as 'Women are becoming more independent and, consequently, adopting less-traditional lifestyles. One symbol of their newly discovered freedom may well be cigarettes' (Zimmerman 1990). Thus we have seen in Japan Virginia Slims advertisements urging women to 'Be you'. Capri advertisements have encouraged them to have their own opinions and have featured 'real life' European female role models such as a dress designer stating that 'The dress I design represents my own way of life'. Virginia Slims has shown a pair of Caucasian male and female rugby players with the by-line 'the locker rooms are separate but the playground and the goal are common'. Smoking among Japanese women in their twenties more than doubled between 1986 and 1999, from 10% to 23%.

Low- and middle-income countries

UPBEAT. Amid the gloomy environment, Tobacco Reporter continued to look for the positive in Asia. And guess what! There are reasons for optimism; 'The situation does not fundamentally change the underlying strengths of the market,' an Indonesian source assures us. Rising per-capita consumption, a growing population and an increasing acceptance of women smoking continue to generate new demand.

Tobacco Reporter editorial about the Asian market (Tuinstra 1998)

Until the 1980s, there was relatively little tobacco promotion in low- and middle-income countries. The national monopolies did not, in general, promote their products, or did so only minimally. But from the 1980s, when young women in some countries were starting to become more independent and were copying western fashion and trends, the transnational tobacco industry introduced tobacco advertisements into developing countries. Many of these initial advertisements were very 'masculine' like the Marlboro cowboy, but gradually a whole range of advertisements were produced, moving from 'men-only' advertisements; through 'neutral' advertisements showing, for example, a pleasant mountain scene or a blue lagoon; advertisements where both men and women appeared, for example, enjoying the outdoors in a group; to women-only advertisements.

By the mid-1980s, examples of these latter advertisements specifically targeting women were beginning to emerge, in particular advertisements for Virginia Slims. Smoking was promoted as being glamorous, sophisticated, fun, romantic, sexually attractive, healthy, sporty, sociable, relaxing, calming, emancipated, feminine, rebellious, and an aid to slimming. Designer cigarettes then appeared: in 1989, the Yves St Laurent brand of cigarettes was launched in Malaysia and other countries throughout Asia, with elegant packing appealing to women. Some of the monopolies and national companies, such as in Indonesia, then began to copy promotion targeting women. The tobacco industry used seductive but false images of health, emancipation, slimness, modernity, glamour, sophistication, fun, romance, sexual attractiveness, health, sport, sociability, femininity, and rebelliousness. Concurrently, feminized cigarettes appeared – long, extra-slim, low-tar, light-coloured, menthol.

In South Africa, for example, Benson and Hedges have produced advertisements which feature young black women. One advertisement showed a young dark skinned woman in aerobics gear smoking a cigarette with a young black male. In another a black woman wearing traditional head-gear was shown seated with a black man accepting a cigarette from a white man. The copy line was 'Share the feeling, share the taste'. In the Middle East a Gauloise advertisement featured a young woman in western dress with the copyline 'Always Freedom' (Simpson 2001).

Not only do these advertising images and messages echo those seen in the 1930s advertisements in the United States and United Kingdom, but so do other elements of the social marketing strategies. For example, in Sri Lanka in a modern version of the 1929 New York Easter Parade march, the Ceylon Tobacco Company hired young women to drive around in 'Players Gold Leaf' cars handing out free cigarettes and promotional items (Seiman and Mehl 1998). These women also handed out free merchandise at popular shopping malls and university campuses. In a country where only 1% of women smoke, this seemed to be part of a wider strategy to challenge the social taboo that respectable women in Sri Lanka should not smoke and certainly not in the street.

Other forms of marketing

Other forms of marketing are also being targeted at women. For example, tobacco companies have produced a range of brands aimed at women. Most notable are the 'women-only' brands such as Kim, Virginia Slims, Capri, Vogue, MS, and More. These are feminized cigarettes – long, extra-slim, low-tar, light-coloured, menthol. In India in 1990 the Golden Tobacco Company attempted to target women with a new brand, 'MS Special Filter' (Gupta and Ball 1990). Advertisements featured Indian women in Western clothing and affluent settings, symbols of liberation for Indian women who are gaining financial and professional independence. In 2003, the same company launched the cigarette brand Platinum in Mumbai with an insert entitled 'Understanding Women' in the top selling magazine Mid Day (Bansal et al. 2005). The insert included articles on women's issues, interspersed with different advertisements for Platinum on every page. In China the first ever brands to be developed by the Chinese tobacco industry were aimed at women (Hui 1998). Some companies have also produced special gift packs and offers designed to appeal to women. In Taiwan, tobacco companies launched gift packs for the Lunar New Year, with the Yves St Laurent luxurious gift pack containing two cartons of cigarettes plus one crystal item. The 555 gift packs had either a tea set or an ashtray and the Virginia Slim Lights gift packs stylish lighters suitable for women smokers.

Tobacco companies also sponsor popular sport and leisure events in an attempt to reach young women. A recent analysis of tobacco industry documents found that the companies used six vehicles and themes to develop a tobacco culture among Asian young women and men (Knight and Chapman 2004). These were: music, entertainment (including nightclubs, discos, films), adventure, sport (including motor sports, soccer, tennis), glamour (beauty and fashion), and independence. For example, in 1997 in an attempt to get around advertising bans, Philip Morris ran the 'My Journey' fashion competition in Hong Kong with prizes including shopping trips to Milan and New York. Although mainly men's sports are sponsored in low- and middle-income countries, these are watched by many women. For example, 46% of spectators at the Hong Kong Salem Tennis in 1993 were women. There are also sponsored women's events. In 1989, British American Tobacco Co decided to add the Viceroy Women Football Competition on to the final match of Viceroy Cup in Hong Kong. In 1995, Benson and Hedges ran whole page advertisements in newspapers in Malaysia featuring a female climber Lum Yuet Mei, suspended from a rock face, provocatively saying 'Tonight cling on to me as I attempt to conquer the amazing Dolomite cliffs' in an advertisement entitled 'She took the challenge and realised her golden dream.' Malaysia is a prime example in the world of brand-stretching – for example, travel holidays and bistros. RJ Reynolds designed 'Salem Attitude' clothing stores for the Asian market specifically to circumvent restrictions on tobacco promotion (Kaufman and Nichter 2001).

Arts sponsorship provides the tobacco industry with culture, glamour, and respectability, sponsoring events that appeal to women as well as men. Events in Asia include the Philip Morris Philippine Art Awards competition (2007); Tony Bennett Jazz concerts (Thailand 1993); Central Ballet of China (1994); Andrew Lloyd Webber's 'The Phantom of the Opera' sponsored by Philip Morris (Hong Kong 1995); ASEAN Arts Awards (Asia 1994).

Events and activities popular with the young also receive sponsorship. Admission to films and pop or rock concerts has been either free, or through the exchange of empty cigarette packets for free tickets (Taiwan 1988; Hong Kong 1994). In Nepal tobacco companies have sponsored music nights in top hotels with names such as Surya Lights Musical Nights and Surya Lights Bollywood nights with young women featured in the advertising and clearly a key target group (Simpson 2007). Singers, such as Alanis Morissette and Madonna, who would not promote tobacco in the United States, have allowed their names to be associated with cigarettes in other countries. Film stars such as Sylvester Stallone have accepted money from the tobacco industry for product placement in their films. However, Philip Morris had to withdraw its sponsorship of a concert by Alicia Keys in Indonesia in 2008 after criticism that this targeted children, and the singer herself called for the sponsorship to be withdrawn (Simpson 2008).

Action

Tobacco control strategies targeted at decreasing smoking uptake and increasing cessation are much more cost-effective than treating patients with lung cancer and other tobacco-related illnesses. There is therefore an urgent need to develop effective gender-sensitive and gender-specific tobacco control strategies, and to allocate sufficient funds for tobacco control programmes that reach women and girls (INWAT Europe 2000; WHO 2007). Public policy, legislation, research, and education therefore need to be geared specifically towards preventing girls from initiating smoking and helping women quit. Over the past ten years there has been a growing recognition, at both the international and national levels, of the increasing impact of smoking on women's health around the world. However, action on this issue has tended to be restricted to those countries with the longest history of female cigarette smoking.

International level
WHO

WHO has given high priority to strengthening global action on women and tobacco issues, for example:

- WHO has secured funding for a major initiative on women and tobacco currently underway in the Southern African Development Commission (14 Southern African countries).
- An international meeting on Women and Tobacco took place in Kobe, Japan in November 1999. This drew in, for the first time, women's organizations beyond the traditional tobacco control groups, culminating in The Kobe Declaration on Women and Tobacco.
- In the Western Pacific Region, all three five-year Action Plans on Tobacco or Health since 1990 have emphasized the importance of preventing a rise in smoking among women as a high priority, including the 2005–2009 Plan.
- In 2007 it published 'Gender and Tobacco Control – a policy brief' and in 2009 the updated WHO monograph on 'Women and the Tobacco Epidemic' will be published.

♦ The WHO Framework Convention on Tobacco Control (FCTC). The FCTC specifically highlights the importance of women and tobacco. The FCTC Preamble states:

Alarmed by the increase in smoking and other forms of tobacco consumption by women and young girls worldwide and keeping in mind the need for full participation of women at all levels of policy-making and implementation and the need for gender-specific tobacco control strategies,

Emphasizing the special contribution of nongovernmental organizations and other members of civil society not affiliated with the tobacco industry, including health professional bodies, women's, youth, environmental and consumer groups, and academic and health care institutions, to tobacco control efforts nationally and internationally and the vital importance of their participation in national and international tobacco control efforts,

Recalling that the Convention on the Elimination of All Forms of Discrimination against Women, adopted by the United Nations General Assembly on 18 December 1979, provides that States Parties to that Convention shall take appropriate measures to eliminate discrimination against women in the field of health care,

In addition in the Guiding Principles, Article 4 on of the FCTC, specifically mentions gender:

2. Strong political commitment is necessary to develop and support, at the national, regional and international levels, comprehensive multisectoral measures and coordinated responses, taking into consideration:

   (d) the need to take measures to address gender-specific risks when developing tobacco control strategies.

The Director General of the World Health Organization, Dr Margaret Chan, stated in her address to the World Health Assembly in 2007:

Chronic diseases, long considered the companions of affluent societies, now impose their greatest burden in low- and middle-income countries … For the treatment of chronic diseases, we now have packages of interventions that are effective and affordable in every part of the world. The Framework Convention on Tobacco Control is supported by more than 140 countries, making it one of the most widely embraced treaties in the history of the United Nations. This is really primary prevention at its best.

♦ WHO MPower Report, 2008

This WHO report is the first-ever comprehensive analysis of global tobacco use and control efforts, using sex-disaggregated data compiled from 179 Member States. The report is important because it sets out a road map with guideposts helping every country in the world to act. The report outlines a six-prong strategy to stem the epidemic:

- **M**onitor tobacco use and prevention policies
- **P**rotect people from tobacco smoke
- **O**ffer help to quit tobacco use
- **W**arn about the dangers of tobacco
- **E**nforce bans on tobacco advertising, promotion and sponsorship
- **R**aise taxes on tobacco.

WHO is also working with many UN organizations, such as UNICEF, IMF, World Bank, and others to form partnerships to reduce the epidemic.

The World Bank

The World Bank's report 'Curbing the Epidemic' marked the first time a major financial institution had supported policies designed to reduce tobacco demand (World Bank 1999). This document argued that tobacco control is good for the wealth as well as the health of nations; that it does not lead to loss of taxes or jobs; and that tobacco control measures (e.g. price increases, advertising bans, smoke-free areas, health education, pharmaceutical assistance in quitting) are cost-effective in both industrialized and developing countries. Men and women are not specifically indexed, but the findings have relevance to both.

International NGOs

The International Network of Women Against Tobacco (INWAT) was founded in 1990 to address the issues around tobacco and women (www.INWAT.org). It has members in over 90 countries and produces a regular newsletter, The Net, and publications on specific issues around women and tobacco. Other NGOs involved with tobacco maintain a gender awareness, like the International Union Against Cancer (UICC), the International Union Against Tuberculosis and Lung Disease (IUATLD), the World Heart Federation, the Framework Convention Alliance and The International Non-Government Coalition Against Tobacco (INGCAT). They encourage their member organizations to take a public stand on tobacco, and some fund projects, research, and meetings. GLOBALink, the internet network based at the UICC Headquarters in Geneva, links tobacco control advocates all over the world, and has a specific website devoted to tobacco and women.

The Chest Foundation, based in the United States developed a Speaker's Kit for Women, which was then adapted and produced in many Asian languages during 2002–2004. Philanthropic donations and grants, such as The Bloomberg Global Initiative to Reduce Tobacco Use, and American Cancer Society projects, involve women and tobacco issues either directly or indirectly.

Journals and conferences

Many authoritative articles have been published on women and tobacco in health journals such as the WHO Bulletin (2000), Respirology (2003), National Cancer Institute (USA) (2004), Tobacco Control (2007), and the US Surgeon General Released a new Report on Impact of Smoking on US Women and Girls in 2001. In 2007, the Rio Declaration on women and tobacco was issued. World and regional conferences on Tobacco or Health now strive for gender equality in terms of committees, chairs, speakers, and include the topic of women in the programmes.

International conferences

The 10th World Conference on Tobacco or Health in Beijing in 1997, pioneered gender equity in World Conferences. Fifty percent of all committee members, chairs, and invited speakers were women. When funding was offered to developing countries for two delegates, it was suggested that one be a female. Each speaker was asked to incorporate the twin themes of 'developing countries' and 'women' into his or her presentation on whatever topic. This has become a goal for all subsequent conferences. In 1998 the European Union, through Europe Against Cancer, organized the first European conference on women and tobacco in Paris.

Regional level

APACT

The Asia Pacific Association for the Control of Tobacco (APACT), first established by the late Dr David Yen in Taipei, organizes biennial regional meetings. Delegates from the poorer countries find the smaller regional meetings more supportive than the large, international conferences, and it facilitates delegates, especially women, speaking out.

INWAT Europe

The INWAT Europe Development Project was a pilot project funded by the European Union (Europe Against Cancer) which ran from 1997 to 2002. It aimed to contribute to reducing tobacco use among women in Europe by developing a strong, effective, and sustainable network which raises awareness about this issue, promoting communication and exchange of information and support, and developing consensus on a women-centred tobacco control strategy for Europe. Since the end of the pilot project, the Board of INWAT Europe has been successful in gaining funding to hold several European expert seminars and produce publications on key issues including women-centred tobacco control policies (INWAT Europe 2000); women, smoking and inequalities in Europe (Bostock 2003); women and secondhand smoking in Europe (Amos *et al.* 2008).

National level

At the national level, governments have the central and crucial role in tobacco control, especially in the areas of legislation and tobacco tax increases. Without government leadership and commitment, tobacco control measures – especially in low- and middle-income countries – are unlikely to succeed. Because the full impact of tobacco-related deaths is not yet apparent in low- and middle-income countries, many governments are still not convinced of the degree of the harmfulness of smoking. They are preoccupied with other problems, such as high infant mortality, communicable diseases, economic difficulties, or political conflict, they lack funds, and have little experience in dealing with the tactics of the transnational tobacco companies. In addition they may be reluctant to act because of the mistakenly perceived economic 'benefits' of tobacco.

The lead government ministry is the Ministry of Health, but with the issue of tobacco and women, women's commissions or ministries should be active. There is no government department that does not have some role. Many low- and middle-income countries have implemented tobacco control programmes, including legislation, far ahead of many western countries, and without any severe economic consequences. For example, legislation in Singapore, Fiji, Mongolia, Hong Kong, South Africa, Thailand, and Vietnam is far ahead of many western countries. Many tobacco control measures cost little other than political will – for example, legislation requiring health warnings on cigarette packets; or the creation of smoke-free areas public places. However many tobacco control programmes countries continue to take a gender neutral or gender blind approach.

NGOs, including women's groups, also have a crucial role to play. For example, they can:

- lobby, advise or pressure governments, to make sure that all legislation and other tobacco control action is gender-sensitive
- make sure that ministries or commissions on women address tobacco as a woman's issue and uphold the principle of women's right to health as a basic human right, building on the progress made at the Fourth World Conference on Women and the Convention to Eliminate All Forms of Discrimination Against Women (CEDAW)
- demand a total ban on direct and indirect advertising, promotion, and sponsorship by the tobacco industry, especially that targeting girls and women
- ask for increased public funding for research and advocacy on women and girls and tobacco
- promote women's leadership in tackling tobacco
- lobby women's magazines and other media to better inform women about the issue and not to promote positive images of smoking

- recruit the entertainment industry, especially female movie and pop stars
- counter the claims of the tobacco industry that tobacco is a freedom for women
- support cessation
- join the International Network of Women Against Tobacco (INWAT).

Individual women can act in an exemplar role by not smoking themselves, by discouraging their own children from starting smoking, and by encouraging their partners, parents, children, friends, and co-workers to quit.

Research gaps

Developing more effective tobacco control programmes for women, particularly in low- and middle-income countries, is hampered by the lack of research on women and smoking. Recent national and international reviews on women and smoking have identified a range of research questions, including biomedical, social, economic, policy, intervention, and evaluation, which need addressing. For example, the first INWAT Europe seminar (INWAT Europe 2000) outlined key research questions in relation to:

- understanding the determination of tobacco use among women across the life-course and in different countries
- a biomedical research agenda which looked at the impact of smoking in relation to sex-specific biological factors (developmental and reproductive) across the life-course, including nicotine addiction
- extending and deepening current understanding of the effectiveness and cost-effectiveness of tobacco control policies, particularly by providing a gender-sensitive perspective that takes into account socioeconomic status.

Similarly the Kobe report on women and tobacco identified the need for 'prospectively designed research studies to further elucidate the complexity of the relationships between failure to quit, nicotine withdrawal symptoms, level of addiction to nicotine, cigarette smoking relapse, depression, alcohol use, eating and fear of weight gain in girls and women' (Hunter 2001). Among the other research issues highlighted was the importance of researching the differential impact of tobacco control polices and the health consequences of such policies on girls, women and disadvantaged women, particularly in low- and middle-income countries, given that the burden of the tobacco epidemic is shifting to these population groups (Jacobs 2001). More recently, INWAT Europe has highlighted the limited research data and evidence on issues around women and secondhand smoke and made recommendations for future research in this area (Amos *et al.* 2008). The need to incorporate gender into tobacco control research and planning, using gender and diversity-based analysis (Johnson *et al.* 2007), has been recognized and supported by the WHO (WHO 2007).

Conclusion

At the beginning of the twentieth century few people could have imagined how such a stigmatized behaviour as female smoking would be transformed, through judicious marketing by the tobacco companies, into a socially acceptable and desirable behaviour in high-income countries. The challenge facing us in the twenty-first century is to how stem the second wave of the tobacco epidemic, particularly in low- and middle-income countries and among disadvantaged women in high-income countries. There needs to be wider recognition that women's tobacco use is a global health problem and that effective women-centred tobacco control programmes should be implemented at international as well as national levels. Clearly there is a need to ban all tobacco promotion. But building support for women-centred tobacco control programmes through partnerships will also be vital to achieve success. In particular there is a need to work with and involve both women's organizations and women themselves, and to broaden the agenda to encompass other social and economic factors that work against girls and women breaking free from this fatal addiction.

References

Aghi, M., Gupta, P.C., and Mehta, F.S. (1988). Impact of intervention on the reverse smoking habit of rural Indian women. In: Aoki M *et al.*, ed. *Smoking and Health. Proceedings of the 6th World Conference on Smoking and Health.* Amsterdam: Excerpta Medica, 255.

Anderson, S.J., Glantz, S.A., and Ling, P.M. (2005). Emotions for sale: cigarette advertising and women's psychosocial needs. *Tobacco Control*, **14**: 127–35.

Amos, A. (1996). Women and smoking. *British Medical Bulletin*, **52**: 74–89.

Amos, A. (2001). Women, smoking and cessation – meeting the challenge. *Promoting Health*, **12**: 24–5.

Amos, A. and Bostock, Y. (2007). Young people, smoking and gender- a qualitative exploration. *Health Education Research*, **22**: 770–81.

Amos, A. and Haglund, M. (2000). From social taboo to 'torch of freedom' – the marketing of cigarettes to women. *Tobacco Control*, **9**: 3–8.

Amos, A., Sanchez, S., Skar, M., and White, P. (2008). *Exposing the evidence- women and secondhand smoke in Europe.* Brussels, INWAT Europe/ENSP.

Bansal, R., John, S., and Ling, P.M. (2005). Cigarette advertising in Mumbai, India: targeting different socioeconomic groups, women and youth. *Tobacco Control*, **14**: 201–06.

Borland, R., Yong, H.-H., Cummings, M., Hyland, A., Anderson, S., and Fong, S. (2006). Determinants and consequences of smoke-free homes: findings from the International Tobacco Control (ITC) four country survey. *Tobacco Control*, **15**: 42–50.

Bostock, Y. (2003). Women, smoking and inequalities in Europe. London, INWAT Europe/HDA. http://www.inwat.org

British Medical Association (BMA) (2004). *Smoking and Reproductive Life.* London, BMA.

Bridgwood, A., Lilly, R., Thomas, M., Bacon, J., Sykes, W., and Morris, S. (2000). *Living in Britain 1998.* London, Stationery Office.

Cavelaars, A., Kunst, A., Geurts, J., Crialesi, R., Grotvedt, L., Helmert, U. *et al.* (2000). Educational differences in smoking: international comparison. *BMJ*, **320**: 1102–7.

Chinese Academy of Preventive Medicine (1999). *Smoking and Health in China: 1996 National Prevalence Survey of Smoking Patterns.* Beijing, China Science and Technology Press.

Corrao, M.A., Guidon, G.E., Sharma, N., and Shokoohi, D.F. (2000). *Tobacco Control Country Profiles.* Atlanta, American Cancer Society.

Currie, C., Nic Gabhainn, S., Godeau, E., Roberts, C., Smith, R., Currie, D. *et al.*, eds. (2008). *Inequalities in Young People's Health: HBSC International Report from the 2005/2006 Survey.* Copenhagen, WHO Regional Office for Europe.

Department of Health (2002). *Tackling Health Inequalities: Cross-cutting Review.* London, The Stationery Office.

Efroymson, D. Ahmed, S., Townsend, J., Mahbubul Alam, S., Ranjan Dey, A., Saha, R. *et al.* (2001). Hungry for tobacco: an analysis of the economic impact of tobacco consumption on the poor in Bangladesh. *Tobacco Control*, **10**: 212–17.

Elegbeleye, O.O. and Femi-Pearse, D. (1976). Incidence and variables contributing to the onset of cigarette smoking among secondary school children and medical students in Lagos, Nigeria. *Br J Prev Soc Med*, **30**: 66–70.

Ernster, V. (2001). Impact of tobacco use on women's health. In: J.M. Samet and S.-Y. Yoon (eds) *Women and the Tobacco Epidemic- Challenges for the 21st Century*, p1–16. Geneva, WHO.

Ezzati, M., Lopez, A.D., Rodgers, A., and Murray, C.J.L. (eds), (2004). Smoking and Oral tobacco use, *Comparative Quantification of Health Risks, Global and Regional Burden of Disease Attributable to Selected Major Risk Factors*. WHO: Geneva; http://www.who.int/publications/cra/chapters/volume1/part4/en/index.html

Ezzati, M. and Lopez, A. D. (2003). Estimates of global mortality due to smoking. *Lancet*, **362**: 847–52.

Gaunt-Richardson, P., Amos, A., Howie, G., McKie, L., and Moore, M. (1999). *Women, low income and smoking – breaking down the barriers*. Edinburgh, ASH Scotland/Health Education Board for Scotland.

Global Partnerships (2001). Global partnerships for Tobacco Control, Essential Action Survey. www.essential.org/tobacco

Gong, L.Y., Koplan, J.P., Feng, W., Chen, C.H., Zheng, P., and Harris, J.R. (1995). Cigarette smoking in China. *JAMA*, **274**: 1232–4.

Goddard, E. (2008). *Smoking and Drinking in Adults, 2006*. Newport, Office for National Statistics.

Graham, H. (1993). *When Life's a Drag*. London, HMSO.

Graham, H., Francis, B., Inskip, H.M., Harman, J., and SWS Study Group (2006). Socioeconomic lifecourse influences on women's smoking status in early adulthood. *Journal of Epidemiology and Community Health*, **60**: 228–33.

Graham, H. (1998). Promoting health against inequality: using research to identify targets for intervention – a case study of women and smoking. *Health Education Journal*, **57**: 292–302.

Greaves, L., Jategaonkar, N., and Sanchez, S. (eds) (2006). *Turning a New Leaf: Women, Tobacco and the Future*. Vancouver, BC Centre of Excellence for Women's Health. http://www.inwat.org

Greaves, L. (1996). *Smokescreen – Women's Smoking and Social Control*. Halifax, Fernwood Publishing.

Gupta, P. C. and Ball, K. (1990). India: a tobacco tragedy. *Lancet*, **335**: 594–5.

Huisman, M., Kunst, A.E., and Mackenbach, J.P. (2005). Educational inequalities in smoking among men and women aged 16 years and older in 11 European countries. *Tobacco Control*, **14**: 106–13.

Hunter, S.M. (2001). Quitting. In: J.M. Samet and S.-Y. Yoon (eds) *Women and the Tobacco Epidemic-Challenges for the 21st Century*, p121–46. Geneva, WHO.

Hole, D. (2005). Passive Smoking and Associated Causes of Death in Adults in Scotland. NHS Health Scotland. http://www.healthscotland.com/uploads/documents/MortalityStudy.pdf

Hu, T. and Mao, Z. (2002). Effects of Cigarette Tax on Cigarette Consumption and the Chinese Economy. *Tobacco Control*, **11**: 105–08.

Hui, L. (1998). Chinese smokers take to slim cigarettes. *Word Tobacco*, 11 July.

INWAT Europe (2000). *Part of the Solution? Tobacco Control Policies and Women*. London, Health Development Agency/Cancer Research Campaign. www.inwat.org

International Network of Women against Tobacco. (2005). INWAT Factsheets. www.inwat.org.

Jarvis, J.M. (1997). Health behaviour interventions in the context of lifestyles and influences: cigarette smoking and inequalities. MRC/ESRC meeting on health behavioural interventions, London, 30 April – 1 May.

Jacobs, R. (2001). Economic policies, taxation and fiscal measures. In: J.M. Samet and S.-Y. Yoon (eds) *Women and the Tobacco Epidemic- Challenges for the 21st Century*, p177–200. Geneva, WHO.

Jha, P. Jacob, B., Gajalakshmim, V., Gupta, P.C., Dhingra, N., Kumar, R. *et al.* (2008). A Nationally Representative Case–Control Study of Smoking and Death in India. *New England Journal of Medicine*, **358**: 1137–47.

Johnson, J., Greaves, L., and Repta, R. (2007). *Better science with sex and gender – a primer for health research*. Vancouver, Women's Health Research Network.

Joossens, L. and Sasco, A.J. (1999). Some Like it 'Light' – Women and Smoking in the European Union. Brussels, European Union Europe Against Cancer/ENSP.

Kaufman, N. and Nichter, M. (2001). The marketing of tobacco to women: global perspectives. In: J.M. Samet and S.-Y. Yoon (eds) *Women and the Tobacco Epidemic – Challenges for the 21st Century*, pp 69–98. Geneva, WHO.

Knight, J. and Chapman, S. (2004). 'Asian yuppies … are always looking for something new and different': creating a tobacco culture among young Asians. *Tobacco Control*, **13**: ii22–ii29.

Lewit, E.M., Hyland, A., Kerrebrock, N., and Cummings, K.M. (1997). Price, public policy, and smoking in young people. *Tobacco Control*, **6** (Suppl 2): S17–24.

Lewit, E.M., Coate, J.L., and Grossman, M. (1981). The effects of government regulation on teenage smoking. *J Law Econ*, **24**: 545–69.

Lewit, E.M. and Coate, J.L. (1982). The potential for using excise taxes to reduce smoking. *J Health Econ*, **1**: 121–45.

Liu, B.-Q., Peto, R., Chen, Z.-M., Boreham, J., Wu, Y.-P., Li, J.-Y. *et al.* (1998). Emerging tobacco hazards in China: 1. Retrospective proportional mortality study of one million deaths. *British Medical Journal*, **317**: 1411–22.

Lopez, A.D., Collishaw, N.E., and Piha, T. (1994). A descriptive model of the cigarette epidemic in developed countries. *Tobacco Control*, **3**: 242–7.

Lum, K.L., Polansky, J.R., Jackler, R.K., and Glantz, S.A. (2008). Signed, sealed and delivered: 'big tobacco' in Hollywood, 1927–1951. *Tobacco Control*, **17**: 313–23.

Marsh, A. (1997). Tax and spend: a policy to help poor smokers. *Tobacco Control*, **6**: 5–6.

Mackay, J. and Eriksen, M. (2002). *The Tobacco Atlas*. Geneva, WHO.

Muller, T. (2007). *Breaking the cycle of children's exposure to tobacco smoke*. London: British Medical Association. http://www.bma.org.uk/ap.nsf/AttachmentsByTitle/PDFbreakingthecycle/$FILE/Breakingcycle.pdf

NHS Information Centre (2008). Statistics on NHS Stop Smoking Services: England April 2007 to March 2008. NHS Information Centre.

NICE (2008). *Smoking cessation services in primary care, pharmacies, local authorities and workplaces, particularly for manual working groups, pregnant women and hard to reach communities*. London, NICE. http://www.nice.org.uk/Guidance/PH10

Perkins, K.A. and Scott, J. (2008). Sex differences in long-term cessation rates due to nicotine patch. *Nicotine and Tobacco Research*, **10**: 1245–51.

Perlman, F., Bobak, M., Gilmore, A., and McKee, M. (2007). Trends in the prevalence of smoking in Russia during the transition to a market economy. *Tobacco Control*, **16**: 299–305.

Poetschke-Langer, M. and Schunk, S. (2001). Germany: tobacco industry paradise. *Tobacco Control*, **10**: 300–3.

Roth, L.K. and Taylor, H.S. (2001). Risks of smoking to reproductive health: assessment of women's knowledge. *American Journal of Obstetrics and Gynaecology*, **184**: 934–9.

Samet, J.M. and Yang, G. (2001). Passive smoking, women and children. In: J.M. Samet and S.-Y. Yoon (eds) *Women and the Tobacco Epidemic- Challenges for the 21st Century*, pp 17–48. Geneva, WHO.

Samet, J.M. and Yoon, S.-Y. (2001). *Women and the Tobacco Epidemic- Challenges for the 21st Century*. Geneva, WHO.

Seimon, T. and Mehl, G.L. (1998). Strategic marketing to young people in Sri Lanka: 'Go ahead – I want to see you smoke it now'. *Tobacco Control*, **7**: 429–33.

Shafey, O., Eriksen, M., Ross, H., and Mackay, J. (2009). *The Tobacco Atlas* (3rd edn). The American Cancer Society, The World Lung Foundation.

Simpson, D. (2008). Philippines: bad year for PM's PR. *Tobacco Control*, **17**: 300.

Simpson, D. (2007). Nepal: ad peak overshadows law drafters. *Tobacco Control*, **16**: 78.

Simpson, D. (2007). USA: Camel for women. *Tobacco Control*, **16**: 167–8.

Simpson, D. (2001). Gauloises: to Oxford and the Middle East. *Tobacco Control*, **10**: 92–3.

Thuy, T.T. (1998). Activities for Tobacco Control in Vietnam. 4th Working Group on TOH, Manila, Philippines, November 1998.

Tinkler, P. (2006). *Smoke Signals – Women, Smoking and Visual Culture*. New York, Berg.

Toll, B.A. and Ling, P.M. (2005). The Virginia Slims identity crisis: an inside look at tobacco industry marketing to women. *Tobacco Control*, **14**: 172–80.

Townsend, J., Roderick, P., and Cooper, J. (1994). Cigarette smoking by socio-economic group, sex and age: effects of price, income and health publicity. *British Medical Journal*, **309**: 923–7.

Tuinstra, T. (1998). The end of the tunnel. *Tobacco Reporter*, Summer, 4.

Tuomilehto, J., Zimmet, P., Taylor, R., Bennet, P., Wolf, E., and Kankaapaa, J. (1986). Smoking rates in Pacific islands. *Bulletin of the World Health Organisation*, **64**: 447–56.

US Department of Health and Human Services (USDHHS) (1998). Responses to increases in cigarette prices by race/ethnicity, income and age groups – United States, 1976–1993. *MMWR*, **47**: 605–9.

USSG (2001). Women and Smoking: A Report of the Surgeon General. Department of Health and Human Services. www.cdc.gov/tobacco/sgr_forwomen.htm

Warren, C.W., Jones, N.R., Peruga, A., *et al.* (2008). Global youth tobacco surveillance, 2000–2007. CDC MMWR Surveillance Summaries, 25, 57, 1–28. www.cdc.gov/mmwr/preview/mmwrhtml/ss5701a1.htm.

WHO (1997). *Tobacco or Health – a Global Status Report*. Geneva, WHO. http://www.cdc.gov/tobacco/who/whofirst.htm

WHO (1999). *Report of the WHO International Conference on Tobacco and Health. Kobe- Making a Difference in Tobacco and Health*. Geneva, WHO.

WHO (2007). *Gender and Tobacco Control: A Policy Brief*. Geneva, WHO.

WHO (2008). *Mpower – a policy package to reverse the tobacco epidemic*. Geneva, WHO.

WHO Europe (2007). *The European Tobacco Control Report 2007*. http://www.euro.who.int/document/e89842.pdf

Wiltshire, S., Bancroft, A., Amos, A., and Parry, O. (2001). 'They're doing people a service'- qualitative study of smoking, smuggling and social deprivation. *British Medical Journal*, **323**: 203–7.

Wold, B., Holstein, B., Griesbach, D., and Currie, C. (2000). *Control of Adolescent Smoking*. Bergen, University of Bergen Research Centre for Health Promotion.

World Bank (1999). *Curbing the Epidemic. Governments and the Economics of Tobacco Control*. Washington DC, The World Bank.

Zimmerman, C. (1990). Growth is the watchword for the Asian tobacco industry. *Tobacco Reporter*, **117**: 4.

Chapter 19

Cancer of the prostate

Fabio Levi and Carlo La Vecchia

Prostate is the second site for cancer incidence worldwide in men, and the first one in developed countries, followed by lung and colon-rectum (Parkin *et al.* 2005). Considerable changes in incidence rates from prostate carcinoma have been observed in the United States, the European Union, and in most other developed countries, suggesting that an epidemic of this neoplasm occurred in the late 1980s or early 1990s, followed by a fall in rates. A critical appraisal of the descriptive epidemiology of prostate cancer indicates, however, that most trends were attributable to changes in diagnostic procedures (mainly, the introduction of prostate-specific antigen–PSA–blood test), rather than substantial changes in risk factor exposure (Levi *et al.* 2000).

The descriptive epidemiology of prostate cancer is in any case inconsistent with a major role of tobacco on prostate cancer risk, given its time trends and geographic pattern. Thus, while mortality rates from lung and other tobacco-related neoplasms have substantially changed in various countries following the spread of cigarette smoking in subsequent generations, only minor long-term changes have been observed in prostatic cancer mortality rates (Levi *et al.* 2004).

Nonetheless, a possible relation between prostate cancer and cigarette smoking has been considered in several studies (Schwartz *et al.* 1961; Hammond 1966; Kahn 1966; Weir and Dunn 1970; Wynder *et al.* 1971; Kolonel and Winkelstein 1977; Schuman *et al.* 1977; Williams and Horm 1977; Hirayama 1979; Niijima and Koiso 1980; Rogot and Murray 1980; Mishina *et al.* 1985; Whittemore *et al.* 1985; Carstensen *et al.* 1987; Checkoway *et al.* 1987; Ross *et al.* 1987; Honda *et al.* 1988; Yu *et al.* 1988; Mills *et al.* 1989; Newell *et al.* 1989; Oishi *et al.* 1989; Severson *et al.* 1989; Elghany *et al.* 1990; Fincham *et al.* 1990; Hsing *et al.* 1990; Ross *et al.* 1990; Slattery *et al.* 1990; Hsing *et al.* 1991; Mills and Beeson 1992; Slattery and West 1993; Talamini *et al.* 1993; Doll *et al.* 1994; Hayes *et al.* 1994; Hiatt *et al.* 1994; Tavani *et al.* 1994; Van der Gulden *et al.* 1994; De Stefani *et al.* 1995; McLaughlin *et al.* 1995; Siemiatycki *et al.* 1995; Adami *et al.* 1996; Andersson *et al.* 1996; Coughlin *et al.* 1996; Ilic *et al.* 1996; Pawlega *et al.* 1996; Cerhan *et al.* 1997; Key *et al.* 1997; Lumey *et al.* 1997; Rodriguez *et al.* 1997; Rohan *et al.* 1997; Giovannucci *et al.* 1999; Parker *et al.* 1999; Sung *et al.* 1999; Villeneuve *et al.* 1999; Lotufo *et al.* 2000; Lund Nilsen *et al.* 2000; Putnam *et al.* 2000; Giles *et al.* 2001; Sharpe and Siemiatycki 2001; Plaskon *et al.* 2003; Crispo *et al.* 2004; Doll *et al.* 2005; Cox *et al.* 2006; Darlington *et al.* 2007; Pourmand *et al.* 2007; Strom *et al.* 2008). Among these, only three case-control (Schuman *et al.* 1977; Honda *et al.* 1988; Plaskon *et al.* 2003) and four prospective studies (Kahn 1966; Rogot and Murray 1980; Hsing *et al.* 1990, 1991; Hiatt *et al.* 1994; McLaughlin *et al.* 1995; Rodriguez *et al.* 1997) showed a positive relation between prostate cancer and tobacco smoking. This relationship, if real, may be mediated by hormonal factors, since male cigarette smokers have elevated levels of serum testosterone and androstenedione (Dai *et al.* 1988). However, one review on the health effects of cigarette smoking (IARC 1986) and two other on major risk factors for prostate cancer (Nomura and Kolonel 1991; Boyle *et al.* 1997) did not support the association between cigarette smoking and increased risk for prostate cancer.

Table 19.1 Summary of results of case-control studies on prostate cancer in relation to cigarette smoking

Investigator(s)	Location	No. of subjects	Major findings
Schwartz et al. 1961	Paris, France	139 cases 139 hospital controls	No association. 79% and 73% of smokers among cases and controls, respectively.
Wynder et al. 1971	New York, US	300 cases 400 hospital controls	No association. 40% and 39% of cigarettes smokers among cases and controls, respectively.
Kolonel and Winkelstein 1977	New York, US	176 cases 269 hospital controls	No significant association.[a] Ever-smokers: OR = 1.1 (non-cancer controls), OR = 1.0 (cancer controls)
Schuman et al. 1977	Minneapolis US	40 cases 43 hospital 35 neighbourhood controls	Direct association, when neighbourhood, but not hospital controls, were used.
Williams and Horm 1977	US, (Third Nat. Cancer controls Survey)	257 cases 1 116 population controls	No association. No of cigarette smoked: 1–400/year, OR = 0.7; 401–800/year, OR = 0.7; >800/year, OR = 0.9.
Niijima and Koiso 1980	Japan	187 cases 200 hospital controls	No association.
Mishina et al. 1985	Kyoto, Japan	111 cases 100 population controls	No significant association.[a] Ever-smokers RR = 1.6.
Checkoway et al. 1987	Chapel Hill, US	40 cases 64 hospital controls	No association.
Ross et al. 1987	Los Angeles US	284 cases (142 blacks and 142 whites) 284 population controls (142 blacks and 142 whites)	No association.[a] Ever-smokers: Whites, RR = 1.1; Blacks, RR = 0.9.
Honda et al. 1988	California, US	216 cases 212 population controls	Ever-smokers RR = 1.9; years of smoking: >40, RR = 2.6.
Yu et al. 1988	US	1162 cases (989 whites and 161 blacks) 3 124 hospital controls (2 791 whites and 320 blacks)	No significant association.[a] Whites: ex-smokers OR = 0.9; current-smokers OR = 1.0. Blacks: ex-smokers OR = 1.4; current-smokers OR = 1.7.
Newell et al. 1989	Houston, US	103 cases 220 hospital controls	No association.
Oishi et al. 1989	Kyoto, Japan	117 cases 296 hospital controls	No significant association. Current-smokers: OR = 0.6; former smokers: OR = 1.4.
Fincham et al. 1990	Alberta, Canada	382 cases 625 population controls	No association[a]. Ex-smokers RR = 0.8; current-smokers RR = 0.9.
Slattery et al. 1990	Utah, US	385 cases 679 population controls	No association.

Table 19.1 (continued) Summary of results of case-control studies on prostate cancer in relation to cigarette smoking

Investigator(s)	Location	No. of subjects	Major findings
Slattery and West 1993; Elgany *et al.* 1990	Utah, US	720 cases 1 364 population controls	57% and 58% of ever-smokers among cases and controls.
Talamini *et al.* 1993; Tavani *et al.* 1994	Northern Italy	281 cases 599 hospital controls	No significant association.[a] Ever-smokers: OR = 0.8.
Hayes *et al.* 1994	Atlanta, Detroit, New Jersey, US	981 cases (502 whites, 479 blacks) 1 315 population controls (721 Whites, 594 Blacks)	Whites: current- OR=1.2; former-smokers, OR=1.2. Blacks: current: OR = 1.0; former-smokers: RR=1.1.
Van der Gulden *et al.* 1994	The Netherlands	345 cases 1 346 hospital controls	Significant direct association. Ever-smokers: OR = 2.1. No relation with amount, duration or age started smoking.
De Stefani *et al.* 1995	Uruguay	156 cases 302 hospital (cancer) controls	No significant association.[a] Ever-smokers: OR = 0.7; ex-smokers: OR = 0.6; current: OR = 0.8.
Siemiaticki *et al.* 1995	Montreal, Canada	449 hospital cases, 1266 population controls	No significant association.[a] Ever-(cigarette) smokers: OR = 1.1.
Andersson *et al.* 1996	Sweden	256 cases 252 population controls	Current-smokers: OR = 1.8. No dose–response trend.
Ilic *et al.* 1996	Serbia, Yugoslavia	101 cases 202 hospital controls	No significant difference in smoking habits or in the number or type of smoking.
Pawlega *et al.* 1996	Poland	76 cases 152 controls	No association.
Key *et al.* 1997	U.K.	328 cases 328 population controls	No significant association. Current-smokers: OR = 1.1; former- smokers: OR = 1.1.
Lumey *et al.* 1997	US	1 097 cases 3 250 hospital controls	No association. Current-smokers: OR = 0.9; ex-smokers: OR=0.9; No dose–response trend.
Rohan *et al.* 1997	Canada	408 cases 407 population controls	Direct association. Current-smokers: OR = 1.4; ex-smokers: OR=1.7.
Sung *et al.* 1999	Taiwan	90 cases 180 hospital controls	46% and 40% of smokers in cases and controls, respectively. Ever-smokers: OR = 1.3.
Villeneuve *et al.* 1999	Canada	1 623 cases 1 623 population controls	Nonsignificant inverse association.
Giles *et al.* 2001	Australia	1 476 cases 1 409 population controls	No association.[a] Ever-smoker: OR = 1.0; ex-smoker: OR = 1.0; current-smoker: OR = 0.8
Sharpe and Siemiatycki, 2001	Montreal, Canada	319 cases 476 population controls	No association, with overall OR = 1.1 for ever (cigarette) smokers. Direct relation among obese men (OR = 2.3)

(Continued)

Table 19.1 (continued) Summary of results of case-control studies on prostate cancer in relation to cigarette smoking

Investigator(s)	Location	No. of subjects	Major findings
Plaskon et al. 2003	US	753 cases 703 population controls	OR = 1.0 ex smokers, 1.4 (95% CI, 1.0–2.0) for current-smokers, with direct relation with cigarettes day/pack years of smoking.
Crispo et al, 2004	Italy	1 294 cases 1 451 hospital controls	No association.
Cox et al. 2006	New Zealand	923 cases 1 224 population controls	No association. OR = 1.0 for both ex- and current-smokers.
Darlington et al. 2007	Canada	752 cases 1 613 population controls	OR = 1.1 for ex-, 1.2 for current-smokers. No dose–risk relation.
Pourmand et al. 2007	Iran	130 cases 75 hospital Controls	No significant association.
Strom et al. 2008	US (Mexican Americans)	176 cases 174 population controls	No association. OR = 1.1 for former, 0.9 for current-smokers.

Note

[a] Never-smokers as reference category; RR, relative risk; OR, odds ratio.

The main results from case-control studies are given in Table 19.1. Among 37 case-control studies that examined the role of cigarette smoking on prostate cancer (Schwartz *et al.* 1961; Wynder *et al.* 1971; Kolonel and Winkelstein 1977; Schuman *et al.* 1977; Williams and Horn 1977; Niijima and Koiso 1980; Mishina *et al.* 1985; Checkoway *et al.* 1987; Ross *et al.* 1987; Honda *et al.* 1988; Yu *et al.* 1988; Newell *et al.* 1989; Oishi *et al.* 1989; Elghany *et al.* 1990; Fincham *et al.* 1990; Slattery *et al.* 1990; Slattery and West 1993; Talamini *et al.* 1993; Hayes *et al.* 1994; Tavani *et al.* 1994; Van der Gulden *et al.* 1994; De Stefani *et al.* 1995; Siemiatycki *et al.* 1995; Andersson *et al.* 1996; Ilic *et al.* 1996; Pawlega *et al.* 1996; Key *et al.* 1997; Lumey *et al.* 1997; Rohan *et al.* 1997; Sung *et al.* 1999; Villeneuve *et al.* 1999; Giles *et al.* 2001; Sharpe and Siemiatycki 2004; Plaskon *et al.* 2003; Crispo *et al.* 2004; Cox *et al.* 2006; Darlington *et al.* 2007; Pourmand *et al.* 2007; Strom *et al.* 2008), only three reported a positive association (Schuman *et al.* 1977; Honda *et al.* 1988; Plaskon *et al.* 2003). The study by Honda *et al.* (1988), based on 216 cases and 212 controls, showed a moderate positive relation between prostate cancer and cigarette smoking (smokers vs. non-smokers: RR = 1.9, 95% confidence interval (CI), 1.2–3.0) and a significant direct trend only in the highest level of smoking duration. The study by Schuman *et al.* (1977) also showed some association with cigarette smoking when comparison was made with population controls only, but it was too small (40 cases) to be informative. Furthermore, a study of 345 cases and 1 346 hospital controls from the Netherlands (Van der Gulden *et al.* 1994) found a direct association with ever smoking, but no dose- nor duration–risk relationship. A study including 753 cases and 703 population controls found a RR of 1.0 for former, and 1.4 for current-smokers, of borderline significance, with a direct relation with number of cigarettes per day and pack-years of smoking (Plaskon *et al.* 2003). However, these results also contrast with other case-control studies (Williams and Horm 1977; Mishina *et al.* 1985; Ross *et al.* 1987; Slattery *et al.* 1990; Elghany *et al.* 1990; Fincham *et al.* 1990; Slattery and West 1993; Hayes *et al.* 1994; Siemiatycki *et al.* 1995; Key *et al.* 1997) which, using population controls, did not show any meaningful association between tobacco smoking and prostate cancer. However, a large Canadian population-based case-control study (Villeneuve *et al.* 1999) found a modest and inconsistent inverse association with various measures of cigarette smoking.

A report by Giles *et al.* (2001), based on a uniquely large case-control study, provides further evidence on an absence of excess risk of prostate cancer among current- or former-smokers, including those who smoked the highest number of cigarettes for the longest period of time. There is also a lack of material influence of smoking on prostate cancer in younger or elderly men, with early or advanced, or moderate or high-grade neoplasms.

Thus, most case-control studies found no association between smoking and prostate cancer, with a few reporting direct or other inverse associations, which appear to be attributable to the play of chance, in the absence of any causal association.

Among 23 prospective studies (Hammond 1966; Kahn 1966; Weir and Dunn 1970; Hirayama 1979; Rogot and Murray 1980; Whittemore *et al.* 1985; Carstensen *et al.* 1987; Mills *et al.* 1989; Severson *et al.* 1989; Hsing *et al.* 1990; Ross *et al.* 1990; Hsing *et al.* 1991; Mills and Beeson 1992; Doll *et al.* 1994; Hiatt *et al.* 1994; McLaughlin *et al.* 1995; Adami *et al.* 1996; Coughlin *et al.* 1996; Cerhan *et al.* 1997; Rodriguez *et al.* 1997; Giovannucci *et al.* 1999; Parker *et al.* 1999; Lotufo *et al.* 2000; Lund Nilsen *et al.* 2000; Putnam *et al.* 2000; Doll *et al.* 2005), four (Kahn 1966; Rogot and Murray 1980; Hsing *et al.* 1990, 1991; Hiatt *et al.* 1994; McLaughlin *et al.* 1995; Rodriguez *et al.* 1997) showed some positive relation with cigarette smoking (Table 19.2). Hsing *et al.* (1991), based on incidence, and McLaughlin *et al.* (1995), based on mortality, in the US Veterans Cohort Study found a significantly elevated relative risk among cigarette smokers (RR = 1.18; 95% CI, 1.09–1.28), particularly among heavy smokers (OR = 1.51 in smokers of 40 or more cigarettes per day compared with nonsmokers). Hsing *et al.* (1990) in a report on the Lutheran Brotherhood cohort study, reported significantly elevated relative risk among persons who smoked any type of tobacco (RR = 1.8; 95% CI, 1.1–2.9), as well as among users of smokeless tobacco (RR = 2.1; 95% CI, 1.1–4.1). No clear dose–response relation was however found. Likewise, the data of the Cancer Prevention Study II (CPSII; Rodriguez *et al.* 1997) showed an elevated risk (RR = 1.34; 95% CI, 1.16–1.56) of fatal prostate cancer in cigarette smokers, with a stronger association below age 60, but no trend in risk with number of cigarettes smoked nor duration of smoking. The conclusion was that smoking may adversely affect survival in prostatic cancer patients (Rodriguez *et al.* 1997). Positive results came from the US Kaiser Permanente Study (Hiatt *et al.* 1994), based on 238 cases.

Another prospective study from Norway (Lund Nilsen *et al.* 2000) found a weak positive association with number of cigarettes smoked, and a cohort study of Iowa men (Parker *et al.* 1999; Putnam *et al.* 2000), including only about 100 prostate cancer cases, showed a nonsignificant association with number of cigarettes. Likewise, the multiple risk factor intervention trial (MRFIT) (Coughlin *et al.* 1996) cohort showed a significant excess risk for smokers vs. non-smokers, in the absence of any dose–risk relation (i.e., RR was 1.5 for smokers of <15 cigarettes/day, but 1.2 for smokers of >45 cigarettes/day).

In contrast, no consistent association between smoking and prostate cancer was evident from the British Physicians (Doll *et al.* 1994, 2005), the US Health Professionals' (Giovannucci *et al.* 1999) and the Physicians' Health Study (Lotufo *et al.* 2000). In the 50-year follow-up of the British Physicians Cohort Study, compared to never-smokers the RR of prostate cancer death was 0.8 for moderate smokers, but rose to 1.3 for heavy smokers (Doll *et al.* 2005).

This pattern of risk would suggest that the relation between smoking and prostate cancer diagnosis or death may not be causal, but attributable to other socioeconomic or lifestyle correlates of smoking (IARC 1986; Dai *et al.* 1988; Nomura and Kolonel 1991; La Vecchia *et al.* 1992; Boyle *et al.* 1997), which are likely to be less relevant in studies conducted in health conscious populations like doctors or health professionals. A major problem of cohort studies, in fact, is often the limited number of covariates available in order to allow for potential confounding.

Table 19.2 Summary of results of cohort studies on prostate cancer in relation to cigarette smoking

Investigator(s)	Location	No. of subjects	Major findings (reference)
Hammond 1966	US	440558 (319 cases)	No association.
Kahn 1966;Rogot and Murray 1980;Hsing et al. 1991	US(Veterans)	293916 (4607 cases)	Ex-smokers RR = 1.1; current-smokers RR = 1.2; No. cigarette smoked: 10–20/day, RR = 1.2; 21–39/day, RR = 1.2; >39/day, RR = 1.5.
Weir and Dunn 1970	California, US	68153 (37 cases)	No association.[a] Ever-smokers RR = 0.8; <1–2 pk/day, RR = 0.6; 1 pk/day, RR = 1.0; >1 pk/day, RR = 0.8.
Hirayama 1979	Japan	122261 (63 cases)	No association. Age-standardized death rate per 100000 (6.1) among non-smokers, (3.7) ex-smokers, (5.8) current-smokers.
Whittemore et al. 1985	US (college alumni)	47271 (243 cases)	No association.
Carstensen et al. 1987	Sweden	25129 (193 cases)	No association.[a] Ex-smokers RR = 1.0; No. cigarettes smoked: 1–7/day, RR = 1.1; 8–15/day, RR = 0.8; > 15/day, RR = 0.9.
Mills et al. 1989	California, US	14000 (180 cases)	No association.[a] Ex-smokers RR = 1.2; current-smokers RR = 0.5.
Severson et al. 1989	Honolulu, Japan	7999 (174 cases)	No association.[a] Ex-smokers RR = 0.9; current-smokers RR = 0.9.
Hsing et al. 1990	Minnesota, US, (Lutheran)	17633 (149 cases)	Positive association.[a] Ever used any form of tobacco RR = 1.8; current-smokers RR = 2.0.
Ross et al. 1990	US, California	5105 (138 cases)	No association.[a] Current-smokers: RR = 0.9; former-smokers: RR = 0.8.
Mills and Beeson 1992	US, California (7th Day Adventists)	14000 (180 cases)	No association. Current-smokers: RR = 1.0. No relation with amount or duration of smoking.
Hiatt et al. 1994	US California (Kaiser Perman.)	43432 (238 cases)	Positive association. Compared to never-smokers, =<20 cig/day, RR = 1.0; >20 cig/day, RR = 1.9 (95% CI 1.2–3.1)
McLaughlin et al. 1995	US (Veterans)	293916 (3124 deaths)	Positive association.[a] Ex-smokers, RR = 1.1. 1–9 cig/day, RR = 1.1; 10–20 cig/day, RR = 1.2; 21–39 cig/day, RR = 1.2; 21–39 cig/day, RR = 1.2; =>40 cig/day, RR = 1.5.
Adami et al. 1996	Sweden	135006 (2368 cases)	Current-smokers, RR = 1.1; ex-smokers, RR = 1.1. No trend with amount or duration of smoking.

Table 19.2 (continued) Summary of results of cohort studies on prostate cancer in relation to cigarette smoking

Investigator(s)	Location	No. of subjects	Major findings (reference)
Coughlin et al. 1996	US (MRFIT)	348 874 (826 cases)	Positive association. No. cigarettes smoked, 1–15 cig/day, RR = 1.5; 16–25 cig/day, RR = 1.3; 26–35 cig/day, RR = 1.2; 36–45 cig/day, RR = 1.5; >45 cig/day, RR = 1.2.
Rodriguez et al. 1997	US, (Cancer Prevention Study II)	450 279 (1 748)	Positive association with current smoking for fatal cancers. Ever-smokers, RR = 1.0; current cig. only smokers, RR = 1.3; former cig. only smokers, RR = 1.0. No trend with amount or duration of smoking.
Cerhan et al. 1997	Iowa, US	1 050 (71 cases)	63% and 58% ever-smokers among cases and controls. Current, <20 cig/day, RR = 2.0; current, =>20 cig/day, RR = 2.9. Significant dose-dependent trend.
Giovannucci et al. 1999	US (Health Professionals)	51 529 (1 369 cases)	No association.[a] Current-smokers, RR = 1.1. Impact of recent use on occurrence of fatal cancer (RR = 1.6)
Parker et al. 1999	Iowa, US	1 117 (81 cases)	Former-smokers, RR = 1.3; current, <20 cig/day, RR = 1.7; current, =>20 cig/day, RR = 1.9.
Lotufo et al. 2000	US (Physicians' Health Study)	22 071 (996 cases)	No association.[a] Ex-smokers, RR=1.1; current <20 cig/day, RR = 1.1; current, =>20 cig/day, RR = 1.1. No dose- or duration-dependent trend.
Lund Nilsen et al. 2000	Norway	22 895 (644 cases)	RR = 0.8, 1.1,1.4,1.3 for subsequent levels of cigarette smoking.
Putnam et al. 2000	Iowa, US	1 572 (101 cases)	Non-significant association. Former-smokers, RR = 1.4; current, <20 cig/day, RR = 1.3; current, =>20 cig/day, RR = 1.6
Doll et al. 2005	U.K. (physicians)	34 440 (878 deaths)	RR=0.7,1.1,1.3 in subsequent levels of smoking (1–14.15–24;=>25 cig/day

Note

[a] Never-smokers as reference category; RR, relative risk; OR, odds ratio.

Thus, there is now definite evidence that cigarette smoking is not a relevant risk factor for prostate cancer, even after a long latency period. The issue of a modest association remains open to debate, but it is unclear whether such a modest association can be investigated in observational epidemiological studies, in consideration also of the need for careful allowance for confounding, since some differences in other factors (including dietary, socioeconomic, or other) may account for the apparent inconsistencies observed across studies (Wynder 1990; Colditz 1996).

These factors may also influence prostate cancer diagnosis or prognosis, since smoking has been associated with worse outcomes in patients treated by radical prostatectomy (Pantarotto *et al.* 2006).

These cautions notwithstanding, it is now clear that tobacco smoking is not a relevant risk factor for prostate cancer incidence. A possible role of smoking on prostrate cancer mortality remains open to discussion and interpretation.

References

Adami, H.-O., Bergstrom, R., Engholm, G., Nyrén, O., Wolk, A., Ekbom, A. *et al.* (1996). A prospective study of smoking and risk of prostate cancer. *International Journal of Cancer*, **67**:764–8.

Andersson, S.O., Baron, L., Bergstrom, R., Lindgren, C., Wolk, A., and Adami, H.O. (1996). Lifestyle factors and prostate cancer risk: a case-control study in Sweden. *Cancer Epidemiology Biomarkers and Prevention*, **5**:509–13.

Boyle, P., Maisonneuve, P., and Napalkov, P. (1997). Urological cancers: an epidemiological overview of a neglected problem. *Journal of Epidemiology and Biostatistics*, **2**:125–45.

Carstensen, J.M., Pershagen, G., and Eklund, G. (1987). Mortality in relation to cigarette and pipe smoking: 16 years' observation of 25000 Swedish men. *Journal of Epidemiology and Community Health*, **41**:166–72.

Cerhan, J.R., Torner, J.C., Lynch, C.F., Rubenstein, L.M., Lemke, J.H., Cohen, M.B. *et al.* (1997). Association of smoking, body mass, and physical activity with risk of prostate cancer in the Iowa 65+ Rural Health Study (United States). *Cancer Causes and Control*, **8**:229–38.

Checkoway, H., Di Ferdinando, G., Hulka, B.S., and Mickey, D.D. (1987). Medical, life-style, and occupational risk factors for prostate cancer. *Prostate*, **10**:79–88.

Colditz, G. (1996). Consensus conference: smoking and prostate cancer. *Cancer Causes and Control*, **7**:560–2.

Coughlin, S.S., Neaton, J.D., and Sengupta, A. (1996). Cigarette smoking as a predictor of death from prostate cancer in 348,874 men screened for the Multiple Risk Factor Intervention Trial. *American Journal of Epidemiology*, **143**:1002–6.

Cox, B., Sneyd, M.J., Paul, C., and Skegg, D.C.G. (2006). Risk factors for prostate cancer: a national case-control study. *International Journal of Cancer*, **119**:1690–4.

Crispo, A., Talamini, R., Gallus, S., Negri, E., Gallo, A., Bosetti, C., *et al.* (2004). Alcohol and the risk of prostate cancer and benign prostatic hyperplasia. *Urology*, **64**:717–22.

Dai, W.S., Gutai, J.P., Kuller, L.H., and Cauley, J.A. for the MRFIT Research Group. (1988). Cigarette smoking and serum sex hormones in men. *American Journal of Epidemiology*, **128**:796–805.

Darlington. G.A., Kreiger, N., Lightfood, N., Purdham, J., and Sass-Kortsak, A. (2007). Prostate cancer risk and diet, recreational physical activity and cigarette smoking. *Chronic Diseases in Canada*, **37**: 145–53.

De Stefani, E., Fierro, L., Barrios, E., and Ronco, A. (1995). Tobacco, alcohol, diet and risk of prostate cancer. *Tumori*, **81**:315–20.

Doll, R., Peto, R., Wheatley, K., Gray, R., and Sutherland, I. (1994). Mortality in relation to smoking: 40 years' observations on male British doctors. *British Medical Journal*, **309**:901–10.

Doll, R., Peto, R., Boreham, J., and Sutherland, I. (2005). Mortality from cancer in relation to smoking: 50 years observations on British doctors. *British Journal of Cancer*, **92**:426–9.

Elghany, N.A., Schumacher, M.C., Slattery, M.L., West, D.W., and Lee, J.S. (1990). Occupation, cadmium exposure, and prostate cancer. *Epidemiology*, **1**:107–15.

Fincham, S.M., Hill, G.B., Hanson, J., and Wijayasinghe, C. (1990). Epidemiology of prostatic cancer: a case-control study. *Prostate*, **17**:189–206.

Giles, G.G., Severi, G., McCredie, M.R.E., English, D.R., Johnson, W., Hopper, J.L. *et al.* (2001). Smoking and prostate cancer: findings from an Australian case-control study. *Annals of Oncology*, **12**:761–5.

Giovannucci, E., Rimm, E.B., Ascherio, A., Colditz, G.A., Spiegelman, D., Stampfer, M.J. *et al.* (1999). Smoking and risk of total and fatal prostate cancer in United States Health Professionals. *Cancer Epidemiology Biomarkers and Prevention*, **8**:277–82.

Hammond, E.C. (1966). Smoking in relation to the death rates of one million men and women. *National Cancer Institute Monograph*, **19**:127–204.

Hayes, R.B., Pottern, L.M., Swanson, G.M., Liff, G.M., Schoenberg, J.B., Greenberg, R.S. *et al.* (1994). Tobacco use and prostate cancer in blacks and whites in the United States. *Cancer Causes and Control*, **5**:221–6.

Hiatt, R.A., Armstrong, M.A., Klatsky, A.L., and Sidney, S. (1994). Alcohol consumption, smoking, and other risk factors and prostate cancer in a large health plan cohort in California (United States). *Cancer Causes and Control*, **5**:66–72.

Hirayama, T. (1979). Epidemiology of prostate cancer with special reference to the role of diet. *National Cancer Institute Monograph*, **53**:149–55.

Honda, G.D., Bernstein, L., Ross, R.K., Greenland, S., Gerkins, V., and Henderson, B.E. (1988). Vasectomy, cigarette smoking, and age at first sexual intercourse as risk factors for prostate cancer in middle-aged men. *British Journal of Cancer*, **57**:326–31.

Hsing, A.W., McLaughlin, J.K., Schuman, L.M., Bjelke, E., Gridley, G., Wacholder, S. *et al.* (1990). Diet, tobacco use, and fatal prostate cancer: results from the Lutheran Brotherhood Cohort Study. *Cancer Research*, **50**:6836–40.

Hsing, A.W., McLaughlin, J.K., Hrubec, Z., Blot, W.J., and Fraumeni, J.F. Jr. (1991). Tobacco use and prostate cancer: 26-year follow-up of US veterans. *American Journal of Epidemiology*, **133**:437–41.

IARC Working Group on the Evaluation of the Carcinogenic Risk of Chemicals to Humans. (1986). IARC Monographs on the evaluation of carcinogenic risk of chemicals to humans. *Tobacco Smoking*. Vol. 38, pp. 199–298. International Agency for Research on Cancer, Lyon, France.

Ilic, M., Vlajinac, H., and Marinkovic, J. (1996). Case-control study of risk factors for prostate cancer. *British Journal of Cancer*, **74**:1682–6.

Kahn, H.A. (1966). The Dorn study of smoking and mortality among US veterans: report on eight and one-half years of observation. *National Cancer Institute Monographs*, **19**:1–125.

Key, T.J.A., Silcocks, P.B., Davey, G.K., Appleby, P.N., and Bishop, D.T. (1997). A case-control study of diet and prostate cancer. *British Journal of Cancer*, **76**:679–87.

Kolonel, L. and Winkelstein, W. Jr. (1977). Cadmium and prostatic carcinoma. *Lancet*, **2**:566–7.

La Vecchia, C., Negri, E., Franceschi, S., Parazzini, F., and Decarli, A. (1992). Differences in dietary intake with smoking, alcohol, and education. *Nutrition and Cancer*, **17**:297–304.

Levi, F., La Vecchia, C., and Boyle, P. (2000). The rise and fall of prostate cancer. *European Journal of Cancer Prevention*, **9**:381–5.

Levi, F., Lucchini, F., Negri, E., Boyle, P., and La Vecchia, C. (2004). Leveling of prostate cancer mortality in western Europe. *The Prostate*, **60**:46–52.

Lotufo, P.A., Lee, I.-M., Ajani, U.A., Hennekens, C.H., and Manson, J.E. (2000). Cigarette smoking and risk of prostate cancer in the Physicians' Health Study (United States). *International Journal of Cancer*, **7**:141–4.

Lumey, L.H., Pittman, B., Zang, E.A., and Wynder, E.L. (1997). Cigarette smoking and prostate cancer: no relation with six measures of lifetime smoking habits in a large case-control study among US Whites. *Prostate*, **33**:195–200.

Lund Nilsen, T.I., Johnsen, R., and Vatten, L.J. (2000). Socio-economic and lifestyle factors associated with the risk of prostate cancer. *British Journal of Cancer*, **82**:1358–63.

McLaughlin, J.K., Hrubec, Z., Blot, W.J., and Fraumeni, J.F. Jr. (1995). Smoking and cancer mortality among US veterans; a 26-year follow-up. *International Journal of Cancer*, **60**:190–5.

Mills, P.K. and Beeson, W. (1992). Re: 'Tobacco use and prostate cancer: 26-year follow-up of US veterans'. *American Journal of Epidemiology*, **135**:326–7.

Mills, P.K., Beeson, W.L., Phillips, R.L., and Fraser, G.E. (1989). Cohort study of diet, lifestyle, and prostate cancer in Adventist men. *Cancer*, 64:598–604.

Mishina, T., Watanabe, H., Araki, H., and Nakao, M. (1985). Epidemiological study of prostatic cancer by matched-pair analysis. *Prostate*, **6**:423–36.

Newell, G.R., Fueger, J.J., Spitz, M.R., and Babaian, R.J. (1989). A case-control study of prostate cancer. *American Journal of Epidemiology*, **130**:395–8.

Niijima, T. and Koiso, K. (1980). Incidence of prostatic cancer in Japan and Asia. *Scandinavian Journal of Urology and Nephrology*, **55**(suppl):17–21.

Nomura, A.M.Y. and Kolonel, L.N. (1991). Prostate cancer: a current perspective. *Epidemiologic Reviews*, **13**:200–27.

Oishi, K., Okada, K., Yoshida, O., Yamabe, H., Ohno, Y., Hayes, R.B. *et al.* (1989). Case-control study of prostatic cancer in Kyoto, Japan: demographic and some life-style factors. *Prostate*, **14**:117–22.

Pantarotto, J., Malone, S., Dahrouge, S., Gallant, V., and Eapen, L. (2006). Smoking is associated with worse outcomes in patients with prostate cancer treated by radical prostatectomy. *BJU International*, **99**:564–9.

Parker, A.S., Cerhan, J.R., Putmann, S.D., Cantor, K.P., and Lynch, C.F. (1999). A cohort study of farming and risk of prostate cancer in Iowa. *Epidemiology*, **10**:452–5.

Parkin, D.M., Bray, F., Ferlay, J., and Pisani, P. (2005). Global cancer statistics, 2002. *CA Cancer J Clin*, **55**:74–108.

Pawlega, J., Rachtan, J., and Dyba, T. (1996). Dietary factors and risk of prostate cancer in Poland. Results of case-control study. *Neoplasma*, **43**:61–3.

Plaskon, L.A., Penson, D.F., Vaughan, T.L., and Stanford, J.L. (2003). Cigarette smoking and risk of prostate cancer in middle-aged men. *Cancer Epidemiology, Biomarkers & Prevention*, **12**:604–9.

Pourmand, G., Salem, S., Mehrsai, A., Lotfi, M., Amirzarga, M.A., Mazdak, H., *et al.* (2007). The risk factors of prostate cancer: a multicentric case-control study in Iran. *Asian Pacific Journal of Cancer Prevention*, **8**:422–8.

Putnam, S.D., Cerhan, J.R., Parker, A.S., Bianchi, G.D., Wallace, R.B., Kantor, K.P. *et al.* (2000). Lifestyle and anthropometric risk factors for prostate cancer in a cohort of Iowa men. *Annals of Epidemiology*, **10**:361–9.

Rodriguez, C., Tatham, L.M., Thun, M.J., Calle, E.E., and Heath, Jr. C.W. (1997). Smoking and fatal prostate cancer in a large cohort of adult men. *American Journal of Epidemiology*, **145**:466–75.

Rogot, E. and Murray, J.L. (1980). Smoking and causes of death among US veterans: 16 years of observation. *Public Health Reports*, **95**:213–22.

Rohan, T.E., Hislop, T.G., Howe, G.R., Gallagher, R.P., The C.-Z., and Ghadirian, P. (1997). Cigarette smoking and risk of prostate cancer: a population-based case-control study in Ontario and British Columbia, Canada. *European Journal of Cancer Prevention*, **6**:382–8.

Ross, R.K., Shimizu, H., Paganini-Hill, A., Honda, G., and Henderson. B.E. (1987). Case-control studies of prostate cancer in Blacks and Whites in Southern California. *Journal of the National Cancer Institute*, **78**:869–74.

Ross, R.K., Bernstein, L., and Paganini-Hill, A. (1990). Effects of cigarette smoking on «hormone related diseases» in a southern California retirement community. In N. Wald and J. Baron (eds) *Smoking and Hormone-Related Disorders*, pp. 32–54. Oxford University Press, New York.

Schuman, L.M., Mandel, J., Blackard, C., Bauer, H., Scarlett, J., and McHugh, R. (1977). Epidemiologic study of prostatic cancer: preliminary report. *Cancer Treatment Reports*, **61**:181–6.

Schwartz, D., Flamant, R., Lellouch, J., and Denoix, P.F. (1961). Results of a French survey on the role of tobacco, particularly inhalation, in different cancer sites. *Journal of the National Cancer Institute*, **26**:1085–108.

Severson, R.K., Nomura, A.M.Y., Grove, J.S., and Stemmermann, G.N. (1989). A prospective study of demographics, diet, and prostate cancer among men of Japanese ancestry in Hawaii. *Cancer Research*, **49**:1857–60.

Sharpe, C.R. and Siemiatycki, J. (2001). Joint effects of smoking and body mass index on prostate cancer risk. *Epidemiology*, **12**:546–51.

Siemiatycki, K., Krewski, D., Franco, E., and Kaiserman, M. (1995). Associations between cigarette smoking and each of 21 types of cancer. A multi-site case-control study. *International Journal of Epidemiology*, **24**:504–14.

Slattery, M.L., Schumacher, M.C., West, D.W., Robison, L.M., and French, T.K. (1990). Food-consumption trends between adolescent and adult years and subsequent risk of prostate cancer. *American Journal of Clinical Nutrition*, **52**:752–7.

Slattery, M.L. and West, D.W. (1993). Smoking, alcohol, coffee, tea, caffeine, and theobromine: risk of prostate cancer in Utah (United States). *Cancer Causes and Control*, **4**:559–63.

Strom, S.S., Yamamura, Y., Flores-Sandoval, F.N., Pattaway, C.A., and Lopez, D.S. (2008). Prostate cancer in Mexican-Americans: identification of risk factors. *The Prostate*, **68**:563–70.

Sung, J.F.C., Lin, R.S., Pu, Y.-S., Chen, Y.-C., Chang, H.C., and Lai, M.-K. (1999). Risk factors for prostate carcinoma in Taiwan. A case-control study in a Chinese population. *Cancer*, **86**:484–91.

Talamini, R., Franceschi, S., La Vecchia, C., Guarneri, S., and Negri, E. (1993). Smoking habits and prostate cancer: a case-control study in Northern Italy. *Preventive Medicine*, **22**:400–8.

Tavani, A., Negri, E., Franceschi, S., Talamini, R., and La Vecchia, C. (1994). Alcohol consumption and risk of prostate cancer. *Nutrition and Cancer*, **21**:25–31.

Van der Gulden, J.W.J., Verbeek, A.L.M., and Kolk, J.J. (1994). Smoking and drinking habits in relation to prostate cancer. *British Journal of Urology*, **73**:382–9.

Villeneuve, P.J., Johnson, K.C., Kreiger, N., and Mao, Y. (1999). Risk factors for prostate cancer: results from the Canadian National Enhanced Cancer Surveillance System. The Canadian Cancer Registries Epidemiology Research Group. *Cancer Causes and Control*, **10**:355–67.

Weir, J.M. and Dunn, J.E. Jr. (1970). Smoking and mortality: a prospective study. *Cancer*, **25**:105–12.

Whittemore, A.S., Paffenbarger, R.S. Jr., Anderson, K., and Lee, J.E. (1985). Early precursors of site-specific cancers in college men and women. *Journal of the National Cancer Institute*, **74**:43–51.

Williams, R.R. and Horm, J.W. (1977). Association of cancer sites with tobacco and alcohol consumption and socioeconomic status of patients: Interview study from the Third National Cancer Survey. *Journal of the National Cancer Institute*, **58**:525–47.

Wynder, E.L. (1990). Epidemiological issues in weak associations. *International Journal of Epidemiology*, **19**(Suppl 1):S5–7.

Wynder, E.L., Mabuchi, K., and Whitmore, W.F. Jr. (1971). Epidemiology of cancer of the prostate. *Cancer*, **28**:344–60.

Yu, H., Harris, R.E., and Wynder, E.L. (1988). Case-control study of prostate cancer and socioeconomic factors. *Prostate*, **13**:317–25.

Chapter 20

Laryngeal cancer

Paolo Boffetta

Summary

More than 160 000 new cases of laryngeal cancer are estimated to occur each year worldwide, and 90 000 people die from this disease. Tobacco smoking is the main cause of laryngeal cancer in all populations among which studies have been conducted, and at least two-thirds of cases among men and one-third of cases among women are attributable to tobacco smoking. The risk of laryngeal cancer among heavy smokers is at least 20 times higher than that of non-smokers. The amount of cigarettes smoked per day and the duration of smoking are important determinants of the risk; a protective effect of quitting smoking is clear after five years. Several studies have suggested a higher risk among deep inhalers; smokers of hand-rolled cigarettes and smokers of black-tobacco cigarettes have a higher risk than other smokers. An increased risk has been shown following smoking of cigar and pipe, as well as of bidi and other local tobacco products. Tobacco smoking seems to exert a stronger carcinogenic effect on the supraglottic region of the organ than on the glottis. Tobacco smoking acts synergistically with alcohol drinking in causing laryngeal cancer; a similar interaction with the carcinogenic effect of a diet poor in fruits and vegetables is probable. A genetic susceptibility to tobacco-induced laryngeal cancer in plausible, but specific factors have not yet been identified. Data on p53 mutations in laryngeal cancer are consistent with a major carcinogenic role played by tobacco. Tobacco control remains the main tool to prevent laryngeal cancer.

Epidemiology of laryngeal cancer

More than 90% of cancers of the larynx are squamous cell carcinomas, and the majority originate from the supraglottic and glottic regions of the organs. The incidence in men is high (8/100 000 or more) in Southern and Central Europe, South America, West Asia, and among Blacks in the United States while the lowest rates (in the order of 1/100 000) are recorded in Western and Central Africa. The incidence in women is below 1.5/100 000 in most populations. In most high-income countries rates have declined in men over the last two decades. An estimated 160 000 new cases and 90 000 deaths occurred worldwide in 2002, of which 140 000 cases and 80 000 deaths among men (Ferlay *et al.* 2004).

Up to 80% of cases of laryngeal cancer in high-income countries are attributable to tobacco smoking, alcohol drinking, and the interaction between the two factors (Olshan 2006) [see below]. The risk in smokers relative to never-smokers in the order of 10, and it seems to be higher for glottic than supraglottic neoplasms. Studies in several populations have shown a dose–response relationship and a beneficial effect of quitting smoking. Smoking black-tobacco cigarettes entails a stronger risk than smoking blond-tobacco cigarettes. Studies from India have also reported an effect of chewing tobacco-containing products. The effect of alcohol appears to be stronger for supraglottic tumours than for tumours at other sites; there is no consistent evidence for a different carcinogenic effect of different alcoholic beverages.

There are suggestive evidence for a protective effect exerted by fruits and vegetables and food containing carotenoids, while the evidence is inadequate for other foods and micronutrients (WCRF 2007).

Occupational exposure to mists of strong inorganic acids, in particular of sulphuric acid, and to asbestos are established risk factors for laryngeal cancer (Olshan *et al*. 2006). A possible effect has been suggested for other occupational exposures, including nickel and ionizing radiation, but the evidence is not conclusive. Indoor air pollution from cooking fumes in poorly ventilated houses has been suggested as risk factor in India (Sapkota *et al*. 2008) and Europe (Maier *et al*. 1997).

An aetiological role of HPV infection on the larynx has been suggested by the association of this infection with oropharyngeal cancer and by the observation that laryngeal papillomatosis, a condition characterized by multiple benign papillomas caused by infection with HPV types 6 and 11, entails an increased risk of laryngeal cancer. However, studies aimed at assessing the presence of HPV DNA have provided contrasting results, although some studies reported an association between seropositivity and laryngeal cancer risk (Kreimer *et al*. 2005; Mork *et al*. 2001).

There is no evidence of strong genetic factors in laryngeal carcinogenesis; however, variants involved in the metabolism of alcohol have been shown to play a weak role in laryngeal carcinogenesis (Hashibe *et al*. 2008).

Tobacco smoking

A strong association between tobacco smoking and laryngeal cancer has been reported since the 1950s (Doll and Hill 1954; Schrek *et al*. 1950; Wynder *et al*. 1955). This finding has been replicated in different populations and under different circumstances of tobacco smoking. As early as 1964, public health and scientific authorities considered that the causal association between tobacco smoking and laryngeal cancer was clearly established (USDHEW 1964). Since then, evidence has accumulated on different aspects of the carcinogenic effect of tobacco smoking on the larynx, based on data from both cohort and case-control studies. On the one hand, cohort studies, although they may be considered methodologically superior, are mainly based on mortality data and have primarily been assembled in areas with a low incidence of laryngeal cancer, such as the United States, the United Kingdom, Japan, and the Nordic countries, resulting in a relatively small number of cases, even in the largest cohorts. For example, during the 12-year follow-up of the American Cancer Society Cancer Prevention Study I, which included over one million individuals, a total of 109 deaths from laryngeal cancer was recorded among men and 22 among women (Burns *et al*. 1996). On the other hand, case-control studies are based on incident cases and have often been conducted in high-risk areas, such as Southern Europe and South America.

Cigarette smoking

Among men, the risk of laryngeal cancer is increased 5–10 times among ever cigarette smokers as compared to never-smokers (Gandini *et al*. 2008). In population-based series, the proportion of cases who report not having smoked during their lifetime is in the order of 1–5%. In all studies that have analysed it, a positive trend was found between amount of smoking and risk of laryngeal cancer relative to that of non-smokers. Table 20.1 summarizes the results of the selected case-control studies. Additional studies provided similar results for other populations, for example, Uruguay (De Stefani *et al*. 1995), Spain (Lopez-Abente *et al*. 1992), and Denmark (Olsen *et al*. 1985), but they did not fulfil the criteria for inclusion in Table 20.1. The heterogeneity in the results can be explained by the small number of non-smoking cases in some of the studies, by the type of tobacco smoked, by differences in the interactive effect of alcohol drinking and possibly

Table 20.1 Results of selected cases-control studies of tobacco smoking and laryngeal cancer

Study	Area, period, gender*	Cases**	Controls***	Categories (cig/day)	OR	95% CI	Comments
Graham et al., 1981	USA, 1957–1965, M	374, NA	H, 381, NA	0	1.0	Ref.	controls from cancer institute
				1–10	2.1	p<0.05	
				11–20	4.8	p<0.005	
				21–39	8.8	p<0.005	
				40+	8.5	p<0.005	
Burch et al., 1981	Canada, 1977–1979	204, 79%	N, 204, 77%	0	1.0	Ref.	
				1–14	3.0	1.4–6.3	
				15–24	3.4	1.7–6.8	
				25+	4.5	2.2–9.2	
Tuyns et al., 1988	Italy, Spain, France, Switzerland, 1973–1980, M	696, >80%	P, 3057, 56–75%	0	1.0	Ref.	
				1–7	2.4	1.3–4.3	
				8–15	6.7	4.2–10.7	
				16–25	13.7	8.7–21.6	
				26+	16.4	10.1–26.6	
Zheng et al., 1992	China, 1988–1990	201, 76%	P, 414, 88%	0	1.0	Ref.	
				1–9	1.6	0.5–4.9	
				10–19	7.1	3.1–16.6	
				20	12.4	4.6–33.2	
				21+	25.1	9.9–63.2	

(Continued)

Table 20.1 (continued) Results of selected cases-control studies of tobacco smoking and laryngeal cancer

Study	Area, period, gender*	Cases**	Controls***	Categories (cig/day)	OR	95% CI	Comments
Hedberg et al., 1994	USA, 1983–1987	235, 81%	P, 547, 75%	0	1.0	Ref.	ref. cat. includes ex-smokers > 15 yrs
				1–19	6.3	3.1–11.8	
				20–39	10.6	6.5–18.7	
				40+	23.1	9.4–52.6	
Tavani et al., 1994	Italy, 1986–1992, M	350, NA	H, 1373, NA	0	1.0	Ref.	low exp. cat. includes ex smokers
				1–14	3.5	2.1–6.0	
				15+	10.4	6.2–17.5	
Dosemeci et al., 1997	Turkey, 1979–1984, M	832, NA	H, 829, NA	0	1.0	Ref.	
				1–10	1.6	0.9–2.6	
				11–20	3.5	2.6–4.8	
				21+	6.6	4.2–10.3	
Hashibe et al., 2007	Central Europe, 1998–2002	384, NA	H, 918, NA	0	0.2	0.09–0.4	
				1–9	1.0	Ref.	
				10–19	1.9	1.1–3.2	
				20–29	2.7	1.5–4.7	
				30+	5.6	2.8–11.3	

Selection criteria include publication after 1980, N cases of laryngeal cancer > 200, report of odds ratios for amount of smoking, adjustment for alcohol drinking, separate category of never smokers.

* M if results are restricted to men, no indication if they refer to both sexes.

** number of cases, response rate.

*** source of controls, number of controls, response rate.

NA, not available; H, hospital-based; P, population-based; N, neighbourhood.

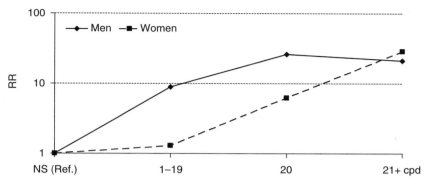

RR, relative risk; NS, non-smoker; Ref, reference category

Figure 20.1 Relative risk of laryngeal cancer by amount of smoking American Cancer Society Cancer Prevention Study I.

Source: Burch *et al*, 1996.

by differences in genetic susceptibility factors, in addition to differences in the quality of the studies and the validity of the results.

Results from cohort studies are comparable to those available from case-control studies (e.g., Burch *et al.* 1981; Doll and Hill 1954; Dorn 1959; Jee *et al.* 2004). As an example, Fig. 20.1 shows the relative risk among white men and women enrolled in the American Cancer Society Cancer Prevention Study I (Burns *et al.* 1996).

Several cohort- and case-control studies reported a positive dose–response according to duration of smoking (Choi and Kahyo 1991; Dosemeci *et al.* 1997; Falk *et al.* 1989; Lopez-Abente *et al.* 1992; Restrepo *et al.* 1989; Sankaranarayanan *et al.* 1990; Zheng *et al.* 1992). For example, in the study by Zheng *et al.* (1992) from China, the odds ratios were 1.4 (95% confidence interval [CI] 0.4–4.6), 4.1 (1.6–11.1), 12.0 (4.8–30.1), and 13.2 (5.6–31.2) for less than 20 years, 20–29 years, 30–39 years, and 40 or more years of smoking.

Selected results on the effect of quitting are summarized in Table 20.2. No significant protective effect is apparent during the first five years after quitting, a phenomenon that can be partially explained by quitting because of early symptoms of the neoplastic lesion. After that time, however, there is strong evidence of a decrease in risk of laryngeal cancer.

A higher relative risk was suggested in several studies for deep inhalation of tobacco smoke, as compared to light or no inhalation (Burns *et al.* 1996; Lewin *et al.* 1998; Lopez-Abente *et al.* 1992; Restrepo *et al.* 1989). In a study from Uruguay, smokers of hand-rolled cigarettes had a higher risk than smokers of manufactured cigarettes (De Stefani *et al.* 1992). Studies from southern Europe and South America have consistently reported a 1.5- to two-fold stronger risk among smokers of black-tobacco cigarettes as compared to blond-tobacco cigarettes (De Stefani *et al.* 1987, 2004; Lopez-Abente *et al.* 1992; Schlecht *et al.* 1999; Tuyns *et al.* 1988).

Smoking of products other than cigarettes

An increased risk of laryngeal cancer from cigar and pipe smoking was noticed in the early epidemiological studies (Wynder *et al.* 1955, 1976) and confirmed in some (Hashibe *et al.* 2007; Henley *et al.* 2004; Schlecht *et al.* 1999; Shapiro *et al.* 2000) but not all (Freudenheim *et al.* 1992) recent investigations. In most studies, the magnitude of the risk is similar to that of light or moderate smokers, possibly reflecting a lower consumption of tobacco in this group of smokers. In large

Table 20.2 Odds ratios of laryngeal cancer among ex-smokers: results of selected case-control studies

Study	Years since quitting	OR	95% CI
Tuyns *et al.*, 1988	< 1*	1.0	Ref.
	1–4	1.5	1.2–2.0
	5–9	0.5	0.3–0.8
	10+	0.3	0.2–0.4
Zatonski *et al.*, 1991	< 5*	1.0	Ref.
	5–10	0.8	0.3–1.8
	11+	0.3	0.1–0.6
Zheng *et al.*, 1992	< 2*	1.0	Ref.
	2–4	1.8	0.6–4.9
	5–9	0.6	0.2–1.5
	10+	0.6	0.3–1.2
Hashibe *et al.*, 2007	< 2*	1.0	Ref.
	2–4	0.7	0.3–1.5
	5–9	0.5	0.3–1.0
	10–19	0.5	0.3–0.9
	20+	0.1	0.03–0.3
Bosetti *et al.*, 2008	<1*	1.0	Ref.
	1–10	0.8	0.6–1.1
	10–19	0.3	0.2–0.5
	20+	0.2	0.1–0.3

* including current smokers.

cohort studies from the United States, however, current-smokers of cigarettes, cigars and pipe experienced a similar increase in risk of laryngeal cancer (Henley *et al.* 2004; Shapiro *et al.* 2000). Smoking of local tobacco products, such as bidis in India (Sankaranarayanan *et al.* 1990; Znaor *et al.* 2003) and yaa muan in Thailand (Simarak *et al.* 1977), also increases the risk of laryngeal cancer. In particular, the effect of bidi smoking seems to be similar to that exerted by cigarette smoking (Fig. 20.2).

Smokeless tobacco products

Use of oral snuff and chewing of tobacco-containing products have been associated with an increased risk in Europe, North America, and India (Jussawalla and Deshpande 1971; Lee *et al.* 2005; Lewin *et al.* 1998; Sapkota *et al.* 2007; Wynder *et al.* 1955; Znaor *et al.* 2003), although some studies did not detect an increased risk (Sankaranarayanan *et al.* 1990). The high prevalence of smokeless tobacco use in South Asia might explain, at least in part, the relatively high incidence of laryngeal cancer as compared to lung cancer (e.g., the ratio of the incidence of lung cancer to that of laryngeal cancer in 2002 was 1.45 among Indian men and 10.5 among US men [Ferlay *et al.* 2004]).

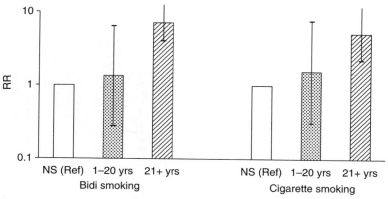

RR, relative risk; NS, non-smoker; Ref, reference category

Figure 20.2 Relative risk of laryngeal cancer from bidi and cigarette smoking – India
Source: Sankaranarayanan *et al*, 1990.

Involuntary smoking

Limited data are available on the risk of laryngeal cancer following involuntary exposure to tobacco smoke. In a study of 59 non-smoking head and neck cancer cases and matched non-smoking controls, cases had higher exposure to involuntary smoking than controls (Tan *et al*. 1997). In a pooled analysis of six studies comprising 78 non-smoking cases of laryngeal cancer and 1 872 non-smoking controls, the relative risk of ever exposure to involuntary smoking at home or at work was 1.71 (95% CI 0.98–3.00) and that of exposure at home for more than 15 years was 2.58 (95% CI 1.20–5.57) (Lee *et al*. 2008). The relative risk was particularly high (2.90, 95% CI 1.09–7.73) among never-smokers who were also never drinkers (26 cases, 896 controls). Studies including smokers confirmed the presence of an increased risk of laryngeal cancer following exposure to involuntary smoking (e.g., Ramroth *et al*. 2008): in such studies, however, it is difficult to completely exclude residual confounding by active smoking. Supportive evidence for a possible carcinogenic role of involuntary smoking on the larynx comes from the similarities of the carcinogenic effect of active smoking on the lung and the larynx, both at the epidemiological and the molecular level (Stewart and Semmler 2002). It can be concluded therefore that an increased risk of laryngeal cancer following involuntary smoking in humans is plausible, although it has not yet been demonstrated.

Interaction with other risk factors

The synergism between tobacco smoking and alcohol drinking in laryngeal carcinogenesis has been noted in the early epidemiological studies (Wynder *et al*. 1976) and analysed in many subsequent reports (Baron *et al*. 1993; Brownson and Chang 1987; Burns *et al*. 1996; Choi and Kahyo 1991; De Stefani *et al*. 1987; Falk *et al*. 1989; Flanders and Rothman 1982; Franceschi *et al*. 1990; Herity *et al*. 1982; Olsen *et al*. 1985; Talamini *et al*. 2002; Tavani *et al*. 1994; Zatonski *et al*. 1991; Zheng *et al*. 1992). Figure 20.3 shows the relative risks for different combinations of tobacco smoking and alcohol drinking estimated in the largest available study (Hashibe *et al*. 2009). An independent effect of the two carcinogens is clearly shown, and the combined relative risk fits well with a multiplicative model of interaction. An interpretation of these results is that tobacco smoking and alcohol drinking act through independent carcinogenic mechanisms on the laryngeal mucosa.

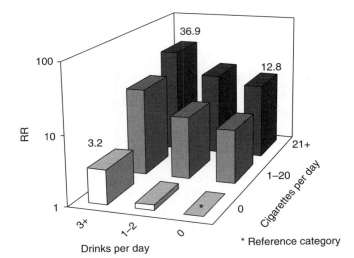

Figure 20.3 Relative risk of laryngeal cancer according to tobacco smoking and alcohol drinking.

Source: Hashibe *et al*, 2009.

The joint effect of tobacco smoking and dietary factors has been studied by several authors. Freudenheim *et al.* (1992) found a greater effect of high fat or retinol intake (but not of low carotenoid intake) among heavy smoker than among light smokers. De Stefani *et al.* (1995) found a similar risk from high intake of salted or fresh meat among heavy and light smokers. A similar lack of synergism was reported for low fruit intake by De Stefani *et al.* (1987), for low intake of β-carotene by Tavani *et al.* (1994), and for low intake of fruits or vegetables by Zheng *et al.* (1992). Overall, the available evidence suggests no interaction in laryngeal carcinogenesis, under a multiplicative model, between tobacco smoking and dietary factors. In one single study, an increased risk from heavy meat intake was found among heavy smokers but not among light smokers (De Stefani *et al.* 1987). No data are available on the joint effect of tobacco smoking and exposure to other known causes of laryngeal cancer, such as occupational exposures.

Effect of gender

Few studies included a sufficiently large number of smoking women to allow a gender-specific analysis of tobacco-related risk of laryngeal cancer. In the most informative studies (e.g., Gallus *et al.* 2003; Wynder and Stellman 1979), higher relative risks have been reported among women than among men for comparable amounts of smoking. Similar findings have been reported for lung cancer: although these results might reflect an increased susceptibility to tobacco carcinogenesis among women compared to men, an alternative explanation is the lower rate of the disease in non-smoking women than men, possibly reflecting the lack of effect of other environmental carcinogens (Bain *et al.* 2004).

Genetic susceptibility

A role of genetic polymorphism of enzymes involved in the metabolism of tobacco carcinogens in modulating tobacco-related risk of laryngeal cancer has been postulated, but the available results do not suggest an important role polymorphisms in genes encoding for phase I (e.g., *CYP2D6*) or phase II (e.g., *GSTM1* or *GSTT1*) enzymes (Benhamou *et al.* 1996; Jourenkova *et al.* 1998; Risch *et al.* 2003). A recent analysis of several variants in alcohol dehydrogenase (*ADH*) genes identified two variants associated with a reduced risk of laryngeal cancer (rs rs1229984 in *ADH1B* and rs1573496 in *ADH7*), whose effect seemed to be more pronounced among smokers than among non-smokers (Hashibe *et al.* 2008). It is unclear however whether this interaction is attributable to residual confounding by alcohol drinking.

Effect of different subsites within the larynx

A number of case-control studies have provided separate estimates of the tobacco-related risk of glottic (or intrinsic laryngeal) cancer and supraglottic (or extrinsic laryngeal) cancer (Brugere *et al.* 1986, Dosemeci *et al.* 1997; De Stefani *et al.* 2004; Elwood *et al.* 1984; Falk *et al.* 1989; Guenel *et al.* 1988; Hashibe *et al.* 2007; Lopez-Abente *et al.* 1992; Maier *et al.* 1992; Menvielle *et al.* 2004; Muscat and Wynder 1992; Tuyns *et al.* 1988). Without exception, relative risks are higher for supraglottic than for glottic cancer, which is compatible with a direct contact mechanism of tobacco carcinogenicity on the organ. As an example, Fig. 20.4 reports the results of the largest available study from four European countries.

Limited data are available on the synergism between tobacco smoking and alcohol drinking on cancer in different parts of the organ (Dosemeci *et al.* 1997; Guenel *et al.* 1988): although risk estimates are often unstable due to small numbers, it is suggested that the combined effect of the two exposures on glottic cancer is compatible with a multiplicative model of interaction, while for supraglottic cancer the combined relative risks are lower than expected according to the multiplicative model, suggesting some overlap in the carcinogenic action of the two agents.

Evidence from mechanistic studies

Mutation in the p53 gene is a common genetic alteration in laryngeal cancer. A distinct pattern of mutations has been reported in cancer of the larynx, and in other tobacco-related cancers, as compared to non-tobacco-related cancers. This includes a higher proportion of tumours harbouring a mutation and a higher proportion in G-T transversions, in particular at codons 157, 158, 179, and 249 (Pfeifer *et al.* 2002). These mutations likely reflect the effect of the interaction of tobacco carcinogens, such as BPDE, the active metabolite of benzo(a)pyrene, on the DNA (Brennan and Boffetta 2002). The evidence directly linking tobacco smoking to p53 mutation in laryngeal carcinogenesis, however, is weak. Out of 171 p53 mutations reported in laryngeal

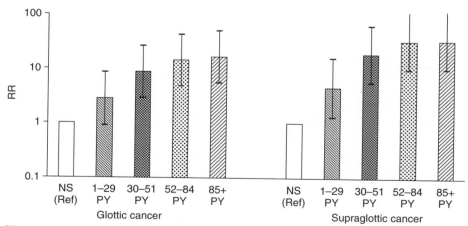

RR, relative risk; NS, non-smoker; PY, pack-years; Ref, reference category

Figure 20.4 Relative risk of glottic and supraglottic cancer from cigarette smoking - Uruguay.
Source: De Stefani *et al.*, 2004.

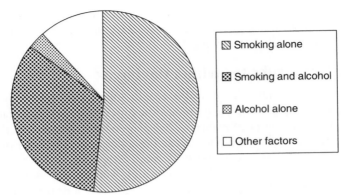

Figure 20.5 Proportion of laryngeal cancers attributable to tobacco smoking and alcohol drinking.
Source: Hashibe *et al.* 2009.

cancers in the IARC p53 database (www.iarc.fr/p53/index.html), data on smoking habit were available for 73 patients, of whom only 3 were non-smokers.

Effect on survival

In a study comprising 931 cases of laryngeal cancer from three European countries, mortality of laryngeal cancer cases was greater among heavy smokers than among non-smokers and light smokers (Dikshit *et al.* 2005). This result mainly reflects the increased risk of other tobacco-related causes of death, and mortality from head and neck cancer was only moderately associated with tobacco smoking.

Public health impact

Tobacco smoking greatly increases the risk of laryngeal cancer. The proportion of male cases of laryngeal cancer attributable to tobacco smoking in Europe and North America is around 80%.

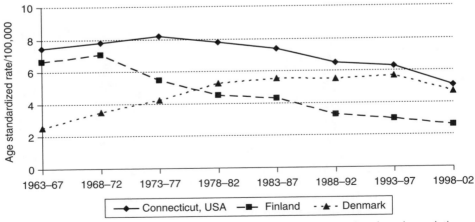

Figure 20.6 Time trends in the incidence of laryngeal cancer among men in selected populations.
Source: Parkin *et al.*, 2005; Curado *et al.*, 2008.

This proportion might be lower in men from other regions of the world where other causes of laryngeal cancer might play an important role, and in women. A study of the burden of tobacco-related cancer worldwide provided conservative estimates of 67% of cases in men and 28% in women, corresponding to 100 600 new cases each year and, assuming no effect of smoking on laryngeal cancer-specific mortality, 55 600 deaths (Parkin *et al.* 1994).

As is shown in Fig. 20.5, tobacco smoking plays by far the largest aetiological role in laryngeal carcinogenesis, either alone or in combination with other factors, and tobacco control remains the main avenue for prevention of this disease. The decline during the recent decades in the incidence of laryngeal cancer among men in some regions in which tobacco control has been implemented more effectively (e.g., the USA and Finland vs. Denmark, Fig. 20.6) suggests that prevention of this disease through the avoidance of its major cause is possible. As for other tobacco-related diseases, the main priority today is tobacco control in low- and medium-income countries.

References

Bain C, Feskanich D, Speizer FE, *et al.* (2004). Lung cancer rates in men and women with comparable histories of smoking. *J Natl Cancer Inst*, 2;96(11): 826–34.

Baron AE, Franceschi S, Barra S, Talamini R, La Vecchia C (1993). A comparison of the joint effects of alcohol and smoking on the risk of cancer across sites in the upper aerodigestive tract. *Cancer Epidemiol Biomarkers Prev*, 2: 519–23.

Benhamou S, Bouchardy C, Paoletti C, Dayer P (1996). Effects of CYP2D6 activity and tobacco on larynx cancer risk. *Cancer Epidemiol Biomarkers Prev*, 5: 683–6.

Bosetti C, Gallus S, Peto R, *et al.* (2008). Negri E, Talamini R, Tavani A, Franceschi S, La Vecchia C. Tobacco smoking, smoking cessation, and cumulative risk of upper aerodigestive tract cancers. *Am J Epidemiol*, **167**(4): 468–73.

Brennan P, Boffetta P (2004). *Mechanisms of carcinogenesis: contributions of molecular epidemiology.* IARC Scientific Publications No. 157. International Agency for research on Cancer, Lyon, France.

Brownson RC, Chang JC (1987). Exposure to alcohol and tobacco and the risk of laryngeal cancer. *Arch Environ Health*, 42: 192–6.

Brugere J, Guenel P, Leclerc A, Rodriguez J (1986). Differential effects of tobacco and alcohol in cancer of the larynx, pharynx, and mouth. *Cancer*, 57: 391–5.

Burch JD, Howe GR, Miller AB, Semenciw R (1981). Tobacco, alcohol, asbestos, and nickel in the etiology of cancer of the larynx: a case-control study. *J Natl Cancer Inst*, 67: 1219–24.

Burns DM, Shanks TG, Choi W, Thun MJ, Heath CW Jr, Garfinkel L (1996). *The American Cancer Society Cancer Prevention Study I: 12-year followup of 1 million men and women* (Smoking and Tobacco Control Monograph No 8). Washington (DC): National Cancer Institute, 113–304.

Choi SY, Kahyo H (1991). Effect of cigarette smoking and alcohol consumption in the aetiology of cancer of the oral cavity, pharynx and larynx. *Int J Epidemiol*, **20**: 878–85.

Curado MP, Edwards B, Shin HR, Storm H, Ferlay J, Heanue M, *et al.* (eds) (2008). *Cancer Incidence in Five Continents*, Vol. IX. IARC Scientific Publications No. 160, Lyon.

De Stefani E, Boffetta P, Deneo-Pellegrini H, *et al.* (2004). Supraglottic and glottic carcinomas: epidemiologically distinct entities? *Int J Cancer*, 20;112(6): 1065–71.

De Stefani E, Correa P, Oreggia F, *et al.* (1987). Risk factors for laryngeal cancer. *Cancer*, 60: 3087–91.

De Stefani E, Oreggia F, Rivero S, Fierro (1992). L. Hand-rolled cigarette smoking and risk of cancer of the mouth, pharynx, and larynx. *Cancer*, 70: 679–82.

De Stefani E, Oreggia F, Rivero S, Ronco A, Fierro L (1995). Salted meat consumption and the risk of laryngeal cancer. *Eur J Epidemiol*, 11: 177–80.

Dikshit RP, Boffetta P, Bouchardy C, *et al.* (2005). Lifestyle habits as prognostic factors in survival of laryngeal and hypopharyngeal cancer: a multicentric European study. *Int J Cancer*, **117**(6): 992–5.

Doll R, Hill AB (1954). The mortality of doctors in relation to their smoking habits; a preliminary report. *Brit Med J*, **1**: 1451–5.

Dorn HF (1959). Tobacco consumption and mortality from cancer and other diseases. *Public Health Rep*, **74**: 581–93.

Dosemeci M, Gokmen I, Unsal M, Hayes RB, Blair A (1997). Tobacco, alcohol use, and risks of laryngeal and lung cancer by subsite and histologic type in Turkey. *Cancer Causes Control*, **8**: 729–37.

Elwood JM, Pearson JCG, Skippen DH, Jackson SM (1984). Alcohol, smoking, social and occupational factors in the aetiology of cancer of the oral cavity, pharynx and larynx. *Int J Cancer*, **34**: 603–12.

Falk RT, Pickle LW, Brown LM, Mason TJ, Buffler PA, Fraumeni JF Jr (1989). Effect of smoking and alcohol consumption on laryngeal cancer risk in coastal Texas. *Cancer Res*, **49**: 4024–9.

Ferlay J, Colombet M, Boniol M, Authier P, Heanue M, Boyle P (2007). Cancer Incidence and Mortality in Europe. *Annal Oncol*, **16**(3): 481–8.

Flanders WD, Rothman KJ (1982). Interaction of alcohol and tobacco in laryngeal cancer. *Am J Epidemiol*, **115**: 371–9.

Franceschi S, Talamini R, Barra S, *et al.* (1990). Smoking and drinking in relation to cancers of the oral cavity, pharynx, larynx, and esophagus in northern Italy. *Cancer Res*, **50**: 6502–7.

Freudenheim JL, Graham S, Byers TE, *et al.* (1992). Diet, smoking, and alcohol in cancer of the larynx: a case-control study. *Nutr Cancer*, **17**: 33–45.

Gallus S, Bosetti C, Franceschi S, Levi F, Negri E, La Vecchia C (2003). Laryngeal cancer in women: tobacco, alcohol, nutritional, and hormonal factors. *Cancer Epidemiol Biomarkers Prev*, **12**(6): 514–7.

Gandini, S., Botteri, E., Iodice, S., Boniol M, Lowenfels AB, Maisonneuve P, *et al.* (2008). Tobacco smoking and cancer: a meta-analysis. *Int J Cancer*, **122**(1): 155–64.

Graham, S., Mettlin, C., Marshall, J., Priore, R., Rzepka, T., and Shedd, D. (1981). Dietary factors in the epidemiology of cancer of the larynx. *Am J Epidemiol*, **113**: 675–80.

Guenel, P., Chastang, J.-F., Luce, D., Leclerc, A., and Brugere, J. (1988). A study of the interaction of alcohol drinking and tobacco smoking among French cases of laryngeal cancer. *J Epidemiol Comm Health*, **42**: 350–4.

Hashibe, M., Boffetta, P., and Zaridze, D. (2007). Contribution of tobacco and alcohol to the high rates of squamous cell carcinoma of the supraglottis and glottis in Central Europe. *Am J Epidemiol*, **165**(7): 814–20.

Hashibe, M., Brennan, P., Benhamou, S. *et al.* (2008). Alcohol drinking in never users of tobacco, cigarette smoking in never drinkers, and the risk of head and neck cancer: pooled analysis in the International Head and Neck Cancer Epidemiology Consortium. *J Natl Cancer Inst*, 2007 May 16;**99**(10): 777–89. Erratum in: *J Natl Cancer Inst*, **100**(3): 225.

Hashibe, M., Brennan, P., Chuang, S.C. *et al.* (2009). Interaction between tobacco and alcohol use and the risk of head and neck cancer: pooled analysis in the International Head and Neck Cancer Epidemiology Consortium. *Cancer Epidemiol Biomarkers Prev*, **18**(2): 541–550.

Hedberg, K., Vaughan, T.L., White, E., Davis, S., and Thomas, D.B. (1994). Alcoholism and cancer of the larynx: a case-control study in western Washington (United States). *Cancer Causes Control*, **5**: 3–8.

Henley, S.J., Thun, M.J., Chao, A., and Calle, E.E. (2004). Association between exclusive pipe smoking and mortality from cancer and other diseases. *J Natl Cancer Inst*, 2;**96**(11): 853–61.

Herity, B., Moriarty, M., Daly, L., Dunn, J., and Bourke, G.J. (1982). The role of tobacco and alcohol in the aetiology of lung and larynx cancer. *Br J Cancer*, **46**: 961–4.

Jee, S.H., Samet, J.M., Ohrr, H., Kim, J.H., and Kim, I.S. (2004). Smoking and cancer risk in Korean men and women. *Cancer Causes Control*, **15**(4): 341–8.

Jourenkova, N., Reinikainen, M., Bouchardy, C., Dayer, P., Benhamou, S., and Hirvonen, A. (1998). Larynx cancer risk in relation to glutathione S-transferase M1 and T1 genotypes and tobacco smoking. *Cancer Epidemiol Biomarkers Prev*, **7**: 19–23.

Jussawalla, D.J. and Deshpande, V.A. (1971). Evaluation of cancer risk in tobacco chewers and smokers: an epidemiologic assessment. *Cancer*, **28**: 244–52.

Kreimer, A.R., Clifford, G.M., Boyle, P., and Franceschi, S. (2005). Human papillomavirus types in head and neck squamous cell carcinomas worldwide: a systematic review.*Cancer Epidemiol Biomarkers Prev*, **14**: 467–75.

Lee, K.W., Kuo, W.R., Tsai, S.M. *et al.* (2005). Different impact from betel quid, alcohol and cigarette: risk factors for pharyngeal and laryngeal cancer. *Int J Cancer*, **117**: 831–6.

Lee, Y.C., Boffetta, P., Sturgis, E.M. *et al.* (2008). Involuntary smoking and head and neck cancer risk: pooled analysis in the International Head and Neck Cancer Epidemiology Consortium. *Cancer Epidemiol Biomarkers Prev*, **17**(8): 1974–81.

Lewin, F., Norell, S.E., Johansson, H. *et al.* (1998). Smoking tobacco, oral snuff, and alcohol in the etiology of squamous cell carcinoma of the head and neck: a population-based case-referent study in Sweden. *Cancer*, **82**: 1367–75.

Lopez-Abente, G., Pollan, M., Monge, V., and Martinez-Vidal, A. (1992). Tobacco smoking, alcohol consumption, and laryngeal cancer in Madrid. *Cancer Detection Prev*, **16**: 265–71.

Maier, H., Gewelke, U., Dietz, A., and Heller, W.-D. (1992). Risk factors of cancer of the larynx: results of the Heidelberg case-control study. *Otolaryngol Head Neck Surg*, **107**: 577–82.

Maier, H. and Tisch, M. (1997). Epidemiology of laryngeal cancer: results of the Heidelberg case-control study. *Acta Oto-Laryngologica*, 160–64.

Menvielle, G., Luce, D., Goldberg, P., Bugel, I., and Leclerc, A. (2004). Smoking, alcohol drinking and cancer risk for various sites of the larynx and hypopharynx. A case-control study in France. *Eur J Cancer Prev*, **13**(3): 165–72.

Mork, J., Lie, A.K., Glattre, E. *et al.* (2001). Human papillomavirus infection as a risk factor for squamous-cell carcinoma of the head and neck. *N Eng J Med*, **12**; 344(15): 1125–31.

Muscat, J.E. and Wynder, E.L. (1992). Tobacco, alcohol, asbestos, and occupational risk factors for laryngeal cancer. *Cancer*, **69**: 2244–51.

Olsen, J., Sabreo, S., and Fasting, U. (1985). Interaction of alcohol and tobacco as risk factors in cancer of the laryngeal region. *J Epidemiol Comm Health*, **39**: 165–8.

Olshan, A.F. (2006). Cancer of the Larynx. In Schottenfeld D, Fraumeni J (eds) *Cancer Epidemiology and Prevention*, third edition, 627–37. Oxford University Press, Oxford.

Parkin, D.M., Pisani, P., Lopez, A.D., and Masuyer, E. (1994). At least one in seven cases of cancer is caused by smoking: global estimates for 1985. *Int J Cancer*, **59**: 494–504.

Parkin, D.M., Whelan, S.L., Ferlay, J., and Storm, H. (2005). *Cancer Incidence in Five Continents, Vol. I to VIII*. IARC CancerBase No. 7, Lyon.

Pfeifer, G.P., Denissenko, M.F., Olivier, M., Tretyakova, N., Hecht, S.S., and Hainaut, P. (2002). Tobacco smoke carcinogens, DNA damage and p53 mutations in smoking-associated cancers. *Oncogene*, **21**(48): 7435–51.

Ramroth, H., Dietz, A., and Becher, H. (2008). Environmental tobacco smoke and laryngeal cancer: results from a population-based case-control study. *Eur Arch Otorhinolaryngol*, **265**(11): 1367–71.

Restrepo, H.E., Correa, P., Haenszel, W., Brinton, L.A., and Franco, A. (1989). A case-control study of tobacco-related cancers in Colombia. *Bull Pan Am Health Organ*, **23**: 405–13.

Risch, A., Ramroth, H., Raedts, V. *et al.* (2003). Laryngeal cancer risk in Caucasians is associated with alcohol and tobacco consumption but not modified by genetic polymorphisms in class I alcohol dehydrogenases ADH1B and ADH1C, and glutathione-S-transferases GSTM1 and GSTT1. *Pharmacogenetics*, **13**(4): 225–30.

Sankaranarayanan, R., Duffy, S.W., Nair, M.K., Padmakumary, G., and Day, N.E. (1990). Tobacco and alcohol as risk factors in cancer of the larynx in Kerala, India. *Int J Cancer*, **45**: 879–82.

Sapkota, A., Gajalakshmi, V., Jetly, D.H., Roychowdhury, S., Dikshit, R.P., Brennan, P. *et al.* (2008). Indoor air pollution from solid fuels and risk of hypopharyngeal/laryngeal and lung cancers: a multicentric case-control study from India. *Int J Epidemiol*, **37**(2): 321–8.

Schlecht, N., Franco, E.L., Pintos, J., and Kowalski, L.P. (1999). Effect of smoking cessation and tobacco type on the risk of cancers of the upper areo-digestive tract in Brazil. *Epidemiology*, **10**: 412–8.

Schrek, R., Baker, L.A., Ballard, G.P., and Dolgoff, S. (1950). Tobacco smoking as an etiologic factor in disease, I, *Cancer. Cancer Res*, **10**: 49–58.

Shapiro, J.A., Jacobs, E.J., and Thun, M.J. (2000). Cigar smoking in men and risk of death from tobacco-related cancers. *J Natl Cancer Inst*, **16**;92(4): 333–7.

Simarak, S., de Jong, U.W., Breslow, N. *et al.* (1977). Cancer of the oral cavity, pharynx/larynx and lung in north Thailand: case-control study and analysis of cigar smoke. *Br J Cancer*, **36**: 130–40.

Stewart, B.W. and Semmler, P.C. (2002). Sharp v Port Kembla RSL Club: establishing causation of laryngeal cancer by environmental tobacco smoke. *Med J Aust*, **176**: 113–6.

Talamini, R., Bosetti, C., La Vecchia, C. *et al.* (2002). Combined effect of tobacco and alcohol on laryngeal cancer risk: a case-control study. *Cancer Causes Control*, **13**(10): 957–64.

Tan, E.-H., Adelstein, D.J., Droughton, M.L., Van Kirk, M.A., and Lavertu, P. (1997). Squamous cell head and neck cancer in nonsmokers. *Am J Clin Oncol*, **20**: 146–50.

Tavani, A., Negri, E., Franceschi, S., Barbone, F., and La Vecchia, C. (1994). Attributable risk for laryngeal cancer in northern Italy. *Cancer Epidemiol Biomarkers Prev*, **3**: 121–5.

Tuyns, A.J., Esteve, J., Raymond, L. *et al.* (1988). Cancer of the larynx/hypopharynx, tobacco and alcohol: IARC international case-control study in Turin and Varese (Italy), Zaragoza and Navarra (Spain), Geneva (Switzerland) and Calvados (France). *Int J Cancer*, **41**: 483–91.

USDHEW Laryngeal cancer. (1964). In: *Smoking and health: Report of the Advisory Committee to the Surgeon General of the Public Health Service*. US Department of Health, Education and Welfare, Public Health Service; pp. 205–12.

WCRF (World Cancer Research Fund). (2007). *Food, Nutrition, Physical Activity, and the Prevention of Cancer: a global perspective*. Washington DC: AICR.

Wynder, E.L., Bross, I.J., and Day, E. (1955). A study of environmental factors in cancer of the larynx. *Cancer*, **9**: 86–110.

Wynder, E.L., Covey, L.S., Mabuchi, K., and Mushinski, M. (1976). Environmental factors in cancer of the larynx: a second look. *Cancer*, **38**: 1591–601.

Wynder, E.L., Stellman, S.D. (1979). Impact of long-term filter cigarette usage on lung and larynx cancer risk: a case-control study. *J Natl Cancer Inst*, **62**: 471–7.

Zatonski, W., Becher, H., Lissowska, J., and Wahrendorf, J. (1991). Tobacco, alcohol, and diet in the etiology of laryngeal cancer: a population-based case-control study. *Cancer Causes Control*, **2**: 3–10.

Zheng, W., Blot, W.J., Shu, X.-O. *et al.* (1992). Diet and other risk factors for laryngeal cancer in Shanghai, China. *Am J Epidemiol*, **136**: 178–91.

Znaor, A., Brennan, P., Gajalakshmi, V. *et al.* (2003). Independent and combined effects of tobacco smoking, chewing and alcohol drinking on the risk of oral, pharyngeal and esophageal cancers in Indian men. *Int J Cancer*, **10**;105(5): 681–6.

Chapter 21

Smoking and cancer of the oesophagus

Eva Negri

It has been estimated that in the year 2002 there were in the world about 315 000 new cases of oesophageal cancer (OC) among men and 145 000 among women [1]. The great majority of these cases (255 000 men and 130 000 women) occur in less developed countries. The age standardized rate in men is two-fold in less developed areas compared to more developed areas of the world (13.8/100 000 vs. 6.8/100 000). In women the ratio between rates in less and more developed areas is 5 (6.5/100 000 vs. 1.3/100 000).

Oesophageal cancer incidence rates show a remarkably large geographical variation, with a difference of over 300-fold between high and low risk areas [2]. Very high rates have been observed in a belt starting in eastern Turkey and extending through the southern states of the former Soviet Union, Iran, and Iraq into Northern China [3, 4]. Large differences in rates can be observed also within small geographical areas [2], and rapid changes of rates over time have been observed [5]. In North America, rates are much higher among African Americans than among whites [2, 6].

The two major histologic types are squamous cell carcinoma of the oesophagus (SCCO) and adenocarcinoma of the oesophagus (ACO), which account for over 90% of OC [6]. Worldwide the vast majority of OC are SCCO. Over recent periods, however, a levelling off or decreases in SCCO incidence rates, and increases in ACO incidence rates have been observed in the United States, Canada, and several European countries, especially Northern European ones, and in a few other areas [7–11]. In white men in the United States, and in men in a few Northern European countries and Australia, ACO incidence rates are now higher than SCCO rates [6, 7, 10, 11].

Squamous cell carcinoma of the oesophagus and ACO differ in geographic distribution, temporal trends, and risk factors, and thus represent two separate epidemiological entities [12]. Thus, they will be considered separately in this chapter.

Squamous-cell carcinoma of the oesophagus

Already in the late 1950s some studies reported an association between tobacco and cancer of the oesophagus [13–15], although the authors still doubted the causality of this association. In the following years, further evidence accumulated, and in 1986 the Working group of the International Agency for Research on Cancer (IARC) Monograph on Tobacco smoking concluded that 'smoking is an important cause of oesophageal cancer' [16]. A further evaluation in 2004 confirmed that 'tobacco smoking is causally associated with cancer of the oesophagus, particularly squamous cell carcinoma' [17].

This conclusion relies on overwhelming evidence derived from case-control and cohort studies conducted in different areas of the world, that – with only very rare exceptions – found higher risks of SCCO in smokers. Table 21.1 shows the results of selected case-control studies of OC/SCCO [15, 18–40]. As it will be discussed later, alcohol consumption is an important confounder/effect modifier of the relation between smoking and risk of SCCO. Thus, only studies that present alcohol-adjusted estimates are included in the table. In most studies, the risk of smokers was two

Table 21.1 Results from selected case-control studies on smoking and risk of squamous-cell carcinoma of the oesophagus

Study (reference) and location	Type of controls #Cases:#controls	OR for current and former-smokers	Dose		Duration	
			Cutpoints	OR[a]	Cutpoints	OR[a]
North America						
Wynder and Bross 1961 [18] – New York, USA	Hospital 99 OC[b]:100 Co[c]		1–9[d]	2.3		
			10–20	2.7		
			21–34	4.1		
			≥35	4.6		
Brown et al. 1988 [19] – Coastal South Carolina, USA	Hospital or deceased (for deceased cases) 207 OC:422 Co Men only	Current OR=1.8 (1.0–3.0) Former (<10years) 2.0 (1.0–3.7) Former (10+years) 1.0 (0.5–2.1)	1–19[e]	0.8 (0.4–2.5)	1–24 years	1.4 (0.6–2.9)
			20–29	2.0 (1.1–3.4)	25–34	1.6 (1.0–2.8)
			≥30	2.6 (1.4–4.7)	≥35	1.8 (1.0–3.3)
Kabat et al. 1993 [20] – 8 US cities	Hospital 212 SCCO[f]: 6772 Co	**Men** Current OR=4.5 (2.5–8.1) Former OR=1.3 (0.7–2.4) **Women** Current OR=6.8 (3.7–12) Former OR=2.2 (1.1–4.3)	1–20[e]	1.9 (1.1–3.5)		
			21–30	2.7 (1.3–5.4)		
			>30	2.7 (1.5–5.0)		
			1–20	3.7 (2.0–6.7)		
			>20	4.8 (2.4–9.5)		

Gammon et al. 1997 [21] – 3 areas of USA	Population 221 SCCO: 695 Co	Current	OR=5.1 (2.8–9.2)	<16^e	2.7 (1.4–5.1)	<20 years	1.8 (0.9–3.7)
				16–20	3.9 (2.1–7.2)	20–31	2.0 (1.0–4.0)
				21–30	5.3 (2.6–11)	32–42	3.3 (1.8–6.1)
		Former	OR=2.8 (1.5–4.9)	>30	3.9 (2.0–7.6)	>42	5.9 (2.0–7.6)

South America

Castellsagué et al. 1999 [22] – Argentina, Brasil, Paraguay, Uruguay	Hospital (5 studies) 830 SCCO: 1779 Co	**Men**					
		Current	OR=5.1 (3.4–7.6)	1–7^e	2.2 (1.3–3.5)	1–29 years	2.6 (1.7–4.2)
				8–14	4.1 (2.6–6.4)	30–39	3.6 (2.3–5.6)
		Former		15–24	5.3 (3.4–8.1)	40–49	4.7 (3.0–7.2)
			OR=2.8 (1.8–4.3)	≥25	5.0 (3.2–7.7)	≥50	6.0 (3.8–9.5)
		Women					
		Current	OR=3.1 (1.8–5.3)	1–14^e	2.1 (1.2–3.7)	1–29 years	.5 (0.8–2.9)
		Former		≥15	2.8 (1.4–5.4)	30–39	2.0 (0.9–4.4)
			OR=1.6 (0.8–3.1)			≥40	4.4 (2.2–9.0)

Australia

Pandeya et al. 2008 [23] Mainland states of Australia	Population309 SCCO: 1580 Co	Current	OR=4.6 (3.0–7.0)	<10^e	1.4 (0.8–2.5)	≤15 years	2.0 (1.2–3.3)
				10–19	2.6 (1.7–4.1)	>15–25	2.3 (1.4–3.8)
		Former		20–25	3.2 (2.1–5.0)	25–35	2.5 (1.5–3.9)
			OR=2.2 (1.5–3.2)	>25	4.7 (2.9–7.6)	>35	4.3 (2.8–6.5)

Europe

Tuyns et al. 1977 [15] – Ille-et-Vilaine, France				0–9^d	1.0 (ref)		
				10–19	1.5		
				20–29	1.6		
				≥30	6.1		

(Continued)

Table 21.1 (continued) Results from selected case-control studies on smoking and risk of squamous-cell carcinoma of the oesophagus

Study (reference) and location	Type of controls #Cases:#controls	OR for current and former-smokers	Dose		Duration	
			Cutpoints	ORa	Cutpoints	ORa
Lagergren et al. 2000 [24] – Sweden	Population 167 SCCO: 820 Co	Current OR=9.3 (5.1–17) Former OR=2.5 (1.4–4.7)	1–9e 10–19 >19	2.3 (1.1–4.6) 2.9 (1.5–5.8) 8.8 (4.9–16)	1–20 years 21–35 >35	2.3 (1.1–4.6) 2.9 (1.5–5.8) 8.8 (4.9–16)
Zambon et al. 2000 [25] – Northern Italy	Hospital 275 SCCO: 593 Co Men only		1–14e 15–24 ≥25	3.2 (1.6–6.4) 5.4 (2.8–10) 7.0 (3.2–15)	1–24 years 25–34 ≥35	1.5 (0.4–6.2) 2.6 (1.2–5.6) 6.4 (3.5–12)
Hashibe et al. 2006. [26] – Multicentric: Romania, Russia, Czech Republic, and Poland	Hospital 192 SCCO:1114 Co	Current OR=7.4 (4.0–14) Former OR=2.4 (1.2–4.9)	1–95e 10–19 20–29 ≥30	4.2 (2.0–8.9) 5.2 (2.8–9.8) 5.9 (3.0–11) 4.8 (1.9–12)	1–9 years 10–19 20–29 30–39 40–49 ≥50	2.6 (0.8–8.4) 3.9 (1.7–8.9) 3.8 (1.8–8.0) 7.4 (3.8–14) 6.2 (3.1–12) 3.7 (1.6–8.6)
Vioque et al. 2008 [27] – Spain	Hospital 160 SCCO: 455 Co	Current OR=2.3 (0.95–5.5) Former OR=1.1 (0.4–2.7)	1–14e 15–29 ≥30	1.4 (0.4–4.5) 2.1 (0.8–5.4) 5.8 (2.0–17)	1–19 years 20–29 ≥30	0.5 (0.1–2.1) 1.6 (0.6–4.7) 2.0 (0.8–4.9)
Asia						
Gao et al. 1994 [28] – Shanghai, China	Population 605 SCCO:1552 Co	Current OR=1.9* Former OR=1.6*	1–9e 10–19 20–29 ≥30	1.1 1.7* 2.5* 4.8*	0.5–19 years 20–29 30–39 ≥40	0.7 1.6* 2.2* 2.5*

Study	Type	Cases : Controls	Smoking status	OR (CI)	Amount	OR (CI)	Duration	OR (CI)
Guo et al. 1994 [29] – Linxian, north-central China	Nested within a cohort	640 OC: 3200 Co (Men only)	Ever	OR=1.8 (1.4–2.4)	<10[e]	1.8[g] (1.3–2.6)	<20 years	1.2 (0.7–2.0)
					10–19	1.8 (1.3–2.5)	20–39	1.8 (1.3–2.5)
					≥20	1.9 (1.3–2.8)	≥40	2.1 (1.4–3.1)
Hu et al. 1994 [30] – North-east China	Hospital	196 OC: 392 Co			1–10[e]	1.7 (1.0–2.9)	1–10 years	1.5[h] (05.–5.2)
					11–20	2.2 (1.3–3.7)	11–20	2.1 (1.1–4.3)
					21–30	1.7 (0.8–3.7)	21–30	2.8 (1.6–5.0)
					≥31	3.3 (1.5–7.4)	≥31	3.3 (2.0–5.3)
Sankaranarayanan et al. 1991 [31] – Kerala, Southern India	Hospital	267 OC: 895 Co			1–10[i]	1.9 (0.8–4.3)	<20[i] years	2.1 (0.8–5.9)
					11–20	3.9 (1.7–8.9)	≥20	4.7 (2.8–7.9)
					≥21	4.8 2.3–9.8		
Takezaki et al. 2000 [32] – Nagoya, Japan	Outpatients	284 OC: 11936 Co (Men only)	Current	OR=3.5 (2.1–5.8)	1–19[e]	3.1 (1.8–5.5)	1–29 years	2.2 (1.1–4.4)
			Former	OR=1.6 (0.9–2.8)	≥20	3.5 (2.1–5.9)	≥30	3.6 (2.1–6.0)
Znaor et al. 2003 [33] – South India	Non tobacco-related cancers (47%) and healthy hospital visitors (53%)	566 OC: 3638 Co	Current	OR=2.8 (2.2–3.7)	1–9[d]	2.1 (1.6–2.8)	<20 years	1.6 (1.1–2.3)
			Former	OR=1.6 (1.1–2.2)	10–19	2.9 (2.2–3.9)	20–29	2.5 (1.8–3.4)
					≥20	2.7 (1.8–4.1)	30–39	2.9 (2.1–3.9)
							≥40	2.9 (2.1–4.0)
Lee et al. 2005 [34] – Taiwan	Hospital	513 SCCO: 818 Co	Current	OR=4.2 (2.7–6.3)	1–20[e]	3.5 (2.2–5.6)	1–15 years	2.3 (1.0–4.9)
			Former	OR=3.4 (2.1–5.3)	21–40	4.0 (2.7–6.1)	16–30	3.8 (2.4–6.1)
					≥41	4.6 (1.5–14)	>30	4.4 (2.9–6.7)
Wu et al. 2006 [35] – Southern Taiwan	Hospital and outpatients	165 SCCO: 255 Co	Current	OR=6.3 (2.8–15)	≤20[e]	4.6 (2.1–11)	<25 years	7.4 (2.4–24)
			Former	OR=2.5 (0.9–7.6)	>20	6.4 (2.5–18)	≥25	4.8 (2.1–12)

(Continued)

Table 21.1 (continued) Results from selected case-control studies on smoking and risk of squamous-cell carcinoma of the oesophagus

Study (reference) and location	Type of controls #Cases:#controls	OR for current and former-smokers	Dose		Duration	
			Cutpoints	OR[a]	Cutpoints	OR[a]
Jiang et al. 2006 [36] 24 major cities and 79 rural communities in China	Living spouses of deceased women. 19,734 male OC deaths: 104,846 Co	**Urban**				
			<20[e]	1.5 (1.4–1.6)	<20 years	1.3 (1.1–1.6)
			20–29	2.0 (1.9–2.2)	20–29	1.7 (1.5–2.0)
			≥30	3.4 (2.9–3.9)	≥30	1.9 (1.8–2.0)
		Rural				
			<20[e]	1.3 (1.2–2.4)	<20 years	1.2 (1.0–1.3)
			20–29	1.4 (1.2–1.5)	20–29	1.3 (1.2–1.5)
			≥30	1.9 (1.5–2.5)	≥30	1.5 (1.3–1.6)
Nasrollahzadeh et al. 2008 [37] – Golestan province northeastern Iran	Population 300 SCCO: 571 Co	Current[k] OR=1.6 (0.97–2.8) Former OR=1.3 (0.8–2.2)	≤11 (median)	0.98 (0.6–1.8)	≤21 (median)	1.3 (0.8–2.1)
			>11	2.0 (1.2–3.3)	>21	1.7 (1.0–2.9)
Africa						
Segal et al. 1988 [38] – Soweto, South Africa	Hospital 200 OC:391 cont		0–19[d]	1.0 (ref)		
			20–39	3.0 (1.5–5.9)		
			≥40	2.2 (1.3–3.7)		
Vizcaino et al. 1995 [39] – Bulawayo, Zimbabwe	Non smoking or alcohol related cancers 826 OC: 3007 Co Men only	Former OR=3.4 (1.9–6.2)	<15[d]	3.5 (2.7–4.5)		
			≥15	5.7 (3.8–8.4)		

| Pacella-Norman et al. 2002 [40] – South Africa | Non smoking or alcohol related cancers 267 OC:804 Co | Current OR=3.8 (2.3–6.1) Former OR= 3.8 (2.3–6.3) | 1–14 [d] ≥15 | 3.3 (2.0–5.5) 6.0 (3.2–11) |

Note

[a] All odds ratios presented were adjusted for age, sex (when required), plus a variable number of other potential confounders. The reference category is set to never-smokers, if not otherwise specified.

[b] OC=oesophageal cancers.

[c] Co=controls.

[d] Grams of tobacco per day.

[e] Cigarettes per day.

[f] SCCO=squamous-cell oesophageal cancer.

[g] Not adjusted for alcohol. Drinking uncommon in controls, 22% of OC cases were drinkers

[h] Not alcohol-adjusted.

[i] Cigarettes+bidi.

[j] Duration of bidi smoking.

[k] Not adjusted for alcohol. Only 2% of cases and controls ever drank alcohol.

to five times that of never-smokers, and the risk of former-smokers was intermediate between the two. The causality of the association is further supported by the fact that the risk of OC increases with increasing daily dose and with duration of the habit in almost all studies. Using spline models, Polesel and colleagues found a significant excess in risk of OC beginning with as low as two cigarettes per day, highlighting the absence of any harmless level of cigarette smoking [41].

The association between smoking and SCCO/OC is somewhat weaker, but still present, in some very high risk areas in China and Iran [37, 42].

Type of cigarettes

De Stefani and colleagues [43] noted that the OR of OC were higher in studies conducted in populations smoking mainly black tobacco, as compared to those in populations smoking predominantly blond tobacco. Consistently, studies presenting ORs separately for smokers of blond and black tobacco cigarettes tended to find higher risks in black tobacco smokers. Compared to blond tobacco cigarette smoker, the risk of OC of black tobacco cigarette smokers was two to four times higher in studies from Uruguay [43] and Spain [27]. Smokers of hand-rolled cigarettes also tend to have higher risks of OC than smokers of commercial cigarettes [30,43–45]. Also high-tar cigarettes convey a higher risk of OC [46, 47].

Bidi, cigars, and pipe smoking

Also cigar and pipe smokers have an increased risk of OC. In the study by Wynder and Bross [18] the OR of OC of cigarette smokers was 2.8, compared to never-smokers, that of cigar and pipe smokers was 6.0, and that of pipe only smokers was 9.0. Other studies also found higher risks of OC in pipe smokers compared to cigarette smokers [43, 44]. The studies that analysed the risk of smokers of cigars only were generally based on small numbers of cases, but they consistently found an increased risk of about four-fold or more for ever cigar smokers [26, 48, 49]. In a case-control from India [33] the OR of smokers of bidis only was 3.3 (95% CI 2.5–4.4), and 3.2 (95% CI 1.2–8.19) for smokers of cigars/cheroots only.

Smokeless tobacco

The association between smokeless tobacco and SCCO risk was recently reviewed in a IARC monograph [50]. The working group reviewed five studies and drew no definite conclusion. One study in Assam, India, found a five-fold increased risk among tobacco leaves chewers [51]. Modest, nonsignificant increases were found in a Norwegian cohort [52] and in two Swedish case-control studies [24, 53], and no association in a study from the United States [19]. All these studies were based on small numbers of exposed cases. A case-control study from Iran published afterwards found an OR of 2.0 (95% CI 1.2–3.3) in nass chewers (a mixture of tobacco, ash and lime), based on 44 exposed cases [37].

Interaction with alcohol

Alcohol is another well-established risk factor for OC, and alcohol and tobacco act synergistically in magnifying the risk. Thus, in countries where both habits are widespread, the effect of tobacco cannot be considered separately from that of alcohol. Some studies have analysed how the joint exposure to alcohol and tobacco influences the risk of OC. Already in 1961 Wynder and Bross [18] noted that both factors were independently associated to oesophageal cancer risk. In 1977 Tuyns and colleagues [15] published the results of their case-control study on cancer of the oesophagus conducted in Ille-et-Vilaine, France. This study of 200 cases of OC and 778 controls has been used in textbooks [54] as an example of how the joint effect of two factors can affect the OR.

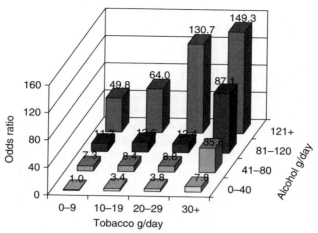

Figure 21.1 Odds ratios of cancer of the oesophagus for various combinations of alcohol and tobacco consumption.

Source: Data from Tuyns et al. 1977, modified by Doll and Peto 1981.

Figure 21.1 shows the odds ratios for the Ille-et-Vilaine study [15], modified by Doll and Peto [55], for the combination of alcohol and tobacco. The reference category is set to those who smoke less than 10 g of tobacco per day, and drink 40 g or less alcohol per day. The risk of OC increases with dose of tobacco for each level of alcohol drinking: in non or light drinkers, the OR is 1.0 in smokers of less than 10 g of tobacco per day (reference category), 3.4 in smokers of 10–19 g/day, 3.8 in smokers of 20–29 g/day, and 7.8 in smokers of 30 or more g/day. In drinkers of 41–80 g/day the corresponding OR in subsequent categories of tobacco consumptions are 7.3, 8.4, 8.8, and 35.5; in drinkers of 81–120 g/day the OR for smoking are 11.7, 13.6, 12.4, and 87.1; and in very heavy drinkers (>120 g/day) the risk for increasing tobacco consumption categories are 49.8, 64.0, 130.7, and 149.3. Likewise, for every category of tobacco consumption, the OR increases as alcohol consumption increases. Heavy smokers and heavy drinkers have a risk of OC which is 150 times that of those who are non or moderate smokers and non or moderate drinkers. This impressive risk would have been higher if only non-smokers had been included in the reference category. This was not possible due to lack of cases not exposed to the two factors: only 9 of the 200 cases were non-smokers, as compared to 57 expected from the control distribution, and none of them drank less than 40 g/day of alcohol. Thus, in the high-risk area of Ille-et-Vilaine, OC is a rare disease in non-smoking moderate drinkers. Further studies have confirmed that the risk of OC in heavy smokers and drinkers, compared to non or light smokers and drinkers, is extremely high [25, 26, 34, 35,18].

Tuyns and colleagues [15] further noted that the risks appeared to follow a multiplicative model, that is, the risk for subjects simultaneously exposed to both alcohol and tobacco is the product of the risks of those exposed to only one factor. Breslow and Day [54] have modelled in detail the relation between alcohol and tobacco consumption and risk of cancer of the oesophagus, using the Ille-et-Vilane data. Also in many other studies, a multiplicative model appeared to describe in the joint ORs for alcohol and tobacco satisfactorily [25]. Moreover, smoking may also interact with other risk factors, for example, betel quid chewing [33], opium use [37] or dietary factors [56], as well as familial factors [57].

Although oesophageal cancer is less frequent in women than in men in many countries, and most of the studies were based only or prevalently on men, smoking and drinking are also risk factors for women [58].

Tobacco in alcohol non-drinkers

The few studies that investigated the effect of smoking in alcohol non-drinkers were generally based on small numbers of cases. Nevertheless, they have consistently reported that smoking is a risk factor for OC also in the absence of alcohol consumption [59–61]. These studies included both never- and former-drinkers. In a case-control study conducted in Hong Kong among never-drinkers, smoking was still a risk factor for OC, and the OR for heavy smokers was increased ten-fold compared to never-smokers [62]. In a case-control study from Taiwan [62] the OR of ever-smokers who were never-drinkers and never-chewers was 2.0 (95% 1.2–3.3). A significant trend with dose and duration of cigarette smoking was also reported in a case-control study from Iran, where only 2% of cases and controls were alcohol users [37].

Smoking and drinking cessation

Several studies have shown that the risk is lower in ex-smokers than in current-smokers, and declines steeply with time since stopping smoking [19, 23, 27, 33, 63–67]. A study conducted in Italy and Switzerland provided convincing evidence that stopping consumption of both alcohol and tobacco leads to a substantial reduction of oesophageal cancer risk [68]. After ten or more years since stopping both habits the risk was only about one-tenth of that of current-smokers and drinkers (Fig. 21.2). Similar results were found also in a combined analysis of five case-control studies conducted in South America [65]. Bosetti and colleagues estimated the effect of smoking cessation on the cumulative incidence of OC in men using ORs from two Italian case-control studies and incidence data for Italian men [69]. They estimated that the cumulative risks of OC by 75 years of age were 1% for men who continued to smoke any type of tobacco, 0.5% and 0.4% for men who stopped smoking at around 50 and 30 years of age, and 0.2% among lifelong non-smokers. Thus, stopping smoking before age 50 years avoided about half the excess risk of OC [69].

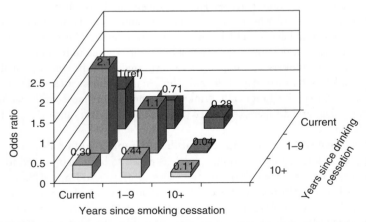

Figure 21.2 Odds ratios of cancer of the oesophagus for various combinations of times since cessation of alcohol and tobacco consumption.

Source: Data from Bosetti et al. 2000.

Anatomical subsite

A few studies consistently reported a higher smoking-associated risk in the middle third of the oesophagus [28, 32, 63, 70, 71]. This has been related to the more abundant blood supply in the middle third, as compared to the lower and upper third [71].

Attributable risks

The proportion of cases of OC attributable to smoking, and to the joint effect of alcohol and tobacco, varies widely between geographical areas. The attributable fraction depends not only on the relative risk but also on the frequency of the exposure in a population. Moreover, as shown above, the effect of smoking is magnified by alcohol (and possibly other risk factors). Thus, even the same amount of smoking may have a different impact in populations with different exposure to alcohol or other factors. In North and South America and Europe alcohol and tobacco explain the vast majority of cases, particularly in men, where the disease is more frequent than in women [15, 18, 22, 56, 72, 73]. Moreover, different smoking and alcohol consumptions have been shown to account for the differences in rates between sexes or urban and rural areas [15, 56].

In some areas of China and Central Asia where the higher incidence rates of the world are observed, and rates in women are comparable to those in men, these two factors appear to play only a limited role, and nutritional deficiencies or other yet not well-identified factors may play an important role [2]. The effect of tobacco, however, is not negligible in some areas of Asia and Africa. Tobacco accounted for between 20% and 50% of OC in various studies from China [28, 36, 74), 63% in Taiwan [34], 54% of cases in Bombay [75], 54% in men in Bulawayo, Zimbabwe [39], and – in combination with opium use – for 30% of cases in Golestan Province in northeastern Iran, one of the regions with the highest OC incidence in the world [37].

Adenocarcinoma of the oesophagus

Adenocarcinoma of the oesophagus is much less frequent worldwide than SCCO. There are thus fewer and smaller studies available. However, the recent increases in ACO incidence rates in several western countries have prompted investigations on its aetiology. This neoplasm resembles under many aspects to the adenocarcinoma of the gastric cardia, and cancers that occur at the oesophageal–gastric junction are difficult to attribute to one site or the other. Although several studies have considered adenocarcinomas of the oesophagus and gastric cardia together, there is evidence that these two cancers differ as concerns their geographic distribution and risk factors [76–78]. Thus, in this review we consider only studies showing separate results for ACO.

Most, if not all ACO arise in areas of Barrett's oesophagus (BO), a columnar-lined metaplasia of the specialized intestinal type of the distal oesophagus. The risk of developing ACO is increased 30–60 times in patients with BO as compared to the general population [79]. Gastro-oesophageal reflux disease, or reflux symptoms are a risk factor for BO and consequently for ACO [79, 80]. Besides studies comparing ACO patients with healthy controls, a few studies have also investigated the role of smoking in the progression from BO to ACO.

Table 21.2 presents the results of selected case-control studies of ACO according to tobacco consumption [21, 23, 24, 26, 28, 81–87]. Most studies have been conducted in North America and Europe, and only few data from other areas of the world are available. The largest case-control study, however, includes 367 ACO cases and has been conducted in Australia [23]. Smoking is quite consistently associated to the risk of ACO (Table 21.2), although the association appears weaker than for SCCO. Across studies with controls without documented BO, the OR of current-smokers ranges between 1.4 and 2.8 as compared to non-smokers, and that of former-smokers between 1.0 and 2.5. In most studies the risk increases with increasing dose and duration.

Table 21.2 Results from selected case-control studies on smoking and risk of adenocarcinoma of the oesophagus

Study (reference) and location	Type of controls #Cases:#controls	OR for current and former-smokers	Dose Cutpoints	Dose OR[a]	Duration Cutpoints	Duration OR[a]
North America						
Brown et al. 1994 [81] – 3 areas of the USA	Population 174 ACO[b,c] 750 Co[d] Men only	Current OR=1.7 (0.9–3.2)	<20[e]	1.1 (0.5–2.4)	<30 years	2.5 (1.3–4.7)
			20–39	2.4 (1.3–4.4)	30–39	2.5 (1.3–4.9)
			≥40	2.6 (1.3–5.0)	≥40	1.6 (0.8–3.2)
Gammon et al. 1997 [21] – 3 areas of USA	Population 293 ACO:695 Co	Current OR=2.2 (1.4–3.3) Former OR=2.0 (1.4–2.9)	<16[e]	1.5 (1.0–2.4)	<20 years	1.4 (0.9–2.2)
			16–20	2.2 (1.4–3.4)	20–31	1.7 (1.0–2.8)
			21–30	3.1 (1.9–5.1)	32–42	2.9 (1.8–4.4)
			>30	2.1 (1.3–3.3)	>42	2.4 (1.5–3.7)
Wu et al. 2001 [82] – Los Angeles county, USA	Population 222 ACO:1356 Co	Current OR=2.8 (1.8–4.3) Former OR=1.5 (1.0–2.2)	Former		≤ 20 years	1.4 (0.9–2.2)
			1–19[e]	1.2 (0.8–2.0)	21–40	2.1 (1.4–3.1)
			≥ 20	1.7 (1.1–2.5)	≥ 41	2.2 (1.3–3.5)
			Current			
			1–	1.6 (0.7–3.3)		
			20–39	2.9 (1.8–4.8)		
			≥ 40	4.5 (2.3–8.7)		
Australia						
Pandeya et al. 2008 [23] – mainland states of Australia	Population 367 ACO:1580 Co	Current OR=2.5 (1.1–2.0) Former OR=1.5(1.0–2.2)	<10[e]	0.9 (0.5–1.5)	≤15 years	1.3 (0.8–2.0)
			10–19	2.1 (1.4–3.1)	16–25	1.4 (0.9–2.2)
			20–25	1.7 (1.2–2.5)	26–35	1.7 (1.2–2.6)
			>25	1.9 (1.2–2.9)	>35	2.2 (1.5–3.3)

Europe

Study	Setting	Cases:Controls	Smoking status	OR	Cigarettes/day	OR	Duration	OR
Garidou et al. 1996 [83] – Athens, Greece.	Hospital	56 ACO: 200 Co			≤20 [e]	1.5 (0.7–3.1)		
					>20	2.7 (1.3–5.8)		
Cheng et al. 2000 [84] – 4 regions of the UK	Population	74 ACO: 74 Co Women only	Current	OR=1.4 (0.5–3.7)			≤ 37.7 years	0.2 (0.02–2.0)
			Former	OR=1.0 (0.5–1.9)			37.7–48.6	2.2 (0.4–12)
							≥ 48.6	3.0 (0.6–16)
Lagergren et al. 2000 [24] – Sweden	Population	189 ACO: 820 Co	Current	OR=1.6 (0.9–2.7)	1–9 [e]	2.3 (1.1–4.6)	1–20 years	2.3 (1.1–4.6)
			Former	OR=1.9 (1.2–2.9)	10–19	2.9 (1.5–5.8)	21–35	2.9 (1.5–5.8)
					>19	8.8 (4.9–16)	>35	8.8 (4.9–16)
Hashibe et al. 2007 [26] – Romania, Russia Czech Republic, and Poland	Hospital	35 ACO:, 1114 Co	Current	OR=2.4 (0.9–7.4)	<10 [e]	1.9 (0.5–8.3)	<10 years	no cases
			Former	OR=2.5 (1.2–2.9)	10–19	2.0 (0.7–6.4)	10–19	2.1 (0.5–9.4)
					20–29	3.2 (1.0–10.2)	20–29	2.6 (0.6–10.6)
					≥30	3.0 (0.7–12.9)	30–39	3.7 (1.2–22.3)
							40–49	2.9 (0.8–10.4)
							>50	0.8 (0.09–7.7)

Asia

Study	Setting	Cases:Controls	Smoking status	OR	Cigarettes/day	OR	Duration	OR
Gao et al. 1994 [28] – Shanghai, China	Population	55 ACO:1552 Co	Current	OR=2.1	1–9 [e]	2.0	0.5–19yrs	1.8
			Former	OR=1.8	10–19	1.1	20–29	1.0
					20–29	2.0	30–39	2.0
					≥30	3.5	≥40	2.0

Studies in patients with Barrett's oesophagus (BE)

Study	Cases:Controls	Cigarettes/day	OR
Levi et al. 1990 [85] – Lausanne, Switzerland	30 ACO in BE: 140 Co with BE	<15 [f]	1.0 (0.3–41)
		15–24	0.6 (0.2–1.9)
		>25	0.9 (0.3–2.9)

(Continued)

Table 21.2 (continued) Results from selected case-control studies on smoking and risk of adenocarcinoma of the oesophagus

Study (reference) and location	Type of controls #Cases:#controls	OR for current and former-smokers	Dose		Duration	
			Cutpoints	OR[a]	Cutpoints	OR[a]
Menke-Pluymers et al. 1993 [86] – Rotterdam, The Netherlands	62 ACO in BE: 96 Co with BE	Current OR=2.3[g] (p<0.05)				
De Jonge et al. 2006 [87] – SW of The Netherlands	91 ACO 244 BE	Current OR=3.7 (1.4–9.9) Former OR=2.6 (1.1–6.4)			≤ 20 years 21–40 ≥ 41	2.2 (0.9–5.5) 1.9 (0.8–4.8) 4.7 (1.7–13)

Note

[a] All odds ratios presented were adjusted for age and sex (when required), plus a variable number of other potential confounders), if not otherwise specified. The reference category is set to never-smokers, if not otherwise specified.

[b] ACO=adenocarcinoma of the oesophagus.

[c] Includes oesophagogastric junction.

[d] Co=controls.

[e] Cigarettes per day.

[f] Grams of tobacco per day.

[g] Former-smokers and smokers of less than 5 cigarettes/day included in the reference category.

Table 21.3 Results from selected cohort studies on smoking and risk of adenocarcinoma of the oesophagus

Study (reference) and location	Subjects # of cases	ORᵃ for current and former-smokers	Dose		Duration	
			Cutpoints	ORᵃ	Cutpoints	ORᵃ
Lindblad et al. 2005 [88] – UK	General Practitioners Research Database, UK (1994–2001) 4,340,000 person-years Nested case-control study on 287 ACO and 10,000 controls	Current OR=1.5 (1.1–2.0) Former OR=1.1 (0.7–1.6)				
Freedman et al. 2007 [67] – 8 States, USA	NIH-AARP Diet and Health Study. 474,4006 respondents from the American Association of Retired Persons. (1995–2000). 2,121,800 person-years; 205 ACO	Current OR=3.7 (2.2–2.0) Former OR=1.1 (0.7–1.6)	≤20ᵇ 21–40 >40	2.6 (1.6–4.0) 3.7 (2.3–5.8) 2.6 (1.5–4.8)		

Note

ᵃ All odds ratios presented were adjusted for age and sex (when required), plus a variable number of other potential confounders), if not otherwise specified. The reference category is set to never-smokers, if not otherwise specified.

ᵇ Cigarettes per day.

Only three small studies compared subjects with BO that progressed to ACO with those who did not, yielding contrasting results. The largest one included 91 ACO cases and 244 BO [87], and found an OR of 3.7 (95% CI 1.4–9.9) for current-smokers, 2.6 (95% CI 1.1–6.4) for former-smokers, and of 4.7 (95% CI 1.7–13) for smokers for over 40 years.

Two cohort studies from the United Kingdom [88] and the United States [67] reported significant ORs of 1.5 and 3.7 for current-smokers, respectively.

The IARC evaluation of tobacco in 2004 concluded that 'tobacco smoking is causally associated with adenocarcinoma of the oesophagus' [17], and studies published thereafter, including two cohort studies, have strengthened this conclusion. In contrast with SCCO, alcohol consumption does not appear to increase the risk of ACO [79, 80], and thus interaction between alcohol and tobacco is not an important issue for this histologic type. While the risk of SCCO decreases steadily after stopping smoking, no clear reduction in ACO risk was observed after cessation of smoking, at least for 20–30 years [23, 26, 66, 67]. This could also partly explain the diverging trends observed for the two histologic types of oesophageal cancer in the United States and some European countries.

In the NIH-AARP Diet and health Study cohort [67], smoking accounted for approximately 58% of ACO (95% CI 38–72%), and in a multi-centre case-control study also from the United States [21, 72] the estimated population attributable risk was 40% (95% CI 26–56%). Thus, though less strongly associated than with SCCO, smoking is an important aetiologic determinant of ACO, too.

References

1. Ferlay, J., Bray, F., Pisani, P., and Parkin, D.M. (2004). *GLOBOCAN 2002: Cancer Incidence, Mortality and Prevalence Worldwide*. IARC CancerBase No. 5. version 2.0, IARC Press, Lyon, France.

2. Munoz, N. and Day, N.E. (1996). Esophageal cancer. In: D. Schottenfeld, J.F. Fraumeni Jr, (eds) *Cancer Epidemiology and Prevention*, second edition, pp 681–706. New York: Oxford University Press.

3. Kmet, J.and Mahboudi, E. (1972). Esophageal cancer in the Caspian littoral of Iran: initial studies. *Science*, **175**: 846–53.

4. Blot WJ (1994). Esophageal cancer trends and risk factors. 46: *Semin Oncol*, **21**: 403–10.

5. Negri, E., La Vecchia, C., Levi, F., Franceschi, S., Serra-Majem, L., and Boyle, P. (1996). Comparative descriptive epidemiology of oral and oesophageal cancers in Europe. *Eur J Cancer Prev*, **5**: 267–79.

6. Curado, M.P., Edwards, B., Shin, H.R., Storm, H., Ferlay, J., Heanue, M. *et al.* (eds) (2007). *Cancer Incidence in Five Continents, Vol. IX*. IARC Scientific Publications No. 160, Lyon, IARC.

7. Blot, W.J. and McLaughlin, J.K. (1999). The changing epidemiology of esophageal cancer. *Semin Oncol*, **26**(Suppl 15): 2–8.

8. Powell, J., McConkey, C.C., Gillison, E.W., and Spychal, R.T. (2002). Continuing rising trend in oesophageal adenocarcinoma. *Int J Cancer*, **102**: 422–7.

9. Fernandes, M.L., Seow, A., Chan, Y.H., and Ho, K.Y. (2006). Opposing trends in incidence of esophageal squamous cell carcinoma and adenocarcinoma in a multi-ethnic Asian country. *Am J Gastroenterol*, **101**: 1430–6.

10. Bosetti, C., Levi, F., Ferlay, J., *et al.* (2008). Trends in osesophageal cancer incidence and mortality in Europe. *Int J Cancer*, **122**: 1118–29.

11. Trivers, K.F., Sabatino, S.A., and Stewart, S.L. (2008). Trends in esophageal cancer incidence by histology, United States, 1998–2003. *Int J Cancer*, **123**: 1422–8.

12. Holmes, R.S. and Vaughan, T.L. (2006). Epidemiology and pathogenesis of esophageal cancer. *Semin Radiat Oncol*, **17**: 2–9.

13. Hammond, E.C. and Horn, D. (1958). Smoking and death rates. Report on 44 months of follow-up of 187 783 men. *J Am Med Ass*, **116**: 1159–72 and 1294–308.

14. Dorn, H.F. (1959). Tobacco consumption and mortality from cancer and other diseases. *Publ Health Rep*, **74**: 581–93.

15. Tuyns, A.J., Pequignot, G., and Jensen, O.M. (1977). Le cancer de l'oesophage en Ille-et-Vilaine en fonction des niveaux de consommation d'alcool et de tabac. Des risques qui se multiplient. *Bull Cancer*, **64**: 45–60.

16. International Agency for Research on Cancer (1986). Tobacco smoking. In *IARC Monographs on the Evaluation of the Carcinogenic Risk of Chemicals to Humans, Vol 38.* Lyon: WHO, IARC.

17. International Agency for Research on Cancer (2004). Tobacco smoking and tobacco smoke. In *IARC Monographs on the Evaluation of the Carcinogenic Risks to Humans, Vol 83.* Lyon: WHO, IARC.

18. Wynder, E.L. and Bross, I.J. (1961). A study of etiological factors in cancer of the esophagus. *Cancer*, **14**: 389–413.

19. Brown, L.M., Blot, W.J., Schuman, S.H., Smith, V.M., Ershow, A.G., Marks, R.D. *et al.* (1988). Environmental factors and high risk of esophageal cancer among men in coastal South Carolina. *J Natl Cancer Inst*, **80**: 1620–5.

20. Kabat, G.C., Ng, S.K., and Wynder, E.L. (1993). Tobacco, alcohol intake, and diet in relation to adenocarcinoma of the esophagus and gastric cardia. *Cancer Causes Control*, **218**: 123–32.

21. Gammon, M.D., Schoenberg, J.B., Ahsan, H., Risch, H.A., Vaughan, T.L., Chow, W.H. *et al.* (1997). Tobacco, alcohol, and socioeconomic status and adenocarcinomas of the esophagus and gastric cardia. *J Natl Cancer Inst*, **89**: 1277–84.

22. Castellsagué, X., Munoz, N., De Stefani, E., Victora, C.G., Castelletto, R., Rolon, P.A., *et al.* (1999). Independent and joint effects of tobacco smoking and alcohol drinking on the risk of esophageal cancer in men and women. *Int J Cancer*, **82**: 657–64.

23. Pandeya, N., Williams, G.M., Sadhegi, S., Green, A.C., Webb, P.M., and Whiteman, D.C. (2008). Associations of duration, intensity, and quantity of smoking with adenocarcinoma and squamous cell carcinoma oft he esophagus. *Am J Epidemiol*, **168**: 105–14.

24. Lagergren, J., Bergstrom, R., Lindgren, A., and Nyren, O. (2000). The role of tobacco, snuff and alcohol use in the aetiology of cancer of the oesophagus and gastric cardia. *Int J Cancer*, **85**: 340–6.

25. Zambon, P., Talamini, R., La Vecchia, C., Dal Maso, L., Negri, E., Tognazzo, S. *et al.* (2000). Smoking, type of alcoholic beverage and squamous-cell oesophageal cancer in northern Italy. *Int J Cancer*, **86**: 144–9.

26. Hashibe, M., Boffetta, P., Janout, V. *et al.* (2007). Esophageal cancer in Central and Eastern Europe: tobacco and alcohol. *Int J Cancer*, **120**: 1518–22.

27. Vioque, J., Barber, X., and Bolumar, F. (2008). Esophageal cancer risk by type of alcohol drinking and smoking: a case-control study in Spain. *BMC Cancer*, **8**: 221.

28. Gao, Y.T., McLaughlin, J.K., Blot, W.J., Ji, B.T., Benichou, J., Dai, Q., *et al.* (1994). Risk factors for esophageal cancer in Shanghai, China. I. Role of cigarette smoking and alcohol drinking. *Int J Cancer*, **58**: 192–6.

29. Guo, W., Blot, W.J., Li, J.Y., Taylor, P.R., Liu, B.Q., Wang, W., *et al.* (1994). A nested case-control study of oesophageal and stomach cancers in the Linxian nutrition intervention trial. *Int J Epidemiol*, **23**: 444–50.

30. Hu, J., Nyren, O., Wolk, A., Bergstrom, R., Yuen, J., Adami, H.O., *et al.* (1994). Risk factors for oesophageal cancer in northeast China. *Int J Cancer*, **57**: 38–46.

31. Sankaranarayanan, R., Duffy, S.W., Padmakumary, G., Nair, S.M., Day, N.E., and Padmanabhan, T.K. (1991). Risk factors for cancer of the oesophagus in Kerala, India. *Int J Cancer*, **49**: 485–9.

32. Takezaki, T., Shinoda, M., Hatooka, S., Hasegawa, Y., Nakamura, S., Hirose, K. *et al.* (2000). Subsite-specific risk factors for hypopharyngeal and esophageal cancer (Japan). *Cancer Causes Control*, **11**: 597–608.

33. Znaor, A., Brennan, P., Gajalakshmi, V. *et al.* (2003). Independent and combined effects of tobacco smoking, chewing and alcohol drinking on the risk of oral, pharyngeal and esophageal cancers in Indian men. *Int J Cancer*, **105**: 681–6.

34. Lee, C.H., Lee, J.M., Wu, D.C. *et al.* (2005). Independent and combined effects of alcohol intake, tobacco smoking and betel quid chewing on the risk of esophageal cancer in Taiwan. *Int J Cancer*, **113**: 475–82.

35. Wu, I.C., Lu, C.J., Kuo, F.C. *et al.* (2006). Interaction between cigarette, alcohol and betel nut use on esophageal cancer risk in Taiwan. *EUR J Clin Invest*, **36**(4): 236–41.

36. Jiang, J.M., Zeng, X.J., Chen, J.S. *et al.* (2006). Smoking and mortality from esophageal cancer in China: a large case-control study of 19 734 male esophageal cancer deaths and 104 846 living spouse controls. *Int J Cancer*, **119**: 1427–32.

37. Nasrollahzadeh, D., Karmangar, F., Aghcheli, K. *et al.* (2008). Opium, tobacco, and alcohol use in relation to oesophageal squamous cell carcinoma in a high-risk area of Iran. *Br J Cancer*, **98**: 1857–63.

38. Segal, I., Reinach, S.G., de Beer, M. (1988). Factors associated with oesophageal cancer in Soweto, South Africa. *Br J Cancer*, **58**: 681–6.

39. Vizcaino, A.P., Parkin, D.M., and Skinner, M.E. (1995). Risk factors associated with oesophageal cancer in Bulawayo, Zimbabwe. *Br J Cancer*, **72**: 769–73.

40. Pacella-Norman, R., Urban, M.I., Sitas, F., Carrara, H., Sur, R., Hale, M. *et al.* (2002). Risk factors for oesophageal, lung, oral and laryngeal cancers in black South Africans. *Br J Cancer*, **86**: 1751–6.

41. Polesel, J., Talamini, R., La Vecchia, C. *et al.* (2008). Tobacco smoking and the risk of upper aero-digestive tract cancers: a reanalysis of case-control studies using spline models. *Int J Cancer*, **122**: 2398–402.

42. Tran, G.D., Sun, X.D., Abnet, C.C. *et al.* (2005). Prospective study of risk factors for esophageal and gastric cancers in the Linxian general Population Trial cohort in China. *Int J Cancer*, **113**: 456–63.

43. De Stefani, E., Barrios, E., and Fierro, L. (1993). Black (air-cured) and blond (flue-cured) tobacco and cancer risk. III: Oesophageal cancer. *Eur J Cancer*, **29A**: 763–6.

44. Tuyns, A.J. and Esteve, J. (1983). Pipe, commercial and hand-rolled cigarette smoking in oesophageal cancer. *Int J Epidemiol*, **12**: 110–3.

45. Launoy, G., Milan, C., Faivre, J., Pienkowski, P., and Gignoux, M. (2000). Tobacco type and risk of squamous cell cancer of the oesophagus in males: a French multicentre case-control study. *Int J Epidemiol*, **29**: 36–42.

46. La Vecchia, C., Liati, P., Decarli, A., Negrello, I., and Franceschi, S. (1986). Tar yields of cigarettes and the risk of oesophageal cancer. *Int J Cancer*, **38**: 381–5.

47. Gallus, S., Altieri, A., Bosetti, C. *et al.* (2003). Cigarette tar yield and risk of upper digestive tract cancers: case-control studies from Italy and Switzerland. *Ann Oncol*, **14**: 209–13.

48. Shanks, T.G. and Burns, D.M. (1998). *Disease consequences of cigar smoking. Smoking and tobacco control monograph 9. Cigars, health effects and trends.* Bethesda (MD): National Institutes of Health; DHHS Publ No 98-4302. pp 105–58.

49. La Vecchia, C., Bosetti, C., Negri, E., Levi, F., and Franceschi, S. (1998). Cigar smoking and cancers of the upper digestive tract. *J Natl Cancer Inst*, **90**: 1670.

50. International Agency for Research on Cancer (2007). Smokeless tobacco. In *IARC Monographs on the Evaluation of the Carcinogenic Risk of Chemicals to Humans, Vol 89.* Lyon: WHO, IARC.

51. Phukan, R.K., Ali, M.S., Chetia, C.K., and Mahanta, J. (2001). Betel nut and tobacco chewing; potential risk factors of cancer of oesophagus in Assam, India. *Br J Cancer*, **85**: 661–7.

52. Boffetta, P., Aagnes, B., Weiderpass, E., and Andersen, A. (2005). Smokeless tobacco use and risk of cancer of the pancreas and other organs. *Int J Cancer*, **114**: 992–5.

53. Lewin, F., Norell, S.F., Johansson, H. *et al.* (1998). Smoking tobacco, oral snuff, and alcohol in the etiology of squamous cell carcinoma of the head and neck: A population-based case-referent study in Sweden. *Cancer*, **82**: 1367–75.

54. Breslow, N.E. and Day, N.E. (1980). *Statistical methods in cancer research, Vol 1: the analysis of case-control studies.* Lyon, International Agency for Research on Cancer, Sci Publ 32.

55. Doll, R.and Peto, R. (1981). Tha causes of cancer. *J Natl Cancer Inst*, **66**: 1191–308.

56. Negri, E., La Vecchia, C., Franceschi, S., Decarli, A., and Bruzzi, P. (1992). Attributable risks for oesophageal cancer in northern Italy. *Eur J Cancer*, **28A**: 1167–71.

57. Garavello, W., Negri, E., Talamini, R. *et al.* (2005). Family history of cancer, its combination with smoking and drinking, and risk of squamous cell carcinoma of the esophagus. *Cancer Epidemiol Biomarkers Prev*, **14**(6): 1390–3.

58. Gallus, S., Bosetti, C., Franceschi, S., Levi, F., Simonato, L., Negri, E. *et al.* (2001). Oesophageal cancer in women: tobacco, alcohol, nutritional and hormonal factors. *Br J Cancer*, **85**: 341–5.

59. Tuyns, A.J. (1983). Oesophageal cancer in non-smoking drinkers and in non-drinking smokers. *Int J Cancer*, **32**: 443–4.

60. La Vecchia, C. and Negri, E. (1989). The role of alcohol in oesophageal cancer in non-smokers, and of tobacco in non-drinkers. *Int J Cancer*, **43**: 784–5.

61. Tavani, A., Negri, E., Franceschi, S., and La Vecchia, C. (1996). Tobacco and other risk factors for oesophageal cancer in alcohol non-drinkers. *Eur J Cancer Prev*, **5**: 313–8.

62. Cheng, K.K., Duffy, S.W., Day, N.E., and Lam, T.H. (1995). Oesophageal cancer in never-smokers and never-drinkers. *Int J Cancer*, **60**: 820–2.

63. Yu, M.C., Garabrant, D.H., Peters, J.M., and Mack, T.M. (1988). Tobacco, alcohol, diet, occupation, and carcinoma of the esophagus. *Cancer Res*, **48**: 3843–8.

64. La Vecchia, C., Bidoli, E., Barra, S. *et al.* (1990). Type of cigarettes and cancers of the upper digestive and respiratory tract. *Cancer Causes Control*, **1**: 69–74.

65. Castellsagué, X., Munoz, N., De Stefani, E., Victora, C.G., Quintana, M.J., Castelletto, R. *et al.* (2000). Smoking and drinking cessation and risk of esophageal cancer (Spain). *Cancer Causes Control*, **11**: 813–8.

66. Bosetti, C., Gallus, S., Garavello, W., and La Vecchia, C. (2006). Smoking cessation and the risk of osesophageal cancer: an overview of published studies. *Oral Oncol*, **42**: 957–64.

67. Freedman, N.D., Abnet, C.C., Leitzmann, M.F. *et al.* (2007). A prospective study of tobacco, alcohol, and the risk of esophageal and gastric cancer subtypes. *Am J Epidemiol*, **162**(12): 1424–33.

68. Bosetti, C., Franceschi, S., Levi, F., Negri, E., Talamini, R., and La Vecchia, C. (2000). Smoking and drinking cessation and the risk of oesophageal cancer. *Br J Cancer*, **83**: 689–91.

69. Bosetti, C., Gallus, S., Peto, R. *et al.* (2007). Tobacco smoking, smoking cessation, and cumulative risk of upper aerodigestive tract cancers. *Am J Epidemiol*, **167**(4): 468–73.

70. Wu, M.T., Wu, D.C., Hsu, H.K., Kao, E.L., and Lee, J.M. (2003). Relationship between site of oesophageal cancer and areca chewing and smoking in Taiwan. *Br J Cancer*, **89**: 1202–4.

71. Lee, C.H., Wu, D.C., Lee, J.M. *et al.* (2007). Anatomical subsite discrepancy in relation to the impact of the consumption of alcohol, tobacco and betel quid on esophageal cancer. *Int J Cancer*, **120**: 1755–62.

72. Engel, L.S., Chow, W.H., Vaughan, T.L. *et al.* (2003). Population attributable risks of esophageal and gastric cancers. *J Natl Cancer Inst*, **95**(18): 1404–13.

73. Anonymous (2005). Annual cancer deaths attributable to smoking in males, 1995–1999. *J Natl Cancer Inst*, **97**(15): 1111.

74. Gu, D., Kelly, T.N., Wu, X. *et al.* (2009). Mortality attributable to smoking in China. *New Engl J Med*, **360**: 150–9.

75. Jayant, K., Balakrishnan, V., Sanghvi, L.D. and Jussawalla, D.J. (1977). Quantification of the role of smoking and chewing tobacco in oral, pharyngeal, and oesophageal cancers. *Br J Cancer*, **35**: 232–5.

76. Lagergren, J., Bergstrom, R., Lindgren, A., and Nyren, O. (1999). Symptomatic gastroesophageal reflux as a risk factor for esophageal adenocarcinoma. *New Engl J Med*, **340**: 825–31.

77. Corley, D.A. and Buffler, P.A. (2001). Oesophageal and gastric cardia adenocarcinomas: analysis of regional variation using the Cancer Incidence in Five Continents datbase. *Int J Epidemiol*, **30**: 1415–25.

78. Eksteen, J.A., Latchford, A., Thomas, S.J., and Jankowski, J.A. (2001). Commentary: regional variations in oesophageal and gastric cardiacancers – implications and practice. *Int J Epidemiol*, **30**: 1425–7.

79. Lagergren, J. (2005). Adenocarcinoma of oesophagus: what exactly is the size of the problem and who is at risk. *Gut*, **54**: i1–i5.

80. Pera, M., Manterola, C., Vidal, O., and Grande, L. (2005). Epidemiology of esophageal adenocarcinoma. *J Surg Oncol*, **92**: 151–9.

81. Brown, L.M., Silverman, D.T., Pottern, L.M., Schoenberg, J.B., Greenberg, R.S., Swanson, G.M. *et al.* (1994). Adenocarcinoma of the esophagus and esophagogastric junction in white men in the United States: alcohol, tobacco, and socioeconomic factors. *Cancer Causes Control*, **5**: 333–40.

82. Wu, A.H., Wan, P., and Bernstein, L. (2001). A multiethnic population-based study of smoking, alcohol and body size and risk of adenocarcinomas of the stomach and esophagus (United States). *Cancer Causes Control*, **12**: 721–32.

83. Garidou, A., Tzonou, A., Lipworth, L., Signorello, L.B., Kalapothaki, V., and Trichopoulos, D. (1996). Life-style factors and medical conditions in relation to esophageal cancer byhistologic type in a low-risk population. *Int J Cancer*, **68**: 295–9.

84. Cheng, K.K., Sharp, L., McKinney, P.A., Logan, R.F., Chilvers, C.E., Cook-Mozaffari, P. *et al.* (2000). A case-control study of oesophageal adenocarcinoma in women: a preventable disease. *Br J Cancer*, **83**: 127–32.

85. Levi, F., Ollyo, J.B., La Vecchia, C., Boyle, P., Monnier. P., and Savary, M. (1990). The consumption of tobacco, alcohol and the risk of adenocarcinoma in Barrett's oesophagus. *Int J Cancer*, **45**: 852–4.

86. Menke-Pluymers, M.B., Hop, W.C., Dees. J., van Blankenstein, M., and Tilanus, H.W. (1993). Risk factors for the development of an adenocarcinoma in columnar-lined (Barrett) esophagus. The Rotterdam Esophageal Tumor Study Group. *Cancer*, **72**: 1155–8.

87. De Jonge, P.J.F., Steyerberg, E.W., Kuipers, E.J. *et al.* (2006). Risk factors for the development of esophageal adenocarcinoma in Barrett's esophagus. *Am J Gastroenerol*, **101**: 1421–9.

88. Lindblad, M., Garcia Rodriguez, L.A., and Lagergren, J. (2005). Body mass, tobacco and alcohol and risk of esophageal, gastric cardia, and gastric non-cardia adenocarcinoma among men and women in a nested case-control study. *Cancer Causes Control*, **16**: 285–94.

Chapter 22

Tobacco use and risk of oral cancer

Tongzhang Zheng, Peter Boyle, Bing Zhang,
Yawei Zhang, Patricia H. Owens, Qing Lan, and
John Wise

Introduction

Epidemiological studies from various populations have consistently shown that tobacco smoking (including filter- and non-filter cigarettes, cigars, and pipe tobacco) increases oral cancer risk. In sum, these results indicate that: ever-smokers experience an increased risk; current smokers have a higher risk than ex-smokers; those who started smoking at younger ages have a higher risk than those that started at later ages; risk increases with amount of cigarettes smoked per day, duration of smoking, and lifetime pack-years of smoking; smokers of filter cigarettes have lower risk than smokers of unfiltered cigarettes. Epidemiological studies have also shown that other factors may also contribute to the effect of smoking on oral cancer risk. For example, alcohol consumption dramatically increases the effect of tobacco smoking on the risk of oral cancer. Similarly, xenobiotic metabolizing enzymes, involved in the metabolism of tobacco carcinogens, have a significant impact on the relationship between tobacco smoking and oral cancer risk. Overall, based on very conservative estimates, about 46% of the cancers of the oral cavity and pharynx in men and 11% in women are attributable to smoking worldwide, with considerable variation by location (Parkin *et al.* 2000).

In this review, we will summarize the results from major epidemiological studies investigating the association between oral cancer and tobacco product use, including cigarette smoking, pipe tobacco and cigar smoking, and smokeless tobacco use (snuff dipping and chewing tobacco). In most of the epidemiological studies, 'oral cancer' includes cancer of the tongue (CD9 141), mouth (ICD9 143–145), and pharynx (ICD146, 148, 149), with a few including larynx (ICD9 161). Cancer of the lip (ICD9 140), salivary glands (ICD9 142), and nasopharynx (ICD9 147) were not included in most of the epidemiological studies of oral cancer, and therefore, cancers of these sites will not be discussed in this review. These cancer sites also appear to have quite different etiological profiles and very distinct natural histories as reviewed by Boyle *et al.* (1995).

Descriptive epidemiology

Cancers of the oral cavity and pharynx combined is the sixth most common cancer site for both sexes (reviewed in Boyle *et al.* 1990a, 1995; La Vecchia *et al.* 1997; Franceschi *et al.* 2000). Combined these cancers account for approximately 220 000 new cases per year in men and 90 000 in women worldwide. Their incidence rates vary approximately 20-fold in both sexes across the world. At present, high incidence rates are found in southern India, Pakistan, northern France, and a few areas of central and eastern Europe, with the highest rate recorded in Bas Rhin, France (49.4/100 000 men) (Franceschi *et al.* 2000).

Men are more likely to be diagnosed with oral cancer than women. Male-to-female ratios for oral and pharyngeal cancers ranged between 4 and 20 in southern, central, and eastern Europe (Franceschi *et al.* 2000). In the United States, the rates for men are 2.5–4 times higher than those for women (Weller *et al.* 1993). Based on the SEER programme, in the US, African-Americans have an overall incidence of oral cancer 13.2/100 000, 65% higher than whites of 8.0/100 000 (Weller *et al.* 1993). The majority of these racial and gender differences in the US is attributable to the effects of tobacco and alcohol (Day 1993).

In many parts of the world (such as India, Puerto Rico, and Colombia), a steady decline in oral cancer incidence in both sexes has been observed while a stable incidence rate was observed in the USA (Franceschi *et al.* 2000). There are, however, reports that oral cancer is increasing, particularly amongst younger persons in the Nordic countries and Europe with the reasons unknown (Boyle *et al.* 1990*b*; Macfarlane *et al.* 1994).

Tobacco use and risk of oral cancer

Cigarette smoking

Oral cancer and smoking has been investigated for many years. The early studies were restricted by the methodologies of their time and have been the subject of numerous other reviews (Boyle *et al.* 1995). Accordingly, this review will focus on more recent studies using newer epidemiological methods. In fact, a large number of studies have explored the relationship of cigarette smoking and oral cancer risk over the past two decades. The methods have varied but largely consist of hospital-based case–control studies, population-based case–control studies, and prospective follow-up studies. The major findings using each method are discussed next (also see Table 22.1) with a brief presentation of the strengths and limitations of each method.

Hospital-based case–control studies

A number of hospital-based case–control studies have been conducted and have clearly shown a strong relationship between oral cancer and cigarette smoking. In interpreting the results from these hospital-based case–control studies, a major concern is whether the control group selected represents the population that produced the cases. Indeed, in some of the hospital-based case–control studies, the control group considered included cancers thought to be unrelated to smoking and drinking, and some with benign neoplastic or non-neoplastic lesions, which may be smoking related. If it turns out that these diseases were actually associated with tobacco smoking, then, the true relationship between tobacco smoking and oral cancer risk would be underestimated. Since most of these studies showed a strong association between cigarette smoking and oral cancer risk, underestimation is less of a concern. But the variation of disease in controls in different studies is still important to note as when considered together with the relatively small sample size in some of the studies, it may explain in large part, the significant variation in the magnitude of the reported association between tobacco smoking and oral cancer risk.

In 1984, Elwood *et al.* reported an alcohol-adjusted OR of 2.8 (95% CI 1.3–6.0) for smoking 50 or more cigarettes per day when compared to never smokers. Additional adjustment for 4 other factors reduced the OR to 2.1 (95% CI 0.9–4.8). A weak association observed in this study could be due to the fact that controls were composed of various cancer patients (including cancer of the prostate, colo-rectum, skin, breast, etc.).

In a case–control study of oral cancer in Brazil, Franco *et al.* (1989) reported that tobacco smoking was, by any measure, the strongest risk factor for oral cancer in this population. The adjusted ORs for ever vs. never smokers were 6.3 (95% CI 2.4–16.3), 5.5 (95% CI 1.2–24.8), 13.9 (95% CI 4.4–44.2), and 7.0 (95% CI 2.7–18.7) for industrial brand cigarettes, cigars, pipe, and

Table 22.1 Tobacco use and risk of oral cancer

Author (year) country (Cases/controls)	Cancer site	Major results			Comments
		Cigarettes	Cigar/pipe	Smokeless	
Hospital-based case-control studies					
Winn DM et al. (1981) Southern United States, US (255/502)	Oral cavity, pharynx	RR = 4.6 (95% CI 1.6–13.4) for oral cavity; RR = 9.6 (95% CI 2.5–37.0) for pharynx among non-users of snuff		RR = 47.5 (95% CI 9.1–249.5) for cancer of the gum and buccal mucosa among snuff use of 50 or more years	The study subjects were women residing in 67 countries in central North Carolina
Elwood et al. (1984), Vancouver, Canada (374/374)	Oral cavity, pharynx, larynx	OR = 2.1 (95% CI 0.9–4.8) for smoking more than 50 cigarettes per day			Controls were cancer patients with tumour sites which were considered to be no strong evidence of association with smoking
Spitz et al. (1988) Houston, US (185/185)	Oral cavity, pharynx, larynx	OR = 7.5 (P_{trend}<0.01) for men OR = 12.0 (P_{trend}<0.01) for women for smoking 50+ pack-years	Men: Cigar: OR = 2.8 (95% CI 1.5–5.5) Pipe: OR = 1.8 (95% CI 1.0–3.4)	Snuff dipping: OR = 3.4 (95% CI 1.0–10.9)	Combined effects of alcohol and tobacco were more than additive, but less than multiplicative
Franco et al. (1989), Brazil (232/464)	Oral cavity	RR = 6.3 for ever vs. never smokers	RR = 13.9 for pipe RR = 5.5 for cigar for ever vs. never smokers	Snuff dipping or tobacco chewing was not associated with oral cancer risk	The RR was 142 for those with >100 pack-years of smoking and >1000 kg of alcohol drinking. Only 9 cases and 13 controls used smokeless tobacco
Kabat et al. (1989), US (125/107)	Oral cavity	OR = 2.0 (95% CI 1.0–4.0) for current vs. never			Women only and the numbers of cases and controls were small
Zheng et al. (1990), Beijing, China (404/404)	Tongue and oral cavity	OR = 1.6 for ever vs. never smokers	Pipe: OR = 5.7 for ever vs. never in men		The combined effects of tobacco and alcohol were approximately multiplicative. Tobacco smoking accounts for about 34% of all cases of oral cancer in this population

(Continued)

Table 22.1 (continued) Tobacco use and risk of oral cancer

Author (year) country (Cases/controls)	Cancer site	Major results			Comments
		Cigarettes	**Cigar/pipe**	**Smokeless**	
Talamini et al. (1990), Northern Italy (336/1652)	Oral cavity, pharynx	OR = 3.8 (95% CI 0.2–58.2) for smokers of <15 cigarettes per day: OR = 12.9 (95% CI 2.3–106.3) for smokers of >15 cigarettes per day			The results are for non-drinkers
La Vecchia et al. (1990), Northern Italy (741/1272)	Oral cavity, pharynx, larynx	Oral cavity/pharynx: RR = 2.3 (95% CI 1.6–3.2) Larynx: RR = 1.8 (95% CI 1.2–2.8)			Reference category is smokers of cigarette brands with less than 22 mg tar yield per cigarette
Franceschi et al. (1990), Northern Italy (741/1272)	Oral cavity, pharynx, larynx	Oral cavity: OR = 11.1 (95% CI 3.4–34.8) for ever vs. never Pharynx: OR = 12.9 (95% CI 3.1–52.9) for ever vs. never Larynx: OR = 4.6 (95% CI 2.2–9.6) for ever vs. never	Oral cavity: OR = 20.7 (95% CI 5.6–76.3) for ever vs. never		The risk of oral cavity and pharyngeal cancer for the highest levels of alcohol and smoking was increased 80-fold relative to the lowest levels of both factors
Nandakumar et al. (1990), Bangalore, India (348/348)	Oral cavity	OR = 2.1 (95% CI 1.1–4.2) for cigarette smoking		OR = 17.7 (95% CI 8.7–36.1) for chewing during sleep	OR = 242.6 (95% CI 52.6–1119.0) for tobacco chewing and ragi consumption
Franceschi et al. (1992), Northern Italy (206/726)	Tongue and mouth	Tongue: OR = 10.5 (95% CI 3.2–34.1) for current vs. never Mouth: OR = 11.8 (95% CI 3.6–38.4) for current vs. never	Mouth: OR = 21.9 (95% CI 3.8–125.6)		Smokers of high tar cigarettes had a 10-fold increased risk of cancer of the tongue and 14-fold increased risk of cancer of mouth compared with non-smokers. Results are for male only.

Study	Site	Risk estimate	Comments
Boffetta et al. (1992), US (359/2280)	Mouth	Floor of the mouth: OR = 4.0 (95% CI 1.5–10.3) for smoking of >35 cigarettes per day Soft palate complex: OR = 4.9 (95% CI 1.1–21.5) for smoking of >35 cigarette per day	Non-significantly increased risk was observed for floor of mouth (OR = 1.8), soft palate (OR = 2.3), buccal mucosa (OR = 1.9)	This study supports the hypothesis of the carcinogenic effect of tobacco smoke on the oral mucosa through direct contact
Negri et al. (1993), Northern Italy (439/2106)	Oral cavity and pharynx	RR = 3.6 for moderate smokers vs. never smokers; RR = 9.4 for heavy smoker vs. never smokers		The single factor with the highest attributable risk was smoking, which account for 81–87% of oral cancers in males and for 42–47% in females
Mashberg et al. (1993), New Jersey, US (359/2280)	Oral cavity and pharynx	OR = 4.0 (95% CI 1.9–8.2) for smoking of >36 cigarettes per day	No increased risk was found for use of snuff (OR = 0.8) or chewing tobacco (OR = 1.0)	The number of subjects using snuff and chewing tobacco was small
Rao et al. (1994) India (713/635)	Lip, oral cavity (excluding base of the tongue and soft palate)	No significantly increased risk for smoking cigarettes	RR = 2.8 (95% CI 2.3–3.6) for tobacco chewers compared to non-chewers	Very few subjects smoked cigarette alone
Kabat et al. (1994), US (1560/2948)	Oral cavity and pharynx	OR = 3.3 (95% CI 2.4–4.3) for current vs. never in males; OR = 4.3 (95% CI 3.2–5.9) for current vs. never in females	Crude OR = 2.3 (95% CI 0.7–7.3) for regular chewer in men. Crude OR = 34.5 (95% CI 8.5–140.1) for snuff users in women	The results for smokeless tobacco use were based on small number of subjects
Macfarlane et al. (1995), US, Italy, China (835/1300)	Oral cavity, tongue, pharynx	OR = 3.8 (95% CI 2.5–5.8) for smoking of >30 pack-years in males; OR = 6.2 (95% CI 3.4–11.2) for smoking of >18 pack-years in females		The risk of oral cancer increased with increasing tobacco consumption among women who never drank alcohol

(Continued)

Table 22.1 (continued) Tobacco use and risk of oral cancer

Author (year) country (Cases/controls)	Cancer site	Major results			Comments
		Cigarettes	Cigar/pipe	Smokeless	
Muscat et al (1996), US (1009/923)	Oral cavity and pharynx	OR = 2.1 (95% CI 1.4–3.2) for cumulative lifetime tar intake of >6.8 kg in males; OR = 4.6 (95% CI 2.5–8.7) for cumulative tar intake of >6.8 kg in females		Oral snuff and chewing tobacco were unrelated to oral cancer risk in this study	Very few subjects used oral snuff and chewing tobacco
Zheng et al (1997), Beijing, China (111/111)	Tongue	OR = 2.7 (95% CI 1.3–5.9) for current vs. never; OR = 2.2 (95% CI 1.1–4.6) for ex-smokers vs. never			The number of cases and controls was small
De Stefani et al. (1998), Uruguay, US (471/471)	Oral cavity and pharynx	OR = 13.4 (95% CI 6.5–27.9) for smoking of >62 pack-years vs. newer smoking			The combined effect for tobacco and alcohol is supramultiplicative
Schlecht et al. (1999), Brazil (784/1578)	Mouth, pharynx, and larynx	OR = 8.0 (95% CI 4.6–13.8) for smoking of >40 cigarettes per day	Pipe: OR = 8.2 (95% CI 3.7–17.8) for smoking of >20 pack years Cigar: OR = 3.9 (95% CI 1.5–10.4) for ever vs. never		Smoking cessation resulted in a significant risk reduction, decreasing nearly to the levels of never smokers after 20 years of abstention
Franceschi et al. (1999), Italy (638/1254)	Oral cavity and pharynx	OR = 10.7 (95% CI 5.0–22.8) for smoking of ≥25 cigarettes per day			Men only
Moreno-Lopez et al. (1999), Spain (75/150)	Oral cavity	OR = 8.3 (95% CI 3.4–20.4) for smoking of >20 cigarettes per day			The number of cases and controls was small
La Vecchia et al. (1999), Italy (1280/4179)	Oral cavity and pharynx	OR = 8.4 (95% CI 6.6–10.6) for current vs. never			Significantly reduced risk was observed for smoking cessation

Reference	Site	Results	Comments
Zavras et al. (2000), Greece (110/115)	Oral cavity and pharynx	OR = 3.3 (95% CI 1.3–8.5) for smoking of >50 pack years during lifetime	OR was 8.3 (95% CI 2.4–29.1) for smoking >50 pack years and drinking 28 drinks per week. The number of cases and controls was small
Talamini et al. (2000), Italy (132/148)	Tongue, mouth, and pharynx	OR = 14.8 (95% CI 3.1–70.4) for smoking of ≥25 cigarette per day	The number of cases and controls was small
Garrote et al. (2001), Havana city, Cuba (200/200)	Oral cavity, pharynx	OR = 20.8 (95% CI 8.9–48.3) for smoking of ≥30 cigarettes per day; OR = 20.45 (95% CI 4.7–89.7) for smoking of >4 cigars/pipes per day	A supra-multiplicative effect for smoking and drinking on oral cancer risk. 82% of oral cancer cases in Cuba attributable to tobacco smoking

Population based case-control studies

Reference	Site	Results	Comments
Blot et al. (1988), US (1114/1268)	Oral cavity and pharynx	OR = 1.9 (95% CI 1.1–3.4) for ever vs. never in males; OR = 3.0 (95% CI 2.0–4.5) for ever vs. never in females; OR = 6.2 (95% CI 1.9–19.8) for non-smoking females	The tobacco smoking and alcohol drinking combine to account for about 75% of all oral and pharyngeal cancers in US
Tuyns et al. (1988), Italy, Spain, Switzerland, and France (1147/3057)	Larynx and pharynx	Endolarynx: RR = 9.9 (95% CI 6.4–15.4) for ever vs. never. Hypopharynx/Epilarynx: RR = 12.4 (95% CI 6.3–24.4) for ever vs. never	Men only. The relative risks for joint exposure to alcohol and tobacco are consistent with a multiplicative model
Merletti et al (1989), Italy (122/606)	Oral cavity and pharynx	OR = 3.9 (95% CI 1.6–94) for ever vs. never; Pipe: OR = 3.8 (95% CI 1.1–12.6) for ever vs. never Cigar: OR = 14.6 (95% CI 4.7–45.6) for ever vs. never	Attributable risks for tobacco in this population were 72% in men and 54% in women. The number of cases was small

(Continued)

Table 22.1 (continued) Tobacco use and risk of oral cancer

Author (year) country (Cases/controls)	Cancer site	Major results			Comments
		Cigarettes	Cigar/pipe	Smokeless	
Marshall et al. (1992), US (290/290)	Tongue, pharynx, and floor of mouth	OR = 5.7 (95% CI 2.7–12.1) for smoking of >70 pack-years			The effects of cigar and pipe smoking as practiced might be much less significant than cigarette smoking in this study. The number of cases and controls were small
Day et al. (1993), US (1065/1182)	Oral cavity, tongue and pharynx	OR = 3.6 (95% CI 2.6–4.8) for ever vs. never in whites OR = 2.3 (95% CI 1.1–4.7) for ever vs. never in blacks	OR = 2.2 (95% CI 1.3–4.0) for ever vs. never in whites: OR = 1.8 (95% CI 0.4–8.5) for ever vs. never in blacks		Smoking–drinking interaction was generally consistent with a multiplicative enhancement of risk following joint exposure to tobacco and alcohol among both whites and blacks
Day et al. (1994), US (83/189)	Oral cavity and pharynx	OR = 4.3 (95% CI 1.6–12) for current vs. never and former	OR = 5.0 (95% CI 0.6–4.4) for ever vs. never		The number of cases and controls was small
Bundgaard et al. (1995), Denmark (161/483)	Oral cavity	OR = 6.3 (95% CI 3.1–12.9) for smoking of >235 kg during lifetime			A multiplicative enhancement of risk for the combination of tobaoco and alcohol exposure was observed in this population. The number of cases was small
Andre et al. (1995), France (299/645)	Oral cavity, pharynx, and larynx	OR = 12.9 (95% CI 5.3–31.5) for smoking of ≥20 cigarettes per day			The combined effect of alcohol and tobacco appeared to follow a multiplicative model
Hung et al. (1997), Taiwan (41/123)	Oral cavity	OR = 5.9 (95% CI 1.9–18.5) for smoking of ≥22.5 pack-years			Men only. The number of cases and controls was small
Lewin et al. (1997), Sweden (605/756)	Oral cavity, pharynx. and larynx	RR = 6.5 (4.4–9.5) for current vs. never		RR = 1.8 (95% CI 0.9–3.7) for ex-users vs. never	The joint effect of high alcohol intake (≥20 grams per day) and current smoking was nearly multiplicative

Reference	Site	Relative risk	Other tobacco	Comments
Schwartz et al. (1998), US (284/477)	Oral cavity and pharynx	OR = 2.5 (95% CI 1.5–4.3) for past smoking of ≥20 pack-years; OR = 5.5 (95% CI 3.5–8.6) for current smoking of ≥20 pack-years	OR = 1.0 (95% CI 0.4–2.3) for smokeless tobacco use in men	Very few subjects used smokeless tobacco in this study
Schildt et al. (1998), Sweden (410/410)	Oral cavity	OR = 1.8 (95% CI 1.1–2.7) for current vs. never	Oral snuff: OR = 1.5 (0.8–2.9) for ex-users vs. never	A potential interaction between smoking and alcohol drinking
Hayes et al. (1999), Puerto Rico (342/521)	Oral cavity and pharynx	OR = 3.9 (95% CI 2.1–7.1) for ever vs. never in men; OR = 4.9 (95% CI 2.0–11.6) for ever vs. never in women	Pipe: OR = 2.0 (95% CI 1.1–3.4) for current vs. never	Cigarette smoking included cigar or pipe smoking. Joint exposure to alcohol and tobacco resulted in risks consistent with independent effects on a multiplicative scale

Prospective follow-up studies

Reference	Site	Relative risk	Other tobacco	Comments
Hammond and Seidman (1980), US (more than 1000000)	Buccal, pharynx, and larynx	Mortality ratio = 6.5 for ever vs. never in men; Mortality ratio = 3.3 for ever vs. never in women	Mortality ratio = 5.1 for ever vs. never in men	
Akiba and Hirayama (1990), Japan (265000)	Oral cavity, larynx	Oral cavity: RR = 2.5 (95% CI 1.3–5.7) for ever vs. never in men; Larynx RR = 23.8 (95% CI 5.3–420) for ever vs. never in men		Non-significantly increased RR found in women
Chyou et al. (1995), Hawaiian, US (7995)	Upper aero-digestive tract	RR = 3.2 (95% CI 1.7–5.9) for current vs. never		Men only. The RR = 14.35 for men who drank 14 or more ounces per month and smoked more than 20 cigarettes per day compared with those who had never drunk or smoked

hand-rolled cigarettes, respectively. The OR for the heaviest vs. the lowest consumption categories (>100 vs. <1 pack-years) was 14.8 (95% CI 4.7–47.3). Smoking cessation also resulted in a significant risk reduction, with levels close to those of never smokers after 10 years stopping smoking. A study by Spitz *et al.* (1988) in Texas, US, also showed a linear increase in risk with increasing pack-years of cigarette smoking (P_{trend}< 0.01 for both males and females). In males, the OR rose from 1.8 (95% CI 0.7–4.4) for those who smoked 1–24 pack-years to 7.5 (95% CI 3.7–15.3) for those who smoked >49 pack-years when compared to non-smokers. In females, the corresponding values were 1.5 (95% CI 0.4–5.1) and 12.0 (95% CI 3.8–38.0), respectively. Site-specific analysis for males also showed a significant increase with increasing pack-years of cigarette smoking for cancer of the larynx (P_{trend}< 0.01), tongue (P_{trend}< 0.01), and floor of mouth (P_{trend}= 0.02), but not for orohypopharynx (P_{trend}= 0.13), and other oral cavity (P_{trend}= 0.15). A significant risk reduction was observed after 15 or more years of smoking cessation.

Zheng *et al.* (1990) conducted a case–control study of oral cancer in Beijing, China, including 404 histologically confirmed incident cases and an equal number of hospital-based controls. The study reported an alcohol-adjusted OR of 2.4 (95% CI 1.5–4.0) for male smokers when compared to never smokers. Three measures of level of exposure— cigarette equivalents smoked per day, years smoked, and lifetime pack-years of smoking—all showed highly significant exposure–response relationships (P_{trend}< 0.001). Among females, while the numbers of smokers is small, the same trends as were seen among males are evident. An OR of 2.1 (95% CI 1.1–4.2) for male cigarette smokers was also reported from a case–control study in India by Nandakumar *et al.* (1990). The ORs were 2.2 (95% CI 1.1–4.3) for those who smoked for more than 25 years, and 2.1 (95% CI 1.0–4.4) for those who smoked more than 20 cigarettes per day. A small study from the United States by Kabat *et al.* (1989) also reported an alcohol-adjusted OR of 2.0 (95% CI 1.0–4.0) for current smokers. Being an ex-smoker was not found to be associated with an increased risk in this study (OR = 1.0, 95% CI 0.5–2.1).

Using the data from the northern Italy study, Talamini *et al.* (1990) further examined the role of tobacco in non-drinkers for oral and pharyngeal cancer. They found that, among non-drinkers, ex-smokers had a risk four times that of never smokers (OR = 4.1, 95% CI 0.5–93.6). For current smokers, ORs for smokers of <15 and ≥15 cigarettes per day were 3.8 (95% CI 0.2–58.2) and 12.9 (95% CI 2.3–106.3), respectively. The test for trend in risk was highly significant (P_{trend}< 0.001). La Vecchia *et al.* (1990) further examined the risk by low/medium or high tar contents of the cigarettes smoked, using only the male subjects of the study. They found that, among ever smokers, the ORs for oral and pharyngeal cancer were 8.5 (95% CI 3.7–19.4) for low to medium tar and 16.4 (95% CI 7.1–38.2) for high tar. The corresponding estimates were 4.8 (95% CI 2.3–10.1) and 7.1 (95% CI 3.2–15.6) for laryngeal cancers. A direct comparison between high vs. low tar cigarettes showed an OR 2.3 for oral cavity and pharyngeal cancers, and 3.8 for laryngeal cancer, and all these estimates were statistically significant.

Franceschi *et al.* (1990) reported the results from a case–control study involving cancer of the tongue and oral cavity, pharynx, and oesophagus. The study found that the alcohol-adjusted ORs for current smokers of cigarettes were 11.1 for oral cavity, 12.9 for pharynx, and 4.6 for larynx. The risks increased significantly with increasing the number of cigarettes smoked per day, duration of smoking, and with younger age started smoking, however, decreased with smoking cessation.

Using the data from a case–control study in northern Italy, Negri *et al.* (1993) reported that, compared to non-smokers, the alcohol-adjusted ORs were 3.6 for moderate smokers, and 9.4 for heavy smokers. In another report from northern Italy, Franceschi *et al.* (1992) reported that, among current smokers, the risk associated with cigarette smoking was similar for cancer of the tongue (OR = 10.5, 95% CI 3.2–34.1) and for cancer of the mouth (OR = 11.8, 95% CI 3.6–38.4). The risks also increased significantly with increasing number of cigarette smoking and duration of smoking for both cancer sites. An early age at starting smoking led to an OR of 7.6 (95% CI 2.3–25.0) for cancer of the tongue and 11.0 (95% CI 3.3–36.4) for cancer of the mouth. Smokers of high-tar cigarettes had a 10-fold increased risk of cancer of the tongue (95% CI 2.9–33.1) and a 14-fold increased risk (95% CI 4.2–49.5) of cancer of the mouth compared with non-smokers. Ex-smokers, who had quit smoking for more than 10 years, had an OR close to unity in this study.

Mashberg *et al.* (1993), in a study of US veterans in New Jersey, reported that smokers of filter cigarettes had a lower risk of oral cancer than that of smokers of unfiltered cigarettes. For smokers of unfiltered cigarettes, the ORs were 7.8 (95% CI 2.4–19.0), 7.7 (3.6–16.5), 12.3 (5.3–28.6), and 7.6 (3.5–16.8) for consumption of 6 to 15, 16 to 25, 26 to 35, and 36 or more cigarettes per day, respectively. The corresponding ORs for smokers of filtered cigarettes were 1.5 (0.5–4.2), 3.6 (1.6–7.7), 1.9 (0.7–5.0), and 2.3 (1.0–5.2), respectively. Using the same dataset, Boffetta *et al.* (1992) showed that soft palate had the highest ORs associated with tobacco smoking (OR = 4.9, 95% CI 1.1–21.5 for those smoking more than 35 cigarettes per day). A similar susceptibility to tobacco was shown for floor of the mouth (OR = 4.0, 95% CI 1.5–10.3, $P_{trend} <$ 0.01 for those smoking more than 35 cigarettes per day). A stronger effect of tobacco on posterior sites of the oral cavity, such as soft palate, is consistent with the earlier studies by Hirayama (1966) and by Jussawalla and Deshpande (1971).

Kabat *et al.* (1994) reported a large hospital-based case–control study in eight US cities, involving 1560 histologically incident cases of oral and pharyngeal cancer and 2948 controls (including both cancerous and non-cancerous controls). The study found that the OR for oral cancer was significantly increased in current smokers for both males (OR = 3.3, 95% CI 2.4–4.3) and females (OR = 4.3, 95% CI 3.2–5.9). Among current smokers of both sexes the OR increased with amount of smoking, and among ever smokers the risk increased with duration of smoking. Compared to lifetime non-filter smokers, lifetime filter smokers or those who switched to filter cigarettes had a reduced risk of oral cancer. Quitting smoking was associated with a substantial reduction of cancer risk which was evident even in the first few years following cessation.

Macfarlane *et al.* (1995) also reported a higher risk of female smokers from tobacco smoking in a combined analysis of three case–control studies from China, US, and Italy. They found that, among men, the ORs were 1.7 (95% CI 1.2–2.5) for those who smoked 33 pack-years or less, and 3.8 (95% CI 2.5–5.8) for those who smoked more than 33 pack years. Among women, the corresponding ORs were 2.7 (95% CI 1.6–4.7) and 6.2 (95% CI 3.4–11.2), respectively. The large sample size of the combined analysis allowed the authors to examine the risk associated with smoking among never alcohol drinkers. They reported that, among those who never consumed alcohol, the risk of oral cancer increased with increasing consumption of tobacco and the risk again was found to be higher for females amongst whom the increases were statistically significant. Smoking cessation resulted in a significant risk reduction, those who had stopped smoking for more than 9 years had a risk half that of current smokers (OR = 0.5, 95% CI 0.3–0.7).

In a case–control study of 1009 oral cancer patients and 923 age-matched controls in the US, Muscat *et al.* (1996) not only found a significant dose-response relationship between oral cancer risk and lifetime cumulative tar intake ($P_{trend} <$ 0.01) or lifetime pack-years of smoking ($P_{trend} <$ 0.01), they also reported a significant gender difference in the smoking-related risks for oral cancer. For example, the adjusted OR for men, according to increasing quartile of cumulative lifetime tar consumption and relative to never smokers, was 1.0, 0.9, 1.6, and 2.1. Among women, the corresponding ORs were 1.8, 2.8, 3.2, and 4.6.

Zheng *et al.* (1997) reported a case–control study of tongue cancer in Beijing, China. They found a significantly increased risk of tongue cancer among ex-smokers (OR = 2.2, 95% CI 1.1–4.6), and among current smokers (OR = 2.7, 95% CI 1.3–5.9). The risk also increased with increasing tobacco smoking, as reflected by both cigarette equivalents smoked per day and lifetime pack-years of tobacco smoking. Quitting smoking was associated with a significant risk reduction for tongue cancer.

In a case–control study in Uruguay, De Stefani et al. (1998) reported an increased risk of squamous-cell carcinoma of the oral cavity and pharynx for ever-smokers (OR = 7.4, 95% CI 3.7–14.8), current smokers (OR = 10.5, 95% CI 5.2–21.3), and former smokers (OR = 4.5, 95% CI 2.2–9.2). The risk increases with the increasing intensity of smoking, smoking duration, and pack-years of smoking. An OR of 13.4 (95% CI 6.5–27.9) was observed for heavy smokers (more than 62 pack-years). Analyses by type of tobacco products showed that risk was higher for black tobacco smokers (OR = 10.2, 95% CI 5.0–20.5) than for blond tobacco smokers (OR = 4.5, 95% CI 2.2–9.2).

A study from Brazil by Schlecht et al. (1999) investigated the relationship between different types of tobacco smoking and oral cancer risk. The study found that smokers of non-filter cigarettes had an OR of 6.9 (95% CI 4.1–11.8), and smokers of filter cigarettes had an OR of 6.2 (3.9–10.0). Smokers of more than 40 pack-years of commercial cigarettes had an OR of 8.0 (95% CI 4.6–13.8), and smokers of more than 40 packyears of black tobacco had an OR of 7.0 (95% CI 4.2–11.5). Current smokers were found to have an alcohol-adjusted RR of 8.1 (95% CI 4.9–13.4) compared to never smokers. As observed in other studies, smoking cessation resulted in a significant risk reduction, decreasing nearly to the levels of never smokers after 20 years of abstention.

Franceschi et al. (1999) also reported a dose-dependent relationship between cigarette smoking per day and oral cancer risk. The alcohol-adjusted OR was 3.3 (95% CI 1.5–7.2) for smoking 1–14 cigarettes daily, 7.7 (95% CI 3.8–15.4) for smoking 15–24 cigarettes daily, and 10.7 (95% CI 5.0–22.8) for smoking 25 or more cigarettes daily. Similarly, a dose–response relationship was observed for daily cigarette smoking by Moreno-Lopez et al. (2000) in Spain. The study reported that the alcoholadjusted OR was 3.1 (95% CI 1.4–6.7) for smoking 1–20 cigarettes/day, and 8.3 (95% CI 3.4–20.4) for smoking more than 20 cigarettes daily.

A study in the south of Greece by Zavras et al. (2001) also reported a significantly increased risk of oral cancer among current smokers (OR = 3.0, 95% CI 1.4–6.6). No increased risk, however, was observed for former smokers (OR = 0.9, 95% CI 0.4–2.1). A strong dose–response relationship was observed for pack-years of tobacco smoking (P_{trend} = 0.01). For those who had more than 50 pack-years of tobacco smoking, the alcohol-adjusted OR was 3.3 (95% CI 1.3–8.5) when compared to never smokers.

In a study from north-eastern Italy, Talamini et al. (2000) reported an OR of 2.4 (95% CI 1.0–5.8) for former smokers compared to never smokers. Among current smokers, risk increased with increasing number of cigarettes smoked per day (P_{trend} < 0.001). An alcohol-adjusted OR of 14.8 (95% CI 3.1–70.4) was observed for those who smoked 25 or more cigarettes per day.

In a combined analysis of two hospital-based case–control studies from Italy and Switzerland involving 1280 oral and pharyngeal cases and 4179 controls, La Vecchia et al. (1999) reported an OR of 8.4 (95% CI 6.6–10.6) for current smokers. A significantly reduced risk was observed following smoking cessation: the ORs were 6.2 for those who had stopped smoking for less than 2 years, 4.5 for those who had stopped for 3–5 years, 3.5 for those who had stopped for 6–9 years, 1.6 for those who had stopped for 10–14 years, and 1.4 for those who had stopped for 15 or more years.

Garrote et al. (2001) reported the results from a case–control study of tobacco smoking and risk of oral and oro-pharyngeal cancers in Cuba. A strong dose–response was reported between cigarette smoking per day and risk of oral cancer among current smokers (P_{trend}< 0.01). The alcohol-adjusted OR for smoking 30 cigarettes or more per day, compared with never smokers, was 20.8 (95% CI 8.9–48.3) among current smokers. Former smokers also had an OR of 6.3 (95% CI 3.0–13.4), but risk was significantly reduced after 10 or more years smoking cessation.

Population-based case–control studies

A potential advantage of population-based case–control study design is that controls are randomly selected from the population which produced the cases, and therefore, more likely to represent the population with regards to the major risk factors. However, the relatively higher refusal rate from potential study subjects may still hamper the interpretation of the study.

In a multicentre study in the four areas of the US, Blot et al. (1988) found that, compared with never smokers, cigarette smokers had twice the risk in males (OR = 1.9, 95% CI 1.3–2.9), and three times the risk in females (OR = 3.0, 95% CI 2.0–4.5). The risks of oral cancer rose with the number of cigarettes smoked per day and with the duration of cigarette smoking. Those who smoked only filter cigarettes had a 50% (95% CI 30–80) of the risk of those who smoked only non-filter cigarettes, and smoking cessation resulted in a rapid decline in risk.

In a multi-centre case–control study in four European countries, Tuyns et al. (1988) reported a clear dose–response relationship between cigarette smoking and risk of cancer of the larynx and hypopharynx. For those who smoked more than 26 cigarettes per day, the ORs were 24.0 (95% CI 11.8–48.7) for cancer of the supraglottic, 10.2 (95% CI 5.4–19.3) for cancer of the glottic and subglottic, 9.4 (95% CI 3.2–28.0) for cancer of the epilarynx, and 20.0 (95% CI 7.9–51.0) for cancer of the hypopharynx. The study also found that earlier age started smoking carried a higher risk. Unlike the study by Merletti et al. (1989), the smokers of exclusively filter cigarettes in this study were found to have only half the risk of laryngeal or hypopharynx/epilarynx cancer as compared with smokers of only plain cigarettes. As reported by Schlecht et al. (1999) and De Stefan et al. (1998), smokers of black tobacco cigarettes had higher risk than smokers of blond tobacco. Smoking cessation resulted in a decrease in risk after 5 years' abstention.

Merletti et al. (1989) from Italy reported a four- to sixfold increased risk among subjects with medium or high tobacco consumption in both males and females. A trend in increasing risk with duration of smoking was observed in men, but not in women. As reported by Franceschi et al. (1990), younger age at start of smoking was found to be associated with a higher risk in this study, and smoking cessation is associated with a sharp risk reduction. Subjects smoking black cigarettes had a higher risk, while use of filter cigarettes showed no clear risk difference.

Marshall et al. (1992) reported the results from a case–control study in western New York, and they found that, while the risk associated with cigarette smoking did not increase in strict dose–response fashion, it was sizably and significantly elevated from those who had 21–30 pack-years of smoking (OR = 2.7, 95% CI 1.2–6.0) to those who had more than 70 pack-years of smoking (OR = 5.7, 95% CI 2.7–12.1).

Using data from a multicentre population-based case–control study of oral cancer risk factors in the US (1065 cases and 1182 controls), Day et al. (1993) examined the black–white differences in the risk of oral cancer associated with tobacco smoking. The study found that the patterns of risk among smokers were generally similar among blacks and whites. After controlling for alcohol consumption, the risk was almost doubled for those who smoked 20–39 cigarettes per day, and tripled for those who smoked 40 or more cigarettes per day. The alcohol-adjusted OR for current smokers was higher among whites (OR = 3.6, 95% CI 2.6–4.8) than among blacks (OR = 2.3, 95% CI 1.1–4.7), but this difference was not statistically significant. The risk declined sharply with cessation of smoking for both racial groups, with little elevation in risk even for those who had quit smoking 1–9 years earlier.

Tobacco smoking was also found to be significantly associated with the risk of second cancers of the oral cavity and pharynx in a nested case–control study by Day et al. (1994). The effects of smoking was found to be more pronounced than those of alcohol in this study. Current smokers relative to never and former smokers had an OR of 4.3 (95% CI 1.6–12). The alcohol-adjusted ORs for smoking rose with duration and intensity of smoking. Risk, however, was significantly reduced 5 years after smoking cessation.

Bundgaard *et al.* (1995) in Denmark also reported an increased risk of oral cancer associated with increasing lifetime kilogram cigarette smoking ($P_{trend}< 0.001$) and with current daily amount of smoking ($P_{trend}< 0.001$). For those who had a lifetime consumption of cigarettes greater than 235 kg, the OR was 6.3 (95% CI 3.1–12.9). The OR was 5.8 (95% CI 3.1–10.9) for those with current consumption of more than 20 cigarettes per day.

A dose–response relationship was observed for daily grams of cigarette smoking in a case–control study by Andre *et al.* (1995) in France. The study found that those who smoked more than one packet of cigarettes a day had a risk that was 13 times higher than that of non-smokers. Subjects who smoked only non-filter cigarettes had a higher risk (OR = 2.0) than those who smoked filter cigarettes, and risk decreaseed after stopping smoking.

A small study by Hung *et al.* (1997) in Taiwan found that, compared with nonsmokers, cigarette smoking had an increased risk of oral cancer (OR = 5.0, 95% CI 1.7–15.1). The risk increased with increasing lifetime pack-years of smoking: the ORs were 4.0 (95% CI 1.2–13.5) for those with less than 22.5 pack-years of smoking, and 5.9 (95% CI 1.9–18.5) for those with more than 22.5 pack-years of smoking.

In a case–control study in Sweden, Lewin *et al.* (1997) reported that men who smoked only cigarettes had an OR of 3.7 (95% CI 2.5–5.5). The risk was considerably lower for ex-smokers (OR = 1.9, 95% CI 1.3–2.8) than for current smokers (OR = 6.5, 95% CI 4.4–9.5). No increased risk was found for men who had stopped smoking for more than 20 years. There was dose-dependent excess risk associated with duration of smoking, total lifetime kilograms of tobacco smoking, and daily grams of tobacco smoking. Analysis by cancer site showed that, for men who smoked 45 years or longer, the ORs were 6.3 (95% CI 3.2–12.4) for cancer of the oral cavity, 10.1 (95% CI 4.6–22.1) for pharynx, 7.6 (95% CI 3.9–14.7) for larynx, and 5.4 (95% CI 2.7–11.0) for oesophagus.

In a case–control study of oral cancer in western Washington state, USA, Schwartz *et al.* (1998) reported a significantly increased risk of oral cancer for both current and past cigarette smokers. For those who smoked greater than or equal to 20 pack-years of cigarettes, the OR was 2.5 (95% CI 1.5–4.3) for past smokers and 5.5 (95% CI 3.5–8.6) for current smokers.

In a case–control study of oral cancer in Sweden, Schildt *et al.* (1998) found a significantly increased risk of oral cancer among the current smokers (OR = 1.8, 95% CI 1.1–2.7), while found no increased risk for ex-smokers (OR = 1.0, 95% CI 0.6–1.6). They found, however, that OR was 1.8 (95% CI 1.2–2.8) for current smokers with more than 124.8 kg cigarette consumption. Analysis by anatomic site showed that the risk appeared to be the highest for cancer of the floor of the mouth (OR = 8.0, 95% CI 1.0–64.0).

Hayes *et al.* (1999) conducted a case–control study in Puerto Rico and found that any cigarette use was associated with an increased risk of oral cancer among men (OR = 3.9, 95% CI 2.1–7.1) and women (OR = 4.9, 95% CI 2.0–11.6). Risks increased with increasing cigarette use, whether estimated by usual daily amount ($P_{trend}< 0.0001$), or by cumulative lifetime consumption ($P_{trend}< 0.0001$). As reported by Macfarlane *et al.* (1995) and Muscat *et al.* (1996), this study also reported that women seemed to have greater risk at a given amount of cigarette consumption. Unlike the study of Mashberg *et al.* (1993), this study did not find a reduced risk associated with smoking filter cigarettes compared to smoking non-filter cigarettes. Smoking cessation was shown to reduce the risk gradually, with the risk remaining elevated up to 19 years after smoking cessation.

Prospective follow-up studies

A prospective follow-up study is conducted based on the presence or absence of exposure of investigation without the information regarding disease status. Therefore, a follow-up study is less prone to selection bias at the start of the study. However, the losses to follow-up may still pose an issue for the interpretation of the study results, especially for diseases, such as cancers, which have long induction and latency periods.

Hammond and Seidman (1980) reported a prospective mortality study of over one million Americans in 1721 counties in 25 states in the US. The study reported that, among men, oral cancer mortality rates were 2.3/100 000 for those who never smoked regularly, 11.7/100 000 for pipe and cigar smokers, and 15.0/100 000 for cigarette smokers. Among women, the oral cancer mortality rates were 2.0/100 000 for those who never smoked regularly and 6.5/100 000 for cigarette smokers.

Another prospective cohort mortality study from Japan by Akiba and Hirayama (1990) examined the site-specific cancer risk associated with cigarette smoking, using the data from 265 000 residents of 29 public health districts in six prefectures throughout Japan. The study reported a statistically significant dose–response relationship between cigarette smoking and mortality rate for cancer of the oral cavity, larynx, oesophagus, bladder, and stomach in men. Compared to never smokers, the RRs were 2.5 (95% CI 1.3–5.7) for cancer of the oral cavity and 23.8 (95% CI 5.3–420.0) for cancer of the larynx among males. Very few women smoked cigarettes in this population.

Chyou et al. (1995) reported a cohort study of upper aerodigestive tract cancer among 7995 Japanese–American men in Hawaii in which they examined the potential impact of smoking and other risk factors on the incidence of upper aerodigestive tract cancer (30 men with oral/pharyngeal cancer, 27 men with laryngeal cancer, and 35 men with oesophageal cancer). The study found that current cigarette smokers at time of examination had a threefold risk for upper aerodigestive tract cancer compared with never-smokers (RR = 3.2, 95% CI 1.7–5.9). A significant positive linear trend in relative risk was observed in number of cigarettes smoked per day (P_{trend}= 0.002), and number of years of smoking (P_{trend}= 0.0006).

Pipe and cigar smoking

Another major source of exposure to tobacco is through cigar and pipe smoking. Similar to the observations for cigarettes smoking and oral cancer risk, the vast majority of studies have identified a strong association between cigar and pipe smoking and oral cancer risk (Blot et al. 1988; Spitz et al. 1988; Franco et al. 1989; Merletti et al. 1989; Franceschi et al. 1990; La Vecchia et al. 1990, 1998; Zheng et al. 1990; Mashberg et al. 1993; Schildt et al. 1998; Hayes et al. 1999; Schlecht et al. 1999; Shapiro et al. 2000; Garrote et al. 2001). With only a few studies, such as the study by Marshall et al. (1992), reporting little or no association. In some studies, the risk of oral cancer was actually found to be higher for pipe and cigar smokers than for cigarette smokers. For example, a case–control study by Franceschi et al. (1990) reported an OR of 20.7 (95% CI 5.6–76.3) for pipe and cigar smokers compared to an OR of 11.1 (95% CI 3.4–34.8) for cigarette smokers.

Zheng et al. (1990) reported an OR of 5.7 (95% CI 2.4–13.3) for male pipe smokers compared to 1.6 (95% CI 1.0–2.6) for male cigarette smokers in their case–control study. Franco et al. (1989) reported a higher risk of oral cancer for pipe smoking compared to other smoking behaviours, particularly for cancer of other parts of the mouth (ICD9 143–145).

Pipe smoking also showed a strong dose-dependent relationship with oral cancer risk in several studies (Blot et al. 1988; Mashberg et al. 1993; Schlecht et al. 1999). For example, the study by Schlecht et al. (1999) reported an OR of 6.7 (95% CI 3.1–14.8) for those who smoked 1–20 pack-years of commercial cigarette equivalents of pipe, and 8.2 (95% CI 3.7–17.8) for those with more than 20 pack-years of commercial cigarette equivalents of pipe smoking. Similarly, in a large case–control study, Blot et al. (1988) reported an OR of 1.9 (9% CI 1.1–3.4) for those exclusively smoking cigars and/or pipes, with a positive trend associated with increasing numbers of cigars/pipes smoked. The OR rose to 16.7 (95% CI 3.7–76.7) for men who smoked 40 or more cigars/week, and to 3.1 (95% CI 1.1–8.7) for those consuming 40+ pipefuls/week.

However, other studies, such as Merletti *et al.* (1989) reported a higher risk of oral cancer for cigar smokers (OR = 14.6, 95% CI 4.7–45.6) than pipe smokers (OR = 3.8, 95% CI 1.1–12.6) and than cigarette smokers (OR = 3.9, 95% CI 1.6–9.4) among male smokers. A strong dose–response relationship has been shown between cigar smoking and risk of oral cancer. In particular, the study by Garrote *et al.* (2001) showed a strong dose–response relationship between cigar smoking and oral cancer risk ($P_{trend} < 0.01$). They found that, compared with never smokers, those who smoked <4 cigars or equivalents per day had an OR of 4.3 (95% CI 1.1–16.4), and those who smoked ≥4 cigars or equivalents per day had an OR of 20.5 (95% CI 4.7–89.7). Shanks and Burns (1998) reported a RR of 7.9 for 'ever' cigar smokers and a RR of 15.9 for heavy cigar smokers (>5 cigars per day) for oral and pharyngeal cancer risk. In a case–control study of oral and oesophageal cancers involving only those who never smoked pipe tobacco or cigarettes, La Vecchia *et al.* (1998) reported an OR of 6.8 (95% CI 2.5–18.5) for ever smokers and 8.9 for smokers of more than 3 cigars per day, and 14.9 (95% CI 4.0–55.9) for current cigar smokers when compared to never cigar smokers.

In either case, pipe and cigar smoking clearly increases the risk of oral cancer. This risk seems to vary by anatomic subsite. Shapiro *et al.* (2000) found that, compared with never smokers, current cigar smokers had an RR of 4.0 (95% CI 1.5–10.3) for cancer of the oral cavity/pharynx compared to 10.3 (95% CI 2.6–41.0) for cancer of the larynx. Former smokers had an OR of 2.4 (95% CI 0.8–7.3) for cancer of the oral cavity/pharynx, but 6.7 (95% CI 1.5–30.0) for cancer of the larynx. In their case– control study of oral and oesophageal cancers, La Vecchia *et al.* (1998) reported an OR 9.0 (95% CI 2.7–30.0) for oral and pharyngeal cancers, compared to 4.1 (95% CI 0.7–23.0) for oesophageal cancer among ever cigar smokers. Boffetta *et al.* (1992) showed that soft palate seems to be more susceptible to cigar and pipe smoking than other sites.

Smokeless tobacco

People are also exposed to smokeless tobacco including snuff and chewing tobacco. Snuff consists of a tobacco that has been cured and grounded into dry snuff (<10% moisture), or moist snuff (up to 50% moisture). Snuff dipping consists of taking a small amount of snuff between the gingival and the lip or the bucca mucosa, and leaving there from a few minutes to several hours. Chewing tobacco includes plug tobacco, loose-leaf tobacco, twist or roll tobacco. Chewing tobacco is held in the mouth where it can be chewed intermittently for several hours (Grasso and Mann 1998).

Since the 1980s, there has been considerable interest in the relationship between smokeless tobacco use and oral cancer risk, and several excellent reviews have summarized the major results linking smokeless tobacco use to oral cancer risk (Winn 1988, 1997; Vigneswaran *et al.* 1995; Gupta *et al.* 1996; Grasso and Mann 1998; Johnson 2001).While the IARC has concluded that 'there is sufficient evidence that oral use of snuff of the types commonly used in North America and western Europe is carcinogenic to humans' (IARC 1985), the relationship between smokeless tobacco use and oral cancer risk is not as consistent as what was observed for tobacco smoking from different populations, ranging from no increased risk from studies in Sweden (Axell *et al.* 1978; Lewin *et al.* 1997; Schildt *et al.* 1998) to an estimated 23-fold (rural women) and 61-fold (urban women) excess in risk associated with snuff use in Atlanta (Vogler *et al.* 1962).

A number of factors may have affected the observed relationship between smokeless tobacco use and oral cancer risk. For example, few studies were designed specifically to examine the relationship. Considering the low prevalence of smokeless tobacco users in most of the populations together with the small sample sizes in many studies, few studies would have the sufficient power to address the issue.

Perhaps a more important factor, which may account for the observed inconsistent association, is that smokeless tobacco products used in different countries contain very different levels of carcinogens. For example, smokeless tobacco used in Sweden is quite different from that used in India or US. In Sweden, where studies have failed to support an association between local snuff use and oral cancer risk, snuff is not fermented and contains much lower nitrosamine levels than fermented tobaccos (Johnson 2001). In India, however, processing of smokeless tobacco is done by individual farmers and small companies with little control over fermentation and curing (Vigneswaran *et al.* 1995); fermentation produces potentially carcinogenic nitrosamines. Also, in India, smokeless tobacco is often used in combination with betel leaf, areca nut, and powdered slaked lime, and these additives make the combination more genotoxic than tobacco alone. Fermentation is also used in the US, though recent improvements in tobacco agriculture and smokeless tobacco processing have resulted in substantial decline in the concentration of several important carcinogens (Brunnemann and Hoffmann 1993).

Since the levels of carcinogens in smokeless tobacco vary considerably from country to country, studies of different populations have reached very different conclusions. In the following, we will review the studies based on the country of origin of the study.

Studies in Sweden Approximately, 15–20% of adult males use moist snuff in Sweden (Lewin *et al.* 1997). In fact, Sweden was the world's largest per capita consumer of smokeless tobacco throughout the twentieth century (Nordgren and Ramstrom 1990). Although an early study by Wynder *et al.* (1957) suggested an increased risk of oral cancer among snuff users, more recent studies from Sweden have found no relationship between use of local snuff and oral cancer risk. The population-based case– control study by Lewin *et al.* (1997) found no increased risk of head and neck cancer with ever using oral snuff. Age started using snuff, total number of years of using snuff, and total amount of snuff used in a lifetime all had little or no impact on the risk of head and neck cancer in this study.

Another recent case–control study by Schildt *et al.* (1998) also showed no increased risk of oral cancer among current snuff users regardless of tobacco smoking habits. Lifetime consumption of snuff also showed no increased risk. While ex-snuff users were found to have an increased risk, but the risk was seen only among those who were also active tobacco smokers. Users of chewing tobacco in this study (5 cases and 8 controls) also did not show an increased risk of oral cancer (OR = 0.6, 95% CI 0.2–2.2).

An early retrospective follow-up study of 200 000 male snuff users in Sweden also failed to find a significantly increased risk of oral cancer (Axell *et al.* 1978). Ecological data from Sweden do not support an association between use of local snuff and oral cancer risk in this population (Lewin *et al.* 1997). Specifically, Geographic areas where consumption of oral snuff is highest, the incidence rate of head and neck cancers is low, and, areas with low consumption of snuff, the incidence for cancer of the head and neck is the highest.

Studies in the US In the US, while the national prevalence rate of smokeless tobacco use is low (about 5% for regular use), the rates are high in some parts of the country. In North Carolina, for example, Winn *et al.* (1981) reported that 46% of the oral cancer cases and 30% of the controls were snuff users. Epidemiological studies from the US have generally indicated an increased risk of oral cancer associated with the use of oral snuff.

The most conclusive study was conducted in North Carolina by Winn *et al.* (1981). The study interviewed 232 female cases and 410 female controls, and found that smokeless tobacco use was a potent risk factor for oral cancer in this population. Among white women without a smoking habit, the oral and pharyngeal cancer cases were 4.2 times (95% CI 2.6–6.7) more likely to have used smokeless tobacco than were controls. Among women with cancer in the cheek or gums, where tissues come in direct contact with the tobacco powder, the relative risks rose from 13-fold for less than 25, and 25 to 49 year of use, to nearly 50-fold for 50 or more years of use. It is estimated that about 31% of the oral cancer in this population could be attributable to snuff dipping alone. While the study was criticized for using hospital-based controls that may not represent the population, which produced the cases with regards to the snuff use, the underlying association would actually be underestimated if the control diseases were in fact associated with the use of smokeless tobacco.

A large population-based case–control study by Blot *et al.* (1988) also reported a significantly sixfold (95% CI 1.9–19.8) increased risk of oral cancer due to use of smokeless tobacco among non-smoking females. Kabat *et al.* (1994) reported a crude OR of 34% (95% CI 8.5–140.1) for using snuff among female never smokers. An early hospital-based case–control study by Vogler *et al.* (1962) also found an increased risk of oral cancer associated with snuff use among both urban women (Crude OR = 60.8) and rural women (crude OR = 22.9). Spitz *et al.* (1988) also reported a significantly increased risk of oral cancer associated with snuff dipping among males (OR = 3.4, 95% CI 1.0–10.9).

There are also several studies of US populations that did not find an increased risk of oral cancer associated with smokeless tobacco use (Mashberg *et al.* 1993; Muscat *et al.* 1996; Schwartz *et al.* 1998). These studies, however, generally involved populations that have a very low prevalence rate for smokeless tobacco use, and none of them were designed specifically to investigate the association between smokeless tobacco use and risk of oral cancer. For example, the study by Schwartz *et al.* (1998) from western Washington State found that, out of 294 female cases and controls, only one female control subject used smokeless tobacco. Among males, prior smokeless tobacco use was reported by only 6.7% of the cases and 5.6% of the controls (OR = 1.0, 95% CI 0.4–2.3). The hospital-based case–control study by Mashberg *et al.* (1993) in New Jersey also found no increased risk of oral cancer for use of snuff (OR = 0.8, 95% CI 0.4–1.9) or chewing tobacco (OR = 1.0, 95% CI 0.7–1.4). The proportion of snuff or chewing tobacco together was found in only 14% of the cases and 11% of the controls.

Muscat *et al.* (1996) also found no increased risk of oral cancer associated with snuff use or chewing tobacco. But only 1.3% of the cases and 1.6% of the controls in males used snuff. Among women, only two cases and one control reported snuff use in this study. About 5% of the cases and controls in men and none of the women reported regularly using chewing tobacco. Sterling *et al.* (1992) evaluated the relationship between smokeless tobacco use and cancer risk based on data from the national mortality followback survey, and found no increased risk of oral or other digestive cancers associated with smokeless tobacco use, either as snuff or chewing tobacco. However, as pointed out by Johnson (2001), a number of limitations have limited the interpretation of the study results, including small number of subjects used the products, and issues related to data collection and presentation.

Studies in India Oral cancer is the most common cancer in India, where large quantities of smokeless tobacco are used (Jayant and Deo 1986). Smokeless tobacco use is considered to be a major risk factor for the high incidence rate of oral cancer in this country. The study by Nandakumar *et al.* (1990) reported an increased risk of oral cancer among pan tobacco chewers in both males and females, and no increased risk among pan chewing without tobacco. A dose–response was observed for years of chewing, number of times of chewing per day, and period of retaining the pan in the mouth. A linear test for trend was statistically significant ($P < 0.001$) in all three instances. Compared to those with no history of chewing tobacco, the ORs were 8.5 (95% CI 4.7–15.2) for those who did not chew during sleep, and 17.7 (95% CI 8.7–36.1) for those with a history of chewing during sleep.

Rao *et al.* (1994) also reported a significant association between tobacco chewing and risk of oral cancer (OR = 3.0, 95% CI 2.3–3.7), and the risk increased with increasing frequency ($P_{trend} < 0.001$). For chewers who chewed tobacco 21–30 times per day, the OR was 10.7 times higher than that for non-chewers. Several other earlier case–control studies (Sanghvi *et al.* 1955; Wahi *et al.* 1965;

Jussawalla and Deshpande 1971; Notani 1988) and follow-up studies (Bhargava *et al.* 1975; Gupta *et al.* 1980) from different parts of India have also provided unequivocal evidence between chewing tobacco and oral cancer risk, and this risk appeared to be even higher among those who began the habit at a younger age (Jayant *et al.* 1971).

Other countries Franco *et al.* (1989) reported no association between use of smokeless tobacco, either as snuff or tobacco chewing, and risk of oral cancer in Brazil. However, the number of subjects who used tobacco in this form was small (9 cases and 13 controls). In Sudan, however, an increased risk of oral cancer was reported among those who used toombak, a coarse powder made of dried tobacco leaves, and the risk was found to be higher for anatomic sites (buccal cavity, floor of mouth, and lip) where tissues come in direct contact with the product (Idris *et al.* 1995).

Tobacco and alcohol interaction

A number of studies from different populations or racial groups have investigated the interaction between tobacco and alcohol on the risk of oral cancer, and most of them have concluded that the effects of tobacco and alcohol are certainly more than additive and seem to be consistent with multiplicative, with some suggesting a supramultiplicative effect (Negri *et al.* 1993; De Stefani *et al.* 1998; Garrote *et al.* 2001). Studies, which presented the joint distribution of cases and controls for each combination of smoking and alcohol consumption with the corresponding ORs, have shown a sharp increase in the risk for those with the heaviest levels of consumption of both products compared to the lowest levels of consumption of both products. The OR for the highest levels of consumption of both products reached as high as 305 (Baron *et al.* 1993).

A strong interaction between tobacco and alcohol in the risk of oral cancer was observed no matter if the relationship is expressed by lifetime consumption of the products (Franco *et al.* 1989; Zheng *et al.* 1990; Bundgaard *et al.* 1994; Schidt 1998), or daily or weekly or monthly consumption of the products (Rothman and Keller 1972; Wynder *et al.* 1976; Elwood *et al.* 1984; Blot *et al.* 1988; Tuyns *et al.* 1988; Merletti *et al.* 1989; Franceschi *et al.* 1990; Day *et al.* 1993; Mashberg *et al.* 1993; Kabat *et al.* 1994; Andre *et al.* 1995; Chyou *et al.* 1995; Franceschi *et al.* 1999; Hayes *et al.* 1999; Garrote *et al.* 2001), or by cumulative tar/amount of alcohol day (Muscat *et al.* 1996), or expressed by other means (Baron *et al.* 1993; Lewin *et al.* 1997; De Stefani *et al.* 1998; Zavras *et al.* 2001).

A strong interaction between smoking and alcohol use on the risk of oral cancer is exemplified from the study by Franceschi *et al.* (1999) in Italy. In this study, the highest level of risk of oral cancer (OR = 227.8, 95% CI 54.6–950.7) was observed among those most heavily consuming both tobacco and alcohol.

Tobacco and gene interaction

It is suggested that functional polymorphisms in genes encoding tobacco carcinogen-metabolizing enzymes may modify the relationship between tobacco smoking and an individual's oral cancer risk. This is biologically plausible since the phase I enzymes (cytochromes P-450) activate many tobacco procarcinogens by forming or exposing their functional groups. For example, CYP1A1 is the major enzyme responsible for the metabolic activation of benzo-(*a*)-pyrene and other polycyclic aromatic hydrocarbons (PAHs), and CYP2E1 is the major enzyme responsible for the metabolic activation of nitrosamines. The activated carcinogens can bind covalently to DNA to form DNA adducts. Accumulation of DNA adducts at critical loci such as oncogenes or tumour suppressor genes can lead to somatic mutation and disruption of the cell cycle (Geisler and Olshan 2001).

The phase II enzymes (such as the glutathione S-transferases (GSTs) and *N*-acetyl transferase (NATs)) are involved in the detoxification of activated metabolites of carcinogens by phase I enzymes. GSTM1, for instance, metabolizes and detoxifies benzo-(*a*)-pyrene-diol epoxides

(Bundgaard *et al*. 1995; Chyou *et al*. 1995), while GSTT1 detoxifies epoxides and other constituents of tobacco smoke, such as alkyl halides (Day *et al*. 1993; Day *et al*. 1994). Therefore, individuals who have high phase I metabolizing activities but have low or lack certain phase II metabolizing activity, may accumulate more DNA adducts, and thus have a particularly high cancer risk after exposure to tobacco smoke (Brunnemann *et al*. 1996; De Stefani *et al*. 1998; Elwood *et al*. 1984).

A few studies have investigated the association between tobacco smoking, genetic polymorphisms, and oral cancer risk (Brenna *et al*. 1995; Franco *et al*. 1999; Franceschi *et al*. 1990, 1992, 1999, 2000; Garrote *et al*. 2001; Geisler *et al*. 2001). For example, Park *et al*. (1999) reported a greater risk for those with the GSTP1 (var/var) genotype who were exposed to low levels of smoking (i.e. ≤20 pack-years, OR= 3.4, 95% CI 1.1–11) than among heavier smokers (i.e. >20 pack-years, OR= 1.4, 95% CI 0.5–4.0), suggesting GSTP1 genotype may play a role in risk for oral cancer particularly among lighter smokers. The studies by Sato *et al*. (1999, 2000) also showed that individuals with a combined genotype of Val/Val and GSTM1(–) were at an increased risk for oral squamous-cell carcinoma compared with other combined genotypes, in particular, at a low dose level of cigarette smoking. These observations are consistent with the suggestion that genetic variations in the ability to metabolize tobacco smoke carcinogens are most important in determining cancer risk at low levels of exposure, and may be less relevant at higher smoking doses where high levels of carcinogen exposure overwhelm polymorphism-induced differences in enzyme activity and/or expression (London *et al*. 1995).

It should be pointed out, however, that epidemiological results linking, smoking, gene and oral cancer risk have been inconsistent. In their recent review of 24 published studies that evaluated the risk of squamous-cell carcinoma of the head and neck in relation to GSTM1 and GSTT1 genetic polymorphisms, Geisler and Olshan (2001) reported that some of the studies reported weak-to-moderate associations and others finding no elevation in risk for the main effect of the gene. Few studies have directly evaluated the interaction with tobacco. As pointed out by Geisler and Olshan (2001) none of the studies conducted to date have been able to assess gene–environment interaction with precision due to limited statistical power. Lack of accurate and detailed measurement of exposure in many of the studies may have also contributed to the inconsistent results. It is obvious that well-designed studies with large sample size are needed to better understand the relationship between smoking, gene, and risk of oral cancer.

Attributable risk

The International Agency for Research on Cancer has classified cancer of the oral cavity, pharynx, and larynx as tobacco-related cancers. A number of case–control studies have estimated the proportion of oral cancer cases attributable to tobacco smoking, but the estimated proportion depends on the validity of the estimation of the prevalence of smoking in the population and the relative risk from the exposure. A number of factors may affect the estimation: for example, hospital-based studies with patients as controls, population-based studies with high refusal rate, or lack of adequate control for major confounding factors (such as alcohol consumption). Since smoking and drinking are highly correlated, some studies calculated estimates of the population attributable risk (PAR) of oral cancer due to smoking and/or drinking rather than due to smoking alone. In most of the studies, the reported PAR from smoking did not include the impact from smokeless tobacco use, or even pipe and cigar smoking.

Parkin *et al*. (2000) have estimated that about 46% of the cancer of the oral cavity and pharynx in men and 11% of these diseases in women are attributable to smoking worldwide. Estimates vary for specific countries and are presented below.

In Italy, Merletti *et al*. (1989) estimated that 72.4% of oral cancer cases in men and 53.9% of the cases in women are attributable to smoke of more than 7 g of tobacco/day. The study by Negri *et al.* (1993) reported that, for both sexes, the single factor with the highest attributable risk was smoking, which in males accounted for 81–87% of oral cancer cases and in females for 42–47%.

In the US, Mashberg *et al.* (1993) estimated that 74% of oral cancer in this population was attributable to smoking 6 or more cigarette equivalents per day, and 97% of the disease was attributable to the combination of smoking and drinking. In a population-based case–control study of oral cancer involving 4 states in the US, Blot *et al.* (1988) estimated that 80% of the oral and pharyngeal cancer cases in men and 61% in women were attributable to smoking and alcohol drinking. Using the data from this population-based case–control study, Day *et al.* (1993) estimated that 83% of blacks and 73% of whites developed oral cancer as a result of alcohol and/or tobacco consumption, with most tumours arising from the combined effect of drinking and smoking. Almost half of all oral cancer (48%) among black men was attributed to smoking one pack or more daily in combination with heavy drinking (≥30 drinks per week). For white men, 36% of oral cancers were accounted for by this level of smoking and drinking. Tobacco and alcohol consumption account for bulk of the racial and gender differences in oral cancer in the US.

In Beijing, China, Zheng *et al.* (1990) found that tobacco smoking accounts for about 34% of all cases of oral cancer in the Chinese population (45% among males and 21% among females) and 44% of all oral squamous-cell carcinoma. In Bombay, it is estimated that 70% of oral cancer cases were attributable to smoking and chewing tobacco.

Biological plausibility

Tobacco smoke is a complex mixture of compounds. Over 300 carcinogens have been identified in cigarette smoke. Polycyclic aromatic hydrocarbons (PAHs) have long been recognized as carcinogens present in tar. There are about 20–40 ng of benz-pyrene per cigarette and substantial levels of carcinogenic metals such as hexavalent chromium (Johnson 2001). The most important and abundant carcinogenic agents in tobacco smoke are the tobacco-specific *N*-nitrosamines (TSNA), including nitrosonornicotine (NNN) and 4-(methylnitrosamino)-1-(3-pyridyl)-1-butanone (NNK).

About 30 carcinogens have been identified in smokeless tobacco. Again, the TSNAs are major contributors to the carcinogenic activity of these types of tobacco (Hoffman and Djordjevic 1997). TSNAs are formed exclusively from nicotine and from the minor tobacco alkaloids, primarily formed after harvesting the leaves, during drying, curing, aging, and especially during fermentation (Hoffmann *et al.* 1994; Brunnemann *et al.* 1996).

The absorbed PAHs, TSNA, and aromatic amines from tobacco use can be metabolically activated to form electrophilic intermediates, which have the ability to react with DNA to form covalently bound DNA adducts, which interfere with DNA replication and initiate the carcinogenesis process. Oral swabbing of a low concentration of a mixture of NNN plus NNK in water induces oral tumours in rats (Hoffman and Djordjevic 1997).

In vitro assays have shown that human buccal mucosa has the capability to metabolize NNK and NNN to alkyldiazohydroxides that can react with DNA as reviewed by Gupta *et al.* (1996). DNA adducts play a crucial role in tobacco-induced carcinogenesis and studies have demonstrated a positive correlation between DNA adduct levels and patient smoking status. Jones *et al.* (1993) have shown that the mean adduct levels in isolated oral tissue DNA from smokers were significantly higher than in non-smokers, and adduct levels in ex-smokers (1–12 years since cessation) were similar to those in non-smokers.

Studies have suggested that the p53 tumour suppressor gene is a likely target for tobacco carcinogens (Jones 1998; Ralhan *et al.* 1998; Saranath *et al.* 1999; Hsieh *et al.* 2001). p53 tumour suppressor gene mutations are the most frequently found genetic errors in oral cancer (Jones 1998). Brennan *et al.* (1995) have shown that p53 mutation were more common in tumours from patients who were exposed to both tobacco and alcohol than in tumours from patients who were not exposed to these risk factors. As discussed previously, genetic polymorphism of drug-metabolizing enzymes may affect the susceptibility to oral cancer from exposure to tobacco carcinogens.

Conclusion

In 1986 an IARC Working Party concluded that there was sufficient evidence that tobacco was carcinogenic to humans and that the occurrence of malignant tumours of the upper digestive tract was causally related to the smoking of different forms of tobacco. IARC has also concluded that there is sufficient evidence that oral use of snuff of the types commonly used in North America and western Europe is carcinogenic to humans, and there was sufficient evidence that the habit of chewing betel quid containing tobacco was carcinogenic in humans (IARC 1985). More recent epidemiological studies and experimental studies further support these conclusions. There is convincing evidence that a large attributable risk can be ascribed to the joint habits of cigarette smoking and alcohol consumption.

References

Akiba, S. and Hirayama, T. (1990). Cigarette smoking and cancer mortality risk in Japanese men and women—results from reanalysis of the Six-Prefecture Cohort Study data. *Environ Health Perspect*, **87**: 19–26.

Andre, K., Schraub, S., Mercier, M., and Bontemps, P. (1995). Role of alcohol and tobacco in the aetiology of head and neck cancer: A case-control study in the Doubs Region of France. *Oral Oncol, Eur J Cancer*, **31B**: 301–9.

Axell, T., Mornstad, H., and Sundstrom, B. (1978). Snuff and cancer of the oral cavity: A retrospective study. *Lakartidningen*, **75**: 1224–6.

Baron, A.E., Franceschi, S., Barra, S., Talamini, R., and La Vecchia, C. (1993). A comparison of the joint effects of alcohol and smoking on the risk of cancer across sites in the upper aerodigestive tract. *Cancer Epidemiol Biomark Prevent*, **2**: 519–23.

Bhargava, K., Smith, L.W., Mani, N.J., Silverman, S., Malaowalla, A.M., and Billimoria, K.F. (1975). A follow-up study of oral cancer and precancerous lesions in 57,518 industrial workers of Gujarat, India. *Indian J Cancer*, **12**: 124–32.

Blot, W.J., McLaughlin, J.K., Winn, D.M., Austin, D.F., Greenberg, R.S., Preston-Martin, S., *et al.* (1988). Smoking and drinking in relation to oral and pharyngeal cancer. *Cancer Res*, **48**: 3282–7.

Boffetta, P., Mashberg, A., Winkelmann, R., and Garfinkel, L. (1992). Carcinogenic effect of tobacco smoking and alcohol drinking on anatomic sites of the oral cavity and oropharynx. *Int J Cancer*, **52**: 530–33.

Boyle, P., Macfarlane, R., McGinn, R., Zheng, T., La Vecchia, C., Maisonneuve, P., and Scully, C. (1990a). International epidemiology of head and neck cancer. In: N. de Vries, and J.L. Gluckman (ed.) *Multiple Primary Tumors in the Head and Neck*, pp. 80–138. Thieme Medical Publishers, Inc.

Boyle, P., Macfarlane, G.J., Maisonneuve, P., Zheng, T., Scully, C., and Tedesco, B. (1990b). Epidemiology of mouth cancer in 1989. *J Royal Soc Med*, **83**: 724–729.

Boyle, P., La Vecchia, C., Maisonneuve, P., Zheng, T., and Macfarlane, G.J. (1995). Cancer epidemiology and prevention. In: U. Veronesi, M.J. Peckham, and R. Pinedo (ed.) *Oxford Textbook of Oncology*. Oxford University Press, Oxford.

Brenna, J.A., Boyle, J.O., Koch,W.M. (1995). Association between cigarette smoking and mutation of the p53 gene in squamous-cell carcinoma of the head and neck. *N Engl J Med*, **332**: 712–7.

Brunnemann, K.D. and Hoffmann, D. (1993). Chemical composition of smokeless tobacco products. Monograph 2. Smokeless tobacco or health: An international perspective. NIH publication No. 93-3461:96-1.5.

Brunnemann, K.D., Prokopczyk, B., Djordjevic, M.V., and Hoffmann, D. (1996). Formation and analysis of tobacco-specific N-nitrosamines. *Crit Rev Toxicol*, **26**: 121–37.

Bundgaard, T., Wildt, J., Frydenberg, M., Elbrond, O., and Nielsen, J.E. (1995). Case-control study of squamous cell cancer of the oral cavity in Denmark. *Cancer Causes Control*, **6**: 57–67.

Chyou, P.H., Momura, A.M.Y., and Stemmermann, G.N. (1995). Diet, alcohol, smoking and cancer of the upper aerodigestive tract: A prospective study among Hawaii Japanese men. *Int J Cancer*, **60**: 616–21.

Day, G.L., Blot, W.J., Shore, R.E., McLaughlin, J.K., Austin, D.F., and Greenberg, R.S. (1994). Second cancers following oral and pharyngeal cancers: Role of tobacco and alcohol. *JNC*, **86**: 131–7.

Day, G.L., Blot, W.J., Austin, D.F., Bernstein, L., Greenberg, R.S., Preston-Martin, S. *et al.* (1993). Racial differences in risk of oral and pharyngeal cancer: Alcohol, tobacco, and other determinants. *JNCI*, **85**: 465–73.

De Stefani, E., Boffetta, P., Oreggia, F., Fierro, L., and Mendilaharsu, M. (1998). Hard liquor drinking is associated with higher risk of cancer of the oral cavity and pharynx than wine drinking. A case-control study in Uruguay. *Oral Oncol*, **34**: 99–104.

Elwood, J.M., Pearson, J.C.G., Skippen, D.H., and Jackson, S.M. (1984). Alcohol, smoking, social and occupational factors. The aetiology of cancer of the oral cavity, pharynx and larynx. *Int J Cancer*, **34**: 603–12.

Franco, E.L., Kowalski, L.P., Oliveira, B.V., Curado, M.P., and Pereira, R.N. (1989). Risk factors for oral cancer in Brazil: A case-control study. *Int J Cancer*, **43**: 992–1000.

Franceschi, S., Levi, F., La Vecchia, C., Conti, E., Maso, L.D., Barzan, L. *et al.* (1999). Comparison of the effect of smoking and alcohol drinking between oral and pharyngeal cancer. *Int J Cancer*, **83**: 1–4.

Franceschi, S., Barra, S., La Vecchia, C., Bidoli, E., Negri, E., and Talamini, R. (1992). Risk factors for cancer of the tongue and the mouth. *Cancer*, **70**: 2227–33.

Franceschi, S., Talamini, R., Barra, S., Baron, A.E., Negri, E., Bidoli, E., *et al.* (1990). Smoking and drinking in relation to cancers of the oral cavity, pharynx, larynx, and esophagus in Northern Italy. *Cancer Res*, **50**: 6502–7.

Franceschi, S., Bidoli, E., Herrero, R., and Munoz, N. (2000). Comparison of cancers of the oral cavity and pharynx worldwide: Etiological clues. *Oral Oncol*, **36**: 106–15.

Garrote, L.F., Herrero, R., Reyes, R.O., Vaccarella, S., Anta, J.L., Ferbeye, L. *et al.* (2001). Risk factors for cancer of the oral cavity and oro-pharynx in Cuba. *Br J Cancer*, **85**: 46–54.

Geisler, S.A. and Olshan, A.F. (2001). GSTM1, GSTT1, and the risk of squamous cell carcinoma of the head and neck: A Mini-HuGE review. *Am J Epidemiol*, **154**: 95–105.

Grasso, P. and Mann, A.H. (1998). Smokeless tobacco and oral cancer: An assessment of evidence derived from laboratory animals. *Food Chem Toxicol*, **36**: 1015–29.

Gupta, P.C., Murti, P.R., and Bhonsle, R.B. (1996). Epidemiology of cancer by tobacco products and the significance of TSNA. *Crit Review Toxicol*, **26**: 183–8.

Gupta, P.C., Mehta, F.S., Daftary, D.K., Pindborg, J.J., Bhonsle, R.B., Jalnawalla, P.N. *et al.* (1980). Incidence rates of oral cancer and natural history of oral precancerous lesions in a 10-year follow-up study of India villagers. *Community Dent Oral Epidemiol*, **8**: 287–93.

Hammond, E.C. and Seidman, H. (1980). Smoking and cancer in the United States. *Prevent Med*, **9**: 169–73.

Hayes, R.B., Bravo-Otero, E., Kleinman, D.V., Brown, L.M., Fraumeni, J.F., Jr., Harty L.C. *et al.* (1999). Tobacco and alcohol use and oral cancer in Puerto Rico. *Cancer Causes Control*, **10**: 27–33.

Hirayama, T. (1966). An epidemiological study of oral and pharyngeal cancer in Central and South- East Asia. *Bull WHO*, **34**: 41–69.

Hoffman, D., Brunnemann, K.D., Prokopczyk, B., and Djordjevic, M.V. (1994). Tobacco-specific N-nitrosamines and areca-derived N-nitrosamines: Chemistry, biochemistry, carcinogenicity, and relevance to humans. *J Toxicol Environ Hlth*, **41**: 1–52.

Hoffman, D. and Djordjevic, M.V. (1997). Chemical composition and carcinogenicity of smokeless tobacco. *Adv Dent Res*, **11**: 322–9.

Hsieh, L.L., Wang, P.F., Chen, I.H., Liao, C.T., Wang, H.M., Chen, M.C. *et al.* (2001). Characteristics of mutations in the p53 gene in oral squamous cell carcinoma associated with betel quid chewing and cigarette smoking in Taiwanese. *Carcinogenesis*, **22**: 1497–503.

Hung, H.C., Chuang, J., Chien, Y.C., Chern, H.D., Chiang, C.P., Kuo, Y.S. *et al.* (1997). Genetic polymorphisms of CYP2E1, GSTM1, and GSTT1, environmental factors and risk of oral cancer. *Cancer Epidemiol Biomark Prevent*, **6**: 901–5.

Idris, A.M., Ahmed, H.M., and Malik, M.O.A. (1995). Toomak dipping and cancer of the oral cavity in the Sudan: A case-control study. *Int J Cancer*, **63**: 477–80.

International Agency for Research on Cancer (1986).Monograph 38, Tobacco Smoking. International Agency for Research on Cancer, Lyon, France.

International Agency for Research on Cancer (1985). IARC monographs on the evaluation of the carcinogenic risk of chemicals to humans: Tobacco habits other than smoking: betel-quid and areca-nut chewing; and some related nitrosamines. Vol. 37, p. 116. International Agency for Research on Cancer, Lyon, France.

Jayant, K. and Deo, M.G. (1986). Oral cancer and cultural practices in relation to betel quid and tobacco chewing and smoking. *Cancer Detect Prevent*, **9**: 207–13.

Jayant, K., Balakrishnan,V., and Sanghvi, L.D. (1971). A note on the distribution of cancer in some endogamous groups in Western India. *Br J Cancer*, **25**: 611–9.

Johnson, N. (2001). Tobacco use and oral cancer: A global perspective. *J Dent Educat*, **65**: 328–39.

Jones, A. (1998). A general review of the p53 gene and oral squamous cell carcinoma. *Ann Roy Australas Coll Dent Surg*, **14**: 66–9.

Jones, N.J., McGregor, A.D., and Waters, R. (1993). Detection of DNA adducts in human oral tissue: Correlation of adduct levels with tobacco smoking and differential enhancement of adducts using the butanol extraction and nuclease P1 versions of 32p postlabeling. *Cancer Res*, **53**: 1522–8.

Jussawalla, D.J. and Deshpande,V.A. (1971). Evaluation of cancer risk in tobacco chewers and smokers: An epidemiologic assessment. *Cancer*, **28**: 244–52.

Kabat, G.C., Chang, C.J., and Wynder, E.L. (1994). The role of tobacco, alcohol use, and body mass index in oral and pharyngeal cancer. *Int J Epidemiol*, **23**: 1137–44.

Kabat, G.C., Hebert, J.R., and Wynder, E.L. (1989). Risk factors for oral cancer in women. *Cancer Res*, **49**: 2803–6.

La Vecchia, C., Franceschi, S., Bosetti, C., Levi, F., Talamini, R., and Negri, E. (1999). Time since stopping smoking and the risk of oral and pharyngeal cancers. *JNCI*, **91**: 726–7.

La Vecchia, C., Bosetti, C., Negri, E., Levi, F., and Franceschi, S. (1998). Cigar smoking and cancers of the upper digestive tract. *JNCI*, **90**: 1670.

La Vecchia, C., Bidoli, E., Barra, S., D'Avanzo, B., Negri, E., Talamini, R., *et al.* (1990). Type of cigarette and cancers of the upper digestive and respiratory tract. *Cancer Causes Control*, **1**: 69–74.

La Vecchia, C., Tavani, A., Franceschi, S., Levi, F., Corrao, G., and Negri, E. (1997). Epidemiology and prevention of oral cancer. *Oral Oncol*, **33**: 302–12.

Lewin, F., Norell, S.E., Johansson, H., Gustavsson, P., Wennerberg, J., Biorklund, A., Rutqvist, L.E. (1997). Smoking tobacco, oral snuff, and alcohol in the etiology of squamous cell carcinoma of the head and neck. *Cancer*, **82**: 1367–75.

London, S.J., Daly, A.K., Cooper, J., Navidi, W.C., Capenter, C., Idle, J.R. *et al.* (1995). Polymorphism of gluathione S-transferase M1 and lung cancer risk among African Americans and Caucasians in Los Angeles County, California. *JNCI*, **87**: 1246–53.

Macfarlane, G.J., Boyle, P., Evstifeeva, T.V., Robertson, C., and Scully, C. (1994). Rising trends of oral cancer mortality among males worldwide: The return of an old public health problem. *Cancer Causes Control*, **5**: 259–65.

Macfarlane, G.J., Zheng, T., Marshall, J.R., Boffetta, P., Niu, S., Brasure, J., *et al.* (1995). Alcohol, tobacco, diet and risk of oral cancer: A pooled analysis of three case-control studies. *Oral Oncol, Eur J Cancer*, **31B**: 181–7.

Marshall, J.R., Graham, S., Haughey, B.P., Shedd, D., O'Shea, R., Brasure, J., *et al.* (1992). Smoking, alcohol, dentition and diet in the epidemiology of oral cancer. *Oral Oncol, Eur J Cancer*, **28B**: 9–15.

Mashberg, A., Boffetta, P., Winkelman, R., and Garfinkel, L. (1993). Tobacco smoking, alcohol drinking, and cancer of the oral cavity and oropharynx among U.S. veterans. *Cancer*, **72**: 1360–75.

Merletti, F., Boffetta, P., Cicone, G., Msshberg, A., and Terracini, B. (1989). Role of tobacco and alcoholic beverages in the etiology of cancer of the oral cavity/oropharynx in Torino, Italy. *Cancer Res*, **49**: 4919–24.

Moreno-Lopez, L.A., Esparza-Gomez, G.C., Gonzalez-Navarro, A., Cerero-Lapiedra, R., Gonzalez-Henandez, M.J., and Dominguez-Rojas,V. (2000). Risk of oral cancer associated with tobacco smoking, alcohol consumption and oral hygiene: A case-control study in Madrid, Spain. *Oral Oncol*, **36**: 170–4.

Muscat, J.E., Richie, J.P., Thompson, S., and Wynder, E.L. (1996). Gender differences in smoking and risk for oral cancer. *Cancer Res*, **56**: 5192–7.

Nandakumar, A., Thimmasetty, K.T., Sreeramareddy, N.M., Venugopal, T.C., Rajanna, Vinutha, A. T. *et al.* (1990). A population-based case-control investigation on cancers of the oral cavity in Bangalore, India. *Br J Cancer*, **62**: 847–51.

Negri, E., La Vecchia, C., Franceschi, S., and Tavani, A. (1993). Attributable risk for oral cancer in Northern Italy. *Cancer Epidemiol Biomark Prevent*, **2**: 189093.

Nordgren, P. and Ramstrom, L. (1990). Moist snuff in Sweden: Tradition and evolution. *Br J Addict*, **85**: 1107–12.

Notani, P.N. (1988). Role of alcohol in cancers of the upper alimentary tract: Use of models in risk assessment. *J Epidemiol Commun Hlth*, **42**: 187–92.

Park, J.Y., Schantz, S.P., Stern, J.C., Kaur, T., and Lazarus, P. (1999). Association between glutathione S-transferase π genetic polymorphisms and oral cancer risk. *Pharmacogenetics*, **9**: 497–504.

Parkin, D.M., Pisani, P., and Masuyer, E. (2000). Tobacco-attributable cancer burden: a global review. In: R. Lu, J.Mackay, S. Niu, and R. Peto (ed.) *Tobacco: The Growing Epidemic*, Proceedings of the Tenth World Conference on Tobacco or Health, 24–28 August 1997. Springer-Verlag London Limited, Beijing, China. pages 81–84.

Ralhan, R., Nath, N., Agarwal, S., Mathur, M., Wasylyk, B., and Shukla, N.K. (1998). Circulating p53 antibodies as early markers of oral cancer: Correlation with p53 alterations. *Clin Cancer Res*, **4**: 2147–52.

Rao, D.N., Ganesh, B., Rao, R.S., and Desai, P.B. (1994). Risk assessment of tobacco, alcohol and diet in oral cancer—A case-control study. *Int J Cancer*, **58**: 469–73.

Rothman, K. and Keller, A. (1972). The effect of joint exposure to alcohol and tobacco on risk of cancer of the mouth and pharynx. *J Chron Dis*, **25**: 711–6.

Sanghvi, L.D., Rao, K.C.M., and Khanolkar,V.R. (1955). Smoking and chewing tobacco in relation to cancer of the upper alimentary tract. *BMJ*, **I**: 1111–4.

Saranath, D., Tandle, A.T., Teni, T.R., Dedhia, P.M., Borgens, A.M., Parikh, D. *et al.* (1999). p53 inactivation in chewing tobacco-induced oral cancers and leukoplakias from India. *Oral Oncol*, **35**: 242–50.

Sato, M., Sato, T., Izumo, T., and Amagasa, T. (2000). Genetically high susceptibility to oral squamous cell carcinoma in terms of combined genotyping of CYP1A1 and GSTM1 genes. *Oral Oncol*, **36**: 267–71.

Sato, M., Sato, T., Izumo, T., and Amagasa, T. (1999). Genetic polymorphism of drug-metabolizing enzymes and susceptibility to oral cancer. *Carcinogenesis*, **20**: 1927–31.

Schildt, E.B., Eriksson, M., Hardell, L., and Maonuson, A. (1998). Oral snuff, smoking habits and alcohol consumption in relation to oral cancer in a Swedish case-control study. *Int J Cancer*, **77**: 341–6.

Schlecht, N.F., Franco, E.L., Pintos, J., and Kowalski, L.P. (1999). Effect of smoking cessation and tobacco type on the risk of cancers of the upper aero-digestive tract in Brazil. *Epidemiology*, **10**: 412–8.

Schwartz, S.M., Daling, J.R., Doody, D.R., Wipf, G.C., Carter, J.J., Madeleine, M.M. *et al.* (1998). Oral cancer risk in relation to sexual history and evidence of human papillomavirus infection. *JNCI*, **90**: 1626–36.

Shanks, T.G. and Burns, D.M. (1998). Disease consequences of cigar smoking. Smoking and Tobacco Control Monograph 9 Cigars. Health effects and trends. Bethesda (MD), pp. 105–158. National Institutes of Health, Report No: DHHS Publ No. (NIH) 98-4302.

Shapiro, J.A., Jacobs, E.J., and Thun, M.J. (2000). Cigar smoking in men and risk of death from tobacco-related cancers. *JNCI*, **92**: 333–7.

Spitz, M.R., Fueger, J.J., Goepfert, H., Hong, W.K., and Newell, G.R. (1988). Squamous cell carcinoma of the upper aerodigestive tract. *Cancer*, **61**: 203–8.

Sterling, T.D., Rosenbaum,W.L., and Weinkam, J.J. (1992). Analysis of the relationship between smokeless tobacco and cancer based on data from the national mortality followback survey. *J Clin Epidemiol*, **42**: 223–31.

Talamini, R., Vaccarella, S., Barbone, F., Tavani, A., La Vecchia, C. *et al.* (2000). Oral hygiene, dentition, sexual habits and risk of oral cancer. *Br J Cancer*, **83**: 1238–42.

Talamini, R., Franceschi, S., Barra, S., and La Vecchia, C. (1990). The role of alcohol in oral and pharyngeal cancer in non-smokers and of tobacco in non-drinkers. *Int J Cancer*, **46**: 391–3.

Tuyns, A.J., Esteve, J., Raymond, L., Berrino, F., Benhamou, E., Blanchet, F. *et al.* (1988). Cancer of the larynx/hypopharynx, tobacco and alcohol: IARC International case-control study in Turin and Varese (Italy), Zaragoza and Navarra (Spain), Geneva (Switzerland) and Calvados (France). *Int J Cancer*, **41**: 483–91.

Vigneswaran, N., Dent, M., Tilashalski, K., Rodu, B., and Cole, P. (1995). Tobacco use and cancer. *Oral Surg Oral Med Oral Pathol Oral Radiol Endod*, **80**: 178–82.

Vogler, W.R., Lioyd, J.W., and Milmore, B.K. (1962). A retrospective study of etiological factors in cancer of the mouth, pharynx, and larynx. *Cancer*, **15**: 246–58.

Wahi, P.N., Kehar, U., and Lahiri, B. (1965). Factors influencing oral and oropharyngeal cancers in India. *Br J Cancer*, **19**: 642–60.

Weller, E.A., Blot,W.J., and Feigal, E. (1993). Oral cavity and pharynx. In: B.A. Hiller, L.A.G. Ries, B.F. Hankey, C.L. Kosary, A. Harras, S.S, Devesa, B.K. Edwards (ed.) *SEER Cancer Statistics Review: 1973–1990*, pp. XIX.1–15. National Cancer Institute. NIH Pub. No 932789.

Winn, D.M., Blot,W.J., Shy, C.M., Pickle, L.W., Toledo, A., and Fraumeni, J.F. Jr. (1981). *New Engl J Med*, **304**: 745–9.

Winn, D.M. (1988). Smokeless tobacco and cancer: The epidemiologic evdence. *CA-A Cancer J Clin*, **38**: 236–43.

Winn, D.M. (1997). Epidemiology of cancer and other systemic effects associated with the use of smokeless tobacco. *Adv Dent Res*, **11**: 313–21.

Wynder, E.L., Covey, L.S., Mabuchi, K., and Mushinski, M. (1976). Environmental factors in cancer of the larynx. *Cancer*, **38**: 1591–601.

Wynder, E.L., Hultberg, S., Jacobsson, F., and Bross, I.J. (1957). Environmental factors in cancer of the upper alimentary tract: A Swedish study with special reference to Plummer-Vinson (Paterson-Kelly) syndrome. *Cancer*, **10**: 470–87.

Zavras, A.I., Douglass, C.W., Joshipura, K., Wu, T., Laskaris, G., Petridou, E. *et al.* (2001). Smoking and alcohol in the etiology of oral cancer: Gender-specific risk profiles in the south of Greece. *Oral Oncol*, **37**: 28–35.

Zheng, T., Holford, T., Chen, Y., Jiang, P., Zhang, B., and Boyle, P. (1997). Risk of tongue cancer associated with tobacco smoking and alcohol consumption: A case-control study. *Oral Oncol*, **33**: 82–5.

Zheng, T., Boyle, P., Hu, H., Duan, J., Jiang, P.J., Ma, D.Q. *et al.* (1990). Tobacco smoking, alcohol consumption and risk of oral cancer: A case-control study in Beijing, People's Republic of China. *Cancer Causes Control*, **1**: 173–9.

Chapter 23

Smoking and stomach cancer

David Zaridze

Incidence and mortality from stomach cancer is declining practically in all countries. Nevertheless stomach cancer remains the second most common cause of death from cancer in the world, accounting for 700 000 cases annually. Incidence and mortality from stomach cancer are high in Japan, Korea, China, Russia, in Columbia, and other countries of South America, and are low in North America and Western Europe (Parkin *et al.* 2005). Decline in the incidence of stomach cancer is accompanied by increase in cancer of the gastric cardia (Devesa *et al.* 1998; Botterweck *et al.* 2000; Ward *et al.* 2006).

Helicobacter pylori infection is causally associated with stomach cancer (IARC 1994). It has been shown that type of food storage, namely the lack of refrigeration is a major risk factor for stomach cancer (World Cancer Research Fund 1997). Diets low in fruits and vegetables decrease the risk of stomach cancer (Nomura *et al.* 1990; Kabat *et al.* 1993; World Cancer Research Fund 1997; De Stefani *et al.* 1998; Terry *et al.* 1998; Mathew *et al.* 2000), while high salt intake has been claimed to increase the risk (Nomura *et al.* 1990; World Cancer Research Fund 1997). Alcohol consumption and especially consumption of liquors has been found to increase the risk of gastric cancer and especially cancer of the gastric cardia (Agudo *et al.* 1992; Kabat *et al.* 1993; Hansson *et al.* 1994; Gammon *et al.* 1997; De Stefani *et al.* 1998; Lagergren *et al.* 2000; Zaridze *et al.* 2000).

Smoking has been found to be associated with an increase in the risk of stomach cancer in many cohort and case-control studies reported from Asia, America, and Europe. The majority of cohort studies found a statistically significant association between smoking and the risk of stomach cancer, relative risks ranging from 1.4 to 3.0 in current-smokers. These studies include American Cancer Society study (Hammond 1966), US Veteran's cohort (Kahn 1966), Japanese cohort (Hirayma 1982), British doctors cohort study (Doll *et al.* 1994, 2005), cohort of male Japanese physicians (Kono *et al.* 1987), six prefecture study in Japan (Akiba and Hirayama 1990), cohort of American men of Japanese ancestry (Nomura *et al.* 1990, 1995), cohort of American men of Scandinavian and German descent (Kneller *et al.* 1991), cohort study of inhabitants of Aichi prefecture in Japan (Kato *et al.* 1992*a*), cohort of inhabitants of five areas of Norway (Tverdal *et al.* 1993), cardiovascular risk factor study from Iceland (Tulinius *et al.* 1997), cohort of residents of Taiwan (Liaw and Chen 1998), Cancer Prevention Study II (Chao *et al.* 2002), European prospective investigation into cancer (EPIC) (Gonzalez *et al.* 2003), cohort study of Korean men 30–95 years of age (Jee *et al.* 2004; Yun *et al.* 2005; Sung *et al.* 2007), Japanese collaborative cohort study (Fijino *et al.* 2005), longitudinal study of atomic bomb survivors in Hiroshima and Nagasaki (Sauvaget *et al.* 2005), nested case-control study of persons included in the General Practitioners Research Database in Sweden (Lindblad *et al.* 2005), cohort study of US participants (Freedman *et al.* 2007), prospective study in Nord-Trondelag County in Norway (Sjodal *et al.* 2007), Korean multi-centre cancer cohort study (Kim *et al.* 2007), Whitehall study (Batty *et al.* 2008), and Swedish constructive workers cohort (Zendehdel *et al.* 2008). In some cohort studies the increase in the risk associated with smoking was statistically not significant (Kato *et al.* 1992*b*; Guo *et al.* 1994;

Engeland *et al.* 1996; Yuan *et al.* 1996). Three studies did not find any association between smoking and stomach cancer (Chen *et al.* 1997; Nordlund *et al.* 1997; Terry *et al.* 1998).

In several of the positive cohort studies dose–response relationships were observed between intensity, and/or duration of smoking and the risk of cancer of the stomach. Statistically significant trends between number of cigarettes smoked per day and the risk of stomach cancer were observed in a 16-year follow-up report of Japanese six prefecture study (P for trend < 0.01) (Akiba and Hirayma 1982), a 26-year follow-up report of the cohort of US Veterans (P for trend < 0.01) (McLaughlin *et al.* 1995), in a 20-year follow-up report of the cohort of American men of Scandinavian and German origin (P for trend 0.01) (Kneller *et al.* 1991), in a 40- and 50-year follow-up report of the cohort of British doctors (P for trend < 0.01) (Doll *et al.* 1994, 2005), and in the cohort of inhabitants of Taiwan (P for trend < 0.06) (Liaw and Chen 1998). In Cancer Prevention Study II there was a statistically significant trend between number of cigarettes smoked per day and the risk of stomach cancer among current-smoking women (P for trend = 0.04) and among ex-smoker men (P for trend = 0.06) (Chao *et al.* 2002). The association between duration of smoking and the risk of stomach cancer were reported by Nomura *et al.* (1990), MacLaughlin *et al.* (1995), Liaw and Chen (1998), and Chao *et al.* (2002), with a statistically significant trend between number of years smoked and the increase in relative risk. Age of commencement of smoking was statistically significantly associated with the risk of stomach cancer in the cohort of American men of Japanese ancestry (P for trend < 0.0001) (Nomura *et al.* 1995), in the cohort of the inhabitants of Taiwan (P for trend < 0.02) (Liaw and Chen 1998), and among men in Cancer Prevention Study II (P for trend = 0.03) (Chao *et al.* 2002). Cumulative exposure to smoking expressed as number of pack-years of smoking has also been found to influence the risk of stomach cancer (Kneller *et al.* 1991; Chao *et al.* 2002). In Korean multi-centre cancer cohort significant dose–response relationships were observed between duration of smoking and risk of gastric cancer: men who smoked for 20–30 years had a 2.09-fold (95% CI 1.00–4.38) increase, and those who smoked more than 40 years had 3.13-fold (95% CI 1.59–6.17) increase in risk of gastric cancer (p for trend <0.01) (Kim *et al.* 2007). In cohort study conducted in Norway dose–response relationships were found with earlier age of initiation (p = 0.02), frequency (p = 0.00), and duration of smoking (p = 0.00) (Sjodahl *et al.* 2007). In pooled analysis of two population-based prospective cohort studies from Japan (Koizumi *et al.* 2004) higher number of cigarettes smoked per day among current-smokers was associated with a linear increase in the risk (p < 0.05).

In the systematic review of cohort studies addressing the relationship between smoking and gastric cancer 42 articles were considered (Ladeiras-Lopes *et al.* 2008). Comparing current-smoker with never-smokers the summary RR estimates were 1.62 (95% CI 1.50–1.75) in males and 1.20 (95% CI 1.01–1.43) in females; the relative risk increased from 1.3 for lowest consumption to 1.7 for the smoking of approximately 30 cigarettes per day.

Several cohort studies examined the effect of cessation on the risk of gastric cancer and found lower relative risk among former-smokers than in current-smokers (Kahn *et al.* 1966; Nomura *et al.* 1990, 1995; Kneller *et al.* 1991; Tverdal *et al.* 1993; McLaughlin *et al.* 1995; Engeland *et al.* 1996; Nordlund *et al.* 1997; Tulinius *et al.* 1997; Doll *et al.* 2005; Kouzumi *et al.* 2004; Fujino *et al.* 2005). In Cancer Prevention Study II there was a dose–response relationship between age-quit smoking (P for trend = 0.0015), number of years since smoking cessation (P for trend = 0.0015), and relative risk of gastric cancer (Chao *et al.* 2002).

It should be noted that in most if not all studies the cohorts were followed passively and the information on smoking habit of cohort members was based only on the inter-view at the initial survey, while many cohort members could change their smoking habit during the long follow-up period. Therefore, the risk of stomach cancer associated with smoking in these cohort studies could be underestimated due to misclassification of former-smokers as current-smokers.

About 50 case-control studies, both population-based and hospital-based, investigated the association between tobacco smoking and stomach cancer. In most studies relative risks were adjusted for different variables, such as sex, age, SES, education, income, diet, namely consumption of fruits and vegetables, alcohol consumption.

The majority of case-control studies reported a statistically significant increase in the risk of stomach cancer among smokers (Hoey *et al.* 1981; Correa *et al.* 1985; Risch *et al.* 1985; Hu *et al.* 1988; You *et al.* 1988; De Stefani *et al.* 1990; Kato *et al.* 1990; Lee *et al.* 1990; Wu-Williams *et al.* 1990; Dockerti *et al.* 1991; Saha 1991; Yu and Hsieh 1991; Hoshiyama and Sasaba 1992; Kabat *et al.* 1993; Hansson *et al.* 1994; Inoue *et al.* 1994; Siemiaticky *et al.* 1995; Yu *et al.* 1995; Gajalakshmi and Shanta 1996; Ji *et al.* 1996; Zhang *et al.* 1996; Gammon *et al.* 1997; De Stefani *et al.* 1998; Liu *et al.* 1998; Chow *et al.* 1999; Innoue *et al.* 1999; Ye *et al.* 1999; Lagergren *et al.* 2000; Mathew *et al.* 2000; Zaridze *et al.* 2000; Wu *et al.* 2001; Phukan *et al.* 2005; Crane *et al.* 2008).

In few case-control studies smoking was found not to have any influence on the risk of stomach cancer (Haenszel *et al.* 1972, 1976; Armijo *et al.* 1981; Jedrychowski *et al.* 1993; Buatti *et al.* 1989; Ferraroni *et al.* 1989; Boeing *et al.* 1991; Agudo *et al.* 1992; Guo *et al.* 1994; Mao *et al.* 2002; Hamada *et al.* 2002; Rao *et al.* 2005).

Statistically significant dose–response trend between number of cigarettes smoked per day and/or duration of smoking and/or age of commencement of smoking and/or pack-years smoked and the risk of gastric cancer was demonstrated in the studies of Hu *et al.* (1988), You *et al.* (1988), De Stefani *et al.* (1990), Kato *et al.* (1990), Lee *et al.* (1990), Wu-Williams *et al.* (1990), Yu and Hsieh (1991), Kabat *et al.* (1993), Hansson *et al.* (1994), Gajalakshmi and Shanta (1996), Ji *et al.* (1996), Zhang *et al.* (1996), Gammon *et al.* (1997), De Stefani *et al.* (1998), Liu *et al.* (1998), Ye *et al.* (1999), Lagergren *et al.* (2000), Mathew *et al.* (2000), Zaridze *et al.* (2000), Wu *et al.* (2001), and Phukan *et al.* (2005). For example, a population-based case-control study from China which included 1 124 stomach cancer cases and 1 452 community controls (Ji *et al.* 1996) showed statistically significant dose–response relationship between number of cigarettes smoked per day and risk of stomach cancer (*P* for trend = 0.0002), with highest risk observed in men who smoked 20–29 cigarettes per day (RR = 1.77, 95% CI 1.35–2.33); statistically significant trend in the risk was observed for duration of smoking (*P* for trend = 0.002), with highest risk seen in men who smoked for more than 40 years (RR = 1.64, 95% CI 1.21–2.24) and for cumulative lifelong exposure to smoking expressed as pack-years smoked (*P* for trend = 0.0002), with highest risk estimates in the highest exposure group (RR = 1.68, 95% CI 1.22–2.30). Statistically significant dose–response relationships between duration of smoking (*P* for trend < 0.001), pack-years smoked (*P* for trend < 0.001), age at start smoking (*P* for trend < 0.01), and relative risks of stomach cancer were observed in hospital-based case-control study from Uruguay which included 330 male cases and 622 controls drawn from the same hospitals as cases (De Stefani *et al.* 1998). In the population-based study in the United States (Gammon *et al.* 1997) statistically significant dose–response was observed for number of cigarettes smoked per day (*P* for trend < 0.05), duration of smoking in years (*P* for trend < 0.05), and cumulative exposure to tobacco smoke, or pack-years (*P* for trend <0.05).

Cessation of smoking affected the risk of cancer of the stomach. Risk was lower in ex-smokers than in current-smokers (Correa *et al.* 1985; De Stefani *et al.* 1990, 1998; Kato *et al.* 1990; Wu-Williams *et al.* 1990; Saha 1991; Kabat *et al.* 1993; Hansson *et al.* 1994; Inoue *et al.* 1994, 1999; Gammon *et al.* 1997; Gajalakshmi and Shanta 1996; Chow *et al.* 1999; Ye t al. 1999; Lagengren *et al.* 2000; Zaridze *et al.* 2000; Wu *et al.* 2001). In the population-based case-control study from Sweden which included 338 cases of stomach cancer and 678 community controls (Hansson *et al.* 1994), there was a statistically significant association between number of years since quitting and the risk of stomach cancer (*P* for trend = 0.02). In the study of De Stefani *et al.* (1998) relative risk of stomach cancer among men who gave up smoking 10–14 years ago was 1.0 (95% CI 0.5–2.1), while in those who gave up smoking 1–4 years ago the relative risk was 2.4 (95% CI 1.3–3.6), and in current-smokers it was 2.6 (95% CI 1.6–4.1). In the study reported by De Stefani *et al.* in 1990, quitting for more than ten years resulted in the decrease of relative risk (RR = 0.6, 95% CI 0.3–1.0) in comparison with individuals who gave up smoking 1–4 years ago (*P* for trend = 0.028).

Several case-control studies presented results separately for gastric cardia (or for adenocarcinoma of distal oesophagus and gastric cardia) and distal stomach (Wu-Williams *et al.* 1990; Kabat *et al.* 1993; Zhang *et al.* 1996; Gammond *et al.* 1997; De Stefani *et al.* 1998; Ye *et al.* 1999; Zaridze *et al.* 2000; Wu *et al.* 2001; Crane *et al.* 2008). In all these studies effects of smoking on the risk have been seen for cancers of both sites. In some studies association was somewhat stronger for distal stomach (Wu-Williams *et al.* 1990; Zhang *et al.* 1996; Wu *et al.* 2001; Crane *et al.* 2008), in others with cancer of the gastric cardia (Kabat *et al.* 1993; Zaridze *et al.* 2000). Dose–response relationship was observed between number of cigarettes smoked per day, duration of smoking, pack-years of smoking, age started smoking, and the risk of cancer of the gastric cardia (Zhang *et al.* 1996; Gammon *et al.* 1997; De Stefani *et al.* 1998; Ye *et al.* 1999; Zaridze *et al.* 2000; Wu *et al.* 2001), and distal stomach (Zhang *et al.* 1996; Gammon *et al.* 1997; De Stefani *et al.* 1998; Wu *et al.* 2001). Case-control study from Sweden reported similar trends in relative risk of stomach cancer related to number of cigarettes smoked per day – for cancer of the distal stomach (*P* for trend = 0.005) and gastric cardia (*P* for trend = 0.04), duration of smoking – for cancer of the distal stomach (*P* for trend = 0.002) and gastric cardia (*P* for trend = 0.03) (Lagergren *et al.* 2000)

Smoking cessation significantly decreased the risk of cancer of gastric cardia. In a population-based case-control study reported from Sweden which included 262 cases of cancer of gastric cardia and 820 community controls, the increase in number of years since smoking cessation was associated with statistically significant decrease in the risk (*P* for trend < 0.0001). Those individuals who gave up smoking for more than 25 years had relative risk of 1.9 (95% CI 1.1–3.1), while those who quit 0–2 years ago had relative risk of 4.2 (95% CI 2.8–6.4) (Lagergren *et al.* 2000). Similar trend was observed by Wu *et al.* (2001), both for cancer of gastric cardia (*P* for trend < 0.0002) and cancer of the distal stomach (*P* for trend < 0.002).

Significant association between smoking and risk persisted when relative risks were computed separately for intestinal and diffuse types of stomach cancer (Kato *et al.* 1990; Ye *et al.* 1999).

Number of cases of stomach cancer in women was generally small and the increases in risks associated with smoking were less than for men and statistically not significant (Kato *et al.* 1990; Ji *et al.* 1996; Zaridze *et al.* 2000). However, in the studies where sufficient number of cases of stomach cancer in women were included the size of relative risks were comparable with relative risk in men. For example, in the study from Japan which included 995 cases of stomach cancer of which 344 were women showed statistically significant increase in relative risk among current-smoking women (RR = 1.74, 95% CI 1.28–2.36). Risk estimates were higher in women in the age of 60 years or more (RR = 1.99, 95% CI 1.24–3.21) (Innoue *et al.* 1994). In the study of Kabat *et al.* (1993) current-smoking women were at increased risk of adenocarcinoma of distal oesophagus and the gastric cardia (RR = 4.8, 95% CI 1.7–5.4) and cancer of the distal stomach (RR = 4.8, 95% CI 1.9–11.9). Highest relative risks were for those women who smoked for more than 21 years. Ever-smoking Polish women were also at increased risk of stomach cancer (RR = 1.8, 95% CI 1.1–3.0) (Chow *et al.* 1999). Risk was increased in current-smokers (RR = 1.8, 95% CI 1.0–3.3), as well as in former-smokers (RR = 1.8, 95% CI 0.9–3.7).

Of special interest is the mortality-based case-control study carried out in China (Liu *et al.* 1998). In this study 27 710 deaths (20 195 men and 7 515 women) from stomach cancer were identified. The reference group included individuals who died from causes not related to smoking. Information on smoking habit was obtained from proxy interviews. It has been shown that in men smoking increases the risk of stomach cancer by 30%, while current-smoking in women was associated with only 17% increase in the risk. According to this study 18% of death from stomach cancer in Chinese men and only 1.7% in women could be attributed to smoking. These figures reflect present not very high smoking rates in Chinese, specially in Chinese women, which unfortunately inevitably will rise. Similar trends will be seen in other countries, where smoking epidemics in women have not yet reached its maximum. Increase in smoking rates in women will be followed by rise of smoking-related relative risks of cancers, including stomach cancer and proportion of death attributable to smoking.

Diet and alcohol consumption, all associated with the risk of stomach cancer could be major confounding factors of the effect of smoking on the risk of cancer of this site. However, adjustment for alcohol drinking (De Stefani *et al.* 1990; Yu and Hsieh 1991; Kabat *et al.* 1993; Ji *et al.* 1996; Simieticky *et al.* 1995; Zhang *et al.* 1996; Gammon *et al.* 1997; De Stefani *et al.* 1998; Innoue *et al.* 1999; Ye *et al.* 1999; Lagergren *et al.* 2000; Zaridze *et al.* 2000), as well as for consumption of fresh fruits and vegetables (De Stefani *et al.* 1990; Yu and Hsieh 1991; Inoue *et al.* 1994; Semiaticki *et al.* 1995; Gajalakshmi and Shanta 1996; De Stefani *et al.* 1998; Innoue *et al.* 1999; Lagergren *et al.* 2000), did not materially effect the risk estimates associated with smoking.

Positive association between smoking and the risk of stomach cancer could be confounded by the effect of *H. pylori* infection status. A large body of evidence supports a causative role for *H. pylori* in stomach cancer. In 1994, IARC recognized *H. pylori* as a class 1 human carcinogen (IARC 1994). Several surveys have shown that *H. pylori* infection status is not associated with the smoking habit. Limburg *et al.* (2001) examined association between seropositivity for *H. pylori* with different risk factors in Linxian prospective study. The proportion of seropositive individuals was similar in non-smokers (58%) and in smokers (61%). Moreover, the prevalence of CagA seropositive individuals was higher in non-smokers (32%), than in smokers (24%). Another study in China looked at association between prevalence of *H. pylori* infection and smoking, drinking, and diet. Prevalence of *H. pylori* positivity was higher among never-smokers, relative risk for ever smoking being 0.9 (0.7–1.0). In highest category of smokers of more than 14 235 pack-years OR was 0.8 (0.6–1.1) (Brown *et al.* 2002). Similar evidence is observed in Europe. Prevalence of seropositive subjects is similar among never (50.9%), former (48.7%), and current-smokers (45.1%). In fact, among never-smokers proportion of *H. pylori* seropositives is somewhat higher than among current-smokers (OR = 0.8, CI 0.7–0.9) (The Eurogast Study Group 1993). In only one study conducted in north England smoking of more than 35 cigarettes/day turned to be associated with higher risk of *H. pylori* positivity. However, it should be noted that the proportion of subjects infected were identical in all lower smoking intensity categories. Overall there is no association between *H. pylori* infection status and smoking (Moaygedy *et al.* 2002).

Zaridze *et al.* (2000) computed the interaction between *H. pylori* seropositivity and smoking in relation to the risk of stomach cancer. *H. pylori* infection did not affect significantly smoking-associated risk of stomach cancer. However, relative risk of stomach cancer was higher among *H. pylori* positive men. Similar results were obtained by Siman *et al.* (2001). The results of these analyses suggest that smoking potentiates the effect of *H. pylori* infection on the risk of stomach cancer.

In the recently published prospective study of 17 071 men 40+ years of age followed for 14 years on the risk of stomach cancer was significantly higher in those men who smoked and were *H. pylori* positive compared with those who did not have both risk factors (OR 11.41, 95% CI 1.54–84.67), while OR for highest category of tobacco consumption not stratified by *H. pylori* status was 1.88 (95% CI 1.02–3.43) (Shikata *et al.* (2008).

Camargo *et al.* (2007) examined the effect of smoking on failure of *H. pylori* therapy in Columbia. Multivariate logistic regression showed that smokers had a two-fold higher probability of failure in *H. pylori* eradication than non-smokers (OR 2.00, 95% CI 1.01–3.95).

The relative risk of gastric cancer associated with smoking is most probably underestimated in hospital-based case-control studies, due to substantial proportion of patient with smoking-related diseases in control groups. Of special concern are the studies in which prevalence of smoking was higher in controls than in cases and in which controls with smoking-associated diseases were recruited (Jedrychowski *et al.* 1986; Lee *et al.* 1990; Boeing *et al.* 1991; Agudo *et al.* 1992).

According to the widely accepted model of gastric carcinogenesis development of cancer in stomach is preceded by several stages, including chronic atrophic gastritis, intestinal metaplasia, and dysplasia. Relative risk of developing these lesions have been shown to be associated with smoking. Risk of both metaplasia ($P = 0.03$) and dysplasia ($P < 0.001$) increased significantly with increasing tobacco consumption, but the magnitude of association was much stronger for dysplasia. The odds ratio for dysplasia among heavy smokers (> 20 cigarettes/day) compared with lifelong non-smokers exceeded two and was statistically significant (OR = 2.2, 95% CI 1.5–3.3). The risks of metaplasia and dysplasia also increased with increasing duration of smoking. P values for trend were 0.02 and < 0.001 for metaplasia and dysplasia, respectively. The risk of dysplasia also rose with increasing pack-years of smoking (Kneller *et al.* 1992). You *et al.* (2000) assessed the effect of smoking on progression of gastric precursor lesions to dysplasia and cancer. Smoking duration for more than 25 years was associated with significant increase in the risk of progression to gastric cancer and dysplasia (OR = 1.6, 95% CI 1.0–2.1; P for trend = 0.04). The risk was also increased in those who smoked more than 20 cigarettes/day (OR = 1.4 95% CI 0.9–2.3).

Few studies have reported on cigar, pipe, or smokeless tobacco use in relation to stomach cancer. In most recent analyses of CPS II cohort, current-smokers of exclusively cigars had significantly higher stomach cancer mortality than non-users of any tobacco (OR = 2.29, CI 1.49–3.41) (Chao *et al.* 2002). In a cohort study of American men of German and Scandinavian origin regular pipe users were at very high risk (RR = 4.4, CI 1.84–10.72). Relative risk remained marginally significant after stratification for pack-years of cigarette smoking (RR = 2.3, CI 0.98–5.22). In case-control studies reported by Correa *et al.* (1985), Wu-Williams *et al.* (1990), and Lagergren *et al.* (2000) significant association between cigar and/or pipe smoking and risk of stomach cancer was observed. In case-control study conducted in India smoking of bidi (RR = 3.3, CI 1.8–5.67) and chutta (RR = 2.4, CI 1.18–4.93) was associated with statistically significant increase in the risk of gastric cancer, with dose–response relationship between intensity and duration of smoking and relative risk (Gajalakshmi and Shanta 1996). Chewing tobacco increased risk of stomach cancer in cohort study reported from America by Kneller *et al.* (1991). However after adjusting for cigarette smoking increase in the risk lost statistical significance. The early Swedish studies reported no association between snus (snuff) dipping and stomach cancer incidence (Hansson *et al.* 1994; Ye *et al.* 1999; Lagergren *et al.* 2000), while the recently published retrospective cohort study of Swedish construction workers observed excess risks for oesophageal squamous cell carcinoma (RR = 3.5, 95% CI 1.6–7.6) and non-cardia gastric cancer (RR = 1.4, 95% CI 1.1–1.9) among snus users who never smoked (Zendehdel *et al.* 2008).

Worldwide, it has been estimated that the smoking-attributable proportion of stomach cancer is 11% among men and 4% among women in developing countries, and 17% among men and 11% among women in developed countries (Tredaniel *et al.* 1997). According to Liu *et al.* (1998) 18% death from stomach cancer in men and 1.8% in women in China are caused by smoking. The proportion of incident cases of stomach cancer attributable to smoking has been estimated to be 20% in Poland (Chow *et al.* 1999) and 31% in India (Gajalakshmi and Shanta (1996). In the United States, 28% of stomach cancer death in men and 14% in women are attributable to tobacco smoking (Chao *et al.* 2002). According to estimates of Siemieticky *et al.* (1995) smoking causes 35% of incidence cases of stomach cancer in the United States. Adding stomach cancer to the list of cancers caused by smoking would increase the total number of smoking-attributable death by at least 84 000 per year worldwide (Tredaniel *et al.* 1997) not accounting for recent increases in smoking prevalence or the expected rise in stomach cancer incidence due to ageing in the developing world.

In summary, the existing scientific evidence suggests a causal association between smoking and stomach cancer.

References

Agudo, A., Gonzalez, C.A., Marcos, G., Sanz, M., Saigi, E., Verge, J. *et al.* (1992). Consumption of alcohol, coffee, and tobacco, and gastric cancer in Spain. *Cancer Causes Control*, **3**: 137–43.

Akiba, S. and Hirayama, T. (1990). Cigarette smoking and cancer mortality risk in Japanese men and women – results from reanalysis of the six-prefecture cohort study data. *Environ. Health Perspect*, **87**: 19–26.

Armijo, R., Orellana, M., Medina, E., Coulson, A.H., Sayre, J.W., and Detels, R. (1981). Epidemiology of gastric cancer in Chile: Case-control study. *Int. J. Epidemiol*, **10**: 53–6.

Batty, G.D., Kivimaki, M., Gray L., Smith, G.D., Marmot, M.G., and Shipley, M.J. (2008). Cigarette smoking and site-specific cancer mortality: testing uncertain associations using extended follow-up of the original Whitehall study. *Ann. Oncol*, **19**: 996–1002.

Boeing, H., Frentzel-Beyme, R., Berger, M., Berdt, V., Gores, W., Korner, M. *et al.* (1991). Case-control study on stomach cancer in Germany. *Int. J. Cancer*, **47**: 858–64.

Botterweck, A.A., Schouten, L.J., Volovics, A., Dorant, E., and van Den Brandt, P.A. (2000). Trends in incidence of adenocarcinoma of the oesophagus and gastric cardia in ten European countries. *Int. J. Epidemiol*, **29**, (4): 645–54.

Brown, L.M., Thomas, T.L., Ma, J., Chang, Y., You, W., Liu, W. *et al.* (2002). Helicobacter pylori infection in rural China: demographic, lifestyle and environmental factors. *Int. J. Epidemiol*, **31**: 638–46.

Buiatti, E., Palli, D., Decarli, A., Amadori, D., Avellini, C., Bianchi, S. *et al.* (1989). A case-control study of gastric cancer and diet in Italy. *Int. J. Cancer*, **44**: 611–6.

Camargo, M.C., Piazuelo M.B., Mera, R.M., Fontham, E.T., Delgado, A.G. *et al.* (2007). Effect of smoking on failure of H. pylori therapy and gastric histology in a high gastric cancer risk area of Colomdia. *Acta Gastroenterol Latinoam*, **37**: 238–45.

Chao, A., Thun, M.J., Henley, S.J., Jacobs, E.J., McCullough, M.L., and Calle, E.E. (2002). Cigarette smoking, use of other tobacco products and stomach cancer in US adults: the cancer prevention study II. *Int. J. Cancer*, **101**: 380–9.

Chen, Z.M., Xu, Z., Collins, R., Li, W.X., and Peto, R. (1997). Early health effects of the emerging tobacco epidemic in China: a 16-year prospective study. *J. Am. Med. Assoc*, **278**: 1500–04.

Chow, W.H., Swanson, C.A., Lissowska, J., Groves, F.D., Sobin, L.H., Nasierowska-Guttmejer, A. *et al.* (1999). Risk of stomach cancer in relation to consumption of cigarettes, alcohol, tea and coffee in Warsaw, Poland. *Int. J. Cancer*, **81**: 871–6.

Correa, P., Fontham, E., Pickle, L.W., Chen, V., Lin, Y., and Haenszel, W. (1985). Dietary determinants of gastric cancer in South Louisiana. *J. Natl. Cancer Inst*, **75**: 645–54.

Crane S.J., Locke G.R., III, Harmsen, W.S., Diehl, N.N., Zinsmeister, A.R., Melton, L.J., III, *et al.* (2008). Subsite-specific risk factors for esophageal and gastric adenocarcinoma. *Am. J. Gastroenterol*, **102**: 1596–602.

De Stefani, E., Boffetta, P., Carzoglio, J., Mendilaharsu, S., and Deneo-Pellegrini, H. (1998). Tobacco smoking and alcohol drinking as risk factors for stomach cancer: a case-control study in Uruguay. *Cancer Causes Control*, **9**: 321–9.

De Stefani, E., Correa, P., Fierro, L., Carzoglio, J., Deneo-Pellegrini, H., and Zavala, D. (1990). Alcohol drinking and tobacco smoking in gastric cancer. A case-control study. *Rev. Epidemiol. Santé Publique*, **38**: 297–307.

Devesa, S.S., Blot, W.J., and Fraumeni J.F. Jr. (1998). Changing patterns in the incidence of esophageal cancer and gastric carcinoma in the United States. *Cancer*, **83**: 2049–53.

Dockerty, J.D., Marshall, S., Fraser, J., and Pearce, N. (1991). Stomach cancer in New Zealand: time trends, ethnic group differences and a cancer registry-based case-control study. *Int. J. Epidemiol*, **20**: 45–53.

Doll, R., Peto, R., Wheatey, K., Gray, R., and Sutherland, E. (1994). Mortality in relation to smoking: 40 years' observation on male British doctors. *Br. Med. J*, **309**: 901–12.

Doll. R., Peto. R., Boreham. J., and Sutherland, I. (2005). Mortality from cancer in relation to smoking: 50 years observation on British doctors. *Br. J. Cancer*, **92**: 426–9.

Engeland, A., Andersen, A., Haldorsen, T., Tretli, S. (1996). Smoking habits and risk of cancers other than lung cancer: 28 years' follow-up of 26 000 Norwegian men and women. *Cancer Causes Control*, 7: 497–506.

Ferraroni, M., Negri, E., La Vecchia, C., D'Avanzo, X., and Franceschi, S. (1989). Socioeconomic indicators, tobacco and alcohol in the aetiology of digestive tract neoplasms. *Int. J. Epidemiol*, **18**: 556–62.

Freedman, N.D., Abnet, C.C., Leitzmann, M.F., Mouv, T., Subar, A.F., Hollenbeck, A.R. et al. (2007). A prospective study tobacco, alcohol, and the risk of esophageal and gastric cancer subtypes. *Am. J. Epidemiol*, **165**: 1424–33.

Fujino, Y., Mizoue, T., Tokui, N., Kikuchi, S., Hoshiyama, Y., Toyoshima, H., et al. (2005). Cigarette smoking and mortality due to stomach cancer: findings from the JACC Study. *J. Epidemiol*, **15**Suppl 2: S 113–9.

Gajalakshmi, C.K. and Shanta, V. (1996). Lifestyle and risk of stomach cancer: a hospital-based case-control study. *Int. J. Epidemiol*, **25**: 1146–53.

Gammon, M.D., Schoenberg, J.B., Ahsan, H., Risch, H.A., Vaughan, T.L., Chow, W.H. et al. (1997). Tobacco, alcohol, and socioeconomic status and adenocarcinomas of the esophagus and gastric cardia. *J. Natl. Cancer Inst*, **89**: 1277–84.

Gonzales, C.A., Pera, G., Agudo, A., Palli, D., Krogh, V., Vineis, P. et al. (2003). Smoking and the risk of gastric cancer in Europe. Prospective Investigation into Cancer and Nutrition (EPIC). *Int. J. Cancer*, **20**, **107**: 629–34.

Guo, W., Blot, W.J., Li, J.Y., Taylor, P.R., Liu, B.Q., Wang, W. et al. (1994). A nested case-control study of oesophageal and stomach cancers in the Linxian Nutrition Intervention Trial. *Int. J. Epidemiol*, **23**: 444–50.

Haenszel, W., Kurihara, M., Segi, M., and Lee, R.K.C. (1972). Stomach cancer among Japanese in Hawaii. *J. Natl. Cancer Inst*, **49**: 968–88.

Haenszel, W., Kurihara, M., Locke, F.B., Shimuzu, X., and Segi, M. (1976). Stomach cancer in Japan. *J. Natl. Cancer Inst*, **56**: 265–78.

Hamada, G.S., Kowalski, L.P., Nishimoto, I.N., Rodrigues, J.J., Iriya, K. et al. (2002). Sao Paulo–Japan Cancer Project Gastric Cancer Study Group. Risk factors for stomach cancer in Brazil(II): a case control study among Japanese Brazilians in Sao Paulo. *Jpn. J. Clin. Oncol*, **32**: 275–6.

Hammond, E.C. (1966). Smoking in relation to the death rates of one million men and women. *Natl. Cancer Inst. Monogr*, **19**: 127–204.

Hansson, L.E., Baron, J., Nyren, O., Bergstrom, R., Wolk, A., and Adami, H. (1994). Tobacco, alcohol and the risk of gastric cancer: a population-based case-control study in Sweden. *Int. J. Cancer*, **57**: 26–31.

Hirayma, T. (1982). Smoking and cancer in Japan. A prospective study on cancer epidemiology based on census population in Japan. Results of 13 years follow-up. In: S. Tominaga, and K. Aoki (ed.), *The UICC Smoking Control Workshop, Nagoya, Japan, 24–25 August 1981*. The University of Nagoya Press, Nagoya.

Hoey, J., Montvernay, C., and Lambert, R. (1981). Wine and tobacco: risk factors for gastric cancer in France. *Am. J. Epidemiol*, **113**: 668–74.

Hoshiyama, Y. and Sasaba, T. (1992). A case-control study of stomach cancer and its relation to diet, cigarettes, and alcohol consumption in Saitama Prefecture, Japan. *Cancer Causes Control*, 3: 441–8.

Hu, J.F., Zang, S., Jia, E., Wang, Q., Liu, S., Liu, Y. et al. (1988). Diet and cancer of the stomach: case-control study in China. *Int. J. Cancer*, **41**: 331–5.

IARC Monographs on the evaluation of carcinogenic risks to humans (1994). Schistosomes, liver flukes and Helicobacter pylori, Vol. 61, pp. 177–241, IARC, Lyon.

Inoue, M., Tajima, K., Hirose, K., Kuroishi, T., Gao, C. M., and Kitoh, T. (1994). Life-style and subsite of gastric cancer – Joint effect of smoking and drinking habits. *Int. J. Cancer*, **56**: 494–9.

Inoue, M., Tajima, K., Yamamura, Y., Hamajima, N., Hirose, K., Nakamura, S. *et al.* (1999). Influence of habitual smoking on gastric cancer by histologic subtype. *Int. J. Cancer*, **81**: 39–43.

Jee, S.H., Samet, J.M., Ohrr, H., Kim, J.H., and Kim, I.S. (2004). Smoking and cancer risk in Korean men and women. *Cancer Causes Control*, **15**: 341–8.

Jedrychowski, W., Boeing, H., Wahrendorf, J., Popila, T., Tobiasz-Adamczyk, B., and Kulig, J. (1993). Vodka consumption, tobacco smoking and risk of gastric cancer in Poland. *Int. J. Epidemiol*, **22**: 606–13.

Ji, B.T., Chow, W.H., Yang, G., McLaughlin, J.K., Gao, R.N., Zheng, W. *et al.* (1996). The influence of cigarette smoking, alcohol, and green tea consumption on the risk of carcinoma of the cardia and distal stomach in Shanghai. *China. Cancer*, **77**: 2449–57.

Kabat, G.C., Ng, S.K., and Wynder, E.L. (1993). Tobacco, alcohol intake, and diet in relation to adenocarcinoma of the esophagus and gastric cardia. *Cancer Causes Control*, **4**: 123–32.

Kahn, H.A. (1966). The Dorn study of smoking and mortality among US veterans: report of eight and one-half years of observation. *Natl. Cancer Inst. Monogr*, **19**: 1–125.

Kato, I., Tominaga, S., Ito, Y., Kobayshi, S., Yoshii, Y., and Matsuura, A. (1990). A comparative case-control analysis of stomach cancer and atrophic gastritis. *Cancer Res*, **50**: 6559–64.

Kato, I., Tominaga, S., and Matsumoto, K. (1992a). A prospective study of stomach cancer among a rural Japanese population: a 6-year survey. *Jpn. J. Cancer Res*, **83**: 568–75.

Kato, I., Tominaga, S., Ito, Y., Kobayashi, S., Yoshii, Y., Matsuura, A. *et al.* (1992b). A prospective study of atrophic gastritis and stomach cancer risk. *Jpn. J. Cancer Res*, **83**: 1137–42.

Kim, Y., Shin, A., Gwack, J., Jun, J.K., Park, S.K., Kang, D. *et al.* (2007). Cigarette smoking and gastric cancer risk in a community-based cohort study in Korea. *J. Prev. Med. Public. Health*, **40**: 467–74.

Kneller, R.W., McLaughlin, J.K., Bjelke, E., Schuman, L.M., Blot, W.J., Wacholder, S. *et al.* (1991). A cohort study of stomach cancer in a high-risk American population. *Cancer*, **68**: 672–8.

Kneller, R.W., You, W.C., Chang, Y.S., Liu, W.D., Zhang, L., Zhao, L. *et al.* (1992). Cigarette smoking and other risk factors for progression of precancerous stomach lesions. *J. Natl Cancer Inst*, **84**: 1261–6.

Koizumi, Y., Tsubono, Y., Nakaya, N., Kuriyama, S., Shibuya, D., Matsuoka, H. *et al.* (2004). Cigarette smoking and the risk of gastric cancer: a pooled analysis of two prospective studies in Japan. *Int. J. Cancer*, **112**: 1049–55.

Kono, S., Ikeda, M., Tokudome, M., and Keratsune, M. (1987). Cigarette smoking, alcohol consumption and mortality: a cohort study of male Japanese physicians. *Jpn. J. Cancer Res*, **78**: 1323–8.

Ladeiras-Lopes, R., Pereira, A.K., Nogueira, A., Pinheiro-Torres, T., Pinto, I., Santos-Pereira, R. *et al.* (2008). Smoking and gastric cancer: systematic review and meta-analysis of cohort studies. *Cancer Causes Control*, **19**: 689–701.

Lagergren, J., Bergstrom, R., Lindgren, A., and Nyren, O. (2000). The role of tobacco, snuff and alcohol use in the aetiology of cancer of the oesophagus and gastric cardia. *Int. J. Cancer*, **85**: 340–6.

Lee, H.H., Wu, H.Y., Chuang, Y.C., Chang, A.S., Chao, H.H., Chen, K.Y. *et al.* (1990). Epidemiologic characteristics and multiple risk factors of stomach cancer in Taiwan. *Anticancer Res*, **10**: 875–8.

Liaw, K.M. and Chen, C.J. (1998). Mortality attributable to cigarette smoking in Taiwan: a 12-year follow-up study. *Tob. Control*, **7**: 141–8.

Lindblad, M., Rodriguez, L.A., and Lagergren, J. (2005). Bode mass, tobacco and alcohol and risk of esophageal, gastric cardia, and gastric non-cardia, adenocarcinoma among men women in a nested case-control study. *Cancer Causes Control*, **16**: 285–94.

Linburg, P.J., Qiao, Y., Mark, S.D., Wang, G., Perez-Perez, G.I., Blaser, M.J. *et al.* (2001). Helicobacter pylori seropositivity and subsite specific gastric cancer risks in Linxian, China. *J. Natl. Cancer Inst*, **93**: 226–33.

Liu, B.Q., Peto, R., Chen, Z.M., Boreham, J., Wu, Y.P., Li, J.Y. *et al.* (1998). Emerging tobacco hazards in China: 1 Retrospective proportional mortality study of one million death. *BMJ*, **317**: 1411–22.

Mathew, A., Gangadharan, P., Vargese, C., and Nair, M.K. (2000). Diet and stomach cancer: case-control study in South India. *Eur. J. Cancer Prev*, **9**: 89–97.

McLaughlin, J.K., Hrubec, Z., Blot, W.J., and Fraumeni, J.F. (1995). Smoking and cancer mortality among US veterans: a 26-year follow-up. *Int. J. Cancer*, **60**: 190–3.

Moaygedi, P., Axon A.T.N., Feltbower, R., Duffet S., Crocombe, W., Braunholtz, D. *et al.* (2002). For the Leeds HELP Study Group. Relation of adult lifestyle and socioeconomic factors to the prevalence of Helicobacter pylori infection. *Int. J. Epidemiol*, **31**: 624–31.

Nomura, A., Grove, J.S., Stemmermann, G.N., and Severson, R.K. (1990). A prospective study of stomach cancer and its relation to diet, cigarettes, and alcohol consumption. *Cancer Res*, **50**: 627–31.

Nomura, A.M., Stemmermann, G.N., and Chyou, P.H. (1995). Gastric cancer among the Japanese in Hawaii. *Jpn. J. Cancer Res*, **86**: 916–23.

Nordlund, L.A., Carstensen, J.M., and Pershagen, G. (1997). Cancer incidence in female smokers: a 26-year follow-up. *Int. J. Cancer*, **73**: 625–8.

Parkin, D.M., Bray, F., Ferlay, J., and Pisani, P. (2005). Global cancer statistics, 2002. *CA Cancer J. Clin*, **55**: 74–108.

Phukan, R.K., Zomavie, E., Narain, K., Hazarica, N.C., and Mahanta, J. (2005). Tobacco use and stomach cancer in Mizoram, India. *Cancer Epidemiol Biomarkes Prev*, **14**: 1892–6.

Rao, D.H., Ganesh, B., Dinshaw, K.A., and Mohandas, K.M. (2002). A case-control study of stomach cancer in Mumbai, India. *Int. J. Cancer*, **99**: 727–31.

Risch, H.A., Jain, M., Choi, N.W., Fodor, J.G., Pfeffer, C.L., Howe, G.R. *et al.* (1985). Dietary factors and incidence of cancer of the stomach. *Am.J.Epidemiol*, **122**: 947–59.

Saha, S. K. (1991). Smoking habits and carcinoma of the stomach: a case-control study. *Jpn. J. Cancer Res*, **82**: 497–502.

Sauvaget, C., Lagarde. F., Nagano, J., Soda, M., Koyama, K., and Kodama, K. (2005). Lifestyle factors, radiation and gastric cancer in atomic-bomb survivors (Japan). *Cancer Causes Control*, **16**: 773–80.

Shikata, K., Doi, Y., Yonemoto, K., Arima, H., Ninomiya, T., Kubo, *et al.* (2008). Population-based prospective study of the combined influence of cigarette smoking and Helicobacter pylori infection on gastric cancer incidence: the Hisayama Study. *Am. J. Epidemiol*, **168**: 1409–15.

Siemiatycki, J., Krewski, D., Franco, E., and Kaiserman, M. (1995). Association between cigarette smoking and each of 21 types of cancer: a multi-site case-control study. *Int. J. Epidemiol*, **24**: 504–14.

Siman, J.H., Forsgren, A., Berglund, G., and Floren, C.H. (2001). Tobacco smoking increases the risk for gastric adenocarcinoma among Helicobacter pylori-infected individuals. *Scand. J. Gastroenterol*, **36**: 208–13.

Sjodahl, K., Lu, Y., Nilsen, T.I., Ye, W., Hveem, K., Vatten, L. *et al.* (2007). Smoking and alcohol drinking in relation to risk of gastric cancer: a population-based, prospective cohort study. *Int. J. Cancer*, **120**: 128–32.

Sung, N.V., Choi, K.S., Park, E.C., Park. K., Lee. S.Y., Lee. A.K. *et al.* (2007). Smoking, alcohol and gastric cancer risk in Korean men: the National Health insurance Corporation Study. *Br. J. Cancer*, **97**: 700–04.

Terry, P., Nyren, O., and Yuen, J.K. (1998). Protective effect of fruits and vegetables on stomach cancer in a cohort of Swedish twins. *Int. J. Cancer*, **76**: 35–7.

The Eurogast Study Group (1993). Epidemiology of, and risk factors for, Helicobacter pylori infection among 3 194 asymptomatic subjects in 17 populations. *Gut*, **34**: 1672–6.

Tredaniel, J., Boffetta, P., Buiatti, E., Saracci, R., and Hirsch, A. (1997). Tobacco smoking and gastric cancer: review and meta-analysis. *Int. J. Cancer*, **72**: 565–73.

Tulinius, H., Sigfusson, N., Sigvaldason, H., Bjarnadottir, K., and Tryggvadottir, L. (1997). Risk factors for malignant diseases: a cohort study on a population of 22 946 Icelanders. *Cancer Epidemiol. Biomarkers Prev*, **6**: 863–73.

Tverdal, A., Thelle, D., Stensvold, I., Leren, P., and Bjartveit, K. (1993). Mortality in relation to smoking history: 13 years' follow-up of 68 000 Norwegian men and women 35–49 years. *J. Clin. Epidemiol*, **46**: 475–87.

Ward, E.M., Thun, M.J., Hannan, L.M., and Jemal, A. (2006). Interpreting cancer trends. *Ann. N. Y. Acad Sci*, **1076**: 29–53.

World Cancer Research Fund/American Institute for Cancer Research (1997). *Food, Nutrition And The Prevention of Cancer: A Global Perspective*. pp. 148–75, Washington, D.C.

Wu, A., Wan, P., and Bernstein, L. (2001). A multicentric population based case-control study of smoking, alcohol and body size and risk of adenocarcinoma of the stomach and esophagus (United States). *Cancer Causes Control*, **12**: 721–32.

Wu-Williams, A.H., Yu, M.C., and Mack, T.M. (1990). Life-style, work-place, and stomach cancer by subsite in young men of Los Angeles County. *Cancer Res*, **50**: 2569–76.

Ye, W., Ekstrom, A.M., Hansson, L.E., Bergstrom, R., and Nyren, O. (1999). Tobacco, alcohol and the risk of gastric cancer by sub-site and histologic type. *Int. J. Cancer*, **83**: 223–9.

You, W., Zhang, L., Gail, M.H., Chang, Y., Liu, W., Ma, J. *et al.* (2000). Gastric dysplasia and gastric cancer: Helicobacter pylori, serum vitamin C, and other risk factors. *J. Natl. Cancer Inst*, **92**: 1607–12.

You, W.C., Blot, W., Chang, Y.S., Ershow, A.G., Yang, Z.T., An, Q. *et al.* (1988). Diet and high risk of stomach cancer in Shandong, China. *Cancer Res*, **48**: 3518–23.

Yu, G.P. and Hsieh, C.C. (1991). Risk factors for stomach cancer: a population-based case-control study in Shanghai. *Cancer Causes Control*, **2**: 169–74.

Yuan, J.M., Ross, R.K., Wang, X.L., Gao, Y.T., Henderson, B.E., and Yu, M.C. (1996). Morbidity and mortality in relation to cigarette smoking in Shanghai, China: a prospective male cohort study. *J. Am. Med. Assoc*, **275**: 1646–50.

Yun, Y.H., Jung, K.W., Bae. J.M., Lee, J.S., Shin, S.A., Min Park, S. *et al.* (2005). Cigarette smoking and cancer incidence risk in adult men: National Health Insurance Corporation Study. *Cancer Detect Prev*, **29**: 15–24.

Zaridze, D., Borisova, E., Maximovitch, D., Chkhikvadze, V. (2000). Alcohol consumption, smoking and risk of gastric cancer: case-control study from Moscow, Russia. *Cancer Causes Control*, **11**: 363–71.

Zendehdel, K., Nyren, O., Luo, J., Dickman, P.W., Boffetta, P., Englund, A. *et al.* (2008). Risk of gastroesophageal cancer among smokers and users of Scandinavian moist snuff. *Int. J. Cancer*, **122**: 1095–9.

Zhang, Z.F., Kurtz, R.C., Sun, M., Karpeh, M., Yu, G.P., Gargon, *et al.* (1996). Adenocarcinomas of the esophagus and gastric cardia: medical conditions, tobacco, alcohol, and socioeconomic factors. *Cancer Epidemiol. Biomarkers Prev*, **5**: 761–8.

Chapter 24

Cigarette smoking and colorectal cancer

Edward Giovannucci

Introduction

Our understanding of the potential association between tobacco and risk of colorectal cancer has had an interesting history. The landmark early studies, which covered the 1950s and 1960s, consistently did not support an association between tobacco and colorectal cancer risk (Hammond and Horn 1958; 1960; Higginson 1966; Kahn 1966; Staszewski 1969; Weir and Dunn 1970; Doll and Peto 1976; Williams and Horm 1977; Graham *et al.* 1978; Doll *et al.* 1980; Haenszel *et al.* 1980; Rogot and Murray 1980). Many of these studies had been instrumental in demonstrating important associations with other cancer sites. Generally, by the 1970s, tobacco was not considered an important risk factor for colorectal cancer. However, around this time colorectal adenomas had become established as cancer precursors through careful pathologic studies (Morson 1974; Lev 1990). When epidemiologists began studying risk factors for colorectal adenomas in studies conducted in the 1980s and 1990s, smokers were consistently found to have an appreciably elevated risk. In 1994, a hypothesis, attempting to reconcile the apparent paradoxical findings between colorectal adenomas and cancers, stated that carcinogens from cigarette smoke cause irreversible genetic damage in colorectal epithelial cells, but several decades are required for completion of all the carcinogenic events following this initiating event (Giovannucci *et al.* 1994a, 1994b). This hypothesis predicted that an association would be observed initially in adenomas, and then in cancers, after a certain period of time. Thus, the early studies may not have considered a sufficiently long time lag between smoking exposure and time of risk.

In recent years, the association between tobacco and colorectal cancer has been re-evaluated, including in studies that initially did not support an association but that had additional follow-up (Giovannucci 2001). In this chapter, the results for an association between tobacco and colorectal adenoma and cancer are summarized. Evidence addressing the likelihood of a causal association, and the implications of the findings, are then addressed.

Cigarette smoking and colorectal adenoma

Beginning in the 1980s, a number of studies have addressed the association between tobacco use and risk of colorectal adenoma. In almost every study, smokers had a higher risk of colorectal adenoma (Hoff *et al.* 1987; Demers *et al.* 1988; Kikendall *et al.* 1989; Cope *et al.* 1991; Monnet *et al.* 1991; Zahm *et al.* 1991; Honjo *et al.* 1992; Kune *et al.* 1992b; Lee *et al.* 1993; Olsen and Kronborg 1993; Giovannucci *et al.* 1994a, 1994b; Jacobson *et al.* 1994; Boutron *et al.* 1995; Martinez *et al.* 1995; Longnecker *et al.* 1996; Terry and Neugut 1998; Nagata *et al.* 1999; Potter *et al.* 1999; Almendingen *et al.* 2000; Breuer-Katschinski *et al.* 2000). Typically, the studies have demonstrated dose–response relationships between adenoma risk with cigarettes per day among current-smokers, and associations with duration of smoking, and with total cigarette pack-years. Generally, individuals who smoked one to two packs (20–40 cigarettes) daily, or who have accumulated 20–40 cigarette pack-years of smoking, have approximately a two- to three-fold higher risk than non-smokers. The studies are remarkable in their consistency in both men and women; in stark contrast to these studies, relatively few case-control studies found no or equivocal relationships. One of these studies, conducted in the US (Sandler *et al.* 1993), found a non-significant but suggestive two-fold increased risk in women with higher numbers of pack-years, but no association was apparent in men. A Japanese study, based on only 86 cases, showed no association (Kono *et al.* 1990), but with 116 additional cases that occurred with continued follow-up, a strong positive association emerged (Honjo *et al.* 1992).

Several important observations are noteworthy. First, while smoking intensity is important, duration also appears to be critical. For example, a Japanese study (Nagata *et al.* 1999) found a higher risk among those who had smoked for 30+ years (relative risk (RR) = 1.60; 95% confidence interval (CI) = 1.02–2.62) but not less (RR = 1.10, 95% CI = 0.69–1.84). In two US studies of men (Giovannucci *et al.* 1994b) and women (Giovannucci *et al.* 1994a), elevated risks for large adenoma were observed only among individuals, who had smoked for at least 20 years. Other studies also tend to indicate that several decades of smoking may be required for a clear association to emerge for adenomas (Monnet *et al.* 1991; Zahm *et al.* 1991; Terry and Neugut 1998). This finding is noteworthy because adenomas typically arise a decade or more before malignancies; thus, this pattern would suggest at least several decades to elapse between smoking exposure and colorectal cancer risk. Second, the findings generally held for risk of large (>1 cm) adenoma (Zahm *et al.* 1991; Honjo *et al.* 1992; Kune *et al.* 1992b; Lee *et al.* 1993; Giovannucci *et al.* 1994a; Giovannucci *et al.* 1994b; Jacobson *et al.* 1994; Boutron *et al.* 1995; Longnecker *et al.* 1996; Terry and Neugut 1998; Nagata *et al.* 1999; Potter *et al.* 1999). Thirdly, an association has been observed relatively consistently among past-smokers (Hoff *et al.* 1987; Monnet *et al.* 1991; Zahm *et al.* 1991; Honjo *et al.* 1992; Giovannucci *et al.* 1994a; Giovannucci *et al.* 1994b; Jacobson *et al.* 1994; Martinez *et al.* 1995; Longnecker *et al.* 1996). Finally, the association between tobacco and risk of colorectal adenoma persisted and was not appreciably attenuated in every study after controlling for potential confounders, including diet and alcohol in many of the studies. The presence of an association is incontrovertible, suggesting that this association is causal, or represents a consistent bias or uncontrolled confounding. Arguing against confounding is the consistency of the findings in males and females in diverse populations, including the United,States, Norway, France, and Japan, the strength of the association, and the dose–response pattern for intensity and duration of smoking, and the similar results for age-adjusted and multivariate analyses (Hill 1965). A second possibility is that the results were due to some consistent bias. Of note, most studies were based on endoscopied individuals, it is plausible that smokers are more likely to undergo endoscopy for indications related to an underlying polyp as compared with non-smokers, creating a bias whereby smokers with adenomas would be preferentially entered into the study population. However, even in studies or sub-groups in which all in the defined population are screened regardless of symptoms (Hoff *et al.* 1987; Demers *et al.* 1988; Monnet *et al.* 1991; Zahm *et al.* 1991; Honjo *et al.* 1992; Giovannucci *et al.* 1994a, 1994b), smokers are at higher risk. Another possibility is that adenomas might be more easily detectable during endoscopy for smokers, perhaps because of a relaxing effect of nicotine on the large bowel. However, this bias is more plausible for small adenomas but less so for large adenomas (Zahm *et al.* 1991; Honjo *et al.* 1992; Kune *et al.* 1992b; Lee *et al.* 1993; Giovannucci *et al.* 1994a, 1994b; Jacobson *et al.* 1994; Boutron *et al.* 1995; Longnecker *et al.* 1996; Terry and Neugut 1998; Nagata *et al.* 1999; Potter *et al.* 1999); moreover, associations have been observed consistently in past-smokers, where the putative relaxing influence of nicotine would no longer be present.

The findings for smoking and adenoma risk were recently evaluated in a meta-analysis, which included 42 independent studies (Botteri *et al.* 2008b). The pooled risk estimates for current-, former-, and ever-smokers in comparison with never-smokers were 2.14 (95% CI, 1.86–2.46),

1.47 (95% CI, 1.29–1.67), and 1.82 (95% CI, 1.65–2.00), respectively. Of note, the association was stronger for high-risk adenomas than for low-risk adenomas. Further, the studies in which all controls underwent full colonoscopy showed a higher relative risk compared with studies in which some or all controls underwent partial colon examination. The results from this meta-analysis strongly support an association between smoking and adenoma risk.

Smoking and colorectal cancer
Summary of studies in the United States

In general, the early studies on tobacco and colorectal cancer did not support an association (Hammond and Horn 1958, 1960; Higginson 1966; Kahn 1966; Staszewski 1969; Weir and Dunn 1970; Doll and Peto 1976; Williams and Horm 1977; Graham *et al.* 1978; Doll *et al.* 1980; Haenszel *et al.* 1980; Rogot and Murray 1980). For example, in the earliest report based on data from the Veterans Administration by Hammond and Horn (1958), 187 783, men were followed from 1952 to 1955 and accrued 667 753 person-years. Compared to never-smokers, cigarette smokers had a two-fold excess risk of all cancers combined but not for cancers of the colon (84 cases observed, 108.4 expected) or rectum (55 observed, 58.8 expected). Following publication of data suggesting a 35- to 40-year induction period between smoking and risk for colorectal cancer (Giovannucci *et al.* 1994a, *et al.* 1994b), Heineman *et al.* (1994) further studied the Veterans Administration population for the period covering 1954 to 1980. In this new analysis, based on 3 812 colon cancer deaths and 1 100 rectal cancer deaths, risk increased with earlier age of initiating smoking (about a 40–50% increase for both colon and rectal cancers among those who began before the age of 15 years). This study offered strong support for the hypothesis that smoking primarily influences the early stages of colorectal cancers.

In contrast to the earlier published studies of US men, studies that have had follow-up time after 1970 have almost universally supported an association (Wu *et al.* 1987; Slattery *et al.* 1990; Giovannucci *et al.* 1994b; Heineman *et al.* 1994; Chyou *et al.* 1996; Le Marchand *et al.* 1997; Slattery *et al.* 1997; Hsing *et al.* 1998; Chao *et al.* 2000; Sturmer *et al.* 2000). A study of male health professionals (Giovannucci *et al.* 1994b) demonstrated a two-fold elevated risk in men who had accumulated at least ten cigarette pack-years more than 35 years previously, even among those who had subsequently quit decades previously. In a cohort study of US males followed from 1980 to 1985, Wu *et al.* (1987) reported an elevated risk of colorectal cancer among current-smokers (RR = 1.80), past-smokers who stopped <20 years (RR = 2.63) and ≥20 years (RR = 1.71). In a study of Hawaiian-Japanese men (Chyou *et al.* 1996), the results were not statistically significant up until 30 pack-years, but the RR = 1.48 (95% CI = 1.13–1.94) for colon cancer and RR = 1.92 (95% CI = 1.23–2.99) for rectal cancer for 30+ pack years. In the prospective Lutheran Brotherhood Study, a linear dose–response was observed between cigarettes/day in current-smokers at baseline and colon cancer risk, although the number of cases was limited ($n = 120$) (Hsing *et al.* 1998). Relative to never-smokers, the RR for past-smokers was 1.45 (95% CI = 0.8–2.7); for current-smokers (1–19 cigarettes per day), 1.1 (95% CI = 0.5–2.5); current-smokers (20–29 cigarettes per day), 1.6 (95% CI = 0.7–3.4); current-smokers (≥ 30 cigarettes per day), 2.3 (95% CI = 0.9–5.7).

Two recent cohorts have added further support. In the Physicians' Health Study, smoking status was examined in 1982 and men were followed for more than twelve years (Sturmer *et al.* 2000). In a multivariate model, the RR for colorectal cancer was elevated for current-smokers (RR = 1.81; 95% CI = 1.28–2.55) and past-smokers (RR = 1.49; 95% CI = 1.17–1.89). Smoking up to twenty years before baseline ($p = 0.05$) and smoking up to and including age 30 years ($p = 0.01$) were statistically significantly related to risk, even controlling for subsequent smoking history. The results indicated that smoking in the distant past is most critical, but recent past smoking may also be important. In the Cancer Prevention II Study (CPS II), a prospective study of mortality of 312 332 men and 469 019 women begun in 1982, smoking for ≥ 20 years after baseline increased risk of colorectal cancer in men (Chao *et al.* 2000). Dose–response relations were observed for cigarettes per day, pack-years smoked and earlier age started smoking for current- and past-smokers. In this study, risk was not elevated for those who quit smoking > 20 years before baseline.

An association between smoking and risk of colorectal or colon cancer in men has also been observed in case-control studies (Dales *et al.* 1979; Slattery *et al.* 1990; Le Marchand *et al.* 1997; Slattery *et al.* 1997). The study by Le Marchand *et al.* (1997) was notable in finding a positive association between smoking and colorectal cancer risk with a generally increasing risk with time since smoking. In the study by Slattery *et al.* (1997), the risk increased with number of cigarettes per day and remained elevated even in men who had quit for ≥15 years. A case-control study of US blacks conducted on 1973–76, which also included women, found an elevated risk of colorectal cancer with 20+ years of smoking (Dales *et al.* 1979).

Less relevant information is available for women, but the data also tend to suggest a long lag between smoking history and risk for colorectal cancer. Because women began smoking substantially in the United States only during the late 1940s and 1950s (Pierce *et al.* 1989), a rise in the incidence of colorectal cancer would not have been expected until approximately the late 1980s assuming a 35–40 year induction period (Giovannucci *et al.* 1994a, 1994b). In fact, up to around 1990, there do not appear to be studies that found a positive association between smoking and colorectal cancer risk among women in the United States, but some supportive data have emerged recently. The first study to show a clear association was based on data from the Nurses' Health Study (Giovannucci *et al.* 1994a). This analysis found a two-fold elevated RR among long-term smokers, including past smokers. Interestingly, an earlier analysis from this cohort, which included cases diagnosed from June of 1976 to May of 1984, found only a weak, statistically non-significant association between smoking and colon cancer, although past smoking was significantly associated with risk of rectal carcinoma (Chute *et al.* 1991). These results were confirmed for colorectal cancer mortality for women in the Cancer Prevention Study II (Chao *et al.* 2000). In that study, elevated risks of colorectal cancer mortality were observed after 20–30 years of smoking duration before baseline both in current-smokers (RR = 1.41; 95% CI = 1.26–1.58) and past-smokers (RR = 1.22; 95% CI = 1.09–1.37).

Case-control studies have tended to support an association between long-term tobacco use and colorectal cancer risk. Newcomb *et al.* (1995) found among women who smoked for at least 31 years, but not less, a dose–response relation with cigarettes per day. In addition, earlier age at smoking initiation was associated with an increased risk. Past smokers had a moderately increased risk. Slattery *et al.* (1997) found that >35 pack-years of smoking was associated with an elevated risk (RR = 1.38; 95% CI = 1.11–1.71) in women. Also, Le Marchand *et al.* (1997) also found an elevated risk of colorectal cancer for smokers; in this study, risk was particularly strong for women who had smoked for >30–40 years in the past.

Summary of studies in other countries

In recent years, a number of studies reporting on colorectal cancer risk and smoking have been conducted outside the United States. Almost all of these have been in European countries, except for a few studies in Japan. One of the landmark studies on tobacco and cancer is a long-term follow-up study of British male doctors (Doll *et al.* 1994). In recent analyses, smokers of 25+ cigarettes per day had a 4.4-fold higher rate of rectal cancer ($P < 0.001$), based on 168 cases. Colon cancer, based on 437 cases, exhibited only weak evidence of an increased risk (not statistically significant; RR = 1.44). This study had follow-up of 40 years, but did not present time-lagged analyses.

In a population-based case-control study of 174 colorectal cancer cases in Great Britain (Welfare *et al.* 1997), male and female smokers were at increased risk (OR = 1.77; 95% CI = 1.03–3.14).

A Norwegian cohort study of 68 825 men and women documented 51 fatal colon cancers and 40 fatal rectal cancers from 1972–1988 (Tverdal *et al.* 1993). Males who had smoked in the past had a moderately increased risk for fatal colon cancer (RR = 1.2) and fatal rectal cancer (RR = 1.4), and male current-smokers, but not female smokers, were at elevated risk from fatal colon cancer (RR = 1.5) and rectal cancer (RR = 1.8).

In a cohort study in Finland (Knekt *et al.* 1998), 56 973 men and women were followed from 1966–1972 to 1994. A non-statistically significant overall association was observed, but for follow-up periods of between 11 and 20 years, a significant increase risk was observed for smokers (RR = 1.57; 95% CI = 1.09–2.24). At baseline, smokers had smoked for 20 years on average. This association was limited to men (RR = 1.94; 95% CI = 1.25–2.24), who smoked more than women. In a comparison of colorectal cancer risk for persons recorded as smokers in both of two baseline examinations, a significant increase in risk was observed in the consistent smokers (RR = 1.71; 95% CI = 1.09–2.68).

An Icelandic cohort study documented 145 colorectal cancers in 11 580 women and 193 cases in 11 366 men followed from 1968 to 1995 (Tulinius *et al.* 1997). In this cohort, the prevalence of current smoking at baseline was higher in women than in men (1–14 cigarettes/day: 11% of men, 20% of women; 15–24 cigarettes/day: 13% of men, 16% of women; 25+ cigarettes/day: 6% of men, 3% of women). Among women, risk of colorectal cancer increased with increasing level of cigarette smoking (multivariate RRs = 1.37, 1.53, 2.48). Results were not presented for men (Tulinius *et al.* 1997).

In a Yugoslavian hospital-based case-control study over 1984–1986 (Jarebinski *et al.* 1988, 1989), risk of colorectal cancer was not elevated among men and women who had smoked for 1–30 years (RR = 1.0), but risk was elevated for total colorectal (RR = 2.0) and rectal cancer (RR = 2.7) among long-term smokers (30+ years).

A large non-supportive study of the relationship between smoking and colorectal cancer risk was a hospital-case control study of 955 cases of colon cancer and 629 cases of rectal cancer in northern Italy (D'Avanzo *et al.* 1995). Cancers of the colon and rectum were not associated with number of cigarettes smoked, number of pack-years, duration, time since initiation, and time since quitting.

Several studies of smoking and colorectal cancer risk were conducted in Sweden, producing mixed results. A random sample of 26 000 Swedish women were asked about their smoking status in the early 1960s and then were followed for 26 years (Nordlund *et al.* 1997). No significant association was observed, except for a slight increase in smokers of 16+ cigarettes per day at baseline (RR = 1.42; 95% CI = 0.77–2.60). However, this study was conducted before 1990. A case-control study (Baron *et al.* 1994) of 352 colon cancer cases and 217 rectal cancer cases found no association with tobacco, even among long-term smokers (40+) years. A cohort study of Swedish construction workers did not find any association among 713 men with colon cancer, and only a weak association with 505 rectal cancer cases (Nyren *et al.* 1996). Among men with 30+ years of smoking at the start of follow-up, the RR was 1.03 (95% CI = 0.85–1.25) for colon cancer and 1.21 (95% CI = 0.96–1.53) for rectal cancer. However, in a prospective cohort study of 17 118 Swedish twins, long-term heavy tobacco use was associated with an increased risk of colorectal cancer (RR=3.1, 95% CI = 1.4–7.1) (Terry *et al.* 2001).

Several studies were conducted in Japan. A Japanese study of 59 male and 34 female colorectal cancer cases yielded no results (Tajima and Tominaga 1985), but smoking became prevalent in Japan only in the 1950s and this study was conducted from 1982–1983. A hospital-based case-control study in Nagoya, Japan (Inoue *et al.* 1995), examined 'habitual' smoking (both past and current) and risk of colon cancer ($n = 231$) and rectal cancer ($n = 201$) over the years 1988–1992. No relationship was observed for colon cancer, but 'habitual' smoking was associated with an increased risk of rectal cancer for both males (odds ratio = 1.9; 95% CI = 1.1–3.2) and females (odds ratio = 1.7; 95% CI = 1.0–3.1). A case-control study in Tokyo (Yamada et al. 1997) of 129 colorectal carcinoma-in-situ cases, 66 colorectal cancers and 390 controls from 1991 to 1993 found that cumulative exposure (pack years) to cigarette smoking within the prior 20 years was significantly associated with risk for colorectal carcinoma-in-situ (RR = 3.7; 95% CI = 1.6–8.4 for ≥31 versus 0 pack-years; p(trend) = 0.0003), whereas smoking until 20 years before the diagnosis was associated with risk for colorectal cancer (RR = 5.0; 95% CI = 1.3–18.3; for ≥31 versus 0 pack-years; p(trend) = 0.005).

Results from recent meta-analyses

Two recent meta-analyses have evaluated studies of smoking and colorectal cancer. In one of the meta-analyses, which evaluated all cohort and case-control studies, the authors identified 106 studies of colorectal cancer incidence (Botteri et al. 2008a). Twenty-six studies provided adjusted risk estimates for ever-smokers versus never-smokers, leading to a pooled relative risk of 1.18 (95% CI, 1.11–1.25). Results were similar in cohort studies and case-control studies, and in Europe, North America, and Asia. Both the colon and rectum were affected, though the associations seemed stronger for rectal cancer, and the associations were stronger in former-smokers compared to current-smokers, especially for colon cancer. A linear increase was observed for increasing number of cigarettes smoked per day, and the risk increased by duration of smoking. Only after 30 years of smoking was statistical significance attained.

The results from the second meta-analysis, which focused on 36 cohort studies, largely confirmed those of the other meta-analysis (Liang et al. 2009). The analysis showed that relative to non-smokers, current- and former-smokers had a significantly increased risk of colorectal incidence. All four dose–response variables examined were significantly associated with colorectal cancer incidence (all p-values < 0.0001): daily cigarette consumption (RR = 1.38 for an increase of 40 cigarettes/day), duration (RR = 1.20 for an increase of 40 years of duration), pack-years (RR = 1.51 for an increase of 60 pack-years), and age of initiation (RR = 0.96 for a delay of ten years in smoking initiation). Among the subset of studies that distinguished cancer by site, a higher risk was seen for rectal cancer than for colon cancer for all analyses.

Assessment of evidence that smoking causally increases risk of colorectal cancer

The evidence summarized earlier strongly implicates long-term smoking as causally related to risk of cancers of the colon and rectum. Particularly if one examines the more recent studies, which can better study the impact of long-term smoking, the results are remarkably consistent with few exceptions. The following characteristics of the results support that this association is causal.

First, in studies of US men with follow-up time exclusively after 1970, published studies generally report a positive association (Wu et al. 1987; Slattery et al. 1990; Giovannucci et al. 1994b; Heineman et al. 1994; Chyou et al. 1996; Le Marchand et al. 1997; Slattery et al. 1997; Hsing et al. 1998; Chao et al. 2000; Sturmer et al. 2000). In addition, studies for US women with follow-up time in the 1990s report statistically significant positive associations (Giovannucci et al. 1994a; Newcomb et al. 1995; Le Marchand et al. 1997; Slattery et al. 1997; Chao et al. 2000). In studies conducted outside of the United States, although there have been several notable non-supportive studies (Baron et al. 1994; D'Avanzo et al. 1995; Nyren et al. 1996; Nordlund et al. 1997), most recent studies (Jarebinski *et al.* 1988, 1989; Tverdal *et al.* 1993; Inoue *et al.* 1995; Tulinius *et al.* 1997; Welfare *et al.* 1997; Yamada *et al.* 1997; Knekt *et al.* 1998; Terry *et al.* 2001) found long-term smokers to be at elevated risk. A recent meta-analysis found that risk of colorectal cancer was statistically significant only after 30 years of smoking (Botteri *et al.* 2008a). Even accounting for possible publication bias, it is implausible that these findings are all due to chance.

Second, the studies of cancers are complemented by studies of adenomas, for which almost all have supported an association with long-term smoking history. Perhaps, associations with small adenomas are less compelling, because only a small percentage progress to cancer and these are more prone to detection biases. However, studies that examined large adenomas have found a positive association with smoking history (Zahm *et al.* 1991; Honjo *et al.* 1992; Kune *et al.* 1992b; Lee *et al.* 1993; Giovannucci *et al.* 1994a, 1994b; Jacobson *et al.* 1994; Boutron *et al.* 1995; Longnecker *et al.* 1996; Terry and Neugut 1998; Nagata *et al.* 1999; Potter *et al.* 1999). A recent meta-analysis actually showed a stronger association between tobacco and advanced adenoma than with non-advanced adenoma (Botteri *et al.* 2008b). Large adenomas have acquired many genetic alterations observed in malignancies (Vogelstein *et al.* 1988), and the epidemiology for these lesions closely parallels that of cancers.

Third, given the diversity of study designs for cancer, prospective, retrospective and endoscopy-controlled studies for adenomas, for men and for women in different populations, it is unlikely that some consistent detection bias could account for all these observations. In addition, some of the theoretical biases should be opposing for adenomas and cancers. For example, if there is a stronger likelihood of smokers with adenomas being more likely to be diagnosed than non-smokers with adenomas, this should produce a positive detection bias for adenomas but a negative detection bias for cancers because their precursors would be removed preferentially. Also, while current-smokers tend to have lower screening rates than the non-smokers, past-smokers (especially in populations such as physicians, health professionals, and nurses) may have similar or even enhanced screening than never-smokers, but both current- and past-smokers are at increased risk for colorectal cancer.

Fourth, in every study of cancer or large adenoma that has adjusted for various potential confounders, results for smoking have not been appreciably attenuated. This pattern exists even in studies that adjusted for numerous potential lifestyle factors (e.g. physical activity, alcohol, diet) that could be plausibly related to tobacco use (Wu *et al.* 1987; Slattery *et al.* 1990; Giovannucci *et al.* 1994b; Newcomb *et al.* 1995; Chyou *et al.* 1996; Le Marchand *et al.* 1997; Slattery *et al.* 1997; Chao *et al.* 2000; Sturmer *et al.* 2000). Results from a recent meta-analysis suggested that alcohol was unlikely to be a major confounding factor in the studies (Botteri *et al.* 2008a). Moreover, past-smokers, especially those who quit long in the past would tend to have different covariate patterns than continuing smokers, yet associations with tobacco use have been seen for both groups. Finally, the relatively consistent findings for men and women in diverse populations from various countries argue against confounding.

Fifth, the association has a high degree of biologic plausibility. Cigarette smoking is judged unequivocally to be causally related to at least eight different cancers, including those not directly related to smoke, such as the pancreas, kidney, and bladder (Anonymous 1979). The burning of tobacco produces numerous genotoxic compounds, including polynuclear aromatic hydrocarbons, heterocyclic amines, nitrosamines, and aromatic amines (Anonymous 1986; Manabe *et al.* 1991; Alexandrov *et al.* 1996; Hoffmann and Hoffmann 1997). The large intestine is exposed to these compounds either through the circulatory (Yamasaki and Ames 1977) or digestive system (Kune *et al.* 1992a). DNA adducts to metabolites of benzo(*a*)pyrene, a carcinogenic polycyclic aromatic hydrocarbon, are detected more frequently in the colonic mucosa of smokers compared to non-smokers (Alexandrov *et al.* 1996). DNA adduct levels in the normal-appearing colonic epithelium of colorectal cancer patients are at a higher frequency than in non-cancer patients (Pfohl-Leszkowicz *et al.* 1995). The apparently long induction period of at least three or four decades between the presumably genotoxic event and ultimately diagnosis of malignancy is consistent with the natural history of colorectal cancer (Giovannucci and Martinez 1996).

Unresolved issues and implications

The data just summarized strongly support an association between smoking and risk of colorectal cancer. Dose–response relations have been reported for pack-years, smoking duration, smoking intensity, smoking history in the distant past, and younger age at initiation of smoking. Relative risk comparing the high versus low categories of these factors have generally been in the range of 1.3–1.8. As most of these variables tend to be correlated, teasing out which are the most relevant factors is difficult, although clearly those who began early and smoked most intensely for many years are at highest risk. To what degree and how quickly risk drops after one ceases smoking remains somewhat in question, but most data suggest that part of the excess risk persists indefi-nitely in past-smokers (Wu *et al.* 1987; Giovannucci *et al.* 1994a, 1994b; Slattery *et al.* 1997; Sturmer *et al.* 2000). Only one study (Chao *et al.* 2000) found that the excess risk appears to approach zero after about 20 years since quitting. While smoking at any age has numerous health benefits, for colorectal cancer the avoidance of smoking at early ages appears particularly important.

Generally, associations have been observed for both colon and rectal cancers, although, in several studies (Doll and Peto 1976; Chute *et al.* 1991; Inoue *et al.* 1995; Nyren *et al.* 1996), an association was observed or suggestive only with rectal cancer. However, in one of these studies (Chute *et al.* 1991), with additional follow-up (Giovannucci *et al.* 1994a), an association emerged for colon cancer. In most studies that have distinguished among colon and rectal cancer, the association has been stronger for rectal cancer (Tverdal *et al.* 1993; Doll *et al.* 1994; Giovannucci *et al.* 1994a; Heineman *et al.* 1994; Newcomb *et al.* 1995; Chyou 1996; Chao *et al.* 2000), though present for both. In a recent meta-analysis, former-smokers had similar relative risks for colon and rectal cancer but among current-smokers, risk was elevated only for rectal cancer (Botteri *et al.* 2008a), suggesting some heterogeneity by rectal versus colon cancer. Overall, whether differences exist between the proximal and distal colon has not been adequately addressed.

It is unclear whether smoking may preferentially increase risk of some molecular sub-types of colorectal cancer, though some early evidence is provocative. For example, smoking history may be an important risk factor for the sub-type of colorectal cancer characterized by microsatellite instability (MSI) (Slattery *et al.* 2000; Chia *et al.* 2006), and by CpG island methylator phenoptype (CIMP) status and BRAF mutations (Samowitz *et al.* 2006). An additional study found a higher risk of mismatch repair-deficient colorectal cancer in cigarette smokers (Yang *et al.* 2000). In addition, smoking history has been associated with an increased risk of hyperplastic polyps (Kearney *et al.* 1995), particularly when they coexist with adenomas (Morimoto *et al.* 2002; Ji *et al.* 2006; Yeoman et al. 2007). Interestingly, hyperplastic polyps have been linked to BRAF mutations and CIMP positivity (O'Brien *et al.* 2004). Overall, this evidence suggests that smoking may be associated primarily with a molecular sub-type of colorectal cancer that is characterized by a pathway involving hyperplastic (serrated) polyps, BRAF mutations, and CIMP positivity status. Future studies focused on such sub-types of colorectal cancer may yield much stronger associations with smoking compared to studies pooling all sub-types of colorectal cancer. If the association with a sub-type of colorectal cancer is confirmed, that would increase the plausibility of a causal association between tobacco use and colorectal cancer.

Most studies have focused on cigarette smoking, whereas relatively few have examined cigar or pipe smoking. In the large CPS II study, current-smokers who had smoked exclusively cigars or pipes were at elevated risk of colorectal cancer mortality (multivariate RR = 1.34; 95% = 1.11–1.62) (Chao *et al.* 2000). Other studies have also indicated that cigar/pipe smoking may increase risk of colorectal cancer (Hammond and Horn 1960; Heineman *et al.* 1994; Slattery *et al.* 1997). As smoking of these products has increased in some segments of the population, further work in defining the association for pipe and cigar smoking is important.

Another area where further work would be of interest is determining whether specific individuals would be at higher risk because of their genetic background or other modifiable behaviour. While there have been a number of studies of polymorphic genes encoding xenobiotic metabolizing enzymes in colorectal cancer, potential interactions with tobacco have been examined in a relatively small proportion of these (Brockton *et al.* 2000). This is a relatively untapped area of research. Only a few reports have considered whether there are smokers at relatively higher or lower risk of colorectal cancer based on behaviours or characteristics.

In conclusion, the overall body of evidence indicates that colorectal cancer is a smoking-related malignancy. Two factors probably have contributed to the fact that this has not been appreciated until relatively recently. First, there appears to be a relatively long time lag between onset of smoking and period of risk, and second, colorectal cancers are common even in non-smokers so the population attributable risk has been moderate compared to other malignancies. In the United States, estimates of the population attributable risk due to smoking have been 21% of colorectal cancer in men (Giovannucci *et al.* 1994b), 16% of colon cancer and 22% of rectal cancer in men (Heineman *et al.* 1994); 12% of colorectal cancer mortality in men and women (Chao *et al.* 2000), and 11% of colon cancer and 17% of rectal cancer in women (Newcomb *et al.* 1995). In a recent study of colorectal cancer in Norwegian women, 12% were attributed to smoking (Gram *et al.* 2009 Mar 10 [Epub ahead of print]). From these estimates, approximately 7 000 to 10 000 deaths from colorectal cancer per year would be attributable to cigarette smoking in the United States (Chao *et al.* 2000). Because at least part of the excess risk appears to be permanent, the prevention of smoking in the young is especially important for this malignancy.

References

Alexandrov, K., Rojas, M., Kadlubar, F.F., Lang, N.P., and Bartsch, H. (1996). Evidence of *anti*-benzo[a]pyrene diolepoxide-DNA adduct formation in human colon mucosa. *Carcinogenesis*, **17**: 2081–2.

Almendingen, K., Hofstad, B., Trygg, K., Hoff, G., Hussain, A., and Vatn, M.H. (2000). Smoking and colorectal adenomas: a case-control study. *European Journal of Cancer Prevention*, **9**: 193–203.

Anonymous. (1979). *Smoking and Health: A Report of the Surgeon General.* Rockville, Md: US Department of Health, Education and Welfare, Public Health Service.

Anonymous. (1986). Tobacco smoking. *IARC Monographs on the Evaluation of Carcinogenic Risks to Humans*, **38**: 397.

Baron, J.A., Gerhardsson de Verdier, M., and Ekbom, A. (1994). Coffee, tea, tobacco, and cancer of the large bowel. *Cancer Epidemiology, Biomarkers and Prevention*, **3**: 565–70.

Botteri, E., Iodice, S., Bagnardi, V., Raimondi, S., Lowenfels, A.B., and Maisonneuve, P. (2008a). Smoking and colorectal cancer: a meta-analysis. *JAMA*, **300**: 2765–78.

Botteri, E., Iodice, S., Raimondi, S., Maisonneuve, P., and Lowenfels, A.B. (2008b). Cigarette smoking and adenomatous polyps: a meta-analysis. *Gastroenterology*, **134**: 388–95.

Boutron, M.C., Faivre, J., Dop, M.C., Quipourt, V., and Senesse, P. (1995). Tobacco, alcohol, and colorectal tumors: a multistep process. *American Journal of Epidemiology*, **141**: 1038–46.

Breuer-Katschinski, B., Nemes, K., Marr, A., Rump, B., Leiendecker, B., and Breuer, N. (2000). Alcohol and cigarette smoking and the risk of colorectal adenomas. *Digestive Diseases and Sciences*, **45**: 487–93.

Brockton, N., Little, J., Sharp, L., and Cotton, S.C. (2000). N-acetyltransferase polymorphisms and colorectal cancer: a HuGE review. *American Journal of Epidemiology*, **151**: 846–61.

Chao, A., Thun, M.J., Jacobs, E.J., Henley, S.H., Rodriguez, C., and Calle, E.E. (2000). Cigarette smoking and colorectal cancer mortality in the Cancer Prevention Study II. *Journal of the National Cancer Institute*, **92**: 1888–96.

Chia, V.M., Newcomb, P.A., Bigler, J., Morimoto, L.M., Thibodeau, S.N., and Potter, J.D. (2006). Risk of microsatellite-unstable colorectal cancer is associated jointly with smoking and nonsteroidal anti-inflammatory drug use. *Cancer Research*, **66**: 6877–83.

Chute, C.G., Willett, W.C., Colditz, G.A., Stampfer, M.J., Baron, J.A., and Rosner, B. (1991). A prospective study of body mass, height, and smoking on the risk of colorectal cancer in women. *Cancer Causes and Control*, **2**: 117–24.

Chyou, P.H., Nomura, A.M.Y., and Stemmermann, G.N. (1996). A prospective study of colon and rectal cancer among Hawaii Japanese men. *Annals of Epidemiology*, **6**: 276–82.

Cope, G.F., Wyatt, J.I., Pinder, I.F., Lee, P.N., Heatley, R.V., and Kelleher, J. (1991). Alcohol consumption in patients with colorectal adenomatous polyps. *Gut*, **32**: 70–2.

D'Avanzo, B., La Vecchia, C., Franceschi, S., Gallotti, L., and Talamini, R. (1995). Cigarette smoking and colorectal cancer: a study of 1,584 cases and 2,879 controls. *Preventive Medicine*, **24**: 571–9.

Dales, L.G., Friedman, G.D., Ury, H.K., Grossman, S., and Williams, S.R. (1979). A case-control study of relationships of diet and other traits to colorectal cancer in American blacks. *American Journal of Epidemiology*, **109**: 132–44.

Demers, R.Y., Neale, A.V., Demers, P., Deighton, K., Scott, R.O., and Dupuis, M.H. (1988). Serum cholesterol and colorectal polyps. *Journal of Clinical Epidemiology*, **41**: 9–13.

Doll, R. and Peto, R. (1976). Mortality in relation to smoking: 20 years' observations on male British doctors. *British Medical Journal*, **2**: 1525–36.

Doll, R., Gray, R., Hafner, B., and Peto, R. (1980). Mortality in relation to smoking: 22 years' observations on female British doctors. *British Medical Journal*, **280**: 967–71.

Doll, R., Peto, R., Wheatley, K., Gray, R., and Sutherland, I. (1994). Mortality in relation to smoking: 40 years' observations on male British doctors. *British Medical Journal*, **309**: 901–11.

Giovannucci, E. (2001). An updated review of the epidemiological evidence that cigarette smoking increases risk of colorectal cancer. *Cancer Epidemiology, Biomarkers and Prevention*, **10**(7): 725–31.

Giovannucci, E. and Martinez, M.E. (1996). Tobacco, colorectal cancer, and adenomas: a review of the evidence. *Journal of the National Cancer Institute*, **88**: 1717–30.

Giovannucci, E., Colditz, G.A., Stampfer, M.J., Hunter, D., Rosner, B.A., and Willett, W.C. (1994a). A prospective study of cigarette smoking and risk of colorectal adenoma and colorectal cancer in US women. *Journal of the National Cancer Institute*, **86**: 192–9.

Giovannucci, E., Rimm, E.B., Stampfer, M.J., Colditz, G.A., Ascherio, A., and Kearney, J. (1994b). A prospective study of cigarette smoking and risk of colorectal adenoma and colorectal cancer in US men. *Journal of the National Cancer Institute*, **86**: 183–91.

Graham, S., Dayal, H., Swanson, M., Mittelman, A., and Wilkinson, G. (1978). Diet in the epidemiology of cancer of the colon and rectum. *Journal of the National Cancer Institute*, **61**: 709–14.

Gram, I.T., Braaten, T., Lund, E., Le Marchand, L., and Weiderpass, E. (2009 Mar 10 [Epub ahead of print]). Cigarette smoking and risk of colorectal cancer among Norwegian women. *Cancer Causes and Control.*

Haenszel, W., Locke, F.B., and Segi, M. (1980). A case-control study of large bowel cancer in Japan. *Journal of the National Cancer Institute*, **64**: 17–22.

Hammond, E.C. and Horn, D. (1958). Smoking and death rates: report on forty-four months of followup of 187,783 men. II. Death rates by cause. *JAMA*, **166**: 1294–308.

Hammond, E.C. and Horn, D. (1966). Smoking in relation to the death rates of one million men and women. *Journal of the National Cancer Institute. Monographs*, **19**: 127–204.

Heineman, E.F., Zahm, S.H., McLaughlin, J.K., and Vaught, J.B. (1994). Increased risk of colorectal cancer among smokers: results of a 26-year follow-up of US veterans and a review. *International Journal of Cancer*, **59**: 728–38.

Higginson, J. (1966). Etiological factors in gastrointestinal cancer in man. *Journal of the National Cancer Institute*, **37**: 527–45.

Hill, A.B. (1965). The environment and disease: association or causation? *Proceedings of the Royal Society of Medicine*, **58**: 295–300.

Hoff, G., Vatn, M.H., and Larsen, S. (1987). Relationship between tobacco smoking and colorectal polyps. *Scandinavian Journal of Gastroenterology*, **22**: 13–16.

Hoffmann, D. and Hoffman, I. (1997). The changing cigarette, 1950–1995. *Journal of Toxicology and Environmental Health*, **50**: 307–64.

Honjo, S., Kono, S., Shinchi, K., Imanishi, K., and Hirohata, T. (1992). Cigarette smoking, alcohol use and adenomatous polyps of the sigmoid colon. *Japanese Journal of Cancer Research*, **83**: 806–11.

Hsing, A.W., McLaughlin, J.K., Chow, W.H., Schuman, L.M., Co Chien, H.T., and Gridley, G. (1998). Risk factors for colorectal cancer in a prospective study among US white men. *International Journal of Cancer*, **77**: 549–53.

Inoue, M., Tajima, K., Hirose, K., Hamajima, N., Takezaki, T., and Hirai, T. (1995). Subsite-specific risk factors for colorectal cancer: a hospital-based case-control study in Japan. *Cancer Causes and Control*, **6**: 14–22.

Jacobson, J.S., Neugut, A.I., Murray, T., Garbowski, G.C., Forde, K.A., and Treat, M.R. (1994). Cigarette smoking and other behavioral risk factors for recurrence of colorectal adenomatous polyps (New York City, NY, USA). *Cancer Causes and Control*, **5**: 215–20.

Jarebinski, M., Vlajinac, H., and Adanja, B. (1988). Biosocial and other characteristics of the large bowel cancer patients in Belgrade (Yugoslavia). *Archiv fur Geschwulstforschung*, **58v**: 411–17.

Jarebinski, M., Adanja, B., and Vlajinac, H. (1989). Case-control study of relationship of some biosocial correlates to rectal cancer patients in Belgrade, Yugoslavia. *Neoplasma*, **36**: 369–74.

Ji, B.T., Weissfeld, J.L., Chow, W.H., Huang, W.Y., Schoen, R.E., and Hayes, R.B. (2006). Tobacco smoking and colorectal hyperplastic and adenomatous polyps. *Cancer Epidemiology, Biomarkers and Prevention*, **15**(5): 897–901.

Kahn, H.A. (1966). The Dorn study of smoking and mortality among US Veterans on 8 years of observation. In W. Haenszel (Ed.), *National Cancer Institute Monograph No. 19* (pp. 1–125). Bethesda, MD: National Cancer Institute.

Kearney, J., Giovannucci, E., Rimm, E.B., Stampfer, M.J., Colditz, G.A., and Ascherio, A. (1995). Diet, alcohol and smoking and the occurrence of hyperplastic polyps of the colon and rectum (United States). *Cancer Causes and Control*, **6**: 45–56.

Kikendall, J.W., Bowen, P.E., Burgess, M.B., Magnetti, C., Woodward, J., and Langenberg, P. (1989). Cigarettes and alcohol as independent risk factors for colonic adenomas. *Gastroenterology*, **97**: 660–64.

Knekt, P., Hakama, M., Järvinen, R., Pukkala, E., and Heliövaara, M. (1998). Smoking and risk of colorectal cancer. *British Journal of Cancer*, **78**: 136–39.

Kono, S., Ikeda, N., Yanai, F., Shinchi, K., and Imanishi, K. (1990). Alcoholic beverages and adenomatous polyps of the sigmoid colon: a study of male self-defence officials in Japan. *International Journal of Epidemiology*, **19**: 848–52.

Kune, G.A., Kune, S., Vitetta, L., and Watson, L.F. (1992a). Smoking and colorectal cancer risk: data from the Melbourne Colorectal Cancer Study and brief review of literature. *International Journal of Cancer*, **50v**: 369–72.

Kune, G.A., Kune, S., Watson, L.F., and Penfold, C. (1992b). Smoking and adenomatous colorectal polyps (letter). *Gastroenterology*, **103**: 1370–1.

Le Marchand, L., Wilkens, L.R., Kolonel, L.N., Hankin, J.H., and Lyu, L.C. (1997). Associations of sedentary lifestyle, obesity, smoking, alcohol use, and diabetes with the risk of colorectal cancer. *Cancer Research*, **57**: 4787–94.

Lee, W.C., Neugut, A.I., Garbowski, G.C., Forde, K.A., Treat, M.R., and Waye, J.D. (1993). Cigarettes, alcohol, coffee, and caffeine as risk factors for colorectal adenomatous polyps. *Annals of Epidemiology*, **3**: 239–44.

Lev, R. (1990). *Adenomatous Polyps of the Colon.* New York: Springer-Verlag.

Liang, P.S., Chen, T.Y., and Giovannucci, E. (2009). Cigarette smoking and colorectal cancer incidence and mortality: systematic review and meta-analysis. *International Journal of Cancer,* **124**(10): 2406–15.

Longnecker, M.P., Chen, M.J., Probst-Hensch, N.M., Harper, J.M., Lee, E.R., and Frankl, H.D. (1996). Alcohol and smoking in relation to the prevalence of adenomatous colorectal polyps detected at sigmoidoscopy. *Epidemiology,* **7**: 275–80.

Manabe, S., Tohyama, K., Wada, O., and Aramaki, T. (1991). Detection of a carcinogen, 2-amino-1-methyl-6-phenylimidazo[4,5-b]pyridine (PhIP), in cigarette smoke condensate. *Carcinogenesis,* **12**: 1945–7.

Martinez, M.E., McPherson, R.S., Annegers, J.F., and Levin, B. (1995). Cigarette smoking and alcohol consumption as risk factors for colorectal adenomatous polyps. *Journal of the National Cancer Institute,* **87**: 274–9.

Monnet, E., Allemand, H., Farina, H., and Carayon, P. (1991). Cigarette smoking and the risk of colorectal adenoma in men. *Scandinavian Journal of Gastroenterology,* **26**: 758–62.

Morimoto, L.M., Newcomb, P.A., Ulrich, C.M., Bostick, R.M., Lais, C.J., and Potter, J.D. (2002). Risk factors for hyperplastic and adenomatous polyps: evidence for malignant potential? *Cancer Epidemiology, Biomarkers and Prevention,* **11**(10 Pt 1): 1012–18.

Morson, B.C. (1974). Evolution of cancer of the colon and rectum. *Cancer,* **34** (suppl): 845–9.

Nagata, C., Shimizu, H., Kametani, M., Takeyama, N., Ohnuma, T., and Matsushita, S. (1999). Cigarette smoking, alcohol use, and colorectal adenoma in Japanese men and women. *Diseases of the Colon and Rectum,* **42**: 337–42.

Newcomb, P.A., Storer, B.E., and Marcus, P.M. (1995). Cigarette smoking in relation to risk of large bowel cancer in women. *Cancer Research,* **55**: 4906–9.

Nordlund, L.A., Carstensen, J.M., and Pershagen, G. (1997). Cancer incidence in female smokers: a 26-year follow-up. *International Journal of Cancer,* **73**: 625–8.

Nyren, O., Bergstrom, R., Nystrom, L., Engholm, G., Ekbom, A., and Adami, H.O. (1996). Smoking and colorectal cancer: a 20-year follow-up study of Swedish construction workers. *Journal of the National Cancer Institute,* **88**: 1302–7.

O'Brien, M.J., Yang, S., Clebanoff, J.L., Mulcahy, E., Farraye, F.A., and Amorosino, M. (2004). Hyperplastic (serrated) polyps of the colorectum: relationship of CpG island methylator phenotype and K-ras mutation to location and histologic subtype. *American Journal of Surgical Pathology,* **28**: 423–34.

Olsen, J. and Kronborg, O. (1993). Coffee, tobacco and alcohol as risk factors for cancer and adenoma of the large intestine. *International Journal of Epidemiology,* **22**: 398–402.

Pfohl-Leszkowicz, A., Grosse, Y., Carriere, V., Cugnenc, P.H., Berger, A., and Carnot, F. (1995). High levels of DNA adducts in human colon are associated with colorectal cancer. *Cancer Research,* **55**: 5611–16.

Pierce, J.P., Fiore, M.C., Novotny, T.E., Hatziandreu, E.J., and Davis, R.M. (1989). Trends in cigarette smoking in the United States. Projections to the year 2000. *JAMA,* **261**: 61–5.

Potter, J.D., Bigler, J., Fosdick, L., Bostick, R.M., Kampman, E., and Chen, C. (1999). Colorectal adenomatous and hyperplastic polyps: smoking and N-acetyltransferase 2 polymorphisms. *Cancer Epidemiology, Biomarkers and Prevention,* **8**: 69–75.

Rogot, E. and Murray, J.L. (1980). Smoking and causes of death among US Veterans: 16 years of observation. *Public Health Reports,* **95**: 213–22.

Samowitz, W.S., Albertsen, H., Sweeney, C., Herrick, J., Caan, B.J., and Anderson, K.E. (2006). Association of smoking, CpG island methylator phenotype, and V600E BRAF mutations in colon cancer. *Journal of the National Cancer Institute,* **98**(23): 1731–8.

Sandler, R.S., Lyles, C.M., McAuliffe, C., Woosley, J.T., and Kupper, L.L. (1993). Cigarette smoking, alcohol, and the risk of colorectal adenomas. *Gastroenterology,* **104**: 1445–51.

Slattery, M.L., West, D.W., Robison, L.M., French, T.K., Ford, M.H., and Schuman, K.L. (1990). Tobacco, alcohol, coffee, and caffeine as risk factors for colon cancer in a low-risk population. *Epidemiology,* **1**: 141–5.

Slattery, M.L., Potter, J.D., Friedman, G.D., Ma, K.N., and Edwards, S. (1997). Tobacco use and colon cancer. *International Journal of Cancer*, **70**: 259–64.

Slattery, M.L., Curtin, K., Anderson, K., Ma, K.N., Ballard, L., and Edwards, S. (2000). Associations between cigarette smoking, lifestyle factors, and microsatellite instability in colon tumors. *Journal of the National Cancer Institute*, **92**: 1831–36.

Staszewski, J. (1969). Smoking and cancer of the alimentary tract in Poland. *British Journal of Cancer*, **23**: 247–53.

Sturmer, T., Glynn, R.J., Lee, I.-M., Christen, W.G., and Hennekens, C.H. (2000). Lifetime cigarette smoking and colorectal cancer incidence in the Physicians' Health Study I. *Journal of the National Cancer Institute*, **92**: 1178–81.

Tajima, K. and Tominaga, S. (1985). Dietary habits and gastro-intestinal cancer. A comparative case-control study of stomach and large intestinal cancers in Nagoya, Japan. *Japanese Journal of Cancer Research*, **76**: 705–16.

Terry, M.B, and Neugut, A.I. (1998). Cigarette smoking and the colorectal adenoma-carcinoma sequence: a hypothesis to explain the paradox. *American Journal of Epidemiology*, **147**: 903–10.

Terry, P., Ekbom, A., Lichtenstein, P., Feychting, M., and Wolk, A. (2001). Long-term tobacco smoking and colorectal cancer in a prospective cohort study. *International Journal of Cancer*, **91**: 585–7.

Tulinius, H., Sigfusson, N., Sigvaldason, H., Bjarnadottir, K., and Tryggvadottir, L. (1997). Risk factors for malignant diseases: a cohort study on a population of 22,946 Icelanders. *Cancer Epidemiology Biomarkers and Prevention*, **6**: 863–73.

Tverdal, A., Thelle, D., Stensvold, I., Leren, P., and Bjartveit, K. (1993). Mortality in relation to smoking history: 13 years' follow-up of 68,000 Norwegian men and women 35–49 years. *Journal of Clinical Epidemiology*, **46**: 475–87.

Vogelstein, B., Fearon, E.R., Hamilton, S.R., Kern, S.E., Preisinger, A.C., and Leppert, M. (1988). Genetic alterations during colorectal-tumor development. *New England Journal of Medicine*, **319**: 525–32.

Weir, J.M. and Dunn, J.E., Jr. (1970). Smoking and mortality: a prospective study. *Cancer*, **25**: 105–12.

Welfare, M.R., Cooper, J., Bassendine, M.F., and Daly, A.K. (1997). Relationship between acetylator status, smoking, and diet and colorectal cancer risk in the north-east of England. *Carcinogenesis*, **18**: 1351–4.

Williams, R.R. and Horm, J.W. (1977). Association of cancer sites with tobacco and alcohol consumption and socioeconomic status of patients: interview study from the Third National Cancer Survey. *Journal of the National Cancer Institute*, **58**: 525–47.

Wu, A.H., Paganini-Hill, A., Ross, R.K., and Henderson, B.E. (1987). Alcohol, physical activity and other risk factors for colorectal cancer: a prospective study. *British Journal of Cancer*, **55**: 687–94.

Yamada, K., Araki, S., Tamura, M., Sakai, I., Takahashi, Y., and Kashihara, H. (1997). Case-control study of colorectal carcinoma *in situ* and cancer in relation to cigarette smoking and alcohol use (Japan). *Cancer Causes and Control*, **8**: 780–5.

Yamasaki, E. and Ames, B. N. (1977). Concentration of mutagens from urine by absorption with the nonpolar resin XAD-2: cigarette smokers have mutagenic urine. *Proceedings of the National Academy of Sciences of the United States of America*, **74**: 3555–9.

Yang, P., Cunningham, J.M., Halling, K.C., Lesnick, T.G., Burgart, L.J., and Wiegert, E.M. (2000). Higher risk of mismatch repair-deficient colorectal cancer in alpha1-antitrypsin deficiency carriers and cigarette smokers. *Molecular Genetics and Metabolism*, **71**: 639–45.

Yeoman, A., Young, J., Arnold, J., Jass, J., and Parry, S. (2007). Hyperplastic polyposis in the New Zealand population: a condition associated with increased colorectal cancer risk and European ancestry. *New Zealand Medical Journal*, **120**(1266): U2827.

Zahm, S.H., Cocco, P., and Blair, A. (1991). Tobacco smoking as a risk factor for colon polyps. *American Journal of Public Health*, **81**: 846–9.

Chapter 25

Smoking and cervical neoplasia

Maribel Almonte, Anne Szarewski, and Jack Cuzick

Squamous cell cervical cancer is primarily related to sexual activity (reviewed by Brinton 1992). Important risk factors are the number of lifetime sexual partners, early age at first intercourse and multiple sexual partners of a woman's husband. Use of barrier methods of contraception appears to be protective, whereas long-term use of the combined oral contraceptive pill appears to increase risk. Overwhelming evidence now implicates the human papillomaviruses, particularly certain so-called 'high-risk' types (e.g. 16, 18, 31, 33, 35, 39, 45, 51, 52, 56, 58, 59 and 68) as the causal sexually transmitted agents although other sexually transmitted infections such as chlamydia, herpes simplex virus (HSV), and human immunodeficiency virus (HIV) may also have a role. The high frequency of infection with human papillomavirus (HPV) and the relative rarity of cervical cancer suggest that other factors are needed to facilitate the carcinogenic process.

Winkelstein (1977) first drew attention to a possible role of cigarette smoking as a cofactor. Several studies had previously reported an association but it had been dismissed as a confounding factor for sexual variables, assumed to be either unmeasured or recorded inaccurately. Cigarette smoking and sexual behaviour are frequently related and the strong link between sexual behaviour and cervix cancer makes the evaluation of any relationship with smoking very difficult. However, as demonstrated below, the overall epidemiologic evidence supports the hypothesis that smoking is a cofactor or risk factor in its own right, even after controlling for sexual variables. In addition, there is now a substantial body of evidence from studies which have controlled for the effect of HPV, and which still show a significant effect of smoking. Three possible biological mechanisms have been proposed to explain the association, namely a direct carcinogenic effect on the cervix of cigarette smoke metabolites, an indirect effect mediated by an alteration of the host immune response, and an effect on antioxidants. These will be discussed later in this review.

We reviewed this topic extensively in the past and in this chapter we update these reviews. Readers are referred to the previous publications for details of studies not fully covered or referenced here. We have included a series of forest plots of the individual studies, which allow simple visualization of the data. We have focused on the impact of current smoking where the data were available, but if not, have used ever smoking as the exposure variable. No specific attempt has been made to summarize information on dose–response and duration.

Cohort studies

We are aware of twenty three cohort studies in this field. Two cohorts in Taiwan were pooled and reported together by Wen *et al.* (2004), another two American cohorts were reported separately by Trimble *et al.* (2005). Greenberg *et al.* (1985) evaluated the risk for cervical intraepithelial neoplasia or cancer incidence among smokers who participated in the Oxford Family Planning Association contraceptive study, and more recently risks for cervical cancer mortality. No individual estimates from the Million Women study in the UK were available, although the data were previously used in a pooled analysis.

Four cohorts studied the relationship between smoking and cervical cancer incidence. Three of them reported a significant increased risk of developing cervical cancer among smokers and a recent fourth study showed no effect. However the combined results were highly significant indicating a 54% increase risk (OR: 1.54, 95% CI 1.33–1.78, $p<0.001$). Three of six reports on cancer mortality showed significant increased risk of dying of cervical cancer among smokers (including the one study with no effect on incidence) and again the overall results were highly significant indicating a 68% increase (OR: 1.68, 95% CI 1.40–2.03, $p<0.001$).

Nine cohort studies have used incidence of cervical intraepithelial neoplasia (CIN) (different grades) or abnormal cytology as endpoints, only two of them did not show significant increased risk (Fig. 25.1). In general, however, these studies did not adjust for sexual behaviour variables and this limits their value for assessing an independent effect of smoking. Four cohorts included HPV testing, only one of them had low-grade squamous intraepithelial lesion(LSIL) as an endpoint, the others concentrated in HPV prevalence, acquisition or clearance and will be discussed in detail later.

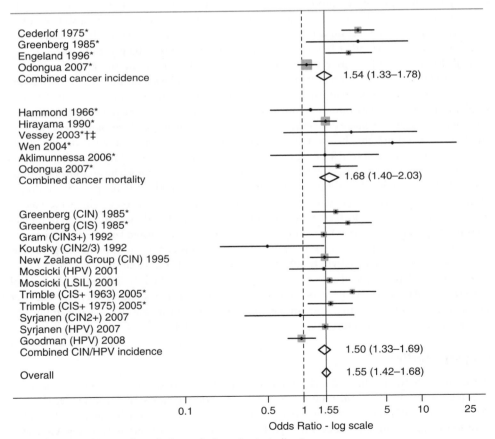

Figure 25.1 Smoking and cervical neoplasia: cohort studies [a].

[a] Numbers are odds ratios and (95% confidence intervals).

[*] Unadjusted. [†] Heavy exposure group. [‡] Mortality analysis of Greenberg study (Greenberg et al. 1985).

Case-control studies

We have previously reviewed case-control studies in detail. In the last 10 years, the majority of new studies published have included HPV testing and have therefore been of greater interest. Later in this chapter, we will therefore concentrate on those studies.

There are 38 case-control studies which have addressed the relationship between smoking and invasive cervical cancer, summarized in Fig. 25.2. Three of them specifically looked at risk associated with adenocarcinomas and two showed a positive although not significant relationship. There were no smokers in the control group of one IARC case-control study so no risk estimates were available. All but one of the remaining 37 studies reported elevated risks; however, only 21 of them were significant with odds ratios for current smokers mostly between 1.6 and 3.0, leading to an overall 56% increase risk (OR 1.56 95% CI 1.47–1.65, $p<0.001$).

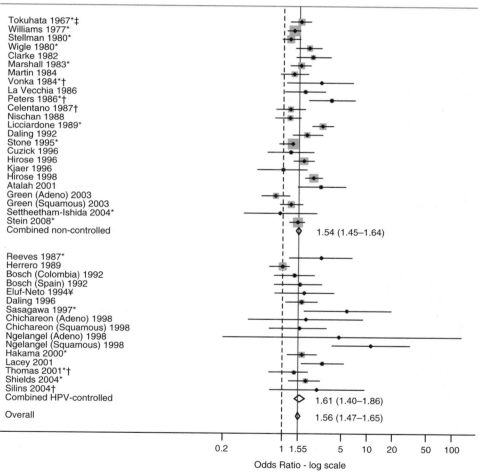

Figure 25.2 Smoking and cervical neoplasia: case-control studies – cancer [a].

[a] Numbers are odds ratios and (95% confidence intervals).

* Unadjusted. [†] Heavy exposure group. [‡] Cervical cancer mortality.

[¥] OR obtained from Plummer's meta-analysis (Plummer et al., 2003).

Twenty-three case-control studies have looked at carcinoma in situ (CIS) or CIN3. Sixteen made some adjustment for sexual behaviour, all but one of them show a significant increased risk among smokers, and 12 of them show a dose–response relationship (Fig. 25.3). The adjusted ORs for current smokers are generally higher than those reported for invasive cancer, hence, the overall OR of 2.45 (95% CI 2.25–2.67). The reasons for this are unclear, but could reflect a younger age group where current smoking is more prevalent.

Eighteen studies report data on both CIN and invasive cancer. These studies generally encompass CIS, CIN3, or CIN2 and worse lesions and separate odds ratios for CIN and cancer are usually not given. All but two of these studies (both in adenocarcinoma) showed a positive relationship with smoking, with an overall increase risk of 89% (OR 1.89, 95% CI 1.71–2.10) (Fig. 25.4).

Twenty-eight studies have reported data on different grades of CIN, some of them had evaluated the association between smoking and a variety of endpoints separately. Additionally, four

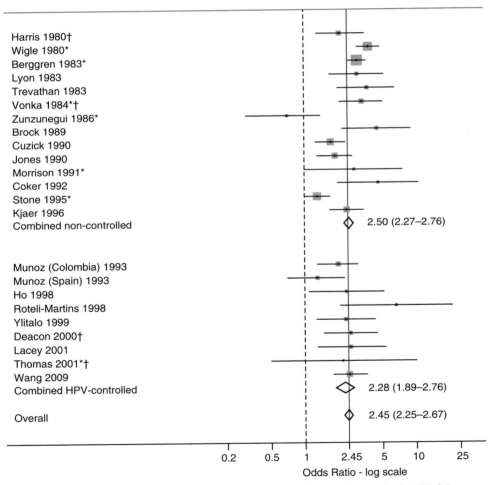

Figure 25.3 Smoking and cervical neoplasia: case-control studies – carcinoma in situ/CIN 3 [a].

[a] Numbers are odds ratios and (95% confidence intervals).

* Unadjusted. [†] Heavy exposure group.

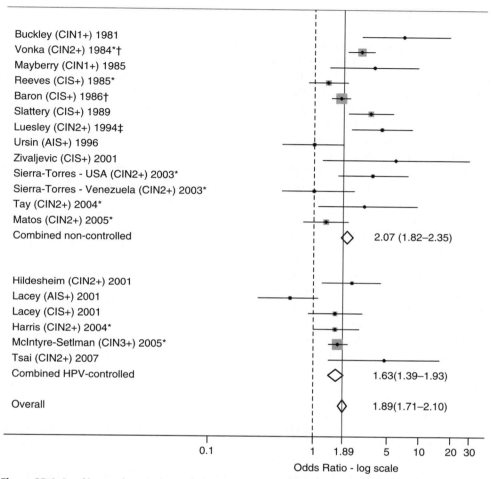

Figure 25.4 Smoking and cervical neoplasia: case-control studies – both cancer and CIN [a].

CIN: cervical intraepithelial neoplasia, CIN+: CIN (each grade) or worse cervical lesions, CIS+: carcinoma in situ and cancer, AIS+: in situ and invasive adenocarcinoma.

[a] Numbers are odds ratios and (95% confidence intervals).

* Unadjusted. [†] Heavy exposure group. [‡] Controls were women with CIN1 or less histology.

addressed the association on CIN2 and CIN3 combined, six on CIN1 and CIN3 combined, and four on abnormal cytology, and Brisson (1994) and Derchain (1999) reported risks associated with CIN1 alone, as well as CIN2 and CIN3 combined, but not on cancer. Of 17 studies that included CIN3, 12 showed significant increased risks among smokers, with an overall odds ratio of 2.44 (95% CI 2.16–2.75).

It is of interest that some studies which have looked separately at low and high grades of CIN have found that the relationship with smoking tends to be stronger for the higher grades. For example, in the study by Cuzick et al. (1990), the adjusted OR for women with CIN1 was 1.21 (95% CI 0.8–1.6), whereas for CIN3 it was 1.72 (1.3–2.3). Similar results were reported by Brisson et al. (1994), Kjaer et al. (1996), Derchain et al. (1999), Morrison et al. (1991), and Vonka et al. (1984) in which the percentage of smokers increased steadily from controls to CIN1, to high grade CIN or cancer (test for heterogeneity between studies on CIN1 only vs. studies on CIN3 only: $p<0.001$).

Luesley *et al.* (1994) studied 167 women referred to a colposcopy clinic with cervical smears showing mild dyskaryosis. Histological outcome was made on the basis of a large loop excision of the transformation zone (LLETZ). Current smoking was associated with an OR of 4.35 (CI 2.25–8.43) for high-grade disease (CIN2 or worse compared to CIN1 or less). In addition, lesion size was found to be significantly larger in smokers ($p = 0.007$). Similar results were reported by Daly *et al.* (1998) among 173 women with mildly abnormal smears. High-grade disease on colposcopy was the outcome of the study, and was compared to low-grade or less colposcopy result. The authors also reported a dose–response relationship between the number of cigarettes smoked and the risk of high-grade disease (OR 5.85 95% CI 1.92–17.80 for women who smoked more than 20 cigarettes per day). Unfortunately, these studies did not include testing for HPV and did not adjust for sexual variables other than parity and contraceptive status.

Harris *et al.* (2004) conducted a screening study in Seattle. Women were screened with cytology and HPV testing (PCR L1 consensus primer and reverse line blot hybridization). Women with abnormal cytology or with negative cytology and positive HPV test, and a random sample of women negative on both tests were referred to colposcopy, where second cervical samples were collected. Among 461 women with high-risk HPV infection, 181 had negative histology and were considered controls, 137 had CIN1, 53 CIN2, and 90 CIN3+ (only 2 cancer cases). Current-smokers were at higher risk of having CIN1 (OR 1.8 95% CI 1.1–3.1) or CIN2+ (OR 1.6 95% CI 1.0–2.7). There was a dose–response relationship between smoking intensity and CIN1 and CIN2+ and the strength of the effects was similar.

Tay and Tay (2004) evaluated the association of cigarette smoking and spouse's cigarette smoking with low-grade (LSIL: HPV changes or CIN1) or high-grade squamous intraepithelial lesions (HSIL: CIN2, CIN3, or invasive cancer) in 623 women referred to colposcopy after abnormal cytology in Singapore. Current cigarette smoking was associated with HSIL (OR 3.0 95% CI 1.2–7.8) but not with LSIL (OR 0.9 95% CI 0.2–39.1). Women whose spouses were current smokers were also at higher risk of having HSIL (OR 2.3 95% CI 1.5–3.5) but there was no significant elevated risk for LSIL (OR 1.5 95% CI 0.9–2.4). After controlling for reproductive and sexual behaviour factors, the risk of developing HSIL was also increased by every additional cigarette that the women's spouse smoked in a day (OR 1.046 95% CI 1.013–1.080), suggesting that the woman's risk would be doubled if the husband smoked 22 cigarettes a day. Unfortunately these results are not adjusted for HPV infection as no HPV testing was carried out.

Tsai *et al.* (2007) carried a community case-control study in Taiwan to evaluate the association between HPV infection and CIN. Cases were women with inflammation or worse histology after abnormal cytology. Six women with negative histology and 507 women in the same community who had two previous consecutive negative smears were considered controls. HPV testing was done by HC-II. There was a significant association between smoking and CIN2+ (OR 4.7 95% CI 1.4–15.7) after adjusting for HPV status and other risk factors, while the effects were not significant for inflammation (OR 2.2 95% CI 0.6–8.2) or CIN1 (OR 2.9 95% CI 0.8–10.1).

Moscicki *et al.* (2008) studied 622 adolescents and young women aged 13–24 years referred to colposcopy because of abnormal cytology. Biopsies were obtained at time of colposcopy yielding 157 CIN1s, 81 CIN2s, and 41 CIN3s, no cancers were diagnosed. Patients were interviewed for risk factors. HPV testing was done by polymerase chain reaction (PCR). Smoking was measured as the number of cigarettes smoked in the 24 hours before the interview and was only weakly associated with risk of CIN3 (compared to CIN1 or less, $p = 0.05$). But no significant association was found with CIN3 (OR 2.29 95% CI 0.35–15.03), or CIN2 (OR 1.50 95% CI 0.32–7.06) after adjusting for age, use of oral contraception, sexual behaviour, and HPV positivity.

Wang *et al.* (2009) evaluated risk factors for CIN2, CIN3, and cancer in the SUCCEED (Study to Understand Cervical Cancer Early Endpoints and Determinants) study of 1 899 women enrolled in a colposcopy centre. The Linear Array HPV Genotyping Test (Roche Diagnostics) was used for HPV typing of 37 genotypes. Among 1 378 high-risk HPV positive women without cancer, current smoking was associated with CIN3 (OR 2.5 95% CI 1.8 3.6) but not CIN2 (OR 1.3 95% CI 0.9–1.8) after adjusting for sexual behaviour, reproductive health, and demographic factors. When the analysis was restricted to women with HPV16 or HPV16/18 infections, current-smokers were at higher risk of CIN2 and CIN3. The authors also found increasing risk for both CIN2 and CIN3 for 10 or more years of smoking and there was a dose–response relationship with number of pack-years. All associations were stronger for CIN3.

Interaction with the human papillomavirus HPV

In 1982, zur Hausen suggested that the HPV might be the primary cause of cervical cancer. Although it appears to be one of the few complete carcinogens (i.e. not necessarily requiring other cofactors) it is clear that carcinogenicity is greatly accelerated when cofactors are present. He postulated that, in the case of cervical cancer, both smoking and HSV were possible cocarcinogens. Since then, the evidence implicating HPV as the major causal agent has become overwhelming, with a number of high-risk types identified, in particular types 16 and 18.

The number of studies which have included information both on smoking and presence of HPV infection has increased considerably in recent years. Early studies used assays of limited accuracy but more recent studies have mostly used a consensus PCR system or hybrid capture II (HC-II). After adjustment for HPV positivity, the majority of odds ratios were reduced but remained significant (Figs. 25.2–25.5). These studies will now be considered in greater detail.

Reeves *et al.* (1987) were the first to use HPV typing in a case-control study of cervical cancer cases in Latin America. Unfortunately, the method chosen was filter in situ hybridization (FISH) which is now known to be of low sensitivity and specificity. There was no dose–response information from this study, but the unadjusted OR for current smoking (number/day not specified) was 2.88 (95% CI 1.2–6.6). The results from this study are of limited value in view of the lack of a sexual behaviour adjusted OR.

Herrero *et al.* (1989) reported another Latin American study of cancer cases, again using FISH for HPV detection. In this study, only 30% of cases and controls had ever smoked for more than six months, and over half of these (in both groups) had smoked less than 10 cigarettes per day. This study did not show an overall effect of smoking (relative risk [RR] 1.7 95% CI 0.8–3.6), but it is interesting that within the subgroup of women who were positive for HPV 16/18 there was some additional increased risk with smoking (RR 6.3 95% CI 4.3–9.2), after adjustment for other sexual variables, and also a dose–response relationship (RR for > 10/day 8.4 95% CI 4.4–16.2).

Morrison *et al.* (1991) used a combination of Southern blotting and PCR techniques to assess HPV status in a study conducted in New York. This case-control study did not include cancer cases, restricting itself to CIN (of any grade). Once again, a high proportion of both cases (53%) and controls (44%) were of Hispanic origin and relatively few women (20% of cases and 9% of controls) smoked more than 10 cigarettes per day. The study showed an increased risk in smokers (OR 3.0 95% CI 1.1–8.1) and a dose–response relationship, but the association was no longer significant after adjustment for HPV.

Bosch *et al.* (1992) reported a Spanish/Colombian study of invasive cancer cases, using a consensus PCR technique to evaluate HPV status. The results were presented separately for Spain and Colombia, as there were some differences between the two countries. In Spain, only 26% of the cases and 17% of the controls had ever smoked, while in Colombia 50% of the cases and 40%

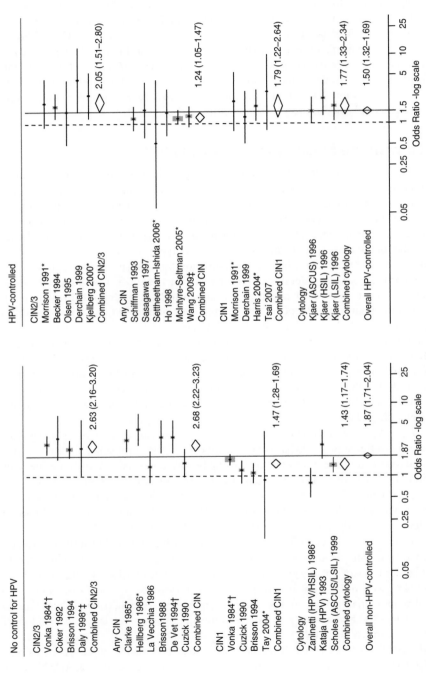

Figure 25.5 Smoking and cervical neoplasia: case-control studies – CIN of all grades [a].

[a] Numbers are odds ratios and (95% confidence intervals).

* Unadjusted. † Heavy exposure group.

of the controls had ever smoked. No information was available regarding the amount smoked. After adjusting for HPV and sexual variables smoking was only marginally significant in this study (combined OR 1.5 (95% CI 1.0–2.2).

A study by Munoz et al. (1993) was carried out in parallel with the one by Bosch et al. (1992), this time looking specifically at cases with CIN3/carcinoma in situ rather than invasive cancer. In Spain 59% of cases and 34% of controls were current-smokers; in Colombia 38% of cases and 14% of controls were current-smokers. However, in Spain 19% of cases and 46% of smoking controls had smoked for less than five pack-years and in Colombia the figures were 60% of cases and 49% of controls. Thus, even if the women smoked, they tended to be relatively light smokers. In Spanish women, although a significant overall association with current smoking was not found, there was a dose–response relationship ($p = 0.003$), with an OR of 3.1 (95% CI 2.0–4.7) for smokers of more than 5 pack-years. In Colombia, there was an association with current smoking, OR 2.0 (95%-CI 1.3–3.0), but no clear dose–response ($p = 0.09$).

Schiffman et al. (1993) reported a case-control study from a health screening clinic in Oregon, using consensus PCR for determination of HPV status. Cases and controls were chosen on the basis of cytology results, which introduced misclassification problems in both case and control groups. Although not all cases had colposcopy and biopsy, of those who did, the majority were low-grade lesions. Based on cytology, there were 450 low-grade lesions and 50 of high grade. Thirty-five percent of cases and 20% of controls were current-smokers; no data were presented regarding amount or duration of smoking. An increased risk in current smokers was observed (RR 1.7, $p < 0.05$), but this was no longer significant after adjustment for HPV (RR 1.2 95% CI 0.8–1.8). However, an ancillary analysis showed that among HPV positive women, current-smokers were almost three times as likely to have CIN2/3 as non-smoking women (RR 2.7 95% CI 1.1–6.5).

The International Agency for Research on Cancer (IARC) has carried out a series of studies in developing countries. These studies [Eluf-Neto et al. 1994] have had a similar design and so will be discussed together. Women with invasive cancer were recruited, with controls from the same hospital. HPV testing was performed by the G5+/G6+ consensus PCR. A common problem in these studies is that relatively few women smoked, reducing their statistical power. In addition, smokers tended to smoke fewer than 10 cigarettes per day. Both squamous and adenocarcinoma were included, but not always reported separately (because of small numbers). The studies which looked at adenocarcinoma separately did not find a significant association with smoking. Three studies present results only from HPV positive cases and controls. This reduces the number of women still further and although all show an elevated OR for smoking, none is statistically significant. IARC recognized that the individual studies lacked power and has recently published a meta-analysis (using only HPV positive cases and controls), which shows a significant association with smoking (OR 2.04 95% CI 1.32–3.14) and a dose-response effect (Plummer et al. 2003).

Becker et al. (1994) compared Hispanic with non-Hispanic women in a university gynaecology clinic in New Mexico. HPV status was determined by a consensus PCR. Incident cases of CIN2/3 were included, with the majority of both cases and controls (64%) being of Hispanic origin. The women were relatively young, with a median age of 26 and a range of 18–40 years. An increased risk of CIN2/3 in current smokers persisted, even after adjustment for HPV (OR 1.8 95% CI 1.2–2.8). Interestingly, a separate analysis by ethnic group showed that current smoking was significant only in non-Hispanic women (OR 2.7 95% CI 1.3–5.7), though the difference between the ethnic groups was not statistically significant.

Olsen et al. (1995) reported on women with CIN2/3 in Norway, using PCR methods for HPV assessment. The women were relatively young (median age 31–32 years, range 20–44 years). They found a very strong association between HPV 16 and high-grade disease (adjusted OR 182.4 95%

CI 54.0–616.1). Information on smoking status was limited to ever vs. never smokers; the crude OR of 4.1 (95% CI 2.1–8.1) was reduced to 1.5 (95% CI 0.5–4.3) after adjustment for HPV status and sexual behaviour. A further analysis of these data (Olsen *et al.* 1998) confirmed these results for HPV 16 status (OR 4.6 95% CI 0.9–22.9). In addition, statistical testing showed that 74% of cases were attributable to the joint effect of smoking and HPV positivity.

Kjaer *et al.* (1996) showed that even after adjustment for sexual behaviour and the presence of HPV (detected by consensus PCR), among young women aged 20–29 years, smoking remained an independent risk factor for both low- and high-grade cervical abnormalities (as measured by cytology). The adjusted relative risks (RR) were 1.8 (95% CI 1.1–2.8) for low-grade abnormalities and 2.3 (95% CI 1.3–4.2) for high-grade abnormalities. The study also showed that current smoking was a significant risk factor in both HPV positive (OR 1.9 95% CI 1.2–3.2) and HPV negative women (OR 2.4 95% CI 1.3–4.6).

Sasagawa *et al.* (1997) in Japan found that smoking was a significant risk factor for invasive cancer after adjustment for HPV (OR 5.8 95% CI 1.8–19.0), but not for CIN (OR 1.6 95% CI 0.63–4.0). Smoking significantly elevated the risk of having an HPV infection (by PCR) in controls (OR 2.7 95% CI 1.1–6.9) but not cases (OR 1.4 95% CI 0.38–5.4), most of whom were in any case HPV positive.

Roteli-Martins *et al.* (1998) compared risk factors in 54 women with biopsy-proven CIN1 with 23 who had high-grade CIN, in their study in Brazil. HPV testing was performed by Hybrid Capture I. All women had abnormal Pap smears and were between 20 and 35 years of age. Smokers were significantly more likely to have high grade CIN (35% of women with CIN1 smoked vs. 78% of those with CIN2/3, $p < 0.001$) and there was a trend towards an increasing risk with increasing duration of smoking ($p = 0.07$). In addition, smokers were significantly more likely to test positive for high-risk HPV types ($p = 0.046$).

Ho *et al.* (1998) also used women with CIN1 as controls for those with high-grade CIN in their study from New York. In this larger study of 348 women, 90% were Hispanic or black. HPV testing was performed by PCR and Southern blotting. It was found that the risk of having CIN3 was significantly greater in smokers (OR 2.37 95% CI 1.09–5.15) and increased with the number of cigarettes smoked per day ($p = 0.03$) and duration of smoking ($p = 0.02$). However, this was not the case for CIN2 (OR for current smoking 1.46 95% CI 0.67–3.19).

Derchain *et al.* (1999) compared women with biopsy proven CIN with those whose biopsies were normal (despite an abnormal colposcopy). After adjustment for the presence of HPV (by Hybrid Capture I) smoking was still associated with in increased risk of high-grade CIN (OR 4.37 95% CI 1.48–12.92).

Ylitalo *et al.* (1999) in Sweden used all women without CIN3 as controls for those with CIN3 (thus the control group included even those with CIN2). This was a case-control study nested in a screening cohort, so HPV testing for types 16 and 18 was performed only on archival smears by PCR. A doubling of risk for CIN3 was found in current smokers (OR 1.94 95% CI 1.32–2.85). The effect of smoking remained significant in women who were HPV positive (OR 2.34 95% CI 1.28–4.27), but not in those who were HPV negative.

A similar nested case control study was carried out by Deacon *et al.* (2000), and once again any women without CIN3 were used as controls for those who had CIN3. There were 199 HPV positive cases (by PCR), 181 HPV positive controls, and 203 HPV negative controls. The risk factors for HPV positivity and having CIN3 were different, with smoking significant (with a dose response) for CIN3 (OR 2.57 95% CI 1.49–4.45) but not for HPV infection. The authors suggest that this provides evidence for a synergism of smoking with HPV to cause cervical neoplasia.

Kjellberg *et al.* (2000) in Sweden looked at 137 women with high-grade CIN and 253 age-matched controls. HPV testing was performed by PCR. Smoking was significantly associated with high-grade CIN even after adjustment for the presence of HPV (OR 2.6 95% CI 1.2–5.6). In addition, there was a dose response for both duration and amount of smoking (adjusted OR for > 15/day 6.0 95% CI 2.7–13.3).

Lacey et al. (2001) presented results for both adenocarcinoma (in situ and invasive) and squamous cancer (in situ and invasive) from a multi-centre study in the United States. Interestingly, there was a suggestion that current smoking was inversely related with adenocarcinoma, with an OR of 0.6 (95% CI 0.3–1.1), though only 18% of the 124 cases and 22% of the 307 controls smoked. Numbers for the squamous cancer analysis were also small, with 91 invasive and 48 in situ cases, of whom 43% smoked. There was a positive, though non-significant, association with current smoking (OR 1.6 95% CI 0.9–2.9). HPV testing (by consensus PCR) was not carried out on all women and some only had post-treatment samples, which may have reduced the power of the study further.

Hildesheim et al. (2001) included both cancer and CIN in their Costa Rican study. The analysis was restricted to HPV positive cases and controls (using both hybrid capture II and PCR). Despite the fact that only 12% of cases and 6% of controls were smokers, a significant association was found with current smoking (OR 2.3 95% CI 1.20–4.3) and there was a dose–response relationship for those smoking more than six cigarettes per day, having an OR of 3.1 (95% CI 1.2–7.9).

Thomas et al. (2001) carried out a hospital-based case-control study to identify risk factors for progression of intraepithelial cervical lesions. Two groups of cases and controls were selected: 190 invasive cancer and 291 controls, and 75 CIN3 or carcinomas in situ and 124 controls from the same hospital. HPV testing was done by PCR. Smoking was weakly associated with carcinoma in situ (age-adjusted OR 2.2 95% CI 0.5–1.0) and invasive carcinoma (age-adjusted OR 1.4 95% CI 0.7–2.0). The authors also evaluated risk of invasive cancer relative to risk of carcinoma in situ and found no significant increase (OR 1.2 95% CI 0.4–3.7) after adjusting for HPV infection.

Coker et al. (2002) have looked at both active and passive smoking as risk factors for CIN on cytology, using hybrid capture I as their HPV test. Current smoking was associated with a non-significant increase in risk of high-grade CIN (OR 1.81 95% CI 0.71–4.6), with a similar, but again non-significant OR for passive smoking exposure (OR 2.05 95% CI 0.77–6.2).

Sierra-Torres et al. (2003) carried out a hospital-based case-control study to evaluate the association between HPV infection, other co-factors and cervical cancer in 121 women from Caracas, Venezuela (38 cases and 83 controls) and 151 women from Texas (76 cases, 75 controls). The same protocol was used in both populations. Cases were women with histologically confirmed CIN2 or worse lesions. Age-matched controls were recruited from benign clinics in each country. HPV testing was done by PCR on biopsies at colposcopy (cases) or Hybrid Capture II (controls). High-risk HPV infection was significantly associated with CIN2+ in both populations, but there were more HPV positive controls in Venezuela (25% compared to 13% in Texas). Venezuelan women who started sexual relations before 18 and those with more than one lifetime sexual partner were at higher risk of CIN2+, but not those currently smoking. In contrast, among Americans, smoking was associated with higher risk of CIN2+ (OR 3.6 95% CI 1.7–7.7) but not with sexual behaviour.

Brinton et al. (1987) carried out a case-control in five cities of the United States. Cases were 481 women aged 20–74 years recently diagnosed with invasive cancer in 24 hospitals of these cities during April 1982 to January 1984. Two community controls per case were selected and individually matched to cases. There was an increased risk of cervical cancer in current-smokers when compared to never-smokers (OR 1.7 95% CI 1.4–2.3) after adjusting for sexual behaviour and other risk factors and a dose–response relationship with increasing number of cigarettes smoked per day. Shields et al. (2004) reanalysed the data after determining HPV status (seropositivity for types 16, 18, 31, 45, and 52) in 235 cases (156 were HPV positive to any of five types) and 486 (209 HPV positive) controls who donated blood samples at the time of recruitment. On the basis of data of 235 cases and 209 HPV positive controls, the original association between smoking and cervical cancer and the dose-response effect with smoking intensity and duration were confirmed (new OR 1.9 95% CI 1.2–2.8).

Studies examining the relationship between smoking and HPV infection

Nineteen studies have addressed the association between smoking and HPV positivity on women (Fig. 25.6). Four of them have reported estimates for both high-risk and low-risk HPV types separately. Five studies have evaluated the risk only for different high-risk HPV types and 10 for low- and high-risk types combined. Only seven studies reported positive associations, three with

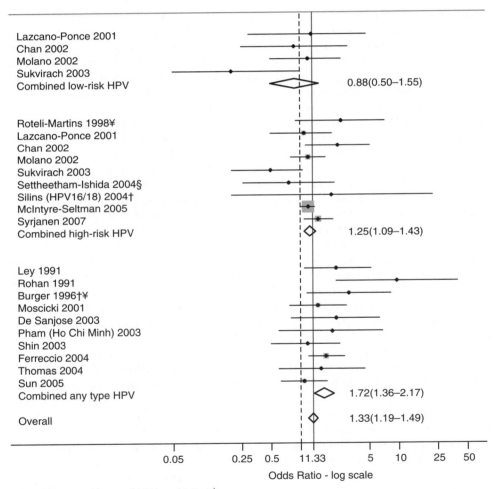

Figure 25.6 Smoking and HPV positivity [a,b].

[a] HPV positivity: HPV prevalence (cross-sectional studies) or HPV acquisition (follow-up studies).

[b] Numbers are odds ratios and (95% confidence intervals).

† Heavy exposure group. ¥ Study on women with CIN. § Estimates include women with cervical cancer.

high-risk types and four with any risk HPV. The overall odds ratios were 1.25 (95% CI 1.09–1.43) for high-risk types, 1.72 (1.36–2.17) for high- and low-risk types combined and non-significant for low-risk HPV (OR 0.88, 95% CI 0.50–1.55). Additionally, four longitudinal studies have evaluated associations between smoking with HPV persistence and two with HPV clearance. None of them showed significant associations.

Ley *et al.* (1991) investigated HPV prevalence in a screening population, using PCR methods for HPV detection. The study consisted of a cross-sectional sample of 467 women attending a university health clinic in California for routine screening. The women were young (median age 22 years), mostly white (72%) and non-Hispanic (87%). On initial analysis, current smoking was correlated with presence of HPV (OR 2.3 95% CI 1.1–5.2). The study did not investigate the women further and therefore no information is available regarding cervical abnormality in the two groups.

Rohan *et al.* (1991) conducted a similar cross-sectional university health clinic screening study, in Toronto. In this study, 105 women attending for routine cervical screening had samples taken for HPV typing (types 6, 11, 16, 18, and 33) by PCR. Once again, these women were young, with a mean age of 23 (range 20–27 years). Current smokers were more likely to have HPV infection of any type (OR 9.5 95% CI 2.3–39.5). Ever-smokers were also more likely to be infected with HPV of any type (OR 4.8 95% CI 1.6–14.2) and of HPV 16 (OR 5.8 95% CI 1.5–22.3). None of the women had an abnormal smear and no further investigations were performed.

Burger *et al.* (1993) in a study of 181 women with abnormal cervical smears, found that the prevalence of HPV types 16, 18, and 33 (as measured by PCR) increased in accordance with the number of cigarettes smoked (χ^2trend =10.75 1df, p = 0.001) even after adjustment for sexual variables. In a separate, though overlapping study, Burger *et al.* (1996) found that the likelihood of women with CIN being HPV positive (by PCR) again increased significantly as their smoking intake increased (OR for > 20/day 3.11 95% CI 1.16–8.29).

Fairley *et al.* (1995) looked at the effect of stopping smoking in 49 women who originally tested positive for HPV. Based only on self-reports, no significant difference in HPV positivity (measured by PCR in material collected from tampons) at one year was found between the women who reported to have stopped smoking completely and the remaining women, some of whom were reported as 'partial quitters'.

Four studies have looked at factors affecting persistence of HPV infections. Of these, one showed no effect of smoking and one did not collect enough information on smoking behaviour for analysis. Liu *et al.* (1995) carried out a six-month intervention trial of folate supplementation, in which they found that heavy smokers had a lower risk of progression of dysplasia (RR 0.79, 95% CI 0.66–0.94). Hildesheim *et al.* (1994) also found a lower risk of persistent HPV infection in current-smokers compared to never-smokers (OR 0.22 95% CI 0.06–0.79). None of these studies was specifically designed to look at the effect of smoking and all had little information on smoking behaviour (indeed, too little for analysis in the case of Remmink *et al.*). Several ongoing cohort studies should provide more definitive evidence on this important question.

Bosch and Munoz have published further analyses of the studies carried out in Spain (Bosch *et al.* 1996) and Colombia (Munoz *et al.* 1996). They have looked at the effect of male sexual behaviour and penile HPV carriage on the risk of cervical cancer and CIN3 in the wives. In Spain, the presence of HPV DNA in the male (measured by PCR) conveyed a five-fold risk of cervical cancer for the wives (OR 4.9 95% CI 1.9–12.6). However, even after controlling for the presence of HPV DNA, other infections, sexual behaviour and the wife's smoking habit, smoking by the male partner was still a significant risk factor for cervical cancer (OR 2.8 95% CI 1.8–4.4) and showed a dose–response relationship (OR for >26 pack years 3.3 95% CI 2.0–5.5). In Colombia, by contrast, the presence of penile HPV DNA was not a significant factor (OR 1.2 95%

CI 0.6–2.3). However, after adjustment for the presence of HPV DNA and sexual behaviour, smoking was once again a significant factor, though less strongly than in the Spanish study, (OR 1.7 95% CI 1.1–2.5), with a suggestion of a dose–response relationship (OR for > 26 pack-years 2.0 95% CI 1.0–3.9).

In a similar effort to that of case-control studies, the IARC has carried out a series of HPV prevalence population-based surveys in 11 countries worldwide. These studies were carried out between 1993 and 2005, shared the same protocols and questionnaires, which included smoking habits and so will be discussed together. HPV testing was performed by the G5+/G6+ consensus PCR. The studies in Thailand (Lampang survey), Argentina, and Chile reported prevalences of smoking of 29% or more, but in the other sites few women smoked (less than 10%) and in three sites almost no woman smoked. The studies in Korea (OR 2.35 95% CI 1.2–4.6) and Chile (OR 1.8 95% CI 1.2–2.8) reported a significant positive association for ever smoking, while the study in Thailand reported an inverse association (OR 0.4 95% CI 0.2–0.9). These contradictive results suggested lack of power due to the low prevalence of smoking and so IARC decided to do a pooled-analysis, which allowed to evaluate not only the effect of ever smoking, but also its intensity and to adjust for sexual behaviour factors. The pooled estimate for ever smoking was 1.18 (95% CI 1.01–1.39) and there was a dose–response relationship with smoking intensity among current smokers. The authors analysed the association separately for one, two and three or more lifetime number of sexual partners and found that among women who reported only one sexual partner, the risk of being HPV positive increased with smoking intensity (OR 3.03 95% CI 1.58–5.82 for smoking 15 or more cigarettes compared with never-smokers), but no significant trends were found in women with more than one sexual partner.

The survey in Colombia became the platform of a cohort study in Bogota which has reported on factors associated with clearance of HPV incident infections. A total of 1 728 women aged 15–85 years with normal cytology at baseline were followed every six months for an average of 9 years. There was no association between ever smoking and clearance of HPV infection at baseline (OR 1.0 95% CI 0.7–1.3) or when duration of incident infections including all new infections in every visit was used to define persistence (OR for clearance of HPV16: 0.7 95% CI 0.4–1.1, OR for HPV18: 0.6 95% CI 0.2–1.4).

Moscicki et al. (2001) carried out a longitudinal study in women aged 13 to 20 years in San Francisco. Women who were HPV negative at the beginning of the study were followed up for a median of 50 months. Smoking was not associated with development of incident HPV infection (OR 1.5 95% CI 0.77–2.94), but was a significant risk factor for development of low-grade CIN, in women who were HPV positive (OR 1.67 95% CI 1.12–2.48), suggesting that HPV infections are more likely to lead to CIN in smokers.

Chan et al. (2002) in a study of over 2 000 women attending for routine screening, found that current smoking was significantly associated with the presence of high-risk, but not low-risk HPV types (by PCR). The adjusted OR for current smoking were 0.87 (95% CI 0.25–3.06) for low-risk and 2.40 (95% CI 1.13–5.09) for high-risk HPV types.

Settheetham-Ishida et al. (2004) carried out a case-control study in Thailand. Cases were 90 women with histological confirmed squamous cell carcinoma and controls were 100 volunteers with normal histopathological appearance of the cervix. Information on risk factors was collected by self-reporting or interview. HPV testing was done by PCR, for detection of HPV types 16, 18, 31, 35, 52b and 58. PCR was also used to detect the *p53* codon 72 polymorphism. Smoking was not associated with cervical cancer (OR 0.93 95% CI 0.35–2.52). In a separate report, using data from 181 women, irrespectively of disease status (cases or controls), there was no association between HPV positivity and current smoking (OR 0.76 95% CI 0.26–2.21). But these results are limited because of including women with invasive cervical cancer. The same authors conducted a parallel study with similar HPV and *p53* detection protocols in 103 women with histologically confirmed CIN and 105 healthy controls to evaluate risk factors for CIN including HPV infection, the *p53* codon 72 polymorphism, sexual behaviour, and smoking. No significant association was found between current smoking and CIN (OR 0.53 95% CI 0.06–4.35) after adjusting for age, p53 genotypes, and HPV status.

Silins *et al.* (2004) evaluated risk factors including HPV infection for cervical cancer in Latvia. Cases were 223 women with incident invasive cancer and 239 healthy controls were selected from the Latvian population registry. HPV testing was done by PCR. After adjusting for HPV, age, screening history, and area of residence, heavy smoking (more than ten cigarettes per day) was not associated with cervical cancer (OR 2.6 95% CI 0.72–9.37). The same results were obtained for risk of HPV types 16/18 DNA positivity among population controls (OR 2.08 95% CI 0.20–22.23). But the proportion of smokers, and hence, heavy smokers in the study was very small.

McIntyre-Seltman *et al.* (2005) evaluated the associations of smoking with HPV positivity, CIN2 and CIN3+ (CIN3 and cancer) in the ALTS (ASCUS and LSIL Triage Study) trial. HPV status was determined by a stringent combination of results of Hybrid Capture II (HC2) and a consensus PCR method. Controls were women with histology less than CIN2. Among controls, former smoking was associated with decreased risk of HPV infection (OR 0.6 95% CI 0.5–0.8) while current smoking was positively but weakly associated with HPV infection (OR 1.2 95% CI 1.0–1.4). Among HPV positive women, current smoking was associated with CIN3+ (OR 1.7 95% CI 1.4–2.1) but not with CIN2 (OR 1.2 95% CI 0.95–1.06). Former smoking was associated with both CIN2 (OR 1.5 95% CI 1.0–2.1) and CIN3+ (OR 1.7 95% CI 1.2–2.4). Among HPV positive current-smokers, there was a dose–response relationship between smoking intensity and duration and CIN3+ but not with CIN2. When the analysis was restricted to HPV 16 DNA positive women, the effect of current smoking was similar for CIN3+ (OR 2.0 95% CI 1.4–2.8) and stronger for CIN2 (OR 1.7 95% CI 1.1–2.8) but showed no dose–response relationship. The authors also reported on the association of smoking and detection of oncogenic HPV DNA in control women. There was a positive although not significant association with current smoking (OR 1.2 95% CI 1.0–1.4) and inversely, a protective effect of former smoking (OR 0.6 95% CI 0.5–0.8).

Sun *et al.* (2005) explored factors affecting HPV prevalence in all grades of cervical neoplasia among 1 264 Chinese women with abnormal cytology in Taiwan. After colposcopy and biopsy, 477 women were diagnosed with low-grade cervical lesions, 453 with high-grade lesions, and 16 with cervical cancer. HPV testing was done with HC-II. Information on risk factors was collected through interviews at enrolment. There was no association between smoking and HPV prevalence at entry (adjusted OR 1.08 95% CI 0.63–1.84), estimates were based on data of all women independently of their disease status. This study has been the platform for a cohort study organized by the Taiwan Cooperative Oncology Group (TCOG) which will report on risk factors associated with HPV persistence.

Syrjanen *et al.* (2007) explored predictors of HPV infection and CIN2 or worse lesions (CIN2+) in a cohort of 3 187 women from three New Independent States of the former Soviet Union. HPV testing was done by both HC-II and PCR. Cases were women with histologically confirmed CIN2+, although the cohort was only followed-up for two years at the time of analysis. Women were stratified according to their smoking history in never, past, and current smokers and predictors were evaluated within categories for both endpoints. Further analysis included evaluation of predictors of each endpoint independently in all women. After adjusting for several risk factors, smoking was associated with HPV positivity (OR 1.52 95% CI 1.09–2.14) but not with CIN2+ (OR 0.94 95% CI 0.32–2.67).

Goodman *et al.* (2008) evaluated the association between smoking and HPV acquisition and clearance within the Hawaiian Human Papillomavirus Cohort Study. Participants were asymptomatic women aged 18–85 years who attended five gynaecological clinics in Hawaii between 1998 and 2003 underwent a gynaecological exam, had cervical samples for cytology and HPV testing collected and gave information on demographics, reproductive history, sexual behaviour, tobacco, and alcohol use in an interview at entry and at each follow-up visit (every four months). HPV testing was done by PCR. Among 972 women who had at least two clinical visits, 243 high-risk HPV incident infections occurred and 134 of them cleared during follow-up (the median infection duration was 224 days). The authors did not find associations between ever smoking and acquisition or clearance of high-risk HPV infections (OR for HPV acquisition 0.96 95% CI 0.74–1.26, OR for HPV clearance 0.94 95% CI 0.67–1.33) after adjusting for age at entry to the study.

Intervention studies

An intervention study (Szarewski *et al.* 1996) found a significant correlation between the extent of smoking reduction and reduction in the size of minor-grade lesions over a six-month period. This study also looked at the effect of smoking reduction on immunological parameters (see below).

Possible mechanisms

Direct effects

Evidence has accumulated to support a direct biological mechanism for the association of smoking with cervical neoplasia. It has been shown that nicotine and cotinine are both found in cervical mucus possibly at concentrations that are higher than in serum (Sasson *et al.* 1985, Hellberg *et al.* 1988). It has also been reported that the mucus concentrations correlate with reported cigarette consumption (Schiffman *et al.* 1987; McCann *et al.* 1992; Prokopczyk *et al.* 1997). Nicotine can be converted to nitrosamines, which are known to be carcinogenic (Hoffman *et al.* 1985) but polycyclic aromatic amines in cigarette smoke are thought to be more important for other sites. Studies have shown malignant transformation of HPV 16-immortalized human endocervical cells by cigarette smoke condensate (Nakao *et al.* 1996; Yang *et al.* 1996, 1997, 1998). Alam *et al.* (2008) have shown that high cervical mucus concentrations of Benzo[a]pyrene (BaP), resulted in a ten-fold increase in HPV type 31 viral titers, whereas treatment with low concentrations of BaP resulted in an increased number of HPV genome copies but not an increase in virion morphogenesis. This might enhance viral persistence and thus cancer progression. In addition, DNA adducts (Simons *et al.* 1995; Mancini *et al.* 1999) and other evidence of genotoxic damage (Cerqueira *et al.* 1998) are detectable in cervical exfoliated cells. A recent study has shown that N7-MedG adduct levels were significantly correlated with number of cigarettes smoked per day and pack years of cigarette smoking in current smokers (Harrison 2006). Differences in genotype may affect susceptibility to the effects of smoking: in a study by Singh *et al.* (2008) carriers of the AA genotype of GSTM3 (part of the glutathione S-transferase gene family) among tobacco users were at elevated risk of cervical cancer ($p = .024$, OR 2.1 95% CI 1.0–4.1) as compared with AB and BB genotypes. These enzymes play an active role in the detoxification and elimination of carcinogens by conjugating reduced glutathione to genotoxic intermediates.

Another mechanism may be inactivation of tumour suppression genes, such as p16 (Lea *et al.* 2004), FHIT (Holschneider *et al.* 2005), p53 (Lindström *et al.* 2007), and LRIG1 (Lindström *et al.* 2008). In the study by Lea *et al.*, aberrant p16 methylation was associated with active tobacco use in patients with squamous carcinoma (OR 20.6 95% CI 3.6–118; P<.001) and high-grade

CIN (OR 4.57 95% CI 1.63–12.78; $P=0.002$). The fragile histidine triad (FHIT) gene is a tumour suppressor gene that is altered in 80% of tobacco-associated lung cancers. Holschneider et al. (2005) found that loss of FHIT expression, homozygous deletions, hemizygous deletions, and microsatellite alterations at the FHIT/FRA3B locus occurred significantly more commonly in cervical cancers of smokers. The tumour suppressor gene p53 is activated in response to DNA damage; it has been shown that the E6 oncogene of HPV is able to promote p53 degradation. Lindström et al. (2007), while investigating ten different tumour markers found a significant association between an absence of p53 staining and smoking ($p = 0.008$). Lindström et al. (2008) also demonstrated diminished expression of LRIG1 in advanced stages of cervical cancer and an inverse correlation with smoking.

Winkelstein (1977) has pointed out that smoking is strongly associated with squamous cell carcinoma at other sites (lung, bladder) and that the vast majority of cervical carcinomas are of this type.

Immunologic effects

Immunosuppression is associated with an increased risk of cervical neoplasia and smoking is associated with a number of immunological changes in the cervix. Women who are on immuno-suppressive therapy are known to be at increased risk of developing condylomas, CIN, and cervical carcinoma (Porecco et al. 1975; Schneider et al. 1983; Sillman et al. 1984; Penn et al. 1986; Sillman et al. 1987; Alloub et al. 1989). In addition, a recent study (Alloub et al. 1989) has shown that these women are more likely to show positivity for HPV 16/18; in this study, 27% of the immunosuppressed women vs. 6% of the controls were positive for HPV 16/18, ($p < 0.005$).

Women infected with the HIV virus have been shown to be at higher risk of developing both HPV infection and CIN (Byrne et al. 1989; Maiman et al. 1990; Schafer et al. 1991; Vermund et al. 1991; Johnson et al. 1992; Mandelblatt et al. 1992; Maggwa et al. 1993). Since these conditions share many of the same risk factors, confounding is always a possibility. However, it does appear that the degree of immunosuppression (as measured by CD4/CD8 ratio) in HIV positive women is related to the risk of CIN (Schafer et al. 1991; Conti et al. 1993) and also to the risk of recurrence of CIN after treatment (Maiman et al. 1993). It has been suggested that, by virtue of its immuno-suppressive effects, HIV infection may facilitate infection with HPV and may also promote the effect of HPV in cervical carcinogenesis (Vermund et al. 1991; Matorras et al. 1991; Conti et al. 1993).

There is still controversy as to which immune parameters might be affected by smoking. In 1978 Rasp reported an impairment in adhesion of alveolar macrophages in smokers, which appeared to be reversible on cessation of smoking. Miller et al. (1982) found a reduced CD4/CD8 ratio in the blood of heavy smokers compared to non-smokers, and showed that the CD4/CD8 ratio returned to normal six weeks after cessation of smoking.

In recent years, attention has focused on the possible effect of smoking on Langerhans cells, epithelial dendritic cells which appear to have an important role in presenting antigen to T lymphocytes (Stingl et al. 1978; Hauser et al. 1992). It has been shown that application of a known skin carcinogen in mice results in a marked depletion of Langerhans cells (Muller et al. 1985). Smokers have been shown to have a reduced cutaneous inflammatory response to standard test irritants (Mills et al. 1993).

A number of studies have assessed the relationship between cervical neoplasia, human papillomavirus, and Langerhans cells. There is general agreement that Langerhans' cell density is reduced in the presence of HPV infection (Morris et al. 1983, Vayrynen et al. 1984, Caorsi et al. 1986, McArdle et al. 1986, Tay et al. 1987, Hawthorn et al. 1988, Morelli et al. 1993). However, some studies show that Langerhans' cell density is also reduced in CIN (Tay et al. 1987,

Morelli *et al.* 1993, Szarewski *et al.* 2001) while others suggest that it is increased (Morris *et al.* 1983, Vayrynen *et al.* 1984, Caorsi *et al.* 1986, McArdle *et al.* 1986, Hawthorn *et al.* 1988). Interestingly, Morelli *et al.* (1993) compared Langerhans' cell density across the grades of CIN and found a decrease in CIN 1 (comparable to that seen with HPV infection) and an increase in the higher grades. A contrasting pattern was found by Spinillo *et al.* (1993), who showed a significant reduction in Langerhans' cell counts in HIV positive women who had CIN, compared with HIV negative controls. In this study, Langerhans' cell density was reduced in HIV positive women even after adjusting for the presence of HPV by in situ hybridization. In addition, significantly lower Langerhans' cell counts were found in high-grade compared with low-grade CIN. These studies are complicated by different techniques of measuring Langerhans' cell density, which may, at least in part account for the discrepancies observed.

Daniels *et al.* (1992) studied the effect of smokeless tobacco on Langerhans' cell density in oral mucosal premalignant lesions (leukoplakia) and found it to be significantly reduced. However, Cruchley *et al.* (1994) found no such reduction in the normal oral mucosa of smokers.

Barton *et al.* (1988) showed a reduction in Langerhans' cell counts in cervical biopsies from women with both CIN and HPV infection. In addition, current-smokers had significantly reduced Langerhans' cell counts compared to non-smokers in both normal epithelium ($p = 0.005$) and biopsies showing CIN and/or HPV ($p = 0.03$). Poppe *et al.* (1995, 1996) confirmed these findings (in normal epithelium) and also showed a reduction of CD4 lymphocytes in the normal epithelium of smokers. However, Poppe *et al.* (1996) failed to show a correlation between the number of cigarettes smoked daily and the Langerhans' cell counts. Barton *et al.* (1988) did not distinguish between different smoking levels, differentiating only between current, ex- and non-smokers. Nadais *et al.* (2006) compared the intraepithelial population of Langerhans' cells (in normal cervical epithelium adjacent to CIN3 and found a lower number of Langerhans' cells in smokers than in non-smokers ($p = 0.045$). There was also a lower number of Langerhans' cells in normal areas adjacent to CIN3 than in normal cervix control group ($p = 0.004$). However, they did not show a significant difference in the number of Langerhans' cells in normal areas of the cervix with CIN3 between smokers and non-smokers.

By contrast, Szarewski *et al.* (2001) showed a significant increase in the number of Langerhans' cells with increasing levels of smoking, as measured by salivary cotinine levels. This study assessed changes in both Langerhans' cells and lymphocytes when women attempted to give up smoking: a significant trend towards a reduction in cell count with stopping smoking was found for Langerhans' cells ($p = 0.05$), total lymphocytes ($p = 0.02$), and CD8 lymphocytes ($p = 0.05$). Heavy smoking was also significantly associated ($p = 0.02$) with an increased chance of persistence of HPV in cervical biopsies.

Other immune parameters may also be involved in the aetiology of cervical HPV infection and CIN. A decrease in T cell counts, particularly of the CD4 component, has been reported, resulting in a reversed CD4/CD8 ratio (Tay *et al.* 1987). In the study of HIV positive women by Spinillo *et al.* (1993) both the reduction in Langerhans' cell count and increasing grade of CIN were correlated with a progressively greater reversal of the blood CD4/CD8 ratio. Several studies (Turner *et al.* 1988, Kesic *et al.* 1990, Soutter *et al.* 1994) have shown a lower CD4/CD8 ratio in the peripheral blood of women with CIN, compared to colposcopically normal controls. In the study by Soutter *et al.*, laser treatment of the CIN resulted in a rise in the CD4/CD8 ratio. The specific effects of smoking were not, however, evaluated in these studies.

In recent years it has been suggested that cytokine interactions may be influenced by smoking (Eppel *et al.* 2000) and that these are significant in the immune response to HPV and CIN (Mota *et al.* 1999, Stanley *et al.* 1999). Simhan *et al.* (2005), investigating a population of pregnant women, found an increase of cervical anti-inflammatory cytokines (interleukin-4, -10, and -13) in smokers without a commensurate increase of pro-inflammatory cytokines. Median concentrations of interleukin-4 and -10 were greater among women who smoked > or = 20 cigarettes per day than among non-smokers or less heavy smokers ($P < 0.05$ for both). The authors speculate that higher concentrations of multiple anti-inflammatory cytokines early in pregnancy may indicate a broad immune hypo-responsiveness that may create a permissive environment for ascending infection. By contrast, Lieberman et al. (2008) looking at non-pregnant women, found a significant decrease in the levels of the anti-inflammatory cytokines IFN-gamma, IL-1β, IL-6, and IL-10 in smokers. Also, non-significant trends towards lower cytokine levels were found in the presence of incident and persistent human papillomavirus infection. The authors point out that the cervical mucosal environment is complex, with many endogenous and exogenous factors that may affect cytokine levels. In addition, as with all immunological studies, differences in methodology may influence outcomes. A further complexity has been suggested by Sobti et al. (2008), who showed a significant association between IL-1β+3953 genotype and risk of cervical cancer, which was greater in passive smokers (there were virtually no active smokers in this study, making it impossible to assess this group). The authors suggest that IL-1 may be involved in the early steps of cervical carcinogenesis, and that individual differences in IL-1 secretion may affect individual susceptibility to cervical cancer progression.

Antioxidants

In recent years another aspect of the effect of smoking has come to light. It appears that smokers have a significantly different intake of many nutrients compared to non-smokers, and, in particular, a lower intake of foods providing antioxidants (Cade et al. 1991; Wichelow et al. 1991; Margetts et al. 1993). Smoking itself generates about 10^{15} free radicals with each puff, increasing the requirement for antioxidants which protect cells from damage by free radicals (Church et al. 1985). Smokers have been shown to have lower plasma levels of antioxidants compared with non-smokers (Palan et al. 1996). Not only do smokers have lower intakes of antioxidants such as ß carotene, alpha-tocopherol, and ascorbic acid, but, for a given intake, smokers have lower circulating blood levels of these vitamins compared to non-smokers (Stryker et al. 1988; Margetts et al. 1993). It has been suggested that the dietary intake of smokers and the metabolic effects of smoking on nutrient metabolism increase the risk of oxidative tissue damage in smokers above that which might be expected from the free radicals generated by smoking itself (Halliwell et al. 1993, Margetts et al. 1993). This may be of relevance to cervical neoplasia, where a number of studies have suggested a protective effect of antioxidant vitamins such as vitamin E (alpha-tocopherol), vitamin C (ascorbic acid), and beta-carotene (Marshall et al. 1983; La Vecchia et al. 1988; Slattery et al. 1990; Verreault et al. 1989; Basu et al. 1991; Romney et al. 1985; Wassertheil-Smoller et al. 1981; Cuzick et al. 1990). Although the role of dietary factors in cervical neoplasia is still unclear, it, and the possible link with smoking, merit further investigation.

Adenocarcinoma

Adenocarcinoma of the cervix is relatively rare by comparison with the squamous cell type, accounting for approximately 5–10% of all cervical cancer. However, the incidence appears to be increasing, particularly in young women (Kjaer et al. 1993). Studies in this field are limited by the rarity of the disease, which results in small numbers for comparison. This topic has been well reviewed by Kjaer et al. (1990), however, it is interesting to note that sexual behaviour, in particular, the number of sexual partners, and also HPV types 16 and especially 18 appear to be more strongly linked to adenocarcinoma than has previously been suspected. Seven studies have included estimates for adenocarcinoma (Figs 25.2 and 25.4), none of them have shown significant associations. Ursin et al. (1996), Lacey et al. (2001), and Green et al. (2003) included large number of cases of in situ or invasive adenocarcinomas and still found no association. More recently, the International Collaboration of Epidemiological Studies in Cervical Cancer published a meta-analysis of carcinoma of the cervix and tobacco smoking where individual data from 23 published studies were pooled (13 541 cases including 840 adenocarcinomas in situ and 1 191 adenocarcinomas). Results were reassuring, current-smokers and past-smokers were at higher risk of squamous cell carcinoma of the cervix (RR for current smokers 1.60 95% CI 1.48–1.73, RR for past smokers 1.12 95% CI 1.01–1.25) but not of adenocarcinoma (RR for current smokers 0.89 95% CI 0.74–1.06, RR for past smokers 0.89 95% CI 0.72–1.10). These results did not change when restricting the analysis to HPV positive women (RR for squamous carcinoma 1.95 95% CI 1.43–2.65, RR for adenocarcinoma 1.06 95% CI 0.14–7.96).

Conclusion

Epidemiologic evidence strongly links smoking with squamous cell cervical cancer and high-grade CIN. However, some controversy still exists as to whether the link is causal or in some way reflects residual confounding with unmeasured aspects of sexual behaviour (Phillips *et al.* 1994), although the case for causality has strengthened considerably in the past few years. Attempts to adjust for sexual behaviour through variables such as age at first intercourse and number of sexual partners have generally reduced the strength of the relationship with smoking, but it has not disappeared: it remains at or above two-fold for current-smokers and shows a dose–response relationship in many studies.

Recent studies which have collected data on HPV infection have further complicated the interpretation of the data. This is partly due to the much higher odds ratios found for HPV infection, which is clearly the major risk factor. In general, cases tend to be almost universally HPV positive whereas controls are primarily HPV negative, so that adjustment essentially results in a comparison of (HPV positive) cases to HPV positive controls. This situation leads to difficulties in obtaining an adequate number of HPV positive controls.

This raises the possibility that smoking is important only because it leads to a weakened immune response which in turn increases the likelihood that an HPV infection will become persistent, but itself have no direct carcinogenic effect. If this were true, adjusting for persistent HPV infection as an intermediate endpoint would indicate no effect of smoking on carcinogenesis. This is not the case and adjustment for HPV infection has not substantially reduced the odds ratios for smoking. In particular, the strong relationship shown between smoking and CIN3 after HPV adjustment (Fig. 25.3), the non-significant association between smoking and CIN1 (Fig. 25.5), and the association between smoking and high-risk HPV types but not low-risk HPV types (Fig. 25.6) suggest that smoking is related to both the likelihood that HPV infections will become persistent and that smoking will accelerate the progression of cervical lesions to become CIN3 and cancer.

To further clarify these issues, despite a number of recent pooled analyses, there is a need for further studies with detailed smoking histories and use of validated HPV assays. Controls can provide valuable information as to whether HPV positivity is increased in smokers in the absence of disease, which would shed light on its role in persistence of HPV infection in older women. Ideally HPV positive controls should be tested again after one year to more accurately evaluate this hypothesis. This should be soon reported by a number of ongoing cohorts in young women which examine the factors leading to persistent HPV infections.

References

Alloub, M. I. (1989). Human papillomavirus infection and cervical intraepithelial neoplasia in women with renal allografts. *BMJ*, **298**, 153–6.

Barton, S. E., *et al.* (1988). Effect of cigarette smoking on cervical epithelial immunity: a mechanism for neoplastic change? *Lancet*, **2**, 652–4.

Basu, J., *et al.* (1991). Plasma ascorbic acid and beta-carotene levels in women evaluated for HPV infection, smoking and cervix dysplasia. *Cancer Detect Prev*, **15**, 165–70.

Bosch, F. X., *et al.* (1992). Risk factors for cervical cancer in Colombia and Spain. *Int J Cancer*, **52**, 750–8.

Bosch, F. X., *et al.* (1996). Male sexual behaviour and human papillomavirus DNA: key risk factors for cervical cancer in Spain. *J Natl Cancer Inst*, **88**(15), 1060–7.

Brinton, L. A. (1992). Epidemiology of cervical cancer—overview. *IARC Scientific Publications*, **119**, 3–23.

Brinton, L. A., *et al.* (1987). Epidemiology of cervical cancer by cell type. *Cancer Res*, **47**, 1706–11.

Burger, M. P. M., *et al.* (1993). Cigarette smoking and human papillomavirus in patients with reported cervical cytological abnormality. *BMJ*, **306**, 749–52.

Byrne, M. A., *et al.* (1989). The occurrence of human papillomavirus infection and intraepithelial neoplasia in women infected by HIV. *AIDS*, **3**, 379–82.

Cade, J. and Margetts, B. M. (1991). The relationship between diet and smoking: is the diet of smokers different? *J Epidemiol Community Health*, **45**, 270–2.

Caorsi, I. and Figueroa, C. D. (1986). Langerhan's cell density in the normal cervical epithelium and in cervical intraepithelial neoplasia. *Br J Obstet Gynaecol*, **93**, 993–8.

Cerqueira, E. M. *et al.* (1998). Genetic damage in exfoliated cells of the uterine cervix. Association and interaction between cigarette smoking and progression to malignant transformation? *Acta Cytol*, **42**, 639–49.

Church, D. F. and Pryor, W. A. (1985). Free-radical chemistry of cigarette smoke and its toxicological implications. *Environ Health Perspect*, **64**, 111–26.

Coker, A. L., *et al.* (2002). Active and passive smoking, high-risk papillomaviruses and cervical neoplasia. *Cancer Detection and Prevention*, **26**, 121–8.

Conti, M., *et al.* (1993). HPV, HIV infection and risk of cervical intraepithelial neoplasia in former intravenous drug abusers. *Gynecol Oncol*, **49**, 344–8.

Cruchley, A. T., *et al.* (1994). Langerhans' cell density in normal human oral mucosa and skin: relationship to age, smoking and alcohol consumption. *J Oral Pathol Med*, **23**, 55–9.

Cuzick, J., *et al.* (1990). Vitamin A, vitamin E and the risk of cervical intraepithelial neoplasia. *Br J Cancer*, **62**, 651–2.

Daniels, T. E., *et al.* (1992). Reduction of Langerhans' cells in smokeless tobacco-associated oral mucosal lesions. *J Oral Pathol Med*, **21**, 100–4.

Deacon, J. M., *et al.* (2000). Sexual behaviour and smoking as determinants of cervical HPV infection and of CIN 3 among those infected: a case-control study nested within the Manchester cohort. *Br J Cancer*, **88**(11), 1565–72.

Eluf-Neto, J., *et al.* (1994). Human papillomavirus and invasive cervical cancer in Brazil. *Br J Cancer*, **69**, 114–19.

Eppel, W., *et al.* (2000). The influence of cotinine on interleukin 6 expression in smokers with cervical preneoplasia. *Acta Obstet Gynecol Scand*, **79**, 1105–11.

Fairley, C. K., *et al.* (1995). A cohort study comparing the detection of HPV DNA from women who stop and continue to smoke. *Aust NZ J Obstet Gynaecol*, **35**(2), 181–5.

Halliwell, B. (1993). Cigarette smoking and health: a radical view. *J R Soc Health*, **113**, 91–6.

Hauser, C. (1992). The interaction between Langerhans' cells and CD4+ T cells. *J Dermatol*, **19**, 722–5.

Hawthorn, R. J., *et al.* (1988). Langerhans' cells and subtypes of human papillomavirus in cervical intraepithelial neoplasia. *BMJ*, **297**, 643–6.

Hellberg, D., *et al.* (1988). Smoking and cervical intraepithelial neoplasia: nicotine and cotinine in serum and cervical mucus in smokers and nonsmokers. *Am J Obstet Gynecol*, **158**, 910–13.

Herrero, R., *et al.* (1989). Invasive cervical cancer and smoking in Latin America. *J Natl Cancer Inst*, **81**, 205–11.

Hildesheim, A., *et al.* (2001). HPV co-factors related to the development of cervical cancer: results from a population-based study in Costa Rica. *Br J Cancer*, **84**(9), 1219–26.

Hoffmann, D. and Hecht, S. S. (1985). Nicotine-derived N-nitrosamines and tobacco-related cancer: current status and future directions. *Cancer Res*, **45**, 935–44.

Johnson, J. C. *et al.* (1992). High frequency of latent and clinical human papillomavirus cervical infections in immune compromised human immunodeficiency virus infected women. *Obstet Gynecol*, **72**, 321–7.

Kesic,V., *et al.* (1990). T lymphocytes in non-malignant, pre-malignant and malignant changes of the cervix. *Eur J Gynaecol Oncol*, **11**, 191–4.

Kjaer, K. S. and Brinton, L. (1993). Adenocarcinomas of the uterine cervix: the epidemiology of an increasing problem. *Epidemiologic Reviews*, **15**(2), 486–98.

La Vecchia, C., *et al.* (1988). Dietary vitamin A and the risk of intraepithelial and invasive neoplasia. *Gynecol Oncol*, **30**, 187–95.

Luesley, D., *et al.* (1994). Cigarette smoking and histological outcome in women with mildly dyskaryotic smears. *Br J Obstet Gynaecol*, **101**, 49–52.

Maggwa, B. N., *et al.* (1993). The relationship between HIV infection and cervical intraepithelial neoplasia among women attending two family planning clinics in Nairobi, Kenya. *AIDS*, **7**, 733–8.

Maiman, M., *et al.* (1990). Human immunodeficiency virus infection and cervical neoplasia. *Gynecol Oncol*, **38**, 377–82.

Maiman, M., *et al.* (1993). Recurrent cervical intraepithelial neoplasia in human immunodeficiency virus seropositive women. *Obstet Gynecol*, **82**, 170–4.

Mancini, R., *et al.* (1999). Polycyclic aromatic hydrocarbon-DNA adducts in cervical smears of smokers and non-smokers. *Gynecol Oncol*, **75**, 68–71.

Mandelblatt, J. S., *et al.* (1992). Association between HIV infection and cervical neoplasia: implications for clinical care of women at risk for both conditions. *AIDS*, **6**, 173–8.

Margetts, B. and Jackson, A. (1993). Interactions between people's diet and their smoking habits: the dietary and nutritional survey of British adults. *BMJ*, **307**, 1381–4.

Matorras, R., *et al.* (1991). Human immunodeficiency virus-induced immunosuppression: a risk factor for human papillomavirus infection. *Am J Obstet Gynecol*, **164**, 42–4.

McArdle, J. P. and Muller, H. K. (1986). Quantitative assessment of Langerhans' cells in human cervical intraepithelial neoplasia and wart virus infection. *Am J Obstet Gynecol*, **154**, 509–15.

McCann, M. F., *et al.* (1992). Nicotine and cotinine in the cervical mucus of smokers, passive smokers and nonsmokers. *Cancer Epidemiol, Biomarkers and Prev*, 1, 125–9.

Miller, L. G., *et al.* (1982). Reversible alterations in immunoregulatory T cells in smoking. *Chest*, **5**, 527–9.

Mills, C. M., *et al.* (1993). Altered inflammatory responses in smokers. *BMJ*, **307**, 911.

Morelli, A. E., *et al.* (1993). Relationship between types of human papillomavirus and Langerhans' cells in cervical condyloma and intraepithelial neoplasia. *Am J Clin Path*, **99**, 200–6.

Morris, H. H. B., *et al.* (1983). Langerhans' cells in human cervical epithelium: effects of wart virus infection and intraepithelial neoplasia. *Br J Obstet Gynaecol*, **90**, 412–20.

Morrison, E. A. B., *et al.* (1991). Human papillomavirus infection and other risk factors for cervical neoplasia: A case-control study. *Int J Cancer*, **49**, 6–13.

Mota, F., *et al.* (1999). The antigen-presenting environment in normal and human papillomavirus (HPV)-related premalignant cervical epithelium. *Clin Exp Immunol*, **116**, 33–40.

Muller, H. K., *et al.* (1985). Carcinogen-induced depletion of cutaneous langerhans cells. *Br J Cancer*, **52**, 81.

Munoz, N., *et al.* (1993). Risk factors for cervical intraepithelial neoplasia grade III/carcinoma in situ in Spain and Colombia. *Cancer Epidemiol Biomarkers Prev*, **2**, 423–31.

Munoz, N., *et al.* (1996). Difficulty in elucidating the male role in cervical cancer in Colombia, a high risk area for the disease. *J Natl Cancer Inst*, **88**, 1068–75.

Nakao, Y., *et al.* (1996). Malignant transformation of human ectocervical cells immortalized by HPV 18: in vitro model of carcinogenesis by cigarette smoke. *Carcinogenesis*, **17**(3), 577–83.

Olsen, A.O., *et al.* (1998). Combined effect of smoking and HPV 16 infection in cervical carcinogenesis. *Epidemiology*, **9**, 346–9.

Palan, P., *et al.* (1996). Plasma levels of®-carotene, lycopene, canthaxanthin, retinol and ⟨α- and τ-tocopherol in cervical epithelial neoplasia and cancer. *Clinical Cancer Research*, **2**, 181–5.

Penn, I. (1986). Cancers of the anogenital region in renal transplant recipients. *Cancer*, **58**, 611.

Phillips, A. N. and Davey Smith, G. (1994). Cigarette smoking as a potential cause of cervical cancer: has confounding been controlled? *Int J Epidemiol*, **23**, 42–9.

Plummer, M., *et al.* (2003). IARC Multi-center Cervical Cancer Study Group. Smoking and cervical cancer. *Cancer Causes Control*, **14**, 805–14.

Poppe, W. A., *et al.* (1995). Tobacco smoking impairs the local immunosurveillance in the uterine cervix. An immunohistochemical study. *Gynecol Obstet Invest*, **39**, 34–8.

Poppe, W. A. J., *et al.* (1996). Langerhans' cells and L1 antigen expression in normal and abnormal squamous epithelium of the cervical transformation zone. *Gynecol Obstet Invest*, **41**, 207–13.

Porecco, R., *et al.* (1975). Gynaecological malignancies in immunosuppressed organ homograft recipients. *Obstet Gynecol*, **45**, 359–64.

Prokopczyk, B., *et al.* (1997). Identification of tobacco-specific carcinogen in the cervical mucus of smokers and nonsmokers. *J Natl Cancer Inst*, **89**, 868–73.

Reeves, W. C., *et al.* (1987). Case-control study of human papillomaviruses and cervical cancer in Latin America. *Int J Cancer*, **40**, 450–4.

Romney, S. L., *et al.* (1985). Plasma vitamin C and uterine cervical dysplasia. *Am J Obstet Gynecol*, **151**, 976–80.

Sasson, I. M., *et al.* (1985). Cigarette smoking and neoplasia of the uterine cervix: smoke constituents in cervical mucus. *N Eng J Med*, **312**, 315–16.

Schafer, A., *et al.* (1991). The increased frequency of cervical dysplasia in women infected with the human immunodeficiency virus is related to the degree of immunosuppression. *Am J Obstet Gynecol*, **164**, 593–9.

Schiffman, M. H., *et al.* (1987). Biochemical epidemiology of cervical neoplasia. *Cancer Res*, 3886–8.

Schneider, V., *et al.* (1983). Immunosuppression as a high risk factor in the development of condylomata acuminata and squamous neoplasia of the cervix. *Acta Cytol*, **27**, 220–4.

Sillman, F. H. and Sedlis, A. (1987). Anogenital papillomavirus infection and neoplasia in immunodeficient women. *Obstet Gynecol Clin North Am*, **14**, 537–57.

Sillman, F., *et al.* (1984). The relationship between human papillomavirus and lower genital tract neoplasia in immunosuppressed women. *Am J Obstet Gynecol*, **150**, 300–8.

Simons, A. M., *et al.* (1995). Demonstration of smoking-related DNA damage in cervical epithelium and correlation with human papillomavirus type 16, using exfoliated cervical cells. *Br J Cancer*, **71**, 246–9.

Slattery, M. L., *et al.* (1990). Dietary vitamins A, C and E and selenium as risk factors for cervical cancer. *Epidemiology*, **1**, 8–15.

Soutter,W. P. and Kesic,V. (1994). Treatment of cervical intraepithelial neoplasia reverses CD4/CD8 lymphocyte abnormalities in peripheral venous blood. *Int J Gynecol Cancer*, **4**, 279–82.

Spinillo, A., *et al.* (1993). Langerhans' cell counts and cervical intraepithelial neoplasia in women with Human Immunodeficiency Virus infections. *Gynaecol Oncol*, **48**, 210–13.

Stanley, M. (1999). Mechanism of action of Imiquimod. *Papillomavirus Report*, **10**(2), 23–9.

Stingl, G., *et al.* (1978). Immunologic functions of 1a-bearing epidermal Langerhans cells. *J Immunol*, **121**, 2005–13.

Stryker, W. S., *et al.* (1988). The relation of diet, cigarette smoking and alcohol consumption to plasma beta-carotene and alpha tocopherol levels. *Am J Epidemiol*, **127**, 283–95.

Szarewski, A., *et al.* (1996). The effect of smoking cessation on cervical lesion size. *Lancet*, **347**, 941–3.

Szarewski, A., *et al.* (2001). The effect of stopping smoking on cervical Langerhans' cells and lymphocytes. *Br J Obstet Gynaecol*, **108**, 295–303.

Tay, S. K., *et al.* (1987). Subpopulations of Langerhans' cells in a cervical neoplasia. *Br J Obstet Gynaecol*, **94**, 10–15.

Turner, M. J., *et al.* (1988). T lymphocytes and cervical intraepithelial neoplasia. *Irish J Med Science*, **81**, 184.

Vayrynen, M., *et al.* (1984). Langerhans' cells in human papillomavirus (HPV) lesions of the uterine cervix identified by the monoclonal antibody OKT6. *Int J Gynaecol Obstet*, **22**, 375–83.

Vermund, S. H., *et al.* (1991). High risk of human papillomavirus infection and cervical intraepithelial lesions among women with symptomatic human immunodeficiency syndrome. *Am J Obstet Gynecol*, **165**, 392–400.

Verreault, R., *et al.* (1989). A case-control study of diet amd invasive cervical cancer. *Int J Cancer*, **48**, 34–8.

Wassertheil-Smoller, S., *et al.* (1981). Dietary vitamin C and uterine cervical dysplasia. *Am J Epidemiol*, **114**, 714–24.

Wichelow,M. J., *et al.* (1991). A comparison of the diets of non-smokers and smokers. *Br J Addict*, **86**, 71–81.

Winkelstein,W. Jr. (1977). Smoking and cancer of the uterine cervix. *Am J Epidemiol*, **106**, 257–9.

Yang, X., *et al.* (1996). Malignant transformation of HPV 16-immortalized human endocervical cells by cigarette smoke condensate and characterization of multistage carcinogenesis. *Int J Cancer*, **65**, 338–44.

Yang, X., *et al.* (1997). Expression of cellular genes in HPV 16-immortalised and cigarette smoke condensate-transformed human endocervical cells. *J Cellular Biochem*, **66**, 309–21.

Yang, X., *et al.* (1998). Enhanced expression of anti-apoptotic proteins in human papillomavirus immortalized and cigarette smoke condensate-transformed human endocervical cells. *Molecular Carcinogenesis*, **22**, 95–101.

zur Hausen, H. (1982). Human genital cancers: synergism between two virus infections or synergism between a virus infection and initiating events? *Lancet*, **II**, 1370–2.

Chapter 26

Tobacco and pancreatic cancer

Patrick Maisonneuve

Introduction

In developed countries, pancreas cancer is the 10th most common form of cancer in men and the 9th most common form of cancer in women, but because of its very poor prognosis, it ranks as the fourth most common cause of cancer deaths in both sexes (Ferlay *et al.* 2001).

The risk of pancreatic cancer increases rapidly with age, with 80% of the cases being diagnosed after age 60. Pancreatic cancer has been predominantly a male disease, presumably because of past differences in smoking habits, but the sex ratio decreases with increasing age. Blacks are 50% more likely to contract pancreatic cancer than whites (Coughlin *et al.* 2000). The cause for this racial difference is poorly understood. There is little evidence to suggest that blacks smoke more than whites, but suggestive evidence support the fact that there are racial differences in the ability to degrade carcinogens contained within tobacco smoke (Richie *et al.* 1997).

Risk factors for pancreatic cancer comprise a diet rich in meat and fat, past medical history of pancreatitis or diabetes, exposure to certain chemicals, and hereditary factors, but tobacco smoking remains the major recognized risk factor for pancreatic cancer.

Tobacco smoking

Cigarette smoking

The strongest evidence of the association between cigarette smoking and pancreatic cancer comes from series of large prospective studies: In 1966, Hammond investigated the relation between smoking and death rates in a large prospective study of one million US men and women (Hammond 1966). Between October 1959 and February 1960, 1 078 894 men and women were enrolled in the study and completed a detailed questionnaire including smoking habits. After three years of follow-up, the pancreatic cancer mortality ratio for men who ever smoked regularly compared to men who never smoked regularly was 2.69 for subjects aged 45–64 and 2.17 for subjects over 65 years of age. For women aged 45–64, the mortality ratio was 1.81 for women who ever smoked regularly and 2.58 for women classified as 'Heavier' cigarette smokers. (At that time, many female cigarette smokers smoked only a few cigarettes a day, did not inhale, and had been smoking for only few years.)

Since then, the association between tobacco smoking and pancreatic cancer risk has been subject of numerous studies. To summarize the association between tobacco smoking and pancreatic cancer risk and assess sources of heterogeneity, Iodice *et al.* (2008) conducted a meta-analysis of all published studies. They performed a literature search using the Ovid MEDLINE® database (1950 to March 2007), ISI Web of Science® Science Citation Index Expanded™, and PUBMED and identified 82 independent reports satisfying a series of inclusion and eligibility criteria (42 case-control studies, 35 cohort studies, and 5 nested case-control studies): The overall risk of pancreatic cancer estimated from the combined results was RR = 1.74 (95% CI = 1.61–1.87) for current or ever smokers and 1.29 (0.68–2.45) for former-smokers implying that, in a population where the prevalence of smoking is 30%, the population's attributable risk – the proportion of pancreatic cancer explained by smoking – is about 20% (Iodice *et al.* 2008).

The risk of pancreatic cancer increases with both smoking intensity (RR = 1.62; 95% CI = 1.51–1.75 for an increase consumption of 20 cigarettes per day) and duration of smoking (RR = 1.16; 95% CI = 1.12–1.19 for an increase duration of ten years) and remained elevated during the ten years following smoking cessation (RR = 1.48 1.25–1.76). After ten years of smoking cessation the association is no more statistically significant. The summary risk estimates based on cohort studies and case-control studies were similar (RR = 1.70 and 1.77, respectively) (Iodice *et al.* 2008).

At least nine new studies have been published since the publication of the meta-analysis by Iodice *et al.* including five case-control or nested case-control studies (Hassan *et al.* 2007; Lindkvist *et al.* 2008; De Martel *et al.* 2008; Anderson *et al.* 2009; Li *et al.* 2009), three cohort studies (Andreotti *et al.* 2009; Batty *et al.* 2009; Stevens *et al.* 2009), and a pooled analysis from the Pancreatic Cancer Cohort Consortium (Lynch *et al.* 2009). The risk estimates for current-smokers, ever-smokers, and former-smokers from these recent studies are comparable to the pooled risk estimates from the meta-analysis (Fig. 26.1).

Pipe and cigars

While cigarette smoking remains the most common form of tobacco in westernized countries, alternative forms of tobacco are available. In particular, cigars became increasingly fashionable since mid-1990s in the United States and later in Western Europe. The number of cigars consumed in the United States increased by approximately 50% between 1993 and 1998

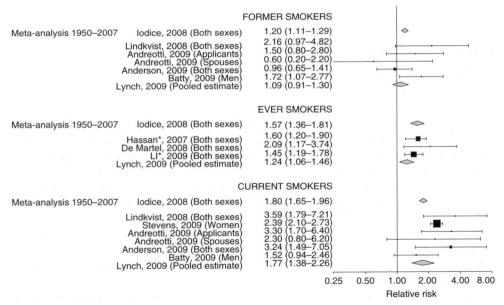

Figure 26.1 Association between cigarette smoking and pancreatic cancer risk based on study reports published between 1950 and 2009.

Note

The summary risk estimates of the meta-analysis of studies published between 1950 and 2007 (data from Iodice *et al.* 2008) are based on 41 studies for current-smokers, 18 studies for ever-smokers, and 39 studies for former-smokers.

(US Department of Agriculture 1996, 1999). Still, little is known about the health hazard of cigar smoking, possibly because cigars were not required to carry a health warning from the Surgeon General until 26 June 2000 (US Department of Health and Human Services 2000)

In the previous meta-analysis, Iodice *et al.* also assessed the association between pipe and cigar consumption and pancreatic cancer risk. Based respectively on estimates from nine studies, the summary relative risk of pancreatic cancer was 1.56 (1.02–2.28) for exclusive cigar smokers and 1.39 (0.94–2.07) for exclusive pipe smokers. When either pipe or cigar smoking was considered, the association was limited to current-smokers (RR = 1.57; 95% CI = 1.29–1.91) while no association was present for ex-smokers (Iodice *et al.* 2008). In conclusion, pipe and cigar smoking have the same detrimental effect on pancreas than cigarette smoking.

Smokeless tobacco

Because of the relatively low incidence of pancreatic cancer, the limited use of smokeless tobacco worldwide, and the confounding effect of other forms of tobacco use, only few studies were able to assess the association between smokeless tobacco and pancreatic cancer. Results from two recent systematic reviews provide different conclusion. Based on results from six studies, Boffetta *et al.* reported a summary relative risk of 1.6 (1.1–2.2) of pancreatic cancer for ever use of smokeless tobacco with limited evidence of heterogeneity. The risk was somewhat higher in studies conducted in Nordic countries than in those conducted in the United States (Boffetta *et al.* 2008). In a subsequent meta-analysis based on seven studies from North America and Scandinavia, Sponsiello-Wang *et al.* concluded that, at most, the data suggest a possible effect of smokeless tobacco on pancreatic cancer risk (Sponsiello-Wang *et al.* 2008). Undoubtedly, the risk associated with smokeless tobacco is lower than that from tobacco smoking and needs to be further assessed as current risk estimates are based on small number of exposed cases and residual confounding by tobacco smoking cannot be completely ruled out.

Tobacco smoking as a potential confounder

Many of the risk factors for pancreatic cancer are themselves associated with tobacco smoking. Tobacco smoking could therefore act as an important confounding factor and the lack of adjustment or inadequate adjustment for tobacco smoking could lead to spurious associations. Some conditions such as long-term diabetes or periodontal disease have been associated with modest increased risk of pancreatic cancer, but are themselves conditions which are more frequent among smokers (Huxley *et al.* 2005; Johnson *et al.* 2007; Willi *et al.* 2007; Meyer *et al.* 2008). While, until recently, alcohol drinking was not thought to be associated with pancreatic cancer risk (Hart *et al.* 2008), some recent studies have identified a possible association with very high levels of alcohol consumption (Genkinger *et al.* 2009; Jiao *et al.* 2009). Because of the strong correlation between alcohol and cigarette consumption, residual confounding by tobacco smoking could not be discarded.

Gene–environment interaction

Research in the area of gene–environment interaction is an important topic for various cancers because minimizing exposure to environmental risk factors could reduce the impact of inherited genetic susceptibility factors. A positive family history of pancreatic cancer and smoking are two independent risk factors, each of which approximately doubles the risk of pancreatic cancer but Schenk *et al.* found an interaction between these two risk factors (Schenk *et al.* 2001).

Smokers who are related to a person who develops pancreatic cancer before the age 60 have eight times the risk of pancreatic cancer as individuals lacking these two risk factors.

In familial pancreatic cancer, Rulyak *et al.* (2003) found that smokers developed cancer one decade earlier than nonsmokers. In patients with hereditary pancreatitis, which is caused by a mutation in the trypsinogen gene and is associated with a 50- to 70-fold increased risk of pancreatic cancer smoking doubles the risk of pancreatic cancer, as it does in the general population, but pancreatic cancer developed in average 20 years earlier in smokers than in non-smokers (Lowenfels *et al.* 1997, 2001).

It was hypothesized that polymorphisms in genes that encode carcinogen-metabolizing enzymes could also affect the risk of smoking-related pancreatic cancer. In particular, it has been shown that the glutathione S-transferase T1 (GSTT1) enzyme protects pancreatic cells from the damaging effects of tobacco smoking and that lacking this enzyme may increase the risk of smoking-related pancreatic cancer (Duell *et al.* 2002). Using biological material collected in a large case-control study in the San Francisco Bay Area, it was shown that the XRCC1 (X-ray repair cross-complementing group 1) 399Gln allele, which has been associated with elevated biomarkers of DNA damage in human cells, is also a potentially important determinant of susceptibility to smoking-induced pancreatic cancer (Duell *et al.* 2002). Still, previous smaller studies did not found significant associations between GSTM1, GSTT1, NAT1 or CYP1A1 polymorphisms and pancreatic cancer susceptibility (Bartsch *et al.* 1998; Liu *et al.* 2000). With the advances of genomic, an increasing number of studies have investigated and detected candidate single nucleotide polymorphisms associated with pancreatic cancer. Gene–gene and gene-smoking interaction between various candidate metabolic gene polymorphisms (MTHFR, GSTP1, NAT1, NAT2, TS, and UGT1A7) or DNA repair gene polymorphisms (ATM, LIG3, XPF, and XRCC3) have been described but need further confirmations (Duell *et al.* 2008; Jiao *et al.* 2008; Suzuki *et al.* 2008; Zhao *et al.* 2009).

Histological and experimental studies

There is also strong evidence that smoking is associated with histologic alterations and molecular damages of the pancreas. In a large autopsy study based on 22 344 slides from 560 autopsied subjects, histological alterations in the ductal epithelium was strongly associated with smoking habits. Only 5.4% of the nonsmokers had medium to high percentages of ductal cells with atypical nuclei. This rose to 50.7% in light smokers and to 74.9% in smokers of more than 40 cig./day. Advanced findings (increased numbers) of cells with atypical nuclei were found in the acinar cells of the parenchyma in only 1.8% of nonsmokers; 11.4% in smokers of less than 20 cig./day; 29.2% in smokers of 20–39 cig./day; and 69.1% in smokers of more than 40 cig./day. Moderate or advanced hyaline thickening of arterioles in 12.8% of the non-smokers increased to 74.4% in the heaviest smoking group. A similar relationship was observed for fibrous thickening in the arteries (Auerbach and Garfinkel 1986).

The nicotine-derived nitrosamine, nitrosamine 4-(methylnitrosamino)-1-(3-pyridyl)-1-butanone (NNK), is known to cause adenocarcinomas of the lung and pancreas in laboratory animals (Hoffmann *et al.* 1993; Schuller *et al.* 1993), and is thought to be largely responsible for the development of these cancers in smokers. In particular, NNK has genotoxic effects on cells, such as the formation of DNA adducts and mutations in the RAS gene. Experimental studies have demonstrated that aromatic amines and nitroaromatic hydrocarbons are metabolized by the pancreas and may be involved in the aetiology of human pancreatic cancer (Anderson *et al.* 1997), and that DNA damage derived from carcinogen exposure is involved in pancreatic carcinogenesis and in particular that smoking was positively correlated to the level of total DNA adducts in pancreatic cancer tissue (Wand *et al.* 1998).

The recent sequencing of the pancreatic cancer genome provided an unprecedented opportunity to identify mutational patterns associated with smoking. Comparing the somatic mutations in the cancers obtained from individuals who ever smoked cigarettes to the somatic mutations in the cancers obtained from individuals who never smoked cigarettes Blackford *et al.* found that pancreatic carcinomas from cigarette smokers harbour more mutations than do carcinomas from never-smokers providing insight into the mechanisms by which cigarette smoking causes pancreatic cancer (Blackford *et al.* 2009).

Conclusion

Overall, tobacco smoking is associated with a two-fold increased risk of pancreatic cancer and is responsible for approximately 20% of all pancreatic tumours. The risk is increasing with the amount of cigarette smoked and ten to fifteen years have to pass from quitting smoking until the risk fell to the level of a non-smoker. The risk seems to be higher for younger subjects and decreases to non-significant values among elderly peoples. Among individuals at high risk of pancreatic cancer such as patients with hereditary pancreatitis, smoking further advances the age at which cancer develops. Smoking has also been associated with histopathological alterations of the epithelial cells of the pancreas and the tobacco-related carcinogens NNK induces adenocarcinoma of the pancreas in laboratory animals. Still, smoking remains the strongest risk factor amenable to preventive intervention.

References

Anderson, K.E., Hammons, G.J., Kadlubar, F.F., Potter, J.D., Kaderlik, K.R., Ilett, K.F. *et al.* (1997). Metabolic activation of aromatic amines by human pancreas. *Carcinogenesis*, **18**: 1085–92.

Anderson, L.N., Cotterchio, M., and Gallinger, S. (2009). Lifestyle, dietary, and medical history factors associated with pancreatic cancer risk in Ontario, Canada. *Cancer Causes Control*, **20**: 825–34.

Andreotti, G., Freeman, L.E., Hou, L., Coble, J., Rusiecki, J., Hoppin, J.A. *et al.* (2009). Agricultural pesticide use and pancreatic cancer risk in the Agricultural Health Study Cohort. *Int J Cancer*, **124**: 2495–500.

Auerbach, O., Garfinkel, L. (1986). Histologic changes in pancreas in relation to smoking and coffee-drinking habits. *Dig Dis Sci*, **31**: 1014–20.

Bartsch, H., Malaveille, C., Lowenfels, A.B., Maisonneuve, P., Hautefeuille, A., and Boyle, P. (1998). Genetic polymorphism of N-acetyltransferases, glutathione S-transferase M1 and NAD(P)H:quinone oxidoreductase in relation to malignant and benign pancreatic disease risk. The International Pancreatic Disease Study Group. *Eur J Cancer Prev*, **7**: 215–23.

Batty, G.D., Kivimaki, M., Morrison, D., Huxley, R., Smith, G.D., Clarke, R. *et al.* (2009). Risk factors for pancreatic cancer mortality: extended follow-up of the original Whitehall Study. *Cancer Epidemiol Biomarkers Prev*, **18**: 673–5.

Batty, G.D., Kivimaki, M., Morrison, D., Huxley, R., Smith, G.D., Clarke, R. *et al.* (2009) Risk factors for pancreatic cancer mortality: extended follow-up of the original Whitehall Study. *Cancer Epidemiol Biomarkers Prev*, **18**: 673–5.

Blackford, A., Parmigiani, G., Kensler, T.W., Wolfgang, C., Jones, S., Zhang, X. *et al.* (2009). Genetic mutations associated with cigarette smoking in pancreatic cancer. *Cancer Res*, **69**: 3681–8.

Boffetta, P., Hecht, S., Gray, N., Gupta, P., and Straif, K. (2008). Smokeless tobacco and cancer. *Lancet Oncol*, **9**: 667–75.

Coughlin, S.S., Calle, E.E., Patel, A.V., Thun, M.J. (2000). Predictors of pancreatic cancer mortality among a large cohort of United States adults. *Cancer Causes Control*, **11**: 915–23.

de Martel, C., Llosa, A.E., Friedman, G.D., Vogelman, J.H., Orentreich, N., Stolzenberg-Solomon, R.Z. *et al.* (2008). Helicobacter pylori infection and development of pancreatic cancer. *Cancer Epidemiol Biomarkers Prev*, **17**: 1188–94.

Duell, E.J., Bracci, P.M., Moore, J.H., Burk, R.D., Kelsey, K.T., and Holly, E.A. (2008). Detecting pathway-based gene-gene and gene-environment interactions in pancreatic cancer. *Cancer Epidemiol Biomarkers Prev*, **17**: 1470–9.

Duell, E.J., Holly, E.A., Bracci, P.M., Liu, M., Wiencke, J.K., and Kelsey, K.T. (2002). A population-based, case-control study of polymorphisms in carcinogen-metabolizing genes, smoking, and pancreatic adenocarcinoma risk. *J Natl Cancer Inst*, **94**: 297–306.

Duell, E.J., Holly, E.A., Bracci, P.M., Wiencke, J.K., and Kelsey, K.T. (2002). A population-based study of the Arg399Gln polymorphism in X-ray repair cross-complementing group 1 (XRCC1) and risk of pancreatic adenocarcinoma. *Cancer Res*, **62**: 4630–6.

Ferlay, J., Bray, F., Pisani P., and Parkin, D.M. (2001). GLOBOCAN 2000: Cancer Incidence, Mortality and Prevalence Worldwide, Version 1.0. IARC CancerBase No. 5. Lyon, IARCPress.

Genkinger, J.M., Spiegelman, D., Anderson, K.E., Bergkvist, L., Bernstein, L., van den Brandt, P.A. *et al.* (2009). Alcohol intake and pancreatic cancer risk: a pooled analysis of fourteen cohort studies. *Cancer Epidemiol Biomarkers Prev*, **18**: 765–76.

Hammond, E.C. (1966). Smoking in relation to the death rates of one million men and women. *Natl Cancer Inst Monogr*, **19**: 127–204.

Hart, A.R., Kennedy, H., and Harvey, I. (2008). Pancreatic cancer: a review of the evidence on causation. *Clin Gastroenterol Hepatol*, **6**: 275–82.

Hassan, M.M., Bondy, M.L., Wolff, R.A., Abbruzzese, J.L., Vauthey, J.N., Pisters, P.W. *et al.* (2007). Risk factors for pancreatic cancer: case-control study. *Am J Gastroenterol*, **102**: 2696–707.

Hoffmann, D., Djordjevic, M.V., Rivenson, A., Zang, E., Desai, D., and Amin, S. (1993). A study of tobacco carcinogenesis. LI. Relative potencies of tobacco-specific N-nitrosamines as inducers of lung tumours in A/J mice. *Cancer Lett*, **71**: 25–30.

Huxley, R., Ansary-Moghaddam, A., Berrington, dG., Barzi, F., and Woodward, M. (2005). Type-II diabetes and pancreatic cancer: a meta-analysis of 36 studies. *Br J Cancer*, **92**: 2076–83.

Iodice, S., Gandini, S., Maisonneuve, P., and Lowenfels, A.B. (2008). Tobacco and the risk of pancreatic cancer: a review and meta-analysis. *Langenbecks Arch Surg*, **393**: 535–45.

Jiao, L., Hassan, M.M., Bondy, M.L., Wolff, R.A., Evans, D.B., Abbruzzese, J.L. *et al.* (2008). XRCC2 and XRCC3 gene polymorphism and risk of pancreatic cancer. *Am J Gastroenterol*, **103**: 360–7.

Jiao, L., Silverman, D.T., Schairer, C., Thiébaut, A.C., Hollenbeck, A.R., Leitzmann, M.F. *et al.* (2009). Alcohol use and risk of pancreatic cancer: the NIH-AARP Diet and Health Study. *Am J Epidemiol*, **169**: 1043–51.

Johnson, G.K. and Guthmiller, J.M. (2007). The impact of cigarette smoking on periodontal disease and treatment. *Periodontol 2000*, **44**: 178–94.

Lindkvist, B., Johansen, D., Borgström, A., and Manjer, J. (2008). A prospective study of Helicobacter pylori in relation to the risk for pancreatic. *BMC Cancer*, **8**: 321.

Li, D., Suzuki, H., Liu, B., Morris, J., Liu, J., Okazaki, T., *et al.* (2009). DNA repair gene polymorphisms and risk of pancreatic cancer. *Clin Cancer Res*, **15**: 740–6.

Liu, G., Ghadirian, P., Vesprini, D., Hamel, N., Paradis, A.J., Lal, G. *et al.* (2000). Polymorphisms in GSTM1, GSTT1 and CYP1A1 and risk of pancreatic adenocarcinoma. *Br J Cancer*, **82**: 1646–9.

Lowenfels, A.B., Maisonneuve, P., DiMagno, E.P., Elitsur, Y., Gates, L.K. Jr, Perrault, J. *et al.* (1997). Hereditary pancreatitis and the risk of pancreatic cancer. International Hereditary Pancreatitis Study Group. *J Natl Cancer Inst*, **89**: 442–6.

Lowenfels, A.B., Maisonneuve, P., Whitcomb, D.C., Lerch, M.M., and DiMagno, E.P. (2001). Cigarette smoking as a risk factor for pancreatic cancer in patients with hereditary pancreatitis. *JAMA*, **286**: 169–70.

Lynch, S.M., Vrieling, A., Lubin, J.H., Kraft, P., Mendelsohn, J.B., Hartge, P. *et al.* (2009). Cigarette smoking and pancreatic cancer: a pooled analysis from the pancreatic cancer cohort consortium. *Am J Epidemiol* [Advance access published June 26, 2009].

Meyer, M.S., Joshipura, K., Giovannucci, E., and Michaud, D.S. (2008). A review of the relationship between tooth loss, periodontal disease, and cancer. *Cancer Causes Control*, **19**: 895–907.

Richie, J.P. Jr, Carmella, S.G., Muscat, J.E., Scott, D.G., Akerkar, S.A., and Hecht, S.S. (1997). Differences in the urinary metabolites of the tobacco-specific lung carcinogen 4-(methylnitrosamino)-1-(3-pyridyl)-1-butanone in black and white smokers. *Cancer Epidemiol Biomarkers Prev*, **6**: 783–90.

Rulyak, S.J., Lowenfels, A.B., Maisonneuve, P., and Brentnall, T.A. (2003). Risk factors for the development of pancreatic cancer in familial pancreatic cancer kindreds. *Gastroenterology*, **124**: 1292–9.

Schenk, M., Schwartz, A.G., O'Neal, E., Kinnard, M., Greenson, J.K., Fryzek, J.P. *et al.* (2001). Familial risk of pancreatic cancer. *J Natl Cancer Inst*, **93**: 640–4.

Schuller, H.M., Jorquera, R., Reichert, A., and Castonguay, A. (1993). Transplacental induction of pancreas tumors in hamsters by ethanol and the tobacco-specific nitrosamine 4- (methylnitrosamino)-1-(3-pyridyl)-1-butanone. *Cancer Res*, **53**: 2498–501.

Sponsiello-Wang, Z., Weitkunat, R., and Lee, P.N. (2008). Systematic review of the relation between smokeless tobacco and cancer of the pancreas in Europe and North America. *BMC Cancer*, **8**: 356.

Stevens, R.J., Roddam, A.W., Spencer, E.A., Pirie, K.L., Reeves, G.K., Green, J. *et al.* (2009). Factors associated with incident and fatal pancreatic cancer in a cohort of middle-aged women. *Int J Cancer*, **124**: 2400–5.

Suzuki, H., Morris, J.S., Li, Y., Doll, M.A., Hein, D.W., Liu, J. *et al.* (2008). Interaction of the cytochrome P4501A2, SULT1A1 and NAT gene polymorphisms with smoking and dietary mutagen intake in modification of the risk of pancreatic cancer. *Carcinogenesis*, **29**: 1184–91.

US Department of Agriculture. (1996). Tobacco situation and outlook report. TBS-237. Washington DC: US Department of Agriculture, Commodity Economics Division, Economic Research Service.

US Department of Agriculture. (1999). Tobacco situation and outlook reportm. TBS-243. Washington DC: US Department of Agriculture, Commodity Economics Division, Economic Research Service.

US Department of Health and Human Services. (2000). Reducing Tobacco Use: A Report of the Surgeon General. Atlanta, Georgia: US Department of Health and Human Services, Centers for Disease Control and Prevention, National Center for Chronic Disease Prevention and Health Promotion, Office on Smoking and Health.

Wang, M., Abbruzzese, J.L., Friess, H., Hittelman, W.N., Evans, D.B., Abbruzzese, M.C. *et al.* (1998). DNA adducts in human pancreatic tissues and their potential role in carcinogenesis. *Cancer Res*, **58**: 38–41.

Willi, C., Bodenmann, P., Ghali, W.A., Faris, P.D., and Cornuz, J. (2007). Active smoking and the risk of type 2 diabetes: a systematic review and meta-analysis. *JAMA*, **298**: 2654–64.

Zhao, D., Xu, D., Zhang, X., Wang, L., Tan, W., Guo, Y. *et al.* (2009). Interaction of cyclooxygenase-2 variants and smoking in pancreatic cancer: a possible role of nucleophosmin. *Gastroenterology*, **136**: 1659–68.

Chapter 27

Smoking and lung cancer

Graham G. Giles and Peter Boyle

Summary

The establishment of the causal link between smoking and lung cancer was an epidemiological triumph won against considerable resistance marshalled by the tobacco industry. This chapter reviews how the evidence that smoking causes lung cancer was accumulated and weighed against criteria adopted to establish the causal significance of epidemiological associations between an exposure and disease. The history of elucidating the association between lung cancer and smoking is now fundamental to modern epidemiological thinking and practice but in the early to mid-twentieth century the science of epidemiology was new and in the making, and the research on smoking and lung cancer contributed to the development of epidemiology as a discipline (White 1990). In addition to the evaluation of epidemiological evidence, the case for causality was strengthened by evidence from human pathology and by evidence from experimental studies using animal models. Much of this material has been reviewed previously elsewhere (IARC 1986) to which the interested reader is referred for more detail than can be given here.

Introduction

The last century has witnessed a remarkable epidemic of lung cancer. The words of Adler (1912), today make salutatory reading. *'Is it worthwhile to write a monograph on the subject of primary malignant tumours of the lung? In the course of the last two centuries an ever-increasing literature has accumulated around this subject. But this literature is without correlation, much of it buried in dissertations and other out-of-the-way places, and, with but a few notable exceptions, no attempt has been made to study the subject as a whole, either the pathological or the clinical aspect having been emphasised at the expense of the other, according to the special predilection of the author. On one point, however, there is nearly complete consensus of opinion, and that is that primary malignant neoplasms of the lungs are among the rarest forms of the disease. This latter opinion of the extreme rarity of primary tumours has persisted for centuries.'*

The lung is the principal body organ susceptible to tobacco carcinogenesis and, apart from non-melanocytic skin cancer, in many populations it has been or remains the most commonly diagnosed cancer in men and an increasingly common cancer in women (Gilliland and Samet 1994). The smoking of tobacco is the principal cause of lung cancer. The IARC Monograph on Tobacco Smoking (IARC 1986) estimated the proportion of lung cancer deaths attributable to tobacco smoking in five developed countries (Canada, England and Wales, Japan, Sweden, and the United States) to range between 83% and 92% for men and 57% and 80% for women. Historically, the incidence of lung cancer has waxed and waned to a greater or lesser degree in different populations related to the timing, prevalence, and intensity of the smoking epidemic and the different local dose of carcinogens delivered per cigarette. In some countries, especially those in which the epidemic struck early and was supplied with high tar cigarettes, age-standardized annual incidence and mortality rates exceeded 100 per 100 000 men and subsequently declined with the falling prevalence of men smoking. In the same populations the uptake of smoking in women was delayed by one or two decades. This delay, and a contemporaneous marketing of the filter tipped and lower dose cigarettes, resulted in a slower rise in rates. Consistent with the historical rise and fall in the prevalence of smoking in men, in several populations lung cancer rates in men have now peaked or are falling. The prevalence of smoking in women has either continued to grow or has declined only slowly. There is evidence from some countries that lung cancer rates in women may be stabilizing but the scenario in most countries is one of continuing increases in incidence and mortality. In 2000 it was estimated globally that 1.2 million people were diagnosed with lung cancer (Parkin 2001). This number is expected to grow. Many countries of Europe, Asia, Africa, and South America have only recently achieved a high prevalence of smoking, especially in women. In terms of lung cancer alone, these populations will generate millions of additional deaths over the next few decades.

In men in all European countries, except Portugal, lung cancer is now the leading cause of cancer death. In the United States (and in all except a few Scandinavian countries) it is the commonest tumour in terms of incidence as well (although the recent inflation of prostate cancer incidence figures with very early cases is taking prostate cancer above lung cancer in terms of the incidence of the disease). The range of geographical variation in lung cancer mortality in Europe is three-fold in both sexes, the highest rates being observed in the United Kingdom, Belgium, the Netherlands, and Czechoslovakia, and lowest rates reported in southern Europe and also in Norway and Sweden (Levi *et al.* 1989). This overall pattern of age-standardized lung cancer mortality rates does not reveal the important and diverging cohort effects occurring in various countries: for instance, some of the countries in which there are now low rates such as those in southern Europe and parts of eastern Europe, experienced a later uptake and spread of tobacco use, and now appear among the most elevated rates in the younger age groups. This suggests that these same countries, including Italy, Greece, France, Spain, and several countries in eastern Europe, will have the highest lung cancer rates in men at the beginning of the next century in the absence of rapid intervention.

The importance of adequate intervention is shown by the low lung cancer rates in Scandinavian countries which have adopted, since the early 1970s, integrated central and local policies and programs against smoking (Bjartveit 1986; Della-Vorgia *et al.* 1990). These policies may have been enabled by the limited influence of the tobacco lobby in these countries. The experience in Finland provides convincing evidence of the favourable impact, after a relatively short delay, of well-targeted large-scale interventions on the most common cause of cancer death and of premature mortality in general.

With specific reference to women, current rates in most European countries (except the United Kingdom, Ireland, and Denmark) are still substantially lower than in the United States, where lung cancer is now the leading cause of cancer death in women. In several countries, including France, Switzerland, Germany, and Italy, where smoking is now becoming commoner in young and middle-aged women, overall national mortality rates are still relatively low, although appreciable upward trends have been registered over the last two decades. This is particularly worrisome in perspective, since smoking prevalence has continued to increase in subsequent generations of young women in these countries. Thus, the observation that lung cancer is still relatively rare in women, with smoking at present accounting only for approximately 40–60% of all lung cancer deaths cannot constitute a reason for delaying efficacious interventions against smoking by women. The currently more favourable situation in Europe compared with the United States, together with the observation that smoking cessation reduces lung cancer risk after a delay of several years, should in the presence of adequate intervention, enable a major lung cancer epidemic in European women to be avoided.

A proportion of lung cancers, varying in various countries and geographical areas, may be due to exposures at work, and a small proportion to atmospheric pollution (Tomatis 1990). The effect of atmospheric pollution in increasing lung cancer risk appears to be chiefly confined to smokers. Lung cancer risk is elevated in atomic bomb survivors (Shimizu *et al.* 1987), patients treated for ankylosing spondylitis (Smith and Doll 1982), and in underground miners whose bronchial mucosa was exposed to radon gas and its decay products: this latter exposure was reviewed and it was concluded that there was 'sufficient evidence' that this occupational exposure caused lung cancer (IARC 1988). A greater risk of lung cancer is generally seen for individuals who are exposed at an older age. Investigation of the interaction with cigarette smoking among atomic bomb survivors suggests that it is additive (Kopecky *et al.* 1987) but the data from underground miners in Colorado are consistent with a multiplicative effect (Whittemore and McMillan 1983).

The overwhelming role of tobacco smoking in the causation of lung cancer has been repeatedly demonstrated over the past 50 years.Current lung cancer rates reflect cigarette smoking habits of men and women over past decades (Boyle and Robertson 1987; La Vecchia and Franceschi 1984; La Vecchia *et al.* 1988) but not necessarily current smoking patterns, since there is an interval of several decades between the change in smoking habits in a population and its consequences on lung cancer rates. Over 90% of lung cancer may be avoidable simply through avoidance of cigarette smoking. Rates of lung cancer in central and eastern Europe at the present time are higher than those ever before recorded elsewhere; lung cancer has increased 10-fold in men and 8-fold in women in Japan since 1950; there is a worldwide epidemic of smoking among young women (Chollat-Traquet 1992) which will be translated in increasing rates of tobacco-related disease, including cancer, in the coming decades; there is another epidemic of lung cancer and tobacco-related deaths building up in China as the cohorts of men in whom tobacco smoking became popular reach ages where cancer is an important hazard (Boyle 1993). Many solutions have been attempted to reduce cigarette smoking and increasingly many countries are enacting legislation to curb this habit (Roemer 1993).

The epidemiology of smoking and lung cancer

From the perspective of the early twenty-first century, a causal relationship between smoking and lung cancer is taken as self evident, but this was not always the case. An early observer of the then rare respiratory cancer (Rottman 1898) considered it an occupational hazard, possibly from exposure to tobacco dust. The association between tobacco smoking and the development of lung cancer appears to have been suggested in the United Kingdom in 1927 (Tylecote 1927). The first interview study on tobacco smoking and lung cancer seems to have been reported from Vienna (Fleckseder 1936) where lung cancer rates had risen dramatically. Fleckseder (1936) found 51 smokers among 54 patients he found with lung cancer. Thirty seven of these smoked between 20 and 90 cigarettes daily while excessive smoking of pipes, cigars, or both was rarer.

The same association was alluded to in a report from the United States (Ochsner and Debakey 1939) in a study primarily of a series of 79 patients treated by total pneumonectomy. A report from Cologne followed one year later (Muller 1940) based on the post-mortem records of 96 patients. The patient, or more usually the relatives of fatal cases, was interviewed as to their occupation, tobacco consumption, and exposure to specific 'inhalants'. Re-analysis of Muller's data provides relative risk of 3.1 among *moderate* smokers, 2.7 among *heavy* smokers, 16.8 among *very heavy* smokers and 29.2 among *excessive* smokers.Within the limitations of the study (e.g. small numbers, especially among non-smoking cases, possible inaccuracies in elucidation of precise smoking histories) these results were noticeably similar to results obtained from later case–control studies in the United States and, apart from a lack of increase among heavy smokers, there is the possible appearance of a dose–response relationship.

A study of smoking habits and occupation based on 195 post-mortem records of cases of lung cancer at the Pathology Institute at Jena for the years 1930–1941 was reported: useable replies were obtained from relatives of 93 men and 16 women. Of the women, 13 were non-smokers (Schairer and Schoniger 1943). The authors attempted to collect control information by interviewing 700 men in Jena between the ages of 53 and 54, the average age of the lung cancer patients at death (53.9 years). It was a study performed in Germany towards the end of the Second World War and only 270 men from Jena responded to the questionnaire. The authors showed great insight in concluding that wartime conditions (particularly the rationing system) may have favoured results from non-smokers. They reported a statistically significant difference in non-smokers and heavy smokers among lung cancer patients on the one hand and normal patients on the other. Realizing the possible errors in their material they concluded that there was a considerable probability that lung cancer was far more frequent among heavy smokers and far less frequent among non-smokers than expected. Their data is such that an approximate relative risk can be calculated and the risk relative to non-smokers was 1.9 among *light* smokers; 9.1 among *moderate* smokers, and 11.3 among *heavy/excessive* smokers. Again there appears to be a moderate dose–response relationship. A further study from the Netherlands (Wassink 1948) identified very similar associations between smoking and lung cancer.

Over the first few decades of the twentieth century, reports began not only to admit that the incidence of lung cancer was increasing (Clemmeson and Buck 1947) but also to associate the increase with smoking rather than better diagnosis or increased longevity of the population (Anon 1942). These findings were largely ignored until 1950, when five case–control studies of the topic were published (Doll and Hill 1950; Levin *et al.* 1950; Mills and Porter 1950; Schrek *et al.* 1950; Wynder and Graham 1950) that included altogether over 2000 cases, the two largest studies having over 600 cases each and an equivalent numbers of controls (Doll and Hill 1950; Wynder and Graham 1950). Their conclusions were virtually identical—that smoking, particularly cigarette smoking, was an important factor in the production of lung cancer. The evidence from these studies, however, failed to gain wide acceptance. Instead it attracted opposition, not only from the tobacco industry but also from some other scientists because, although an association between smoking and lung cancer had been demonstrated, few were willing to accept it as evidence of a causal relationship, as at this time the case–control design was considered by many to have too many defects for it to produce reliable, unbiased findings (Sadowsky *et al.* 1953; Hammond 1954).

The methodological problems of case–control studies were to be overcome by using another epidemiological design, and shortly after the publication of the first case–control studies, the results of two prospective cohort studies came to hand (Doll and Hill 1954; Hammond and Horn 1958). These two cohort studies essentially confirmed the strong associations that had been shown between cigarette smoking and lung cancer by the case–control studies, and gave additional information; e.g. with respect to the dose–response relationship between the amount smoked and the risk of lung cancer and the decrease in risk in those who were able to stop the habit.

The proof that smoking tobacco causes lung cancer

The evidence described above was not enough to satisfy powerful critics which, as well as tobacco industry apologists such as Todd, included two other well-respected statisticians – Berkson and Fisher. Their criticisms of these epidemiological studies, however frustrating they might have been at the time, ultimately helped to refine the criteria used to assess whether epidemiological associations are causal. Causal reasoning in epidemiology had been developed from considerations of infectious diseases and, in hindsight, the application of Koch's postulates was unlikely to provide a comfortable fit with chronic disease causation. Although elaborated upon further by others, the criteria with which to assess causality were laid down by the mid-1960s (USPHS 1964; Hill 1966) as follows: the consistency, strength, specificity, temporal sequence and coherence of the association.

It is salutary to review the criticisms of the causal hypothesis made at the time. Todds's criticisms included the low correlation between national lung cancer mortality and tobacco consumption ($r = 0.5$), the unreliability of smoking histories, and that the increase in mortality was more likely to be due to pollution (Anon 1991). Hill and Doll were able to dismiss the first criticism as, given the crudeness of the measures, a coefficient of this size strengthened their conclusions. In regard to the second criticism, if smoking histories were in fact unreliable, measurement error would have diluted the strength of the measured association. Furthermore, smoking histories were later found by Todd himself (White 1990) to be remarkably precise. In regard to pollution as a cause, there was simply no evidence to support the proposition.

Berkson's principal criticisms (Berkson 1958) were based on three observations; the first was the lack of specificity of action, the second was lack of biological evidence of a carcinogen and the third was the lower than expected death rates in the cohorts compared with their respective general populations. He was concerned that the studies found too many disease outcomes to be associated with smoking, rather than just with lung cancer that was the subject of investigation, and concluded that the findings were the result of many subtle and complicated biases. He supported his opinion with the failure of the attempts to produce cancer experimentally and to isolate the responsible carcinogen. The lower than expected rates experienced in the early years of the cohort he argued were also evidence of biased sampling.

The concept of specificity of action has limited utility when dealing with a complex mix of more than 4000 carcinogenic substances administered to the whole body rather than a single microorganism. In making this criticism Berkson also failed to take account of the extraordinary strength of the association between smoking and lung cancer and the wide range of relative risks associated with different diseases. Hill's rejoinder was that it was as if he said that milk could not be a cause of any disease because it spread tuberculosis, diptheria, scarlet fever, undulant fever, dysentery etc. (Hill 1966). On the other hand, his request to identify the active carcinogen was appropriate but it unfortunately hindered the widespread acceptance of the epidemiological evidence by some eminent authorities (Anon 1962). The 'healthy' cohort effect that gave rise to the early reduced risks compared with the general population was soon to disappear as the relative risk between smokers and non-smokers in the cohort increased.

Fisher, on the other hand, emphasized Doll and Hill's finding from their case–control study (Doll and Hill 1950), that smokers who developed lung cancer inhaled less often than smokers who remained free of the disease (Fisher 1958), to suggest that inhalation was protective against lung cancer. He also pointed to an apparent inconsistency in the secular trends by sex—that lung cancer rates were increasing more in men than women while the increase in smoking prevalence had recently been greatest in women (Fisher 1957). He did not comment on the cohort study findings. Because of his scientific interests, and possibly because of his smoking habit, he was interested in pursuing studies of genetic susceptibility but these plans were curtailed by his death in 1962.

The paradoxical findings with respect to inhalation patterns were a valid point of criticism that resisted clarification for some time. It is now known that the deposition of particulate matter in the bronchi differs by the depth of inhalation, deep inhalers depositing less in the bronchi and more particulates deep in the lungs (Wald et al. 1983). The concern about trends by gender was misplaced, as it failed to take into account the long latency period between exposure and the diagnosis of lung cancer and the strong cohort effects in the uptake of the smoking habit that differed between the sexes.

The consistency of the association

The consistency of the findings shown by the early case–control and cohort studies has been maintained in numerous additional studies since that time that have been conducted in many different populations (IARC 1986). The consistency of the evidence from these analytical studies has been reinforced further by ecological studies of lung cancer trends in populations that have shown a high correlation between smoking rates and lung cancer rates both within populations and internationally (Doll 1954; Doll and Peto 1981). Analysis of lung cancer mortality trends over time have shown pronounced cohort effects associated with the prevalence of smoking (USDHHS 1982), and in some populations where male smoking prevalence has fallen, so too is lung cancer mortality (Gilliland and Samet 1994).

The strength of the association

Strength of association is perhaps the single most important criterion in establishing causation. It is usually expressed as the ratio of the incidence of disease in those exposed to the causal agent (in this case smoking) to the incidence of the disease in the unexposed. In cohort studies this ratio is termed the relative risk, which is approximated in case–control studies by the odds ratio. In cohort studies, the estimates of relative risk of lung cancer comparing cigarette smokers with non-smokers range from 9 to 14-fold (Doll and Hill 1954; Hammond and Horn 1954; Hammond 1966; Cederlof et al. 1975; Doll and Peto 1976; Lund and Zeiner-Henriksen 1981).

Associations of this strength are likely to reflect a causal relationship and the likelihood is increased when a dose–response relationship can be demonstrated. Evidence of dose–response also supports the biological coherence of the association. In regard to lung cancer, several cohort studies have illustrated dose–response in several ways; in terms of the daily amount smoked, the duration of smoking, the age at onset of smoking, and the cumulative amount smoked. For example, in terms of number of cigarettes smoked, the mortality ratio compared with non-smokers for those who smoked 25 or more a day exceeded 25 for men and 29 for women in the British Physician's Study (Doll and Hill 1950). For age at onset less than 15 years the mortality ratio exceeded 16 for men in the ASC 25 state study (Hammond 1966) and 18 for men in the US Veteran's study (Rogot and Murray 1980).

The specificity of the association

As mentioned already, the specificity criterion for causality is a relict from Koch's postulates with respect to causal agents for infectious diseases. The specificity criterion, however, only reinforces a causal hypothesis and is not considered a necessary criterion (USPHS 1964; Hill 1966). Although tobacco smoke is measured epidemiologically as a single exposure, it is a complex mixture of carcinogenic chemicals that act together in a variety of ways to cause cancers in several organs and tissues. Of all the cancer types that can be at least partly attributed to smoking, the specificity for lung cancer is the greatest as evidenced by the strength of the association already noted above. The relative risks observed for smoking and lung cancer are much larger than those observed for cancers occurring in other organs, especially for cancers in tissues that are not directly exposed to tobacco smoke such as the kidney and the uterine cervix.

The temporal relationship of the association

Obviously, to be causally associated with the disease the suspect aetiological exposure has to antedate the diagnosis. One reason why the findings from major prospective cohort studies have been most useful in establishing a causal relationship between smoking and lung cancer is because the exposure to smoking was measured in advance of diagnosis in thousands of subjects who were free of disease at entry to the studies.

The coherence of the association

The coherence criterion links the epidemiological observations with other knowledge in regard to the biology and natural history of the disease. This takes into account other criteria, for example those of temporal sequence and dose–response relationship discussed above. Another piece of supportive evidence is the diminution of risk after smoking cessation, which shows a negative dose–response relationship with increasing time since quitting. In the British Physician's Study after quitting for 15 years or more the mortality ratio was 2 compared with 16 in those who had quit for less than 5 years (Doll and Peto 1976). This was similar to the mortality ratio for US Veterans who had quit for 20 years or more (Rogot and Murray 1980). Evidence from human pathology was also useful in establishing causality. Auerbach (Auerbach *et al.* 1979) examined pre-malignant changes in the bronchial epithelium from 402 male autopsies and discovered that atypical cells were more prevalent in the bronchial epithelium of smokers compared with non-smokers and that their prevalence increased in a dose–response fashion with the amount habitually smoked, the prevalence of atypical cells in non-smokers being very low.

Experimental evidence

A large amount of supportive evidence has been produced from experimental animal models of smoking carcinogenesis (IARC 1986). Some of this work faced difficulties especially in regard to the development of appropriate inhalation models. Unlike man, experimental animals avoid inhaling tobacco smoke and the delivery of carcinogenic doses of smoke to the lung can also be perturbed by anatomical differences in the animals' upper respiratory tracts compared with humans. It was also commonly observed that the loss of weight experienced by animals that were chronically exposed to smoke often extended their lives (Wynder and Hoffman 1967). Despite these inconsistencies, informative data were obtained on the carcinogenic effect of smoke in its gaseous phase. Further proof of carcinogenic potential was obtained by topical application of cigarette smoke condensate to mouse skin (Wynder and Hoffman 1967) and the injection of cigarette smoke condensate directly into rodents' lungs (Stanton *et al.* 1972).

Passive smoking and lung cancer risk

Having established a strong and consistent causal association between direct smoking and an increased risk of lung cancer, tobacco research turned recently to the association between exposure to environmental tobacco smoke (passive smoking) and a diversity of adverse health events, including lung cancer (Burns 1992; EPA 1992; Stockwell *et al.* 1992). On the basis of 30 epidemiological studies, the United States Environmental Protection Agency (EPA) concluded that environmental tobacco smoke (ETS) was a human lung carcinogen. It has been estimated that each year in the United States, 434 000 deaths are attributable to tobacco use, in particular cigarette smoking (CDC 1991), 112 000 of these smoking-related deaths from lung cancer (USDHHS 1989). There are an estimated 1500 deaths in non-smoking women due to passive smoking and 500 deaths in non-smoking men annually. The basis for these conclusions is a group of epidemiological studies that took spouse smoking as a measure of exposure to ETS (EPA 1992). The overall relative risk obtained from 11 studies conducted in the United States was 1.19; there was a tendency for a positive trend in risk to be found with increasing dose of smoking (EPA 1992). All the spousal smoking was assessed by questionnaire and the group of studies, with notable exceptions

(Garfinkel *et al.* 1985; Fontham *et al.* 1991), is characterized by low statistical power and small increased relative risks with large confidence intervals frequently extending over unity.

Small increased risks such as this are below that which can be reliably detected by epidemiological methods and the exposure assessment in these studies is poor. The use of biomarkers for analysing and quantifying the role of ETS is much more complex for cancer than asthma, given the much longer interval between exposure and clinical manifestation of the disease. The critical reviewer could find shortcomings in the majority of the published studies of ETS and lung cancer. However, as was recognized by an IARC Working Party (IARC 1986) given current knowledge of the chemical constituents of both side stream and mainstream smoke, of the materials absorbed during passive smoking and of the quantitative relationships between dose and effect that are commonly observed from exposure to carcinogens, it could be concluded that passive smoking gives rise to some risk of lung cancer. The great deal that is known about the carcinogenic effects of active smoking (IARC 1986) has undoubtedly bolstered the interpretation of the epidemiological data on passive smoking.

Despite nearly half a century of careful epidemiological study and the scientific certainty that tobacco is carcinogenic there is still a need to quantify the risks of low level exposure.

Public health failure, 1960s onwards

It has been clear for the entire second half of the twentieth century that cigarette smoking causes lung cancer. Current low levels of smoking among physicians and research scientists, in many countries, have led many of them unconsciously to overlook tobacco smoking as an important cause of cancer (Boyle 1993*b*). There is, however, a very substantial body of evidence from many sources which indicates the carcinogenicity of tobacco smoking. Not only does cigarette smoking greatly increase the risk of lung cancer in smokers, but the risk of oral cavity cancer, larynx cancer, oesophageal cancer, bladder cancer, pancreas cancer, cervix cancer, stomach cancer, kidney cancer, and colorectal cancer are also increased (Boyle 1997).

There is at present a worldwide epidemic of tobacco-related diseases: not only does smoking cause increased levels of many different common forms of cancer, but it also increases the risk of cardiovascular disease. Deaths from lung cancer, the cancer site most strongly linked to cigarette smoking, have increased in Japan by a factor of 10 in men and 8 in women since 1950. In central and eastern Europe, more than 400 000 premature deaths are currently caused each year by tobacco smoking. In young men in all countries of central and eastern Europe, currently there are levels of lung cancer which are greater than anything seen before in the western countries and these rates are still rising. In Poland, a country severely hit by the tobacco epidemic, life-expectancy of a 45-year-old man has been falling for over a decade now due to the increasing premature death rates from tobacco-related cancers and cardiovascular disease (Zatonski and Boyle 1996). Tragically, cigarette smoking is still increasing in central and eastern Europe and also in China, where an epidemic of tobacco-related deaths is building up quickly. Tobacco smoking is also the most easily avoided risk factor for cancer.

The most important determinant of risk of lung cancer is the duration of smoking: long-term cigarette smokers have a one hundred-fold increased risk compared with never-smokers (Peto 1986). The content of cigarettes (low tar) produces only a threefold variation in risks between the extremes (Low tar is frequently taken to include a number of features including filtered-tips as well as the active tar yield). Lung cancer is the major tobacco-related site and the leading cause of cancer death in men in almost all developed countries. Incidence rates are around 10–15 per 100 000 in non-smokers, between 80–100 per 100 000 in the highest-incidence population groups such as Afro-Americans and rates exceeding 200 per 100 000 have been reported in cities of central and eastern Europe. Lung cancer being frequently fatal, mortality rates are high and, consequently, the social costs are high.

The early concept that reducing tar and nicotine would reduce cancer risk was well founded on epidemiological studies, which showed a reduction in lung cancer risk, but not cardiovascular disease, of between 20% and 50% in association with the move to filters which occurred over the fifties and sixties (Bross and Gibson 1968; Wynder *et al.* 1970; Dean *et al.* 1977; Hawthorne and Fry 1978; Wynder and Stellman 1979; Rimington 1981; Lubin 1984; Federal Trade Commission 1995). It was therefore logical that public health authorities should press for further reductions. However, the reductions which appeared in the yields as measured by the FTC system do not reflect, in a quantitative way, what passes into the lungs of smokers. That more intensive ('compensatory') smoking patterns are seen in smokers was demonstrated by Russell in 1980 and many others (Russell 1980; Herning *et al.* 1981; Kozlowski *et al.* 1982; United States Surgeon General 1986).

In the absence of systematic on-going analysis of what has been going into smokers lungs, we are left with biological outcomes as an index of what has been happening. There are three potentially important observations in this regard (Gray and Boyle 2000).

First of all, it is very difficult to imagine that the large fall in the tar content of cigarettes sold in the United Kingdom over the last 50 years (Wald *et al.* 1981) has not influenced the lung cancer death rate which has been falling for two decades in men in that country.

Secondly, and paradoxically, mortality from lung cancer in men increased between the first (CPS-I) and second (CPS-II) Cancer Prevention Studies of the American Cancer Society (Thun and Heath 1997; United States Surgeon General 1989): these studies recruited men from birth cohorts approximated 30 years apart. At first glance, the decrease in mortality promised by the yield reductions of the 1950s and 1960s has not been substantial over the 1970s and 1980s. However, this may be too simple an interpretation.

Information of the number of cigarettes smoked at time of enrolment to both studies may not mirror the lifelong patterns of smoking that cause lung cancer (Thun *et al.* 1977): data on smoking in early life, which critically determines duration of smoking, are sparse in both studies. Cigarette consumption during adolescence and early adulthood was probably heavier among smokers in CPS-II for several reasons. Manufactured cigarettes were more readily available in the 1950s than in the 1930s, eras when smoking was likely to be initiated in the CPS-II and CPS-I cohort respectively.

Birth cohort analyses show that a prevalence of smoking among white men increased with each successive birth cohort born from 1900 to 1929 and decreased thereafter (Burns 1994). Age-specific lung cancer death rates have decreased in those born after 1930 (Devesa *et al.* 1989; Gilliland and Samet 1994).

The large increases in lung cancer death rates from CPS-I to CPS-II probably reflect unmeasured heavier smoking among CPS-II during the 1940s and 1950s as well as the measured increase in daily consumption and duration of smoking. In addition, CPS-II may include a more addicted 'hard-core' smokers, who find it virtually impossible to quit smoking, and CPS-II smokers, partly to compensate for lower nicotine content of modern cigarettes, may inhale more deeply, take more puffs per cigarette and retain smoke longer in the lungs than did smokers in the past. The impact of lower tar and nicotine cigarettes is difficult to elucidate with all these other changes in effect.

Thirdly, and what is clear, is that there has been a real swing towards higher rates of adenocarcinoma of the lung both in the United States and elsewhere (Cutler and Young 1975; Vincent *et al.* 1977; Cox and Resner 1979; Young *et al.* 1981; Beard *et al.* 1985; Wu *et al.* 1986; Johnson 1988; El-Torkey *et al.* 1990; Devesa *et al.* 1991; Wynder and Muscat 1995) which is consistent with the hypothesis that qualitative changes in cigarette smoke have led to a change in the observed pattern of lung cancer but not to a substantial decrease in mortality.

Women around the world have taken up cigarette smoking habit with gusto. For many years it appeared that their lung cancer rates were low and that tobacco was not having the same effect on men. This complacency, which crept in during the two decades from the mid-1960s especially, is now exposed as false: neither is there evidence that the effect of cigarette smoking on lung cancer risk is greater in women than in men. The dominance of the effect of duration of smoking means that a long period of time will pass between the exposure (large numbers of women smoking) until the effect (high levels of lung cancer). Lung cancer now exceeds breast cancer as the leading cancer cause of death in women in the United States, Canada, Scotland, and several other countries. In Canada, breast cancer mortality has remained at least constant for nearly four decades while lung cancer death rates have increased between 3 and 4-fold during the same period. While the higher case-fatality of lung cancer may be one factor in the mortality rates overtaking breast cancer, there is increasing evidence that there are regions of the world where the gap in the incidence rate is now closing. For example, in Glasgow, an area where lung cancer has been historically high, by 1990 the incidence rate for lung cancer (115 per 100 000) exceeded that for breast cancer (105 per 100 000) in 1990 (Gillis et al. 1992). In international Cancer Registries, there are some where the incidence of lung cancer now exceeds the incidence of breast cancer and others where there is still a gap. In the SEER (Surveillance Epidemiology and End Results) Programme of the US NCI, the incidence of lung cancer in both black and white women increased by over 90% between 1973–1977 and 1988–1992: the increase in the incidence of breast cancer was around 25% in both racial groups (comparison made between incidence rates age-adjusted using 1970 US population). Of great worry is that there does not appear to be any end in sight to this increase in lung cancer risk internationally: it is programmed to continue for several decades to come.

Part of the complacency over the effect on women was also due to the strong tendency for women to smoke brands of cigarettes which were lower in tar and nicotine content than men: it was assumed that this would have less of a risk on lung cancer than the higher tar cigarettes which men generally smoked. Now marked changes in the rates of the major histological cell types of lung cancer can be seen with particular increases in the risk of adenocarcinoma (Zheng et al. 1994; Levi et al. 1997). The changes seen are compatible with increased risk of adenocarcinoma due to increasing levels of smoking of light cigarettes ('low tar, low nicotine'). It appears that abandoning, high-tar cigarettes (15–45 mg tar) may have had some impact on reducing squamous-cell carcinoma risk, there is now a 'balancing' by light cigarettes increasing risk of adenocarcinoma.

Cigarette smoking kills half of all those who adopt the habit with 50% of these deaths occurring in middle age and each losing an average of 20 years of non-smokers life expectancy (Doll et al. 1994). It kills in over 24 different ways with lung cancer being the commonest cancer-site (Doll et al. 1994). Lung cancer rates have been declining in men and increasing in women: cigarette smoking in men has been declining while it has been increasing in women. These two are closely related. The move to 'light' cigarettes, which is increasingly common, now appears to be linked to increases in adenocarcinoma of the lung and shows no sign of being linked to a reduced risk overall. Clearly cigarettes are different but still seriously harmful after decades of selfregulation. There is no such thing as a safe cigarette. Smokers should be urged and helped to stop smoking, children and young adults should be convinced not to smoke. Tobacco can become an addictive drug: it should be left alone (Boyle et al. 1995).

Acknowledgements

It is a pleasure to acknowledge the support provided by the Cancer Council Victoria and the Italian Association of Cancer Research (*Associazione Italiana per la Ricerca sul Cancro*).

References

Adler, I. (1912). *Primary malignant growths of the lungs and bronchi: A pathological and clinical study*. London: Longmans, Green and Co.

Anon, (1942). Cancer of the lung (editorial). *Br Med J*, **1**: 672–3.

Anon (1962). The cigarette as co-carcinogen (editorial). *Lancet*, **1**: 85–6.

Anon (1991). Conversation with Sir Richard Doll (Journal interview 29). *Br J Addiction*, **86**: 365–77.

Auerbach, O., Hammond, E.C., and Garfinkel, L. (1979). Changes in bronchial epithelium in relation to cigarette smoking, 1955–1960 vs 1970–1977. *N Engl J Med*, **300**: 381–6.

Beard, M.C., Anneges, J.F., Woolner, L.B., and Kurland, L.T. (1985). Bronchiogenic carcinoma in Olmsted County, 1635–1979. *Cancer (Phila.)*, **55**: 2026–30.

Berkson, J. (1958). Smoking and lung cancer: some observations on two recent reports. *J Amer Stat Assoc*, **53**: 28–38.

Bjartveit, K. (1986). Legislation and political activity. In: *Tobacco: a major international health hazard* (ed. DG Zaridze and R Peto), pp. 285–98. IARC, Lyon.

Boyle, P. (1993). The hazards of passive and active smoking. *N Engl J Med*, **329**: 1581.

Boyle, P. (1993b). The hazards of passive and active smoking. *N Engl J Med*, **328**: 1708–9.

Boyle, P. (1997). Cancer, Cigarette smoking and premature death in Europe. A review including the Recommendations of European Cancer Experts Consensus Meeting. Helsinki, October 1996. *Lung Cancer*, **17**: 1–60.

Boyle, P. and Robertson, C. (1987). Statistical modelling of lung cancer and laryngeal cancer incidence data in Scotland, 1960–1979. *Am J Epidemiol*, **125**: 731–44.

Boyle, P., Veronesi, U., Tubiana, M., Alexander, F.E., Calais da Silva, F., Denis, L.J. *et al.* (1995). European School of Oncology Advisory Report to the European Commission for the "Europe Against Cancer Programme" European Code Against Cancer. *Eur J Cancer*, **9**: 1395–405.

Bross, I.D.J. and Gibson, R. (1968). Risks of lung cancer in smokers who switch to filter cigarettes. *Am J Publ Health*, **58**: 1396–403.

Burns, D.M. (1992). Environmental tobacco smoke: the price of scientific certainty. *J Natl Cancer Inst*, **84**: 1387–8.

Burns, D.M. (1994). *Tobacco Smoking. In: Epidemiology of Lung Cancer* (ed. J.M. Somet), pp 15–49. Marcel Dekker, New York.

Centres for Disease Control. (1991). Smoking-attributable mortality and years of potential life lost— United States, 1988. *MMWR*, **40**: 62–71.

Cederlof, R., Friberg, L., Hrubec, Z., and Lorich, U. (1975). *The relationship of smoking and some social covariates to mortality and cancer morbidity. A ten year follow-up in a probability sample of 55,000 Swedish subjects age 18–69, Part 1 and Part 2*. Stockholm: The Karolinska Institute.

Chollat-Traquet, C. (1992). *Women and Tobacco*. Geneva:World Health Organization.

Clemmesen, J. and Buck, T. (1947). On the apparent increase in the incidence of lung cancer in Denmark, 1931–1945. *Br J Cancer*, **1**: 253–9.

Cox, J. D. and Resner, R. A. (1979). Adenocarcinoma of the lung: recent results from the Veterans Administration lung group. *Am Rev Resp Dis*, **120**: 1025–9.

Cutler, S.J. and Young, J.L. (1975). Third National Cancer Survey: incidence data. *J Natl Cancer Inst Monogr*, **41**: 1–454.

Dean, G., Lee, P.N., Todd, G.F., and Wicken, A.J. (1977). Report on a second retrosepective study in Northeast England. Part 1. Factors related to mortality from lung cancer, bronchitis, heart disease, and stroke in cleveland county with particular emphasis on the relative risks associated with smoking filter and plain cigarettes. (Research Paper 14) London, Tobacco Research Council.

Della-Vorgia, P., Sasco, A.J., Skalkidis, Y., Katsouyani, K., and Trichopoulos, D. (1990). An evaluation of the effectiveness of tobacco-control legislative policies in European Community countries. *Scand J Soc Med*, **18**: 81–9.

Devesa, S.S., Blot, W.J., and Fraumeni, J.F. (1989). Declining lung cancer rates among young men and women in the United States: A cohort analysis. *J Natl Cancer Inst*, **81**: 1568–71.

Devesa, S.S., Shaw, G.L., and Blot, W.J. (1991). Changing patterns of cancer incidence by histologic type. *Cancer Epidemiol Biomarkers and Prev*, **1**: 29–34.

Doll, R. (1954). Review of: Cancer of the lung (Epidemiology). *Br Med J*, **2**: 1402.

Doll, R. and Hill, A.B. (1950). Smoking and carcinoma of the lung. *Br Med J*, **2**: 739–48.

Doll, R. and Hill, A.B. (1954). The mortality of doctors in relation to their smoking habits; a preliminary report. *Br Med J*, **1**: 1451–5.

Doll, R. and Peto, R. (1976). Mortality in relation to smoking: 20 years observations on male British doctors. *Br Med J*, **2**: 1525–36.

Doll, R. and Peto, R. (1981). The causes of cancer: quantitative estimates of avoidable risks of cancer in the United States today. *J Natl Cancer Inst*, **66**: 1191–308.

Doll, R., Peto, R., Wheatley, K., Gray, R., and Sutherland, I. (1994). Mortality in relation to smoking: 40 years' observations on male British doctors. *Br Med J*, **309**(6959): 901–11.

El-Torkey, M., El-Zeky, F., and Hall, J.C. (1990). Significant changes in the distribution of histological types of lung cancer. A review of 4928 cases. *Cancer (Phila.)*, **65**: 2361–7.

EPA (United States Environment Protection Agency). (1992). *Respiratory health effects of passive smoking: lung cancer and other disorders*. US Environment Protection Agency, Washington, DC.

Federal Trade Commission. (1995). Tar, nicotine and carbon monoxide of the smoke of 1107 varieties of domestic cigarettes. Washington, DC, US Federal Trade Commission.

Fisher, R.A. (1957). Dangers of cigarette smoking. *Br Med J*, **2**: 43.

Fisher, R.A. (1958). Cancer and smoking. *Nature*, **182**: 596.

Fleckseder, R. (1936). Ueber den Bronchialkrebs und einge seiner Entstehungsbedingungen. *Munch Med Wochenschr Nr*, **36**: 1585–93.

Fontham, E.T.H., Correa, P., Wu-Williams, A., Reynolds, P., Greenberg, R.S., Buflier, P.A. *et al.* (1991). Lung cancer in non-smoking women: A multicentre case-control study. *Cancer Epidemiol Biomarkers Prev*, **1**: 35–43.

Garfinkel, L., Auerbach, O., and Hubert, L. (1985). Involuntary smoking and lung cancer: a casecontrol study. *J Natl Cancer Inst*, **75**: 465–9.

Gilliland, F.D. and Samet, J.M. (1994). Lung cancer. In: *Trends in Cancer Incidence and Mortality* (ed. R. Doll, J.F. Fraumeni, and C.S. Muir), pp. 175–95. Cold Spring Harbor Laboratory Press, Plainview, NY.

Gilliland, F.D. and Samet, J. M. (1994). Lung cancer. *Cancer Surveys*, **19**: 175–84.

Gillis, C., Hole, D.J., Lamont, D.W., Graham, A.C., and Ramage, S. (1992). The incidences of lung cancer and breast cancer in women in Glasgow. *Br Med J*, **305**: 1331.

Gray, N. and Boyle P. (2000). The regulation of tobacco and tobacco smoke. *Ann Oncol*, **11**: 909–14.

Hammond, E.C. (1954). Smoking in relation to lung cancer: A follow up study. *Conn State Med J*, **18**: 3–9.

Hammond, E.C. (1966). Smoking in relation to death rates of one million men and women. *Natl Cancer Inst Monogr*, **19**: 127–204.

Hammond, E.C., Garfinkel, L., Seidman, H., and Lew, E.A. (1976). 'Tar' and nicotine content of cigarette smoke in relation to death rates. *Environ Res*, **12**: 263–74.

Hammond, E. C. and Horn, D. (1954). The relationship between human smoking habits and death rates: A follow up study of 187,766 men. *J Amer Med Assoc*, **154**: 1316–28.

Hammond, E.C. and Horn, D. (1958). *Smoking in relation to death rates*. Manuscript distributed at the time of presentation at the meeting of the American Medical Association, New York, June 4, 1957 and subsequently published (Hammond and Horn, 1958).

Hawthorne, V.M. and Fry, J.S. (1978). Smoking and health. The association between smoking behaviour, total mortality and cardiorespiratory disease in West Scotland. *J Epidemiol Commun Health*, **32**: 260–6.

Herning, R.I., Jones, R.T., Bachman, J., and Mines, A.H. (1981). Puff volume increases when low nicotine cigarettes are smoked. *Br Med J Clin Res*, **283**: 187–9.

Hill, A.B. (1966). *Principles of Medical Statistics* (eighth edn), pp. 305–13. The Lancet, London. IARC (International Agency for Research on Cancer). (1988). Man-made Mineral Fibers and Radon. Monogr Eval Carcinog Risk Hum; **43**, Lyon: IARC.

IARC (International Agency for Research on Cancer). (1986). *Tobacco Smoking*. Monogr Eval Carcinog Risk Hum; **38**, Lyon: IARC.

Johnson, W.W. (1988). Histologic and cytologic patterns of lung cancer in 2580 men and women over a 15-year period. *Acta Cytol*, **32**: 163–8.

Kopecky, K.J., Yamamoto, T., Fujikura, T., Tokuoka, S., Monzen, T., Nishimori, I. *et al.* (1987). *Lung cancer, radiation exposure and smoking among A-bomb survivors, Hiroshima and Nagasaki*, 1950–1980. Radiation Effects Research Foundation Technical Report 13-86. Hiroshima: Japan, Radiation Effects Research Foundation.

Kozlowski, L.T., Rickert, W.S., Pope, M.A., Robinson, J.C., and Frecker, R.C. (1982). Estimating the yields to smokers of tar, nicotine, and carbon monoxide from the lowest yield ventilated filter cigarettes. *Brit J Addict*, **77**: 159–165.

La Vecchia, C. and Franceschi, S. (1984). Italian lung cancer death rates in young males (Letter). *Lancet*, I: 406.

La Vecchia, C., Levi, F., Decarli, A., Wietlisbach, V., Negri, E., Gutzwiller, F. (1988). Trends in smoking and lung cancer mortality in Switzerland. *Prev Med*, **17**: 712–24.

Levi, F., Franceschi, S., La Vecchia, C., Randimbison, L., and Van-Cong, T. (1997). Lung carcinoma trends by histologic type in Vaud and Neuchatel, Switzerland, 1974–1994. *Cancer*, **79**: 906–14.

Levin, M.L., Goldstein, H., and Gerhardt, P.R. (1950). Cancer and Tobacco Smoking. *J Am Med Assoc*, **143**: 336–8.

Levi, F., Maisonneuve, P., Filiberti, R., La Vecchia, C., and Boyle, P. (1989). Cancer incidence and mortality in Europe. *Sozial und Praventivmedizin*, **34**(supp 2): 1–84.

Lubin, L.H. (1984). Modifying risk of developing lung cancer by changing habits of cigarette smoking. *Br Med J*, **289**: 1953–6.

Lund, E., Zeiner-Henriksen, T. (1981). Smoking as a risk factor for cancer among 26,000 Norwegian males and Females. *Tiddskv nor laegeforen*, **101**: 1937–40.

Mills, C.A. and Porter, M.M. (1950). Tobacco smoking habits and cancer of the mouth and respiratory system. *Cancer Res*, **10**: 539–42.

Muller, F.H. (1940). Tabaksmisbrauch und Lungenkarzinom. *Z f Krebsforsch*, **49**: 57–85.

Ochsner, A. and Debakey, M. (1939). Primary pulmonary malignancy. Treatment by total pneumonectomy. Analysis of 79 collected cases and presentation of 7 personal cases. *Surg Gynecol Obs*, **68**: 435–51.

Peto, R. (1986). Influence of dose and duration of smoking on lung cancer rates. *IARC Sci Publ*, **74**: 22–33.

Parkin, D.M. (2001). Global cancer statistics in the year 2000. *Lancet Oncol*, **2**: 533–43.

Rimington, J. (1981). The effects of filters on the incidence of lung cancer in cigarette smokers. *Environ Res*, **24**: 162–6.

Roemer, R. (1993). Legislative Action to combat the World Tobacco Epidemic. World Health Organisation, Geneva.

Rogot, E. and Murray J.L. (1980). Smoking and causes of death among US veterans: 16 years of observation. *Publ Health Rep*, **95**: 213–22.

Rottman H. (1898). Der primare lungencarcinoma. Inaugural-dissertation, Universitat Wurzburg.

Russell, M. A.H. (1980). The case for medium-nicotine, low tar, low carbon monoxide cigarettes. *Banbury Rep*, **3**: 297–310.

Sadowsksy, D.A., Gilliam, A.G., and Cornfield, G. (1953). Statistical association between smoking and cancer of the lung. *J Natl Cancer Inst*, **13**: 1237–58.

Schairer, E. and Schoniger E. (1943). Lungenkrebs und Tabaksverbrauch. *Z f Krebsforsch*, **54**: 261–9.

Schrek, R., Baker, L.A., Ballard, G.P., and Dolgoff, S. (1950). Tobacco smoking as an etiologic factor in disease. *Cancer Res*, **10**: 49–58.

Shimizu, Y., Kato, H., Schull, W.J., Preston, D.L., Fujita, S, and Pierce, D.A. (1987). *Life Span Study report 11, Part 1: comparison of risk coefficients for site specific cancer mortality based on the DS86 and T 65DR shielded kerma and organ doses.* Radiation Effects Research Foundation Technical Report 12–87, Radiation Effects Research Foundation, Hiroshima, Japan.

Smith, P.G. and Doll, R. (1982). Mortality among patients with ankylosing spondylitis after a single treatment course with X-rays. *Br Med J*, **284**: 449–54.

Stanton, M.F., Miller, E., Wrench, C., and Blackwell, R. (1972). Experimental induction of epidermoid carcinoma in the lungs of rats by cigarette smoke condensate. *J Natl Cancer Inst*, **49**: 867–77.

Stockwell, H.G., Goldman, A.L., Lyman, G.H., Noss, C.I., Armstrong, A.W., Pinkham, P.A. *et al.* (1992). Environmental tobacco smoke and lung cancer risk in nonsmoking women. *J Natl Cancer Inst*, **84**: 1417–22.

Thun, M.J. and Heath, C.W. Jr. (1997). Changes in mortality from smoking in two American Cancer Society prospective studies since 1959. *Preventive Medicine*, **26**(4): 422–6.

Thun, M.J., Day-Lally, C., Myers, D.G. *et al. Trends in tobacco smoking and mortality from cigarette use in cancer prevention Studies I (1959 through 1965) and II (1982 through 1988). In: Changes in cigarette-*related *disease risks and their implication for prevention and control.* Bethesda, Maryland: National Cancer Institute, 1977: chapter 4. (NCI Monograph No 8).

Tomatis, L. (1990). *Air Pollution and Human cancer.* European School of Oncology Monographs, Springer-Verlag, Berlin.

Tylecote, F.E. (1927). Cancer of the Lung. *Lancet*, **2**: 256–7.

United States Public Health Service. (1964). *Smoking and health.* Report of the Advisory Committee to the Surgeon General of the Public Health Service. U.S. Department of Health, Education and Welfare, Public Health Service, Centre for Disease Control, DHEW Publication no. 1103.

United States Department of Health, Education and Welfare, Public Health Service, Washington D C, HEW Publication number (PHS) 79–50066, 1979.

USDHHS (United States Department of Health and Human Services). (1982). *The health consequences of smoking: Cancer. A report of the Surgeon General.* Washington, DC: US Public Health Service.

USDHHS (United States Department of Health and Human Services). (1989). *Reducing the health consequences of smoking: 25 years of progress.* A report of the Surgeon General. Washington, DC: US Government Printing Office.

United States Surgeon General. (1986). *The Health Consequences of Smoking.* NIH Pub.No. 86–7874, pp.1–639, Bethesda. MD: United States Department of Health and Human Services.

United States Surgeon General. United States Public Health Service. Reducing the Health Consequences of Smoking. (1989). A Report of the Surgeon General. U.S. Department of Health, and Human Services, Public Health Service, Centre for Disease Control, DHSS Publication no. (CDC) 89–8411, pp. 143.

Vincent, R.G., Pickren, J.W., Lane, W.W., Bross, I., Takita, H., Honten, L. *et al.* (1977). The changing histopathology of lung cancer. *Cancer (Phila.)*, **39**: 1647–55.

Wald, N., Doll, R., and Copeland, G. (1981). Trends in tar, nicotine and carbon monoxide yields of UK cigarettes manufactured since 1934. *Br Med J Clin Res ed*, **282**(6266): 763–5.

Wald, N.J., Idle, M., Boreham, J., and Bailey, A. (1983). Inhaling and lung cancer: an anomaly explained. *Br Med J*, **287**: 1273–75.

Wassink, W.F. (1948). Onstaansvoorwarden voor Longkanker. *Med Tijdschr Geneesk*, **92**: 3732–47.

White, C. (1990). Research on smoking and lung cancer: a landmark in the history of chronic disease epidemiology. *The Yale Journal of Biology and Medicine*, **63**: 29–46.

Whittemore, A.S. and McMillan, A. (1983). Lung cancer mortality among US uranium miners: a reappraisal. *J Natl Cancer Inst*, **71**: 489–99.

Wu, A.H., Henderson, B.E., Thomas, D.C., and Mack, T.M. (1986). Secular trends in histologic type of lung cancer. *J Nat Cancer Inst*, **77**: 53–6.

Wynder, E.L. and Graham, E.A. (1950). Tobacco smoking as a possible etiologic factor in bronchiogenic carcinoma. *J Am Med Assoc*, **143**: 329–36.

Wynder, E.L. and Hoffman, D. (1967). *Tobacco and tobacco smoke.* Studies in experimental carcinogenesis, Academic press, New York.

Wynder, E.L. and Stellman, S. D. (1979). The impact of long term filter usage on lung and larynx cancer risk: a case control study. *J Nat Cancer Inst,* **62**: 471–7.

Wynder, E.L. and Muscat, J. E. (1995). The changing epidemiology of smoking and lung cancer histology. *Environmental Health Perspectives,* **103** (8): 143–6.

Wynder, E.L., Mabuchi, K., and Beattie, E. J. Jr. (1970). The epidemiology of lung cancer. Recent Trends. *J Am Med Assoc,* **213**: 2221–8.

Young, J.L., Percy, C.L., and Asire, A.J. (ed.) (1981). Cancer incidence and mortality in the United States, 1973–1977. *Nat Cancer Inst Monogr,* **57**: 1–1082.

Zatonski, W.A. and Boyle, P. (1996). Health transformations in Poland after 1988. *J Epi Bio,* **1**(4): 183–97.

Zheng, T., Holford, T., Boyle, P., Chen, Y., Ward, B.A., Flannery, J. *et al.* (1994). Time trend and age-period-cohort effect on the incidence of histologic types of lung cancer in Connecticut, 1960–1989. *Cancer,* **74**: 1556–1556.

Chapter 28

Active and passive smoking and cancer of the breast

Areti Lagiou and Dimitrios Trichopoulos

Tobacco smoking is the most important human carcinogen and breast cancer is, at least in the developed world, the cancer type that causes more deaths among women in comparison to any other type of cancer [1]. If tobacco smoking were documented to be a factor that increases the risk for breast cancer, the implications would extend beyond the potential prevention of a fraction of breast cancer cases, because this form of cancer has a disproportional emotional impact at the individual and population level. The evidence, however, has been unusually puzzling.

Biologic considerations

It has been reported that active smoking may increase [2–4], reduce [5, 6], or be unrelated to [7–9] the risk of breast cancer. It has also been indicated that passive smoking may increase the risk of this disease [10]. Various biological plausibility arguments have been invoked in support of each of the various possibilities:

♦ *Tobacco smoking may reduce the risk of breast cancer.* Tobacco smoking has established anti-oestrogenic effects [11, 12] and oestrogens are important determinants of breast cancer risk [13]. The anti-oestrogenicity of tobacco smoking is manifested in several associations with oestrogen-dependent diseases or conditions, including associations with earlier menopause [14], higher risk for osteoporosis [15], and lower risk for endometrial cancer [16].

♦ *Tobacco smoking may increase the risk of breast cancer.* Tobacco smoke is an established human carcinogen and causes cancer in several non-respiratory sites, including pancreas and liver [17]. It contains several fat-soluble compounds with carcinogenic potential that can be activated into electrophilic substances by enzymes in the human mammary cells [18, 19]. Nipple aspirates of smokers contain metabolites of compounds of cigarette smoke, which can be genotoxic [19]. As it is true for other breast carcinogens, notably ionizing radiation [13], tobacco smoking could exert its carcinogenic potential particularly among young women or among women who have never been pregnant and whose mammary epithelium has not been terminally differentiated [20].

♦ *Tobacco smoking is unrelated to breast cancer risk.* Tobacco smoking may be unrelated to breast cancer risk or may have dual effects that integrate a detrimental effect during the early life initiation stage and a beneficial anti-oestrogenic effect during the late life tumour progression stage. Dual effects on breast cancer risk are well established with respect to obesity, which acts in a beneficial way before menopause and in a detrimental way after it [13].

♦ *Passive smoking may increase the risk of breast cancer.* At source, environmental tobacco smoke contains high concentrations of most tobacco carcinogens. Although nicotine inhalation (and cotinine excretion) through passive smoking is two orders of magnitude lower than that through active smoking, this may not apply to other agents, including carcinogenic agents. Exposure to environmental tobacco smoke may start shortly after birth and the carcinogenic effects of tobacco smoke depend exponentially on total duration of exposure [21]. Early life exposures, before terminal mammary differentiation induced by a full-term pregnancy, may have higher carcinogenic potential on the breast [22].

◆ *Passive smoking is unrelated to breast cancer risk.* In every instance in which passive smoking has been implicated in disease causation, active smoking has been an established cause of the corresponding disease with a considerably higher relative risk. Paradigms are lung cancer [21] and chronic obstructive lung disease [23]. Even if there is a weak positive association between breast cancer and active smoking, an association of the disease with passive smoking might be too weak to be empirically detectable.

Epidemiological evidence on active smoking and breast cancer

Until the late 1980s, tobacco smoking had not been specifically studied in relation to breast cancer and the available evidence was a side-product of investigations with different primary objectives. MacMahon was the first to critically evaluate this evidence [24]. He noted that hospital-based case-control studies had indicated an inverse association, which was probably due to the fact that many diseases represented among hospital controls are positively associated with tobacco smoking. He further noted that case-control studies relying on population controls, or on controls with diseases unrelated to smoking, pointed to a weakly positive association, as did cohort studies in which selection bias is unlikely.

An additional refinement in epidemiological studies was introduced when the possibility was raised that passive smoking may increase the risk of breast cancer [10]. Non-smokers were subdivided into those genuinely non-exposed to tobacco smoking (that is, non-smokers that have not been passively exposed to tobacco smoke] and those passively exposed to environmental tobacco smoke. In an exhaustive review covering case-control studies until 2001, Morabia [19] identified 11 such studies that evaluated active smoking in relation to breast cancer using as referent women that were not exposed to either active or passive smoking. In all of these studies, the point estimate of the adjusted odds ratio for breast cancer among active smokers was higher than the null value of one and in five of them the odds ratio elevation was statistically significant (Table 28.1).

The results of case-control studies may have been biased because exposure histories were collected after disease onset, and health conscious women, who are generally non-smokers, may have been over-represented among controls. Indeed, there is some evidence, discussed later on, that points to selection bias, and possibly information bias, in case-control studies. However, the fact that smokers have, as a rule, an earlier age at menopause [14] which is associated with lower breast cancer risk [13], tends to introduce negative confounding that has not always been accounted for.

Case-control studies after 2001 have generated more equivocal results in comparison to those previously published. Thus, among 13 studies, 7 were reported as suggestive of a positive association between active smoking and breast cancer [25–31] whereas in another 6 studies the findings were reported as null or even as suggestive of an inverse association [5, 6, 8, 32–34]. Taking into account the inherent methodological weaknesses of some case-control studies and the marginal elevation of risk among smokers in comparison to non-smokers it can be concluded that the evidence from case-control studies for an association between tobacco smoking and breast cancer risk is overall weak. There is a suggestion, however, that tobacco is more detrimental if smoked before the first full-term pregnancy [28] and for pre-menopausal breast cancer [25, 27, 29, 31], whereas a report that smoking during pregnancy is particularly harmful [35] has not been confirmed [36].

Table 28.1 Odds ratios (and 95% confidence intervals) for breast cancer among passive smokers and among active smokers in comparison to neither- active-nor-passive smokers. Results of 11 case-control studies*

Case control studies	Adjusted OR (95% CI)	
	Active smoking	Passive smoking
Wells 1992 [68]	1.2 (0.6–2.5)	1.6 (0.8–3.4)
Morabia et al. 1996 [10]	2.5 (1.6–3.8)**	2.3 (1.5–3.7)
van Leeuwen et al. 1997 [69]	1.2 (0.8–1.6)	1.2 (0.8–1.7)
Wells 1998 [70]	2.0 (0.98–4.1)	1.6 (0.8–3.1)
Lash and Aschengrau 1999 [71]	2.0 (1.1–3.6)	2.0 (1.1–3.7)
Zhao et al. 1999 [72]	3.5 (1.3–9.3)	2.5 (1.7–3.8)
Millikan et al. 1998 [73]; Marcus et al. 2000 [74]	1.1 (0.8–1.6)**	1.3 (0.9–1.9)
Delfino et al. 2000 [75]	1.4 (0.8–2.7)**	1.9 (0.8–4.3)
Johnson et al. 2000 – premenopausal [76]	2.3 (1.2–4.5)	2.3 (1.2–4.6)
Johnson et al. 2000 – postmenopausal [76]	1.5 (1.0–2.3)	1.2 (0.8–1.8)
Chang-Claude et al. 2001 [77]	1.4 (0.9–2.2)	1.5 (1.0–2.3)

Note

* Modified from: Morabia 2002 [19].

** Crude OR.

Several large cohorts studies (average cohort size about 70 000 women) have also been undertaken. In the Nurses's study [37], Egan and colleagues found that the relative risk (and 95% confidence interval [CI]) for breast cancer were 1.04 (0.94–1.15) among current active smokers. In the Californian Teachers Study, active-smokers were at higher breast cancer risk in comparison to never-smokers, particularly among women who started smoking at a younger age and before their first full-term pregnancy [2]. In the Norwegian–Swedish study [3], women who smoked ten or more cigarettes per day for at least 20 years had a relative risk of 1.34 (95% CI 1.06–1.70). In the Iowa Women's Health Study [38], which was restricted to postmenopausal women, women who started smoking before their first full-term pregnancy had a relative risk for breast cancer of 1.21 (95% CI 1.07–1.37). In the Canadian National Breast Screening Study [39], breast cancer risk was associated with several aspects of smoking intensity and duration, with the strongest association found among those who have started smoking early in life and have smoked for more than forty years (for the later group the relative risk was 1.50 with 95% CI 1.19–1.89). Finally, in a cohort of US female radiologic technologists [4], a statistically significant excess of breast cancer risk was found among those who started smoking between menarche and first child birth. Null results have also been reported from cohort studies but the respective cohorts were generally smaller [7].

Epidemiological evidence on passive smoking and breast cancer

The fact that passive smoking was found to be a significant predictor of coronary heart disease among non-smoking women in the Nurses' Health Study [40], even though the relative risk linking active smoking to this disease is rarely more than three-fold, imparts an element of credibility to the hypothesis that passive smoking may increase the risk of breast cancer. At least 11 case-control studies reviewed by Morabia [19] have evaluated passive smoking in relation to breast cancer risk.

In all these studies, the odds ratio estimates were higher than one, and in five of them the excess breast cancer risk among passive smokers was statistically significant. Thus, the evidence from case-control studies is strongly supportive of a weak positive association between passive smoking and breast cancer risk (Table 28.1).

Subsequent case-control studies have generated more equivocal findings. Liu and colleagues [41], Kropp and Chang-Claude [25], and Slattery and colleagues [31] have reported statistically significant associations between passive smoking and breast cancer risk, but Lash and Aschengrau [5], Shrubsole and colleagues [42], Lissowska and colleagues [29], Roddam and colleagues [34], and Rollison and colleagues [43] have interpreted their results as null.

In contrast to case-control studies that tend to suggest, however inconsistently, a positive association between passive smoking and breast cancer risk, all five cohort studies that have examined this association have been reported as null [2, 9, 37, 44, 45] and in four of them, the point estimate of the relative risk was below the null value of 1 [2, 37, 44, 45].

In meta-analyses of all epidemiological studies [19, 46, 47, 48] the collective empirical evidence would suggest a positive association between passive smoking and breast cancer risk, because case-control studies tend to support such an association. The inherently higher validity of cohort investigations, however, forces a re-examination of the results of the case-control studies. Selection bias is a concern in case-control studies, because women who volunteer to be included as controls may be less exposed to active and passive smoking. Moreover, information bias is an issue because exposure histories are generally collected after disease onset. This is particularly true for breast cancer, an emotionally charged disease with largely unknown aetiology, when studied in relation to an exposure (passive smoking) which is subject to misclassification and which can be viewed with suspicion. In situations like these, women with breast cancer, who are not themselves smokers (an exposure which is not likely to be misclassified), may tend to allocate themselves to the category of passive smokers, thus removing themselves from the category of genuinely non-exposed to that of passively exposed to smoking.

Logical as this argument may be, it is still hypothetical. However, there is an indirect way to evaluate it. Most case-control studies that have examined passive smoking in relation to breast cancer risk have also evaluated active smoking in relation to this risk, using as referent women that were genuinely non-exposed to either active or passive smoking. These studies have been termed 'second generation', because they have used a more appropriate referent in comparison to earlier studies of active smoking, in which passive smokers were not excluded from the referent group of non-smoking women [19]. Table 28.1 abstracts information presented by Morabia and colleagues [19]. If some non-smoking women with breast cancer were inclined to incorrectly designate themselves as passive smokers, the odds ratio for breast cancer in relation to passive smoking would be inflated because of an increase at the numerator of the odds ratio formula. Moreover, the odds ratio for breast cancer in relation to active smoking would also be inflated because of a decrease in the denominator of the formula. Under the hypothesis of information bias, the predicted net result would be a positive correlation of the breast cancer odds ratio estimates among active and passive smokers from each of the 11 studies. The Spearman correlation coefficient from the data in Table 28.1 is +0.81 ($p < 0.05$). Compatibility of the empirical evidence with the working hypothesis of information bias does not, of course, establish the validity of this hypothesis, but it lends credibility to it.

Effect modifiers

In several studies of active smoking in relation to breast cancer risk, the apparent detrimental effect of smoking was stronger among women exposed in early life, particularly before their first full-term pregnancy (e.g. 4, 37). However, different definitions of early life have been used in different studies, some using age at first pregnancy or age at first birth as cut-off, some focusing in the years around menarche, others focusing on specific age limits and some indicating that the breast cancer risk is elevated only among pre-menopausal or only post-menopausal women or differentially among women with oestrogen-receptor alpha positive [49] or negative [50] breast cancer. The concern is, of course, that some significant results are generated in the context of a multiple comparison process. Nevertheless, this is a potentially important issue since the mammary gland is not fully differentiated in early life, especially before the first full-term pregnancy and may thus be particularly susceptible during this early period [20]. This is an obvious priority issue for future investigations.

In a similar context, a few investigators have examined whether maternal smoking during pregnancy may affect breast cancer risk in the offspring. In one of these studies, parental smoking during pregnancy was not associated with risk of breast cancer in the adult daughter [51] whereas in the other [52], foetal exposure to maternal cigarette smoke appeared to be significantly inversely associated with breast cancer risk in the offspring, – possibly on account of the anti-oestrogenic effect of tobacco compounds [11, 12].

If an association between tobacco smoking and breast cancer exists it is plausible that it might be conditioned by specific genotypes. Indeed, they have been inconsistent reports that polymorphisms in NAT1 [53, 54], NAT2 [26, 54–56], GSTM1 [53, 54, 57, 58], XRCC1 [59, 60], CYP1A1 [61], DNA repair genes [62, 63], NOS3 and MPO [64] polymorphisms and several others may affect breast cancer risk in smoking women. Detection of interaction between genes and environmental factors can be validly done in both cohort and case-control studies but requires very large numbers [65], particularly when prior probabilities are low [66]. Accordingly the findings of these studies, although valuable as hypothesis generating cannot be considered as documented. Confirmation is also required for a report indicating that cigarette smoking may modify the prevalence and spectrum of p53 mutations in breast tumours [67].

Conclusion

There is little evidence that passive smoking increases the risk of breast cancer, although one cannot reject this possibility. The problem reflects the more general one of distinguishing a null association from a weakly positive one on the basis of epidemiological evidence alone.

With respect to active smoking, the overall epidemiological evidence is weak. There are findings, however, suggestive of interaction of this exposure with early age at exposure and nulliparity, when the mammary gland is not adequately differentiated. There are also reports that active smoking modifies the spectrum of p53 mutations in breast tumours and interacts with particular genetic polymorphisms. These findings cannot be explained by simple forms of selection or information bias but they may still reflect chance or selective reporting. If they were to be replicated and further supported by epidemiological results, these results would indicate that active smoking does affect breast cancer risk. At this stage, and if one were to adopt the International Agency for Research on Cancer terminology [17] concerning the evaluation of carcinogenicity, the likely verdict on active smoking in relation to breast cancer risk would be that it is a 'possible' carcinogen.

References

1. Lagiou, P., Adami, J., and Trichopoulos, D. (2008). Measures and estimates of cancer burden. In: H.O. Adami, D. Hunter, D. Trichopoulos (eds) *Textbook of Cancer Epidemiology*, 2nd edition, pp. 34–60. Oxford University Press, New York.
2. Reynolds, P., Hurley, S., Goldberg, D.E. *et al.* (2004). Active smoking, household passive smoking, and breast cancer: evidence from the California Teachers Study. *J Natl Cancer Inst*, **96**(1): 29–37.
3. Gram, I.T., Braaten, T., Terry, P.D. *et al.* (2005). Breast cancer risk among women who start smoking as teenagers. *Cancer Epidemiol Biomarkers Prev*, **14**(1): 61–6.

4. Ha, M., Mabuchi, K., Sigurdson, A.J. *et al.* (2007). Smoking cigarettes before first childbirth and risk of breast cancer. *Am J Epidemiol*, **166**(1): 55–61.

5. Lash, T.L. and Aschengrau, A. (2002). A null association between active or passive cigarette smoking and breast cancer risk. *Breast Cancer Res Treat*, **75**(2): 181–4.

6. Trentham-Dietz, A., Nichols, H.B., Egan, K.M., *et al.* (2007). Cigarette smoking and risk of breast carcinoma in situ. *Epidemiology*, **18**(5): 629–38.

7. Lawlor, D.A., Ebrahim, S., and Smith, G.D. (2004). Smoking before the birth of a first child is not associated with increased risk of breast cancer: findings from the British Women's Heart and Health Cohort Study and a meta-analysis. *Br J Cancer*, **91**(3): 512–8.

8. Prescott, J., Ma, H., Bernstein, L., *et al.* (2007). Cigarette smoking is not associated with breast cancer risk in young women. *Cancer Epidemiol Biomarkers Prev*, **16**(3): 620–2.

9. Lin, Y., Kikuchi, S., Tamakoshi, K. *et al.* (2008). Active smoking, passive smoking, and breast cancer risk: findings from the Japan Collaborative Cohort Study for Evaluation of Cancer Risk. *J Epidemiol*, **18**(2): 77–83.

10. Morabia, A., Bernstein, M., Heritier, S. *et al.* (1996). Relation of breast cancer with passive and active exposure to tobacco smoke. *Am J Epidemiol*, **143**: 918–28.

11. MacMahon, B., Trichopoulos, D., Cole, P. *et al.* (1982). Cigarette smoking and urinary estrogens. *N Engl J Med*, **307**: 1062–5.

12. Michnovicz, J.J., Hershcopf, R.J., Naganuma, H. *et al.* (1986). Increased 2-hydroxylation of estradiol as a possible mechanism for the anti-estrogenic effect of cigarette smoking. *N Engl J Med*, **315**: 1305–9.

13. Hankinson, S., Tamimi, R., and Hunter, D. (2008). Breast cancer. In: H.O. Adami, D. Hunter, D. Trichopoulos (eds), *Textbook of Cancer Epidemiology*, 2nd edition pp. 403–45. Oxford University Press, New York.

14. van Asselt, K.M., Kok, H.S., van Der Schouw, Y.T. *et al.* (2004). Current smoking at menopause rather than duration determines the onset of natural menopause. *Epidemiology*, **15**(5): 634–9.

15. Ward, K.D. and Klesges, R.C. (2001). A meta-analysis of the effects of cigarette smoking on bone mineral density. *Calcif Tissue Int*, **68**(5): 259–70.

16. Zhou, B., Yang, L., Sun, Q., *et al.* (2008). Cigarette smoking and the risk of endometrial cancer: a meta-analysis. *Am J Med*, **121**(6): 501–08.

17. IARC Monographs on the Evaluation of Carcinogenic Risks (2007). Tobacco Smoking and Involuntary smoking Volume 83. Lyon.

18. Phillips, D.H., Martin, F.L., Grover, P.L. *et al.* (2001). Toxicological basis for a possible association of breast cancer with smoking and other sources of environmental carcinogens. *J Women's Cancer*, **3**: 9–16.

19. Morabia, A. (2002). Smoking (active and passive) and breast cancer: epidemiologic evidence up to June 2001. *Environ Mol Mutagen*, **39**: 89–95.

20. Russo, J., Hu, Y.F., Silva, I.D. *et al.* (2001). Cancer risk related to mammary gland structure and development. *Microsc Res Tech*, **52**: 204–23.

21. Dockery, D.W. and Trichopoulos, D. (1997). Risk of lung cancer from environmental exposures to tobacco smoke. *Cancer Causes and Control*, **8**: 333–45.

22. Trichopoulos, D., Adami, H.O., Ekbom, A., *et al.* (2008). Early life events and conditions and breast cancer risk: from epidemiology to etiology. *Int J Cancer*, **122**(3): 481–5.

23. Jaakkola, M.S. and Jaakkola, J.J.K. (2002). Effects of environmental tobacco smoke on the respiratory health of adults. *Scandinavian Journal of Work Environment and Health*, **28**(2): 52–70.

24. MacMahon, B. (1990). Cigarette smoking and cancer of the breast. In: Wald and Baron, eds. *Smoking and Hormone-Related Disorders* pp. 154–66. Oxford University Press, Oxford.

25. Kropp, S. and Chang-Claude, J. (2002). Active and passive smoking and risk of breast cancer by age 50 years among German women. *Am J Epidemiol*, **156**(7): 616–26.

26. Egan, K.M., Newcomb, P.A., Titus-Ernstoff, L., *et al.* (2003). Association of NAT2 and smoking in relation to breast cancer incidence in a population-based case-control study (United States). *Cancer Causes Control*, **14**(1): 43–51.

27. Wrensch, M., Chew, T., Farren, G., *et al.* (2003). Risk factors for breast cancer in a population with high incidence rates. *Breast Cancer Res*, **5**(4): R88–102.

28. Li, C.I., Malone, K.E., and Daling, J.R. (2005). The relationship between various measures of cigarette smoking and risk of breast cancer among older women 65–79 years of age (United States). *Cancer Causes Control*, **16**(8): 975–85.

29. Lissowska, J., Brinton, L.A., Zatonski, W., *et al.* (2006). Tobacco smoking, NAT2 acetylation genotype and breast cancer risk. *Int J Cancer*, **119**(8): 1961–9.

30. Kruk, J. (2007). Association of lifestyle and other risk factors with breast cancer according to menopausal status: a case-control study in the Region of Western Pomerania (Poland). *Asian Pac J Cancer Prev*, **8**(4): 513–24.

31. Slattery, M.L., Curtin, K., Giuliano, A.R., *et al.* (2008). Active and passive smoking, IL6, ESR1, and breast cancer risk. *Breast Cancer Res Treat*, **109**(1): 101–11.

32. Magnusson, C., Wedrén, S., and Rosenberg, L.U. (2007). Cigarette smoking and breast cancer risk: a population-based study in Sweden. *Br J Cancer*, **97**(9): 1287–90.

33. Mahouri, K., Dehghani Zahedani, M., and Zare, S. (2007). Breast cancer risk factors in south of Islamic Republic of Iran: a case-control study. *East Mediterr Health J*, **13**(6): 1265–73.

34. Roddam, A.W., Pirie, K., Pike, M.C. *et al.* (2007). Active and passive smoking and the risk of breast cancer in women aged 36–45 years: a population based case-control study in the UK. *Br J Cancer*, **97**(3): 434–9.

35. Innes, K.E. and Byers, T.E. (2001). Smoking during pregnancy and breast cancer risk in very young women (United States). *Cancer Causes Control*, **12**: 179–85.

36. Fink, A.K. and Lash, T.L. (2003). A null association between smoking during pregnancy and breast cancer using Massachusetts registry data (United States). *Cancer Causes Control*, **14**(5): 497–503.

37. Egan, K.M., Stampfer, M.J., Hunter, D. *et al.* (2002). Active and passive smoking in breast cancer: prospective results from the Nurses' Health Study. *Epidemiology*, **13**(2): 138–45.

38. Olson, J.E., Vachon, C.M., Vierkant, R.A. *et al.* (2005). Prepregnancy exposure to cigarette smoking and subsequent risk of postmenopausal breast cancer. *Mayo Clin Proc*, **80**(11): 1423–8.

39. Cui, Y., Miller, A.B., and Rohan, T.E. (2006). Cigarette smoking and breast cancer risk: update of a prospective cohort study. *Breast Cancer Res Treat*, **100**(3): 293–9.

40. Kawachi, I., Colditz, G.A., Speizer, F.E. *et al.* (1997). A prospective study of passive smoking and coronary heart disease. *Circulation*, **95**: 2374–9.

41. Liu, L., Wu, K., Lin, X. *et al.* (2000). Passive smoking and other factors at different periods of life and breast cancer risk in Chinese women who have never smoked - a case-control study in Chongqing, People's Republic of China. *Asian Pac J Cancer Prev*, **1**(2): 131–7.

42. Shrubsole, M.J., Gao, Y.T., Dai, Q. *et al.* (2004). Passive smoking and breast cancer risk among non-smoking Chinese women. *Int J Cancer*, **110**(4): 605–9.

43. Rollison, D.E., Brownson, R.C., Hathcock, H.L. *et al.* (2008). Case-control study of tobacco smoke exposure and breast cancer risk in Delaware. *BMC Cancer*, **8**: 157.

44. Nishino, Y., Tsubono, Y., Tsuji, I. *et al.* (2001). Passive smoking at home and cancer risk: a population-based prospective study in Japanese nonsmoking women. *Cancer Causes Control*, **12**(9): 797–802.

45. Pirie, K., Beral, V., Peto. R. *et al.* (2008). Passive smoking and breast cancer in never smokers: prospective study and meta-analysis. *Int J Epidemiol*, **37**(5): 1069–79.

46. Khuder, S.A. and Simon, V.J. Jr (2000). Is there an association between passive smoking and breast cancer? *Eur J Epidemiol*, **16**(12): 1117–21.

47. Johnson, K.C. (2005). Accumulating evidence on passive and active smoking and breast cancer risk. *Int J Cancer*, **117**(4): 619–28.

48. Lee, P.N. and Hamling, J. (2006). Environmental tobacco smoke exposure and risk of breast cancer in nonsmoking women: a review with meta-analyses. *Inhal Toxicol*, **18**(14): 1053–70.

49. Al-Delaimy, W.K., Cho, E., Chen, W.Y. *et al.* (2004). A prospective study of smoking and risk of breast cancer in young adult women. *Cancer Epidemiol Biomarkers Prev*, **13**(3): 398–404.

50. Manjer, J., Malina, J., Berglund, G. *et al.* (2001). Smoking associated with hormone receptor negative breast cancer. *Int J Cancer*, **91**: 580–4.

51. Titus-Ernstoff, L., Egan, K.M., Newcomb, P.A. *et al.* (2002). Early life factors in relation to breast cancer risk in postmenopausal women. *Cancer Epidemiol Biomarkers Prev*, **11**(2): 207–10.

52. Strohsnitter, W.C., Noller, K.L., Titus-Ernstoff, L., *et al.* (2005). Breast cancer incidence in women prenatally exposed to maternal cigarette smoke. *Epidemiology*, **16**(3): 342–5.

53. van der Hel, O.L., Peeters, P.H., Hein, D.W. *et al.* (2003). NAT2 slow acetylation and GSTM1 null genotypes may increase postmenopausal breast cancer risk in long-term smoking women. *Pharmacogenetics*, **13**(7): 399–407.

54. van der Hel, O.L., Bueno-de-Mesquita, H.B., van Gils, C.H., *et al.* (2005). Cumulative genetic defects in carcinogen metabolism may increase breast cancer risk (The Netherlands). *Cancer Causes Control*, **16**(6): 675–81.

55. Chang-Claude, J., Kropp, S., Jäger, B., *et al.* (2002). Differential effect of NAT2 on the association between active and passive smoke exposure and breast cancer risk. *Cancer Epidemiol Biomarkers Prev*, **11**(8): 698–704.

56. Sillanpää, P., Hirvonen, A., Kataja, V., *et al.* (2005). NAT2 slow acetylator genotype as an important modifier of breast cancer risk. *Int J Cancer*, **114**(4): 579–84.

57. Zheng, T., Holford, T.R., Zahm, S.H. *et al.* (2002). Cigarette smoking, glutathione-s-transferase M1 and t1 genetic polymorphisms, and breast cancer risk (United States). *Cancer Causes Control*, **13**(7): 637–45.

58. Van Emburgh, B.O., Hu, J.J., Levine, E.A. *et al.* (2008). Polymorphisms in CYP1B1, GSTM1, GSTT1 and GSTP1, and susceptibility to breast cancer. *Oncol Rep*, **19**(5): 1311–21.

59. Metsola, K., Kataja, V., Sillanpää, P. *et al.* (2005). XRCC1 and XPD genetic polymorphisms, smoking and breast cancer risk in a Finnish case-control study. *Breast Cancer Res*, **7**(6): R987–97.

60. Patel, A.V., Calle, E.E., Pavluck, A.L. *et al.* (2005). A prospective study of XRCC1 (X-ray cross-complementing group 1) polymorphisms and breast cancer risk. *Breast Cancer Res*, **7**(6): R1168–73.

61. Li, Y., Millikan, R.C., Bell, D.A. *et al.* (2004). Cigarette smoking, cytochrome P4501A1 polymorphisms, and breast cancer among African-American and white women. *Breast Cancer Res*, **6**(4): R460–73.

62. Terry, M.B., Gammon, M.D., Zhang, F.F., *et al.* (2004). Polymorphism in the DNA repair gene XPD, polycyclic aromatic hydrocarbon-DNA adducts, cigarette smoking, and breast cancer risk. *Cancer Epidemiol Biomarkers Prev*, **13**(12): 2053–8.

63. Mechanic, L.E., Millikan, R.C., Player, J. *et al.* (2006). Polymorphisms in nucleotide excision repair genes, smoking and breast cancer in African Americans and whites: a population-based case-control study. *Carcinogenesis*, **27**(7): 1377–85.

64. Yang, J., Ambrosone, C.B., Hong, C.C. *et al.* (2007). Relationships between polymorphisms in NOS3 and MPO genes, cigarette smoking and risk of post-menopausal breast cancer. *Carcinogenesis*, **28**(6): 1247–53.

65. Clayton, D. and McKeigue, P.M. (2001). Epidemiological methods for studying genes and environmental factors in complex diseases. *Lancet*, **358**: 1356–60.

66. Wacholder, S., Chanock, S., Garcia-Clossas, M. *et al.* (2004). Assessing the probability that a positive report is false: an approach for molecular epidemiology studies. *J Natl Cancer Inst*, **96**: 434–42.

67. Conway, K., Edmiston, S.N., Cui, L. *et al.* (2002). Prevalence and spectrum of p53 mutations associated with smoking in breast cancer. *Cancer Res*, **62**: 1987–95.

68. Wells, A.J. (1992). Re: 'Breast cancer, cigarette smoking, and passive smoking' [reply]. *Am J Epidemiol*, **135**: 710–12.

69. Van Leeuwen, F.E., de Vries, F., van der Kooy, K., *et al.* (1997). Smoking and breast cancer risk [abstract]. *Am J Epidemiol*, **145**: S29.

70. Wells, A.J. Re (1998). 'Breast cancer, cigarette smoking, and passive smoking'. *Am J Epidemiol*, **147**: 991–2.

71. Lash, T.L. and Aschengrau, A. (1999). Active and passive cigarette smoking and the occurrence of breast cancer. *Am J Epidemiol*, **149**: 5–12.

72. Zhao, Y., Shi, Z., and Liu, L. (1999). [Matched case-control study for detecting risk factors of breast cancer in women living in Chengdu] (in Chinese). *J Epidemiol*, **20**: 91–4.

73. Millikan, R.C., Pittman, G.S., Newman, B., *et al.* (1998). Cigarette smoking, N-acetyltransferases 1 and 2, and breast cancer risk. *Cancer Epidemiol Biomarkers Prev*, **7**: 371–8.

74. Marcus, P.M., Newman, B., Millikan, R.C. *et al.* (2000). The associations of adolescent cigarette smoking, alcoholic beverage consumption, environmental tobacco smoke, and ionizing radiation with subsequent breast cancer risk (United States). *Cancer Causes Control*, **11**: 271–8.

75. Delfino, R.J., Smith, C., West, J.G. *et al.* (2000). Breast cancer, passive and active cigarette smoking and N-acetyltransferase 2 genotype. *Pharmacogenetics*, **10**: 461–9.

76. Johnson, K.C., Hu, J., Mao, Y. (2000). Passive and active smoking and breast cancer risk in Canada, 1994–97. The Canadian Cancer Registries Epidemiology Research Group. *Cancer Causes Control*, **11**: 211–21.

77. Chang-Claude, J., Kropp, S., Bartsch, H. *et al.* (2001). Active and passive smoking, N-acetyltransferase 2 genotype and breast cancer risk [abstract]. *AACR annual meeting*.

Chapter 29

Smoking and ovarian cancer

Crystal N. Holick and Harvey A. Risch

Epidemiology

Ovarian cancer causes more deaths than any other cancer of the female reproductive system and ranks second in incidence among gynaecologic malignancies, accounting for 3% of all cancers, with 21 600 new cases estimated among women in the United States in 2008 (American Cancer Society 2008). Risk of ovarian cancer increases with age and peaks in the late 1970s. Mutations in the genes *BRCA1* and *BRCA2* account for about 10% of all epithelial ovarian cancers (Risch *et al.* 2006). Pregnancies and use of oral contraceptives are known to reduce the risk of developing ovarian cancer, and nulliparous women are more likely to develop it (Daly and Obrams 1998). In addition to female reproductive factors, personal and environmental exposures including diet practices (Cramer *et al.* 1984; Risch *et al.* 1994), coffee consumption (La Vecchia *et al.* 1984), alcohol intake (Polychronopoulou *et al.* 1993), and smoking history (Doll *et al.* 1980) may also modify the risk of ovarian cancer. Recently, evidence has emerged that risk factors for ovarian cancer – including tobacco smoking (Kuper *et al.* 2000; Marchbanks *et al.* 2000; Green *et al.* 2001), parity (Kvale *et al.* 1988; Risch *et al.* 1996), and oral contraceptive use (The WHO Collaborative Study of Neoplasia and Steroid Contraceptives 1989; Risch *et al.* 1996) – may vary by tumour histologic type.

Hypotheses of ovarian carcinogenesis

The carcinogenic process of epithelial ovarian cancer is not fully understood. Several mechanisms of ovarian pathogenesis have been hypothesized, each of which could have involvement of tobacco smoking.

Incessant ovulation

Increased cell division, stimulated by internal and external factors, increases the accumulation of genetic errors and is thought to enhance the risk of neoplastic transformation (Preston-Martin *et al.* 1990). Fathalla, in 1971, theorized that regularly repeated ovulation in women may increase the likelihood of ovarian malignancy (Fathalla 1971). According to this hypothesis, repeated ovulation-induced disruption and repair of the ovarian surface epithelium increases epithelial cell proliferation and risk of DNA damage, leading to neoplastic transformation and thus to ovarian cancer. Casagrande *et al.* (1979) extended this concept by suggesting that anovulation, resulting from oral contraceptive use, reduces the risk of ovarian cancer. Epithelial clefts and inclusion cysts frequently form within the ovarian stroma as part of ovulatory repair. Cells lining the clefts or inclusion cysts may undergo metaplasia to resemble serous, mucinous, or endometrioid epithelium, as well as neoplastic transformation to produce tumours of serous, mucinous, or endometrioid histologic varieties.

The incessant-ovulation hypothesis is supported by inferences from epidemiologic studies of ovarian cancer (Risch *et al.* 1983; The Cancer and Steroid Hormone Study 1987; Whittemore *et al.* 1992; Schildkraut *et al.* 1997). Hormonal, reproductive, and environmental factors, such as oral contraceptive use, pregnancy, and tobacco smoking, may modify risk of ovarian cancer via an impact on ovulation. A dose–response decrease in risk with increasing parity (Hankinson *et al.* 1995) and with increasing duration of oral contraceptive use (Gross and Schlesselman 1994) is consistently observed in most studies. Evidence also suggests that tobacco smoking may impair ovulation, since smoking is observed to be associated with delayed conception (Baird and Wilcox 1985) and with reduced ovulatory response to gonadotropin stimulation (Van Voorhis *et al.* 1992). Furthermore, ovarian atresia, caused by exposure to polycyclic aromatic hydrocarbons contained in cigarette smoke, has been observed in other species (e.g., rodents) (Mattison and Thorgeirsson 1978). Cigarette smoking also results in earlier age at natural menopause (Cooper *et al.* 1999; Hardy *et al.* 2000). Cigarette smokers thus may average fewer lifetime ovulations than non-smokers, the repeated ovulation model thereby predicting lower risk of ovarian cancer among smokers.

Although the incessant ovulation hypothesis is supported by the above evidence as well as by animal studies showing the proliferative behaviour of the ovarian epithelium following ovulation (Godwin *et al.* 1992), it is unable to explain appreciable discrepancies between the amount of anovulation and the magnitude of effect on risk for several ovulation-related factors (Risch 1998). Tobacco smoking may therefore influence the risk of ovarian cancer through additional biologic mechanisms, unrelated to ovulation, for example involving hormonal factors.

Gonadotropin–oestrogen theory

Stimulation of the ovary by steroid hormones may play a causative role in the pathogenesis of ovarian cancer. Under the gonadotropin–oestrogen (hormonal) theory, the initial stage in the development of epithelial ovarian cancer, as in the incessant-ovulation hypothesis, involves repeated proliferation and invagination of the ovarian surface epithelium to form clefts and inclusion cysts within the ovarian stroma. Subsequent events including differentiation, further proliferation, and eventual malignant transformation are mediated through hormonal stimulation (Cramer and Welch 1983). Specifically, increased pituitary gonadotropin (follicle-stimulating hormone [FSH] or luteinizing hormone [LH]) action and the resulting excessive oestrogen (or oestrogen precursor) stimulation of ovarian epithelial cells is responsible for the increased risk of ovarian cancer development. Factors that affect oestrogen regulation influence gonadotropin stimulation and risk indirectly (Cramer and Welch 1983).

The gonadotropin–oestrogen hypothesis predicts that higher concentrations of FSH and LH, generally associated with greater ovarian oestrogen synthesis, would increase the risk of developing ovarian cancer. This observation is consistent with some reports showing increased risk associated with exogenous menopausal oestrogen use (Hoover *et al.* 1977; Parazzini *et al.* 1994; Rodriguez *et al.* 1995; Purdie *et al.* 1996; Risch 1996; Rossing *et al.* 2007). A number of common chemicals or drugs are believed to enhance hepatic oestrogen degradation or metabolism (Helzlsouer *et al.* 1995). It is possible therefore that tobacco smoking may influence the risk of epithelial ovarian cancer through hormonal mechanisms by altering the levels of circulating oestrogens. Women who smoke appear to have lower levels of urinary oestrogens, and other evidence of endogenous oestrogen-deficiency (Wynder *et al.* 1969; Van Voorhis *et al.* 1992). The reduced circulating oestrogens in smokers could thus result in a decreased risk of ovarian cancer.

There is very little direct evidence bearing on the gonadotropin–oestrogen hypothesis. The site distribution of ovarian epithelial tumours shows a larger fraction arising within epithelial inclusion cysts, compared with the epithelial cells on the ovarian surface, and the smallest fraction in the histogenetically related peritoneal mesothelium which has the greatest surface area (Godwin *et al.* 1992; Resta *et al.* 1993). This suggests a hormonal influence on neoplastic transformation. Studies evaluating the presence of ovarian epithelial cell steroid-hormone receptors show at least low levels of oestrogen receptors (al-Timimi *et al.* 1985). Ovarian cancers mostly arise in the post-menopausal years, after the large perimenopausal rise in gonadotropin levels. However, a nested case-control study of prediagnostic serum gonadotropin and steroid hormone levels showed that women with lower FSH levels were at increased risk of subsequently developing ovarian cancer; there was no association with oestrogen levels (Helzlsouer *et al.* 1995).

Beyond oestrogens: progesterone and androgens

The presence of progesterone and androgen receptors within ovarian epithelial cells (al-Timimi *et al.* 1985; Zeimet *et al.* 1994) suggests that the epithelial cells are exposed to and respond to both of these hormones, and this has led to speculation on the involvement of these hormones in the aetiology of ovarian carcinogenesis (Risch 1998). It has been suggested that the progestin exposure in oral contraceptive use (and in pregnancy, for that matter) may be responsible for the protective effect, independent of or in addition to anovulation (Risch 1998). One mechanism underlying the progestin hypothesis may involve enhanced apoptosis of the ovarian epithelium (Rodriguez *et al.* 1998). The degree of protection associated with oral-contraceptive use may be related to the progestin potency of the formulation (Schildkraut *et al.* 2002).

Various epidemiologic and other studies support a role for androgens in the aetiology of ovarian cancer (reviewed in Risch 1998). In postmenopausal women, smoking appears to be related to increased levels of adrenal androgens. In premenopausal women, smoking increases the androgen–oestrogen ratio of follicular fluid (Van Voorhis *et al.* 1992), to which the ovarian epithelium is exposed. It seems reasonable that smoking could thus act on the ovarian epithelium through hormonal effects, but more studies are needed.

Tobacco smoking and risk of ovarian cancer

Several mechanisms support the biologic plausibility of an association between tobacco smoking and ovarian cancer, however given the above discussion, it is uncertain in which direction, to increase or decrease risk, the association should be. Results from early studies evaluating the association between cigarette smoking and risk of ovarian cancer lead IARC in 1987 to conclude that ovarian cancer was not tobacco-related (IARC 1987). With the exception of a British cohort study (Doll *et al.* 1980), no association has been found between tobacco smoking and risk of ovarian cancer in prospective studies (Engeland *et al.* 1996; Tworoger *et al.* 2008), and additional case-control studies have found null or inconsistent results (Trichopoulos *et al.* 1981; Smith *et al.* 1984; Tzonou *et al.* 1984; Baron *et al.* 1986; Franks *et al.* 1987; Hartge *et al.* 1989; Franceschi *et al.* 1991; Polychronopoulou *et al.* 1993; Riman *et al.* 2004). Some studies have observed non-significant reductions in risk among smokers (Byers *et al.* 1983; La Vecchia *et al.* 1984). Evaluating several reproductive, dietary, genetic, or environmental factors on the development of ovarian cancer, studies by Whittemore *et al.* (1988), Mori *et al.* (1988), and Slattery *et al.* (1989) reported no significant differences in tobacco use between cases and controls. An increase in ovarian cancer risk associated with tobacco smoking has also been observed (Cramer *et al.* 1984; Stockwell and Lyman 1987). Cramer *et al.* (1984) conducted a population-based case-control study of dietary factors and ovarian cancer that found a non-significant increased relative risk of 1.8 (95% CI: 0.54–5.97) for smokers versus non-smokers. Those authors found no significant trends in risk in relation to lifetime pack-years of cigarette smoking (Cramer *et al.* 1984). Several of the studies

(Cramer *et al.* 1984; Mori *et al.* 1988; Slattery *et al.* 1989; Polychronopoulou *et al.* 1993) did not control for all of the most potentially important confounding factors including age, parity, and oral contraceptive use, and this is a limitation in considering their results.

Risk differences according to histologic subtype

We have suggested that various risk factors involved in the development of epithelial ovarian cancer – including parity and oral contraceptive use – vary by the histologic type of the tumour (Risch *et al.* 1996). Germline *BRCA1* and *BRCA2* mutations essentially are not found in women with mucinous tumours (Risch *et al.* 2006). A follow-up study of more than 60 000 women in Norway showed a protective effect of increasing parity among serous, endometrioid, and other epithelial tumours but not for mucinous tumours (Kvale *et al.* 1988). In The WHO Collaborative Study of Neoplasia and Steroid Contraceptives, oral contraceptive use was significantly inversely associated with epithelial ovarian cancer risk for all the principal histologic types except for mucinous tumors (The WHO Collaborative Study of Neoplasia and Steroid Contraceptives 1989). Similarly, Risch *et al.* (1996) reported a population-based study of dietary and reproductive factors and epithelial ovarian cancer, which found decreasing oral contraceptive – and parity-related trends in risk for all of the particular histologic varieties of ovarian tumours except mucinous ones. These studies, as well as others (Collaborative Group on Epidemiological Studies of Ovarian Cancer 2008), consistently demonstrated odds ratios closer to (or even above) unity associated with ever use of oral contraceptives in mucinous tumours compared to serous, endometrioid, clear cell, or other (nonmucinous) epithelial tumours.

A number of studies have evaluated relationships between tobacco smoking and risks of the different histologic subtypes of ovarian cancer. There is now fairly clear evidence for an increase in risk of mucinous ovarian cancer with tobacco smoking. An early report by Franks *et al.* (1987), using data from The Cancer and Steroid Hormone Study, found no association between epithelial ovarian cancer overall and smoking dose or duration, age started smoking, time since started smoking, or latency of smoking. A re-examination of the association in that study according to histologic subtype found current cigarette smoking to be a risk factor for mucinous epithelial ovarian cancer (odds ratio (OR) = 2.9; 95% CI: 1.7–4.9), but not for the other histologic types (Marchbanks *et al.* 2000). This association remained significantly elevated regardless of age started smoking and number of years since first use of cigarettes (Marchbanks *et al.* 2000). Risk of mucinous epithelial ovarian cancer for current-smokers increased slightly with increasing cumulative pack-years of smoking; this same pattern was not observed for serous, endometrioid, or other histologic types (Marchbanks *et al.* 2000). Investigating the association between cigarette smoking and risk of ovarian cancer in a large case-control study, Green *et al.* (2001) concluded that current cigarette smoking was a risk factor for ovarian cancer, but especially for mucinous borderline and invasive types. Significantly elevated risks for mucinous epithelial tumours were seen among both current-smokers (OR = 3.2; 95% CI: 1.8–5.7) and past-smokers (OR = 2.3; 95% CI: 1.3–3.9) compared to never-smokers (Green *et al.* 2001). Similar findings occurred in follow-up of the Canadian National Breast Screening Study participants (Terry *et al.* 2003). While two studies have not shown increased risk of mucinous ovarian cancer among smokers (Goodman *et al.* 2003; Baker *et al.* 2006), the majority of recent studies have indeed provided support for this association (Kuper *et al.* 2000; Modugno *et al.* 2002; Zhang *et al.* 2004; Pan *et al.* 2004; Soegaard *et al* 2007; Gram *et al.* 2008; Tworoger *et al.* 2008; Rossing *et al.* 2008).

If steroid hormones are involved in the aetiology of ovarian cancer, variation in hormone metabolism and degradation could affect disease risk, and exposures such as tobacco smoking may modify these associations through induction effects on enzymes that activate or detoxify both polycyclic hydrocarbons and other (pro)carcinogens found in tobacco smoke, as well as steroid hormones. Thus, it has been suggested that tobacco smoking may affect the relationships between several genetic polymorphic variants and risk of ovarian cancer (Goodman *et al.* 2001). A common high-activity variant in the gene for microsomal epoxide hydrolase (EPHX1), which protein detoxifies endogenous steroids and exogenous xenobiotics, was observed in one study to be associated with increased risk of ovarian cancer (Lancaster *et al.* 1996). Spurdle *et al.* (2001) evaluated the effect of both this variant and smoking on risk of ovarian cancer, taking into account histologic classification. They found smoking to be associated with increased risk of mucinous tumours, regardless of EPHX1 genotype, and that the heterozygote and fast variants of this polymorphism were associated with decreased risk of mucinous tumours among non-smokers (Spurdle *et al.* 2001). These results appear to suggest that smoking may be associated with risk of mucinous ovarian tumours, that this risk may not be mediated through effects on induction of microsomal epoxide hydrolase, but that this enzyme might still be involved in the metabolism of other substances that could be associated with risk.

Histology: mucinous ovarian tumours

The various findings above are consistent with our suggestion that mucinous ovarian tumours comprise a distinct etiologic entity, separate from the other types of epithelial ovarian neoplasms (Risch *et al.* 1996). Differing from most types of ovarian cancer, mucinous tumours are thought to reflect a neoplastic morphologic continuum, from benign cystadenomas, through low-malignant potential (borderline) tumours, to invasive cancers, and many cases show the coexistence of these features within a single neoplasm (Rodriguez and Prat 2002). It has been speculated that the major effect of smoking may occur in the early stages of the mucinous cystadenoma-to-carcinoma sequence (Green *et al.* 2001). Mucinous tumours of the ovary, as well as serous and endometrioid ones, share common histogenetic ancestry with other structures of the reproductive tract, with morphologic similarities to endocervical (or intestinal), endosalpingeal, and endometrial tumours, respectively (Parmley and Woodruff 1974). The resemblance of mucinous ovarian tumour cells to tumour cells of the endocervix or colon, or even pancreas, leads to two possibilities, that (a) risk factors for these tumour types might be shared, or (b) that mucinous ovarian tumours are frequently improperly diagnosed as such but are metastatic from unrecognized intestinal primaries. The latter issue is a recognized problem in diagnosing mucinous ovarian primaries (Lash and Hart 1987; Young and Hart 1989), and it is unclear to what degree the various epidemiologic studies showing positive associations with mucinous neoplasms resolved the true origin of these tumours. Nicotine, benzo[*a*]pyrene, and other metabolites of cigarette smoke have been found in the cervical mucus of smokers (Feyerabend *et al.* 1982; Sasson *et al.* 1985), so it is possible that these substances are also present in the local environment of the ovary. Though cigarette smoking does not appear to be associated with risk of cervical adenocarcinoma (International Collaboration of Epidemiological Studies of Cervical Cancer *et al.* 2006), it is related to risk of both colon cancer (Giovannucci 2001) and pancreas cancer (Muscat *et al.* 1997), and at least the enteric variety of mucinous ovarian tumours might reflect the same association.

Summary

Several possible mechanisms by which various factors may affect the risk of developing epithelial ovarian cancer have been hypothesized. It is possible that the incessant ovulation and gonadotropin–oestrogen hypotheses may work together in the aetiology of this disease. However, evidence points to additional hormonal influences on the behaviour of ovarian epithelial cells. The harmful effects of tobacco smoking may not be limited to these proposed mechanisms of ovarian carcinogenesis. Cigarette smoke contains polycyclic aromatic hydrocarbons, *N*-nitrosamines, and other carcinogenic substances, and it is unknown if these constituents of the smoke reach the epithelium of the ovary to exert a local effect, as has been suggested elsewhere (Mattison and Thorgeirsson 1978; Hellberg and Nilsson 1988). Early studies reported no association between tobacco smoking and risk of epithelial ovarian cancer, but more recent studies looking at the particular histologic varieties of ovarian cancer show fairly consistent associations between tobacco smoking and increased risk of mucinous ovarian tumours. Ovarian cancer may very well be a heterogeneous disease with several distinct pathways that comprise the disease pathogenesis.

References

al-Timimi, A., Buckley, C.H., and Fox, H. (1985). An immunohistochemical study of the incidence and significance of sex steroid hormone binding sites in normal and neoplastic human ovarian tissue. *Int. J. Gynecol. Pathol.*, **4**: 24–41.

American Cancer Society. (2008). *Cancer facts and figures.* American Cancer Society, Inc., Atlanta.

Baird, D.D. and Wilcox, A.J. (1985). Cigarette smoking associated with delayed conception. *JAMA*, **253**: 2979–83.

Baker, J.A., Odunuga, O.O., Rodabaugh, K.J., Reid, M.E., Menezes, R.J., and Moysich, K.B. (2006). Active and passive smoking and risk of ovarian cancer. *Int. J. Gynecol. Cancer Suppl.*, 1, **16**: 211–8.

Baron, J.A., Byers, T., Greenberg, E.R., Cummings, K.M., and Swanson, M. (1986). Cigarette smoking in women with cancers of the breast and reproductive organs. *J. Natl. Cancer Inst.*, **77**: 677–80.

Byers, T., Marshall, J., Graham, S., Mettlin, C., and Swanson, M. (1983). A case-control study of dietary and nondietary factors in ovarian cancer. *J. Natl. Cancer Inst.*, **71**: 681–6.

Casagrande, J.T., Louie, E.W., Pike, M.C., Roy, S., Ross, R.K., and Henderson, B.E. (1979). 'Incessant ovulation' and ovarian cancer. *Lancet*, **2**: 170–3.

Collaborative Group on Epidemiological Studies of Ovarian Cancer (2008). Ovarian cancer and oral contraceptives: collaborative reanalysis of data from 45 epidemiological studies including 23 257 women with ovarian cancer and 87 303 controls. *Lancet*, **371**: 303–14.

Cooper, G.S., Sandler, D.P., and Bohlig, M. (1999). Active and passive smoking and the occurrence of natural menopause. *Epidemiology*, **10**: 771–3.

Cramer, D.W. and Welch, W.R. (1983). Determinants of ovarian cancer risk. II. Inferences regarding pathogenesis. *J. Natl. Cancer Inst.*, **71**: 717–21.

Cramer, D.W., Hutchison, G.B., Welch, W.R., Scully, R.E., and Knapp, R.C. (1982). Factors affecting the association of oral contraceptives and ovarian cancer. *N. Engl. J Med.*, **307**: 1047–51.

Cramer, D.W., Welch, W.R., Hutchison, G.B., Willett, W., and Scully, R.E. (1984). Dietary animal fat in relation to ovarian cancer risk. *Obstet. Gynecol.*, **63**: 833–8.

Daly, M. and Obrams, G.I. (1998). Epidemiology and risk assessment for ovarian cancer. *Semin. Oncol.*, **25**: 255–64.

Doll, R., Gray, R., Hafner, B., and Peto R. (1980). Mortality in relation to smoking: 22 years' observations on female British doctors. *Br. Med. J.*, **280**: 967–71.

Engeland, A., Andersen, A., Haldorsen, T., and Tretli, S. (1996). Smoking habits and risk of cancers other than lung cancer: 28 years' follow-up of 26 000 Norwegian men and women. *Cancer Causes Control*, 7: 497–506.

Fathalla, M.F. (1971). Incessant ovulation – a factor in ovarian neoplasia? *Lancet*, **2**: 163.

Feyerabend, C., Higenbottam, T., and Russell, M.A. (1982). Nicotine concentrations in urine and saliva of smokers and non-smokers. *Br. Med. J. (Clin. Res. Ed.)*, **284**: 1002–4.

Franceschi, S., La Vecchia, C., Booth, M., Tzonou, A., Negri, E., Parazzini, F., *et al.* (1991). Pooled analysis of 3 European case–control studies of ovarian cancer: II. Age at menarche and at menopause. *Int. J. Cancer*, **49**: 57–60.

Franks, A.L., Lee, N.C., Kendrick, J.S., Rubin, G.L., and Layde, P.M. (1987). Cigarette smoking and the risk of epithelial ovarian cancer. *Am.J.Epidemiol.*, **126**: 112–7.

Giovannucci, E. (2001). An updated review of the epidemiological evidence that cigarette smoking increases risk of colorectal cancer. *Cancer Epidemiol. Biomarkers Prev.*, **10**: 725–31.

Godwin, A.K., Perez, R.P., Johnson, S.W., Hamaguchi, K., and Hamilton, T.C. (1992). Growth regulation of ovarian cancer. *Hematol. Oncol. Clin. North Am.*, **6**: 829–41.

Godwin, A.K., Testa, J.R., Handel, L.M., Liu, Z., Vanderveer, L.A., Tracey, P.A., *et al.* (1992). Spontaneous transformation of rat ovarian surface epithelial cells: association with cytogenetic changes and implications of repeated ovulation in the etiology of ovarian cancer. *J. Natl. Cancer Inst.*, **84**: 592–601.

Goodman, M.T., McDuffie, K., Kolonel, L.N., Terada, K., Donlon, T.A., Wilkens, L.R., *et al.* (2001). Case-control study of ovarian cancer and polymorphisms in genes involved in catecholestrogen formation and metabolism. *Cancer Epidemiol. Biomarkers Prev.*, **10**: 209–16.

Goodman, M. T. and Tung, K. H. (2003). Active and passive tobacco smoking and the risk of borderline and invasive ovarian cancer (United States). *Cancer Causes Control*, **14**: 569–77.

Gram, I.T., Braaten, T., Adami, H.O., Lund, E., and Weiderpass, E. (2008). Cigarette smoking and risk of borderline and invasive epithelial ovarian cancer. *Int. J. Cancer*, **122**: 647–52.

Green, A., Purdie, D., Bain, C., Siskind, V., and Webb, P.M. (2001). Cigarette smoking and risk of epithelial ovarian cancer (Australia). *Cancer Causes Control*, **12**: 713–9.

Gross, T.P. and Schlesselman, J.J. (1994). The estimated effect of oral contraceptive use on the cumulative risk of epithelial ovarian cancer. *Obstet. Gynecol.*, **83**: 419–24.

Hankinson, S.E., Colditz, G.A., Hunter, D.J., Willett, W.C., Stampfer, M.J., Rosner, B., *et al.* (1995). A prospective study of reproductive factors and risk of epithelial ovarian cancer. *Cancer*, **76**: 284–90.

Hardy, R., Kuh, D., and Wadsworth, M. (2000). Smoking, body mass index, socioeconomic status and the menopausal transition in a British national cohort. *Int. J. Epidemiol.*, **29**: 845–51.

Hartge, P., Schiffman, M.H., Hoover, R., McGowan, L., Lesher, L., and Norris, H.J. (1989). A case-control study of epithelial ovarian cancer. *Am. J. Obstet. Gynecol.*, **161**: 10–6.

Hellberg, D. and Nilsson, S. (1988). Smoking and cancer of the ovary. *N. Engl. J. Med.*, **318**: 782–3.

Helzlsouer, K.J., Alberg, A.J., Gordon, G.B., Longcope, C., Bush, T.L., Hoffman, S.C. *et al.* (1995). Serum gonadotropins and steroid hormones and the development of ovarian cancer. *JAMA*, **274**: 1926–30.

Hoover, R., Gray, L.A., Sr., and Fraumeni, J.F., Jr. (1977). Stilboestrol (diethylstilbestrol) and the risk of ovarian cancer. *Lancet*, **2**: 533–4.

IARC (1987). Overall evaluations of carcinogenicity: an updating of IARC Monographs volumes 1 to 42. *IARC Monogr. Eval. Carcinog. Risks. Hum. Suppl.*, **7**: 1–440.

International Collaboration of Epidemiological Studies of Cervical Cancer, Appleby, P., Beral, V., Berrington de Gonzalez, A., Colin, D., Franceschi, S., *et al.* (2006). Carcinoma of the cervix and tobacco smoking: collaborative reanalysis of individual data on 13 541 women with carcinoma of the cervix and 23 017 women without carcinoma of the cervix from 23 epidemiological studies. *Int. J. Cancer*, **118**: 1481–95.

Kuper, H., Titus-Ernstoff, L., Harlow, B.L., and Cramer, D.W. (2000). Population based study of coffee, alcohol and tobacco use and risk of ovarian cancer. *Int. J. Cancer*, **88**: 313–8.

Kvale, G., Heuch, I., Nilssen, S., and Beral, V. (1988). Reproductive factors and risk of ovarian cancer: a prospective study. *Int. J. Cancer*, **42**: 246–51.

Lancaster, J.M., Brownlee, H.A., Bell, D.A., Futreal, P.A., Marks, J.R., Berchuck, A., *et al.* (1996). Microsomal epoxide hydrolase polymorphism as a risk factor for ovarian cancer. *Mol. Carcinog.*, **17**: 160–2.

Lash, R.H. and Hart, W.R. (1987). Intestinal adenocarcinomas metastatic to the ovaries. A clinicopathologic evaluation of 22 cases. *Am. J. Surg. Pathol.*, **11**: 114–21.

La Vecchia, C., Franceschi, S., Decarli, A., Gentile, A., Liati, P., Regallo, M., *et al.* (1984). Coffee drinking and the risk of epithelial ovarian cancer. *Int. J. Cancer*, **33**: 559–62.

Marchbanks, P.A., Wilson, H., Bastos, E., Cramer, D.W., Schildkraut, J.M., and Peterson, H.B. (2000). Cigarette smoking and epithelial ovarian cancer by histologic type. *Obstet. Gynecol.*, **95**: 255–60.

Mattison, D.R. and Thorgeirsson, S.S. (1978). Smoking and industrial pollution, and their effects on menopause and ovarian cancer. *Lancet*, **1**: 187–8.

Modugno, F., Ness, R.B., and Cottreau, C.M. (2002). Cigarette smoking and the risk of mucinous and nonmucinous epithelial ovarian cancer. *Epidemiology*, **13**: 467–71.

Mori, M., Harabuchi, I., Miyake, H., Casagrande, J.T., Henderson, B.E., and Ross, R.K. (1988). Reproductive, genetic, and dietary risk factors for ovarian cancer. *Am. J. Epidemiol.*, **128**: 771–7.

Muscat, J.E., Stellman, S.D., Hoffmann, D., and Wynder, E.L. (1997). Smoking and pancreatic cancer in men and women. *Cancer Epidemiol. Biomarkers Prev.*, **6**: 15–9.

Pan, S.Y., Ugnat, A.-M., Mao, Y., Wen, S.W., Johnson, K.C., and Canadian Cancer Registries Epidemiology Research Group (2004). Association of cigarette smoking with the risk of ovarian cancer. *Int. J. Cancer*, **111**: 124–30.

Parazzini, F., La Vecchia, C., Negri, E., and Villa, A. (1994). Estrogen replacement therapy and ovarian cancer risk. *Int. J. Cancer*, **57**: 135–6.

Parmley, T.H. and Woodruff, J.D. (1974). The ovarian mesothelioma. *Am. J. Obstet. Gynecol.*, **120**: 234–41.

Polychronopoulou, A., Tzonou, A., Hsieh, C.C., Kaprinis, G., Rebelakos, A., Toupadaki, N., *et al.* (1993). Reproductive variables, tobacco, ethanol, coffee and somatometry as risk factors for ovarian cancer. *Int. J. Cancer*, **55**: 402–7.

Preston-Martin, S., Pike, M.C., Ross, R.K., Jones, P.A., and Henderson, B.E. (1990). Increased cell division as a cause of human cancer. *Cancer Res.*, **50**: 7415–21.

Purdie, D., Green, A., Bain, C., Siskind, V., Ward, B., Hacker, N., *et al.* (1996). Estrogen replacement therapy and risk of epithelial ovarian cancer [abstract]. *Am. J. Epidemiol.*, **143**: S43.

Resta, L., Russo, S., Colucci, G.A., and Prat, J. (1993). Morphologic precursors of ovarian epithelial tumors. *Obstet. Gynecol.*, **82**: 181–6.

Riman, T., Dickman, P.W., Nilsson, S., Nordlinder, H., Magnusson, C.M., and Persson, I.R. (2004). Some life-style factors and the risk of invasive epithelial ovarian cancer in Swedish women. *Eur. J. Epidemiol.*, **19**: 1011–9.

Risch, H.A. (1996). Estrogen replacement therapy and risk of epithelial ovarian cancer. *Gynecol. Oncol.*, **63**: 254–7.

Risch, H.A. (1998). Hormonal etiology of epithelial ovarian cancer, with a hypothesis concerning the role of androgens and progesterone. *J. Natl. Cancer Inst.*, **90**: 1774–86.

Risch, H.A., Jain, M., Marrett, L.D., and Howe, G.R. (1994). Dietary fat intake and risk of epithelial ovarian cancer. *J. Natl. Cancer Inst.*, **86**: 1409–15.

Risch, H.A., Marrett, L.D., Jain, M., and Howe, G.R. (1996). Differences in risk factors for epithelial ovarian cancer by histologic type. Results of a case–control study. *Am. J. Epidemiol.*, **144**: 363–72.

Risch, H.A., McLaughlin, J.R., Cole, D.E., Rosen, B., Bradley, L., Fan, I. *et al.* (2006). Population BRCA1 and BRCA2 mutation frequencies and cancer penetrances: a kin-cohort study in Ontario, Canada. *J. Natl. Cancer Inst.*, **98**: 1694–706.

Risch, H.A., Weiss, N.S., Lyon, J.L., Daling, J.R., and Liff, J.M. (1983). Events of reproductive life and the incidence of epithelial ovarian cancer. *Am. J. Epidemiol.*, **117**: 128–39.

Rodriguez, I.M. and Prat, J. (2002). Mucinous tumors of the ovary: a clinicopathologic analysis of 75 borderline tumors (of intestinal type) and carcinomas. *Am. J. Surg. Pathol.*, **26**: 139–52.

Rodriguez, C., Calle, E.E., Coates, R.J., Miracle-McMahill, H.L., Thun, M.J., and Heath, C. W., Jr. (1995). Estrogen replacement therapy and fatal ovarian cancer. *Am. J. Epidemiol.*, **141**: 828–35.

Rodriguez, G.C., Walmer, D.K., Cline, M., Krigman, H., Lessey, B.A., Whitaker, R.S. *et al.* (1998). Effect of progestin on the ovarian epithelium of macaques: cancer prevention through apoptosis? *J. Soc. Gynecol. Investig.*, **5**: 271–6.

Rossing, M.A., Cushing-Haugen, K.L., Wicklund, K.G., Doherty, J.A., and Weiss N.S. (2007). Menopausal hormone therapy and risk of epithelial ovarian cancer. *Cancer Epidemiol. Biomarkers Prev.*, **16**: 2548–56.

Rossing, M.A., Cushing-Haugen, K.L., Wicklund, K.G., and Weiss N.S. (2008). Cigarette smoking and risk of epithelial ovarian cancer. *Cancer Causes Control*, **19**: 413–20.

Sasson, I.M., Haley, N.J., Hoffmann, D., Wynder, E.L., Hellberg, D., and Nilsson, S. (1985). Cigarette smoking and neoplasia of the uterine cervix: smoke constituents in cervical mucus. *N. Engl. J. Med.*, **312**: 315–6.

Schildkraut, J.M., Bastos, E., and Berchuck, A. (1997). Relationship between lifetime ovulatory cycles and overexpression of mutant p53 in epithelial ovarian cancer. *J. Natl. Cancer Inst.*, **89**: 932–8.

Schildkraut, J.M., Calingaert, B., Marchbanks, P.A., Moorman, P.G., and Rodriguez, G.C. (2002). Impact of progestin and estrogen potency in oral contraceptives on ovarian cancer risk. *J. Natl. Cancer Inst.*, **94**: 32–8.

Slattery, M.L., Schuman, K.L., West, D.W., French, T.K., and Robison, L.M. (1989). Nutrient intake and ovarian cancer. *Am. J. Epidemiol.*, **130**: 497–502.

Smith, E.M., Sowers, M.F., and Burns, T.L. (1984). Effects of smoking on the development of female reproductive cancers. *J. Natl. Cancer Inst.*, **73**: 371–6.

Soegaard, M., Jensen, A., Hogdall, E., Christensen, L., Hogdall, C., Blaakaer, J., *et al.* (2007). Different risk factor profiles for mucinous and nonmucinous ovarian cancer: results from the Danish MALOVA study. *Cancer Epidemiol. Biomarkers Prev.*, **16**: 1160–6.

Spurdle, A.B., Purdie, D.M., Webb, P.M., Chen, X., Green, A., and Chenevix-Trench, G. (2001). The microsomal epoxide hydrolase Tyr113His polymorphism: association with risk of ovarian cancer. *Mol. Carcinog.*, **30**: 71–8.

Stockwell, H.G. and Lyman, G.H. (1987). Cigarette smoking and the risk of female reproductive cancer. *Am. J. Obstet. Gynecol.*, **157**: 35–40.

Terry, P.D., Miller, A.B., Jones, J.G., and Rohan, T.E. (2003). Cigarette smoking and the risk of invasive epithelial ovarian cancer in a prospective cohort study. *Eur. J. Cancer*, **39**: 1157–64.

The Cancer and Steroid Hormone Study of the Centers for Disease Control and the National Institute of Child Health and Human Development (1987). The reduction in risk of ovarian cancer associated with oral-contraceptive use. *N. Engl. J. Med.*, **316**: 650–5.

The WHO Collaborative Study of Neoplasia and Steroid Contraceptives (1989). Epithelial ovarian cancer and combined oral contraceptives. *Int. J. Epidemiol.*, **18**: 538–45.

Trichopoulos, D., Papapostolou, M., and Polychronopoulou, A. (1981). Coffee and ovarian cancer. *Int. J. Cancer*, **28**: 691–3.

Tworoger, S.S., Gertig, D.M., Gates, M.A., Hecht, J.L., and Hankinson, S.E. (2008). Caffeine, alcohol, smoking, and the risk of incident epithelial ovarian cancer. *Cancer*, **112**: 1169–77.

Tzonou, A., Day, N.E., Trichopoulos, D., Walker, A., Saliaraki, M., Papapostolou, M. *et al.* (1984). The epidemiology of ovarian cancer in Greece: a case-control study. *Eur. J. Cancer Clin. Oncol.*, **20**: 1045–52.

Van Voorhis, B.J., Syrop, C.H., Hammitt, D.G., Dunn, M.S., and Snyder, G.D. (1992). Effects of smoking on ovulation induction for assisted reproductive techniques. *Fertil. Steril.*, **58**: 981–5.

Whittemore, A.S., Harris, R., and Itnyre, J. (1992). Characteristics relating to ovarian cancer risk: collaborative analysis of 12 US case-control studies. II. Invasive epithelial ovarian cancers in white women. Collaborative Ovarian Cancer Group. *Am. J. Epidemiol.*, **136**: 1184–203.

Whittemore, A.S., Wu, M.L., Paffenbarger, R.S., Jr., Sarles, D.L., Kampert, J.B., Grosser, S., *et al.* (1988). Personal and environmental characteristics related to epithelial ovarian cancer. II. Exposures to talcum powder, tobacco, alcohol, and coffee. *Am. J. Epidemiol.*, **128**: 1228–40.

Wynder, E.L., Dodo, H., and Barber, H.R. (1969). Epidemiology of cancer of the ovary. *Cancer*, **23**: 352–70.

Young, R.H. and Hart, W.R. (1989). Metastases from carcinomas of the pancreas simulating primary mucinous tumors of the ovary. A report of seven cases. *Am. J. Surg. Pathol.*, **13**: 748–56.

Zeimet, A.G., Muller-Holzner, E., Marth, C., and Daxenbichler, G. (1994). Immunocytochemical versus biochemical receptor determination in normal and tumorous tissues of the female reproductive tract and the breast. *J. Steroid. Biochem. Mol. Biol.*, **49**: 365–72.

Zhang, Y., Coogan, P.F., Palmer, J.R., Strom, B.L., and Rosenberg, L. (2004). Cigarette smoking and increased risk of mucinous epithelial ovarian cancer. *Am. J. Epidemiol.*, **159**: 133–9.

Chapter 30

Smoking, hormone concentrations, and endometrial cancer

Paul D. Terry, Thomas E. Rohan, and
Elisabete Weiderpass

Endometrial adenocarinoma accounts for approximately one of every ten cancers diagnosed among women worldwide, with incidence rates varying at least ten-fold between areas of low incidence (such as North Africa and China) and high incidence (such as North America) [1]. The use of exogenous oestrogens, and of oestrogen replacement therapy in particular, has been strongly related to increased risk in epidemiological studies [2, 3]. Exogenous oestrogens unopposed by progesterone have been hypothesized to increase the risk of this malignancy through increased mitotic activity of endometrial cells, increased number of DNA replication errors, and somatic mutations resulting in the malignant phenotype [3]. Hence, factors associated with oestrogen absorption or metabolism may alter the risk of this malignancy. In this regard, investigators have hypothesized that cigarette smoking might be associated with anti-oestrogenic effects, and through this mechanism reduce the risk of endometrial cancer [4–7]. Our aim here is to update our previous review [6] on cigarette smoking and endometrial cancer risk and changes in urinary hormone concentrations that may underlie this smoking-cancer association. In addition, we review recent studies that have included expanded measures of cigarette smoking and those that have examined the smoking-endometrial cancer association according to specific gene polymorphisms. We review published studies identified through searches of the Medline, Web of Science, and EMBASE databases and cross-matching the references of relevant articles. Virtually all published reports are in the English language, and we have restricted our review to those.

Studies of cigarette smoking and endometrial cancer risk

To date, at least 42 epidemiological studies have examined the association between smoking and endometrial cancer risk [8–50], 17 of which were published in the five years since the first edition of this book was published [34–50]. These studies have been categorized according to their basic design (case-control or cohort) and the type of smoking measures used (qualitative or quantitative). Studies that have used both qualitative (e.g., 'ever', 'current', or 'former' smoker) and quantitative measures (e.g., number of cigarettes per day or years of smoking duration) are reviewed in both sections.

Current-, former-, ever-, and never-smokers
Cohort studies

To date, there have been 13 prospective cohort studies [12, 26, 31, 34–40, 45, 48, 50] of the association between cigarette smoking and endometrial cancer risk (Table 30.1). The majority of these studies suggest a decreased risk among current-smokers, including the largest study with over 9 000 cases [35]. Overall, however, these studies do not clearly support a reduction in endometrial cancer risk among current-, ever-, or former-smokers compared with never-smokers. One prospective cohort study suggested the possibility of effect modification according to menopausal status [34], although this finding is not consistent with the overall results of epidemiological studies that considered menopausal status (discussed in greater detail later).

Case-control studies

The results of 17 population-based case-control studies [10, 11, 13, 14, 21–24, 27, 28, 32, 33, 41, 42, 46, 47, 51], that have included between 46 and 1 304 endometrial cancer cases, generally have shown reductions in risk among current-smokers compared with never-smokers (although the magnitude of the reduction in risk has varied somewhat), with equally variable results (albeit somewhat weaker overall) among former-smokers compared with never-smokers (Tables 30.1 and 30.4). The results of eight hospital-based case-control studies [8, 15, 16, 19, 20, 25, 43, 44], that have included between 83 and 1 374 endometrial cancer cases, are somewhat consistent with those of population-based studies in showing moderate (e.g., 30–40%) lower risks among current- compared with never-smokers, but do not show altered risks (or perhaps small 10–20% reduced risks) in former- compared with never-smokers (Table 30.1). The largest of the hospital-based studies [25], with 1 374 cases and 3 921 controls, found both former- and current-smokers to be at moderately (approximately 30%) reduced risk of endometrial cancer.

Quantitative measures of smoking

Cohort studies

Five [26, 31, 34, 40, 48] of the 13 [12, 26, 31, 34–40, 45, 48, 50] prospective cohort studies mentioned in the previous section have examined quantitative smoking measures in relation to endometrial cancer risk (Tables 30.2 and 30.3). The direction and magnitude of the association with quantitative measures is similar to that of the association with 'current' smoking status in the case-control studies. Of these five studies, one [26] found a 50% reduced risk among current-smokers in the highest level of intensity (11 cigarettes per day or more) compared with non-smokers, but the number of cases was low and the confidence intervals correspondingly wide (Table 30.2). A more recent and larger cohort study [31] found a statistically significant 40% reduced risk among current-smokers of more than 20 cigarettes per day, but showed somewhat weaker and statistically non-significant reductions in risk with smoking of long duration or high cumulative consumption (i.e., pack-years). In contrast, the risk among former-smokers was similar to that among never-smokers. The largest and most recent prospective cohort study generally showed decreasing risk of endometrial cancer with increasing smoking intensity, duration, and pack-years of consumption [48]. This latter study [48], along with two other prospective cohort studies [34, 40], did not show a clear association between age at smoking initiation and endometrial cancer risk (Table 30.3). The results of one of these studies suggest that smoking initiation among very young women (<16 years old) may actually increase risk of premenopausal endometrial cancer [34], although this was not shown in the other two studies that examined smoking initiation among those < 19 years old [40] and < 18 years old [48]. In addition, three studies examined the association between time since smoking cessation and endometrial cancer risk (Table 30.3). Two of these studies suggested a positive association with time since quitting (compared with non-smokers) [40, 48], whereas one suggested the opposite among premenopausal women (compared with current-smokers). However, most of these findings were based on relatively small numbers of cases in the specific smoking categories.

Table 30.1 Epidemiological studies of cigarette smoking and endometrial cancer risk: current, former, and never smokers

First author, study year	Study design	# Cases/controls (# in cohort)	Age range at recruitment	Ever smoking vs. never OR (95% CI)	Former smoking vs. never OR (95% CI)	Current smoking vs. never OR (95% CI)	Adjustment for:*
Engeland, 1996	Prospective cohort	140/26,000	32–72	-------	1.2 (0.6–2.2)	1.1 (0.7–1.6)	Not specified
Terry, 1999	Prospective cohort	123/11,659	42–82	-------	0.7 (0.3–2.0)	0.9 (NO CI)†	Age, weight, parity
Terry, 2002	Prospective cohort	403/70,591	40–59	-------	1.0 (0.8–1.3)	0.8 (0.6–1.1)	Age, BMI, HRT, parity
Furberg, 2003	Prospective cohort	130/24,460	20–49	0.8 (0.5–1.1)**	-------	-------	Age
Folsom, 2003	Prospective cohort	415/23,335	55–69	-------	0.8 (0.6–1.1)	0.5 (0.4–0.8)	Age
Viswanathan, 2005	Prospective cohort	702/96,704	30–55	-------	0.8 0.7 (0.6–0.9) 0.7 (0.6–0.9)	0.6 0.6 (0.5–0.8) 0.7 (0.6–0.9)	Age Age, OC use, HRT use, parity, age at menarche, hypertension, diabetes Age, OC use, HRT use, parity, age at menarche, hypertension, diabetes, BMI
Bjørge, 2006	Prospective cohort	9,227/1,038,018	20–74	-------	1.1 (0.8–1.7)†† 1.1(0.7–1.5)‡‡	0.5 (0.4–0.8)†† 0.7 (0.5–1.0)‡‡	Age at measurement, year of birth, BMI, height
Loerbroks, 2006	Prospective cohort	280/62,573	5–69	0.7 (0.5–1.0)	0.8 (0.6–1.2)	0.6 (0.4–0.9)	Age, BMI, parity, OC use, non-occupational physical activity, hypertension, age at first child birth, age at menopause, alcohol consumption

(Continued)

Table 30.1 (continued) Epidemiological studies of cigarette smoking and endometrial cancer risk: current, former, and never smokers

First author, study year	Study design	# Cases/controls (# in cohort)	Age range at recruitment	Ever smoking vs. never OR (95% CI)	Former smoking vs. never OR (95% CI)	Current smoking vs. never OR (95% CI)	Adjustment for:*
Setiawan, 2007	Prospective cohort	321/46,933	45–75	—	1.2 (0.9–1.5)	0.7 (0.5–1.1)	Adjusted for race/ethnicity, BMI, age at menarche, age at natural menopause, parity, HRT use per 5 years, OC- use, diabetes, hypertension, family history of endometrial cancer
Al-Zoughool, 2007	Prospective cohort	619/249,986	NA	—	Premenopausal 0.8 (0.5–2.8) Postmenopausal 0.9 (0.7–1.1)	Premenopausal 1.8 (1.2–2.8) Postmenopausal 0.8 (0.6–1.0)	Stratified for age and center Adjusted for BMI, total physical activity, OC-use, parity, educational level, alcohol consumption; in postmenopausal: further HRT use and age at menopause
Lacey, 2007	Prospective cohort	433/73,211	50–71	—	0.8 (0.7–1.0)	0.7 (0.5–0.9)	Age, OC-use, BMI, race, menopausal status
Lindemann, 2008	Prospective cohort	222/36,761	20–101	—	1.1 (0.7–1.6)	0.6 (0.4–0.9)	Age, physical activity, hypertension, alcohol consumption, BMI, diabetes
Brinton, 1993	Population case-control	405/297	20–74	0.8 (0.5–1.1)	1.1 (0.7–1.6)	0.4 (0.2–0.7)	Age, weight, HRT, parity, diabetes, age at menopause
Elliot, 1990	Population case-control	46/138	—	—	1.4 (0.6–3.5)	0.2 (0.1–0.6)	Age, BMI, HRT, parity, diabetes
Franks, 1987	Population case-control	79/416	20–55	0.5 (0.3–0.8)	—	—	Age, BMI, HRT, parity, diabetes, age at menopause
Goodman, 1997	Population case-control	332/511	18–84	0.8 (0.6–1.2)	—	—	Age, BMI, HRT, parity, diabetes
Jain, 2000	Population case-control	220/223	30–79	1.0 (0.8–1.3)	—	—	None
McCann, 2000	Population case-control	236/639	40–85	0.6 (0.4–0.8)	—	—	Age

Study	Design	Cases/Controls	Age				Adjustments
Newcomer, 2001	Population case-control	740/2,372	40–79	0.8 (0.7–0.9)	0.8 (0.7–1.0)	0.8 (0.6–1.0)	Age, BMI, HRT, parity, diabetes
Rubin, 1990	Population case-control	196/986	20–54	--------	0.8 (0.5–1.2)	0.7 (0.5–1.0)	Age, BMI, treatment for diabetes
Shields, 1999	Population case-control	553/752	45–64	--------	0.8 (0.6–1.2)‡	0.6 (0.4–0.8)‡	Age, BMI
Smith, 1984	Population case-control	70/612	20–54	0.8 (0.4–1.5)	--------		Age, BMI, HRT, parity, age at menopause
Tyler, 1985	Population case-control	437/3,200	20–54	0.9 (0.7–1.1)	1.0 (0.7–1.4)	0.8 (0.7–1.1)	Age, Weight, HRT, age at menopause
Weiderpass, 2001	Population case-control	709/3,368	50–74	--------	0.9 (0.7–1.1)	0.6 (0.5–0.8)	Age, BMI, HRT, parity, diabetes, age at menopause
Newcomb, 2003	Population case-control	591/2045	40–79	--------	0.8 (0.7–1.1)	0.6 (0.4–0.8)	Age
Matthews, 2005	Population case-control	832/846	30–69	--------	--------	0.3 (0.1–0.7)§§	Age, education, family income, age at menarche, OC-use, number of pregnancies, menopausal status, age at menopause, height, body mass index, waist-to-hip ratio, family history of cancer
Trentham-Dietz, 2006	Population case-control	740/2,342	40–79	0.9 (0.7–1.1)	0.9 (0.7–1.1)	0.6 (0.4–0.7)	Age
Weiss, 2006	Population case-control	1,304/1,779	45–74		Low tumour aggressiveness 0.7 (0.5–0.8) Moderate tumour aggressiveness 0.6 (0.5–0.8) High tumour aggressiveness 0.4 (0.3–0.7)	Low tumour aggressiveness 0.7 (0.5–0.9) Moderate tumour aggressiveness 0.5 (0.4–0.6) High tumour aggressiveness 1.0 (0.6–1.5)	Age, postmenopausal hormone use, BMI, county of residence, referent year

(Continued)

Table 30.1 (continued) Epidemiological studies of cigarette smoking and endometrial cancer risk: current, former, and never smokers

First author, study year	Study design	# Cases/controls (# in cohort)	Age range at recruitment	Ever smoking vs. never OR (95% CI)	Former smoking vs. never OR (95% CI)	Current smoking vs. never OR (95% CI)	Adjustment for:*
Strom, 2006	Population case-control	511/1,412	50–79	-------	0.8 (0.6–1.0)	0.4 (0.2–0.5)	Age, educational level, BMI during the age decade of 40's, number of full-time pregnancies, years of menses, menopause type, years of smoking, OC-use
Austin, 1993	Hospital case-control	168/334	40–82	-------	0.8 (0.5–1.5)	0.7 (0.4–1.2)	Age, BMI, HRT, parity, diabetes
Kelsey§	Hospital case-control	167/903	45–74	0.8 (NO CI)	-------	-------	Age, HRT, age at menopause
Koumantaki, 1989	Hospital case-control	83/164	40–79	-------	-------	0.5 (0.2–1.3)¶	Age, height, weight, HRT, parity, age at menopause
Lesko, 1985	Hospital case-control	510/727	18–69	-------	0.9 (0.6–1.2)	0.8 (NO CI)†	Age, BMI, HRT, age at menopause, parity, diabetes
Levi, 1987	Hospital case-control	357/1,122	31–74	-------	0.9 (0.5–1.5)	0.5 (0.3–0.7)	Age, BMI, HRT, parity, age at menopause
Stockwell, 1987	Hospital case-control	1,374/3,921	-------	-------	0.6 (0.5–0.8)	0.7 (NO CI)†	Age
Petridou, 2002	Hospital case-control	84/84	-------	-------	-------	1.3 (0.5–3.8)§§	Age, education, height, BMI, age at menarche, pregnancies and abortions, menopausal status, alcohol drinking, cholecystectomy
Okamura, 2006	Hospital case-control	155/96	20–80	1.3 (0.7–2.6)	-------	-------	Age

* Covariates considered here are: age, body mass index (BMI), hormone replacement therapy (HRT), age at menopause, parity, diabetes.
† Crude measures of association were calculated from the data provided.
‡ Results shown are for women not taking unopposed estrogens. Among estrogen users, smokers were also at higher risk than non-smokers.
§ Results reported in Baron[5].
¶ Former smokers were combined with never smokers in this analysis.
** Daily smoking (yes/no).
†† Cancers of Uterine Corpus Type I (mostly endometrial adenocarcinomas with subgroups).
‡‡ Cancers of Uterine Corpus Total (Type I: mostly endometrial adenocarcinomas with subgroups and Type II: papillary, serous, and clear cell adenocarcinomas and poorly differentiated carcinomas).
§§ current smokers vs. non-current.

Table 30.2 Epidemiological studies of cigarette smoking and endometrial cancer risk: smoking frequency, duration, and pack-years

First author, study year	Study design	# Cases/controls (# in cohort)	Age range	Smoking intensity (cigarettes/day)		Smoking duration (years)		Pack years (Packs/day*years)	
				Comparison	OR (95% CI)	Comparison	OR (95% CI)	Comparison	OR (95% CI)
Terry, 1999	Prospective cohort	123/11,659	42–82	Current 11+ vs. never	0.5 (0.1–2.0)				
Terry, 2002	Prospective cohort	403/70,591	40–59	Former > 20 vs. never	0.9 (0.6–1.3)	Former > 20 vs. never	1.1 (0.8–1.6)	Former > 20 vs. never	1.0 (0.7–1.5)
				Current > 20 vs. never	0.6 (0.4–0.9)*	Current > 20 vs. never	0.8 (0.6–1.1)	Current > 20 vs. never	0.7 (0.5–1.1)
Viswanathan, 2005	Prospective cohort	702/96,704	30–55	Ever smokers vs. never smokers		Ever smokers vs. never smokers		Ever smokers vs. never smokers	
				1–4	0.9 (0.7–1.2)†	> 0–10	0.8 (0.6–1.0)†	> 0–10	0.8 (0.6–1.0)†
				5–14	0.7 (0.5–0.8)†	> 10–20	0.7 (0.5–0.9)†	> 10–20	0.6 (0.4–0.8)†
				15–24	0.7 (0.6–0.9)†	> 20–30	0.7 (0.6–1.0)†	> 20–30	0.9 (0.7–1.1)†
				25–34	0.7 (0.5–1.0)†	> 30–40	0.7 (0.6–0.9)†	> 30–40	0.8 (0.6–1.1)†
				35+	0.6 (0.4–1.0)†	> 40	0.6 (0.4–0.8)†	> 40–50	0.6 (0.4–0.8)†
								> 50	0.5 (0.3–0.7)†
				1–4	1.0 (0.7–1.3)‡	> 0–10	0.8 (0.6–1.1)‡	> 0–10	0.8 (0.7–1.0)‡
				5–14	0.7 (0.6–0.9)‡	> 10–20	0.7 (0.5–0.9)‡	> 10–20	0.6 (0.4–0.8)‡
				15–24	0.7 (0.6–0.9)‡	> 20–30	0.7 (0.6–1.0)‡	> 20–30	0.9 (0.7–1.2)‡
				25–34	0.7 (0.5–1.0)‡	> 30–40	0.7 (0.6–0.9)‡	> 30–40	0.8 (0.6–1.1)‡
				35+	0.6 (0.4–0.9)‡	> 40	0.6 (0.5–0.9)‡	> 40–50	0.6 (0.4–0.9)‡
								> 50	0.5 (0.3–0.7)‡

(Continued)

Table 30.2 (continued) Epidemiological studies of cigarette smoking and endometrial cancer risk: smoking frequency, duration, and pack-years

First author, study year	Study design	# Cases/controls (# in cohort)	Age range	Smoking intensity (cigarettes/day)		Smoking duration (years)		Pack years (Packs/day*years)	
				Comparison	OR (95% CI)	Comparison	OR (95% CI)	Comparison	OR (95% CI)
						Ever smokers vs. ever smokers			
				1–4	1.0 (0.7–1.3)§	0–10			
				5–14	0.7 (0.6–0.9)§	> 10–20	0.9 (0.6–1.2)§		
				15–24	0.7 (0.6–0.9)§	> 20–30	0.9 (0.6–1.3)§	Pack years before age 30¶	
				25–34	0.7 (0.5–1.0)§	> 30–40	0.9 (0.6–1.3)§	1 to < 5	0.8 (0.7–1.0)†
				35+	0.6 (0.4–0.9)§	> 40	0.8 (0.5–1.2)§	5 to < 10	0.8 (0.6–1.0)†
								10 +	0.9 (0.5–0.9)†
				Former smokers vs. never smokers		Former smokers vs. never smokers			
				1–14	0.8 (0.6–0.9)†	> 0–20	0.7 (0.6–0.9)†	1 to < 5	0.9 (0.7–1.1)‡
				15–24	0.7 (0.6–0.9)†	> 20–30	0.7 (0.5–1.0)†	5 to < 10	0.8 (0.6–1.1)‡
				25+	0.7 (0.5–1.0)†	> 30	0.8 (0.6–1.0)†	10 +	0.7 (0.5–0.9)‡
								Pack years after age 30¶	
				1–14	0.8 (0.6–1.0)‡	> 0–20	0.7 (0.6–0.9)‡	1 to 10	0.7 (0.4–1.2)†
				15–24	0.7 (0.6–0.9)‡	> 20–30	0.7 (0.5–0.9)‡	> 10 to 20	0.6 (0.3–1.1)†
				25+	0.7 (0.5–1.0)‡	> 30	0.7 (0.6–1.0)‡	20 +	0.6 (0.3–1.1)†
				Former smokers vs. ever smokers		Former smokers vs. former smokers > 0–20		1 to < 5	0.6 (0.4–1.1)‡
				1–14				5 to < 10	0.6 (0.3–1.1)‡
				15–24	1.0 (0.7–1.3)§	> 20–30	0.9 (0.7–1.3)§	10 +	0.6 (0.3–1.1)‡
				25+	0.9 (0.6–1.3)§	> 30	1.0 (0.7–1.4)§		
				Current smokers vs. never smokers					
				1–14	0.7 (0.5–1.0)†				

QUANTITATIVE MEASURES OF SMOKING | 521

				15–24	0.6 (0.4–0.9)†			
				25+	0.6 (0.4–1.0)†			
				1–14	0.8 (0.5–1.1)‡			
				15–24	0.7 (0.5–1.0)‡			
				25+	0.7 (0.4–1.0)‡			
				Current smokers vs. ever smokers				
				1–14	1.0 (0.6–1.6)§			
				15–24	0.9 (0.5–1.6)§			
Loerbroks, 2006	Prospective cohort	280/62,573	55–69	Ever smokers vs. never sm.	0.1–19 1.1 (0.6–2.0)**	Ever smokers vs. never sm.	0.1–19 0.8 (0.4–1.4)**	
					10–19 1.3 (0.7–2.5)**		20–39 0.9 (0.5–1.6)**	
					20+ 1.3 (0.6–3.0)**		40+ 0.4 (0.2–0.9)**	
				Ever smokers vs. never sm.	0.1–19 0.9 (0.5–1.5)††	Ever smokers vs. never sm.	0.1–19 0.7 (0.4–1.2)††	
					10–19 1.0 (0.5–1.9)††		20–39 0.8 (0.5–1.3)††	
					20+ 1.3 (0.5–2.3)††		40+ 0.4 (0.2–1.0)††	
Al-Zoughool, 2007	Prospective cohort	619/249,986	NA	Premenopausal		Premenopausal		Lifetime number of cigarettes per day Premenopausal
				Former <10 vs. never	0.9 (0.4–2.1)	Former <10 vs.never	0.6 (0.2–1.6)	Former < 10 vs. never 0.9 (0.4–2.1)
				10+ vs. never	0.6 (0.2–1.8)	10–19 vs. never	0.7 (0.3–1.6)	10+ vs. never 0.6 (0.2–1.8)
				Current<15 vs. never	1.7 (0.9–3.1)	20–29 vs. never	1.2 (0.5–2.7)	

(Continued)

Table 30.2 (continued) Epidemiological studies of cigarette smoking and endometrial cancer risk: smoking frequency, duration, and pack-years

First author, study year	Study design	Age range	# Cases/controls (# in cohort)	Smoking intensity (cigarettes/day) Comparison	OR (95% CI)	Smoking duration (years) Comparison	OR (95% CI)	Pack years (Packs/day*years) Comparison	OR (95% CI)
				15+ vs. never	2.4 (1.0–5.6)	Current < 25 vs. never	1.6 (0.8–3.2)	Current < 15 vs. never	1.7 (0.9–3.1)
						25–29 vs. never	1.9 (1.0–3.8)	15+ vs. never	2.4 (1.0–5.6)
				Postmenopausal		30–39 vs. never	2.3 (1.1–5.0)	Postmenopausal	
				Former <10 vs. never	0.6 (0.4–0.9)	Postmenopausal		Former < 10 vs. never	0.6 (0.4–0.9)
				10+ vs. never	0.6 (0.4–0.9)	Former <10 vs.never	0.6 (0.4–1.1)	10+ vs. never	0.6 (0.4–0.9)
				Current<15 vs. never	0.5 (0.3–0.8)	10–19 vs. never	1.0 (0.7–1.5)	Current < 15 vs. never	0.5 (0.3–0.8)
				15+ vs. never	0.7 (0.4–1.3)	20–29 vs. never	0.8 (0.6–1.3)	15+ vs. never	0.7 (0.4–1.3)
						30+ vs. never	0.7 (0.5–1.1)	France and Sweden excluded (information not collected)	
						Current < 25 vs. never	0.8 (0.4–1.4)		
						25–29 vs. never	0.7 (0.4–1.1)		
						30–39 vs. never	0.7 (0.5–1.1)		
Brinton, 1993	Population case-control	20–74	405/297	Ever 30+ vs. never	0.7 (0.4–1.4)	Ever 40+ vs. never	0.5 (0.3–0.9)*	------	
				Former 30+ vs. never	1.4 (NO CI)	Former 40+ vs. never	0.5 (NO CI)		
				Current 30+ vs. never	0.3 (NO CI)	Current 40+ vs. never	0.5 (NO CI)		

Study	Type	Cases/Controls	Age	Measure	OR (CI)	Measure	OR (CI)
Lawrence, 1987	Population case-control	301/289	40–69	Former > 20 vs. never; Current > 20 vs. never	0.6 (NO CI); 0.5 (NO CI)		
Lawrence, 1989	Population case-control	84/168	40–69	Former > 20 vs. never; Current > 20 vs. never	1.0 (NO CI); 1.0 (NO CI)		
Newcomer, 2001	Population case-control	740/2,372	40–79	--------		Ever 80+ vs. never	0.9 (0.5–1.4)
Tyler, 1985	Population case-control	437/3,200	20–54	--------		Ever 15+ vs. never	1.0 (0.7–1.2)
Weiderpass, 2001	Population case-control	709/3,368	50–74	Maximum 20+ vs. never; Lifelong 45+ vs. never	0.7 (0.4–1.3); 0.6 (0.3–0.9)	--------	
Baron, 1986	Hospital case-control	476/2,128	40–89	--------		Ever 15+ vs. never	0.6 (0.4–0.9)*
Koumantaki, 1989	Hospital case-control	83/164	40–79	20+ (continuous variable)	0.5 (0.3–0.9)*	--------	
Lesko, 1985	Hospital case-control	510/727	18–69	Current 25+ vs. never	0.5 (0.3–0.8)	--------	
Levi, 1987	Hospital case-control	357/1,122	31–74	Current 15+ vs. never	0.4 (0.2–0.9)*	--------	
Stockwell, 1987	Hospital case-control	1,374/3,921	--------	Current > 40 vs. never	0.5 (0.3–0.9)	--------	
Williams, 1977	Hospital case-control	358/3,189	25–76	--------		Ever 40+ vs. never	0.7 (NS)

* Statistically significant test of trend reported.
† Adjusted for age, OC use, HRT use, parity, age at menarche, hypertension, diabetes.
‡ Adjusted for age, OC use, HRT use, parity, age at menarche, hypertension, diabetes, BMI.
§ Adjusted for age, OC use, HRT use, parity, age at menarche, hypertension, diabetes, BMI and smoking duration or amount cigarettes smoked per day.
¶ Adjusted additionally for pack years after age 30 or for pack years before age 30.
** Adjusted for age, current smoking, duration, BMI, parity, use of OC, non-occupational physical activity, hypertension, age at first child birth, age at menopause, alcohol consumption.
†† Adjusted for age, current smoking status, frequency and duration of smoking.

Table 30.3 Epidemiological studies of cigarette smoking and endometrial cancer risk: age of initiation and time since cessation

First author, study year	Study design	# Cases/controls (# in cohort)	Age range	Age of initiation (years)		Time since cessation (years)	
				Comparison	RR (95% CI)	Comparison	RR (95% CI)
Viswanathan, 2005	Prospective cohort	702/96,704	30–55	vs. never smokers		vs. never smokers	
				13 to < 18	0.8 (0.6–1.0)*	20+	0.7 (0.6–0.9)*
				18 to < 20	0.7 (0.6–0.8)*	15 to < 20	0.9 (0.6–1.2)*
				20 to < 22	0.7 (0.6–0.9)*	10 to < 15	0.9 (0.6–1.2)*
				≥ 22	0.7 (0.5–0.9)*	5 to < 10	0.6 (0.4–0.9)*
						< 5	0.6 (0.4–0.9)*
				13 to < 18	0.8 (0.6–1.0)†	20+	0.8 (0.6–1.0)†
				18 to < 20	0.7 (0.6–0.9)†	15 to < 20	0.9 (0.6–1.2)†
				20 to < 22	0.7 (0.6–0.9)†	10 to < 15	0.8 (0.6–1.2)†
				≥ 22	0.7 (0.6–1.0)†	5 to < 10	0.6 (0.4–0.9)†
						< 5	0.6 (0.4–0.9)†
				vs. 13 to < 18		vs. 20+	
				18 to < 20	0.9 (0.6–1.2)‡	15 to < 20	1.1 (0.8–1.7)‡
				20 to < 22	0.9 (0.7–1.3)‡	10 to < 15	1.1 (0.7–1.6)‡
				≥ 22	0.9 (0.6–1.3)‡	5 to < 10	0.8 (0.5–1.2)‡
						< 5	0.8 (0.6–1.3)‡
Loerbroks, 2006	Prospective cohort	280/62,573	55–69	vs. never smokers		vs. never smokers	
				< 19	0.7 (0.5–1.1)§	20+	1.1 (0.7–1.8)§
				19–24	0.5 (0.3–0.9)§	10–19	0.6 (0.4–1.1)§
				25+	0.7 (0.5–1.1)§	0.1–9	0.6 (0.3–1.1)§
				< 19	0.8 (0.3–1.8)¶	20+	0.8 (0.4–1.6)¶
				19–24	0.6 (0.3–1.3)¶	10–19	0.4 (0.1–1.0)¶
				25+	0.8 (0.5–1.5)¶	0.1–9	0.3 (0.1–1.1)¶

				< 19	0.9 (0.4–2.2)**	1.1 (0.5–2.4)**
				19–24	0.9 (0.4–2.0)**	0.5 (0.2–1.5)**
				25+	1.0 (0.5–1.9)**	0.5 (0.1–2.0)**
Al-Zoughool, 2007	Prospective cohort	619/249,986	NA			

Premenopausal

Premenopausal vs. current smokers

Current smokers vs. never smokers

<16	5.1 (2.4–10.9)††	20+	0.3 (0.1–1.1)††
16–25	1.7 (1.0–2.8)††	10–19	0.4 (0.1–1.0)††
26+	0.8 (0.2–3.2)††	<10	0.7 (0.3–1.4)††

Former smokers vs. never smokers

Postmenopausal

vs. current smokers

<18	0.9 (0.2–3.6)††	20+	1.0 (0.7–1.6)††
18–24	0.7 (0.4–1.3)††	10–19	0.9 (0.6–1.5)††
25+	1.3 (0.3–5.2)††	<10	1.1 (0.7–1.7)††

Postmenopausal

Current smokers vs. never smokers

<16	0.6 (0.2–1.5)††
16–25	0.7 (0.5–1.0)††
26+	0.7 (0.4–1.2)††

Former smokers vs. never smokers

<18	0.8 (0.4–1.7)††
18–24	0.8 (0.6–1.1)††
25+	0.7 (0.4–1.2)††

* Adjusted for age, OC use, HRT use, parity, age at menarche, hypertension, diabetes.
† Adjusted for age, OC use, HRT use, parity, age at menarche, hypertension, diabetes, BMI.
‡ Adjusted for age, OC use, HRT use, parity, age at menarche, hypertension, diabetes, BMI and age at smoking initiation or time since cessation.
§ Adjusted for age.
¶ Adjusted for age, current smoking status, frequency and duration of smoking.
** Adjusted for age, current smoking, duration, BMI, parity, use of OC, non-occupational physical activity, hypertension, age at first child birth, age at menopause, alcohol consumption.
†† Adjusted for BMI, total physical activity, OC-use, parity, educational level, alcohol consumption; in postmenopausal: further HRT use and age at menopause.

Case-control studies

To date, six population-based case-control studies [10, 17, 18, 27, 28, 33] have examined quantitative measures of smoking in relation to endometrial cancer risk, generally showing inverse associations to be strongest among current-smokers of high intensity or long duration (Tables 30.2 and 30.4). However, one population-based study of late-stage endometrial cancer [18] did not show an association with any measure of smoking (although the number of cases in that study was relatively small); in another small study [17], the same investigators found that smoking more than 20 cigarettes per day was associated with a reduced risk of early-stage endometrial cancer among both current- and former-smokers. Whereas the majority of these studies adjusted their relative risk estimates for potentially confounding variables, such as body mass index (BMI) (weight (kg)/height (m)^2), hormone replacement therapy (HRT), parity, diabetes, and age at menopause (Table 30.1), studies that did not adjust for these variables tended to show similar inverse associations. Within individual studies, statistical adjustment for the effects of BMI and other covariates often made little difference, although some attenuation of relative risk estimates has been noted [28, 31].

Six hospital-based case-control studies of endometrial cancer that examined quantitative measures of smoking have mostly shown statistically significant 30–60% reduced risks with current or recent smoking of high intensity [19, 20, 25], with smoking of long duration [16], or with a relatively large number of pack-years (Table 30.2) [9, 30]. However, the fact that the various smoking measures are correlated with each other complicates the differentiation of their independent effects. For example, smokers of high intensity also tend to be smokers of long duration [31], and the latter also tend to have commenced smoking at an early age.

Effect modification

A number of studies have examined the association between smoking and endometrial cancer risk according to factors that are known determinants of endogenous hormone concentrations, and which may counteract or augment possible tobacco-related hormonal changes. These factors include menopausal status, HRT, and BMI. Effect modification can reflect true underlying differences in the association across strata (e.g., if cigarette smoking acts to reduce or modify oestrogen concentrations differently in one group compared with another), but can also reflect methodological factors, such as differences that occur by chance or through the varying prevalence of confounding variables.

Menopausal status

Although endometrial cancer is rare among premenopausal women, several studies have examined the association between cigarette smoking and endometrial cancer risk according to menopausal status, because the effect of smoking (if any) might vary according to the underlying hormonal milieu. The studies have included two prospective cohort studies [31, 34], five population-based case-control studies [10, 13, 17, 24, 28], and four hospital-based case-control studies [16, 19, 20, 25] (Table 30.4). In all but one of these studies, a study of early stage endometrial cancer [17], the inverse association was (to varying degrees) stronger among postmenopausal than premenopausal women. Among premenopausal women, the relative risk estimates for cigarette smoking have been inconsistent, sometimes showing increased risks with certain measures of cigarette smoking [10, 16, 24, 25, 34], sometimes showing decreased risks [10, 17, 20, 31], and sometimes showing practically no association [19, 28, 34]. In analyses limited to postmenopausal women, however, all showed between 10% and 80% reduced risks of endometrial cancer with the various smoking measures.

Table 30.4 Epidemiological studies of cigarette smoking and endometrial cancer risk according to menopausal status

First author, study year	Study design	# Cases/controls (# in cohort)	Comparison	Premenopausal OR (95% CI)	Postmenopausal OR (95% CI)
Terry, 2002	Prospective cohort	403/70,591	Current > 20 cigarettes/day vs. never	0.7 (0.4–1.3)	0.6 (0.3–1.1)
Al-Zoughool, 2007	Prospective cohort	619/249,986	Former vs. never smokers	0.8 (0.5–2.8)	0.9 (0.7–1.1)
			Current vs. never smokers	1.8 (1.2–2.8)	0.8 (0.6–1.0)
Brinton, 1993	Population case-control	405/297	Former vs. never smokers	3.0 (1.2–7.4)	0.8 (0.4–1.2)
			Current vs. never smokers	0.5 (0.1–1.7)	0.4 (0.2–0.7)
			Ever 30+ years vs. never	6.2 (0.9–42.3)	0.6 (0.4–1.0)*
			Ever 30+ cigarettes/day vs. never	1.3 (0.2–7.1)	0.6 (0.3–1.3)*
Franks, 1987	Population case-control	79/416	Ever vs. never smokers	———	0.5 (0.3–0.8)
Lawrence, 1987	Population case-control	301/289	Current vs. never smokers	0.6 (NO CI)	0.6 (NO CI)
Smith, 1984	Population case-control	70/612	Ever vs. never smokers	1.3 (0.7–2.5)	0.4 (0.2–1.0)
Weiderpass, 2001	Population case-control	709/3,368	Current (highest level of duration)	0.9 (0.4–2.0)	0.4 (0.2–0.8)
Koumantaki, 1989	Hospital case-control	83/164	Current vs. former + non-smokers	2.3 (NO CI)	0.2 (NO CI)
Lesko, 1985	Hospital case-control	510/727	Current 25+ vs. never smokers	0.9 (0.4–2.2)	0.5 (0.2–0.9)
Levi, 1987	Hospital case-control	357/1,122	Current vs. never smokers	0.5 (0.2–0.9)	0.4 (0.3–0.7)
Stockwell, 1987†	Hospital case-control	1,374/3,921	Current > 40 vs. never smokers	1.9 (0.5–7.8)	0.4 (0.2–0.8)

* Statistically significant test of trend reported.
† In this study the stratification categories were < 50 vs. 50 + years.

Hormone replacement therapy

Given the possibility that cigarette smoking is associated with hormone concentrations mostly among women who are taking HRT [52–54], one might speculate that an inverse association between smoking and endometrial cancer risk would be stronger among HRT users than among non-users. However, the results of studies that have examined the association between smoking and endometrial cancer risk according to HRT use [13, 17, 20, 29, 31, 50] have been equivocal in showing such a pattern (Table 30.5). Whereas two studies [13, 20] observed a larger reduction in risk among smokers taking HRT than among smokers not taking HRT, two other studies [17, 31] found no difference in the association according to HRT status, including a large prospective cohort study [31]. Finally, a prospective cohort study that examined associations only among women using HRT [50] showed no clear association among users of continuous combined HRT and cyclic combined HRT, and showed some suggestion of increased risk among smokers who used tibolone (perhaps more clearly among former-smokers). Thus, although effect modification by HRT status is biologically plausible, the available epidemiological evidence is equivocal.

Relative body weight

Obesity is an established risk factor for endometrial cancer [55]. Given the fact that smokers tend to have lower body mass indices than non-smokers (although former-smokers tend to have a higher BMI than current- or never-smokers) [4], two case-control studies have examined the association between cigarette smoking and endometrial cancer risk according to BMI [11, 20] (data not shown). Neither of these studies, one hospital-based [20] and one population-based [11], found any clear differences in the association between smoking and endometrial cancer risk according to BMI. Another study [17], a population-based case-control study of early stage endometrial cancer, observed that the inverse association with cigarette smoking tended to become stronger with increasing absolute rather than relative body weight.

Gene polymorphisms

Cigarette smoking and oestrogen are both thought to influence cancer risk through pathways that are under the control of specific genes, such as those involved in the formation of bulky DNA adducts by oestrogen metabolites [56] and both bulky and non-bulky adducts formed by carcinogens in tobacco smoke [57]. Therefore, studies have begun to examine the association between smoking and endometrial cancer risk according to genes that repair these types of DNA damage (Table 30.6). A moderately sized population-based case-control study found no clear effect modification according to certain polymorphisms in the Xeroderma pigmentosum group A (XPA) and Xeroderma pigmentosum group C (XPC) genes, both of which are involved in the nucleotide excision repair (NER) of bulky DNA adducts and may influence endometrial cancer risk [58]. A nested case-control study also showed no clear effect modification according to three polymorphisms in *cytochrome P-450 1A1* (*CYP1A1*) [59], a gene that encodes microsomal CYP1A1, which contributes to aryl hydrocarbon hydroxylase activity, catalyzing the metabolism of PAHs and other carcinogens found in tobacco smoke [60]. Finally, another nested case-control study showed some evidence that the association between smoking and endometrial cancer may vary according to a polymorphism (Ile143Val) in O^6-methylguanine DNA methyl-transferase (*MGMT*), which encodes a protein involved in the direct reversal repair (DRR) of DNA damage at the O^6-position of guanine, which can be caused by various exogenous alkylating agents including tobacco-specific nitrosamines [61]. MGMT may also bind with oestrogen receptors (ERs) and thereby inhibit ER-mediated cell proliferation [62]. Overall, studies that address the

Table 30.5 Epidemiological studies of cigarette smoking and endometrial cancer risk according to hormone replacement therapy (HRT) use

First author, study year	Study design	# Cases/controls (# in cohort)	Comparison	NO HRT OR (95% CI)	HRT OR (95% CI)
Terry, 2002	Prospective cohort	403/70,591	Current > 20 cigarettes/day vs. never	0.6 (0.4–1.0)*	0.6 (0.3–1.3)
Million women study collaborators; Beral, 2005	Prospective cohort	1320/716,738	Current smokers who last used continuous combined HRT	-------	1.1 (0.6–2.1)
			Non-current smokers who last used continuous combined HRT	-------	0.6 (0.5–0.8)
			Current smokers who last used cyclic combined HRT	-------	1.1 (0.7–1.7)
			Non-current smokers who last used cyclic combined HRT	-------	1.0 (0.9–1.2)
			Current smokers who last used tibolone	-------	1.6 (0.7–3.5)
			Non-current smokers who last used tibolone	-------	1.8 (1.4–2.3)
Al-Zoughool, 2007	Prospective cohort	619/249,986	Current vs. never smokers	0.6 (0.4–0.9)	0.8 (0.5–1.2)
Franks, 1987	Population case-control	79/416	Ever vs. never smokers	0.5 (0.3–0.9)	0.3 (0.1–0.8)
Lawrence, 1987	Population case-control	301/289	Current vs. never smokers	0.6 (NO CI)	0.6 (NO CI)
Weiss, 1980	Population case-control	322/289	Ever vs. never smokers	0.4 (0.2–0.7)	-------
Levi, 1987	Hospital case-control	357/1,122	Current vs. never smokers	0.5 (0.3–0.7)	0.2 (0.1–0.7)

* Statistically significant test of trend reported.

Table 30.6 Gene polymorphism, cigarette smoking and endometrial cancer risk

First author, study year	Study design	# Cases/controls (# in cohort)	Age range	Gene/genotype	Type polymorphism	Comparison	Smoking OR (95% CI)
Weiss, 2006	Case-control	371/420	50–69	XPA g23a genotype	gg	Never smokers	1.0 (ref)
					ga/aa		0.8 (0.5–1.2)*
					gg	Ever smokers	1.0 (ref)
					ga/aa		0.6 (0.4–0.9)*
					gg		0.7 (0.5–1.0)†
					ga/aa		0.4 (0.3–0.7)†
				XPC (A499V and K939Q)	0	Never smokers	1.0 (ref)
					1		0.9 (0.5–1.6)*
					2		0.6 (0.3–1.2)*
					0	Ever smokers	1.0 (ref)
					1		0.6 (0.3–1.0)*
					2		0.6 (0.3–1.1)*
					0		0.8 (0.4–1.8)†
					1		0.5 (0.3–0.9)†
					2		0.5 (0.2–1.0)†

Study	Design	Cases/Controls	Age	Gene/enzyme	Genotype	Smoking	OR (95% CI)
Han, 2006	Case-control (nested)	456/1,134	30–55	O⁶-methylguanine DNA methyltransferase (MGMT)	**Leu84Phe** non-carries	Never smokers	1.0 (ref)‡
						>0–30	0.9 (0.7–1.2)
						>30	0.7 (0.5–1.0)
					Leu84Phe carries	Never smokers	0.8 (0.5–1.2)
						>0–30	0.6 (0.4–0.9)
						>30	0.9 (0.4–1.7)
					Ile143Val non-carries	Never smokers	1.0 (ref)
						>0–30	0.8 (0.6–1.1)
						>30	0.9 (0.6–1.4)
					Ile143Val carries	Never smokers	1.1 (0.8–1.7)
						>0–30	0.9 (0.6–1.5)
						>30	0.4 (0.2–0.9)
McGrath, 2007	Case-control (nested)	456/1,134	30–55	Cytochrome P450 1A1 (CYP1A1) **MspI**	Wt/wt	Never smokers	1.0 (ref)§
						Former smokers	0.8 (0.6–1.0)
					Vt carrier		0.8 (0.4–1.4)
					Wt/wt	Current smokers	0.6 (0.4–0.9)
					Vt carrier		0.9 (0.4–2.0)
					Wt/wt	Never smokers	1.0 (ref)
						< 30 pack-year	0.7 (0.5–1.0)
					Vt carrier		0.8 (0.4–1.4)
						≥ 30 pack-year	

(Continued)

Table 30.6 (continued) Gene polymorphism, cigarette smoking and endometrial cancer risk

First author, study year	Study design	# Cases/controls (# in cohort)	Age range	Gene/genotype	Type polymorphism	Smoking Comparison	Smoking OR (95% CI)
					Wt/wt		0.7 (0.5–1.0)
					Vt carrier		0.9 (0.4–2.0)
					Thr461Asn	Never smokers	1.0 (ref)
						Former smokers	
					Ile/Ile		0.8 (0.6–1.1)
					Ile/Val + Val/Val		0.8 (0.3–2.0)
						Current smokers	
					Ile/Ile		0.7 (0.5–1.0)
					Ile/Val + Val/Val		0.5 (0.1–2.9)
						Never smokers	1.0 (ref)
						< 30 pack-year	
					Ile/Ile		0.8 (0.6–1.1)
					Ile/Val + Val/Val		0.6 (0.2–1.6)
						≥ 30 pack-year	
					Ile/Ile		0.7 (0.5–1.0)
					Ile/Val + Val/Val		1.5 (0.4–6.2)
					Ile462Val	Never smokers	1.0 (ref)
						Former smokers	
					Thr/Thr		0.9 (0.7–1.1)
					Thr/Asn + Asn/Asn		0.4 (0.2–0.9)
						Current smokers	
					Thr/Thr		0.7 (0.5–1.0)

Thr/Asn + Asn/Asn	0.5 (0.2–1.6)
Never smokers	1.0 (ref)
< 30 pack-year	
Thr/Thr	0.8 (0.6–1.1)
Thr/Asn + Asn/Asn	0.4 (0.2–1.0)
≥ 30 pack-year	
Thr/Thr	0.8 (0.5–1.1)
Thr/Asn + Asn/Asn	0.5 (0.2–1.3)

* Adjusted for age at reference date and county of residence.

† Postmenopausal estrogen use represents use for at least 6 months of unopposed oestrogens or oestrogens opposed by progestogens for < 10 days per month; women with at least 6 months use of other forms of postmenopausal hormone therapy are excluded from this analysis.

‡ Unconditional logistic regression adjusted for matching variables (age, menopausal status at blood draw, postmenopausal hormone use at blood draw, date at blood draw, time at blood draw, and fasting status at blood draw), and age at menarche, age at menopause, weight gain since 18, postmenopausal hormone use at diagnosis, parity, age at first birth, first-degree family history of endometrial cancer and colorectal cancer.

§ Unconditional logistic regression adjusted for matched factors: age, menopausal status at blood draw, postmenopausal hormone use at blood draw, date at blood draw, time at blood draw, and fasting status at blood draw.

association between smoking and endometrial cancer risk according to genotype are scarce, and these preliminary findings shown in Table 30.2 have yet to be confirmed by other studies.

Studies of cigarette smoking and blood hormone concentrations

Whether mediated through changes in the amount of adipose tissue, altered age at menopause, or anti-oestrogenic effects, blood hormone concentrations might be an important link between smoking and the reduced risk of endometrial cancer observed in most of the studies discussed above. The oestrogens that have typically been studied in relation to cigarette smoking include oestrone, sex hormone binding globulin (SHBG)-bound oestradiol, and estriol. Blood concentrations of androgens, typically androstenedione and dehydroepiandrosterone (DHEAS), have also been studied, because these are biological precursors of oestrone. Studies that have examined blood concentrations of SHBG are less common, and studies of unbound (free) oestradiol are scarce.

Smoking and blood oestrogen concentrations

Studies of cigarette smoking and blood hormone concentrations have been conducted mostly among postmenopausal women who were not taking HRT (Table 30.7). Of these studies, nine examined serum [8, 63–68] or plasma [69, 70] oestrone, ten examined serum [8, 63–68, 71] or plasma [69, 70] oestradiol, and two examined serum [63] or plasma [70] free oestradiol. As shown in Table 30.7, these studies have been consistent in showing little or no association between smoking and blood oestrogen concentrations among postmenopausal women who were not taking hormone replacement therapy. Among pre-menopausal women, three studies [70–72] found no clear association between cigarette smoking and oestrogen concentrations. Studies that adjusted hormone measurements for the effects of BMI (and other covariates) showed similar results to those that did not, suggesting that BMI is not a strong confounding variable in this association.

Two studies examined the association between cigarette smoking and blood oestrogen concentrations after randomization of women to groups receiving either oestradiol or placebo (Table 30.7) [52, 54]. In a small study of 25 postmenopausal women [52], unbound oestradiol was significantly lower among smokers than non-smokers both at baseline and shortly after taking micronized oestradiol orally. No important differences were observed between smokers and non-smokers in serum concentrations of either oestrone or bound oestradiol. In contrast, a study in which 110 postmenopausal women were randomized to take hormones (either orally or percutaneously) or a placebo [54], found that smokers had lower concentrations of both oestrone and bound oestradiol than non-smokers after oral (but not percutaneous) hormone treatment for at least one year (concentrations of free oestrogens were not examined). These results indicate that smoking might affect the absorption or metabolism of hormones used in replacement therapy.

Smoking and blood sex-hormone binding globulin concentrations

Of the five studies that have examined the association between cigarette smoking and serum [63, 67, 73] or plasma [69, 70] SHBG, none found any clear association (Table 30.7). However, one of these studies [69] found an inverse association between smoking and the ratio of bound oestradiol to SHBG, a measure of oestrogen activity. In this context, it is interesting to note that Cassidenti and colleagues [52] found that unbound (but not SHBG-bound) oestradiol was significantly lower among smokers than non-smokers both at baseline and after taking oral oestradiol, suggesting an increased SHBG-binding capacity in the women who smoked.

Table 30.7 Studies of cigarette smoking and blood hormone levels

First author, study year	Study population	Sex hormones examined	Major differences in blood hormone levels between smokers and non-smokers	Additional adjustment for BMI
Austin, 1993	209 postmenopausal women not taking HRT	Serum E1, E2, Δ⁴A	No major differences	Yes
Berta, 1992	694 premenopausal women with BMI < 25	Plasma E1, E2	No major differences	No
Cassidenti, 1990	25 postmenopausal women randomized to take 1 or 2 mg micronized E2	Serum E1, E2, unbound E2, SHBG	Unbound E2 (lower) and SHBG-binding capacity (higher) in smokers.	Randomization
Cassidenti, 1992	38 postmenopausal women not taking HRT	Serum E1, E2, SHBG, non-SHBG-bound E2, Δ⁴A, DHEAS	Δ⁴A (higher) and DHEAS (higher) in smokers	Yes
Cauley, 1989	143 postmenopausal women not taking HRT	Serum E1, E2, Δ⁴A	Δ⁴A (higher) in smokers	Yes
Friedman, 1987	25 postmenopausal women not taking HRT	Serum E1, E2, Δ⁴A, DHEAS	Δ⁴A (higher) and DHEAS (higher) in smokers	Yes
Jensen, 1985	136 postmenopausal women randomized to 4mg, 2 mg, or 1 mg E2, or placebo	Serum E1, E2	E1 (lower) and E2 (lower) in smokers	Randomization
Jensen, 1988	110 postmenopausal women randomized to oral or percutaneous E2 or placebo	Serum E1, E2	E1 (lower) and E2 (lower) in smokers after oral E2	Randomization
Key, 1991	147 pre- and postmenopausal women not taking HRT	Serum E2, DHEAS	No major differences	Yes
Khaw, 1988	233 postmenopausal women not taking HRT	Plasma DHEAS, Δ⁴A, E1, E2, SHBG	Δ⁴A (higher) and DHEAS (higher) in smokers	Yes
Lapidus, 1986	253 postmenopausal women not taking HRT	Serum SHBG	No major differences	Yes
Law, 1997	1,219 pre- and postmenopausal women not taking HRT	Serum E1, E2, Δ⁴A, DHEAS, SHBG	No major differences	Yes
Longcope, 1988	88 pre- and postmenopausal women not taking HRT	Plasma Δ⁴A, E1, E2, free E2, SHBG	Δ⁴A (higher) in smokers	Yes
Michnovicz, 1986	27 premenopausal women not taking HRT, BMI < 25	2-hydroxylation of injected radiolabelled E2	2-hydroxylation of E2 (higher) in smokers	No
Schlemmer, 1990	267 women in the early postmenopause	Serum E1, E2, Δ⁴A	Δ⁴A (higher) in smokers	No
Slemenda, 1989	84 peri- and postmenopausal women	Serum E1, E2, Δ⁴A	Δ⁴A (higher) in smokers	No

Abbreviations: E1 (oestrone), E2 (oestradiol), Δ⁴A (androstenedione), DHEAS (dehydroepiandrosterone), SHBG (sex-hormone binding globulin), HRT (hormone replacement therapy), BMI (body mass index).

Smoking and blood androgen concentrations

In postmenopausal women, androgens are the major source of oestrone, converted through an aromatization process in fat deposits. Thus, adiposity is positively correlated with oestrogen concentrations in postmenopausal women. Of the nine studies that examined blood concentrations of androstenedione in smokers [8, 63–70], all found higher circulating concentrations among current- than never- or former-smokers (Table 30.7). However, these same studies did not show clear variation in blood oestrone concentrations by smoking status, perhaps suggesting a reduced conversion of androstenedione to oestrone among smokers. Of the five studies that have examined cigarette smoking and DHEAS concentrations, three [63, 65, 69] found increased blood concentrations among current-smokers, whereas the other two [67, 71] found no clear differences according to smoking status.

Studies of cigarette smoking and urinary hormone concentrations

Seven studies have examined cigarette smoking and urinary oestrogen concentrations [72, 74–79] (Table 30.8), and of these, three found no major differences according to smoking status [72, 76, 79]. The remaining four studies each showed lower urinary estriol concentrations among smokers than non-smokers, but mixed results for urinary oestrone and oestradiol [74, 75, 77, 78]. The results of two of these studies [76, 78] showed lower concentrations of 2-hydroxyestrone among smokers than non-smokers.

Studies of cigarette smoking and age at menopause

Age at natural menopause varies substantially under the influence of genetic and environmental factors [80]. A relatively early age at menopause has been associated with reduced risk of endometrial cancer [3–5, 15]. For example, a one year decrease in age at menopause has been associated approximately with a 7% decrease in risk [15]. In this regard, it has been proposed that cigarette smoking decreases the age at natural menopause [4], and might reduce endometrial cancer risk through reduced exposure to endogenous oestrogens. A recent review of this literature suggests that smoking does indeed decrease the age at natural menopause, more clearly with qualitative than qualitative smoking measures [81]. Although this review did not provide a summary estimate of the difference in age at menopause, we previously noted that studies have shown that, on average, smokers have menopause approximately 1–1.5 years earlier than non-smokers [6]. We also note that there have been no clear differences in the results of studies that adjusted estimates for obesity (and other covariates) compared with those that did not.

Comments

The results of at least 42 epidemiological studies to date suggest that current or recent smoking is associated with a small to moderate decreased risk of endometrial cancer, particularly among postmenopausal women who smoked for many years at high intensity. Associations between cigarette smoking and increased risk of osteoporosis [4, 5, 53, 54], and attenuated effects of HRT among smokers [54], suggest an 'anti-oestrogenic' effect of smoking [4, 5]. However, circulating concentrations of oestrogen generally do not differ according to categories of cigarette smoking.

Regarding the effects of smoking on oestrogenic profiles, the type, rather than the absolute concentrations, of circulating oestrogens may be important. In particular, smoking may increase oestradiol 2-hydroxylation, which has been observed to decrease mammary epithelial proliferation rates in experimental studies [82]. Although active smokers and non-smokers may have the

Table 30.8 Studies of cigarette smoking and urinary hormone levels

First author, study year	Study population	Sex hormones examined	Differences in urinary hormone excretion levels between smokers and non-smokers	Additional adjustment for BMI
Bernstein, 2000	16 postmenopausal women before and after taking 2 mg per os/d E2	Urinary E1, E2, E3, 16αOHE$_1$, 2OHE$_1$	E1 and E3 (lower), E2 and 2OHE$_1$ (higher) in smokers after treatment	No
Berta, 1992	694 premenopausal women, BMI < 25	Urinary E1, E2, E3	No major differences	No
Key, 1996	367 pre- and postmenopausal women	Urinary E1, E2, E3	E3 (lower) in postmenopausal smokers	Yes
MacMahon, 1982	106 premenopausal women not taking HRT	Urinary E1, E2, E3	E1, E2, E3 (lower) in smokers in the luteal phase of the menstrual cycle	No
Michnovicz, 1988	29 premenopausal women not taking HRT, BMI < 25	Urinary E1, E2, E3, 16αOHE$_1$, 2OHE$_1$	E3 (lower) and 2OHE$_1$ (higher) in smokers	No
Michnovicz, 1986	27 premenopausal women not taking HRT, BMI < 25	Urinary E1, E3	E3 (lower) and the ratio of E3 to E1 (lower) in smokers	No
Trichopoulos, 1987	220 postmenopausal women not taking HRT	Urinary E1, E2, E3	No major differences	Height and Weight

Abbreviations: E1 (oestrone), E2 (oestradiol), E3 (oestriol), 16α-OEH1 (16alpha-hydroxyoestrone), 2-OEH1 (2-hydroxyoestrone), HRT (hormone replacement therapy), BMI (body mass index).

same concentrations of oestrogens overall, smokers might have a lower concentration of more biologically active oestrogens (primarily 16-alpha-hydroxyestrone). One study [75] has directly examined 2-hydroxylation in relation to cigarette smoking, finding a 50% increased oestradiol 2-hydroxylation in premenopausal women who smoked at least 15 cigarettes per day compared with non-smokers. Although based on relatively small sample sizes, the findings of lowered concentrations of urinary estriol, and increased urinary 2-OEH1, among smokers observed in two studies [76, 78] may support the hypothesis that smoking decreases the formation of active oestrogen metabolites along the 16-alpha-hydroxylation pathway.

Because adipose tissue is the main determinant of oestrogen concentrations among postmenopausal women, and is inversely associated with smoking, BMI may partly mediate the inverse association between cigarette smoking and oestrogen. Most studies have adjusted for current BMI, although more relevant measures may include changes in body weight over time, waist-to-hip ratio, or duration of obesity. In addition, smoking appears to lower the age at which women reach menopause by an average of about 1–1.5 years, an association that seems to weaken with time since smoking cessation. Statistical adjustment for the effects of age at menopause generally has not altered the inverse associations between smoking and endometrial cancer risk. Whereas a lower average body weight and earlier age at menopause among current-smokers compared with non-smokers certainly mediates some of the inverse association between smoking and endometrial cancer risk, the extent of this mediation remains unclear.

Effect-modification may provide clues to the mechanisms underlying associations observed in epidemiological studies. However, the data regarding effect modification of the association between cigarette smoking and endometrial cancer risk by other factors remain equivocal. On the one hand, 11 studies have shown a reduced endometrial cancer risk with current smoking that is stronger among, or limited to, postmenopausal women [10, 19, 24, 28, 34], women using HRT [13, 20, 29], parous women [31], and women who are obese [10, 17]. On the other hand, nine studies have failed to demonstrate important differences in the association according to menopausal status [17, 20, 31], obesity [20, 31], or HRT use [10, 17, 28, 31].

In summary, the available data suggest that cigarette smoking is associated with reduced risk of endometrial cancer among current-smokers, mainly among postmenopausal women, and that the association weakens with time since quitting. Studies that examined quantitative measures of exposure to cigarette smoke have shown greater reductions in risk among women who were current-smokers and smoked either more intensely or for a longer duration than women who smoked relatively less. The mechanisms by which this association may be driven remain unclear.

References

1. Parkin, D.M., Bray, F., Ferlay, J. and Pisani, P. (2002). Global cancer statistics, *CA Cancer J Clin* 2005, **55**: 74–108.

2. IARC, (1999). *IARC monograph on the evaluation of carcinogenic risks to humans, vol. 72. Hormonal contraception and postmenopausal hormonal therapy*. IARC, Lyon.

3. Akhmedkhanov, A., Zeleniuch-Jacquotte, A. and Toniolo, P. (2001). Role of exogenous and endogenous hormones in endometrial cancer: review of the evidence and research perspectives. *Ann N Y Acad Sci*, **943**: 296–315.

4. Baron, J.A., La Vecchia, C. and Levi, F. (1990). The antiestrogenic effect of cigarette smoking in women. *Am J Obstet Gynecol*, **162**: 502–514.

5. Baron, J.A. (1984). Smoking and estrogen-related disease. *Am J Epidemiol*, **119**: 9–22.

6. Terry, P., Rohan, T.E., Franceschi, S. and Weiderpass, E. (2004). Endometrial cancer. In: P. Boyle, N. Gray, J. Henningfield, J. Seffrin, W. Zatonski (eds) *Tobacco: Science, Policy and Public Health*. Oxford University Press.

7. Terry, P.D., Rohan, T.E., Franceschi, S. and Weiderpass, E. (2002). Cigarette smoking and the risk of endometrial cancer. *Lancet Oncol*, **3**: 470–480.

8. Austin, H., Drews, C. and Partridge, E.E. (1993). A case-control study of endometrial cancer in relation to cigarette smoking, serum estrogen levels, and alcohol use. *Am J Obstet Gynecol*, **169**: 1086–1091.

9. Baron, J.A., Byers, T., Greenberg, E.R., Cummings, K.M. and Swanson, M. (1986). Cigarette smoking in women with cancers of the breast and reproductive organs. *J Natl Cancer Inst*, **77**: 677–680.

10. Brinton, L.A., Barrett, R.J., Berman, M.L., Mortel, R., Twiggs, L.B. and Wilbanks, G.D. (1993). Cigarette smoking and the risk of endometrial cancer. *Am J Epidemiol*, **137**: 281–291.

11. Elliott, E.A., Matanoski, G.M., Rosenshein, N.B., Grumbine, F.C. and Diamond, E.L. (1990). Body fat patterning in women with endometrial cancer. *Gynecol Oncol*, **39**: 253–258.

12. Engeland, A., Andersen, A., Haldorsen, T. and Tretli, S. (1996). Smoking habits and risk of cancers other than lung cancer: 28 years' follow-up of 26 000 Norwegian men and women. *Cancer Causes Control*, **7**: 497–506.

13. Franks, A.L., Kendrick, J.S. and Tyler, C.W., Jr. (1987). Postmenopausal smoking, estrogen replacement therapy, and the risk of endometrial cancer. *Am J Obstet Gynecol*, **156**: 20–23.

14. Goodman, M.T., Hankin, J.H., Wilkens, L.R., Lyu, L.C., McDuffie, K., Liu, L.Q. *et al.* (1997). Diet, body size, physical activity, and the risk of endometrial cancer. *Cancer Res*, **57**: 5077–5085.

15. Kelsey, J.L., LiVolsi, V.A., Holford, T.R., Fischer, D.B., Mostow, E.D., Schwartz, P.E. *et al.* (1982). A case-control study of cancer of the endometrium. *Am J Epidemiol*, **116**: 333–342.

16. Koumantaki, Y., Tzonou, A., Koumantakis, E., Kaklamani, E., Aravantinos, D. and Trichopoulos, D. (1989). A case-control study of cancer of endometrium in Athens. *Int J Cancer*, **43**: 795–799.

17. Lawrence, C., Tessaro, I., Durgerian, S., Caputo, T., Richart, R., Jacobson, H. *et al.* (1987). Smoking, body weight, and early-stage endometrial cancer. *Cancer*, **59**: 1665–1669.

18. Lawrence, C., Tessaro, I., Durgerian, S., Caputo, T., Richart, R.M. and Greenwald, P. (1989). Advanced-stage endometrial cancer: contributions of estrogen use, smoking, and other risk factors. *Gynecol Oncol*, **32**: 41–45.

19. Lesko, S.M., Rosenberg, L., Kaufman, D.W., Helmrich, S.P., Miller, D.R., Strom, B. *et al.* (1985). Cigarette smoking and the risk of endometrial cancer. *N Engl J Med*, **313**: 593–596.

20. Levi, F., la Vecchia, C. and Decarli, A. (1987). Cigarette smoking and the risk of endometrial cancer. *Eur J Cancer Clin Oncol*, **23**: 1025–1029.

21. Jain, M.G., Howe, G.R. and Rohan, T.E. (2000). Nutritional factors and endometrial cancer in Ontario, Canada. *Cancer Control*, **7**: 288–296.

22. McCann, S.E., Freudenheim, J.L., Marshall, J.R., Brasure, J.R., Swanson, M.K. and Graham, S. (2000). Diet in the epidemiology of endometrial cancer in western New York (United States). *Cancer Causes Control*, **11**: 965–974.

23. Rubin, G.L., Peterson, H.B., Lee, N.C., Maes, E.F., Wingo, P.A. and Becker, S. (1990). Estrogen replacement therapy and the risk of endometrial cancer: remaining controversies. *Am J Obstet Gynecol*, **162**: 148–154.

24. Smith, E.M., Sowers, M.F. and Burns, T.L., (1984). Effects of smoking on the development of female reproductive cancers. *J Natl Cancer Inst*, **73**: 371–376.

25. Stockwell, H.G. and Lyman, G.H., (1987). Cigarette smoking and the risk of female reproductive cancer. *Am J Obstet Gynecol*, **157**: 35–40.

26. Terry, P., Baron, J.A., Weiderpass, E., Yuen, J., Lichtenstein, P. and Nyren, O., (1999). Lifestyle and endometrial cancer risk: a cohort study from the Swedish Twin Registry. *Int J Cancer*, **82**: 38–42.

27. Tyler, C.W., Jr., Webster, L.A., Ory, H.W. and Rubin, G.L., (1985). Endometrial cancer: how does cigarette smoking influence the risk of women under age 55 years having this tumor? *Am J Obstet Gynecol*, **151**: 899–905.

28. Weiderpass, E. and Baron, J.A., (2001). Cigarette smoking, alcohol consumption, and endometrial cancer risk: a population-based study in Sweden. *Cancer Causes Control*, **12**: 239–247.

29. Weiss, N.S., Farewall, V.T., Szekely, D.R., English, D.R. and Kiviat, N. (1980). Oestrogens and endometrial cancer: effect of other risk factors on the association. *Maturitas*, **2**: 185–190.

30. Williams, R.R. and Horm, J.W. (1977). Association of cancer sites with tobacco and alcohol consumption and socioeconomic status of patients: interview study from the Third National Cancer Survey. *J Natl Cancer Inst*, **58**: 525–547.

31. Terry, P., Miller, A. B., Rohan, T.E. (in press). A prospective cohort study of cigarette smoking and the risk of endometrial cancer. *Br J Cancer*.

32. Shields, T.S., Weiss, N.S., Voigt, L.F. and Beresford, S.A. (1999). The additional risk of endometrial cancer associated with unopposed estrogen use in women with other risk factors. *Epidemiology*, **10**: 733–738.

33. Newcomer, L.M., Newcomb, P.A., Trentham-Dietz, A. and Storer, B.E. (2001). Hormonal risk factors for endometrial cancer: modification by cigarette smoking (United States). *Cancer Causes Control*, **12**: 829–835.

34. Al-Zoughool, M., Dossus, L., Kaaks, R., Clavel-Chapelon, F., Tjonneland, A., Olsen, A. *et al.* (2007). Risk of endometrial cancer in relationship to cigarette smoking: results from the EPIC study. *Int J Cancer*, **121**: 2741–2747.

35. Bjorge, T., Engeland, A., Tretli, S. and Weiderpass, E. (2007). Body size in relation to cancer of the uterine corpus in 1 million Norwegian women. *Int J Cancer*, **120**: 378–383.

36. Folsom, A.R., Demissie, Z. and Harnack, L. (2003). Glycemic index, glycemic load, and incidence of endometrial cancer: the Iowa women's health study. *Nutr Cancer*, **46**: 119–124.

37. Furberg, A.S. and Thune, I. (2003). Metabolic abnormalities (hypertension, hyperglycemia and overweight), lifestyle (high energy intake and physical inactivity) and endometrial cancer risk in a Norwegian cohort. *Int J Cancer*, **104**: 669–676.

38. Lacey, J.V., Jr., Leitzmann, M.F., Chang, S.C., Mouw, T., Hollenbeck, A.R., Schatzkin, A. *et al.* (2007). Endometrial cancer and menopausal hormone therapy in the National Institutes of Health-AARP Diet and Health Study cohort. *Cancer*, **109**: 1303–1311.

39. Lindemann, K., Vatten, L.J., Ellstrom-Engh, M. and Eskild, A. (2008). Body mass, diabetes and smoking, and endometrial cancer risk: a follow-up study. *Br J Cancer*, **98**: 1582–1585.

40. Loerbroks, A., Schouten, L.J., Goldbohm, R.A. and van den Brandt, P.A. (2007). Alcohol consumption, cigarette smoking, and endometrial cancer risk: results from the Netherlands Cohort Study. *Cancer Causes Control*, **18**: 551–560.

41. Matthews, C.E., Xu, W.H., Zheng, W., Gao, Y.T., Ruan, Z.X., Cheng, J.R. *et al.* (2005). Physical activity and risk of endometrial cancer: a report from the Shanghai endometrial cancer study. *Cancer Epidemiol Biomarkers Prev*, **14**: 779–785.

42. Newcomb, P.A. and Trentham-Dietz, A. (2003). Patterns of postmenopausal progestin use with estrogen in relation to endometrial cancer (United States). *Cancer Causes Control*, **14**: 195–201.

43. Okamura, C., Tsubono, Y., Ito, K., Niikura, H., Takano, T., Nagase, S. (2006). Lactation and risk of endometrial cancer in Japan: a case-control study. *Tohoku J Exp Med*, **208**: 109–115.

44. Petridou, E., Koukoulomatis, P., Dessypris, N., Karalis, D., Michalas, S. and Trichopoulos, D. (2002). Why is endometrial cancer less common in Greece than in other European Union countries? *Eur J Cancer Prev*, **11**: 427–432.

45. Setiawan, V.W., Pike, M.C., Kolonel, L.N., Nomura, A.M., Goodman, M.T. and Henderson, B.E. (2007). Racial/ethnic differences in endometrial cancer risk: the multiethnic cohort study. *Am J Epidemiol*, **165**: 262–270.

46. Strom, B.L., Schinnar, R., Weber, A.L., Bunin, G., Berlin, J.A., Baumgarten, M. *et al.* (2006). Case-control study of postmenopausal hormone replacement therapy and endometrial cancer. *Am J Epidemiol*, **164**: 775–786.

47. Trentham-Dietz, A., Nichols, H.B., Hampton, J.M. and Newcomb, P.A. (2006). Weight change and risk of endometrial cancer. *Int J Epidemiol*, **35**: 151–158.

48. Viswanathan, A.N., Feskanich, D., De Vivo, I., Hunter, D.J., Barbieri, R.L., Rosner, B. *et al.* (2005). Smoking and the risk of endometrial cancer: results from the Nurses' Health Study. *Int J Cancer*, **114**: 996–1001.

49. Weiss, J.M., Weiss, N.S., Ulrich, C.M., Doherty, J.A. and Chen, C. (2006). Nucleotide excision repair genotype and the incidence of endometrial cancer: effect of other risk factors on the association. *Gynecol Oncol*, **103**: 891–896.

50. Beral, V., Bull, D. and Reeves, G. (2005). Endometrial cancer and hormone-replacement therapy in the Million Women Study. *Lancet*, **365**: 1543–1551.

51. Weiss, J.M., Saltzman, B.S., Doherty, J.A., Voigt, L.F., Chen, C., Beresford, S.A. *et al.* (2006). Risk factors for the incidence of endometrial cancer according to the aggressiveness of disease. *Am J Epidemiol*, **164**: 56–62.

52. Cassidenti, D.L., Vijod, A.G., Vijod, M.A., Stanczyk, F.Z. and Lobo, R.A. (1990). Short-term effects of smoking on the pharmacokinetic profiles of micronized estradiol in postmenopausal women. *Am J Obstet Gynecol*, **163**: 1953–1960.

53. Jensen, J., Christiansen, C. and Rodbro, P. (1985). Cigarette smoking, serum estrogens, and bone loss during hormone-replacement therapy early after menopause. *N Engl J Med*, **313**: 973–975.

54. Jensen, J. and Christiansen, C. (1988). Effects of smoking on serum lipoproteins and bone mineral content during postmenopausal hormone replacement therapy. *Am J Obstet Gynecol*, **159**: 820–825.

55. IARC (2002). *IARC handbook of cancer prevention, vol. 6. Weight control and physical activity.* IARC Press, International Agency for Research on Cancer, Lyon.

56. Cavalieri, E., Frenkel, K., Liehr, J.G., Rogan, E. and Roy, D., (2000). Estrogens as endogenous genotoxic agents–DNA adducts and mutations. *J Natl Cancer Inst Monogr*, 75–93.

57. Terry, P.D. and Rohan, T.E., (2002). Cigarette smoking and the risk of breast cancer in women: a review of the literature. *Cancer Epidemiol Biomarkers Prev*, **11**: 953–971.

58. Weiss, J.M., Weiss, N.S., Ulrich, C.M., Doherty, J.A., Voigt, L.F. and Chen, C. (2005). Interindividual variation in nucleotide excision repair genes and risk of endometrial cancer. *Cancer Epidemiol Biomarkers Prev*, **14**: 2524–2530.

59. McGrath, M., Hankinson, S.E. and De Vivo, I., (2007). Cytochrome P450 1A1, cigarette smoking, and risk of endometrial cancer (United States). *Cancer Causes Control*, **18**: 1123–1130.

60. Masson, L.F., Sharp, L., Cotton, S.C. and Little, J. (2005). Cytochrome P-450 1A1 gene polymorphisms and risk of breast cancer: a HuGE review. *Am J Epidemiol*, **161**: 901–915.

61. Margison, G.P., Santibanez Koref, M.F. and Povey, A.C. (2002). Mechanisms of carcinogenicity/chemotherapy by O6-methylguanine. *Mutagenesis*, **17**: 483–487.

62. Teo, A.K., Oh, H.K., Ali, R.B. and Li, B.F. (2001). The modified human DNA repair enzyme O(6)-methylguanine-DNA methyltransferase is a negative regulator of estrogen receptor-mediated transcription upon alkylation DNA damage. *Mol Cell Biol*, **21**: 7105–7114.

63. Cassidenti, D.L., Pike, M.C., Vijod, A.G., Stanczyk, F.Z. and Lobo, R.A. (1992). A reevaluation of estrogen status in postmenopausal women who smoke. *Am J Obstet Gynecol*, **166**: 1444–1448.

64. Cauley, J.A., Gutai, J.P., Kuller, L.H., LeDonne, D. and Powell, J.G. (1989). The epidemiology of serum sex hormones in postmenopausal women. *Am J Epidemiol*, **129**: 1120–1131.

65. Friedman, A.J., Ravnikar, V.A. and Barbieri, R.L., (1987). Serum steroid hormone profiles in postmenopausal smokers and nonsmokers. *Fertil Steril*, **47**: 398–401.

66. Schlemmer, A., Jensen, J., Riis, B.J. and Christiansen, C. (1990). Smoking induces increased androgen levels in early post-menopausal women. *Maturitas*, **12**: 99–104.

67. Law, M.R., Cheng, R., Hackshaw, A.K., Allaway, S. and Hale, A.K. (1997). Cigarette smoking, sex hormones and bone density in women. *Eur J Epidemiol*, **13**: 553–558.

68. Slemenda, C.W., Hui, S.L., Longcope, C. and Johnston, C.C., Jr. (1989). Cigarette smoking, obesity, and bone mass. *J Bone Miner Res*, **4**: 737–741.

69. Khaw, K.T., Tazuke, S. and Barrett-Connor, E., (1988). Cigarette smoking and levels of adrenal androgens in postmenopausal women. *N Engl J Med*, **318**: 1705–1709.

70. Longcope, C. and Johnston, C.C., Jr. (1988). Androgen and estrogen dynamics in pre- and postmenopausal women: a comparison between smokers and nonsmokers. *J Clin Endocrinol Metab*, **67**: 379–383.

71. Key, T.J., Pike, M.C., Baron, J.A., Moore, J.W., Wang, D.Y., Thomas, B.S. *et al.* (1991). Cigarette smoking and steroid hormones in women. *J Steroid Biochem Mol Biol*, **39**: 529–534.

72. Berta, L., Frairia, R., Fortunati, N., Fazzari, A. and Gaidano, G., (1992). Smoking effects on the hormonal balance of fertile women. *Horm Res*, **37**: 45–48.

73. Lapidus, L., Lindstedt, G., Lundberg, P.A., Bengtsson, C. and Gredmark, T., (1986). Concentrations of sex-hormone binding globulin and corticosteroid binding globulin in serum in relation to cardiovascular risk factors and to 12-year incidence of cardiovascular disease and overall mortality in postmenopausal women. *Clin Chem*, **32**: 146–152.

74. MacMahon, B., Trichopoulos, D., Cole, P. and Brown, J., (1982). Cigarette smoking and urinary estrogens. *N Engl J Med*, **307**: 1062–1065.

75. Michnovicz, J.J., Hershcopf, R.J., Naganuma, H., Bradlow, H.L. and Fishman, J., (1986). Increased 2-hydroxylation of estradiol as a possible mechanism for the anti-estrogenic effect of cigarette smoking. *N Engl J Med*, **315**: 1305–1309.

76. Michnovicz, J.J., Naganuma, H., Hershcopf, R.J., Bradlow, H.L. and Fishman, J., (1988). Increased urinary catechol estrogen excretion in female smokers. *Steroids*, **52**: 69–83.

77. Key, T.J., Pike, M.C., Brown, J.B., Hermon, C., Allen, D.S. and Wang, D.Y., (1996). Cigarette smoking and urinary oestrogen excretion in premenopausal and post-menopausal women. *Br J Cancer*, **74**: 1313–1316.

78. Berstein, L.M., Tsyrlina, E.V., Kolesnik, O.S., Gamajunova, V.B. and Adlercreutz, H., (2000). Catecholestrogens excretion in smoking and non-smoking postmenopausal women receiving estrogen replacement therapy. *J Steroid Biochem Mol Biol*, **72**: 143–147.

79. Trichopoulos, D., Brown, J. and MacMahon, B., (1987). Urine estrogens and breast cancer risk factors among post-menopausal women. *Int J Cancer*, **40**: 721–725.

80. McKinlay, S.M., (1996). The normal menopause transition: an overview. *Maturitas*, **23**: 137–145.

81. Parente, R.C., Faerstein, E., Celeste, R.K. and Werneck, G.L., (2008). The relationship between smoking and age at the menopause: A systematic review. *Maturitas*, **61**: 287–298.

82. Bradlow, H.L., Telang, N.T., Sepkovic, D.W. and Osborne, M.P., (1996). 2-hydroxyestrone: the 'good' estrogen. *J Endocrinol*, **150** Suppl: S259–265.

Chapter 31

Tobacco and cardiovascular disease

Konrad Jamrozik

Introduction

At the level of the whole population, tobacco causes far more harm via its contribution to cardio-vascular disease (CVD) than it does through its effects on either the risk of lung cancer or of chronic obstructive pulmonary disease (COPD). This occurs because, in the absence of smoking, lung cancer and COPD are both very rare conditions. CVD, by contrast, is now the commonest cause of death of *Homo sapiens* (World Health Organization 1999). Thus, for a given prevalence of smoking in a population, the small increase in risk of CVD, in relative terms, that is associated with smoking generates many additional cases of CVD. By contrast, the much larger relative risks for lung cancer and COPD associated with smoking generate fewer additional cases of these conditions because these risks are applied to 'background' incidence rates that are much lower than the lifetime risk of CVD in non-smokers (Wald 1978).

Nevertheless, and despite some relationship between smoking and heart disease having been described for at least a century (Bruce 1901), more than twenty years elapsed between publication of the original report on the effects of smoking and health by the Royal College of Physicians of London (1962), which concentrated on lung cancer, and the appearance of a report from the Surgeon-General of the United States dedicated to the adverse effects of smoking on the cardio-vascular system (United States Department of Health and Human Services 1983). Even the latter report is remarkable for the number of aspects of CVD about which information on the impact of smoking was either entirely lacking or inadequate to draw firm conclusions. This emphasizes how much more was learnt about active smoking and CVD in the last two decades of the twentieth century. That picture is now very close to complete, although, as this chapter will show, some significant questions remain unanswered and, arguably, we have yet to distil all of the lessons that might be taught by the knowledge that we have available.

To some extent, history has repeated itself in relation to passive smoking. The first reports of an increased incidence of major respiratory illness in infants and children who were passive smokers appeared in the English-language literature in 1974 (Colley *et al.* 1974; Harlap and Davies 1974), and data implicating passive smoking as a cause of lung cancer in adults were first published in 1981 (Hiryama 1981; Trichopoulos *et al.* 1981). However, another four years elapsed before equivalent studies of CVD appeared (Garland *et al.* 1985), even though a literature on the short-term consequences of passive smoking for cardiovascular function had been amassing since at least 1969 (Ayres *et al.* 1969). This chapter will demonstrate that after more than three decades of research, the epidemiological picture of passive smoking and CVD is still far from complete.

Scope of this chapter

Although the cardiovascular system has both arterial and venous sides, the emphasis here is on arterial disease related to smoking, and on the similarities and differences of the effects of smoking on disease in the four principal arterial 'territories'—those in the head (cerebrovascular tree), heart (coronary arterial tree), abdomen (principally the aorta, but also the mesenteric arteries supplying the gut), and legs (peripheral arterial tree). The corresponding conditions of principal interest are: cerebrovascular disease (CeVD), including stroke and transient cerebral ischaemic attack (TIA); ischaemic heart disease (IHD), including acute myocardial infarction (AMI); abdominal aortic aneurysm (AAA); and peripheral arterial disease (PAD).

The coronary equivalent of TIA is angina pectoris, transient chest pain that is classically brought on by exercise and relieved by rest before permanent damage is done to the muscle of the heart (which is what does occur in AMI, commonly known as 'heart attack'). The peripheral arterial equivalent of TIA and angina is intermittent claudication (IC), cramping pain in the muscles of the calf, thigh, or buttock that also is brought on by exercise, and specifically walking, and is relieved by rest. In contrast to angina and IC, the precipitants of TIA are not well understood, but the syndrome is analogous insofar as there is a temporary disruption of neurological function that is ascribed to a shortterm inadequacy in the supply of blood to part of the brain, relative to its needs, and the symptoms resolve before obvious permanent damage is done to the underlying tissue.

One approach to this chapter would be to consider smoking and disease in each of the four principal arterial territories in turn. However, the material has instead been organized according to the criteria proposed by Sir Austin Bradford Hill for assessing whether statistical associations are likely to reflect underlying causal relationships (Hill 1965). As will become apparent, this allows us to see quickly not only areas of research where the volume of knowledge is such that we can safely regard a particular question as definitively answered, but also where unanswered questions remain or where persisting inconsistencies should cause us to think again about what we hold to be the underlying biological mechanisms. In addition, the Bradford Hill criteria have proved very useful as a framework for evaluating the emerging evidence regarding passive smoking and disease where, in general, the effects of exposure on risk are much smaller than for active smoking (National Health and Medical Research Council 1997) but the policy response throws into sharp focus issues surrounding the right of society to curtail the 'private' behaviour of individuals in public places and workplaces.

With the literature on smoking and health now running to tens of thousands of scientific papers, any review, even one restricted to a particular subset of diseases, is necessarily selective. In the case of active smoking, the references cited here are a mixture of citations of some of the best-known studies and of work conducted by the author in Perth, Western Australia. At first sight, the latter might seem an obscure choice, but it has been made for two reasons. First, Perth is one of few communities worldwide where the same methods have been used to assess the impact of active smoking on disease in each of the four principal arterial territories identified above, ascertainment of all of the cases and selection of control subjects have both been population-based, and internationally agreed criteria have been used to define cases. Framingham, Massachusetts, is another such community (Dawber 1980), but after more than fifty years of study, the numbers of events of the more uncommon arterial syndromes experienced by an inception cohort of just 5209 individuals is still too small to be statistically meaningful. Application of the same methods of enquiry to mathematically informative numbers of events in the different arterial territories in members of the same population provides a firmer basis on which to judge similarities and differences in relationships than does drawing together information from different communities that are widely dispersed in space and time.

The second reason for giving prominence to work from Western Australia is that the context of the investigations, in terms of prevailing patterns and trends in smoking, is well documented. Many of the 'classical' studies of health and smoking were begun, if not also completed, in settings where unfiltered cigarettes dominated the local market and the prevalence of smoking was very high in men and still rising sharply in women. This might beg the question as to how relevant are the findings now when, internationally, filtered cigarettes are completing their takeover of virtually all markets for tobacco products. Set against a background of stable or rising prevalences of smoking, the 'classical' studies probably are relevant to many developing countries now, where the uptake of smoking by both sexes still continues. However, for some time the prevalence of smoking has been falling significantly in many developed countries, especially in the Englishspeaking world and Scandinavia (Molarius *et al.* 2001). Perth is representative of such settings (Macfarlane and Jamrozik 1993), and therefore potentially much more informative as to the risks associated with modern patterns of smoking of modern cigarettes.

After examining the evidence regarding active and passive smoking and arterial disease, this chapter briefly considers effects of smoking on the venous system before closing with a section identifying a relatively small number of areas where further research on smoking and CVD might be worthwhile.

The Bradford Hill criteria

The decision having been taken to organize the information on smoking and arterial disease according to the Bradford Hill criteria, it becomes necessary to introduce those criteria in their own right.

Sir Austin Bradford Hill was an eminent statistician whose long list of accomplishments includes involvement in the original Medical Research Council trial of streptomycin for tuberculosis (Medical Research Council 1948), publication, with Sir Richard Doll, of the first English case–control studies of smoking and lung cancer (Doll and Hill 1950, 1952), and establishment, again with Doll, of the long-running cohort study of smoking in British doctors (Doll *et al.* 1980, 1994). His criteria for assisting judgements about the likelihood of causal relationships explaining associations seen in observational data were published in 1965, with the original paper emphasizing that, as a true experiment, a randomized controlled trial involving human subjects should always provide the best evidence for answering such questions (Hill 1965). The criteria are listed and briefly explained in Table 31.1. Various other individuals and groups have proposed extensions and embellishments to the list of criteria, but Hill's formulation has the claim of simplicity as well as precedence, and therefore has been adopted here.

In relation to diseases purportedly caused by tobacco, the weight of evidence available by at least the early 1960s had made such experiments unethical, even if they were practical, while experimental studies conducted in laboratory animals could contribute only to Hill's criterion of biological plausibility because the potential for between-species differences limited their applicability to humans. Nevertheless, so-called 'natural experiments', in which the incidence of cardiovascular and other diseases are tracked as the smoking habits of a given population change, have contributed important information bearing on the criteria of temporal sequence and reversibility. These observations fall into a category known to epidemiologists as 'ecological studies' because the data on both exposure and disease are collected at the level of an entire community rather than for individuals, and care must be taken that some other factor that influences the pattern of the disease of interest more directly, quickly, or profoundly has not also changed during the period under study. In the case of Australia, for example, the evidence suggests that smoking among men peaked either during or soon after World War II (Hyndman *et al.* 1991) (see Fig. 31.1), which might have contributed to the unprecedented downturn in mortality from IHD that occurred in the late 1960s and has continued since (Dwyer and Hetzel 1980) (see Fig. 31.2). However, the same change in the epidemiology of the disease also 'fits' with the major shift from plain to filter

Table 31.1 The Bradford Hill criteria for judgements about causation

Criterion	Test and its interpretation
Strength	Is the statistical relationship strong? Does it show a dose-response relationship—is a higher level of exposure to the putative cause associated with a greater risk of the disease?
Consistency	Is the relationship seen consistently in studies conducted at different historical periods, in different places, in different people (for example, in men as well as in women, in young people as well as in older ones, in different ethnic groups), and using different epidemiological methods (such as case-control and cohort studies)?
Temporal sequence	Do at least some of the studies provide incontrovertible evidence that exposure to the putative cause preceded development of the alleged effect?
Reversibility	Is a reduction in exposure followed by a reduced risk of the disease of interest? This question is best answered in data from individuals, but indicative information may also be derived from studies of whole populations
Specificity	Is exposure to the putative causal factor associated with development of an outcome that is unique to that exposure?
Biological plausibility	Is there supportive evidence from experimental studies in other species and from laboratory work on relevant organs, tissues, and other physiological systems? A systematic search for, and failure to find, evidence that would not support a conclusion of biological plausibility can be very useful here in demonstrating that the overall body of evidence is 'coherent'.

cigarettes that occurred from the late 1950s onwards. On the other hand, neither the change in level of smoking nor the type of cigarette smoked would explain why mortality from stroke, the more lethal manifestation of CeVD, began falling in the early 1950s (Jamrozik 1997), unless the time-trend for reduction of risk, specifically after cessation of smoking, was significantly faster for CeVD than for IHD. Development of effective pharmacological treatments for high blood pressure might conceivably have triggered the downturn in mortality from CeVD, even though hypertension is also a major independent and modifiable risk factor for IHD. Data on other potentially important factors, such as changes in dietary patterns consequent on the arrival of significant numbers of migrants from continental Europe and on developments in kitchen appliances, are extremely scant (Jamrozik *et al.* 1992), and those on levels of blood lipids and patterns of physical activity virtually non-existent.

The example of secular trends in mortality from arterial disease in Australia serves to illustrate several important points. While application of the Bradford Hill criteria to observational data on individuals itself requires considerable judgement, interpretation of secular trends in these diseases in whole communities, and the role that changes in smoking habits play in initiating and maintaining those trends, is even more difficult. Secondly, as the foregoing discussion makes clear, smoking is just one of several major, independent, and potentially modifiable risk factors for development of CVD, which has direct implications for Bradford Hill's criterion of specificity. Thirdly, if both cigarettes and patterns of their use change simultaneously, it may be close to impossible to discern, at least retrospectively, how much, if any, each change contributed to a population's experience of CVD.

But all of this is to run before we can walk. Let us first consider the individual criteria proposed by Bradford Hill and how they apply to the data on active smoking. Table 31.2 summarizes such a survey.

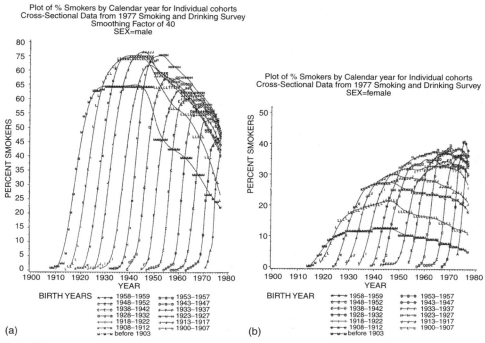

Figure 31.1 Retrospective cohort analyses of smoking habits of Australian (a) men and (b) women.

Footnote, Each line on a graph plots the evolution of smoking habits in the set of men or women born in a particular five-year period. The peak prevalence occurred among men in their twenties at the time of World War II, and far preceded and exceeded that among women, as did the rate of decline once the peak was passed. Overall, Australian women have been slower to stop starting and to start stopping than their male counterparts.

Source: Hyndman *et al.* (1991)

Copyright: Health Department of Western Australia

Strength and dose–response

As may be seen from Table 31.2, active smoking of cigarettes is a strong risk factor for disease in each of the four principal arterial territories, and shows an obvious dose–response in each. The dose–response relationships shown in Tables 31.3 and 31.4 are representative of those seen internationally, and those for IHD in Perth are further supported by data from cohort studies conducted in the same population (see Table 31.5). Unexpectedly, follow-up of healthy subjects recruited to the earlier case–control study of stroke (Jamrozik *et al.* 1994) revealed an inverse relationship between current smoking and major cardiovascular events (Jamrozik *et al.* 2000*b*).

Apart from the long-running studies in Framingham (Dawber 1980) and of British doctors (Doll *et al.* 1980, 1994) that have already been mentioned, new cohorts continue to be established in a wide variety of countries. Individual studies take some time to 'mature', although much useful information has already been obtained from the very large cohorts under follow-up in the Nurses Health Studies (Hu *et al.* 2000) and Health Professionals Study (Verhoef 1998) and from men screened for participation in the Multiple Risk Factor Intervention Trial (MRFIT) (Stamler *et al.* 1986). In addition, patients with AMI who participated in the ISIS-2 trial of aspirin and streptokinase have now been included in one of the largest case–control comparisons ever conducted for a non-communicable disease (Parish *et al.* 1995). Once again, the results show a strong and dose-related increase in risk of major coronary events associated with active smoking.

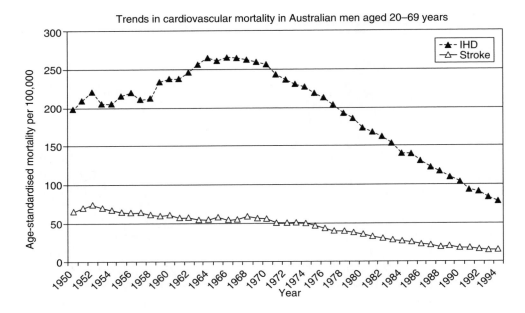

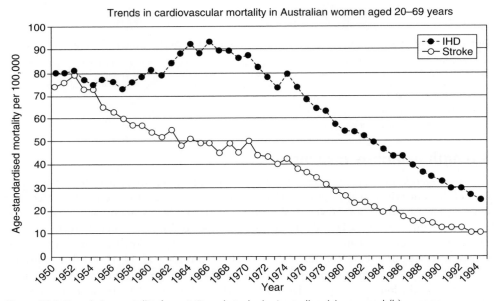

Figure 31.2 Trends in mortality from IHD and stroke in Australian (a) men and (b) women.

Footnote: In both sexes, mortality from stroke began falling early in the 1950s, while that from IHD continued to increase until the late 1960s before beginning to fall sharply and continuously. Taken together, the two patterns are not entirely consistent with the graphs shown in Fig. 31.1, suggesting that factors other than changes in smoking habits are also at play.

Source: National Heart Foundation of Australia (1996)

Copyright: National Heart Foundation of Australia

Table 31.2 Application of Bradford Hill criteria to the evidence on ACTIVE smoking and arterial disease

Criterion	Manifestation of arterial disease			
	Ischaemic heart disease	Cerebrovascular disease	Abdominal aortic aneurysm	Peripheral arterial disease
Strength	✓	✓	✓	✓
dose–response	✓	✓	✓	✓
Consistency				
time	✓	✓	✓	✓
place	✓	✓	✓	✓
person	✓	✓	✓	✓
epidemiological method	✓	✓	?	✓
Temporal sequence	✓	✓	?	✓
Reversibility				
individual	✓	✓	✗	✗
population	✓	?	?	?
Specificity	✗	✗	✗	✗
Biological plausibility	✓	✓	✓	✓

✓ = Evidence Available and supports criterion.
✗ = Available evidence does not support criterion.
? = Evidence either not available or inconclusive.

A recent, large case–control study of stroke in New Zealand (Bonita *et al.* 1999) stands out from all of these studies for two reasons apart from its focus on events in the cerebral rather than the coronary arteries. The first is that ascertainment of cases was population-based and therefore less subject to bias related to either the selected nature of the participants or the fact that, to be included, those suffering an event had to survive to reach hospital alive. Secondly, it has been one of the first studies deliberately to exclude passive smokers from the control group, a problem that may have affected many of the 'classical' studies and that, as Bonita *et al.* demonstrate, serves to underestimate the effects of active smoking on risk of disease (1999). The difference between their two sets of estimates, seen in Table 31.6, is sufficiently large to support a recommendation that exclusion of passive smokers should now be the 'gold standard' in such studies, especially since the spread of smoke-free policies has reached a point where large proportions of many communities are now able to live, travel, work, and relax in smoke-free environments if they so choose.

Smoking has long been accepted as a risk factor for both AAA and particularly PAD, but, as we shall see later, the relative lack of systematic study of these conditions appears to have contributed to a delay in our learning some important lessons about them.

Consistency

As has already been intimated, that active smoking is an important risk factor for the development of IHD is now supported by close to fifty years of research that includes both men and women, both case–control and cohort investigations, and evidence from a wide variety of geographical settings. Much the same is true of stroke, with one important proviso to which we

Table 31.3 Case-control studies of active smoking and ischaemic heart disease in Berth, Western Australia

Type of arterial disease (Period of study) [Reference] Sex and age-groups	Definition and source of cases	Daily consumption of cigarettes	Cases	Controls	Odds ratio	95% Confidence limits	Adjusted for:
Ischaemic heart disease (1989) (Liew 1989) Men only; 25–64 years	AMI: Perth MONICA Register	Never smoked	*n* = 174	*n* = 843	1.0	–	age, history of hypertension, maternal history of IHD, vigorous exercise
		Ex-smoker					
		1–24			1.71	0.87, 3.37	
		25+			2.37	1.14, 4.96	
		Current smoker					
		1–24			2.07	1.06, 4.05	
		25+			6.65	3.27, 13.5	
Ischaemic heart disease (1994) (Spencer et al. 1999) Men only; 25–64 years	AMI: Perth MONICA Register	Never smoked	*n* = 336	*n* = 735	1.0	–	age, dietary salt, fat, meat, alcohol, exercise, obesity, diabetes, history of hypertension, angina, low cholesterol diet
		Ex-smoker			2.0	1.25, 3.33	
		Current smoker			2.5	1.67, 3.33	
Ischaemic heart disease (1990–1993) (Lambert 2000) Women only; 25–64 years	AMI: Perth MONICA Register	Never smoked	*n* = 416	*n* = 935	1.0	–	age, marital status, source of income alcohol, exercise,
		Ex-smoker			1.34	0.94, 1.91	
		Current smoker			3.87	2.67, 5.61	dietary fat, diabetes

Table 31.4 Case-control studies of active smoking and other arterial disease in Perth, Western Australia

Type of arterial disease (Period or study) [Reference] Sex and age-groups	Definition and source of case	Daily consumption of cigarettes	Cases	Controls	Odds ratio	95% Confidence limits	Adjusted for:
Cerebrovascular disease (1989–1990) (Jamrozik et al 1994) Both sexes; ages ≥ 18 years	Stroke: Perth Community Stroke Study		n=295	n =553			history of hypertension, alcohol, claudication, previous CeVD, dietary milk, meat, salt, fish: matched for age and sex
		Never smoked			1.0	-	
		Ex-smoker			0.75	0.46, 1.24	
		1–20			1.99	1.04, 3.79	
		21+			3 52	1.35, 9.14	
Abdominal aortic aneurysm (1996–1998) (Jamrozik et al. 2000a) Men only: 65–83 years	AAA ≥ 30mm WA*		n =875	n =11 328			age, place of birth, height, family history of AAA, dietary salt. exercise, waist: hip ratio
		Never smoked			1.0	-	
	AAA	Ex-smoker			2.5	2.0, 3.1	
	Program	1–24			4.5	3.5, 5.8	
		25+			6.0	4.0, 9.0	
Peripheral arterial disease (1996–1998) (Fowler et al. 2002) Men only: 65–83 years	IC or ABI ≤ 0.9		n=744	n =3726			age, diabetes, exercise, history of hyperlipidaemia
		Neva smoked			1.0	-	
	WA	Ex-smoker			2.1	1.6, 2.6	
	AAA	1–14			3.9	2.7, 5.6	
	Program	15–24			6.6	4.2, 10.5	
		25+			7.3	4.2, 12.8	

*WA=Western Australia; AAA= abdominal aortic aneurysm: IC=intermittent claudication: ABI=ankle brachial index of systolic blood pressure.

Table 31.5 Cohort studies of active smoking and arterial disease in Perth, Western Australia

Type of arterial disease (Period of study) [Reference] Sex and age-groups	Definition and source of data	Daily consumption of cigarettes	Events	Size of cohort	Odds ratio	95% confidence-limits	Adjusted for:
Ischaemic heart disease (1978–1994) [unpublished data] Men only, ages ≥ 18 years Five years of follow-up	First AMI*: Perth Cohort Study	Never smoked	n=72	n =4805	1.0	-	age, diastolic blood pressure, cholesterol, diabetes (men with CVD excluded)
		Ex-smoker			0.99	0.53, 1.88	
		1–14			1.42	0.61, 3.33	
		15–24			1.68	0.67, 4.12	
		25–34			4.10	1.98, 8.49	
		35+			2.83	0.79, 10.1	
Cerebrovascular disease (1989–1994) (Jamrozik et al. 2000b) Both sexes; ages ≥ 18 years Five years of follow-up	Major CVD*: Perth Community Strobe study	Never smoked	n =141	n =931	1.0	-	age, sex, history of AMI, diabetes, intake of meat, use of full fat milk
		Current smoker			0.43	0.19, 0.995	

* AMI= acute myocardial infarction; † major CVD' = death from IHD, CeVD, AAA, PAD or mesenteric thrombosis, plus non-fatal AMI or stroke.

Table 31.6 Effect of exclusion of passive smokers from the control group on the apparent risk of stroke associated with active smoking

Smoking status	With passive smokers INCLUDED				With passive smokers EXCLUDED			
	Cases n=521 (%)	Controls n=1851 (%)	odds ratio*	95% CLs	Cases n=521 (%)	Controls n = 1851(%)	Odds ratio*	95% CLs
Never smoked	31.1	48.7	1.0**	–	21.1	35.7	1.0§	–
					29.8	36.5	1.82¶	1.34, 2.49
Current smoker	31.5	13.8	4.14	3.04, 5.63	31.5	13.8	6.33	4.50, 8.91
1–4 per day	5.2	2.1	2.56	1.35, 4.88	5.2	2.1	3.89	2.03, 7.47
5–14 per day	8.1	3.4	4.37	2.61, 7.32	8.1	3.4	6.63	3.89, 11.3
15+ per day	18.2	8.3	4.59	3.17, 6.63	18.2	8.3	7.06	4.75, 10.5
Ex-smoker	33.4	36.2	1.0	0.75, 1.32	13.6	12.7	2.21	1.50, 3.27
<2 years	4.2	2.4	2.30	1.24, 4.27	4.2	2.4	3.45	1.84, 6.46
2–10 years	9.4	10.3	1.23	0.80, 1.88	9.4	10.3	1.89	1.21, 2.93
>10 years	19.8	23.5	0.79	0.57, 2.51				

Source: Adapted from Bonita *et al.* (1999).

* Adjusted for age, sex, diabetes, hypertension, and history of heart disease.

** Includes never smokers who were passively exposed.

§ Unexposed never smokers and unexposed ex-smokers of more than 10 years' standing.

¶ Passively exposed never smokers and ex-smokers of more than 10 years' standing.

will return. The more limited data on PAD and AAA demonstrate the same features, although both of these tend to be disproportionately diseases of men, the former possibly because men took up smoking much sooner than women, the latter at least partly because of a genetic component.

The outstanding issue with regard to stroke is that it consists of three different pathological syndromes: subarachnoid haemorrhage (SAH), accounting for about 4% of all strokes and due in 85% of cases to rupture of a saccular aneurysm of an artery at the base of the brain external to the brain tissue (van Gijn and Rinkel 2001); primary intracerebral haemorrhage (PICH), responsible for about 11% of strokes in populations of European origin (Jamrozik *et al.* 1999) and due to haemorrhage from a small blood vessel within the brain tissue; and occlusive stroke, accounting for most of the remaining cases and due to thrombosis or to an embolus from the heart or neck, blocking a blood vessel in the brain. That the risk factors for these in general, and the role of smoking in particular, are not necessarily the same has received only limited attention, at least partly because routine CT examination to establish the pathological basis of stroke has become available only relatively recently. In fact, a case–control study conducted as part of the Perth Community Stroke Study (PCSS) was one of the first to provide evidence that active smoking is a risk factor for both occlusive stroke and PICH, although it did point to intriguing differences between these syndromes in regard to their associations with certain other risk factors (Jamrozik *et al.* 1994).

The PCSS alone included too few cases of SAH to permit separate analysis of risk factors for this form of stroke, but a large population-based series amassed retrospectively in the southwest of England suggests that smokers are more likely to survive an episode of SAH than are non-smokers (Pobereskin 2001*a*). As an editorial accompanying this report noted, such a finding is unexpected and potentially controversial (Juvela 2001). Of itself, it provides no clues as to the role of smoking in the *aetiology* of SAH, and Pobereskin concedes that it has not been consistently reported from other series. Most of those have not examined either question or not published the results if they have done so, and few are individually large enough to have a reasonable chance of seeing the effect on survival if it exists. Pobereskin is also open in acknowledging that data on smoking habits are most difficult to collect for patients who do not survive to reach hospital or who die soon after being admitted. Potentially this could lead to a bias in which smoking was apparently associated with better survival, but Pobereskin is confident that this problem has not affected his data (Pobereskin 2001*b*). If his original observation is correct, it may be one of several hints that the relationship between smoking and aneurysmal disease differs fundamentally from that with occlusive, atherosclerotic arterial disease.

Temporal sequence

In practice, the question of temporal sequence—exposure to the putative cause (smoking) preceding development of the alleged outcome (arterial disease)—is rarely a problem in relation to major non-communicable diseases related to tobacco because most smokers acquire the habit in their teens and the consequent diseases usually do not manifest themselves before later middle age. Nevertheless, the issue of temporal sequence is readily addressed by cohort studies to which recruitment is limited to subjects with no evidence of the relevant disease at baseline. With the proviso that any screening test almost certainly generates some false negatives, such cohort studies are certainly available for IHD and CeVD. This is of critical importance as 'temporal sequence' is the only one of the criteria proposed by Bradford Hill that *must* be fulfilled if one is to conclude that a causal relationship does explain the statistical associations observed between an exposure of interest and its putative effect.

Very large studies would be required in the case of AAA, where the prevalence of surgically significant lesions is still less than 1% in men in early old age (Jamrozik *et al.* 2000*a*). The prevalence of PAD, diagnosed either by symptoms (IC) or a reduced ankle: brachial index of systolic blood pressure, is at least six times higher in the same age–sex group (Fowler *et al.* 2002), making cohort studies more feasible. For example, Bowlin *et al.* found that current smokers of more than 20 cigarettes daily doubled their risk of developing IC within five years relative to never smokers (1994).

Reversibility

Good evidence was already available at the time of the 1983 report from the Surgeon-General (United States Department of Health and Human Services 1983) that after an individual stops smoking his or her excess risk of IHD associated with active smoking dissipates rapidly, compared with the equivalent pattern for lung cancer, and probably has disappeared entirely within seven to ten years. While much of the research available at that time was dominated by studies of men whose careers as smokers spanned the change from plain to filter cigarettes, more recent confirmatory evidence of the same pattern is available from the Nurses' Health Study for women (Kawachi *et al.* 1994) and from two of the Australasian centres in the World Health Organization MONICA Project for men (McElduff 1998*a*). The Nurses' Health Study has demonstrated a very similar pattern of reduction of excess risk of stroke after cessation of smoking (Kawachi *et al.* 1993), and the same findings are evident for both the coronary and cerebral arterial territories in studies conducted in Western Australia (Liew 1989; Jamrozik *et al.* 1994; Spencer *et al.* 1999; Lambert 2000) (see Tables 31.3 and 31.4).

In the case of AAA and PAD, however, there is evidence from Western Australia of long persistence of residual excess risk after a man gives up smoking. The sets of data for these conditions displayed in Table 31.4 both come from cross-sectional case–control comparisons based on a large randomized controlled trial of screening for AAA involving men aged 65–83 years selected at random from electoral rolls, enrolment to vote being compulsory for all adult Australian citizens (Jamrozik *et al.* 2000). Information on smoking habits was collected via a self-completed questionnaire that was answered by the men before the screening examinations for AAA and PAD were undertaken. However, claims to have stopped smoking were not verified biochemically, although many men were accompanied to the screening examination by a wife or partner who was all too willing to act as their 'conscience'.

Table 31.7 shows that stratification of ex-smokers, who constituted some 60% of all men screened, by reported time since cessation of smoking did reveal an inverse relationship with apparent risk of PAD, but the excess risk of each condition was still statistically significant among men who claimed to have stopped smoking more than twenty years previously. Misclassification of continuing smokers as ex-smokers could conceivably contribute to these findings, despite the overall pattern of responses regarding smoking status being consistent with the retrospective cohort analysis mentioned previously (Hyndman *et al.* 1991). At the same time, calculations showed that if the apparent excess risk in those who had ever smoked was correct and causal, some 40% of cases of PAD in this population were attributable to previous smoking and a further 32% to current smoking (Fowler *et al.* 2002). Thus, while there is no uncertainty surrounding the reversibility of the excess risk of IHD and stroke if a smoker gives up the habit before overt disease develops in these arterial territories, the same may not be true of the aorta and arteries of the lower limb. Since AAA is, by definition, aneurysmal disease, while PAD is occlusive disease, the explanation for the contradiction cannot lie in a different pathological process affecting arteries below the diaphragm compared with that above it. In any case, the puzzle is compounded further when one considers that atherosclerosis plays a role in all four arterial syndromes.

Table 31.7 Long-term persistence of excess risk of PAD in ex-smokers (Fowler *et al.* 2002)

Smoking status	Odds ratio	95% CLs
Never smoked	1.0	-
Ex-smoker	2.1	1.6, 2.6
20+ years	1.3	1.0, 1.7
10–19 years	2.7	2.0, 3.6
5–9 years	3.7	2.5, 5.3
1–4 years	3.8	2.5, 5.7
<1 year	5.4	2.4, 11.9
Current smoker		
1–14/day	3.9	2.7, 5.6
15–24 per day	6.6	4.2, 10.5
25+ per day	7.3	4.2, 12.8

CLs = confidence limits; odds ratios adjusted for age, physical activity, diabetes and history of high triglyceride and cholesterol levels.

Fewer analyses are available of the relationships between population-wide trends in smoking and those for the incidence or mortality from arterial disease, but, as discussed earlier, the interpretation of such data is fraught with hazard because all of the cigarettes themselves, patterns of smoking, the medical management of cardiovascular risk factors and events, and the epidemiology of the diseases changed rapidly and significantly over the last five decades of the twentieth century.

Specificity

The entries in Table 31.2 for 'specificity', meaning exposure to the putative causal factor being associated with development of an outcome that is unique to that exposure, stand out as the one row for which the evidence on smoking and CVD currently available does not support the criterion proposed by Bradford Hill. The explanation for this lies in the fact that many factors increase the risk of atherosclerotic CVD and, with a final pathological process that is common to all of them, it is very difficult to discern epidemiologically whether any given risk factor makes a contribution that is unique to itself. As is discussed further below, the apparent lack of specificity for smoking in the genesis of CVD has been a matter of scientific note for at least twenty years (Anonymous 1980), and the whole issue has been re-examined very thoroughly more recently in the context of evidence that, relative to active smoking, passive smoking seems to carry a risk for IHD that is disproportionately high compared with its contribution to the development of lung cancer in non-smokers.

Biological plausibility

Randomized, blinded controlled trials have provided incontrovertible evidence that smoking, exposure to tobacco smoke, or exposure to components of tobacco smoke such as carbon monoxide, produce clinically observable effects on various parts of the cardiovascular system including the electrical system of the heart (Sheps *et al.* 1987), the coronary circulation (Ayres *et al.* 1969; Aronow and Rokaw 1971; Sumida *et al.* 1998; Otsuka *et al.* 2001), and the peripheral arteries (Celermajer *et al.* 1996). This evidence is supported by cross-sectional studies demonstrating increased asymptomatic thickening of the lining 'intima' layer of the carotid arteries in both active and passive smokers (Howard *et al.* 1994), with follow-up of the same individuals showing greater rates of evolution of these 'plaques' in smokers (Diez-Roux *et al.* 1995; Howard *et al.* 1998). Since the carotid arteries are the main blood vessels supplying the brain, greater degrees of occlusion at the anatomical sites examined in these studies are associated with neurological symptoms, and surgical clearance of such obstructions reduces the risk of stroke, these findings clearly are of direct relevance to the role purportedly played by smoking in the aetiology of CeVD.

These studies in intact humans are complemented by a wealth of laboratory research on other species (Penn and Snyder 1996; Penn *et al.* 1996, 2001) and on human tissues (Davis *et al.* 1989; Kritz *et al.* 1995). Glantz and Parmley (1995) provide a wide-ranging review of the evidence that passive smoking, in particular, could plausibly cause an increase in risk of CVD in non-smokers and point to a number of mechanisms through which this could occur. It is true that there are differences in chemical and other characteristics between the smoke inhaled directly from cigarettes by smokers and that inhaled from ambient air by non-smokers. However, the overall exposure of the latter to particular constituents of the smoke is so obviously lower that, taken with the evidence of direct, potentially harmful effects of active smoking on parts of the cardiovascular system, the convincing argument regarding the biological plausibility of passive smoking as a cause of CVD means that the case in regard to active smoking must be even more compelling. Significantly, the identification of a number of different mechanisms via which tobacco smoke could harm the arterial tree makes it very difficult to modify cigarettes to make them 'safer' in regard to the risk of CVD in smokers.

Passive smoking and arterial disease

The evidence that passive smoking increased the incidence of severe respiratory infections in infants and young children (Colley *et al.* 1974; Harlap and Davies 1974) was not seriously challenged when it emerged. This is probably because it was known by the 1970s that active smoking caused COPD (Fletcher and Peto 1976) and was associated with increased mortality from pneumonia in adults (Doll and Peto 1976), it was obvious that children of this age could be heavily exposed if their parents smoked around them, and the implications for policy were limited because the majority of that exposure occurred in private homes, a domain that most communities are loathe to regulate. However, the tobacco industry having been alerted in 1978 to the threat to its well-being posed by the issue of passive smoking (Roper Organization 1978), the publication, in 1981, of evidence (Hirayama 1981; Trichopoulos *et al.* 1981) that passive smoking was associated with lung cancer in adults was accompanied by very considerable controversy. The possible contribution of passive smoking to IHD, first identified epidemiologically in 1985 (Garland *et al.* 1985), has proved even more contentious because it appears to be similar in magnitude to the effect of passive smoking on the risk of lung cancer, whereas the multiplying effect of active smoking on the risk of lung cancer is at least five times its effect on IHD.

The National Heart Foundation of Australia was one of the first health organizations to react to the paper from Garland *et al.* (1985), publishing a pamphlet on passive smoking and heart disease entitled, "So you think you're a non-smoker" (National Heart Foundation of Australia 1985) in the same year. More systematic reviews of the scientific evidence on passive smoking generally were published by the Surgeon-General in the United States in 1986 (United States Department of Health and Human Services 1986) and the National Health and Medical Research Council (NHMRC) in Australia in 1987 (National Health and Medical Research Council 1987), but neither body was persuaded at that time that passive smoking caused CVD. When the NHMRC visited the question of passive smoking again (1997), many more epidemiological and laboratory reports on the issue of CVD had been published, leading that body to a conclusion that the evidence for a causal relationship was 'strongly suggestive'. In Britain, the Scientific Committee on Tobacco and Health was unambiguous in its report published in 1998 that passive smoking is a cause of IHD (Department of Health 1998), and Law *et al.*, working in the same country, had been persuaded by the evidence available in the preceding year (1997), as had the California Environmental Protection Agency (Office of Environmental Health Hazard Assessment 1997).

The epidemiological evidence implicating passive smoking as a cause of IHD continues to mount (Ciruzzi *et al.* 1998; McElduff *et al.* 1998*b*; Thun *et al.* 1999; Irabarren *et al.* 2001; Rosenlund *et al.* 2001), with new meta-analyses appearing at frequent intervals (He *et al.* 1999), and the data on stroke are also growing (Bonita *et al.* 1999). However, as may be seen from Table 31.8, little attention has been afforded to the role of passive smoking in the genesis of AAA and PAD, and the question of whether the risk of any of the arterial diseases falls when a non-smoking individual stops being passively exposed to tobacco smoke has not been studied systematically.

Although the elevation in risk of IHD associated with passive smoking is modest, both coronary disease and exposure to tobacco smoke are so common among nonsmokers that the aggregate number of additional cases of heart attack potentially attributable to passive smoking is very large indeed (Wells 1994). The sceptics, some of whom openly acknowledge support from the tobacco industry, regularly advance arguments about misclassification of continuing smokers as

Table 31.8 Application of Bradford Hill criteria to the evidence on passive smoking and arterial disease

Criterion	Manifestation of arterial disease			
	Ischaemic heart disease	Cerebrovascular disease	Abdominal aortic aneurysm	Peripheral arterial disease
Strength	✗	✗	?	?
dose-response	✓	✓	?	?
Consistency				
time	✓	✓	?	?
place	✓	✓	?	?
person	✓	?	?	?
epidemiological method	✓	?	?	?
Temporal sequence	✓	✗	?	?
Reversibility				
individual	?	?	?	?
population	?	?	?	?
Specificity	✗	✗	?	?
Biological plausibility	✓	✓	✓	✓

✓ = Evidence available and supports criterion.
✗ = Available evidence does not support criterion.
? = Evidence either not available or inconclusive.

ex-smokers, publication bias (LeVois and Layard 1995)—the tendency for studies showing no association not to be submitted or accepted for publication—and confounding—systematic differences in the lifestyles of non-smokers who are and are not passive smokers that render the former more prone to development of IHD—as possible explanations for pattern of positive findings in the available literature. These objections are theoretical and largely speculative, but each has been examined systematically and discounted (Steenland *et al.* 1998;Wells *et al.* 1998).

Two further papers, both including authors who are associated with the tobacco industry, proffer elaborate but slightly different arguments about the overall dose–response relationship between tobacco smoke and CVD. Gori (1995) calculates that a pooled estimate of the epidemiological data on the excess risk of IHD associated with active smoking of five cigarettes daily is not statistically significant and therefore that there is a threshold of exposure to tobacco smoke, whether through active or passive smoking, below which individuals suffer no adverse cardiovascular consequences. Smith *et al.* (2000) argue that combining the epidemiological data for active and passive smoking produces a non-linear dose–response curve that is biologically implausible. The best counter to both these observations is a simple experiment that showed that exposure to tobacco smoke in the corridor of a hospital for just 20 minutes resulted in significant 'activation' of the platelets of non-smokers but not those of smokers, platelets being small cells in the bloodstream that play a critical role in thrombosis, including coronary thrombosis and occlusive stroke (Kritz *et al.* 1995).

In summary, the epidemiological association between passive smoking and at least IHD is definitely real, and the available evidence points to it being both based on a causal relationship and of considerable public health significance, even though the excess risk in individual passive smokers is small.

Active smoking and venous disease

Smokers have significantly increased mortality from the most lethal form of venous disease, pulmonary embolism (PE) secondary to deep vein thrombosis (DVT) (Doll *et al.* 1994), which is perhaps a consequence of the higher levels of fibrinogen and activation of platelets in smokers, as well as their increased risk of cancer. Beyond the known interaction with use of the oral contraceptive pill (Farmer *et al.* 2000), it is uncommon to see smoking cited as increasing the risk of DVT and PE. Nevertheless, smoking does appear to be an independent risk factor for these conditions (Hansson *et al.* 1999). Interest in this association may be increased following publication of evidence that cessation of smoking before major elective surgery reduces post-operative complications, of which DVT and PE are among the most serious (Moller *et al.* 2002).

One might also predict a relationship between smoking and varicose veins, perhaps mediated through the 'smoker's cough', but this is evident in some (Brand *et al.* 1988) but not all (Fowkes *et al.* 2001) of the studies that have sought such an association.

Unanswered questions

The case against active smoking as an avoidable cause of major diseases in each of the four principal arterial territories is overwhelming. However, as well as the issue of passive smoking and the somewhat limited investigation of the role of smoking in diseases of the venous system mentioned above, a number of questions surrounding smoking and arterial CVD remain unanswered. Some of these are of considerable significance in terms of public health, others suggest novel lines of enquiry into the biology of vascular disease, and yet others potentially have ramifications in both these spheres.

Type of tobacco product

The great bulk of the evidence concerning the impact of smoking on CVD is derived from studies of users of manufactured cigarettes. When pipes and cigars receded from the tobacco markets in most developed countries in the 1970s and 1980s, epidemiological interest in these products also waned, but it has been rekindled by a recent resurgence in the smoking of cigars. There is little doubt that use of such products is associated with significant hazard (Hein *et al.* 1992; Jacobs *et al.* 1999). Much less information is available concerning hazards potentially associated with traditional forms of smoking in other communities.

Changes over time in manufactured cigarettes raise a related set of questions, especially as it is not clear which component or components of tobacco smoke are responsible for the increased risk of arterial disease in smokers. In practice, with the epidemiology at least of IHD also changing rapidly, it would be very difficult to detect whether changes in the source and blend of tobacco, other additives, cigarette papers or filters affected the risk of vascular events in smokers. Nevertheless, because manufacturers attempt to tailor their products to particular markets, divergences between the patterns of vascular disease in otherwise similar countries might potentially provide clues as to which aspects of tobacco products or their use are particularly relevant to the development of atherosclerosis.

On the other hand, there is little uncertainty regarding one question relating to type of tobacco product and risk of CVD. The evidence already cited suggests that smokers of cigarettes should not be encouraged to change to other tobacco products in an attempt to reduce their risk of CVD. Direct support for this inference is available from a long-term prospective study of 'switching'. Former smokers of cigarettes who changed to pipes and cigars experienced a significant reduction in risk compared with men who continued smoking cigarettes but also a 57% excess risk of dying from one of IHD, lung cancer, and COPD compared with those who stopped smoking entirely (Wald and Watt 1997). The explanation almost certainly lies in the fact that former smokers of cigarettes continue to inhale the smoke when they change to other forms of tobacco product (Goldman 1977).

Lack of reversibility in AAA and PAD

As already noted, case–control studies from Western Australia suggest that the elevation in risk of AAA and PAD persists long after the individual stops smoking, in contrast to the rapid declines in excess risk of IHD and CeVD. Wilmink *et al.* (1999) reported a relative risk for AAA of 3.0 (95% CL 1.4–6.4) in ex-smokers, but Blanchard *et al.* (2000), who summarized a history of smoking in terms of pack-years, did not draw attention to this phenomenon. A major review of the literature by English *et al.* (1995) considered all non-coronary and non-cerebral arterial disease as a single category and therefore does not permit examination of the question. Whether arterial disease related to smoking behaves differently in different anatomical territories bears further investigation as this may provide new insights into the basic biology of atherosclerosis. Any new studies should include independent verification of claims by affected individuals to have stopped smoking before development of their symptoms.

Aneurysmal disease

There is growing evidence that smoking has a protective effect in regard to development of retinopathy in patients with diabetes mellitus (Janghorbani *et al.* 2001; Keen *et al.* 2001; Stratton *et al.* 2001). As the key lesion in this condition is an arterial microaneurysm, there is a sharp contrast with the elevated risk in smokers of macroaneurysmal disease in the cerebral (Shinton and Beevers 1989) and aortic circulations (Jamrozik *et al.* 2000). Again, further investigation of this paradox might reveal new lessons about the pathogenesis of arterial disease.

Smoking and survival from major vascular events

While smoking has a strong influence on the incidence of major arterial disease events, its relationship to survival after such events is less clear. One Australian population-based study of middle-aged patients with AMI who reached hospital alive suggested that case fatality at 28 days was significantly lower in current smokers (Nidorf *et al.* 1990), while another, which included all major coronary events in a defined population, found no significant association in either direction between smoking and short-term survival (McElduff and Dobson 2001). Apparently protective effects of current smoking have also been observed in major trials of acute coronary care (Barbash *et al.* 1995), but careful work in New Zealand suggests that the reduced case-fatality of smokers after they are admitted to hospitals with an AMI is balanced by worse out-of-hospital survival, with no significant relationship apparent overall (Sonke *et al.* 1997). This does not appear to be the explanation for the observation, cited earlier (Pobereskin 2001*a*), that smokers fare better, in terms of survival, after subarachnoid haemorrhage. However, it does underline the importance of taking a population-wide view of rapidly fatal phenomena, lest artefacts related to differential survival to reach hospital alive be accepted at face value.

In the overall picture, sorting out the details of the relationships between smoking and the outcome of major vascular events is not a high priority compared with the need to reduce the contribution of smoking to the incidence of such episodes. Nevertheless, the availability of clear answers would permit unambiguous advice to be given to patients and their families.

Conclusion

The smoking of tobacco is a major independent risk factor for life-threatening diseases in all four principal arterial territories. The totality of the evidence indicates that this relationship goes beyond statistical association to one of cause-and-effect. Most importantly, compared with other factors such as hypertension, hypercholesterolaemia, and lack of physical activity, cessation of smoking requires a once-only change on the part of the individual, and a change to non-smoking is followed by a rapid and complete disappearance of the excess risk of IHD and stroke, the two most common fatal manifestations of arterial disease. *How* smoking harms the arterial tree is not completely clear, but several plausible candidate mechanisms have been identified. A number of other scientifically intriguing questions about smoking and both arterial and venous diseases also remain open. But it is beyond any doubt that smoking does most of its harm in terms of deaths, not through cancer or COPD, but through vascular disease.

Acknowledgements

The author's interest in tobacco was originally kindled by Godfrey Fowler and fostered by Nicholas Wald, Sir Richard Peto, and Sir Richard Doll. Michael Hobbs and Bruce Armstrong designed the Perth MONICA Project, which formed the framework for the Western Australian studies of ischaemic heart disease cited in this chapter, while Ted Stewart-Wynne, Craig Anderson, Sue Forbes, and Graeme Hankey have been pillars of the Perth Community Stroke Study. Robyn Broadhurst has not only managed most of the data for that project, but also is prime mover for the Perth Cohort Study, also cited here. Paul Norman, Michael Lawrence-Brown, Raywin Tuohy, Carole Spencer, and Jim Dickinson have played vital roles in the Western Australian Abdominal Aortic Aneurysm Program, and Bess Fowler made a memorable contribution to the work on peripheral arterial disease. Financial support for these projects has been provided, in various combinations, by the National Health and Medical Research Council, the National Heart Foundation of Australia, Healthway—the Western Australian Health Promotion Foundation, and State and Federal Governments in Australia.

References

Anonymous (1980). How does smoking harm the heart? *Br Med J*, **281**: 573–4.

Aronow,W.S., and Rokaw, S.N. (1971). Carboxyhaemoglobin caused by smoking non-nicotine cigarettes. *Circulation*, **44**: 782–8.

Ayres, S.M., Mueller, H.S., Gregory, J.J., Gianelli, S., and Penny, J.L. (1969). Systemic and myocardial haemodynamic response to relatively small concentrations of carboxyhaemoglobin (COHb). *Arch Environ Health*, **18**: 699–709.

Barbash, G.I., Reiner, J., White, H.D., Wilcox, R.G., Armstrong, P.W., Sadowski, Z. *et al.* (1995). Evaluation of paradoxic beneficial effects of smoking in patients receiving thrombolytic therapy for acute myocardial infarction: mechanism of the "smoker's paradox" from the GUSTO-I trial, with angiographic insights. *J Am College Cardiol*, **26**: 1222–9.

Blanchard, J.F., Armenian, H.K., and Friesen, P.P. (2000). Risk factors for abdominal aortic aneurysm: results of a case-control study. *Am J Epidemiol*, **151**: 575–83.

Bonita, R., Duncan, J., Truelsen, T., Jackson, R.T., and Beaglehole, R. (1999). Passive smoking as well as active smoking increases the risk of acute stroke. *Tob Control*, **8**: 156–60.

Bowlin, S.J., Medalie, J.H., Flocke, S.A., Zyzanski, S.J., and Goldbourt, U. (1994). Epidemiology of intermittent claudication in middle-aged men. *Am J Epidemiol*, **140**: 418–30.

Brand, F.N., Dannenberg, A.L., Abbott, R.D., and Kannel, W.B. (1988). The epidemiology of varicose veins: the Framingham Study. *Am J Prev Med*, **4**: 96–101.

Bruce, J.M. (1901). Diseases and disorders of the heart and arteries in middle life and advanced age. *Lancet*, **i**: 844–8.

Celermajer, D.S., Adams, M.R., Clarkson, P. *et al.* (1996). Passive smoking and impaired endothelium-dependent arterial dilatation in healthy young adults. *N Eng J Med*, **334**: 150–4.

Ciruzzi, M., Pramparo, P., Esteban, O., *et al.* (1998). Case-control study of passive smoking at home and risk of acute myocardial infarction. *J Am Coll Cardiol*, **31**: 797–803.

Colley, J.R.T., Holland, W.W., and Corkhill, R.T. (1974). Influence of passive smoking and parental phlegm on pneumonia and bronchitis in early childhood. *Lancet*, **ii**: 1031–4.

Davis, J., Shelton, L., Watanabe, I.S., and Arnold, J. (1989). Passive smoking affects endothelium and platelets. *Arch Intern Med*, **149**: 386–9.

Dawber, T.R. (1980). The Framingham Study: The epidemiology of atherosclerotic disease. Cambridge, Mass.: Harvard University Press.

Department of Health. (1998). Report of the Scientific Committee on Tobacco and Health. London: Stationery Office.

Diez-Roux, A.V., Nieto, F.J., Comstock, G.W., Howard, G., and Szklo, M. (1995). The relationship of active and passive smoking to carotid atherosclerosis 12–14 years later. *Prev Med*, **24**: 48–55.

Doll, R. and Hill, A.B. (1950). Smoking and carcinoma of the lung: preliminary report. *Br Med J*, **ii**: 739–48.

Doll, R. and Hill, A.B. (1952). A study of the aetiology of carcinoma of the lung. *Br Med J*, **ii**: 1271–86.

Doll, R. and Peto, R. (1976). Mortality in relation to smoking: 20 years' of observations in male British doctors. *Br Med J*, **ii**.

Doll, R., Gray, R., Hafner, B., and Peto, R. (1980). Mortality in relation to smoking: 22 years' observations on female British doctors. *Br Med J*, **280**: 967–71.

Doll, R., Peto, R.,Wheatley, K., Gray, R., and Sutherland, I. (1994). Mortality in relation to smoking: 40 years' observations on male British doctors. *Br Med J*, **309**: 901–11.

Dwyer, T. and Hetzel, B.S. (1980). A comparison of coronary heart disease mortality in Australia, USA and England and Wales with reference to three major risk factors—hypertension, cigarette smoking and diet. *Intl J Epidemiol*, **9**: 65–71.

English, D.R., Holman, C.D.J., Milne, E. et al. (1995). The quantification of drug caused morbidity and mortality in Australia 1995 edition. Canberra: Commonwealth Department of Human Services and Health.

Farmer, R.D., Lawrenson, R.A., Todd, J.C., Williams, T.J., MacRae, K.D., Tyrer, F., and Leydon, G.M. (2000). A comparison of the risks of venous thromboembolic disease in association with different combined oral contraceptives. *Br J Clin Pharmacol*, **49**: 580–90.

Fletcher, C.M. and Peto, R. (1977). The natural history of chronic airflow obstruction. *Br Med J*, **i**: 1654–8.

Fowkes, F.G., Lee, A.J., Evans, C.J., Allan, P.L., Bradbury, A.W., and Ruckley, C.V. (2001). Lifestyle risk factors for lower limb venous reflux in the general population: Edinburgh Vein Study. *Int J Epidemiol*, **30**: 846–52.

Fowler, B.V., Jamrozik, K., Allen, Y., and Norman, P.E. (2002). Prevalence of peripheral arterial disease: Persistence of excess risk in former smokers. *ANZ J Public Health*, **26**: 219–24.

Garland, C., Barrett-Connor, E., Suarez, L., *et al.* (1985). Effects of passive smoking on ischaemic heart disease mortality of nonsmokers. *Am J Epidemiol*, **121**: 645–9.

Glantz, S.A. and Parmley, W.W. (1995). Passive smoking and heart disease. Mechanisms and risk. *JAMA*, **273**: 1047–53.

Goldman, A.L. (1977). Carboxyhemoglobin levels in primary and secondary cigar and pipe smokers. *Chest*, **72**: 33–5.

Gori, G.B. (1995). Environmental tobacco smoke and coronary heart syndromes: Absence of an association. *Regul Toxicol Pharmacol*, **21**: 281–95.

Hansson, P.O., Eriksson, H., Welin, L., Svardsudd, K., and Wilhelmsen, L. (1999). Smoking and abdominal obesity: risk factors for venous thromboembolism among middle-aged men: "the study of men born in 1913". *Arch Intern Med*, **159**: 1886–90.

Harlap, S. and Davies, A.M. (1974). Infant admissions to hospital and maternal smoking. *Lancet*, **i**: 529–32.

He, J., Vupputuri, S., Allen, K., Prerost, M.R., Hughes, J., and Whelton, P.K. (1999). Passive smoking and the risk of coronary heart disease – a meta-analysis of epidemiologic studies. *N Eng J Med*, **340**: 920–6.

Hein, H.O., Suadicani, P., and Gyntelberg, F. (1992). Ischaemic heart disease incidence by social class and form of smoking: the Copenhagen Male Study—17 years' follow-up. *J Intern Med*, **231**: 477–83.

Hill, A.B. (1965). The environment and disease: association or causation. *Proc Roy Soc Med*, **58**: 295–300.

Hirayama, T. (1981). Non-smoking wives of heavy smokers have a higher risk of lung cancer: a study from Japan. *Br Med J*, **282**: 183–5.

Howard, G., Burke, G.L., Szklo, M., Tell, G.S., Eckfeldt, J., Evans, G., and Heiss, G. (1994). Active and passive smoking are associated with increased carotid wall thickness. The Atherosclerosis Risk in Communities (ARIC) Study. *Arch Intern Med*, **154**: 1277–82.

Howard, G., Wagenknecht, L.E., Burke, G.L., *et al.* (1998). Cigarette smoking and progression of atherosclerosis: The Atherosclerosis Risk in Communities (ARIC) Study. *JAMA*, **279**: 119–24.

Hu, F.B., Stampfer, M.J., Manson, J.E., Grodstein, F., Colditz, G.A., Speizer, F.E., and Willett,W.C. (2000). Trends in the incidence of coronary heart disease and changes in diet and lifestyle in women. *N Engl J Med*, **343**: 530–7.

Hyndman, J., Hobbs, M., Jamrozik, K., Hockey, R., and Parsons, R. (1991). A retrospective cohort study of smoking habits in Australia. In: B. Durston, and K. Jamrozik (eds) *Proceedings of the 7th World Conference on Tobacco and Health*. Perth: Health Department of Western Australia, 264–7.

Irabarren, C., Friedman, G.D., Klatsky, A.L., and Eisner, M.D. (2001). Exposure to environmental tobacco smoke: association with personal characteristics and self reported health conditions. *J Epidemiol Community Health*, **55**: 721–8.

Jacobs, E.J., Thun, M.J., and Apicella, L.F. (1999). Cigar smoking and death from coronary heart disease in a prospective study of US men. *Arch Intern Med*, **159**: 2413–8.

Jamrozik, K., Jamieson, R., and Fitzgerald, C. (1992). An oral history of changes in the Australian diet. *Med J Aust*, **157**: 759–61.

Jamrozik, K., Broadhurst, R.J., Anderson, C.S., and Stewart-Wynne, E.G. (1994). The role of lifestyle factors in the aetiology of stroke: A population-based case-control study in Perth, Western Australia. *Stroke*, **25**: 51–9.

Jamrozik, K. (1997). Stroke—a looming epidemic? *Aust Fam Physician*, **26**: 1137–43.

Jamrozik, K., Broadhurst, R.J., Lai, N., Hankey, G.J., Burvill, P.W., and Anderson, C.S. (1999). Trends in the incidence, severity and outcome of stroke in Perth,Western Australia. *Stroke*, **30**: 2105–11.

Jamrozik, K., Norman, P., Spencer, C.A., Parsons, R.W., Tuohy, R., Lawrence-Brown, M.M., and Dickinson, J.A. (2000a). Screening for abdominal aortic aneurysm: lessons from a population based study. *Med J Aust*, **173**: 345–50.

Jamrozik, K., Broadhurst, R.J., Forbes, S., Hankey, G.J., and Anderson, C.S. (2000b). Predictors of death and vascular events in the elderly: The Perth Community Stroke Study. *Stroke*, **31**: 863–8.

Janghorbani, M., Jones, R.B., Murray, K.J., and Allison, S.P. (2001). Incidence of and risk factors for diabetic retinopathy in diabetic clinic attenders. *Ophthalmic Epidemiol*, **8**: 309–25.

Juvela, S. (2001). Cigarette smoking and death following subarachnoid haemorrhage. *J Neurosurg*, **95**: 551–4.

Kawachi, I., Colditz, G.A., Stampfer, M.J. *et al.* (1993). Smoking cessation and decreased risk of stroke in women. *JAMA*, **269**: 232–6.

Kawachi, I., Colditz, G.A., Stampfer, M.J., *et al.* (1994). Smoking cessation and time course of decreased risks of coronary heart disease in middle-aged women. *Arch Intern Med*, **154**: 169–75.

Keen, H., Lee, E.T., Russell, D., Miki, E., Bennett, P.H., and Lu, M. (2001). The appearance of retinopathy and progression to proliferative retinopathy: the WHO Multinational Study of Vascular Disease in Diabetes. *Diabetologia*, **44** Suppl 2: S22–30.

Kritz, H., Schmid, P., and Sinzinger, H. (1995). Passive smoking and cardiovascular risk. *Arch Intern Med*, **155**: 1942–8.

Lambert L.J. (2000). Hysterectomy, hormones and coronary heart disease. Doctor of Philosophy thesis. University of Western Australia, Perth.

Law, M.R., Morris, J.K., and Wald, N.J. (1997). Environmental tobacco smoke exposure and ischaemic heart disease: an evaluation of the evidence. *Br Med J*, **315**: 973–80.

LeVois, M.E. and Layard, M.W. (1995). Publication bias in the environmental tobacco smoke/coronary heart disease epidemiologic literature. *Regul Toxicol Pharmacol*, **21**: 184–91.

Liew, D. (1989). Bachelor of Medical Science Honours thesis. Melbourne: Monash University.

McElduff, P., Dobson, A., Beaglehole, R., and Jackson, R. (1998a). Rapid reduction in coronary risk for those who quit cigarette smoking. *Aust NZ J Public Health*, **22**: 787–91.

McElduff, P., Dobson, A.J., Jackson, R., Beaglehole, R., Heller, R.F., and Lay-Yee, R. (1998b). Coronary events and exposure to environmental tobacco smoke: a case-control study from Australia and New Zealand. *Tob Control*, **7**: 41–6.

McElduff, P. and Dobson, A.J. (2001). Case fatality after an acute cardiac event: the effect of smoking and alcohol consumption. *J Clin Epidemiol*, **54**: 58–67.

Macfarlane, J.E. and Jamrozik, K. (1993). Tobacco in Western Australia: an examination of patterns of tobacco smoking among adults in Western Australia from 1974 to 1991. *Aust J Public Health*, **17**: 350–8.

Medical Research Council (1948). Streptomycin treatment of pulmonary tuberculosis. *Br Med J*, **ii**: 769–82.

Molarius, A., Parsons, R.W., Dobson, A.J., Evans, A., Fortmann, S.P., Jamrozik, K. *et al.* (2001). for the WHO MONICA Project. Trends in cigarette smoking in 36 populations from the early 1980s to the mid 1990s: Findings from the WHO MONICA Project. *Am J Pub Health*, **91**: 206–12.

Moller, A.M., Villebro, N., Pedersen, T., and Tonnesen, H. (2002). Effect of preoperative smoking intervention on postoperative complications: a randomised clinical trial. *Lancet*, **359**: 114–7.

National Health and Medical Research Council (1987). Effects of passive smoking on health – Report of the NHMRC Working Party on the Effects of Passive smoking on Health. Canberra: Australian Government Publishing Service.

National Health and Medical Research Council (1997). The health effects of passive smoking: A scientific information paper. Canberra: Australian Government Publishing Service.

National Heart Foundation of Australia (1985). So you think you're a non-smoker. Canberra: National Heart Foundation.

National Heart Foundation of Australia (2000). Heart Facts Report – 1996. Canberra: National Heart Foundation of Australia.

Nidorf, S.M., Parsons, R.W., Thompson, P.L., Jamrozik, K., and Hobbs, M.S.T. (1990). Reduced risk of death at 28 days in patients taking a beta-blocker before admission to hospital with myocardial infarction. *Br Med J*, **300**: 71–4.

Office of Environmental Health Hazard Assessment. (1997). Health effects of exposure to environmental tobacco smoke. Sacramento: California Environmental Protection Agency.

Otsuka, R.,Watanabe, H., Hirata, K., *et al.* (2001). Acute effects of passive smoking on the coronary circulation in healthy young adults. *JAMA*, **286**: 436–41.

Parish, S., Collins, R., Peto, R., *et al.* (1995). Cigarette smoking, tar yields, and non-fatal myocardial infarction: 14,000 cases and 32,000 controls in the United Kingdom. The International Studies of Infarct Survival (ISIS) Collaborators. *Br Med J*, **311**: 471–7.

Penn, A., Keller, K., Snyder, C., Nadas, A., and Chen, L.C. (1996). The tar fraction of cigarette smoke oes not promote arteriosclerotic plaque development. *Environ Health Perspect*, **104**: 1108–13.

Penn, A., and Snyder, C.A. (1996). Butadiene inhalation accelerates atherosclerotic plaque development in cockerels. *Toxicology*, **113**: 351–4.

Penn, A., Nath, R., Pan, J., Chen, L., Widmer, K., Henk, W., and Chung, F.L. (2001). 1, N(2)-propanodeoxyguanosine adduct formation in aortic DNA following inhalation of acrolein. *Environ Health Perspect*, **109**: 219–24.

Pobereskin, L.H. (2001a). Influence of premorbid factors on survival following subarachnoid haemorrhage. *J Neurosurg*, **95**: 555–9.

Pobereskin, L.H. (2001b). Incidence and outcome of subarachnoid haemorrhage, a retrospective population-based study. *J Neurol Neurosurg Psychiatry*, **70**: 340–3.

Roper Organization. (1978). A study of public attitudes toward cigarette smoking and the tobacco industry. (Vol 1) Roper Organization Inc.

Rosenlund, M., Berglind, N., Gustaavsson, A., *et al.* (2001). Environmental tobacco smoke and myocardial infarction among never-smokers in the Stockholm Heart Epidemiology Program (SHEEP). *Epidemiology*, **12**: 558–64.

Royal College of Physicians of London (1962). Smoking and health: a report of the Royal College of Physicians of London on smoking in relation to cancer of the lung and other diseases. London: Pitman Medical.

Sheps, D.S., Adams, K.S., Bromberg, P.A. *et al.* (1987). Lack of effect of low levels of carboxyhaemoglobin on cardiovascular function in patients with ischaemic heart disease. *Arch Environ Health*, **42**: 108–16.

Shinton, R., and Beevers, G. (1989). Meta-analysis of relation between cigarette smoking and stroke. *Br Med J*, **298**: 789–94.

Smith, C.J., Fischer, T.H., and Sears, S.B. (2000). Environmental tobacco smoke, cardiovascular disease, and the non-linear dose-response hypothesis. *Toxicol Sci*, **54**: 462–72.

Sonke, G.S., Stewart, A.W., Beaglehole, R., Jackson, R., and White, H.D. (1997). Comparison of case fatality in smokers and non-smokers after acute cardiac event. *Br Med J*, **315**: 992–3.

Spencer, C.A., Jamrozik, K., Lambert, L.J. (1999). Do simple prudent health behaviours protect men from myocardial infarction? *Intl J Epidemiol*, **28**: 846–52.

Stamler, J., Wentworth, D., and Neaton, J.D. (1986). Is relationship between serum cholesterol and risk of premature death from coronary heart disease continuous and graded? Findings in 356,222 primary screenees of the Multiple Risk Factor Intervention Trial (MRFIT). *JAMA*, **256**: 2823–8.

Stratton, I.M., Kohner, E.M., Aldington, S.J., Turner, R.C., Holman, R.R., Manley, S.E., and Matthews, D.R. (2001). UKPDS 50: risk factors for incidence and progression of retinopathy in Type II diabetes over 6 years from diagnosis. *Diabetologia*, **44**: 156–63.

Steenland, K., Sieber, K., Etzel, R.A., Pechacek, T., and Maurer, K. (1998). Exposure to environmental tobacco smoke and risk factors for heart disease among never smokers in the Third National Health and Nutrition Examination Survey. *Am J Epidemiol*, **147**: 932–9.

Sumida, H., Watanabe, H., Kugiyama, K., Ohgushi, M., Matsumura, T., and Yasue, H. (1998). Does passive smoking impair endothelium-dependent coronary artery dilation in women? *J Am Coll Cardiol*, **31**: 811–5.

Thun, M., Henley, J., and Apicella, L. (1999). Epidemiologic studies of fatal and nonfatal cardiovascular disease and ETS exposure from spousal smoking. *Environ Health Perspect*, **107** Suppl 6: 841–6.

Trichopoulos, D., Kalandidi, A., Sparros, L., and MacMahon, B. (1981). Lung cancer and passive smoking. *Intl J Cancer*, **27**: 1–4.

United States Department of Health and Human Services (1986). The health consequences of involuntary smoking. Washington DC: US Government Printing Office.

United States Department of Health and Human Services (1983). The health consequences of smoking: cardiovascular disease. Washington DC: US Government Printing Office.

van Gijn, J., and Rinkel, G.J.E. (2001). Subarachnoid haemorrhage: diagnosis, causes and management. *Brain*, **124**: 249–78.

Verhoef, P., Rimm, E.B., Hunter, D.J., Chen, J., Willett,W.C., Kelsey, K., and Stampfer, M.J. (1998). A common mutation in the methylenetetrahydrofolate reductase gene and risk of coronary heart disease: results among U.S. men. *J Am Coll Cardiol*, **32**: 353–9.

Wald N.J. (1978). Smoking in relation to lung cancer and coronary heart disease. *Bull Intl Union Against TB*, **53**: 325–33.

Wald, N.J. and Watt, H.C. (1997). Prospective study of effect of switching from cigarettes to pipes or cigars on mortality from three smoking related diseases. *Br Med J*, **314**: 1860–3.

Wells, A.J. (1994). Passive smoking as a cause of heart disease. *J Am Coll Cardiol*, **24**: 546–54.

Wells, A.J., English, P.B., Posner, S. F., Wagenknecht, L.E., and Perez-Stable, E.J. (1998). Misclassification rates for current smokers misclassified as nonsmokers. *Am J Public Health*, **88**: 1503–9.

Wilmink, T.B., Quick, C.R., and Day, N.E. (1999). The association between cigarette smoking and abdominal aortic aneurysms. *J Vasc Surg*, **30**: 1099–105.

World Health Organization (1999). The world health report 1999: Making a difference. WHO: Geneva.

Chapter 32

Chronic obstructive pulmonary disease

David M. Burns

Introduction

Tobacco use is largely driven by the need to ingest sufficient amounts of nicotine. When smoking pipes and cigars, and obviously with a variety of smokeless tobacco products, that need can be satisfied without inhaling large amounts of tobacco smoke into the lung. The vast majority of cigarette smokers do inhale large amounts of tobacco smoke and this difference in inhalation is responsible for the substantially higher risks of chronic obstructive pulmonary disease (COPD) observed in cigarette smokers compared with cigar and pipe smokers (Shanks and Burns 1998; Baker *et al.* 2000).

Most flue cured and blended cigarettes use tobaccos which produce a milder more acid smoke than the tobacco used for pipes and cigars (IARC 1986). Nicotine is less readily absorbed across the oral mucosa from this more acid smoke and the smoke must be inhaled into the much larger surface area of the lung to allow sufficient nicotine absorption. It is this obligatory inhalation of cigarette smoke by the addicted smoker that makes cigarette smoking the most hazardous form of tobacco use.

An extensive body of literature has examined the relationship between tobacco smoke inhalation and chronic lung disease, and that literature is reviewed elsewhere (USDHHS 1984, 1990, 2001, 2004, In Press; IARC 2007). This chapter presents a synthesis of the available information, but it does not attempt to provide an exhaustive set of references to this substantial body of literature.

Patterns of lung injury

Lung damage from tobacco smoke inhalation is described using a variety of terms including chronic bronchitis, emphysema, chronic obstructive lung disease (COLD), chronic obstructive pulmonary disease (COPD), and chronic airflow obstruction. These terms have technical definitions that differ from one another, but they are commonly used synonymously in the medical and scientific literature. In this chapter we will use the term COPD to encompass all of the patterns of lung injury produced by cigarette smoking.

The pathophysiological pattern of tobacco smoke injury is often separated into three overlapping pictures which are each present to a variable extent in most long-term cigarette smokers. The first pattern consists of inflammatory changes in the larger airways and bronchi down to 2–4 mm in diameter. It is characterized by inflammation and hypertrophy of the airway lining with an increased number of mucus secreting glands. It commonly presents with the clinical symptom of a chronic cough productive of small amounts of sputum. This pattern does not predict future progression to clinically significant chronic airflow obstruction on lung function testing when present in individuals with normal lung function (Vestbo and Lange 2002), but does predict a more rapid decline in function for those individuals who already have evidence of significant abnormality in their lung function testing (Vestbo *et al.* 1996).

A second pathophysiological pattern is that of inflammatory changes in the smaller and more distal airways of the lung (2 mm in diameter and smaller) which narrows these airways and increases their resistance to airflow. It is these airways which contribute the largest fraction of the increased resistance to airflow that characterizes COPD (Hogg *et al.* 1968). The inflammatory changes can progress to fibrosis in the airway walls as clinically significant COPD develops.

Inflammatory cells present in the peribronchiolar spaces release digestive enzymes that ultimately damage and disrupt the alveolar walls producing emphysema, the third pathophysiological pattern of injury. As the alveolar walls rupture, the lung becomes composed of a smaller number of much larger airspaces with a reduced surface area and decreased elastic recoil. When examined at autopsy, this digested lung appears full of holes of various sizes. During life, it functions poorly for gas exchange and ventilation. The decreased elastic recoil of an emphysematous lung reduces the pressure available to drive expiratory airflow and allows the airways to collapse during expiration, further worsening the rate of expiratory airflow produced by the inflammatory changes in the small airways described above.

Most smokers will have all three of these patterns of injury to some extent, but it is not unusual for one of the patterns to predominate in a single individual.

Composition of tobacco smoke

Tobacco smoke is a complex aerosol with particles largely within the range of 0.1–1.0 microns in diameter (Bernstein 2004). These particles are small enough that they are poorly removed in the upper airway and deposit largely on the alveolar and airway surfaces of the lung. The pattern of lung deposition is consistent with particles of a somewhat larger size since there is more deposition in the airways and on the alveolar surfaces than would be expected from extrapolations based on particle size alone (Stratton *et al.* 2001). The difference in deposition location is likely due to aggregation of particles in the very dense aerosol of mainstream smoke and because the particles may grow in size as they are humidified in the airway.

Tobacco smoke contains over 4 000 individual constituents and the composition of the smoke undergoes rapid chemical change as it is inhaled (IARC 1986, 2004). Biologically active free radicals are generated as tobacco is burned, and they persist long enough to interact with lung tissue following inhalation. The constituents of smoke have at least three toxicities important for causing injury to the lung in COPD. Tobacco smoke as whole smoke and several of its constituents are potent irritants to the airways capable of creating an inflammatory response in the airways even with initial use. This acute irritant response disappears as the airway adapts to repetitive exposure to smoke. It is replaced by a chronic low-grade inflammation of the airways. Many constituents in both the gas phase and the particulate phase of smoke also paralyze the cilia lining the airways. Cilia are the hair-like structures on the surface of airway cells that rhythmically beat to move mucus up and out of the lung aiding in the removal of particles deposited on the surface of the airways. Paralysis interferes with the clearance process of the lung and results in a longer residence time in the airway for toxic smoke constituents. Lastly, smoke can oxidatively inactivate some of the protective proteins in the blood, most notably the anti-proteases that prevent lung digestion.

Early responses of the lung to cigarette smoking

Acute cough and bronchoconstriction are common reactions to the first inhalation of cigarette smoke. When this protective warning of the airways is ignored and regular smoking is begun, inflammatory changes appear in the small (less than 2 mm) airways of the lung. These changes are evident in some smokers within the first few years of smoking; and, after smoking for 10–15 years, the majority of smokers have evidence of abnormal function in these small airways. Unfortunately, this development of inflammatory changes in the small airways early in the smoking experience is not a useful predictor of the likelihood of subsequently developing clinically significant COPD. These early changes are likely a nearly universal response to the inhaled irritants in the smoke, and it is other biologic or genetic determinants of how the lung responds to chronic irritation that define which smokers will go on to develop COPD.

Even during adolescence and early adulthood, cigarette smoking is associated with a lower level of lung function and an increased frequency of respiratory symptoms, particularly cough (USDHHS 1994, 2004, In Press). Adolescent smokers have a lower rate of increase in lung function as they grow into adulthood when compared to non-smoking adolescents, and there is evidence that they reach a lower level of peak lung function (Tager *et al.* 1988; USDHHS 2004). There is also concern that their decline in lung function may begin at an earlier age. The changes in lung development in actively smoking adolescents are likely superimposed on similar changes produced by exposure to environmental tobacco smoke during infancy and early childhood.

Changes in lung function in smokers and non-smokers

The most widely used measure of lung function abnormality in COPD is the volume of air that can be expired during the first second with a maximal effort (FEV_1). Among populations of heavy smokers, an excess decline in the FEV_1 is seen by ages 25–34 for both males and females in comparison with never-smokers. An excess decline in FEV_1 is seen among both light and heavy-smokers by ages 35–44 (Beck *et al.*, 1981). This excess decline in lung function is greater among those who smoke more cigarettes per day and worsens with increasing duration of smoking (Burrows *et al.*, 1977; DHHS, 1984, 2004). When more than 70% of lung function is lost, it is common for smokers to have symptoms from their ventilatory limitation, most notably shortness of breath on exertion. Once 90% of lung function has been lost ventilatory limitation can compromise survival and death from ventilatory failure becomes an increasingly likely and unavoidable outcome.

The relationship between smoking and lung function as measured by FEV_1 at various ages is presented in Fig. 32.1. Among normal individuals who do not smoke, and who do not have substantive exposure to environmental tobacco smoke, lung function increases as a child grows and the FEV_1 reaches a peak between ages 20 and 25 years. Thereafter, it slowly declines. This experience is presented as a thick solid line in Fig. 32.1.

Children who are exposed to environmental tobacco smoke have a lower rate of lung growth. That effect of environmental tobacco smoke exposure is portrayed by the dotted line prior to age 20 in Fig. 32.1. This lower rate of growth in lung function may be worsened, and the age of peak lung growth may be reached earlier, if the adolescent begins to actively smoke cigarettes. There is also considerable concern that these changes in the developing lung may predispose the adult lung to a more rapid decline in function with increasing age, particularly if smoking continues during adulthood.

When the entire population of adult smokers is examined, their rate of lung function decline with age is substantially steeper than that for non-smokers, reflecting progressive damage to the airways and alveoli of their lungs. This change with advancing age and duration of smoking is presented in Fig. 32.1 as a dashed line labelled 'all smokers'. However, the rate of decline for all smokers as a group is not sufficient to cause respiratory disability for the majority of smokers, in part because of the large ventilatory reserve of the lung.

Not all smokers develop abnormal lung function or clinically evident COPD (Fletcher *et al.* 1976). When an abnormal FEV_1 is used as the criteria for diagnosis of COPD, approximately one

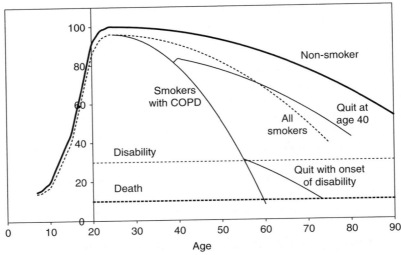

Figure 32.1 FEV$_1$ as a percent of the value at age 25 for smokers, non-smokers and those who quit.

Source: Modified from Fletcher CM, Peto R (1977) with permission from the BMJ Publishing Group Ltd.

Note

The values presented are the FEV$_1$ as a percentage of the value for an individual at age 25 years. The heavy solid line represents those who have never smoked, the dashed line represents the entire population of smokers including those exposed to environmental tobacco smoke as children, the thin solid line represents those smokers who are going to develop COPD, thin solid lines also represent those who quit at age 40 years and when symptoms develop. See text for description.

third of smokers over age 55 (Sherrill *et al.* 1994) have COPD, and that percentage increases to over 45% when smokers over age 65 are examined (Higgins *et al.* 1993). This relatively high prevalence of abnormal lung function is supported by autopsy studies which show evidence of at least some emphysema in the lungs of approximately 90% of long term cigarettes smokers (Auerbach *et al.* 1972; Sutinen *et al.* 1978).

Many smokers with abnormal lung function may be unaware of the presence of lung injury and may have no symptoms related to their lung damage. A minority of cigarette smokers, in the range of 15–25%, will have a more rapid decline in lung function and will develop clinically significant COPD (Fletcher *et al.* 1976). These smokers are more likely to have smoked more cigarettes per day and to have smoked for a longer duration, but known characteristics of smoking behaviour do not fully explain why some smokers develop COPD and others with similar smoking patterns do not. Differences in genetic susceptibility or differences in response to inflammation have been postulated as reasons for the differences in the rate of progression to clinically significant disease.

The thin solid line in Fig. 32.1 represents this fraction of smokers with rapidly declining lung function who go on to develop COPD. Having an abnormal FEV$_1$ by early middle age (age 45) is a strong predictor of developing COPD, but it is less clear that the rate of decline over one period of time is a good predictor of the future rate of decline or of the likelihood of developing COPD. Identification of smokers with abnormal lung function in early middle age offers the opportunity to intervene with smoking cessation assistance before clinically significant ventilatory limitation develops. Those who quit smoking are likely to have a small improvement in lung function during the first year of abstinence, and their rate of decline in lung function slows to that of the never-smoker (Anthonisen *et al.* 1994; Scanlon *et al.* 2000; USDHHS 2004; IARC 2007). This pattern of change is depicted by the thin solid line in Fig. 32.1 labelled 'quit at age 40'. If smokers quit before there is extensive lung damage and remain abstinent, it is likely that most of them will never develop clinically significant COPD (IARC 2007).

In contrast to interventions early in the course of lung injury from smoking, getting smokers to quit once they have developed disease extensive enough to be disabling has more limited benefits. Even for this group with extensive damage, there is a slowing in the rate of decline in lung function with cessation of smoking; but the individuals usually remain symptomatic (Anthonisen *et al.* 1994; IARC 2007). The effect of cessation is simply to prolong the interval between the onset of symptoms and death rather than to eliminate the disability. This effect is depicted by the thin solid line in Fig. 32.1 labelled 'Quit with onset of disability'.

Chronic cough is a less disabling but far more common result of cigarette smoking than is ventilatory limitation. Increased prevalence of chronic cough is evident even among adolescent and young adult smokers. The prevalence increases with increasing duration of smoking and is present in the majority of moderate to heavy smokers over age 60 years (Lebowitz and Burrows 1977). This cough begins as a dry cough but progresses with longer duration of smoking to become productive of small amounts of mucus.

Mechanisms of lung injury

Airway inflammation and enzymatic digestion of lung structural proteins (elastin and collagen) are mechanisms that define the injury to the lung in COPD. Early in the smoking exposure, the changes are edema and inflammatory cell (cytotoxic T lymphocytes and macrophages) infiltration in the walls of the small airways of the lung. Inflammation is due to epithelial cell injury that increases permeability and releases proinflammatory mediators. These mediators draw in neutrophils, and the result is a pathological picture typical of chronic inflammation. The vast majority of smokers develop these changes, and many develop them within the first year or two of smoking. These early changes can reverse within one year following cessation among smokers with a short smoking duration (Buist *et al.* 1976, 1979). With longer duration of smoking, epithelial hyperplasia, smooth muscle hypertrophy, and peribronchiolar fibrosis are commonly found in most smokers (Cosio *et al.* 1978, 1980) and these changes may not fully reverse with cessation.

The neutophils and macrophages that are part of the inflammatory response to cigarette smoke in the lung release enzymes capable of digesting the elastin and collagen that make up the structural elements of the lung. Anti-proteases, released from macrophages and found in the blood, block the action of these enzymes (Barnes 2000). The result is a balance that preserves the integrity of normal lung while allowing the lung to respond to external infectious agents by releasing digestive enzymes. Oxidants in cigarette smoke and generated by cellular inflammatory responses inactivate the anti-proteases unbalancing this relationship and leading to digestion of lung tissue, rupture of alveolar walls, and emphysematous dilation of the alveolar spaces (Barnes 2000; USDHHS In Press).

At least a modest degree of emphysema is found in most continuing smokers over the age of 60 years (Auerbach *et al.* 1972; Sutinen *et al.* 1978), and the severity of the emphysematous change increases with the number of cigarettes smoked per day. In contrast to the inflammatory changes in the small airways, emphysema is usually manifest later in life (over age 50) and is not reversible.

Death rates from COPD in smokers and non-smokers

Death from infection, respiratory failure, or other complications of COPD is an end result of the slowly accumulating lung damage produced by smoking. Because symptoms and disability may be present for a decade or more before death from COPD, and because individuals may die with COPD without it being the cause of death, death rates from COPD underestimate both the extent of cigarette induced lung injury among smokers and the prevalence of COPD for the general population. Comparisons of mortality rates between smokers and non-smokers (e.g. relative risks) yield very high values at most ages, since the occurrence of COPD is largely limited to smokers and very low rates of disease or death from COPD occur among never-smokers. Mortality based relative risks increase with increasing number of cigarettes smoked per day and increasing duration of smoking (USDHHS 1984, 2004).

The effect of smoking on rates of death from COPD can also be examined using the excess death rate in smokers. An excess death rate is simply the age and disease-specific death rates in never-smokers subtracted from the same age and disease specific death rate in smokers, and it offers a different perspective on the absolute risks of the diseases due to smoking at different ages.

Figure 32.2 presents excess death rates for lung cancer, coronary heart disease and COPD for male smokers examined in the American Cancer Society Cancer Prevention Study II (Thun *et al.* 1997). It is evident that coronary heart disease results in substantial excess mortality among smokers by age 40 years, and excess death rates from lung cancer increases rapidly after age 50. However death from COPD is largely confined to ages over 60–65 years. This later onset of excess death rates from COPD is due to the slowly progressive nature of the disease process and the large ventilatory reserve of the lung, but it is also the reason why morbidity and health care costs from COPD are much larger than one might expect from comparisons based solely on numbers of deaths from different causes.

The late rise in smoking attributable death rate from COPD also helps to explain why national death rates from heart disease and lung cancer rise more rapidly than do death rates from COPD as cigarette smoking is first adopted by the population of a country, and correspondingly why death rates from COPD decline more slowly than those of heart disease and cancer as the prevalence of smoking declines.

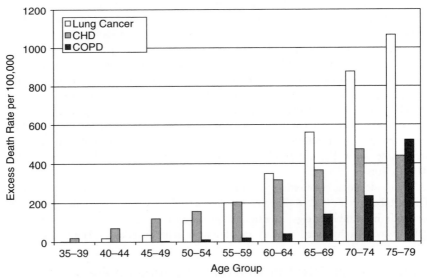

Figure 32.2 Male excess death rates* from smoking caused diseases. (*Rates in smokers minus the rate in never smokers).

Source: CPS II Data (Thun *et al.* 1997).

Note

Excess rates are calculated by subtracting the age specific death rate for a given disease experienced by smokers from that for never smokers in the American Cancer Society Cancer Prevention II study as published by Thun *et al.* 1997. Rates are presented for male smokers.

Changes with cessation of smoking

The risk of dying from COPD declines following cessation of cigarette smoking when compared to that of continuing smokers (USDHHS 1990; IARC 2007; Godtfredsen *et al.* 2008). The decline in risk is slower than that for heart disease and lung cancer, and there remains a small increase in risk even after prolonged abstinence (NCI 1997; IARC 2007). The fraction of the excess risk of dying of COPD, lung cancer, and coronary heart disease that remains after abstinence of various durations is presented in Fig. 32.3. It takes longer for the excess risk of death from COPD to decline following cessation, and the death rate remains substantially elevated in former smokers even after 20 years of abstinence (IARC 2007).

As described above, lung function may improve slightly following cessation probably due to a decrease in airway inflammation once the exposure to the irritants in tobacco smoke ceases. The rate of lung function decline with advancing age also slows following cessation and the rate of decline returns to that of the never-smoker within five years of quitting (Anthonisen *et al.*, 1994; Scanlon *et al.*, 2000; IARC 2007). However, the emphysema present in the lung at the time of cessation does not repair, and lung function rarely returns to normal among smokers with substantial lung injury at the time of cessation.

Respiratory symptoms, most notably a chronic productive cough, often improve following cessation and may disappear altogether with long term abstinence.

Pipe and cigar smoking

Cigarette smokers are much more likely to inhale tobacco smoke than are those who have only smoked pipes and cigars, and this distinction is evident in the pattern of disease risks found

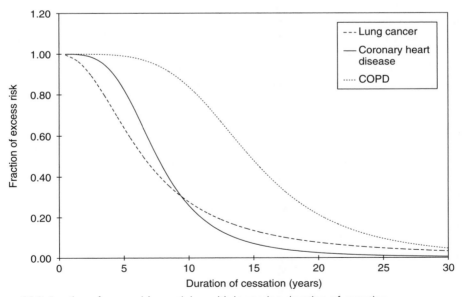

Figure 32.3 Fraction of excess risk remaining with increasing duration of cessation.

Source: Modified from Burns 2000.

Note

The data presented are the fraction of the excess death rate (rate in smokers minus the rate in never smokers of the same age) that remains after different numbers of years following successful smoking cessation. Data are modeled from the American Cancer Society Cancer Prevention Study I as described in Burns 2000.

among smokers of different forms of tobacco. Pipe and cigar smokers have risks similar to those of cigarettes smokers for cancers of the oral cavity where exposure to smoke is similar whether the smoker inhales or not; but cancer of the lung and COPD are much less common among pipe and cigar smokers than among cigarettes smokers (Shanks *et al.* 1998; Baker *et al.* 2000). These distinctions in disease risks disappear if pipe and cigar smokers inhale more deeply, an observation of considerable concern since cigarette smokers who have switched to pipes or cigars are much more likely report that they inhale the smoke than are smokers who have only used these forms of tobacco.

Cigarettes with lower machine-measured yields of tar and nicotine

The yield of tar and nicotine as measured by machine has declined substantially for commercial cigarettes sold over the past 50 years, and these newer and filtered cigarettes have been presented to the public as safer alternatives to unfiltered and higher tar cigarettes (Pollay and Dewhirst 2002). Smokers of these types of cigarettes report them as being 'smoother on the throat and lighter on their chest' (Shiffman *et al.* 2001), and there is some evidence to suggest that smokers of these products may have a lower prevalence of chronic cough (Higenbottam *et al.* 1980). However, the evidence does not suggest a difference in the extent of lung function impairment or mortality from COPD with use of these cigarettes (NCI 2001).

Summary

Cigarette smoking is the dominant cause of chronic obstructive pulmonary disease for both men and women. Changes in the lungs of smokers can be demonstrated within a few years of beginning to smoke. By the age 25–34 years, evidence of functional loss is evident in populations of heavy-smokers. The risks of developing ventilatory impairment and of dying of COPD increase with increasing number of cigarettes smoked per day and increased duration of smoking. Cessation of smoking alters the rate of lung function decline and risk of dying from COPD, but the benefits of cessation are greatest when cessation can be achieved early before substantial lung injury has occurred.

References

Anthonisen, N.R., Connett, J.E., Kiley, J.P., Altose, M.D., Bailey, W.C., Buist, A.S. *et al.* (1994). Effects of smoking intervention and the use of inhaled anticholinergic bronchodilator on the rate of decline in FEV1: the Lung Health Study. *Journal of the American Medical Association*, **272**: 1497–1505.

Auerbach, O., Hammond, E.C., Garfinkel, L., and Benante, C. (1972). Relation of smoking and age to emphysema. Whole-lung section study. *New England Journal of Medicine*, **286**: 853–857.

Baker, F., Ainsworth, S.R., Dye, J.T., Crammer, C., Thun, M.J., Hoffmann, D. *et al.* (2000). Health risks associated with cigar smoking. *JAMA*, Aug 9; **284**(6): 735–740.

Barnes, PJ. (2000). Chronic obstructive pulmonary disease. *New England Journal of Medicine*, **343**: 269–280.

Beck, G.J., Doyle, C.A., and Schachter, E.N. (1981). Smoking and lung function. *American Review of Respiratory Disease*, **123**: 149–155.

Bernstein, D. (2004). A review of the influence of particle size, puff volume, and inhalation pattern on the deposition of cigarette smoke particles in the respiratory tract. *Inhal Toxicol.*, Sep; **16**(10): 675–689.

Buist, A.S., Nagy, J.M., and Sexton, G.J. (1979). The effect of smoking cessation on pulmonary function: a 30-month follow-up of two smoking cessation clinics. *American Review of Respiratory Disease*, **120**: 953–957.

Buist, A.S., Sexton, G.J., Nagy, J.M., and Ross, B.B. (1976). The effect of smoking cessation and modification on lung function. *American Review of Respiratory Disease*, **114**: 115–122.

Burns, D.M. (2000). Primary prevention, smoking, and smoking cessation — implications for future trends in lung cancer prevention. *Cancer* 89, No. 11(Suppl): 2506–2509.

Burrows, B., Knudson, R.J., Cline, M.G., and Lebowitz, M.D. (1977). Quantitative relationships between cigarette smoking and ventilatory function. *American Review of Respiratory Disease*, **115**: 195–205.

Cosio, M.G., Chezzo, H., Hogg, J.C., Corbin, R., Lovelnd, M., Dosman, J. *et al.* (1978). The relations between structural changes in the small airways and pulmonary function tests. *New England Journal of Medicine*, **298**: 1277–1281.

Cosio, M.G., Hale, K.A., and Niewoehner, D.E. (1980). Morphologic and morphometric effects of prolonged cigarette smoking on the small airways. *American Review of Respiratory Disease*, **122**: 265–271.

Fletcher, C.M., Peto, R., Tinker, C., and Speizer, F.E. (1976). *The Natural History of Chronic Bronchitis and Emphysema: an Eight-Year Study of Chronic Obstructive Lung Disease in Working Men in London.* New York: Oxford University Press.

Fletcher, C.M. and Peto, R. (1977). The natural history of chronic airflow obstructions. *Br Med J*, 1: 1645–1648.

Godtfredsen, N.S., Lam, T.H., Hansel, T.T., Leon, M.E., Gray, N., Dresler, C. *et al.* (2008). COPD-related morbidity and mortality after smoking cessation: status of the evidence. *Eur Respir J.*, Oct; **32**(4): 844–853.

Higenbottam, T., Clark, T.J.H., Shipley, M.J., and Rose, G. (1980). Lung function and symptoms of cigarette smokers related to tar yield and number of cigarettes smoked. *Lancet*, 1(8165): 409–411.

Higgins, M.W., Enright, P.L., Kronmal, R.A., Schenker, M.B., Anton-Culver, H., and Lyles, M. (1993). Smoking and lung function in elderly men and women: the Cardiovascular Health Study. *Journal of the American Medical Association*, **269**: 2741–2748.

Hogg, J.C., Macklem, P.T., and Thurlbeck, W.M. (1968). Site and nature of airway obstruction in chronic lung disease. *New England Journal of Medicine*, **278**: 1355–1360.

International Agency for Research on Cancer (1986). IARC Monographs on the carcinogenic risk of chemicals to humans: tobacco smoking. Volume 38. IARC, Lyon, France.

International Agency for Research on Cancer (IARC) (2004). *Tobacco smoke and involuntary smoking.* IARC Monographs on the Evaluation of Carcinogenic Risks to Humans. Vol. 83. Lyon (France): World Health Organization/IARC.

IARC Working Group (2007). Reversal of Risk After Quitting Smoking. IARC Handbooks of Cancer Prevention, Volume 11. International Agency for Research on Cancer, Lyon, France.

Lebowitz, M.D. and Burrows, B. (1977). Quantitative relationships between cigarette smoking and chronic productive cough. *International Journal of Epidemiology*, **6**: 107–113.

National Cancer Institute (1997). Smoking and Tobacco Control Monograph # 8: Changes in cigarette-related disease risks and their implications for prevention and control. Burns D, Garfinkel L, Samet J, editors. U.S. Department of Health and Human Services, Public Health Service, National Institutes of Health, National Cancer Institute. NIH Publication No. 97-4213.

National Cancer Institute (2001). Smoking and Tobacco Control Monograph No.13. Risks associated with smoking cigarettes with low machine yields of tar and nicotine. Bethesda, US Department of Health and Human Services. NCI, October.

Pollay, R. W. and Dewhirst, T. (2002). The dark side of marketing seemingly 'light' cigarettes: successful images and failed fact. *Tobacco Control*, **11**(Suppl. 1): 118–131.

Scanlon, P.D., Connett, J.E., Waller, L.A., Altose, M.D., Bailey, W.C., Buist, A.S. *et al.* (2000). Smoking cessation and lung function in mild-to-moderate chronic obstructive pulmonary disease: the Lung Health Study. *American Journal of Respiratory and Critical Care Medicine*, **161**: 381–390.

Shanks, T. and Burns, D. (1998). Disease consequences of cigar smoking. In: D. Burns, K.M. Cummings, and D. Hoffman (eds) *Cigar smoking in the United States: Health effects and trends.* Smoking and Tobacco Control Monograph No. 9. USDHHS NIH NCI, Chapter 4.

Sherrill, D.L., Holberg, C.J., Enright, P.L., Lebowitz, M.D., and Burrows, B. (1994). Longitudinal analysis of the effects of smoking onset and cessation on pulmonary function. *American Journal of Respiratory and Critical Care Medicine*, **149**: 591–597.

Shiffman, S., Pillitteri, J.L., Burton, S.L., Rohay, J.M., and Gitchell, J.G. (2001). Smokers beliefs about 'light' and 'ultra light' cigarettes. *Tobacco Control*, **10**(Suppl I): i17–i23.

Speizer, F.E. and Tager, I.B. (1979). Epidemiology of chronic mucus hypersecretion and obstructive airways disease. *Epidemiology Reviews*, **1**: 124–142.

Stratton, K., Shetty, P., Wallace, R., Bondurant, S. (eds) (2001). Clearing the smoke. Assessing the science base for tobacco harm reduction. National Academy Press. Washington D.C.

Sutinen, S., Vaajalahti, P., and Paakko, P. (1978). Prevalence, severity, and types of pulmonary emphysema in a population of deaths in a Finnish city. *Correlation with age, sex and smoking. Scandinavian Journal of Respiratory Disease*, **59**: 101–115.

Tager, I.B., Segal, M.R., Speizer, F.E., and Weiss, S.T. (1988). The natural history of forced expiratory volumes: effect of cigarette smoking and respiratory symptoms. *American Review of Respiratory Disease*, **138**: 837–849.

Thun, M., Myers, D., Day-Lally, C., Namboodiri, M., Calle, E., Flanders, W.D. *et al.* (1997). Age and the Exposure-response relationships between cigarette smoking and premature death in cancer prevention study II, Chapter 5. In: D. Burns, L. Garfinkel, and J. Samet (eds). *Changes in Cigarette-Related Disease Risks and Their Implications for Prevention and Control: Smoking and Tobacco Control Monograph # 8.* US Department of Health and Human Services, Public Health Service, National Institutes of Health, National Cancer Institute. NIH Publication No. 97-4213, P. 383–476.

US Department of Health and Human Services (1984). *The Health Consequences of Smoking: Chronic Obstructive Lung Disease. A Report of the Surgeon General.* US Department of Health and Human Services, Public Health Service, Office on Smoking and Health, DHHS Publication No. (PHS) 84-50205.

US Department of Health and Human Services (1990). The Health Benefits of Smoking Cessation. US Dept of Health and Human Services, Public Health Service, Centers for Disease Control, National Center for Chronic Disease Prevention and Health Promotion, Office on Smoking and Health. DHHS Publication No. (CDC) 90-8416.

US Department of Health and Human Services (1994). *Preventing Tobacco Use Among Young People: A Report of the Surgeon General.* Atlanta, GA: US DHHS, Public Health Service, Centers for Disease Control and Prevention, National Center for Chronic Disease Prevention and Health Promotion, Office on Smoking and Health.

US Department of Health and Human Services (2001). *Women and Smoking: A Report of the Surgeon General.* Atlanta, Georgia: US Department of Health and Human Services, Public Health Service, Centers for Disease Control and Prevention, National Center for Chronic Disease Prevention and Health Promotion, Office on Smoking and Health.

US Department of Health and Human Services (2004). *The Health Consequences of Tobacco Use: A Report of the Surgeon General.* Atlanta, Georgia: US Department of Health and Human Services, Public Health Service, Centers for Disease Control and Prevention, National Center for Chronic Disease Prevention and Health Promotion, Office on Smoking and Health.

US Department of Health and Human Services (in press). *How Tobacco Causes Disease – The Biology and Behavioral Basis for Tobacco Attributable Disease: A Report of the Surgeon General.* Atlanta, Georgia: U.S. Department of Health and Human Services, Public Health Service, Centers for Disease Control and Prevention, National Center for Chronic Disease Prevention and Health Promotion, Office on Smoking and Health.

Vestbo, J. and Lange, P. (2002). Can GOLD Stage 0 provide information of prognostic value in chronic obstructive pulmonary disease? *American Journal of Respiratory and Critical Care Medicine*, Aug 1; **166**(3): 329–332.

Vestbo, J., Prescott, E., and Lange, P. (1996). Association of chronic mucus hypersecretion with FEV1 decline and chronic obstructive pulmonary disease morbidity. Copenhagen City Heart Study Group. *American Journal of Respiratory and Critical Care Medicine*, May; **153**(5): 1530–1535.

Chapter 33

Smoking and other disorders

Allan Hackshaw

Introduction

Given that smoking consists of several thousand chemicals and toxins it is no wonder that it is associated with a wide range of diseases. Since the first epidemiological studies linking smoking with lung cancer, there has been an abundance of studies (epidemiological and biological) that have shown smokers to be at a higher (or in a few cases, lower) risk of developing certain disorders. Smoking is an established cause of several cancers, respiratory disease, and cardiovascular disease; these are described elsewhere in this book. This chapter presents an overview of the effects of smoking on other disorders, using published reviews and the results of published meta-analyses where available. In some cases, the results of cohort studies that are based on incident cases (where possible) are provided, thus aiming to ensure that smoking has preceded the disorder and avoiding some of the possible biases associated with case-control studies. The studies referenced here may not be all that are available, and the disorders reviewed here are by no means all those that are or may be associated with smoking. They represent ones that are relatively common in the population and in which smoking has, in the past, been regarded as a risk factor.

Gastrointestinal system

Smoking is associated with several disorders of the gastrointestinal tract. Table 33.1 shows pooled relative risks of some of the main disorders obtained from meta-analyses.

Peptic ulcer

Peptic ulcers (gastric or duodenal) are relatively common among adults. Many epidemiological studies have shown that smokers are about twice as likely to develop peptic ulcers than non-smokers, including several large cohort studies that looked at incidence of the disease (Table 33.2). Risk increases with increasing cigarette consumption (Paffenberger *et al.* 1974; Anda *et al.* 1990) and it is lower in former-smokers (Anda *et al.* 1990; Vessey *et al.* 1992; Doll *et al.* 1994). Studies have also shown that smoking can delay the healing process once ulcers have developed and it can increase the risk of recurrence. The evidence is consistent with that from biological studies from which several mechanisms have been proposed. Smoking affects factors that can promote the development of ulcers, for example by increasing gastric secretions such as pepsin and causing the reflux of contents in the duodenum back into the stomach. It also has a detrimental effect on the defensive mechanisms in the gastroduodenal mucosa, which in the absence of smoking would aid ulcer healing. There have been several reviews on this topic, for example, see Ashley 1997, Eastwood 1997, and Parasher & Eastwood 2000.

However, with the recent discovery of the micro-organism *Helicobactor pylori* as an important cause of peptic ulcer it is possible that the effect of smoking as an independent risk factor is less than originally thought. It is proposed that smokers are only more susceptible to *H. pylori*

Table 33.1 Published pooled relative risks associated with smoking and gastrointestinal disease

Disorder	Author	Number of epidemiological studies in analysis	Gender	Relative risk (95% CI) in smokers compared to non-smokers
Peptic ulcer	Kurata & Nogawa 1997	20	Men & women	2.2 (2.0–2.3)
Crohn's disease	Logan 1990	7	Men & women	2.4 (2.0–2.9)
	English et al. 1995	7	Men	2.24 (1.45–3.46)
		7	Women	4.76 (3.10–7.31)
Ulcerative colitis	Logan 1990	8	Men & women	0.47 (0.39–0.56)
Gallstone disease	English et al. 1995	4	Men & women	1.24 (1.16–1.32)

infection and that smoking enhances the adverse effects of the infection (Parasher & Eastwood 2000). Furthermore, there is evidence that once the infection has been eradicated smoking has little or no effect on ulcer development or recurrence (O'Connor et al. 1995; Chan et al. 1997; Borody et al. 1992; Kadayifci et al. 1997; Marshall et al. 1988). Whatever the true mechanism may be, smoking is an important risk factor, either by causing some ulcers directly or indirectly by leading to *H. pylori* infection.

Table 33.2 Cohort studies that reported results on peptic ulcer and smoking

Study (first author)	Country	Number of subjects	Total number of ulcers diagnosed	Gender	Relative risk in current-smokers compared to never-smokers (95% CI)
Paffenberger et al. 1974	USA	26 954	487	Men	1.30 (1.07–1.58)
Stemmermann et al. 1989	USA (Hawaii)	5 933	326	Men	2.12 (1.60–2.80)
Anda et al. 1990	USA	2 851	140	Women	1.8 (1.2–2.6)
Kurata et al. 1992	USA	34 198	154	Men	1.50 (0.47–4.81)
				Women	1.48 (0.35–6.24)
Vessey et al. 1992	UK	17 032	175	Women	1.74 (not reported)
Doll et al. 1994	UK	34 439	134*	Men	3.00 (not reported)
Johnsen et al. 1994	Norway	6 864	165	Men	2.66 (1.88–3.77)
		6 907	78	Women	2.28 (1.42–3.67)

Note

*Deaths from peptic ulcer

Inflammatory bowel disease

It is well documented that smoking increases the risk of Crohn's disease but decreases the risk of ulcerative colitis, and this has been consistent between studies, most of which have been case-control studies. Table 33.3 shows the results of these studies, including two cohort studies which allowed for oral contraceptive use (associated with both smoking and inflammatory bowel disease, Vessey *et al.* 1986). Current-smokers have about half the risk of ulcerative colitis compared to never-smokers and more than twice the risk of Crohn's disease, though the risk is higher in women than in men (Table 33.1). It is estimated that about one third of all cases of Crohn's disease could be attributed to smoking (Logan 1990). In former smokers, while the risk for Crohn's disease is lower than that in current-smokers (former vs. never; relative risk 1.5, 95% CI 1.1–1.9 and current vs. never; relative risk 2.4, 95% CI 2.0–2.9) the association with ulcerative colitis is unclear; there seems to be an increased risk. The pooled result in the eight case-control studies is 1.9 (95% CI 1.6–2.3) and it is similarly raised, though not greatly so, in the cohort study by Vessey *et al.* 1986 (relative risk 1.25). If similar results are found in further cohort studies it would indicate that the timing of smoking plays some part in the development of ulcerative colitis.

The biological mechanism for inflammatory bowel disease and its association with smoking are not yet fully understood and it is still unclear why current smoking would have opposite effects on these two disorders, that is, it seems to promote Crohn's disease but protect against ulcerative colitis. Nicotine (in the form of patches or chewing gum) has been proposed as a possible treatment for ulcerative colitis though its effectiveness remains to be confirmed. Reviews of smoking and inflammatory bowel disease can be found in Ashley 1997, Logan 1990, and Rubin & Hanauer 2000.

Table 33.3 Studies that reported results on Crohn's disease and smoking*

Study (first author)	Country	Total number of subjects with Crohn's disease	Gender	Relative risk in current-smokers compared to never-smokers (95% CI)
Case-control				
Logan 1984, 1986	UK	131	Men & women	4.2 (2.5–6.8)
Tobin 1987	UK	127	Men & women	3.2 (1.9–5.5)
Franceschi 1987	Italy	109	Men & women	2.9 (1.8–4.9)
Lindberg 1988	Sweden	144	Men & women	2.2 (1.4–3.3)
Benoni 1987	Sweden	155	Men & women	2.0 (1.3–3.1)
Calkins 1984	USA	132	Men & women	2.1 (1.2–3.5)
Sandler 1988	USA	298	Men & women	1.9 (1.3–2.8)
Combined	–	**1 096**	**Men & women**	**2.4 (2.0–2.9)**
Cohort				
Vessey 1986	UK	18/17,032	Women	3.0 (1.0–9.0)#
Logan 1986, 1989	UK	42/>20,000	Women	1.75 (0.93–3.3)#

Note

* Adapted from Logan 1990 (in which the references to the studies are also given).

Current-smokers compared to never- and former-smokers (relative risk adjusted for age, social class, and oral contraceptive use).

Table 33.4 Studies that reported results on ulcerative colitis and smoking*

Study (first author)	Country	Total number of subjects with ulcerative colitis	Gender	Relative risk in current-smokers compared to never-smokers (95% CI)
Case-control				
Logan 1984, 1986	UK	175	Men & women	0.23 (0.14–0.38)
Tobin 1987	UK	131	Men & women	0.18 (0.10–0.33)
Franceschi 1987	Italy	124	Men & women	0.61 (0.35–1.00)
Lindberg 1988	Sweden	258	Men & women	0.64 (0.45–0.90)
Benoni 1987	Sweden	173	Men & women	0.33 (0.21–0.53)
Calkins 1984	USA	85	Men & women	0.62 (0.29–1.30)
Boyko 1987	USA	212	Men & women	0.64 (0.41–1.00)
Sandler 1988	USA	170	Men & women	0.80 (0.46–1.40)
Combined	**–**	**1 328**	**Men & women**	**0.47 (0.39–0.56)**
Cohort				
Vessey 1986	UK	31/17,032	Women	0.65 (0.25–1.70)[#]
Logan 1986, 1989	UK	78/>20,000	Women	0.68 (0.41–1.1)[#]

Note

* Adapted from Logan 1990 (in which the references to the studies are also given).
[#] Current-smokers compared to never- and former-smokers (relative risk adjusted for age, social class, and oral contraceptive use).

Gallbladder (gallstone) disease

The evidence for smoking as a cause has been less consistent compared to inflammatory bowel disease, partly because there is only a modest increase in risk (about a 30% increase in risk in smokers compared to non-smokers). While cohort studies seem to consistently show an increased risk (Table 33.5), other studies, namely surveys and case-control studies, suggest no association or even a decreased risk. Given the consistency between the cohort studies and that they all allowed for several known or potential confounding factors (e.g. alcohol intake and body mass index), smoking does seem to be a risk factor. The subject is reviewed by Ashley 1997 and Logan & Skelly 2000.

Skin

Psoriasis

The prevalence of psoriasis is somewhat high, about 1 in 50 adults. It is associated with several risk factors, both genetic and environmental, including those that are also strongly associated with smoking (e.g. alcohol and stress). For many years there has been speculation over whether smoking is a cause and few studies have been designed to address the issue directly. Most of the epidemiological studies have had a case-control design (see Naldi 1998 for a summary of several studies) and few have allowed for confounding factors. Findings from such studies and a large cohort study suggest that there is a two- to three-fold (100–200%) increase in risk in women (Table 33.6) and a 30–40% increase in risk in men. There is also a dose–response relationship. In the study by Naldi *et al.* 1999 the conclusion was that smoking was a more important risk factor for psoriasis in women than alcohol, but the opposite may be true in men. This observation is

Table 33.5 Cohort studies that reported results on gallbladder (gallstone) disease and smoking*

Study (first author)	Country	Number of subjects	Total number of subjects with gallstone disease	Gender	Relative risk in current-smokers compared to never-smokers (95% CI)#
Layde 1982	UK	17 000	227	Women	1.63 (p-value <0.004)[b]
Kato 1992	USA (Hawaii)	7 831	471	Men	1.6 (1.2–2.0)[a]
Stampfer 1992	USA	90 3000	2 122	Women	1.3 (1.0–1.7)[a]
Murray 1994	UK	23 000	1 087	Women	1.19 (1.06–1.34)[b]
Misciagna 1996	Italy	2 472	104	Men & women	2.15 (1.3–3.5)[a]
Sahi 1998	USA	16 785	685	Men	1.52 (1.03–2.24)[a]
Leitzmann 1999	USA	42 882	1 016	Men	1.40 (1.14–1.72)[a]

Note

* Partly adapted from Logan & Skelly 2000 with some information taken from the individual publications (which are referenced in Logan & Skelly).
# Adjusted for: (a) age, alcohol, body mass index, and other factors; (b) age, body mass index, oral contraceptive use, and other factors.

consistent with the well-known anti-oestrogenic effects of smoking. However, there is some evidence that once acquired, those who quit smoking do not seem to benefit much (Naldi *et al.* 1999), the risk in former-smokers was still increased.

It is possible that stress plays a part in the observed association. Stress could result in the onset of psoriasis, after which the subject takes up smoking; smoking would therefore not be a risk factor.

Table 33.6 Studies that reported results on psoriasis and smoking

Study (first author)	Country	Total number of subjects with psoriasis	Gender	Cigarette consumption	Relative risk in current-smokers compared to never-smokers (95% CI)
Case-control					
Naldi et al. 1999	Italy	219	Men	1–15 cigs/day	1.3 (0.7–2.0)*
				>15	1.4 (0.9–2.2)*
		185	Women	1–15 cigs/day	1.7 (1.0–2.7)*
				>15	3.9 (1.9–7.9)*
Poikolainen et al. 1994[a]	Finland	55	Women	≥20 cigs/day	3.3 (1.4–7.9)#
Cohort					
Vessey et al. 2000[b]	UK	92/17 032	Women	≥15 cigs/day	1.9 (1.0–3.6)+

Note

[a] Based on smoking habits before onset of psoriasis
[b] Based on first hospital referral for psoriasis.
* Adjusted for age and alcohol.
# Alcohol and smoking had independent effects.

This has, to some extent, been allowed for by basing the results of studies on smoking habits before the onset of disease (Poikolainen *et al.* 1994; Naldi *et al.* 1998); both report an increased risk in smokers.

It is estimated that perhaps one in five cases of psoriasis could be due to smoking. Recent reviews of this topic can be found in Naldi (1998) and Higgins (2000).

Neurological system

Parkinson's disease

Smoking and its possible protective effect on Parkinson's disease was reported as far back as 1959 (Dorn *et al.* 1959) and there have since been numerous studies that have consistently shown smokers to have a lower risk of developing or having this disorder than non-smokers; they have about half the risk. Morens *et al.* 1995 reviewed 35 studies (cohort and case-control) and all showed a decreased risk. A recent meta-analysis of three cohort and eight case-control studies confirm the protective effect of smoking, that is, about a halving of risk among current-smokers compared to never-smokers, based on 2 733 cases of Parkinson's disease among 11 726 subjects in total. Furthermore, there appears to be a clear dose–response relationship between cigarette consumption and risk (Table 33.7). Several mechanisms have been proposed to explain the association; nicotine stimulates an increase in dopamine, the anti-oxidant effect of carbon monoxide in cigarette smoke is protective and smoking offers some protection against neuronal damage. There have been several reviews including Marmot 1990, Morens *et al.* 1995, and Fratiglioni & Wang 2000.

Dementia

Because Alzheimer's disease accounts for most cases of dementia in the elderly, there was interest in the early studies that, like Parkinson's disease, suggested a decreased risk in smokers. In an early meta-analysis (Lee 1994) the estimated risk in ever-smokers was almost half that in never-smokers (relative risk 0.64, 95% CI 0.54–0.76). However, the evidence was not consistent between studies. Many were relatively small case-control studies that relied on information from surrogates and suffered from several limitations (see Doll *et al.* 2000 for a discussion). A systematic review of cohort studies only show increased risks for Alzheimer's disease, vascular dementia, and any dementia (Anstey *et al.* 2007); see Table 33.8. The results of the review also suggests that former-smokers have a lower risk than current-smokers, though further research is needed to clarify the age at which a possible benefit of quitting could be obtained.

Eyes

Studies have suggested that smoking may be a risk factor for several diseases of the eye, some of which can lead to irreversible blindness. However, the evidence for many has not been strong, for

Table 33.7 Systematic review of case-control studies on Parkinson's disease and smoking (Ritz *et al.* 2007)

Pack-years of smoking	Relative risk compared to never-smokers (95% CI)	
	Women	Men
0–8.9	0.82 (0.61–1.11)	0.90 (0.70–1.16)
9–28.9	0.73 (0.47–1.13)	0.68 (0.52–0.88)
29–59.9	0.53 (0.33–0.85)	0.80 (0.60–1.05)
≥60	0.52 (0.31–0.89)	0.64 (0.46–0.89)

Table 33.8 Systematic review of dementia, cognitive decline, and smoking

	Number of studies	Total number of subjects	Smoking status	Relative risk compared to never-smokers (95% CI)
Alzheimer's disease	10	13 786	Current	1.79 (1.43–2.23)
			Former	1.01 (0.83–1.23)
Vascular dementia	2	4 888	Current	1.78 (1.28–2.47)
			Former	1.07 (0.59–1.95)
Any dementia	5	3 767	Current	1.27 (1.02–1.60)
			Former	0.99 (0.81–1.21)

example, glaucoma and diabetic retinopathy. It is likely that smoking has some direct effects on the lens and retina because of its well-known thrombotic and atherosclerotic effects. Discussions of this subject can be found in Solberg *et al.* 1998, Cheng *et al.* 2000, and Evans 2001. As well as cataracts and age-related macular degeneration (see below), there is evidence from two systematic reviews that smoking is associated with thyroid eye disease, or Graves' ophthalmopathy, with a 4.4-fold increase in risk among ever-smokers (95% CI 2.88–6.73), based on six studies (Vestergaard 2002; Thornton *et al.* 2007).

Cataracts

Cataracts are one of the commonest causes of blindness and visual impairment in developed countries and their removal is the most common reason for eye surgery. Table 33.9 shows the results from five cohort studies. There is about a 50% increase in risk in current-smokers compared to never-smokers, with some studies showing clear dose-response relationships. In former-smokers, however, it is unclear whether there is a marked reduction in risk (Hankinson 1992; Christen 2000). A review of 27 cohort, case-control, and cross-sectional studies provided consistent conclusions, and suggested that the risk was greatest for nuclear cataracts (i.e. located in the centre of the eye lens), with a possible three-fold increase in risk (Kelly *et al.* 2005).

Age-related macular degeneration (ARMD)

Like cataracts, this disorder is a major cause of blindness and visual impairment; once acquired there is no cure, so prevention is currently the best approach to reducing the health burden. Table 33.10 shows the results of a systematic review of eight case-control studies and five cohort studies (Cong *et al.* 2008). Both current- and former-smokers had a higher risk of developing ARMD. There is about a two-fold increase in risk in current-smokers compared to never-smokers. The review also indicated that giving up smoking could reduce the risk, though it was not possible to identify whether the benefit applies to any age or stage of disease.

Bones

Hip fracture

Hip fracture is an important disorder in the elderly, particularly in post-menopausal women. Many studies have reported on the association between smoking and bone mineral density and smoking and the risk of hip fracture. A meta-analysis of 29 cross-sectional studies based on a total of 2 156 smokers and 9 705 non-smokers (Law & Hackshaw 1997) showed that there was practically no difference in bone density between smokers and non-smokers before the

Table 33.9 Cohort studies that reported results on cataracts and smoking

Study (first author)	Country	Number of subjects	Total number of subjects with cataracts	Gender	Cigarette consumption	Relative risk* in current-smokers compared to never-smokers (95% CI)
Klein et al. 1993	USA	2 164	261, diagnosis	Men		1.09 (1.05–1.14)
		2 762	547, diagnosis	Women		1.09 (1.04–1.16)
Christen et al. 2000	USA	20 907	1118, diagnosis	Men		1.49 (1.30–1.72)
			662, extraction			1.52 (1.26–1.85)
Hankinson et al. 1992	USA	50 828	480, extraction	Women	1–14 cigs/day	0.71 (0.46–1.11)
					15–24	1.33 (0.99–1.79)
					25–34	1.40 (0.93–2.10)
					≥35	1.58 (0.96–2.60)
Weintraub et al. 2002	USA	77 749	1 900, extraction	Men & women	1–14 cigs/day	1.12 (0.75–1.68)
					≥15	1.53 (1.39–1.69)
Hiller et al. 1997	USA	660	381, diagnosis	Men & women	1–19 cigs/day	1.65 (0.82–3.34)
					≥20	2.84 (1.46–5.51)

Note

Some of the women in Hankinson (1992) are included in Weintraub (2002).

* All adjusted for at least age.

menopause, but post-menopause the extent of bone loss was greater than non-smokers and this increased with age. For every increase in age by 10 years, bone density loss was 2% greater in smokers, so that by age 80 there is a 6% difference between smokers and non-smokers. This is consistent with the evidence that the risk of hip fracture in post-menopausal women also increases with age; these studies are shown in Fig. 33.1 (taken from Law & Hackshaw 1997). At age 60, the

Table 33.10 Systematic review of age-related macular degeneration (ARMD) and smoking (Cong et al. 2008)

Study type	Number of studies	Total number of subjects	Number with ARMD	Smoking status	Relative risk compared to never-smokers (95% CI)
Cohort	5	61 213	699	Current	2.06 (1.12–3.77)
				Former	1.40 (0.96–2.06)
Case-control	8	6 175	3 076	Current	2.38 (1.74–3.26)
				Former	1.66 (1.35–2.04)
				Ever	1.76 (1.56–1.99)

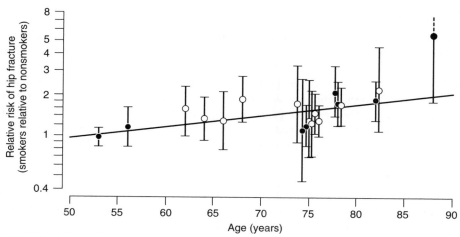

Fig. 33.1 The relative risk of having a hip fracture in smokers compared to non-smokers in 19 studies of postmenopausal women according to age (cohort studies are indicated by solid circles and case-control studies by open circles).

Source: from Law & Hackshaw 1997, with permission from the BMJ publishing group.

excess risk in smokers is 17% rising to 108% at age 90. The limited data in men suggest a similar effect. It is estimated that one in eight hip fractures is attributable to smoking. Several biological mechanisms have been proposed including a direct effect of smoking on bone and that smokers have a reduction in calcium. The studies also suggest that in smokers who quit, further bone loss is prevented. Certainly those who stop at the time of menopause may avoid much of the excess risk associated with smoking.

Reproduction and pregnancy

Despite many attempts to encourage women to quit smoking before conception and during pregnancy there is still a relatively high prevalence of smokers (about 15–20%). Smoking is an established cause of several disorders associated with fertility and complications in pregnancy (UK Department of Health 1988; US Surgeon General 1989; British Medical Association 2004), some of which shall be presented below.

Infertility

About 25% of women of reproductive age experience some degree of infertility. It is defined in several ways, but it is generally accepted to be when conception has not occurred after 12 consecutive months of unprotected intercourse. Women who smoke are less likely to conceive or take longer to conceive. A meta-analysis of eight cohort studies (based on 20 059 women) showed that women who smoked were 42% (95% CI 27–58%) more likely to be infertile than non-smokers (Augood *et al.* 1998). It is likely that such a relationship exists because the risk also increases with increasing cigarette consumption and in several studies the risks were still raised after allowing for several potential confounding factors (such as alcohol and coffee intake and oral contraception use). The subject is reviewed by Augood *et al.* (1998) and Baird (1992), both of which describe the evidence and the limitations to determining causality. There is also evidence that smoking damages sperm and is associated with male sexual impotence (British Medical Association 2004).

Miscarriage

It is well established that women who smoke are more likely to have a miscarriage, and that the association is causal. A meta-analysis of seven cohort studies (based on 86 633 pregnancies) yields a 24% increase in risk (95% CI 19–30%) in smokers compared to non-smokers; all of the individual studies yielded statistically significant results. It is estimated that 3–7.5% of miscarriages can be attributable to smoking (DiFranza & Lew 1995). The results from case-control studies were similar. There is also a dose–response relationship, (the higher the cigarette consumption the higher the risk of miscarriage) and the association remains after allowing for the effects of maternal age, previous miscarriage, alcohol consumption, education, and ethnicity.

Low birthweight

Smoking is also an established cause of low birthweight, an important factor associated with infant morbidity and mortality. Babies in mother who smoke weigh, on average, 150–250 gm less than those from non-smoking mothers (UK Department of Health 1988). From a meta-analysis of 22 studies (based on 347 553 pregnancies) women who smoke were 82% more likely (95% CI 67–97%) to give birth to a baby that weighs <2500 gm compared to non-smokers (DiFranza & Lew 1995); all but one study reported statistically significant results. The results from case-control studies were similar. It was also estimated that 11–21% of babies with low birthweight is due to smoking. The association is certainly causal because randomized trials of smoking cessation during pregnancy have shown that birthweight is increased when the mother quits (UK Department of Health 1988).

Table 33.11 Selected studies (based on study size) showing the effect of maternal active smoking on congenital heart defects and limb reduction defects.

Study (first author)	Country	Total number of babies with the defect/total number of unaffected babies	Adjusted relative risk in current smokers compared to never-smokers (95% CI)
Heart defects			
Kallen 2000	Sweden	13 266/approx 1.39 million	1.15 (1.10–1.20)
McDonald et al. 1992	Canada	318/87 389	1.14 (0.92–1.40)
Woods et al. 2001	USA	260/17 756	1.56 (1.12–2.19)
Morales-Suarez-Varela et al. 2006	Denmark	746/73 001	1.20 (1.00–1.40)
Malik et al. 2008	USA	302/693	1.50 (1.28–1.76)
Limb reduction defects			
Aro et al. 1983	Finland	45/453	1.3 (0.9–2.0)
Shiono et al. 1986	USA	17/28 810	2.2 (0.9–5.8)
Van Den Eeden 1990	USA	35/4500	1.2 (0.6–2.5)
Czeizel et al. 1994	Hungary	537/537	1.68 (1.26–2.24)
Wasserman et al. 1996	USA	175/478	1.19 (0.82–1.74)*
Kallen 2000	Sweden	1023/approx 1.39 million	1.26 (1.11–1.44)

*unadjusted

Congenital birth defects

Many chemicals in tobacco smoke, including nicotine and carbon monoxide, can cross the placental barrier and so may have a direct effect on the fetus. They can restrict blood flow and reduce the amount of oxygen available to the fetus, affecting the development of limbs and organs. Many studies have examined the association between maternal active smoking and the risk of having a baby with a congenital birth defect (see Royal College of Physicians 2010, for a review). There is a 34% (95% CI 25–44%) increase in the risk of having a cleft lip, with or without cleft palate, based on a systematic review of 7.78 million births and 15 200 affected babies (Little *et al* 2004). Congenital heart defects are the most common structural birth abnormality (~8 per 1000 live births in the USA), and several large studies show that maternal smoking increases the chance of having a baby with a heart defect (Table 33.11). The largest indicated a 15% excess risk, though later studies indicated that this could be 50% for septal defects. A consistent association has been observed for babies born with limb reduction defects, in which part or all of one or more limbs fail to develop (Table 33.11), several of which reported dose–response relationships. There is likely to be at least a 30% increase in risk. Furthermore, two of the largest studies based on babies with missing or extra fingers or toes each provided excess risks of about 30%: Honein *et al.* 2001(5573 cases) and Man *et al.* (5171 cases). Finally, two large studies reported that the risk of clubfoot was increased: one from Europe and the other from the USA, each based on 2905 and 3894 affected babies respectively: excess risk of 20% (95% CI 10–30%) (Reefhuis *et al.* 1998), and 62% (95% CI 49–75%) (Honein *et al.* 2001).

Hormonal system

Diabetes

Studies have shown that smokers are more likely to develop type 2 (non-insulin dependent) diabetes than never-smokers. Table 33.12 shows the results from a systematic review of 25 cohort studies based on 1.2 million subjects and 45 844 incident cases of diabetes (Willi *et al.* 2007)). They indicate that smokers have about a 50% increase in risk, and the excess risk remains high after adjustment for other factors that are associated with both smoking and diabetes, such as age, body mass index (an indicator of obesity), and alcohol intake. The risk increases with increasing cigarette consumption. These studies also show that the risk is reduced in former-smokers, indicating the importance of quitting, especially considering that diabetes is itself a risk factor for cardiovascular disease, renal disease, and retinopathy. It has been shown that smoking can promote insulin resistance and that smokers tend to have higher glucose concentrations, both of which can contribute to development of the disorder. Other reviews of this subject can be found in Dierkx *et al.* (1996) and Haire-Joshu *et al.* (1999).

Table 33.12 Systematic review of type 2 (non-insulin dependant) diabetes and smoking (Willi *et al.* 2007)

Smoking status	Number of studies	Number of subjects	Relative risk compared to never-smokers (95% CI)
Active-smoker	25	1.2 million	1.44 (1.31–1.58)
Light-smoker (<20 cigs/day)	6	154 165	1.29 (1.13–1.48)
Heavy-smoker (≥20 cigs/day)	6	154 165	1.61 (1.43–1.80)
Former-smoker	17	1.1 million	1.23 (1.14–1.33)

Graves' disease

This is a disorder of the thyroid characterized by an enlarged thyroid gland (goitre) and hypothyroidism. It is much more common in females than males (ratio 6:1). A systematic review of eight case-control studies, based on 8 458 subjects, of which 952 had Graves' disease, produced an odds ratio of 3.3 (95% CI 2.09–5.22) among current-smokers and 1.41 (95% CI 0.77–2.58) among former-smokers; evidence that quitting reduces the excess risk (Vestergaard 2002).

Oral cavity

There is now much evidence showing that smoking is associated with various oral disorders. As well as the common side effects of halitosis and teeth discolouration there are more serious consequences such as periodontal disease, caries, and acute ulcerative gingivitis (for a review see Allard *et al.* [1999] and Winn [2001]).

Table 33.13 Studies that reported results on periodontitis and smoking

Study (first author)	Country	Number of subjects	Total number of subjects with periodontitis or marker of it	Gender	Cigarette consumption	Relative risk in current-smokers compared to never-smokers (95% CI)
Periodontitis						
Haber *et al.* 1993	USA	95	32	Men & women		8.6 (2.7–27.8)[e]
Tomar & Asma 2000	USA	13 652	1 256	Men & women		3.94 (3.20–4.93) [a]
Ismail *et al.* 1990	USA	165	22	Men & women		6.26 (2.42–16.20)
Marker of periodontitis						
Grossi *et al.* 1995[b]	USA	1361	194	Men & women	≤5.2 pack years	1.48 (1.02–2.14)
					5.3–15	3.25 (2.33–4.54)
					16–30	5.79 (4.08–8.27)
					>30	7.28 (5.09–10.31)
Beck *et al.* 1990[c]	USA	381	–	Black	≥65 years	2.8 (1.71–4.70)
				White	≥65 years	6.7 (3.17–14.02)
Mullaly 1996[d]	Ireland	100	–	Men & women		4.6 (2–10.6)

Note

[a] Adjusted for age, sex, ethnic origin, income, education
[b] Severe alveolar bone loss
[c] Attachment loss and pocket depth
[d] Molar furcation
[e] Adjusted for age

Periodontitis

Periodontitis is a common dental disorder among adults and there have been many studies that have reported on the association with smoking. Although the biological mechanism for the effect of smoking on periodontal disease is uncertain the epidemiological data is clear. The studies, cross-sectional and cohort, have looked at the risk of having a diagnosis of periodontitis or measuring markers of it (such markers are used in diagnosis). Table 33.13 shows some of the studies in which relative risks were reported. Smokers have about a four-fold increase in risk. It has been postulated that smokers only have a poorer oral hygiene (which itself is a cause of periodontitis) and so the observed associations are due to confounding. However, several studies have adjusted for this factor, as well as other confounding factors (such as income) and there is still an effect of smoking. Smoking is also associated with more severe disease and it can delay the healing process. A recent systematic review of eight clinical trials of non-surgical treatment for periodontitis, which reported effects separately for smokers and non-smokers, showed that the treatment-related improvements in the mean pocket probing depth was lower among smokers compared to non-smokers (Labriola *et al.* 2005). The difference was 0.43 mm (95% CI 0.24–0.63). Further discussions can be found in Qandil *et al.* (1997) and Salvi *et al.* (1997).

Caries and tooth loss

Because periodontitis is a cause of tooth loss, a few studies have assessed the effect of smoking on tooth loss, primarily in the elderly. Although the evidence is not as strong as with periodontitis there is a suggestion of an effect (Table 33.14). Among the elderly, smokers are about twice as likely to have no teeth left than non-smokers.

Table 33.15 shows the results from one study that looked at differences between smokers and non-smokers with regards to indicators of caries. There are clear associations; smokers tend to have more missing teeth and more decayed, missing, or filled surfaces.

Table 33.14 Studies that reported on tooth loss and smoking

Study (first author)	Country	Number of subjects	Number of subjects with tooth loss	Gender	Cigarette consumption	Relative risk in current-smokers compared to never-smokers (95% CI)
Holm 1994	Sweden	149	–	Men	1–15 cigs/day	2.07 (1.2–3.5)[a]
					≥15	3.18 (1.9–5.5)[a]
		124		Women	1–15 cigs/day	0.95 (0.5–1.7)[a]
					≥15	1.7 (0.7–4.1)[a]
Locker 1992	Canada	907	137[b]	Men & women[c]	1–9 cigs/day	1.95 (1.2–3.3)
					≥20	2.57 (1.5–4.3)
Jette *et al.* 1993	USA	1156	~433[b]	Men[d]		1.68 (1.16–2.44)
				Women[d]		1.70 (1.12–2.57)

Note

[a] Lost at least 1 tooth during past 10 years
[b] Number that are edentulous
[c] Aged ≥50 years
[d] Aged ≥70 years

Table 33.15 The effect of smoking on tooth health in 808 adults (adapted from Axelsson *et al.* 1998)

Age (years)	Number of subjects	Difference between smokers and non-smokers in relation to:			
		Mean number of missing teeth	Mean number of decayed surfaces	Mean number of missing surfaces	Mean number of filled surfaces
35–49	127	+0.6	+0.6	+2.8	+6.9*
50–64	369	+1.5*	+0.1	+6.8*	+0.7
65–74	190	+3.5*	+0.3	+16.0*	−10.4*
75+	122	+5.8*	+0.07	+26.2*	−11.6*

Note

* Statistically significant (p-value ≤ 0.05).

Conclusion

The literature on smoking and the disorders briefly described in this section is extensive. Many disorders have long been regarded as partly caused by smoking. While most studies have shown an association with smoking, establishing causality has required careful consideration of the evidence. Many studies showed dose–response relationships (risk of the disorder increased with increasing cigarette consumption) and that former-smokers had a lower risk than current-smokers.

Table 33.16 Summary of disorders in which smoking is associated with an increased risk

Disorder	Gender (age if not all ages)	Approximate relative risk in current-smokers compared to never-smokers	Percentage of all affected individuals that may be associated with smoking (%)*	The number of affected individuals associated with smoking among 100 000 smokers#
Gastro-intestinal				
Peptic ulcer	Women	2	20	440
	Men	2	20	800
Crohn's disease	Men	2	20	80
	Women	4.5	47	190
Gallbladder disease	Men & women	1.3	7	100
Skin				
Psoriasis	Men	1.4	9	730
	Women	2.5	27	2 180
Neurological				
Alzheimer's disease	Men & women (≥65)	1.8	17	670
Eyes				
Cataract extraction	Women (≥45)	1.5	11	70
	Men (≥45)	1.5	11	135

Table 33.16 (continued) Summary of disorders in which smoking is associated with an increased risk

Disorder	Gender (age if not all ages)	Approximate relative risk in current-smokers compared to never-smokers	Percentage of all affected individuals that may be associated with smoking (%)*	The number of affected individuals associated with smoking among 100 000 smokers#
Age-related macular degeneration	Women (≥50)	2	20	55
	Men (≥40)	2	20	85
Bones				
Hip fracture	Women (55–64)	1.2	5	10
	Women (≥85)	2.1	22	2 420
Fertility & pregnancy				
Infertility	Women	1.4	10	9 500
Miscarriage	Women	1.25	6	4 700
Low birthweight (<2500 g)	Babies of women who smoke	1.8	17	3 330
Limb reduction defect	Babies of women who smoke	1.5	7	20
Heart defect	Babies of women who smoke	1.15	4	115
Hormonal/endocrine				
Type 2 diabetes	Men (≥40)	1.5	11	130
	Women (30–55)	1.5	11	80
Graves' disease	Men	3.3	36	20
	Women	3.3	36	130
Teeth				
Periodontitis	Men & women	4	43	17 140

Note

* The population attributable proportion. It assumes that 25% of the population are current-smokers. The actual percentage will be less if not all the increased risk observed in smokers is due to smoking.

The absolute excess risk between smokers and non-smokers. Based on the incidence of the disorder (per 100 000 per year), except psoriasis and periodontitis (based on the prevalence) and miscarriage, limb reduction defects, and birthweight (based on 100 000 births).

Allowing for factors that may artificially produce a relationship with smoking and risk has also been addressed, particularly in the more recent and large studies. This has been important when there are established confounding factors, such as alcohol, which is associated with both smoking and several disorders (e.g. psoriasis and gallstones). Study design is also important. Cohort studies of disease incidence can overcome many of the limitations of cross-sectional or case-control studies. Biological plausibility can, in many instances, only be postulated due to the multifactorial nature of the disorders. This is unsurprising given the number of toxins and chemicals in tobacco smoke and the many biological pathways associated with a particular disease.

Table 33.16 provides approximate estimates of the effect of smoking on the population assuming that all the disorders listed are caused by smoking. For disorders, such as Crohn's disease in women and periodontitis, as much as half of all diagnosed cases may be due to smoking. For others, though this proportion is relatively low, smoking can account for several hundred or several thousand extra cases among smokers (e.g. hip fracture and miscarriage). A large number of these affected individuals could be avoided if people quit smoking early.

In summary, smoking is a risk factor for many chronic and non-fatal disorders other than cancer, respiratory, and cardiovascular disease. It is associated with significant morbidity, which significantly impairs quality of life.

References

Allard, *et al.* (1999). Tobacco and oral diseases – Report of EU Working Group, 1999. *J Irish Den Assoc*, **46**(1):12–23.

Anda, R.F., Williamson, D.F., Escobedo, L.G., and Remington, P.L. (1990). Smoking and the risk of peptic ulcer disease among women in the United States. *Arch Intern Med*, **150**:1437–1441.

Anstey, K.J., von Sanden, C., Salim, A., and O'Kearney, R. (2007). Smoking as a risk factor for dementia and cognitive decline: a meta-analysis of prospective studies. *Am J Epidemiol*, **166**(4): 367–378.

Aro, T., (1983). Maternal diseases, alcohol consumption and smoking during pregnancy associated with reduction limb defects. *Early Human Development*, **9**:49–57.

Ashley, M.J. (1997). Smoking and diseases of the gastrointestinal system. An Epidemiological review with special reference to sex differences. *Can J Gastroenterol*, **11**(4):345–352.

Augood C, Duckitt K, Templeton AA (1998). Smoking and female infertility: a systematic review and meta-analysis. *Human Reprod*, **13**(6):1532–1539.

Axelsson, P., Paulander, J., and Lindhe, J. (1998). Relationship between smoking and dental status in 35-, 50-, 65- and 75-year old individuals. *J Clin Periodont*, **25**:297–305.

Baird, D.D. (1992). Evidence for reduced fecundity in female smokers. In Poswillo D, Alberman E. Effects of smoking on the fetus, neonate and child. Oxford University Press, Oxford.

Beck, J.D., Koch, G.G., Rozier, G., and Tudor, G.E. (1990). Prevalence and risk indicators for periodontal attachment loss in a population of older community dwelling blacks and whites. *J Periodonal*, **61**: 521–528.

Borody, T.J., Georg, L.L., Brandl, S., Andrews, P., Jankiewicz, E., and Ostapowicz, N. (1992). Smoking does not contribute to duodenal ulcer relapse after *Helicobactor pylori* eradication. *Am J Gastroenterol*, **87**(10):1390–1393.

British Medical Association (2004). *Smoking and reproductive life: the impact of smoking on sexual, reproductive and child health.* BMJ Publications.

Chan, F.K.L., Sung, J.J.Y., Lee, Y.T., Leung, W.K., Chan, L.Y., Yung, M.Y. *et al.* (1997). Does smoking predispose to peptic ulcer relapse after eradication of Helicobactor pylori? *Am J Gastroenterol*, **92**(3):442–445.

Cheng, A.C.K., Pang, C.P., Chua, J.K.H., Fan, D.S.P., and Lam, D.S.C. (2000). The association between cigarette smoking and ocular diseases. *Hong Kong Med J*, **6**(2): 195–202.

Christen, W.G., Glynn, R.J., Manson, J.E., Ajani, U.A., Buring, J.E., Hennekens, C.H. (1996). A prospective study of cigarette smoking and risk of age-related macular degeneration in men. *JAMA*, **276**:1147–1151.

Christen, W.G., Glynn, R.J., Ajani, U.A., Schaumberg, D.A., Buring, J.E., Hennekens, C.H. *et al.* (2000). Smoking cessation and risk of age-related cataract in men. *JAMA*, **284**:713–716.

Cong, R., Zhou, B., Sun, Q., Gu, H., Tang, N., and Wang, B. (2008). Smoking and the risk of age-related macular degeneration: a meta-analysis. *Annals of Epidemiology*, **18**(8):647–656.

Czeizel, A.E., Kodaj, I., and Lenz, W. (1994). Smoking during pregnancy and congenital limb deficiency. *BMJ*, **308**:1473–1476.

Dierkx, R.I.J., van de Hoek, W., Hoekstra, J.B.L, and Erkelens, D.W. (1996). Smoking and diabetes mellitus. *Neth J Med*, **48**:150–162.

DiFranza, J.R. and Lew, R.A. (1995). Effect of maternal cigarette smoking on pregnancy complications and sudden infant death syndrom. *J Family Practice*, **40**(4):385–394.

Doll, R., Peto, R., Wheatley, K., Gray, R., and Sutherland, I. (1994). Mortality in relation to smoking: 40 years' observations on male British doctors. *BMJ*, **309**:901–911.

Doll, R., Peto, R., Boreham, J., and Sutherland, I. (2000). Smoking and dementia in male British doctors: prospective study. *BMJ*, **320**:1097–1102.

Eastwood, G.L. (1997). Is smoking still important in the pathogenesis of peptic ulcer disease? *J Clin Gastroenterol*, **25**(supp 1):S1–7.

English, D.R., Holman, C.D.J., and Milne, E. (1995). The quantification of drug-caused morbidity and mortality in Australia, 1992. Canberra: Commonwealth Department of Human Services and Health.

Evans, J.R. (2001). Risk factors for age-related macular degeneration. *Progress Retinal Eye Res*, **20**(2): 227–253.

Feskens, E.J.M. and Kromhout, D. (1989). Cardiovascular risk factors and the 25-year incidence of diabetes mellitus in middle-aged men. *Am J Epidemiol*, **130**(6):1101–1108.

Fratiglioni, L. and Wang, H.-X. (2000). Smoking and Parkinson's and Alzheimer's disease: review of the epidemiological studies. *Behav Brain Res*, **113**:117–120.

Gorell, J.M., Rybicki, B.A., Johnson, C.C., and Peterson, E.L. (1999). Smoking and Parkinson's disease: a dose–response relationship. *Neurology*, **52**:115–119.

Grossi, S.G., Genco, R.J., Machtei, E.E., Ho, A.W., Koch, G., Dunford, R. *et al.* (1995). Assessment of risk for periodontal disease. II. Risk indicators for alveolar bone loss. *J Periodontol*, **66**:23–29.

Haber, J., Wattles, J., Crowley, M., and Mandell, R. (1993). Evidence for cigarette smoking as a major risk factor for periodontitis. *J Periodontol*, **64**:16–23.

Haire-Johnson, D., Glasgow, R.E., and Tibbs, T.L. (1999). Smoking and diabetes. *Diabetes Care*, **22**(11):1887–1898.

Hankinson, S.E., Willett, W.C., Colditz, G.A., Seddon, J.M., Rosner, B., Speizer, F.E. *et al.* (1992). A prospective study of cigarette smoking and risk of cataract surgery in women. *JAMA*, **268**:994–998.

Hernan, M.A., Zhang, S.M., Rueda-de Castro, A.M., Colditz, G.A., Speizer, F.E., and Ascherio, A. (2001). Cigarette smoking and the incidence of Parkinson's disease in two prospective studies. *Ann Neurol*, **50**(6):780–786.

Higgins, E. (2000). Alcohol, smoking and psoriasis. *Clin Exp Dermatol*, **25**:107–110.

Hiller, R., Sperduto, R.D., Podger, M.J., Wilson, P.W.F., Ferris, F.L., Colton, T. *et al.* (1997). Cigarette smoking and the risk of development of lens opacities. *Arch Ophthalmol*, **115**:1113–1118.

Holm, G. (1994). Smoking as an additional risk for tooth loss. *J Periodontal*, **65**:996–1001.

Honein, M.A., Paulozzi, L.J., and Watkins, M.L. (2001). Maternal smoking and birth defects: validity of birth certificate data for effect estimation. *Public Health Reports*, **116**:327–335.

Ismail, A.I., Morrison, E.C., Burt, B.A., Caffesse, R.G., and Kavanagh, M.T. (1990). Natural history of periodontal disease in adults: findings from the Tecumseh Periodontal Disease study, 1959–87. *J Dent Res*, **69**(2):430–435.

Jette, A.M., Feldman, H.A., and Tennstedt, S.L. (1993). Tobacco use: a modifiable risk factor for dental disease among the elderly. *Am J Pub Health*, **83**:1271–1276.

Johnsen, R., Forde, O.H., Straume, B., and Burhol, P.G. (1994). Aetiology of peptic ulcer: a prospective study in Norway. *J Epidemiol Comm Health*, **48**:156–160.

Kadayifci, A., and Simsek, H. (1997). Does smoking influence the eradication of *Helicobactor pylori* and duodenal ulcer healing with different regimes. *Int J Clin Pract*, **51**(7):516–517.

Källén, K. (2000). Multiple malformations and maternal smoking. *Paediatric and Perinatal Epidemiology*, **14**:227–233.

Kawakami, N., Takatsuka, N., Shimizu, H., and Ishibashi, H. (1997). Effects of smoking on the incidence of non-insulin-dependent diabetes mellitus. *Am J Epidemiol*, **145**(2):103–109.

Kelly, S.P., Thornton, J., Edwards, R., Sahu, A., and Harrison, R. (2005). Smoking and cataract: review of causal association. *J Cataract Refract Surg*, **31**:2395–2404.

Klein, B.E.K., Linton, K.L.P., Klein, R., and Franke, T. (1993). Cigarette smoking and lens opacities: The Beaver Dam Eye Study. *Am J Prev Med*, **9**:27–30.

Klein, R., Klein, B.E.K., and Moss, S.E. (1998). Relation of smoking to the incidence of age-related maculopathy. The Beaver Dam Eye Study. *Am J Epidemiol*, **147**:103–110.

Kurata, J.H., Nogawa, A.N., Abbey, D.E., and Petersen, F. (1992). A prospective study of risk for peptic ulcer disease in Seventh-Day Adventists. *Gastroenterology*, **102**:909–909.

Kurata, J.H. and Nogawa, A.N. (1997). Meta-analysis of risk factors for peptic ulcer. *J Clin Gastroenterol*, **24**(1):2–17.

Labriola, A., Needleman, I., and Moles, D.R. (2005). Systematic review of the effect of smoking on nonsurgical periodontal therapy. '*Periodontology 2000*', **37**:124–137.

Law, M.R. and Hackshaw, A.K. (1997). A meta-analysis of cigarette smoking, bone mineral density and risk of hip fracture: recognition of a major effect. *BMJ*, **315**:841–846.

Little, J., Cardy, A., and Munger, R.G. (2004). Tobacco smoking and oral clefts: a meta-analysis. *Bulletin of the World Health Organization*, **82**:213–218.

Locker, D. (1992). Smoking and oral health in older adults. *Can J Pub Health*, **83**(6):429–432.

Logan, R.F.A. (1990). Smoking and inflammatory bowel disease. In: N.J. Wald and J. Baron (eds) *Smoking and hormone-related disorders*, 122–133. Oxford University Press, Oxford.

Logan, R.F.A. and Skelly, M.M. (2000). Smoking and hepato-biliary disease. *Eur J Gastroenterol*, **12**: 863–867.

Malik, S., Cleves, M.A., Honein, M.A., Romitti, P.A, Botto, L.D., Yang, S.*et al* (2008). Maternal smoking and congenital heart defects. *Pediatrics*, **121**:e810–e816.

Man, L.X, Chang, B., (2006). Maternal cigarettes smoking during pregnancy increases the risk of having a child with a congenital digital anomaly. *Plastic and Reconstructive Surgery*, **117**:301–308.

Manson, J.E., Ajani, U.A., Liu, S., Nathan, D.M., and Hennekens, C.H. (2000). A prospective study of cigarette smoking and the incidence of diabetes mellitus among US male physicians. *Am J Med*, **109**:538–542.

Marmot, M. (1990). Smoking and Parkinson's disease. In: N.J. Wald and J. Baron (eds) *Smoking and hormone*-related *disorders*, pp. 133–141. Oxford University Press, Oxford.

Marshall, B.J., Goodwin, C.S., Warren, J.R., Murray, R., Blincow, E.D., Blackbourn, S.J. *et al.* (1988). Prospective double-blind trial of duodenal ulcer relapse after eradication of Campylobactor pylori. *Lancet*, **8626**:1437–1441.

McDonald, A.D., Armstrong, B.G., and Sloan, M. (1992). Cigarette, alcohol, and coffee consumption and congenital defects. *American Journal of Public Health*, **82**:91–93.

Morales-Suarez-Varela, M.M., Bille, C., Christensen, K., and Olsen, J. (2006). Smoking habits, nicotine use, and congenital malformations. *Obstetrics & Gynecology*, **107**:51–57.

Morens, D.M., Grandinetti, A., Reed, D., White, L.R., and Ross, G.W. (1995). Cigarette smoking and protection from Parkinson's disease. *Neurology*, **45**:1041–1051.

Mullaly, B.H. (1996). Molar furcation involvement associated with cigarette smoking in periodontal disease. *J Clin Periodont*, **23**:658–661.

Naldi, L. (1998). Cigarette smoking and psoriasis. *Clin Dermatology*, **16**:571–574.

Naldi, L., Peli, L., and Parazzini, F. (1999). Association of early-stage psoriasis with smoking and male alcohol consumption. *Arch Dermatol*, **135**:1479–1484.

O'Connor, H.J., Kanduru, C., Bhutta, A.S., Meehan, J.M., Feeley, K.M., and Cunnane, K. (1995). Effect of *Helicobactor pylori* on peptic ulcer healing. *Postgrad Med J*, **71**:90–93.

Paffenberger, R.S., Wing, A.L., and Hyde, R.T. (1974). Chronic disease in former college students. *Am J Epidemiol*, **100**(4):307–315.

Parasher G, Eastwood GL (2000). Smoking and peptic ulcer in the *Helicobactor pylori* era. *Eur J Gastroenterol Hepatol*, **12**:843–883.

Poikolainen, K., Reunala, T., and Karvonen, J. (1994). Smoking, alcohol and life events related to psoriasis among women. *Br J Dermatol*, **130**:473–477.

Qandil, R., Sandhu, H.S., and Matthews, D.C. (1997). Tobacco smoking and periodontal diseases. *J Canad Den Assoc*, **63**(3):187–195.

Reefhuis, J., de Walle, H.E., and Cornel, M.C. (1998). Maternal smoking and deformaties of the foot: results for the EUROCAT Study. European Registries of Congenital Anomalies. *American Journal of Public Health*, **88**:1554–1555.

Rimm, E.B., Manson, J.E., Stampfer, M.J., Colditz, G.A., Willett, W.C., Rosner, B. *et al.* (1993). Cigarette smoking and the risk of diabetes in women. *Am J Pub Health*, **83**:211–214.

Rimm, E.B., Chan, J., Stampfer, M.J., Colditz, G.A., and Willett, W.C. (1995). Prospective study of cigarette smoking, alcohol use and the risk of diabetes in men. *BMJ*, **310**:555–559.

Ritz, B., Ascherio, A., Checkoway, H., Marder, K.S., Nelson, L.M., Rocca, W.A. *et al.* (2007). Pooled analysis of tobacco use and risk of Parkinson disease. *Archives of Neurology*, **64**(7):990–997.

Royal College of Physicians (2010). Effects of maternal active and passive smoking on fetal and reproductive health. In: J. Britton and R. Edwards (eds) *Passive smoking and children. A report by the Tobacco Advisory Group of the Royal College of Physicians*, Chapter **3**:40–76.

Rubin, D.T. and Hanauer, S.B. (2000). Smoking and inflammatory bowel disease. *Eur J Gastroenterol*, **12**:855–862.

Salvi, G.E., Lawrence, H.P., Offenbacher, S., and Beck, J.D. (1997). Influence of risk factors on the pathogenesis of periodontitis. *Periodontol [2000]*, **14**:173–201.

Seddon, J.M., Willett, W.C., Speizer, F.E., and Hankinson, S.E. (1996). A prospective study of cigarette smoking and age-related macular degeneration in women. *JAMA*, **276**:1141–1146.

Shiono, P.H., Klebanoff, M.A., and Berendes, H.W. (1986). Congenital malformations and maternal smoking during pregnancy. *Teratology*, **34**:65–71.

Solberg, Y., Rosner, M., and Belkin, M. (1998). The association between cigarette smoking and ocular diseases. *Surv Ophthalmol*, **42**:535–547.

Stemmermann, G.N., Marcus, E.B., Buist, A.S., and MacLean, C.J. (1989). Relative impact of smoking and reduced pulmonary function on peptic ulcer risk. *Gastroenterol*, **96**:1419–1424.

Thornton, J., Kelly, S.P., Harrison, R.A., and Edwards, R. (2007). Cigarette smoking and thyroid eye disease: a systematic review. *Eye*, **21**(9):1135–1145.

Tomar, L. and Asma, S. (2000). Smoking-attributable periodontitis in the United States: Findings from NHANES III. *J Periodontol*, **71**:743–751.

UK Department of Health (1988). Fourth Report of the Independent Scientific Committee on Smoking and Health. HMSO, London.

US Surgeon General Report (1989). Reducing the health consequences of smoking: 25 years of progress. US Department of Health & Human Services DHHS Publication number (CDC) 89–8411.

Van den Eeden, S.K., Karagas, M.R., Daling, J.R., and Vaughan, T.L. (1990). A case-control study of maternal smoking and congenital malformations. *Paediatric and Perinatal Epidemiology*, **4**:147–155.

Vessey, M.P., Villard-Mackintosh, L., and Painter, R. (1992). Oral contraceptives and pregnancy in relation to peptic ulcer. *Contraception*, **46**:349–357.

Vessey, M.P., Painter, R., and Powell, J. (2000). Skin disorders in relation to oral contraception and other factors including age, social class, smoking and body mass index. Findings in a large cohort study. *Br J Dermatol*, **143**:815–820.

Vestergaard, P. (2002). Smoking and thyroid disorders – a meta-analysis. *Eur J Endocrin*, **146**:153–161.

Wasserman, C.R., Shaw, G.M., O'Malley, C.D., Tolarova, M.M., and Lammer, E.J. (1996). Parental cigarette smoking and risk for congenital anomalies of the heart, neural tube or limb. *Teratology*, **53**:261–267.

Weintraub, J.M., Willett, W.C., Rosner, B., Colditz, G.A., Seddon, J.M., and Hankinson, S.E. (2002). *Am J Epidemiol*, **155**:72–79.

Willi, C., Bodenmann, P., Ghali, W.A., Faris, P.D., and Cornuz, J. (2007). Active smoking and the risk of type 2 diabetes: a systematic review and meta-analysis. *JAMA*, **298**(22):2654–2664.

Winn, D.M. (2001). Tobacco use and oral disease. *J Dental Educ*, **65**(4):306–312.

Woods, S.E. and Raju, U. (2001). Maternal smoking and the risk of congenital birth defects: a cohort study. *Journal of the American Board of Family Practice*, **14**:330–334.

Chapter 34

Interaction of tobacco with other risk factors

Albert B. Lowenfels and Patrick Maisonneuve

Introduction

Tobacco exposure causes both malignant and non-malignant disease and has been estimated to be the aetiology of approximately 4% of the global burden of disease [1]. Because of the frequency of smoking, it is predictable that smokers will be exposed to other factors that can have an independent deleterious effect on health. In this chapter we will review the interaction of tobacco and four additional substances – alcohol, asbestos, radiation, and arsenic. Of these four exposures, alcohol is the commonest and has the strongest link to smoking. Table 34.1 summarizes some of the salient points with respect to these additional exposures.

Alcohol and tobacco

Throughout the world, tobacco and alcohol abuse are responsible for an appreciable proportion of avoidable deaths. Alcohol has been used in all cultures throughout recorded history, but tobacco became widely available only after the discovery of the New World. At first tobacco use was restricted to the wealthy class, but by the beginning of the seventeenth century, combined exposure to alcohol and tobacco became common (Fig. 34.1). Both agents are addictive, although nicotine, the major addictive compound contained in tobacco, is probably more addictive than alcohol. Both agents are widely used: two-thirds of males and approximately 40% of female Americans over age 12 have consumed alcohol at some time, which is more than the percentage of persons who report ever using tobacco. Consumption of both alcohol and tobacco seems to increase in stressful times [2]. The biologic effects of the two agents tend to overlap: pre-treatment with nicotine shortens the time interval to perceived intoxication [3].

Tobacco use creates an enormous health burden because of its well-known association with numerous diseases, but increased consumption of alcohol is also known to have deleterious health effects and there are several diseases where exposure to both substances can be harmful. Table 34.2 lists background information and societal covariates for these two substances.

Since both substances are so widely used and since tobacco users often consume alcohol, some of the adverse health effects of tobacco may be caused by drinking. Furthermore, it is likely that for many diseases, combined exposure to these two substances is more harmful than exposure to only one of these agents [4].

Combined use of tobacco and alcohol

Epidemiology

The USA National Survey on drug use and health reveals that alcohol consumption is increased in smokers as compared to non-smokers. Recent alcohol use was reported by 67% of current

Table 34.1 Overview of substances that Interact with tobacco

Variable	Alcohol	Asbestos	Radiation	Arsenic
Recommended exposure limits	Suggested limits: Males: 2 drinks/day Females: 1 drink/day	0.1 fibre per cubic centimetre (f/cc) of air averaged over an 8-hour work shift	No federal or state standards. If radon home levels ≥4 pCi/L* remediation suggested	Drinking water: 10 parts per billion
Estimated exposure frequency	50–70%	4% in 1970s. Now decreased	Uncertain	Low except in restricted geographic areas
Gender ratio (M/F)	1.7/1	15–20/1	Uncertain	Males>females
Mode of exposure	Ingestion	Mainly inhalation Also ingestion	Inhalation radiotherapy	Oral
Target organ(s)	Mouth, pharynx, larynx, oesophagus	Lung	Lung breast	Skin, lung, bladder
Occupations or high risk populations	Beverage alcohol industry	Asbestos-cement, insulation, shipyard workers	Miners Occupants of homes with high levels radon; Postmastectomy radiotherapy	Populations exposed to arsenic in well water: Bangladesh

Note

* Picocuries per litre.

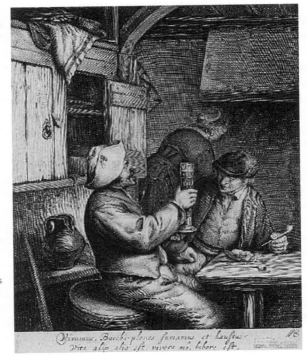

Figure 34.1 By the early seventeenth century exposure to both alcohol and tobacco was common.

Source: Jonas Suyerdof. 'Three peasants in an interior.' With permission, from the print collection, Miriam and Ira D. Wallach Division of Art, Prints and Photgraphs, The New York Public Library, Astor, Lenox and Tilden Foundations.

Table 34.2 Comparison of alcohol and tobacco use in the United States

Variable	Tobacco	Alcohol
Onset of exposure	Widely used in Americas during first century AD. First use in Europe around 1500	Alcohol use as well as intoxication mentioned in Old Testament
Minimum legal age (North America)	18 or 19, depending on locality	18 or 19 in Canada, Commonwealth, Europe. 21 in USA
Taxable	Yes	Yes
Prevalence of current use Persons ≥ 18 yrs in 2006 USA		
Males	24%	67%
Females	18%	39%
Estimated % with addiction	High proportion	5–10%
Warning labels required	Yes	Yes
Recommended 'safe' level for consumption	No 'safe' level	Recommended upper limit: Males ≤ 2 units per day Females ≤ 1 unit per day
Considered to be a carcinogen	Yes	Yes
Impact on fetus	Lowers birth weight	Causes fetal alcohol syndrome
% of global burden of disease [1]	4.1%	4.0%
Number web sites (Google)[1]	Smoking 143 million Tobacco 66 million	Drinking 14 million Alcoholism 15 million
Number medline retrivals[1]	Smoking 141 000 Tobacco 61 000	Drinking 89 000 Alcoholism 65 000

Note

[1] January 2009.

cigarette smokers compared with 46% of persons who were not recent smokers. Binge drinking was reported by 45% of current-smokers compared with 16% of binge drinkers in current non-smokers. Heavy drinking was reported by 16% of current-smokers compared with 3.8% of heavy drinking in non-smokers [5]. These data remind us that the interaction between smoking and drinking persists at all levels of alcohol exposure.

The major effect of alcohol when viewed at the population level relates to increased morbidity and mortality from injuries – usually affecting younger age-groups. It also contributes to a somewhat lesser extent to degenerative diseases and to cancer. The major effect of tobacco is to increase the risk of cardiovascular disease as well as many types of cancer.

Biologic aspects

Experimental and human data are beginning to clarify the damaging effect resulting from combined exposure to these two substances. In animal experiments, tissue-specific DNA alterations have been discovered after combined exposure to alcohol and cigarette smoke. Target organs included the oesophagus, the lung, and the heart. At each organ site, the damage induced by combined exposure to alcohol and cigarette smoke was greater than the DNA damage induced by smoke or alcohol alone [6]. In human studies, both alcohol consumption and tobacco are associated with p53 mutations in non-small cell lung cancer, compatible with the possibility that alcohol enhances mutagenicity induced by tobacco smoke [7].

Alcohol is not considered to be a carcinogen, but more likely acts as a co-carcinogen or a tumour promoter to increase the toxic effects of carcinogens such as NNK contained in tobacco smoke [8]. Another mechanism of action of alcohol metabolism possibly leading to cancer relates to the formation of acetaldehyde and to highly reactive free radicals [9]. Acetaldehyde has greater cellular toxicity than alcohol and could induce DNA damage or interfere with DNA repair mechanisms [10].

For some organs, such as the mouth or the oesophagus, alcohol could increase the permeability of mucous membranes to tobacco-specific carcinogens [11]. Finally, heavy consumption of alcohol can be associated with nutritional deficiencies such as vitamin A or other vitamins and selenium which could enhance tumour development [12]. However a large randomized trial found that neither alpha-tocopherol nor beta-carotene supplements reduced the frequency of upper aerodigestive tract tumours [13].

Genetic factors

There is abundant evidence reminding us that at all levels of consumption smoking patterns correlate with alcohol consumption. This association is especially true for higher consumption categories [14]. A natural question pertains to the reason for this association: Is there a genetic component? If so, how strong are the association, and what gene(s) might be implicated?

Swan and associates in a multivariate analysis of Caucasian male twins identified a genetic factor that explained the link between smoking, alcohol, and coffee use [15]. In a group of adolescent twins, Han et al. [16] estimated the heritable factor for tobacco and alcohol to be, respectively, 59% and 60% in males, and 11% and 10% in females. The data could be explained by a common underlying substance abuse factor. Koopmans and colleagues [17] in a study of 1 266 young adult Dutch twins noted that alcohol and tobacco use were associated due to the same genetic risk factors. A study of monozygotic twins implicated a genetic factor in lifestyle risk factors leading to gastroesophageal reflux which can cause esophageal cancer [13].

Since about 1990, evidence has been accumulating implicating a dopamine receptor gene (DRD2) as a major factor in addictive disorders, including alcohol addiction and smoking [18–20]. The prevalence of the A1 allele of the D_2 dopamine receptor (DRD2) gene appears to be increased in both alcoholics and smokers. DRD2 may act as a reward or 'pleasure' gene; alcohol, tobacco, and other drugs, in conjunction with alterations in the DRD2 gene, might result in an increase in brain dopamine levels, leading to enhanced feelings of reward and satisfaction. These genetic defects could be important because they are potentially associated with early age of onset of smoking or alcoholism [21–23].

Although gene therapy has rarely been successful in humans, Thanos and co-workers report that delivering the DRD2 gene into the brain of rats trained to self-administer alcohol markedly reduces their intake of alcohol [24]. This type of study strengthens the link between the DRD2 gene and sensitivity to alcohol.

Medical consequences

Malignant disease

Cancer of the upper aero-digestive tract (UAT): mouth, oropharynynx, larynx Upper aerodigestive tract tumours provide strong evidence that combined tobacco and alcohol exposure cause an excess risk of cancer in these sites. These agents can produce changes in methylation thereby increasing the risk of cancer [25, 26]. Another mechanism might be that mucosal damage induced by alcohol, acts synergistically with carcinogens contained in tobacco smoke to induce cancer. It is also possible that alcohol and tobacco can interact with human papilloma virus to increase the risk of UAT tumours [27].

Beverages containing higher concentrations of alcohol are more likely to induce epithelial damage than low content beverages. This could explain why some studies have found that fortified wines and spirits yield higher risks of cancer than weaker beverages [28].

Using the World Health Association mortality data base, Macfarlane and co-workers [29] assessed current trends in male mortality from UAT tumours, relating country-specific frequency to past national alcohol consumption and tobacco exposure. Previous alcohol consumption was a strong predictor of deaths from UAT cancer and the increased death rate from these cancers in the 1990s could be explained by increased alcohol consumption during the 1960s and 1970s. We also know that patients after diagnosis of laryngeal or pharyngeal cancer, have an increased risk of other UAT tumours or lung cancer [30].

Oro-pharyngeal cancer

The oral cavity is exposed to high concentrations of both alcohol and tobacco, explaining why these two risk factors are important etiologic factors for oral cancer [31, 32]. Predictably, both agents also are associated with pre-malignant lesions in this area [28, 33–35].

Since oropharyngeal cancers are aggressive lesions with a poor long-term survival, successful efforts to prevent these tumours depends upon recognition of pre-malignant lesions such as leukoplakia and erythroplasia. Both of these lesions are known to be associated with alcohol and tobacco, including the increasingly common used smokeless tobacco – a form of nicotine delivery system that contains the same carcinogens as cigarettes [36]. Effective counselling for managing pre-malignant oropharyngeal cancers must include information about the contributory role of alcohol and all forms of tobacco exposure.

Larynx

Alcohol and tobacco are predictors of risk for laryngeal cancer, but there are site-specific differences in the impact of these two substances. Alcohol is more strongly related to supraglottic laryngeal tumours than to glottic tumours, whereas smoking is related to both types [37]. The probable reason is that both parts of the larynx will be exposed to tobacco smoke, but that the glottis is unlikely to be exposed to ingested alcohol. In laryngeal cancer p53 mutations have been detected after tobacco and alcohol exposure [38].

Oesophageal cancer

Oesophageal cancer is an excellent example of a tumour caused by exposure to tobacco and alcohol. Pioneering work by Tuyns and co-workers [39, 40] carried out over several years have emphasized the importance of both alcohol and tobacco as etiologic agents for this aggressive cancer. Much of this research was carried out in the Northwest of France, where the incidence of oesophageal cancer is exceptionally high. Case-control studies revealed that both alcohol and tobacco are major risk factors and that exposure to both agents produces a greater-than-additive effect. These data imply that control of both smoking and drinking will be required to reduce the burden of oesophageal cancer.

Most patients with oesophageal cancer have been exposed to both tobacco and alcohol, so it is difficult to estimate the independent impact of each single risk factor. But in his study 743 oesophageal cancers from the Calvados region of Normandy, France, Tuyns found 19 non-drinkers and 75 non-smokers [41]. The relative risk of oesophageal cancer in non-drinking smokers was approximately 5, compared to a relative risk of 11 in non-smoking heavy alcohol consumers. It appears that both agents can act independently and that their relative effect will to some extent depend upon the level of population exposure. One report suggests that for tobacco, a moderate intake over a long time period poses a higher risk than a high intake over a short period. For alcohol, high intake over a shorter period is more likely to induce oesophageal cancer than a low intake over a longer period [42]. It also appears that the excess of squamous cell tumours in the mid portion of the oesophagus is related to combined exposure to alcohol and tobacco [43].

Liver cancer

On a global basis, viral infections and heavy alcohol consumption constitute the major risk factors for liver cancer. However, the International Agency for Research on Cancer lists smoking as an additional risk factor for liver cancer where it interacts with alcohol, viral infection, and obesity to increase the frequency of this lethal tumour [44, 45].

Non-malignant disease

Cardiovascular system

Consumption of both alcohol and tobacco have important implications for the heart and for the entire vascular system. There is strong evidence that high levels of exposure to either of these agents damages the heart, leading to both increased morbidity and mortality. The main impact of tobacco relates to the increased risk of atherosclerosis, causing narrowing of coronary arteries and, eventually to myocardial infarcts or to an increased risk of stroke [46]. Large amounts of alcohol are cardiotoxic, causing cardiomyopathy and can lead to fatal cardiac arrhythmias.

The interaction of these agents has been studied in healthy volunteers. Ethanol and nicotine increased heart rate, and the product of heart rate and blood pressure. The combination of exposure to both drugs could contribute to serious arrhythmias and sudden death, especially in persons with pre-existing coronary heart disease [47].

In patients with pre-existing heart disease, both alcohol and tobacco are independent risk factors for disease progression. Evangelista and co-workers [48] conducted a longitudinal study of 753 patients previously hospitalized with heart disease. In a multivariate analysis current smoking (odds ratio 1.8, 95% confidence interval [CI] 1.2–2.8) and current drinking (odds ratio 5.8, 95% CI 3.8–9.1) were independent predictors of readmission for heart disease.

The deleterious effects of tobacco on the heart are dose-related, with no demonstrable 'safe' level of exposure to tobacco. But for alcohol, there are several longitudinal studies suggesting that persons consuming low levels of alcohol – generally about one or perhaps two drinks per day, have a lower risk of cardiac disease than abstainers or than persons consuming larger quantities of alcohol [49, 50]. The overall impact on large populations is questionable and if there is a benefit from light drinking, it is likely to affect males more than females, and older persons rather than younger persons. Most heavy smokers are heavy drinkers, and would be unlikely to derive any benefit from alcohol.

Pancreas

Unlike the upper aerodigestive tract, the oesophagus, and the stomach, the pancreas, does not come into direct contact with ingested alcohol. Alcohol reaches the gland via the blood stream, where it stimulates pancreatic secretion, either directly or via activation of the secreting mechanism. Moderate consumption of alcohol does not usually cause pancreatic injury, but heavy drinking is a major cause of both acute and chronic pancreatitis.

There is evidence from many sources that the combination of heavy drinking and smoking is especially injurious to the pancreas. Individuals who drink heavily tend to be heavy smokers, so it can be difficult to separate the effects of these two agents on the pancreas. However, several studies have now reported that smoking in addition to alcohol is a separate risk factor for pancreatitis [51–56]. Chronic pancreatitis is an example of a digestive tract disorder where exposure to both addictive substances leads to the onset of a debilitating, painful disease.

Trauma

The combination of drinking and smoking can cause serious injury – particularly burns [57]. A frequent scenario is as follows: after two or three drinks, a person smokes a final cigarette in bed, falls asleep with the cigarette still burning, and wakes up only after sustaining a major burn. Warda [58] concluded that smoking and drinking are two modifiable risk factors for the prevention of domestic fires.

Dupuytren's contracture

Dupuytren's contracture, first described by William Dupuytren (1777–1835), a French physician, has long been known to be associated with moderate to heavy alcohol consumption [59, 60]. The lesion, which occurs in the palmar or plantar fascia, is characterized by the development of strong fibrous bands, which restrict digital mobility. Recent studies have demonstrated that smoking, in addition to alcohol is a risk factor for this disease. An English case-control study based on 222 patients operated because of this disease revealed that smoking nearly tripled the risk of developing this disease: adjusted odd ratio 2.8, 95% CI = 1.5–5.2) Alcohol was an additional risk factor, resulting a two-fold increased risk [61]. In an American study, the findings were nearly identical. The mechanism might be related to microvascular occlusion with subsequent development of fibrosis, leading to disabling contractures [62].

Pregnancy, smoking, and drinking

Despite the well-known adverse effects of smoking and drinking during pregnancy, many women continue to smoke and to drink even while they are pregnant [63]. Estimated exposure figures, based on actual interviews, are 34% for tobacco and 25% for alcohol [64].

The main effect of smoking exposure and moderate alcohol intake seems to be a reduction in fetal birthweight [65], whereas heavy alcohol exposure causes fetal alcohol syndrome characterized by distinct facial abnormalities, hyperirritability, and persistent cognitive impairment [66]. Both smoking and drinking may interact with specific genetic alterations to cause cleft lip and/or cleft palate [67, 68]. Clearly, both smoking and drinking have adverse effects on the fetus; efforts at intervention should be included as an integral part of pre-conception planning [69].

Treatment issues and co-dependence

Tobacco is a major factor contributing to the global burden of disease and alcohol plays a role in determining the success of smoking intervention programmes [70]. The evidence strongly suggests that drinking reduces the already low success rate in smoking intervention programmes. This is especially so for heavy drinkers, and less so for light or moderate drinkers. Binge drinking, loosely defined as consuming at least five or more drinks on one or more occasions in the previous month, reduces the probability of success by as much as 50% [71, 72]. The reason might be that binge drinkers are more likely to have a genetic defect leading to a more serious addiction problem to both alcohol and tobacco than moderate drinkers (see earlier).

Prevention of alcohol- and tobacco-related diseases is even more important than treatment, especially in adolescents and young adults. There is solid evidence that the use of both substances begins at an early age, implying that efforts to promote a healthy lifestyle must begin early in life [73].

Asbestos and tobacco

Although Marco Polo may have described asbestos in the thirteenth century, its widespread use only occurred in the twentieth century. Because asbestos has remarkable fire-retardant properties it was widely used as an insulating material and in applications where heat is generated, such as in brake linings. Fibres of asbestos are readily inhaled or ingested and have been linked primarily with lung cancer and with mesothelioma.

Exposure to asbestos

Maximum occupational and population exposure to asbestos has dropped since the 1970s when most asbestos-containing products were banned. At that time about 4–5% of the population may have been exposed to asbestos, with males much more likely to be exposed than females [74]. The mode of exposure is mainly by fibre inhalation, although asbestos fibres can also be ingested. The lung is the primary target organ for asbestos exposure, but asbestos is the major risk factor for mesothelial tumours. Occupational groups with exposure to asbestos include asbestos cement workers, insulation workers, and shipyard workers.

Asbestos, smoking, and lung cancer

Smoking is the major environmental cause of lung cancer, but what is the impact of joint exposure to both asbestos and tobacco products? Lee reviewed the evidence from 23 studies containing information on joint exposure [75]. The main conclusions were: 1) In non-smokers asbestos exposure significantly increases the risk of lung cancer; 2) In smokers there appears to be a multiplicative effect of combined exposure to these two carcinogenic environmental agents. This can be seen graphically in lung cancer mortality data presented in the 1980s in the report of the Surgeon General [76] (Fig. 34.2). Smokers exposed to asbestos have about a 50-fold increased risk of lung cancer. For smokers consuming more than one pack per day, the relative risk is 87 times greater than in the non-smoking, non-asbestos group. In contrast to the synergistic effect of

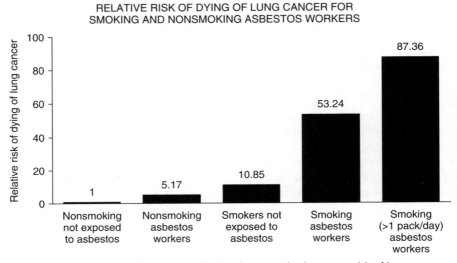

Figure 34.2 Effect of combined exposure to both tobacco and asbestos on risk of lung cancer.
Source: From [76].

smoking and asbestos exposure on lung cancer risk, smoking does not appear to be a risk factor for mesothelioma [77].

Gustavsson and co-workers investigated the risk of lung cancer in a Swedish population that included low-dose asbestos exposure. They found that cumulative risk of joint exposure was greater than predicted by an additive model but less than expected from a multiplicative model [78].

Arsenic

Exposure to arsenic

Arsenic is considered to be a human carcinogen and exposure can occur through occupational exposure to pesticides, but is much more likely to be related to high levels of arsenic in drinking water [79]. A few nutritional supplements may contain arsenic and wine may contain residual amounts of arsenic from spraying. Globally, an estimated 100 million persons are exposed to high levels of arsenic in drinking water, particularly in Bangladesh where over 90% of the population is thought to be exposed to drinking water that exceeds the federal drinking water standard for the allowable amount of arsenic which is 10 parts per billion.

Arsenic and lung cancer

In those areas where levels of arsenic are high, lung cancer rates are also elevated, suggesting a causal link [80]. Since smoking is such a strong risk factor for lung cancer, it is not surprising that the arsenic-related increased risk of lung cancer is increased in smokers [81–83]. In animals, combined exposure to arsenic and tobacco smoke results in synergistic DNA damage [84]. Table 34.3 demonstrates the effect of joint exposure to arsenic and tobacco in a Taiwanese population [81]. A study from Northern Chile also found a synergistic relationship between smoking and arsenic exposure in drinking water and lung cancer [83].

Arsenic and skin cancer

In addition to causing lung cancer, chronic arsenic exposure can lead to skin cancer, usually with a latent period that can last for several decades. Arsenical skin cancer can appear on any dermal

Table 34.3 Relative risk of lung cancer after exposure to tobacco and arsenic[1]

Smoking status	Arsenic exposure	Relative risk (95% CI)
Non-smoker	<10	1
	10–699	1.2 (0.5–2.9)
	≥700	2.2 (0.7–6.9)
<25 Pack-years	<10	2.6 (0.7–9.5)
	10–699	5.5 (2.0–15.5)
	≥700	6.3 (1.5–25.7)
≥25 Pack-years	<10	3.8 (1.3–11.2)
	10–699	5.9 (2.2–16.1)
	≥700	11.1 (3.3–37.2)

Note

[1] From [81] with permission.

site and can be preceded by hyperpigmentation or by Bowen's disease – a pre-malignant condition. As with lung cancer, combined exposure to arsenic and tobacco increases the risk of skin cancer above that seen for exposure to arsenic alone [85, 86].

Arsenic and bladder cancer

In areas where drinking water contains large amounts of arsenic it is a recognized cause of bladder cancer. The level of exposure to arsenic can be approximated by examination of arsenical products in the urine. As with other carcinogens, duration of exposure as well as intensity of exposure are both important risk factors.

Similar to lung and skin cancer, smoking augments the carcinogenic effect of arsenic on the bladder. It is probable that smokers develop arsenic-related bladder cancer at lower levels of arsenic exposure than non-smokers [87, 88]. Chen and co-workers suggest that in persons exposed to environmental tobacco smoke, the risk of bladder cancer is also dependent upon the ability to methylate ingested arsenic [89].

Radiation

Humans are exposed to many sources of radiation including background radiation from the air and the ground, occupational exposure, and exposure resulting from medical therapy.

Radon

Radon, a widely distributed tasteless and colourless element formed during the natural degradation of uranium, is a known carcinogen. Human exposure occurs when radon particles are inhaled with ambient air. Radon can be ingested in drinking water, but little is known about the relationship between ingested radon and gastrointestinal cancer. Radon exposure can come about through occupational exposure as in the case of uranium miners [90], but the major source of exposure for most populations is through the radon content of air that seeps into private dwellings. The Environmental Protection Agency recommends remediation efforts, such as sealing basement cracks to reduce radon exposure along with increasing air circulation, if the ambient air contains more than 4 picocuries of radon per litre of air.

Tobacco, radon, and lung cancer

Since inhalation of radon constitutes the main source of exposure, it is not surprising that the lung is the main target organ. After tobacco exposure, radon is thought to be the second commonest cause of lung cancer [91]. Estimates based on case-control studies in Europe suggest that exposure to radon increases the risk of lung cancer with no minimal threshold level. In the United Kingdom an estimated 3.3% of all deaths from lung cancer are related to radon and in most of these patients smoking is an additional co-factor [92]. Tobacco smoke is estimated to increase the risk of radon-induced lung cancer by a factor of ranging from about 8–25 [93, 94].

Breast cancer, smoking, and radiotherapy

Smoking is not considered a risk factor for breast cancer, but might there be an increased risk of lung cancer in breast cancer patients who are smokers and who have received radiotherapy? The combined effect of smoking and radiotherapy leads to lung cancer risks that are much higher than single exposure to either agent [95, 96]. Again, joint exposure appears to be synergistic.

Summary and conclusions

Tobacco exposure causes a significant proportion of human disease. However there is abundant evidence that several other substances act synergistically with tobacco to increase the risk of disease – particularly malignant disease. Alcohol is especially troublesome because a large proportion of the population has had recent exposure to both agents. For heavy smokers, dual exposure is extremely common. Synergistic effects of alcohol and tobacco exposure are seen for both malignant and non-malignant diseases.

The lungs are major target organ for joint exposure to tobacco and either asbestos, arsenic, or radon. Smokers who are exposed to any of these three agents have a risk of lung cancer that is higher than independent exposure to either agent. Fortunately, asbestos exposure is now much less common than in the latter part of the twentieth century. Arsenic exposure is a special problem mainly in specific geographic areas such as Bangladesh, where well water often contains high levels of arsenic. The combination of smoking and exposure to arsenic leads not only to lung cancer, but also to skin and bladder cancer. Radon is a widely distributed element whose degradation products are carcinogenic. Although miners are exposed, widespread exposure occurs from radon in the ground when it seeps into offices and dwellings. Its main effect is to increase the risk of lung cancer; radon is thought to be the second commonest cause of this tumour.

Effective smoking cessation programmes will be required to reduce the frequency of smoking-related disease. These programmes will be especially important in persons who may also be exposed to any of the agents discussed in this chapter.

Acknowledgement

We thank the C. D. Smithers Foundation, Solvay Pharmaceuticals, and the Italian Association for Cancer Research (AIRC) for their support.

References

1. http://www.who.int/substance_abuse/publications/en/Neuroscience_E.pdf. (2004).

2. Vlahov, D., Galea, S., Ahern, J., Resnick, H., and Kilpatrick, D. (2004). Sustained increased consumption of cigarettes, alcohol, and marijuana among Manhattan residents after September 11, 2001. *Am J Public Health*, **94**(2): 253–254.

3. Kouri, E.M., McCarthy, E.M., Faust, A.H., and Lukas, S.E. (2004). Pretreatment with transdermal nicotine enhances some of ethanol's acute effects in men. *Drug Alcohol Depend*, **75**(1): 55–65.

4. Taylor, B. and Rehm, J. (2006). When risk factors combine: the interaction between alcohol and smoking for aerodigestive cancer, coronary heart disease, and traffic and fire injury. *Addict Behav*, **31**(9): 1522–1535.

5. Substance Abuse and mental Health Services Administration (2008). Results from the 2007 National Survey on Drug Use and Health: National Findings. Office of Applied Studies NSDUH Series H-34, DHHS Publication SMA 084343. 11-19-0008.

6. Izzotti, A., Balansky, R.M., Blagoeva, P.M., Mircheva, Z.I., Tulimiero, L., Cartiglia, C. *et al*. (1998). DNA alterations in rat organs after chronic exposure to cigarette smoke and/or ethanol ingestion. *FASEB J*, **12**(9): 753–758.

7. Ahrendt, S.A., Chow, J.T., Yang, S.C., Wu, L., Zhang, M.J., Jen, J. *et al*. (2000). Alcohol consumption and cigarette smoking increase the frequency of p53 mutations in non-small cell lung cancer. *Cancer Res*, **60**(12): 3155–3159.

8. Hecht, S.S. (1999). DNA adduct formation from tobacco-specific N-nitrosamines. *Mutat Res*, **424**(1-2): 127–142.

9. Salaspuro, V. and Salaspuro, M. (2004). Synergistic effect of alcohol drinking and smoking on in vivo acetaldehyde concentration in saliva. *Int J Cancer*, **111**(4): 480–483.

10. Homann, N., Tillonen, J., Meurman, J.H., Rintamaki, H., Lindqvist, C., Rautio, M. *et al.* (2000). Increased salivary acetaldehyde levels in heavy drinkers and smokers: a microbiological approach to oral cavity cancer. *Carcinogenesis*, **21**(4): 663–668.

11. Du, X., Squier, C.A., Kremer, M.J., and Wertz, P.W. (2000). Penetration of N-nitrosonornicotine (NNN) across oral mucosa in the presence of ethanol and nicotine. *J Oral Pathol Med*, **29**(2): 80–85.

12. Seitz, H.K., Poschl, G., and Simanowski, U.A. (1998). Alcohol and cancer. *Recent Dev Alcohol*, **14**: 67–95.

13. Wright, M.E., Virtamo, J., Hartman, A.M., Pietinen, P., Edwards, B.K., Taylor, P.R. *et al.* (2007). Effects of alpha-tocopherol and beta-carotene supplementation on upper aerodigestive tract cancers in a large, randomized controlled trial. *Cancer*, **109**(5): 891–898.

14. Gulliver, S.B., Rohsenow, D.J., Colby, S.M., Dey, A.N., Abrams, D.B., Niaura, R.S. *et al.* (1995). Interrelationship of smoking and alcohol dependence, use and urges to use. *J Stud Alcohol*, **56**(2): 202–206.

15. Swan, G.E., Carmelli, D., and Cardon, L.R. (1996). The consumption of tobacco, alcohol, and coffee in Caucasian male twins: a multivariate genetic analysis. *J Subst Abuse*, **8**(1): 19–31.

16. Han, C., McGue, M.K., and Iacono, W.G. (1999). Lifetime tobacco, alcohol and other substance use in adolescent Minnesota twins: univariate and multivariate behavioral genetic analyses. *Addiction*, **94**(7): 981–993.

17. Koopmans, J.R., van Doornen, L.J., and Boomsma, D.I. (1997). Association between alcohol use and smoking in adolescent and young adult twins: a bivariate genetic analysis. *Alcohol Clin Exp Res*, **21**(3): 537–546.

18. Noble, E.P. (1998). The DRD2 gene, smoking, and lung cancer. *J Natl Cancer Inst*, **90**(5): 343–345.

19. Noble, E.P. (2000). Addiction and its reward process through polymorphisms of the D2 dopamine receptor gene: a review. *Eur Psychiatry*, **15**(2): 79–89.

20. Noble, E.P. (2000). The DRD2 gene in psychiatric and neurological disorders and its phenotypes. *Pharmacogenomics*, **1**(3): 309–333.

21. Spitz, M.R., Shi, H., Yang, F., Hudmon, K.S., Jiang, H., Chamberlain, R.M. *et al.* (1998). Case-control study of the D2 dopamine receptor gene and smoking status in lung cancer patients. *J Natl Cancer Inst*, **90**(5): 358–363.

22. Comings, D.E., Ferry, L., Bradshaw-Robinson, S., Burchette, R., Chiu, C., and Muhleman, D. (1996). The dopamine D2 receptor (DRD2) gene: a genetic risk factor in smoking. *Pharmacogenetics*, **6**(1): 73–79.

23. Kono, Y., Yoneda, H., Sakai, T., Nonomura, Y., Inayama, Y., Koh, J. *et al.* (1997). Association between early-onset alcoholism and the dopamine D2 receptor gene. *Am J Med Genet*, **74**(2): 179–182.

24. Thanos, P.K., Volkow, N.D., Freimuth, P., Umegaki, H., Ikari, H., Roth, G. *et al.* (2001). Overexpression of dopamine D2 receptors reduces alcohol self-administration. *J Neurochem*, **78**(5): 1094–1103.

25. Chang, H.W., Ling, G.S., Wei, W.I., and Yuen, A.P. (2004). Smoking and drinking can induce p15 methylation in the upper aerodigestive tract of healthy individuals and patients with head and neck squamous cell carcinoma. *Cancer*, **101**(1): 125–132.

26. Smith, I.M., Mydlarz, W.K., Mithani, S.K., and Califano, J.A. (2007). DNA global hypomethylation in squamous cell head and neck cancer associated with smoking, alcohol consumption and stage. *Int J Cancer*, **121**(8): 1724–1728.

27. D'Souza, G., Kreimer, A.R., Viscidi, R., Pawlita, M., Fakhry, C., Koch, W.M. *et al.* (2007). Case-control study of human papillomavirus and oropharyngeal cancer. *N Engl J Med*, **356**(19): 1944–1956.

28. Jaber, M.A., Porter, S.R., Gilthorpe, M.S., Bedi, R., and Scully, C. (1999). Risk factors for oral epithelial dysplasia – the role of smoking and alcohol. *Oral Oncol*, **35**(2): 151–156.

29. Macfarlane, G.J., Macfarlane, T.V., and Lowenfels, A.B. (1996). The influence of alcohol consumption on worldwide trends in mortality from upper aerodigestive tract cancers in men. *J Epidemiol Community Health*, **50**(6): 636–639.

30. Dikshit, R.P., Boffetta, P., Bouchardy, C., Merletti, F., Crosignani, P., Cuchi, T. *et al.* (2005). Risk factors for the development of second primary tumors among men after laryngeal and hypopharyngeal carcinoma. *Cancer*, **103**(11): 2326–2333.

31. Schlecht, N.F., Franco, E.L., Pintos, J., Negassa, A., Kowalski, L.P., Oliveira, B.V. *et al.* (1999). Interaction between tobacco and alcohol consumption and the risk of cancers of the upper aero-digestive tract in Brazil. *Am J Epidemiol*, **150**(11): 1129–1137.

32. Friborg, J.T., Yuan, J.M., Wang, R., Koh, W.P., Lee, H.P., and Yu, M.C. (2007). A prospective study of tobacco and alcohol use as risk factors for pharyngeal carcinomas in Singapore Chinese. *Cancer*, **109**(6): 1183–1191.

33. Macigo, F.G., Mwaniki, D.L., and Guthua, S.W. (1996). Influence of dose and cessation of kiraiku, cigarettes and alcohol use on the risk of developing oral leukoplakia. *Eur J Oral Sci*, **104**(5-6): 498–502.

34. Gupta, P.C. (1984). Epidemiologic study of the association between alcohol habits and oral leukoplakia. *Community Dent Oral Epidemiol*, **12**(1): 47–50.

35. Hashibe, M., Mathew, B., Kuruvilla, B., Thomas, G., Sankaranarayanan, R., Parkin, D.M. *et al.* (2000). Chewing tobacco, alcohol, and the risk of erythroplakia. *Cancer Epidemiol Biomarkers Prev*, **9**(7): 639–645.

36. Hecht, S.S., Carmella, S.G., Murphy, S.E., Riley, W.T., Le, C., Luo, X. *et al.* (2007). Similar exposure to a tobacco-specific carcinogen in smokeless tobacco users and cigarette smokers. *Cancer Epidemiol Biomarkers Prev*, **16**(8): 1567–1572.

37. Brugere, J., Guenel, P., Leclerc, A., and Rodriguez, J. (1986). Differential effects of tobacco and alcohol in cancer of the larynx, pharynx, and mouth. *Cancer*, **57**(2): 391–395.

38. Ronchetti, D., Neglia, C.B., Cesana, B.M., Carboni, N., Neri, A., Pruneri, G. *et al.* (2004). Association between p53 gene mutations and tobacco and alcohol exposure in laryngeal squamous cell carcinoma. *Arch Otolaryngol Head Neck Surg*, **130**(3): 303–306.

39. Tuyns, A.J. (1970). Cancer of the oesophagus: further evidence of the relation to drinking habits in France. *Int J Cancer*, **5**(1): 152–156.

40. Tuyns, A.J., Pequignot, G., and Jensen, O.M. (1977). [Esophageal cancer in Ille-et-Vilaine in relation to levels of alcohol and tobacco consumption. Risks are multiplying]. *Bull Cancer*, **64**(1): 45–60.

41. Tuyns, A.J. (1983). Oesophageal cancer in non-smoking drinkers and in non-drinking smokers. *Int J Cancer*, **32**(4): 443–444.

42. Launoy, G., Milan, C.H., Faivre, J., Pienkowski, P., Milan, C.I., and Gignoux, M. (1997). Alcohol, tobacco and oesophageal cancer: effects of the duration of consumption, mean intake and current and former consumption. *Br J Cancer*, **75**(9): 1389–1396.

43. Lee, C.H., Wu, D.C., Lee, J.M., Wu, I.C., Goan, Y.G., Kao, E.L. *et al.* (2007). Anatomical subsite discrepancy in relation to the impact of the consumption of alcohol, tobacco and betel quid on esophageal cancer. *Int J Cancer*, **120**(8): 1755–1762.

44. Marrero, J.A., Fontana, R.J., Fu, S., Conjeevaram, H.S., Su, G.L, and Lok, A.S. (2005). Alcohol, tobacco and obesity are synergistic risk factors for hepatocellular carcinoma. *J Hepatol*, **42**(2): 218–224.

45. Hassan, M.M., Spitz, M.R., Thomas, M.B., El Deeb, A.S., Glover, K.Y., Nguyen, N.T. *et al.* (2008). Effect of different types of smoking and synergism with hepatitis C virus on risk of hepatocellular carcinoma in American men and women: case-control study. *Int J Cancer*, **123**(8): 1883–1891.

46. Chiuve, S.E., Rexrode, K.M., Spiegelman, D., Logroscino, G., Manson, J.E., and Rimm, E.B. (2008). Primary prevention of stroke by healthy lifestyle. *Circulation*, **118**(9): 947–954.

47. Benowitz, N.L., Jones, R.T., and Jacob, P., III (1986). Additive cardiovascular effects of nicotine and ethanol. *Clin Pharmacol Ther*, **40**(4): 420–424.

48. Evangelista, L.S., Doering, L.V., and Dracup, K. (2000). Usefulness of a history of tobacco and alcohol use in predicting multiple heart failure readmissions among veterans. *Am J Cardiol*, **86**(12): 1339–1342.

49. Thun, M.J., Peto, R., Lopez, A.D., Monaco, J.H., Henley, S.J., Heath, C.W., Jr. *et al.* (1997). Alcohol consumption and mortality among middle-aged and elderly U.S. adults. *N Engl J Med*, **337**(24): 1705–1714.

50. Fuchs, C.S., Stampfer, M.J., Colditz, G.A., Giovannucci, E.L., Manson, J.E., Kawachi, I. *et al.* (1995). Alcohol consumption and mortality among women. *N Engl J Med*, **332**(19): 1245–1250.

51. Lin, Y., Tamakoshi, A., Hayakawa, T., Ogawa, M., and Ohno, Y. (2000). Cigarette smoking as a risk factor for chronic pancreatitis: a case-control study in Japan. Research Committee on Intractable Pancreatic Diseases. *Pancreas*, **21**(2): 109–114.

52. Talamini, G., Bassi, C., Falconi, M., Frulloni, L., Di Francesco, V., and Vaona, B. *et al.* (1996). Cigarette smoking: an independent risk factor in alcoholic pancreatitis. *Pancreas*, **12**: 131–137.

53. Maisonneuve, P., Lowenfels, A.B., Mullhaupt, B., Cavallini, G., Lankisch, P.G., Andersen, J.R. *et al.* (2005). Cigarette smoking accelerates progression of alcoholic chronic pancreatitis. *Gut*, **54**(4): 510–514.

54. Maisonneuve, P., Frulloni, L., Mullhaupt, B., Faitini, K., Cavallini, G., Lowenfels, A.B. *et al.* (2006). Impact of smoking on patients with idiopathic chronic pancreatitis. *Pancreas*, **33**(2): 163–168.

55. Lowenfels, A.B., Zwemer, F.L., Jhangiani, S., and Pitchumoni, C.S. (1987). Pancreatitis in a Native American Indian population. *Pancreas*, **2**: 694–697.

56. Hartwig, W., Werner, J., Ryschich, E., Mayer, H., Schmidt, J., Gebhard, M.M. *et al.* (2000). Cigarette smoke enhances ethanol-induced pancreatic injury. *Pancreas*, **21**(3): 272–278.

57. D'Onofrio, G., Becker, B., and Woolard, R.H. (2006). The impact of alcohol, tobacco, and other drug use and abuse in the emergency department. *Emerg Med Clin North Am*, **24**(4): 925–967.

58. Warda, L., Tenenbein, M., and Moffatt, M.E. (1999). House fire injury prevention update. Part I. A review of risk factors for fatal and non-fatal house fire injury. *Inj Prev*, **5**(2): 145–150.

59. Burke, F.D., Proud, G., Lawson, I.J., McGeoch, K.L., and Miles, J.N. (2007). An assessment of the effects of exposure to vibration, smoking, alcohol and diabetes on the prevalence of Dupuytren's disease in 97,537 miners. *J Hand Surg Eur Vol*, **32**(4): 400–406.

60. Godtfredsen, N.S., Lucht, H., Prescott, E., Sorensen, T.I., and Gronbaek, M. (2004). A prospective study linked both alcohol and tobacco to Dupuytren's disease. *J Clin Epidemiol*, **57**(8): 858–863.

61. Burge, P., Hoy, G., Regan, P., and Milne, R. (1997). Smoking, alcohol and the risk of Dupuytren's contracture. *J Bone Joint Surg Br*, **79**(2): 206–210.

62. An, H.S., Southworth, S.R., Jackson, W.T., and Russ, B. (1988). Cigarette smoking and Dupuytren's contracture of the hand. *J Hand Surg [Am]*, **13**(6): 872–874.

63. Odendaal, H.J., Steyn, D.W., Elliott, A., and Burd, L. (2008). Combined effects of cigarette smoking and alcohol consumption on perinatal outcome. *Gynecol Obstet Invest*, **67**(1): 1–8.

64. Jones-Webb, R., McKiver, M., Pirie, P., and Mine, K. (1999). Relationships between physician advice and tobacco and alcohol use during pregnancy. *Am J Prev Med*, **16**(3): 244–247.

65. Olsen, J., Rachootin, P., and Schiodt, A.V. (1983). Alcohol use, conception time, and birth weight. *J Epidemiol Community Health*, **37**(1): 63–65.

66. Streissguth, A.P., Barr, H.M., Sampson, P.D., and Bookstein, F.L. (1994). Prenatal alcohol and offspring development: the first fourteen years. *Drug Alcohol Depend*, **36**(2): 89–99.

67. Romitti, P.A., Lidral, A.C., Munger, R.G., Daack-Hirsch, S., Burns, T.L., and Murray, J.C. (1999). Candidate genes for nonsyndromic cleft lip and palate and maternal cigarette smoking and alcohol consumption: evaluation of genotype-environment interactions from a population-based case-control study of orofacial clefts. *Teratology*, **59**(1): 39–50.

68. Bille, C., Olsen, J., Vach, W., Knudsen, V.K., Olsen, S.F., Rasmussen, K. *et al.* (2007). Oral clefts and life style factors–a case-cohort study based on prospective Danish data. *Eur J Epidemiol*, **22**(3): 173–181.

69. Barrison, I.G. and Wright, J.T. (1984). Moderate drinking during pregnancy and foetal outcome. Alcohol *Alcohol*, **19**(2): 167–172.

70. Hintz, T. and Mann, K. (2007). Long-term behavior in treated alcoholism: evidence for beneficial carry-over effects of abstinence from smoking on alcohol use and vice versa. *Addict Behav*, **32**(12): 3093–3100.

71. Murray, R.P., Istvan, J.A., Voelker, H.T., Rigdon, M.A., and Wallace, M.D. (1995). Level of involvement with alcohol and success at smoking cessation in the lung health study. *J Stud Alcohol*, **56**(1): 74–82.

72. Dawson, D.A. (2000). Drinking as a risk factor for sustained smoking. *Drug Alcohol Depend*, **59**(3): 235–249.

73. Burke, G.L., Hunter, S.M., Croft, J.B., Cresanta, J.L., and Berenson, G.S. (1988). The interaction of alcohol and tobacco use in adolescents and young adults: Bogalusa Heart Study. *Addict Behav*, **13**(4): 387–393.

74. Rogan, W.J., Ragan, N.B., and Dinse, G.E. (2000). X-ray evidence of increased asbestos exposure in the US population from NHANES I and NHANES II, 1973-1978. National Health Examination Survey. *Cancer Causes Control*, **11**(5): 441–449.

75. Lee, P.N. (2001). Relation between exposure to asbestos and smoking jointly and the risk of lung cancer. *Occup Environ Med*, **58**(3): 145–153.

76. Surgeon General of the United States (1985). The Health Consequences of Smoking. Cancer and chronic lung disease in the workplace. Rockville, Maryland: US Department of Health and Human Services.

77. Muscat, J.E. and Wynder, E.L. (1991). Cigarette smoking, asbestos exposure, and malignant mesothelioma. *Cancer Res*, **51**(9): 2263–2267.

78. Gustavsson, P., Nyberg, F., Pershagen, G., Scheele, P., Jakobsson, R., and Plato, N. (2002). Low-dose exposure to asbestos and lung cancer: dose-response relations and interaction with smoking in a population-based case-referent study in Stockholm, Sweden. *Am J Epidemiol*, **155**(11): 1016–1022.

79. Smith, C.J., Livingston, S.D., and Doolittle, D.J. (1997). An international literature survey of 'IARC Group I carcinogens' reported in mainstream cigarette smoke. *Food Chem Toxicol*, **35**(10–11): 1107–1130.

80. Celik, I., Gallicchio, L., Boyd, K., Lam, T.K., Matanoski, G., Tao, X. *et al.* (2008). Arsenic in drinking water and lung cancer: a systematic review. *Environ Res*, **108**(1): 48–55.

81. Chen, C.L., Hsu, L.I., Chiou, H.Y., Hsueh, Y.M., Chen, S.Y., Wu, M.M. *et al.* (2004). Ingested arsenic, cigarette smoking, and lung cancer risk: a follow-up study in arseniasis-endemic areas in Taiwan. *JAMA*, **292**(24): 2984–2990.

82. Ahsan, H. and Thomas, D.C. (2004). Lung cancer etiology: independent and joint effects of genetics, tobacco, and arsenic. *JAMA*, **292**(24): 3026–3029.

83. Ferreccio, C., Gonzalez, C., Milosavjlevic, V., Marshall, G., Sancha, A.M., and Smith, A.H. (2000). Lung cancer and arsenic concentrations in drinking water in Chile. *Epidemiology*, **11**(6): 673–679.

84. Hays, A.M., Srinivasan, D., Witten, M.L., Carter, D.E., and Lantz, R.C. (2006). Arsenic and cigarette smoke synergistically increase DNA oxidation in the lung. *Toxicol Pathol*, **34**(4): 396–404.

85. Lee, L. and Bebb, G. (2005). A case of Bowen's disease and small-cell lung carcinoma: long-term consequences of chronic arsenic exposure in Chinese traditional medicine. *Environ Health Perspect*, **113**(2): 207–210.

86. Knobeloch, L.M., Zierold, K.M., and Anderson, H.A. (2006). Association of arsenic-contaminated drinking-water with prevalence of skin cancer in Wisconsin's Fox River Valley. *J Health Popul Nutr*, **24**(2): 206–213.

87. Steinmaus, C., Yuan, Y., Bates, M.N., and Smith, A.H. (2003). Case-control study of bladder cancer and drinking water arsenic in the western United States. *Am J Epidemiol*, **158**(12): 1193–1201.

88. Michaud, D.S., Wright, M.E., Cantor, K.P., Taylor, P.R., Virtamo, J., and Albanes, D. (2004). Arsenic concentrations in prediagnostic toenails and the risk of bladder cancer in a cohort study of male smokers. *Am J Epidemiol*, **160**(9): 853–859.

89. Chen, Y.C., Su, H.J., Guo, Y.L., Houseman, E.A., and Christiani, D.C. (2005). Interaction between environmental tobacco smoke and arsenic methylation ability on the risk of bladder cancer. *Cancer Causes Control*, **16**(2): 75–81.

90. Boice, J.D., Jr., Cohen, S.S., Mumma, M.T., Chadda, B., and Blot, W.J. (2008). A cohort study of uranium millers and miners of Grants, New Mexico, 1979-2005. *J Radiol Prot*, **28**(3): 303–325.

91. Frumkin, H. and Samet, J.M. (2001). Radon. *CA Cancer J Clin*, **51**(6): 337–344, 322.

92. Gray, A., Read, S., McGale, P., and Darby, S. (2009). Lung cancer deaths from indoor radon and the cost effectiveness and potential of policies to reduce them. *BMJ*, **338**: a3110.

93. EPA assessment of risks from radon in homes (2003). http://www.epa.gov/radon/pdfs/402-r-03-003.pdf. 2008.

94. Darby, S., Hill, D., Auvinen, A., Barros-Dios, J.M., Baysson, H., Bochicchio, F. *et al.* (2005). Radon in homes and risk of lung cancer: collaborative analysis of individual data from 13 European case-control studies. *BMJ*, **330**(7485): 223.

95. Kaufman, E.L., Jacobson, J.S., Hershman, D.L., Desai, M., and Neugut, A.I. (2008). Effect of breast cancer radiotherapy and cigarette smoking on risk of second primary lung cancer. *J Clin Oncol*, **26**(3): 392–398.

96. Ford, M.B., Sigurdson, A.J., Petrulis, E.S., Ng, C.S., Kemp, B., Cooksley, C. *et al.* (2003). Effects of smoking and radiotherapy on lung carcinoma in breast carcinoma survivors. *Cancer*, **98**(7): 1457–1464.

Chapter 35

Roles of tobacco litigation in societal change

Richard A. Daynard

Litigation plays at least six different roles in tobacco control. First, the most common and least dramatic role is ordinary enforcement of tobacco-control laws. Laws frequently ban sales to minors, smoking in public places, and certain types of advertising. The governments that impose these laws have the burden of enforcing them, which may involve litigation against violators. Second, too frequently governments enforce tobacco-control laws sporadically or not at all, creating the opportunity for NGOs either to bring law enforcement actions directly or to sue their governments to force them to do their job, depending on whether courts will permit NGOs to take such actions. Third, tobacco companies increasingly use litigation to thwart effective tobacco control legislation and programmes, typically arguing that constitutional provisions or other controlling law pre-empts such measures. Fourth, lawsuits and administrative proceedings have been brought by smoke-sensitive individuals against employers and places of public accommodation, seeking protection from secondhand smoke or compensation for illnesses caused or exacerbated by exposure to secondhand smoke. Fifth, many lawsuits have been brought by individuals, groups or classes of individuals, and third-party health care payers against the tobacco companies, seeking compensation for tobacco-caused illness, death, and/or out-of-pocket economic costs. Sixth, governments occasionally attempt to enforce general laws (e.g. against racketeering) against tobacco companies, alleging that deceptive and illegal practices by the industry have harmed the general public. Unlike ordinary law enforcement, these cases seek court orders requiring fundamental changes in the way these companies do business.

Each of these roles has implications for social change. Each will be discussed in turn, with the most attention devoted to the cases against the tobacco industry. We will also look at the role that legislation can play in encouraging or discouraging tobacco litigation. We will conclude with a brief discussion of how tobacco control would have been different in the past in the absence of litigation, and how litigation may affect the course and success of tobacco control in the future.

Law enforcement

While many tobacco-control objectives can be achieved through legislation, legislation is effective only to the extent that it is enforced. This is a major issue because many legislative initiatives seek to change customary social behaviour such as selling to minors and smoking in public places, while the tobacco industry has strong motivation and little compunction about evading legislative restrictions such as advertising bans and counter-smuggling measures on its own behaviour. Both public education and active enforcement are often necessary if these laws are not to be 'dead letters'.

Enforcement can be accomplished through administrative measures (e.g. license suspensions or revocations) or through criminal or quasi-criminal (e.g. traffic summons-type procedures, civil fines) processes. Most enforcement activity does not involve extensive litigation, because the facts are usually easy for the authorities to establish, and the level of sanctions typically low enough that it is not worthwhile for the wrongdoer to fight the charges in court. The principal exceptions are where the defendant, often supported by the tobacco industry, refuses to comply in order to force a legal challenge to the validity of the tobacco-control legislation (discussed below in Section 'Industry counter-attacks'), or in smuggling and tax-avoidance cases where the penalties sought may be very large.

Litigation by NGOs to compel enforcement

Many tobacco-control laws and regulations are rarely if ever formally enforced. Occasionally this is a good sign, as with laws restricting smoking in public places in the United States that are informally but effectively enforced through social pressure. However, where public support has not been mobilized behind the policy underlying the law, the failure of public authorities to enforce the law results in its being flouted by anyone who has incentive to do so. This characterized, for example, the status of sales-to-minors bans in the United States until the 1990s, restrictions on smoking in French restaurants until 2008, and bans on advertising in many countries since their adoption.

In the United States the doctrine of 'prosecutorial discretion' prevents private parties from forcing government action, but state consumer protection laws frequently allow parties to act as 'private attorneys general' in the public interest to require product manufacturers or sellers to obey the law. In Massachusetts, for example, a 1987 lawsuit brought by the Group Against Smoking Pollution of Massachusetts against Store 24, a local convenience store chain, alleging that they had sold cigarettes repeatedly to teenagers in violation of state law, resulted in Store 24 agreeing to demand positive identification from young people before selling them cigarettes as well as monitoring their own stores for compliance with the new policy. This was the first time that such a 'carding' requirement was imposed anywhere in the United States, and set a model for subsequent regulations. A similar approach was used in Bangladesh and in Mali, where NGOs obtained sanctions against tobacco firms that were engaged in illegal promotion and advertising (Rendezvous with Mahamane Cisse 2000).

Some legal systems do permit NGOs to bring 'public interest' actions to require the government to enforce the law, including relevant constitutional provisions. The 1999 pioneering case in the Indian state of Kerala produced a judicial order applying the constitutional right to health protection by requiring the police to enforce a ban on smoking in public places. This was followed by a similar ruling by the Indian Supreme Court in November 2001, which led to action by governmental bodies throughout India banning smoking in public places (Murli S. Deora v Union of India and Others 2001). Another case in Uganda produced a settlement with the government to the same effect (The Environmental Action Network, Ltd. *et al.* 2000).

Industry counter-attacks

While the tobacco industry is quite litigious, it threatens more litigation than it brings. For example, in the United States it typically sends its lawyers to meetings of local legislative bodies that are considering strong tobacco-control measures. They 'inform' the lawmakers that the measures they are considering are beyond their jurisdiction; are unconstitutional; and/or are 'preempted' by higher state or federal law that are expressly or implicitly inconsistent with the proposed regulations, or else that simply 'occupies the regulatory field', leaving no room for local regulation. Sometimes the lawmakers back down and pass ineffective measures instead. Often, they go ahead with the strong measures, and the threatened lawsuits do not materialize. Occasionally the industry (typically acting through local stores, restaurants, or bars, whose legal bills they cover) actually file suit to restrain the enforcement of the measures: these cases have come out both ways, typically depending on nuances of the local and state laws involved, as well as the disposition of the deciding judge.

The industry did score some high-level judicial victories that set back important tobacco control initiatives. In 1995 the Canadian Supreme Court invalidated Canada's cigarette advertising restrictions as a free-speech violation, reasoning that the government had not shown these restrictions to be necessary or effective as a public health measure (MacDonald 1995). The government in 1997 adopted even more sweeping restrictions on the industry's marketing behaviour. In June 2007, the Supreme Court of Canada unanimously upheld the statute, ruling that the protection of public health takes precedence over the rights of cigarette manufacturers. The Supreme Court ruled that the statute does not violate the Charter of Rights. Similarly, a 2000 decision by the European Court of Justice invalidated a European Union (EU) advertising ban on the ground that it was not adopted through the appropriate EU processes. As with Canada, the European Commission tried again, and in December 2006 the European Court of Justice upheld the validity of the new rules in the face of a challenge from Germany.

In the United States, two major Supreme Court decisions based on legal challenges from the tobacco industry have produced substantial though perhaps only temporary damage. In a 2000 decision, the Court invalidated FDA jurisdiction over tobacco products, reasoning that had Congress intended the agency to have such jurisdiction, it would have said so explicitly. As a result, there has been no central regulatory authority in the United States over cigarette design, packaging, or marketing. In 2009 Congress finally passed a law, the Family Smoking Prevention and Control Act, giving the FDA this authority. The second decision, in 2001, cut off state efforts to fill the void in marketing regulation. Massachusetts had attempted to prohibit outdoor tobacco advertising within 1 000 feet of schools and playgrounds. Several cities had adopted similar regulations, which had been upheld by lower courts in the face of tobacco industry challenges. The Supreme Court ruled, however, that the state restrictions were preempted by federal law, and were in any event unconstitutionally violative of the free speech rights of tobacco marketers. The 2009 law imposed substantial marketing restrictions and removed the preemption of state-level restrictions, but it is not yet clear whether the US Supreme Court will overturn these restrictions on free speech grounds.

The tobacco industry also uses litigation and the threat of litigation to harass and discourage tobacco control researchers and activists. The authors of 1991 articles exposing 'Joe Camel's' appeal to young children were required to hand their drafts and research materials over to the tobacco companies as 'discovery' in cases not involving the authors in which these articles were cited, or under state 'freedom of information' acts. Similar orders were issued to authors of landmark studies of the synergy between asbestos and tobacco exposure, and of the adverse effects of secondhand smoke exposure (Sweda and Daynard 1996). The industry has also used the freedom of information acts to harass state and local tobacco control programmes, requiring them to produce voluminous materials for copying by industry lawyers (Aguinaga and Glantz 1995). Defamation actions were filed against advocates and NGOs in several countries including the Netherlands, Sweden, and Switzerland. These actions usually resulted in vindication for the tobacco control supporters, but not until their energies were absorbed for many months in defending the cases, and they had been subjected to 'a good scare'.

Secondhand smoke cases

Two types of cases exert pressure to change social norms in the direction of protecting non-smokers from exposure to secondhand smoke. Some cases, such as those brought under laws protecting disabled individuals, seek judicial orders requiring particular employers or proprietors of places of public accommodation either to ban smoking outright, or at least to ensure that non-smokers can avoid exposure to secondhand smoke. Other judicial or administrative proceedings, such as workers' compensation cases, achieve change indirectly by attaching a high price tag to neglecting to protect employees from secondhand smoke exposure.

In a 1980s case, a non-smoking social worker, supported by an NGO, sued the Commonwealth of Massachusetts to require it to provide her with a safe, that is, smoke-free working environment. A court ruled preliminarily that the common law right to a safe workplace would support injunctive relief: the state settled the case by providing non-smoking workplaces to all its employees. Actions brought under the Americans with Disability Act, the Rehabilitation Act, and various state and federal regulations imposing similar obligations upon governmental bodies and regulated industries, have established that workers and patrons of public accommodations whose medical conditions require smoke-free environments are entitled to them, and have ordered employers and proprietors to change their rules accordingly. Other American decisions have conditioned custody orders in divorce cases upon the custodial spouse not smoking and not permitting smoking, in places where the child is present (Sweda 2004).

Cases seeking financial compensation from employers, whether for illness or disability caused by exposure to secondhand smoke or for lost wages as a result of needing to leave a smoky workplace (or both), are more numerous and widespread. Successful cases have been brought in Sweden, Britain, and Australia, as well as the United States. Even a prior history of smoking has not disqualified claimants, so long as the secondhand smoke exposure was a substantial contributing cause of their illness or disability. In this area a few successful cases can have a broad-scale social impact. A 2001 Australian jury award of Aus$466 000 to a bartender who contracted throat cancer, combined with a handful of earlier less generous awards, led to a movement throughout Australia to ban smoking in restaurants, bars, and casinos. In Britain, a few modest awards led the government to rethink occupational safety rules and mandate protections for non-smokers (Daynard *et al.* 2000). In July 2006, the Supreme Court of Israel accepted an appeal from the Jerusalem Small Claims Court and awarded significant compensation to an individual who was exposed to secondhand smoke in a Jerusalem restaurant. Since then, hundreds of lawsuits have been filed (Siegel 2007). In the United States, the fear of such awards has resulted in insurers, legal counsel for employers, and groups representing building owners and managers urging their insureds, clients, and members to eliminate indoor smoking.

A number of cases have required disability insurers and pension plans to cover employees who were forced to leave the workplace because of smoke-related medical conditions. Others have required employers to pay back wages to employees who were fired for complaining about smoky working conditions or for refusing to work in these conditions. These have added to the impression among employers and their insurers and counsel that prudence requires a smoke-free workplace.

Lawsuits against tobacco companies seeking money damages

The power of the tobacco industry to block most forms of effective tobacco control legislation in the United States led advocates to seek other venues in which the industry could be held accountable and pressured to change its behaviour. Money damage lawsuits at first seemed an odd strategic choice, since the connection with societal change was not obvious. Nonetheless, the Tobacco Products Liability Project began advocating for such lawsuits as a tobacco control strategy in 1984, and gradually persuaded the public health community of its merits (Daynard 1988).

Tobacco products liability suits offer at least six potential social benefits. First, since smoking causes over $100 billion in health care and lost income costs (and untold billions more in suffering by the victims and their families) each year in the United States alone, shifting any substantial fraction of this burden to the manufacturers through successful lawsuits would force them to raise prices dramatically. Since the demand for cigarettes is somewhat price-elastic, especially among children and teenagers, increased prices would result in reduced consumption, especially among youth. This is precisely what has happened as a result of the settlements in 1997 and 1998 of lawsuits against the industry brought by state attorneys general seeking reimbursement of state-borne tobacco-caused health-care expenditures. Consumption among 12th grade students in the United States since 1996 has declined by more than one-third (Fountain 2001).

Second, the publicity from these lawsuits would dramatize for the public the fact that smoking injures and kills real people, not just statistics. This has been enhanced by the industry's public relations response to these cases – that anyone so heedless as to smoke cigarettes after the Surgeon General warned of the dangers has only himself or herself to blame for whatever grave illness ensues. This response has until recently been quite effective for the industry in discouraging adverse jury verdicts, but it severely undercuts their marketing campaign to confuse and distract smokers and potential smokers from thinking about the deadly consequences of using their products.

Third, fear of such lawsuits, and especially of large punitive damage awards, might motivate tobacco executives to change the way they do business. Indeed, the threat of punitive damages is now very real, with for example a $79.5 million award in an Oregon case. Concern about product liability awards is frequently cited by manufacturers of other products as reasons for including graphic warnings, altering product designs, or even withholding particularly dangerous products from the market. In the case of cigarette manufacturers, such concern might lead them to stop denying that smoking causes addiction, disease, and death, or stop targeting their marketing efforts at young people, or perfect and implement cigarette designs that would be somewhat less deadly. Although tobacco liability suits began in 1954, it was not until such cases started winning in 1996 that the industry's behaviour began to change. The 'voluntary' changes to date have been modest and mostly cosmetic, but movement is finally perceptible. The companies no longer deny the connections between smoking and various diseases, and actually admit the connection on their websites, but they do nothing else to publicize these connections. They have refocused their marketing target from children and teenagers to college-age young adults. They have also actively embarked on research and development of less toxic cigarettes.

Fourth, the 'discovery' process, which permits parties in lawsuits to demand copies of relevant internal documents from opposing parties and even non-parties, has unearthed millions of pages of industry documents, many of which are quite incriminating. In particular, they demonstrate that the companies knew since the 1950s that smoking caused cancer and other diseases, yet continued to pretend the contrary, actively suppressing or refuting reports that they believed to be true (Glantz *et al.* 1996). Since these documents became available in the mid-1990s largely as a result of aggressive discovery by the lawyers for the State of Minnesota's case against the industry (as well as the heroic, if illegal, removal and dissemination of documents by a tobacco company paralegal named Merrell Williams), they have been instrumental in persuading juries to focus on the misdeeds of the industry rather than the weakness-of-will of the smokers. Equally important, their wide availability on the Internet and in public depositories and publication in numerous media stories has helped make the industry a political pariah, making anti-tobacco legislation possible in many states. Nor has the effect been limited to the United States: major document-based studies of industry misbehaviour in Britain, the Middle East, and with respect to the World Health Organization, among others, has increased the determination and effectiveness of tobacco control advocates throughout the world (Zeltner *et al.* 2000).

Fifth, the money from verdicts and settlements can be used to reimburse individuals and third-party health-care payers for injuries and expenses caused by the tobacco industry and its products. Some money from the states' settlements of their Medicaid reimbursement cases is being devoted to tobacco-control activities. Although this represents only a small percentage of the approximately $10 billion per year that the states are receiving from the industry, it has nonetheless greatly increased the total amounts that the states are spending for tobacco control. An additional $1.5 billion resulting from the 1998 'Master Settlement Agreement' between 46 states and the industry has gone to the American Legacy Foundation which funds tobacco-control activities on the national level.

Sixth, the fact that, at least in the United States, cigarettes annually produce far more financial harm than revenue creates the ongoing possibility that a flood of individual cases or class actions will bankrupt the industry. While the consequences of bankruptcy are somewhat unpredictable, it is likely that a bankruptcy court would not permit the companies to continue selling cigarettes as part of a reorganization plan if the new cigarettes were likely to create as much liability as the ones that sent the companies into bankruptcy. This would create an important opening for public health organizations, which could advise the court of changes in cigarette design and marketing necessary to reduce the potential for future liability (Gottlieb and Daynard 2002).

While most cases continue to be brought by individuals, class actions and third-party reimbursement cases have also been filed. Class actions permit a large number of similarly situated individuals to be represented by a few named plaintiffs: any legal judgment on the common issues rendered in the case applies equally to the named and unnamed class members. The only tobacco class action settlement thus far was on behalf of a nationwide class of flight attendants who had been exposed on the job to secondhand smoke. The settlement provided $300 million for a foundation to fund medical research on smoke-related illnesses, and eased the legal burden for flight attendants to seek individual damages (Broin Settlement Agreement 1997). Another case, on behalf of Florida smokers who contracted tobacco-caused diseases, produced three landmark jury verdicts: the first found that smoking caused 20 diseases, and held the industry liable on a number of grounds, including conspiracy to defraud their customers and to fraudulently conceal health information (Engle and Reynolds Tobacco Co. 1999); the second awarded an average of $4 million in compensatory damages to each of three named smokers; the third awarded the class $145 billion in punitive damages. While the punitive damages award to the class was overturned, the Florida Supreme Court in 2006 allowed lawsuits by individual plaintiffs to proceed in an expedited manner. While the tobacco industry had successfully discouraged most lawyers from bringing cases in the past by its scorched earth litigation tactics, these two class actions brought by the same husband-and-wife team (Stanley and Susan Rosenblatt) demonstrated that the industry could be defeated by talented, determined, but only modestly funded attorneys.

In another class action, a Louisiana jury ordered tobacco companies to fund a ten-year quit smoking campaign for smokers in that state (Finch 2008). Other class actions have been brought seeking refunds of money spent by smokers who were induced to smoke 'low tar' cigarettes on the fraudulent representation that they were safer. In 2009 the US Supreme Court ruled that federal law did not present an obstacle to the pursuit of these "low tar" consumer fraud cases.

Third party reimbursement cases are predicated on the fact that the tobacco industry knows that most smoking-induced medical costs are not paid by the smokers themselves. Since the companies know that they cause financial injury to third parties (states, health insurers, etc.), they should be liable for the costs that flow from the design of their unreasonably dangerous products and from their deceptive conduct. Litigation pioneered by Mississippi and Minnesota, and later brought by most other US states as well, resulted in mostly favourable judicial decisions and the resulting multi-billion dollar settlements already mentioned (Master Settlement Agreement 1988). Unfortunately, American courts have almost uniformly rejected all subsequent cases brought on the same theory, ruling that the third party's financial injuries were too 'indirect', and distinguishing the opposite decisions in the state cases on unconvincing (but nonetheless authoritative) grounds. Thus, private health insurers, union health and welfare funds, foreign governments, and even the US federal government, have all had their reimbursement claims rejected by US courts. Such litigation brought by the Canadian province of British Columbia is, however, proceeding to trial, as is similar litigation brought by a major private health insurer in Israel.

The tobacco industry has not always been content to take its chances in court. In the United States the industry has been a prime – but usually hidden – sponsor of 'tort reform' efforts, which seek enactment of state or federal laws changing the legal principles applied by the court so as to make lawsuits against the industry more difficult or even impossible. Such a statute prevented tobacco litigation in California for ten years, until it was repealed in 1998. The industry also supports procedural changes with similar effects, such as: (1) laws providing only a modicum of regulation, while 'preempting' claims that could otherwise be brought against the industry; (2) the 'Class Action Fairness Act', which removes class actions against them from state courts, where they have sometimes been successful, to federal courts where they were thought more likely to be dismissed; (3) proposed state legislation to prevent public airing of documents obtained in discovery; (4) proposed bans on the use of class actions or punitive damages in litigation against the industry; and (5) proposed state or federal laws limiting attorneys fees in tobacco litigation so as to discourage competent practitioners from taking these cases.However, laws facilitating the state lawsuits against the industry were passed in Florida, Massachusetts, and Maryland in the mid-1990s. The constitutionality of similar law passed in the Province of British Columbia was upheld by the Canadian Supreme Court in 2005 (Imperial Tobacco Co. Ltd. v. British Columbia 2005).

Enforcement of laws prohibiting deceptive conduct

Tobacco companies, like all other legal entities, are subject to general restrictions against obtaining money dishonestly. In the state context these generally include laws outlawing 'unfair or deceptive acts or practices in commerce'. State attorneys general, and often private litigants as well, may bring lawsuits to enjoin tobacco companies from continuing to engage in such behaviour. Indeed, the state lawsuits, though they principally sought money damages for Medicaid reimbursement, almost all sought injunctive relief under these state consumer protection acts. In response to these claims, the resulting settlements, including the November 1998 Master Settlement Agreement, contained several provisions restricting various tobacco industry marketing techniques. These included bans on outdoor advertising and the distribution of merchandise that advertised tobacco products, as well as limitations on sponsorship of concerts and other public events (Daynard et al. 2001). Similarly, the class actions addressing 'low tar' cigarettes seek, in addition to refunds, injunctions against the companies' continuing the deceptive practice of labelling cigarettes 'low tar' when they are no less dangerous than 'regular' cigarettes.

Federal law has an even more powerful instrument against businesses like the tobacco companies whose success depends on deceiving their customers. The Racketeer-Influenced and Corrupt Organizations Act (RICO) allows the United States Department of Justice to seek judicial orders fundamentally changing the way the industry does business. Private RICO actions are also available to compensate for economic losses but not illness or death. In August 2006, US District Court Judge Gladys Kessler ruled that the tobacco companies did violate RICO, and ordered them to modify their practices in various respects (Guardino et al. 2007). In 2009 her findings were upheld by the US Court of Appeals for the District of Columbia.

Furthermore the discovery, mostly through documents uncovered in the Minnesota litigation, of the industry's deep involvement in smuggling cigarettes to many countries formed the basis for lawsuits by several governments against cigarette manufacturers. In July 2004, Philip Morris

International agreed to pay the European Commission $1 billion, and also agreed to a series of measures to avoid future involvement in smuggling. In July 2008, Rothmans Benson Hedges was fined $100 million under Canada's federal Excise Act, while Imperial Tobacco agreed to pay a $200 million fine.

Going forward

The Framework Convention on Tobacco Control recognizes in Article 4.5 that 'Issues relating to liability, as determined by each Party within its jurisdiction, are an important part of comprehensive tobacco control.' Article 19.1 elaborates on this: 'For the purpose of tobacco control, the Parties shall consider taking legislative action or promoting their existing laws, where necessary, to deal with criminal and civil liability, including compensation where appropriate.' The remainder of Article 19 encourages the parties to share relevant information and provide mutual assistance, as well as suggesting that the Conference of the Parties come up with additional ways to support activities related to liability.

In light of Article 19 and of the widespread publicity that tobacco litigation, especially in the United States, has received, litigation in the twenty-first century is likely to spread worldwide, raising consciousness of the dangers of tobacco use and of exposure to tobacco smoke, and of the nefarious role played by cigarette manufacturers, even in countries where tobacco use and marketing is currently uncontroversial. Litigation will be increasingly used by NGOs to force governments and tobacco companies to take existing laws seriously, and to obtain judicial orders making public places smoke-free. NGOs and health departments will become increasing adept at drafting laws that can withstand industry legal attacks, and defending them when these attacks arrive. Countries other than the United States will begin holding tobacco companies responsible for the health care costs attributable to their products and conduct. As a result, prices will increase, consumption will decline, and some of the damages paid will fund tobacco-control programmes. Some tobacco companies may find their way into bankruptcy court, giving public health authorities and NGOs new opportunities to shape how tobacco products get manufactured and marketed. Finally, more vigorous efforts can be expected to require tobacco manufacturers and their executives to avoid illegal conduct, and a wide range of legal sanctions, civil and criminal, can be anticipated.

References

Aguinaga, S. and Glantz, S. A. (1995). The use of public records acts to interfere with tobacco control. *Tob Control*, **4**: 222–30.

Broin Settlement Agreement (1997). http://www.tobacco.neu.edu/litigation/hotdocs/broin.htm.

Daynard, R. A. (1995). Resisting tobacco industry abuse of the legal process. *Tob Control*, **4**: 209.

Daynard, R. A., Bates, C., and Francey, N. (January 2000). Tobacco Litigation Worldwide, 320 *BMJ*, **111**.

Daynard, R. A., Parmet, W., Kelder, G., *et al.* (2001). Implications for tobacco control of the multistate tobacco settlement. *Am J of Public Health*, **91**: 1967–81.

Daynard, R. A. (2002). Regulating tobacco or why we need a public health judicial decision-making canon. *J. Law, Medicine and Ethics*, **30**: 281–89.

Daynard, R. A. (1988). Tobacco liability litigation as a cancer control strategy. *J National Cancer Institute*, **80**: 9–13.

Efroymson, D. (2000). Bangladesh: voyage of distain sunk without trace. *Tob Control*, **9**: 129.

Engle v. R.J. Reynolds Tobacco Co., Verdict Form For Phase I, 14.3 Tobacco Products Litigation Reporter 2.101 (1999).

Environmental Action Network, Ltd V. Attorney General, *et al.*, Misc. Application No. 39 of 2001 (High Court of Uganda).

Finch, S. (2008). Tobacco companies ordered to pay up. *The Times Picayune*, 22 July. Available at: http://www.nola.com/printer/printer.ssf?/base/news-6/1216705872288820.xml&coll=1.

Fountain, J. W. (2001). Study Finds Teenagers Smoking Less; Campaign Is Cited, *New York Times*, December 20, p. A24.

Glantz, S. A., Slade, J., Bero, L. A. *et al.* (1996). *The Cigarette Papers*. Berkeley, California: University of California Press.

Gottlieb, M. and Daynard, R. A. (2002). Will Big Tobacco Seek Bankruptcy Protection? William and Mary Environmental Policy Review, No. 1.

Guardino, S., Banthin, C., and Daynard, R. (2007). Analysis of Judge Kessler's final order and opinion. Available at: http://tobacco.neu.edu/litigation/cases/DOJ/doj_opinion_summary.pdf.

Imperial Tobacco Co. Ltd. v. British Columbia (2005). 2 S.C.R. 473, 2005 SCC 49, Available at: http://csc.lexum.umontreal.ca/en/2005/2005scc49/2005scc49.html.

MacDonald, R. J. R. Inc. v Attorney General of Canada (1995). 127 DLR 4th, 1 91.

Master Settlement Agreement, November 1998 (Available at: http://www.naag.org/tobac/cigmsa.rtf).

Murli S. Deora v Union of India and Others (2001). Union of India Supreme Court of India Writ Petition No. 316 of 1999, 2 November.

'Rendezvous with Mahamane Cisse', 10 August 2000. Available at: http://www.tobacco.org/News/rendezvous/cisse.html.

Siegel, J. (2007). At 23 Percent, Israel's Smoking Rate Is Lowest Ever, *Jerusalem Post*, 5 November.

Sweda, E. L. and Daynard, R. A. (1996). Tobacco Industry Tactics. *Br Med Bull*, **52**(1): 183–92.

Sweda E, L. Jr. (2004). Summary of Legal Cases Regarding Smoking in the Workplace and Other Places, 18.8 Tobacco Products Litigation Reporter 4.1–4.94.

Zeltner, T. Kessler, D., Martiny, A., and Randera, F. (2000). *Tobacco Industry Strategies to Undermine Tobacco Control Activities at the World Health Organization*. World Health Organization.

Chapter 36

The adoption of smoke-free policies and their effectiveness

Maria Leon-Roux and John P. Pierce

Introduction

Leading health agencies have published authoritative reports evaluating the research on the health risks of secondhand smoke (SHS) (IARC 2004; US Department of Health and Human Services 2006). There is a consensus across these reports that SHS (also called involuntary smoking) causes several diseases in non-smokers including lung cancer, heart disease, and both chronic and acute respiratory disease. Policies to protect against exposure to SHS were first introduced in the 1970s and focused on mandating some buildings (e.g. cinemas) and public transport to be smoke-free and to maintain separate accommodation for non-smokers (e.g. airlines). As the evidence on harm to health mounted in the 1980s, numerous jurisdictions proposed voluntary agreements that were acceptable to, and even promoted by, the tobacco industry (Saloojee & Dagli 2000). In addition, the industry used alternative initiatives to weaken the adoption of stringent smoking restrictions (by promoting ventilation options, separate smoking rooms, or delaying implementation).

   The first jurisdiction to mandate smoke-free workplaces was the state of California in the United States, which passed a smoke-free workplace law in 1994, delaying full implementation for alcohol serving premises until 1998. It was not until 2003 that the next major jurisdiction (New York) introduced a smoke-free policy. This was quickly followed (in 2004) by the first three countries to implement nationwide smoke-free workplace laws (Ireland, Norway, and New Zealand). The World Health Organization (WHO) played an early leadership role when it negotiated the unprecedented Framework Convention on Tobacco Control (FCTC), the first ever public health treaty that achieved widespread support among member nations. Article 8 of the WHO FCTC focuses on the 'protection from exposure to tobacco smoke'. Countries signing the treaty are required to implement policies to protect all people from exposure to SHS by law and not by means of voluntary agreements. Under the WHO FCTC, 'smoke-free' air means that a non-smoker will not be able to see, smell, or sense tobacco smoke, nor will components of tobacco smoke be above detectable levels in the air (WHO 2005). The guidelines for Article 8 delineate the key elements of an effective smoke-free workplace legislation: 100% smoke-free environments (not to include smoking rooms), universal protection by law, public education to reduce second-hand smoke exposure, and implementation and adequate enforcement of the policy (WHO 2007). As of May 2009, 164 countries became Parties to the WHO FCTC and 14 countries (including federated countries such as the United Kingdom, Canada, and Australia) had successfully implemented nationwide smoke-free policies that complied with the WHO FCTC guidelines. Just under half (23) of the states in the United States had implemented smoke-free policies. However, in many jurisdictions, questions about the effectiveness of the proposed policies appeared to be impeding the necessary political consensus to successfully implement a WHO FCTC compliant policy.

To provide better clarification of the benefits of WHO FCTC compliant legislation, in April 2008, the International Agency for Research on Cancer (IARC) convened a group of 17 scientists from 9 countries in Lyon, France to assess the evidence for the effectiveness of smoke-free policies. This Working Group proposed 11 potentially causal statements and summarized the strength of the evidence for each statement using the following five IARC classifications: sufficient, strong, limited, inadequate or no evidence and evidence of lack of an effect (Pierce & Leon 2008). This chapter presents a summary of that evidence and the main conclusions of the report (IARC 2009).

Economic effects of policies

Following a logic model for how smoke-free legislation is implemented, the Working Group first considered evidence of the economic impact of such legislation on the hospitality industry. Jurisdictions considering implementing WHO FCTC compliant legislation frequently express concern with the economic impact of smoke-free policies. The Working Group outlined criteria for what constituted a scientifically rigorous study and noted that many studies did not meet these standards. Frequently, substandard studies were highly publicized when jurisdictions were considering legislation. However, multiple quality studies from many different jurisdictions met the established criteria. These studies used data on several economic indicators, including the following: taxable sales, sales tax revenues, or other sales data; employment; the number of establishments; measures of bankruptcy; and the value of businesses. Most of these robust studies (47 of 49) concluded that smoke-free policies have either no economic impact or a positive economic impact on businesses in the area where the policy is implemented.

In addition, the Working Group examined studies based on surveys of consumer/patron and owner/manager samples and studies sponsored by the tobacco industry. Of the studies reporting survey data, based on convenience samples or information collected on anticipated rather than realized impact, only a minority have been published in a peer-reviewed journal. Nearly all of the peer-reviewed studies (17 of 19) concluded that smoke-free policies had no negative economic effects. The Working Group concluded that existing evidence from high-resource countries indicates that smoke-free workplace policies have no effect or a net positive effect on bar and restaurant businesses, and that the same is likely to be the case in low- and middle-resource countries.

Attitudes and compliance

After jurisdictions implement smoke-free policies, public support for their continuance typically increases into solid majorities. The level of support appears higher when a public education campaign accompanies the implementation. Studies have shown that smoker compliance with smoke-free laws is moderate to high, even with low levels of enforcement (Fong *et al.* 2006).

Studies of jurisdictions with smoke-free workplace policies have observed increases in the percentage of smokers reporting the voluntary introduction of a smoke-free home (Borland *et al.* 1999), suggesting a significant shift in the social norms related to smoking. There are a number of jurisdictions in which the majority of smokers now report smoke-free homes, such as New Zealand (Gillespie *et al.* 2005), Norway (Lund & Lindbak 2007), California (Al-Delaimy *et al.* 2008), and both Finland and Sweden (European Commission 2007). In all countries with data on smoking trends, this proportion has increased over time (IARC 2009). This trend in smoke-free homes started shortly after 1992 following the US Surgeon General's Report (US Department of Health and Human Services 1986) and the 1992 US Environmental Protection Agency declaration of SHS to be a carcinogen as well as the intense media campaign of the California Tobacco Control Programme emphasizing protection of children from SHS in the home (Gilpin *et al.* 1999). Smokers with a smoke-free home were more likely to live with non-smokers, to have young children, to smoke fewer cigarettes, and to be interested in quitting (Borland *et al.* 2006).

Effect on SHS exposure

The Working Group reviewed 30 studies of legislation that prohibits smoking in virtually all indoor workplaces and concluded that such legislation consistently reduced reported exposure to SHS in high-risk settings by 80–90%. Particulate matter (PM) is defined as solid particles or liquid droplets suspended in the atmosphere. The large majority of particles in SHS are smaller than 2.5 microns (Institute of Medicine 2001). A study of the ambient air concentrations of this $PM_{2.5}$ in pubs and restaurants showed the introduction of smoke-free legislation was associated with a reduction from an average of 246 $\mu g/m^3$ to 20 $\mu g/m^3$, an average reduction of 86% (Semple *et al.* 2007). Residual exposure need not indicate non-compliance, as these levels could result from smoking around the boundaries of venues, including designated smoking areas on patios and verandas. As a result, indoor smoke-free workplace laws greatly reduce, but do not remove altogether, the potential for harm to health caused by SHS around bars, restaurants, and similar settings. Evidence from the jurisdiction with ten years of experience with a smoke-free policy indicates that these reductions are maintained over time. A high-quality Scottish study considered the effect of such legislation on population exposure to SHS using an objective biomarker (salivary cotinine) before and one year after the introduction of the WHO FCTC-compliant legislation. This study noted a significant decrease in population level exposure to SHS in non-smoking adults of 39% (95% CI:29%, 47%) (Haw & Gruer 2007).

Protection of children from the harmful effects of SHS is a particular concern for public health, and voluntary smoke-free homes have been associated with smoke-free workplace policies. The Global Youth Tobacco Survey conducted between 1999 and 2005, identified that overall, nearly half of young people aged 13–15 years were exposed to SHS at home (43.9%) in the last 7 days. The WHO region with the highest level of SHS exposure at home was Europe (mean of 78.0%) and the lowest SHS exposure was in Africa (mean of 30.4%) (GTSS Collaborative Group 2006). A large international study used a biomarker of SHS exposure (nicotine in hair samples) and examined children in 1 284 households from 31 countries in Latin America, Asia, and Europe and the Middle East (Wipfli *et al.* 2008). In a multivariate model, hair nicotine concentrations were 2.6 times higher in children residing in non smoke-free households compared to those that were smoke-free.

Changes in smoking behaviour

As smoke-free policies restrict where people can smoke, it is feasible that they might influence a smoker's willingness and ability to quit, as well as the cigarette consumption level among continuing smokers. However, while some smoke-free policies are implemented independently, many are part of an overall coordinated tobacco control programme. Particularly, in these latter instances, partitioning the effect on smoking behaviour that is associated with the smoke-free legislation is not straightforward.

Introducing a smoke-free workplace is associated with a reduction in daily cigarette consumption among smokers, according to a number of reviews of studies of individual worksites. Population surveys of smokers working under different smoking restriction policies are in general agreement with the worksite literature that policies are associated with reduced consumption among continuing smokers. These studies have concluded that implementing a smoke-free workplace consistently leads to a reduction in daily cigarette consumption of two to four cigarettes per day. However, these population studies also suggest that smoke-free policies impact both smoking cessation rates and overall prevalence. One of the highest quality studies suggests that smoke-free workplaces may reduce smoking prevalence by 6% and average daily consumption among smokers by 14%, and that declines in smoking prevalence and intensity occur in all types of workplaces, regardless of size, type of occupation or industry, and health consciousness (Farrelly *et al.* 1999).

Numerous studies have examined the voluntary implementation of a smoke-free home. Less-dependent smokers are more likely to have such a home. Studies investigating the effect of both workplace and home smoking restrictions consistently conclude that voluntary smoke-free homes have a stronger impact on smoking behaviour than smoke-free workplaces. A number of studies have reported on the effect of smoke-free homes on smoking initiation, but additional studies are required to address this effect conclusively. The majority of these studies suggest that adolescents in smoke-free homes are less likely to experiment with cigarettes.

Schools are considered workplaces, and several studies have addressed the effect of a smoke-free school campus (including students, teachers, and visitors) on smoking behaviour, particularly youth initiation. Only a few quality studies used analyses to account for a number of potential confounding factors. The results from these studies suggest that a smoke-free school campus influences smoking behaviour, but the findings are far from definitive.

Changes in health effects

With a single exception, smoke-free policies were implemented after 2000, thus the follow-up time is considerably shorter than the lead time necessary to reveal diseases caused by SHS such as cancer. Accordingly, the growing body of evidence concentrates on the impact of smoke-free policies on acute respiratory illness and cardiovascular disease. Seven studies focused on bar workers, and all showed an improvement in reported respiratory and sensory symptoms irrespective of follow-up period.

Ten studies from five separate countries reported on the incidence of acute myocardial infarction (AMI) and related cardiac conditions, termed acute coronary syndrome (ACS). The findings are based mainly on routine hospital data, and study limitations include inconsistencies in case definition over time and between hospitals, and lack of patient information on smoking status and exposure to SHS. All except one of these studies reported a reduction in the number of admissions for acute events, with the average reduction appearing to be 10–20% (IARC 2009). The New Zealand study reported admission rates for AMI and unstable angina, acute asthma, acute stroke, and chronic obstructive pulmonary disease for the nation between 1997 and 2005 (Edwards *et al.* 2008). After adjusting for underlying trends, they found no discernible change in admissions for AMI, unstable angina, or AMI and unstable angina combined. Further, admissions for respiratory diseases or stroke did not decrease. The design of a Scottish study (Pell *et al.* 2008) reduced many of the limitations of these other studies. In this study, dedicated research nurses collected all data prospectively, using the latest consensus diagnostic criteria. They also collected a blood sample to test for biomarkers of smoking or SHS exposure. Following implementation of smoke-free legislation, the observed drop in admissions was much greater than expected based solely on the underlying trend in ACS admissions. Admissions for ACS decreased by 14% among smokers, 19% among ex-smokers, and 21% among never-smokers. Further, the level of reduction in ACS admissions was of the same order of magnitude expected from applying the known relative risks for SHS to the validated 40% reduction in exposure to SHS.

Conclusions

The effectiveness of smoke-free policies has been reviewed and evaluated by an international group of experts convened by IARC in April of 2008. This Working Group classified the evidence as 'sufficient' to indicate causality if the association was observed in studies in which chance, bias, and confounding could be ruled out with reasonable confidence (IARC 2009). A lesser classification of 'strong evidence' was made when there was consistent evidence of an association, but chance, bias, or confounding could not been ruled out with reasonable confidence. The group concluded there was sufficient evidence to support each of the following six statements

1. Smoke-free policies do not cause a decline in the business activity of the restaurant and bar industry.
2. Implementation of smoke-free policies leads to a substantial decline in exposure to SHS.
3. Implementation of smoke-free legislation decreases respiratory symptoms in workers.
4. Smoke-free workplaces reduce cigarette consumption among continuing smokers.
5. Smoke-free home policies reduce exposure of children to SHS.
6. Smoke-free home policies reduce adult smoking.

For the following five statements the group concluded there was strong evidence because of an inability to rule out chance, bias, or confounding. However, explanations other than causality are thought to be unlikely.

7. Implementation of smoke-free legislation reduces social inequalities in SHS exposure at work.
8. Implementation of smoke-free legislation causes a decline in heart disease morbidity.
9. Smoke-free workplaces lead to increased successful cessation among smokers.
10. Smoke-free policies reduce tobacco use among youth.
11. Smoke-free home policies reduce youth smoking.

References

Al-Delaimy, W.K., White, M.M., Trinidad, D.R. *et al.* (2008). The California Tobacco Program: can we maintain the progress? Results from the California Tobacco Survey, 1990–2005. Sacramento, CA, California Department of Public Health (http://www.cdph.ca.gov/programs/Tobacco/Documents/CTCP-CTSReport1990-2005.pdf).

Borland, R., Mullins, R., Trotter, L. *et al.* (1999). Trends in environmental tobacco smoke restrictions in the home in Victoria, Australia. *Tob Control*, 8(3):266–271.

Borland, R., Yong, H., Cummings, K. *et al.* (2006). Determinants and consequences of smoke-free homes: findings from the International Tobacco Control (ITC) four country survey. *Tob Control*, 15(Suppl 3):iii42–iii50.

Edwards, R., Thomson, G., Wilson, N. *et al.* (2008). After the smoke has cleared: evaluation of the impact of a new national smoke-free law in New Zealand. *Tob Control*, 17(1):e2.

European Commission (2007). Attitudes of Europeans toward tobacco [Special Eurobarometer 272c], European Commission (http://ec.europa.eu/health/ph_publication/eb_health_en.pdf).

Farrelly, M.C., Evans, W.N.,and Sfekas, A.E. (1999). The impact of workplace smoking bans: results from a national survey. *Tob Control*, 8(3):272–277.

Fong, G.T., Hyland, A., Borland, R. *et al.* (2006). Reductions in tobacco smoke pollution and increases in support for smoke-free public places following the implementation of comprehensive smoke-free workplace legislation in the Republic of Ireland: findings from the ITC Ireland/UK Survey. *Tob Control*, 15(Suppl 3):iii51–iii58.

Gillespie, J., Milne, K., and Wilson, N. (2005). Secondhand smoke in New Zealand homes and cars: exposure, attitudes, and behaviours in 2004. *N Z Med J*, 118(1227):U1782.

Gilpin, E.A., White, M.M., Farkas, A.J. *et al.* (1999). Home smoking restrictions: which smokers have them and how they are associated with smoking behavior. *Nicotine Tob Res*, 1(2):153–162.

GTSS Collaborative Group (2006). A cross country comparison of exposure to secondhand smoke among youth. *Tob Control*, 15(Suppl 2):ii4–ii19.

Haw, S.J. and Gruer, L. (2007). Changes in exposure of adult non-smokers to secondhand smoke after implementation of smoke-free legislation in Scotland: national cross sectional survey. *Br Med J (Clin Res Ed)*, **335**(7619):549–552.

IARC (2004). *IARC Monographs on the Evaluation of Carcinogenic Risks to Humans, Vol. 83, Tobacco Smoke and Involuntary Smoking*. Lyon, International Agency for Research on Cancer.

IARC (2009). *IARC Handbooks of Cancer Prevention, Tobacco Control, Vol. 13: Evaluating the Effectiveness of Smoke-free Policies*. Lyon, International Agency for Research on Cancer.

Institute of Medicine (2001). Clearing the smoke: assessing the science base for tobacco harm reduction. Washington DC, National Academy Press.

Lund, M. and Lindbak, R. (2007). Norwegian tobacco statistics 1973–2006. Oslo, Norwegian Institute for Alcohol and Drug Research (SIRUS) (http://www.sirus.no/internett/forsiden?factory=index).

Pell, J.P., Haw, S., Cobbe, S. *et al.* (2008). Smoke-free legislation and hospitalizations for acute coronary syndrome. *N Engl J Med*, **359**(5):482–491.

Pierce, J.P. and Leon, M. (2008). Effectiveness of smoke-free policies. *Lancet Oncol*, **9**(7):614–615.

Saloojee, Y. and Dagli, E. (2000). Tobacco industry tactics for resisting public policy on health. *Bull World Health Organ*, **78**(7):902–910.

Semple, S., Maccalman, L., Naji, A. *et al.* (2007). Bar workers' exposure to second-hand smoke: the effect of Scottish smoke-free legislation on occupational exposure. *Ann Occup Hyg*, **51**(7):571–580.

US Department of Health and Human Services (USDHHS) (1986). The health consequences of involuntary smoking: a report of the Surgeon General. Rockville, MD, US Department of Health and Human Services, Center for Disease Control and Prevention, National Center for Chronic Disease Prevention and Health Promotion, Office on Smoking and Health (http://www.surgeongeneral.gov/library/secondhandsmoke/report/).

US Department of Health and Human Services (USDHHS) (2006). The health consequences of involuntary exposure to tobacco smoke: a report of the Surgeon General. Atlanta, GA, US Department of Health and Human Services, Center for Disease Control and Prevention, National Center for Chronic Disease Prevention and Health Promotion, Office on Smoking and Health.

WHO (2005). WHO Framework Convention on Tobacco Control. Geneva, Switzerland, World Health Organization (http://www.who.int/tobacco/framework/WHO_FCTC_english.pdf).

WHO (2007). Protection from exposure to secondhand tobacco smoke: policy recommendations. Geneva, Switzerland, World Health Organization (http://www.who.int/tobacco/resources/publications/wntd/2007/who_protection_exposure_final_25June2007.pdf).

Wipfli, H., Avila-Tang, E., Navas-Acien, A. *et al.* (2008). Secondhand smoke exposure among women and children: evidence from 31 countries. *Am J Public Health*, **98**(4):672–679.

Chapter 37

Advancing tobacco control by effective evaluation

Ron Borland and K. Michael Cummings

As a result of the World Health Organizations Framework Convention on Tobacco Control (FCTC) there has been a proliferation of policies and associated programmes designed to reduce tobacco use implemented by countries around the globe. These include, but are not restricted to those mandated programmes by the FCTC. Good quality evaluation, including capacity to understand any differential by-country effects is going to be a critical aspect of fulfilling FCTC obligations to deliver the optimum mix of evidence-based policies.

Evaluation of the effectiveness of tobacco control policies at the population level has been limited by inadequate data sources, problems in measurement, and poorly conceptualized evaluation designs borrowed from clinical medicine with insufficient attention to differences in the nature of the interventions. This chapter presents a model for evaluating the evidence for the effects of population-based tobacco control interventions that allows for ongoing improvement and the capacity to build on the accumulated knowledge about intervention effects gathered by others. Much of the material in this chapter is synthesized from a recent IARC handbook on methods for evaluating tobacco control policies (IARC 2008) on which the authors were editors. This chapter also provides some additional discussion of when particular intensities of evaluation are important, both before and after policy implementation, and further consideration of criteria for ranking the quality of evidence.

Nicotine addiction sustains tobacco use in most people and individual variation in response to nicotine has a strong biological basis. However, the great diversity in tobacco use behaviours observed between countries and within countries over time cannot be explained by biology alone. Tobacco use as reflected in population trends are seen as the product of the interaction of agent, host, and environmental factors (Cummings et al. 2009). Tobacco control needs to consider influences that affect the actions of smokers, those vulnerable to uptake, former users, those who produce and sell tobacco products, and governments who determine the parameters of use (Borland et al. in press). There are two key pathways involved in controlling tobacco-related harms: the pathway from policies to tobacco use, and the pathway from tobacco products and their use to levels of exposure to toxic substances and to the harms that result. The pathway from tobacco use to health harms only need to be considered when product changes are involved. For cigarette use, at least, the path from use to harm is among the best established in medical science. This chapter focuses on evaluations of interventions to affect tobacco use (see IARC 2008, section 5.3 for extension of the model to tobacco-related harms).

Policies and the disseminated intervention programmes that result from policy decisions are of particular interest because of their potential to impact large numbers of people, in some cases entire populations. As a result, it is important to be able to both show that they achieve their objectives, and do so in a cost-effective way with any incidental effects ideally having net benefits.

Evaluation allows the most efficient interventions to be maintained (and perhaps improved further), while less effective interventions are either improved or abandoned.

Purpose of evaluation

Intervention evaluation typically involves answering three questions: those of efficacy, effectiveness, and dissemination (Flay *et al.* 2005). 1) Efficacy asks the question: Can this intervention work? Here the double-blinded randomized controlled trial (RCT) is the gold standard, where they can be done, which is almost never for interventions designed to affect behaviour. 2) Effectiveness asks the question: Does the intervention actually work when implemented under real world conditions? Where effectiveness is demonstrated efficacy can be inferred. A key component of effectiveness evaluation is measuring the extent to which an intervention actually reaches the target population. 3) Determining the conditions where an intervention works optimally and/or the populations it works for are critical, both for implementation and equity. Dissemination asks the question: Can we get the intervention to be used by enough of the population who would benefit for it to have an impact? An intervention that few are prepared to offer, or which only reaches a small fraction of the intended target group, or which few in the exposed group are prepared to use, is of limited benefit. A fourth question is also important to address: 4) How does the intervention work (the question of mediation)? Population-level evaluations usually start with interventions that we know can work (at least for some problems under some circumstances) and are asking: 'Does it work here and under what conditions can the desired effects be optimized?' This involves answering questions 2–4.

A focus on evaluating interventions in isolation tends to distract us from what we know and sometimes forget. Some of the things we do know are:

♦ information campaigns can increase knowledge about tobacco
♦ knowledge can change beliefs and attitudes
♦ beliefs and attitudes can affect tobacco use behaviours
♦ advertising can change behaviour independent of conscious awareness of the influence
♦ there are programmes and aids that can help people quit tobacco use
♦ price rises affect levels of consumption of tobacco products
♦ poorly designed and/or executed communications can have boomerang effects.

Tobacco control evaluation efforts up to now have been caught in a framework that does not give adequate value to the accumulation of knowledge or to the benefits of generalizing from findings about similar interventions in other areas. An evaluation framework must be concerned about the form of the intervention, the mechanisms of effect, the ways it is delivered (quality of implementation), and various characteristics of the populations it is provided to, and how it interacts with other interventions. Evaluation should be part of a process of continual improvement, and to do so the study designs need to facilitate the elaboration of causal mechanisms. This requires consideration of awareness, acceptance, and actions taken in response to policies, both immediate and longer term. Awareness is a function of policy implementation, dissemination, and publicity. Engagement is affected by attitudes towards the intervention and ways it is provided. Policies that are unpopular are more likely to be resisted, and forms of assistance seen as inappropriate to the person's needs are unlikely to be adopted. Thus, a smoker who objects to smoke-free rules is more likely to ignore the rules or to seek convenient alternatives, while a smoker who approves and sees this as an opportunity to gain greater control over their smoking, may not only comply, but use the opportunity to either quit altogether or reduce their consumption. Like awareness, acceptance can only really be evaluated at a population level, although it is typically the acceptance of each individual that is critical.[1]

Evaluation of the consequences or outcomes of the intervention is critical, both in terms of intended and unintended, incidental effects. While traditional intervention evaluation restricts its focus on outcomes among those who actually use the interventions, for policy interventions this is not a useful restriction since the evaluator needs to consider the total impact on the population, including those who are not engaged. Outcomes should be considered as a joint function of the potency of the interventions, the ways they are used or responded to (a function of attitudes to them), and the degree of exposure to them.

Characteristics of population-based tobacco control interventions

Tobacco control interventions can be grouped into three categories that describe the primary intent of the intervention. These include: (1) interventions designed to directly influence tobacco users and potential users such as educational campaigns, product warnings, and provision of stop smoking services; (2) interventions that indirectly influence the tobacco user by changing the social contexts that affect incentives for tobacco use such as taxes and rules about where tobacco can be used; and (3) interventions that indirectly influence the tobacco user by constraining the marketing practices of the tobacco industry (IARC 2008). Interventions are needed to influence all three of these general domains to act in ways more consonant with health promotion. The challenge is to apply rigorous evaluation to ensure that the most appropriate and effective mix of strategies for controlling tobacco use are adopted. Typically, policy interventions are designed to have sustained effects, but in some cases this may require designing ongoing programmes to ensure that this happens. Further, there may be short-term onset effects. For example, there is evidence that warning labels on cigarette packs have both an onset effect as well as a sustained effect (Borland *et al.* 2009a), and cessation programmes need to be regularly promoted to attract custom. The form of communication-based interventions may also need to change over time if the effects of the intervention are to be sustained. What is seen as up-to-date, and thus of most relevance for communicating can change rapidly in some communities. Similarly, across cultures, intervention may need to be framed differently to ensure cultural relevance. Under some circumstances it can be useful to conceptually separate the core concepts in an intervention from the mode of communication used to convey them. Thus we might focus our evaluation on the cultural relevance of the intervention or on its underlying potency, or both. Analogous to the way societies and/or people change, interventions need to evolve to maintain their relevance and potency. Thus, tobacco control needs to adopt an approach to intervention that is analogous to what is done in infection control whereby new immunizations are devised to addressing new and emerging strains of infectious agents based on an understanding of the process, not testing each new immunization with randomized trials. This is both because the determinants are sufficiently understood and the rate of change in the problem is too rapid for RCTs to be practical.

The great diversity in tobacco use both between countries and within countries over time creates huge challenges and opportunities for scientific understanding. Changes to interventions may be required as a society progresses through the adoption of innovation cycle (Rogers 2003) for adopting new sets of values and behavioural options for tobacco use. Take, for example, encouraging the adoption of smoke-free homes. This happens first in the face of social disapproval, or at least lack of understanding. Somebody instituting a smoke-free policy will typically be asked to

---

[1] In some collectivist cultures, the views of community leaders are also critical, as they determine what it is acceptable to think and do. These roles are on top of the roles of leaders in all cultures as policy-makers.

justify the policy, and some might see it as unreasonable. However, as such policies become more common, there comes a tipping point, where smoke-free environments become the norm. Since justification is no longer necessary, smokers often just don't smoke when inside and those without such bans feel a need to justify their positions. Before the tipping point, even quite intense interventions may have limited impact (as has been the case for implementing smoke-free homes [Hovell *et al.* 2000]), while after it people may be readily able to change without help (as evidenced by rapid adoption of the practice in some countries [e.g., Borland *et al.* 1999]). The effects of context on intervention effectiveness is one of the reasons why it is important to pre-test the messages used for cultural relevance of even proven interventions when applied in new contexts, as well as conducting ongoing evaluation of disseminated interventions.

However, it is not just trends in tobacco use and tobacco-related knowledge that are likely to impact on policy effects. Broader societal issues may also play a key role. The rapid emergence of China and other countries as economic powerhouses is likely to impact tobacco use, at least in those countries, as more and more people have money to spend on consumer products, such as tobacco, that are marketed to appeal to 'modern' sensibilities. Worldwide concerns about the environment, including the issue of global warming, likewise may affect some of our efforts. Unless we try to understand how tobacco control fits into broader social changes that are sweeping the world, we risk missing out on important determinants of use, with the resultant reduction in our capacity to identify and implement policies and programmes that work.

When do we evaluate?

The evaluation of policy interventions occurs mainly after they are instituted because they first have to be implemented somewhere before we can find out how they actually work. Because the authority of government policy or law may affect compliance as might mass implementation, it is not possible to confidently generalize from the results of analogue studies conducted prior to implementation. This means we cannot in principle be certain of the effectiveness of interventions before they are implemented. As a result, lack of definitive evidence about the effectiveness of an intervention should not be an excuse for delaying needed policy change. The use of rigorous evaluation methods can help to accumulate evidence that will minimize the risk of adopting policies that are not going to work effectively, but such evidence can never fully eliminate the risk. The lack of evidence about a policy impact should not inhibit policy adoption when there is a strong need for action.However, policy-makers should rely on the best available evidence to guide policy decisions so as to maximize the chances of success and minimize the risks of wasting resources. This involves a model in which science plays a role of evaluating interventions once they are disseminated, not just restricting activity to evaluating interventions before they are disseminated. It is a science of evidence *in* action, not just of evidence preceding action. Before we call for more research prior to implementing a policy we need to consider what we would like to know and whether it is feasible to collect it before implementation, and if so, is the inevitable delay worth the wait. For something as harmful as tobacco, the onus of proof should be on showing that plausible interventions will not work or may be counterproductive, instead of a costly search for certainty in expected outcomes at the cost of delaying action. A framework for deciding when more pre-implementation evaluation is required is outlined in Fig. 37.1.

Tobacco control practitioners and policy-makers need to be open to the possibility that data from evaluation efforts will reveal that the assumptions underpinning the intervention are flawed. Such flaws may reveal that assertions about the mechanisms of effect are incorrect and/or incomplete. Evaluation efforts should by designed to force tobacco control practitioners to specify

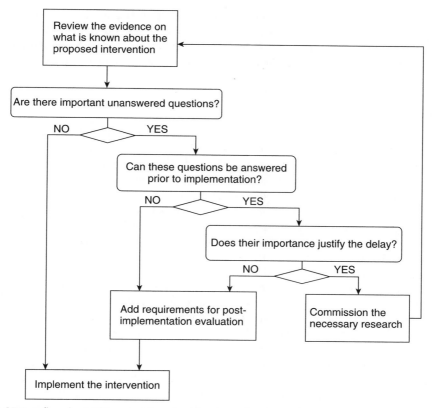

Figure 37.1 A flowchart of key questions to ask prior to implementing a proposed intervention.

assumptions about why and how an intervention will work so that these assumptions can be systematically tested and refined.

Thus, an evaluation model is needed which is designed for the dynamic, ever changing world in which we live. It should use the potential of the world's diversity as a tool to understand, not an obstacle to be overcome. Each action of government is an attempt to influence outcomes in ways consistent with policy goals, which, hopefully, aim to improve the health and well-being of the community. Similarly, the actions of tobacco companies are also designed to affect smoking, in this case in ways that enhance shareholder value, which is why they are almost invariably directed at increasing, or at least maintaining tobacco use. Even the best thought-through interventions sometimes don't work as expected, and policies that work in one context sometimes stop working when the context changes. Because we cannot rely on either past experience or theory to always deliver the best solution to our problems, we need methods to check when and how things are working, and if they are not working, to inform us about why not.

As a basic principle, we need less stringent tests for demonstrating that something has equivalent effects in a new context or when delivered in a new form (where there is no reason to expect changes in efficacy), as compared with evaluation of truly novel interventions or for implementation under conditions where differences in effects are plausible. However, we still need stronger evaluation methods when evidence accumulates to question an assumption of equivalence. Thus it provides an explicit link between the roles of ongoing auditing of programmes to ensure continued effectiveness and more intensive evaluation activity when there are concerns. By basing decisions around clearly articulated theories, the framework is open to scrutiny and should allow the most cost-effective possible evaluation by demanding plausible reasons before testing for differences in effects.

Evaluation framework

From a practical viewpoint population-level effects are what really matters and as these can be highly contextually dependent, the focus of evaluations needs to be on actual performance in the field until moderator effects are sufficiently understood. Practically speaking randomized controlled trials (RCTs) can't be used to evaluate population-based interventions, like government policies to control tobacco use. The lack of an RCT design does not mean that policy evaluations are automatically flawed. Rather, policy evaluation needs to be conceptualized in an analogous way to how epidemiologists inferred causation of smoking and cancer (USDHEW 1964; Hill 1965). This involved triangulating all the available evidence, valuing a diversity of methods, to help rule out alternative explanations of observed effects, rather than focus on attempting to draw conclusions from individual studies or from meta-analyses of studies using the same study design (e.g., RCTs).

Tobacco control practitioners need to maximize the value of studies with individually limited designs by systematically reviewing the findings to determine what they collectively add to knowledge. In isolation such studies may have little to say about intervention effects, but when they are combined in ways that take account of different threats to the internal validity of a conclusion about an effect, collectively a pattern may emerge to allow one to make strong inferences about causality as well as potentially increasing our understanding of the conditions under which the interventions are most effective. The reality is that the best-established influence on tobacco use behaviours is the price of the product, generally manipulated thorough tax increases. The price effect is large enough to observe with crude population measures. By contrast, meta-analyses of RCTs have found that pharmacotherapies increase quit rates (Cummings and Hyland 2005), but such effects have not been easy to detect at a population level (Pierce et al. 2005).

Theory as a guide

Evaluation should be much more than the determination of whether something works and of the effect size. Good evaluation should start with an analysis of the problem, building an understanding of the factors that are or can affect tobacco use and how use relates to the harms. This requires a theory of how the policy is expected to work. As Kurt Lewin noted years ago (1935), 'there is nothing as practical as a good theory.' Theories specify mechanisms or mediating pathways of effects, allowing these pathways to be tested. They also can specify conditions under which interventions will work (i.e., moderators) of intervention impact. We can test whether these factors affect outcomes, and thus be better placed to develop the suite of interventions needed to provide maximal help, or to produce desired structural or cultural changes. While no single theory can encompass the complexity of controlling tobacco use; more can be done to consider how theories that deal with different aspects of the problem interrelate, including different timescales for change (e.g., behaviour change versus change in cultural norms and practices). The set of theories we use should be compatible with each other, even if the nature of the interrelationships is not fully articulated.

Understanding the mechanisms by which interventions have their effects is important for the following reasons: 1) it can provide strong evidence of the causal impact of a particular policy, especially when attempting to differentiate the effects of a specific intervention from other possible causes, including other tobacco policies; 2) it can be used to diagnose the problem in cases where intended effects did not occur, by identifying where in the causal pathway things went wrong; 3) it can help us understand why a policy breaks down for some groups, but not for others (i.e., clarify why moderation occurs); 4) by specifying how a policy works, it may help identify alternative ways of achieving the desired effects; 5) it can be used to identify possible incidental effects and ways of managing them: and 6) it can help define the relative contributions of different interventions which occur together. These understandings can facilitate the development of new, and hopefully improved, ways of targeting key pathways of influence, of tailoring interventions to better reach more resistant or needy groups, and/or working out the best mix of policies.

A general framework for assessing how a policy intervention might affect tobacco use is illustrated in Fig. 37.2. It specifies two levels of mediating variables between a policy intervention and the outcomes, those specific to the policy, and those variables that are part of more general pathways. It also accepts that various other factors (moderators) might affect the size of the effect. Policy-specific mediators involve such things as awareness, policy-specific knowledge, and reactions to specific elements of the intervention. For example, new graphic warning labels should increase salience and noticeability of warnings, and perhaps forgoing of occasional cigarettes. The second set of general mediators are constructs taken from behavioural science which we know mediate effects of behaviour, that is they are means by which changes in tobacco use may occur. They include attitudes, normative beliefs and intentions. Moderators, those things that change the magnitude of the effects of an intervention without necessarily being changed by the intervention include socio-demographic factors (e.g., age, gender, socio-economic status, cultural background) and psychological factors that are either assumed to be stable or which the intervention is not designed to change (e.g., level of dependence). This framework provides a general guide for thinking about policies and their effects on a broad array of important psychosocial and behavioural variables, and for testing how differences in policy implementation relate to effectiveness.

Where we find or theorize moderator effects, it is important to understand where they occur along the proposed mediational pathways, or indeed whether different mediational pathways exist for different groups or situations (see Fig. 37.2). For example, if an intervention is not seen to be relevant to or targeted at a group, this group may not respond to it. Here, making the intervention relevant might be all that is needed to remove the moderating effect. A good example of this is advertisements where the actors are old, which are typically not seen as relevant to young people (the converse is less likely to be true). Something as simple as choice of actor can create moderator effects, which under other conditions would not be present (or be small enough to be ignored).

Knowledge of the mediational pathways that are theorized to explain how policy affects behaviour and environment (or environmental risk) should lead to: an appropriate study design; the

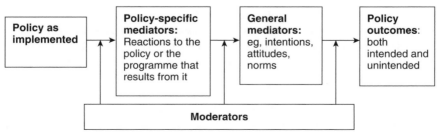

Figure 37.2 A generalized model of mediation making allowance for moderator effects (adapted from IARC 2008; chapter 1 Fig. 4).

inclusion of appropriate constructs and measures; and the selection of analytic tools that are well-suited to estimating the causal impact of policies by providing explanatory pathways and helping to eliminate alternative explanations. Logic models describe these pathways and help identify constructs to measure. Specific measures to use for a range of policy interventions can be found in the Handbook (IARC 2008). It is important to keep the logic models simple to focus attention on key constructs. If a particular challenge in understanding becomes focused within one box in the pathway or in the links between two boxes, the first step is to go to a higher order of magnification and try to spell out in more detail the theoretical pathways, leaving the unproblematic area in 'larger scale' boxes.

Policies are typically implemented with specific goals in mind, often due to the jurisdictional head of power under which they are implemented. Thus, policies to protect workers from exposure to passive smoking, when implemented under occupational health and safety laws to protect non-smokers, cannot explicitly consider the possible benefits of smoke-free places for reducing cigarette consumption or for enhancing quitting. Good evaluation requires consideration of all potentially important outcomes, not just those used to justify the policy. It is also important to consider effects along different theoretical pathways to the intended means of action (that used to justify the policy) as these might be important for analysis of society-wide impacts; e.g., the generally neutral or positive effects on business of smoke-free policies (Scollo *et al.* 2003). Similarly plausible alternative models for the generation of desired effects should be considered; e.g., warning labels having effects through engaging emotional responses not purely due to the propositional content. It should also include effects on other determinants of tobacco use (Borland *et al* 2009b). Consideration of incidental effects is more important in tobacco control than in most other areas of health because the tobacco industry can react to policies in ways that moderate their effects (Cummings *et al.* 2002). This is one reason surveillance of tobacco industry practices is required. Governments have a role in mandating disclosure of this information. The approach taken can be facilitated by a theoretical understanding of the industry's profit motive and marketing practices, as this can guide the selection of data that are most relevant in surveillance for reactive effects.

Tobacco control programme evaluation should provide information about the delivery of the intervention to those who need it in a manner that results in maximal effectiveness, and to determine conditions for any moderators of effectiveness. Some of the key steps in this process are spelled out in Fig. 37.3. It makes a clear distinction between evaluations assessing implementation from those assessing effectiveness once implemented. Near the bottom it allows an option of trying to improve the intervention, something that might not always be possible.

Study designs

To best understand the implications of policy change (including community-wide dissemination of interventions), we need research designs that are as strong as possible. In short, evaluation is strengthened with more observations (both before and after the intervention) within the population an intervention occurs in, the more populations that are studied in parallel, and the more alternative explanations for outcomes that are assessed within each study. In addition, the use of cohorts adds considerable power by allowing mediation and moderation effects to be tested more precisely. Finally, representativeness of the sample to the study population can increase the generalizability of findings. However, repeatability (same sampling frame, questions, and response rates) is more important than representativeness for determination of trends because it requires comparability between estimates over time. The ITC study (Fong *et al.* 2006) is a good example of what can be achieved by attempting to do as many of these things as possible.

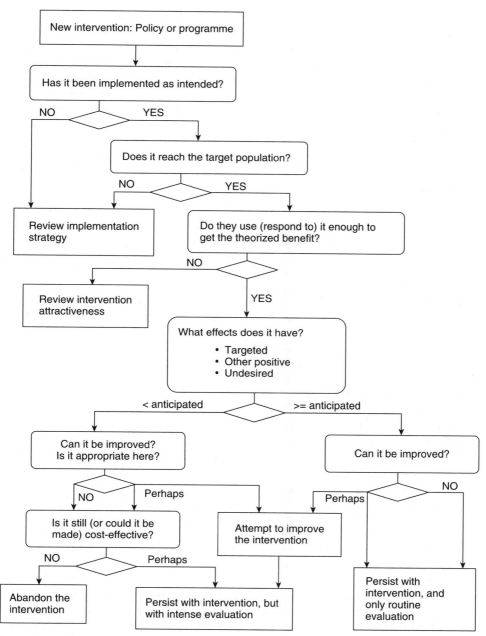

Figure 37.3 A flowchart of key questions to ask after implementing a new intervention.

The core of good evaluation is of designing studies to detect changes in outcomes that might be attributable to a specific intervention, and to put in place measures to rule out alternative explanations. These alternative explanations are of three types, those related to systematic errors of measurement (bias), those related to alternative mechanisms of effect (confounding), and chance effects.

Bias occurs where the measures used to assess the constructs of interest actually measure something different (usually a closely related construct) or are contaminated by some systematic error (e.g., social desirability can affect responses about beliefs and intentions). Confounding occurs when the association with the outcome of interest appears stronger or weaker than it truly is as a result of an uncontrolled association between the intervention and other mechanisms of effect (e.g., a different policy intervention). The contribution of chance is a function of naturally occurring variability in outcomes of interest, and its impact is controlled for by ensuring adequate sample sizes. The quality of evidence from any single study is a joint function of the study design and of the quality of the measures used: that is their reliability and validity for assessing what they are theorized to measure.

Measurement

One's theory about how a programme or policy will influence tobacco use behaviours should help guide the evaluator about what constructs need to measured. Evaluation requires a good description of the problem and its context and of how these are changing. This involves finding appropriate measures of the constructs of interest and of collecting data using the appropriate measures. The goal here is to provide population estimates of what people do and think, focusing on key outcomes. In assessing reports, we need to consider possible meaning changes (due to changing contexts) and effects on response styles (i.e., social desirability) as possible explanations for changes in question responses, especially for questions that have an evaluative component (see IARC 2008 chapter 2.2).

The IARC Handbook (IARC 2008) recommends collecting data in four principal domains: 1) who uses tobacco, what they use, how much, and where and when they use it; as well as any relevant knowledge, beliefs, and attitudes (including those of ex-smokers and non-smokers); 2) tobacco industry behaviour, including characteristics of their products; 3) tobacco control activities to which people are exposed; and 4) aspects of the broader environment that might affect tobacco use or tobacco harm outcomes (cultural norms, controls on activities like alcohol consumption that are linked to tobacco use). To which we would add, information on any relevant policy-specific legislation or regulation. These rules define the context by which the above operate and can moderate their effects (e.g., national smoke-free laws may achieve greater compliance than those voluntarily imposed by proprietors).

High-quality data collections, such as regular cross-sectional surveys are essential to describing the nature of the problem and the quantification of trends in tobacco use and in key determinants of use. More generally, possible incidental effects of policies should always be considered and measured where appropriate. In tobacco control, because the tobacco industry or sections of it might be motivated to moderate the effects of policies, it is important to conduct surveillance of possible counteractions to policies. Governments should be encouraged to collect data from the tobacco industry to help evaluate current and future tobacco control policies, and to assist in identifying tobacco industry actions that might moderate the effects of tobacco control policies. The kind of information that should be readily available from the industry and placed into the public repository includes disaggregated sub-brand specific marketing activities, product sales data, and product content, design, and performance data. It might also include more general information on political contributions, funding of scientists, general sponsorships and other activities of the industry which are designed to affect the environment in which they operate.

Summative evaluation criteria

The evaluation model outline earlier shares more in common with the methods used in epidemiology to determine causes of illness, than with evaluating the efficacy of a clinical intervention using a RCT. As a result, when considering criteria to use in drawing conclusions about the effectiveness of policy interventions we have adapted the criteria used in the epidemiology of disease Hill (1965). The adapted criteria are outlined in Table 37.1.

In providing a summative evaluation of the cause–effect nature of an intervention, the evaluators needs to not only consider the size and nature of effects, but also the possibility that there is no meaningful effect. In particular, of the importance to be able to say something about the absence of effects, separate from the lack of evidence. Science cannot prove the null hypothesis, but it can and should make statements about interventions where there is a consistent failure to find evidence of any meaningful effect.

We need to qualify effects with a statement about generality. Some interventions have similar effects in most contexts, while others can be quite context-specific. This consideration needs to cover cultural adjustments to the intervention itself, as well as factors in the environment that might affect an interventions potency (effect moderators). It is also important to consider the direction of effects. Some interventions might prove counterproductive. Clearly less evidence should be required to stop an intervention where the evidence suggests that it is counterproductive, than if it suggested no effect or only a small positive effect.

The levels of evidence used to evaluate discrete interventions is not appropriate for use in evaluating policy interventions. We see more promise in adapting the criteria used by IARC for its cancer prevention handbooks. This is essentially a four level system: sufficient evidence of an effect, limited evidence of an effect, insufficient evidence, and sufficient evidence suggesting lack of effect. However, such a rating scheme would ideally be augmented by clear ratings of the magnitude of effect, and the generalizability of the effect (see Table 37.2). There is also a need to consider the net societal value of producing the intended effects, taking into account incidental effects, however, this is too complex an issue to readily codify.

Once the effectiveness of an intervention is established, less powerful research designs will be needed to monitor continuation of effects and/or to assess whether similar magnitudes of effect are attained with new populations. It is only when there is reason to believe that there are real differences that stronger research methods might need to be reapplied (see Fig. 37.3).

Table 37.1 Criteria for judging causality

Criteria
Magnitude of the observed effect, particularly in relationship to known naturally occurring variations
Temporal relationship between intervention and change in target outcome
Exposure–response gradient
Biopsychosocial plausibility
Coherence across lines of evidence with different threats to validity, e.g., similar results using aggregate data and self-reported consumption could rule out response biases
Coherence of results from demonstrations of effects on different parts of the theorized causal pathway, or by demonstrating efficacy of components (e.g., the evidence of efficacy of many cessation aids makes more likely that they have effects when delivered as part of programs of help)
Evidence that this type of intervention can have effects on other comparable outcomes (e.g., on other behaviour patterns)
Consistency of observed effects across studies and populations, or clear patterns in the variability to demonstrate limits to generalizability
Elimination of theoretically possible alternative mechanisms for explaining the observed effects

Table 37.2 Proposed ratings to make about evidence on the capacity of interventions to produce intended effects

Certainty of effect	Size of effect	Generalizability of effect
Sufficient evidence: The effect can be taken as established	*Large*: Effect size greater than one standard deviation of usual variation	*High*: Worthwhile levels of effect occur under most or all conditions
Limited evidence: Likely effect, but caution is recommended and further research is needed	*Medium*: Effect size of 0.5–1.0 standard deviations	*Limited*: Some identified conditions where effects may be reduced or not occur
Insufficient evidence: No claims should be made about effect	*Small*: Effect size less than 0.5 standard deviations	*Highly selective*: Effects only occur under special conditions
Sufficient evidence of null effect: Despite considerable research, the intervention has not been shown to contribute anything meaningful towards the desired effect, or there is net evidence that it might be counterproductive		

Finally, we need to accept that much of the evidence we need to be sure policies are working as intended cannot be collected until after they are implemented. This means policies often need to be implemented with some uncertainty about outcomes. The greater this uncertainty, the greater is the requirement for strong post-implementation evaluation of a policy intervention.

Summary

Evaluation requires specific, committed resources. The evaluation framework we have outlined in this chapter highlights the potential value of good evaluation for interventions as it allows for both ongoing improvement and the capacity to build on the accumulated knowledge acquired by others. In 1999, the United States Centers for Disease Control and Prevention (CDC) recommended that 10% of the total budget for a comprehensive tobacco control programme should be allocated for evaluation and surveillance. The CDC recommendation was recently endorsed by WHO and represents a reasonable benchmark for governments to adopt.

The IARC Handbook contains examples of the use of logic models to better understand several key areas in tobacco control. It also provides guidance on study design, choice of measures, and issues involved in translation across cultures. As these models are used they will doubtless be refined, reflecting the stronger understanding of how tobacco control policies and programmes exert their influence on tobacco use behaviours.

For the field of tobacco control to move forward attention and resources need to be provided to knowledge utilization, which in this domain would include appropriate detailed documentation of the results and all the features of evaluation studies, so as to allow the information to be compared and summative evaluations made. Summative evaluations are necessary as many of the key questions about intervention generalizability can only be answered after multiple studies have been conducted. Development of a repository to collect and organize this information is becoming increasingly important. Complementing the repository of evaluations, should be a similar repository of measures, with information as to their validity in the various contexts where they might be useful. The utility of such a repository would be enhanced by the development and agreement upon use of prototype proformas for reporting on the validity data on measures, and on frequently repeated interventions, such as mass media campaigns. This will facilitate their combination into meta-analytic studies, especially important for understanding where and when things work. The continued momentum of the WHO FCTC and of the broader movement to fight against the global tobacco epidemic can be facilitated by the existence of such a repository, with appropriate tools for easy access and utilization of the contents of the repository. Articles 20 and 22 of the WHO FCTC effectively call for such an initiative.

References

Borland, R., Mullins, R., and Trotter, E. (1999). Trends in environmental tobacco smoke restrictions in the home in Victoria, Australia. *Tobacco Control*, **8**:266–271.

Borland, R., Wilson, N., Fong, G.T., Hammond, D., Cummings, K.M., Yong, H.H. *et al.* (2009a). Impact of graphic and text warnings on cigarette packs: Findings from four countries over five years. *Tobacco Control*, **18**: 358–364.

Borland, R., Yong, H.H., Wilson, N., Fong, G.T., Hammond, D., Cummings, K.M. *et al.* (2009b). How reactions to cigarette pack health warnings influence quitting: findings from the ITC Four Country survey. *Addiction*, **104**: 669–675.

Cummings, K.M., Fong, G.T., and Borland, R. (2009). Environmental influences on tobacco use: evidence from societal and community influences on tobacco use and dependence. *Annual Review of Clinical Psychology*, **5**:211–236.

Cummings, K.M. and Hyland, A. (2005). Impact of nicotine replacement therapy on smoking behavior. *Annual Review of Public Health*, **26**:583–599.

Cummings, K.M., Morley, C.P., and Hyland, A. (2002). Failed promises of the cigarette industry and its effects on consumer misperceptions about the health risks of smoking. *Tobacco Control*, **11**(suppl 1):1110–1117.

Flay, B.R., Biglin, A., Boruch, R.F., Castro, F.G., Gottfredson, D., Kellam, S., *et al.* (2005). Standards of evidence: criteria for efficacy, effectiveness and dissemination. *Prevention Science*, **6**:151–175.

Fong, G.T., Cummings, K.M., Borland, R., Hastings, G., Hyland, A., *et al.* (2006). The conceptual framework of the International Tobacco Control (ITC) Policy Evaluation Project. *Tobacco Control*, **15**(Suppl III): iii3–iii11.

Hill, A.B. (1965). The environment and disease: association or causation? *Proceedings of the Royal Society of Medicine*, **58**:295–300.

Hovell, M.F., Zakarian, J.M., Wahlgren, D.R., and Matt, G.E. (2000). Reducing children's exposure to environmental tobacco smoke: the empirical evidence and directions for future research. *Tobacco Control*, **9**:ii40–47.

IARC (2008). *Handbooks of Cancer Prevention Volume 12, Methods for Evaluating Tobacco Control Policies*, Geneva: WHO Press.

Pierce, J.P. and Gilpin, E.A. (2002). Impact of over-the-counter sales on effectiveness of pharmaceutical aids for smoking cessation. *JAMA*, **288**:1260–1264.

Rogers, E.M. (2003). *Diffusion of Innovations (5th edn)*. New York: Free Press.

Scollo, M., Lal, A., Hyland, A., and Glantz, S. (2003). Review of the quality of studies on the economic effects of smoke-free policies on the hospitality industry. *Tobacco Control*, **12**:13–20.

US Department of Health, Education and Welfare (1964). *Smoking and Health report of the advisory committee to the Surgeon General of the Public Health Service*. Washington, D.C., DHEW, Public Health Service.

Chapter 38

Global tobacco control policy

Nigel Gray

Introduction

Tobacco control policy has evolved over time and will continue to do so. To every action by the tobacco industry there has been a reaction by public health authorities and vice versa. As a result there has been a continuing struggle between those committed to market expansion (the industry) and those committed to market shrinkage (public health authorities). As a result the market is shrinking in most developed countries while it expands in many, but not all, developing countries. Between 1997 and 1999 world tobacco leaf sales went down from 7 975 360 tonnes to 6 341 430 tonnes (United States Department of Agriculture 2001), while world cigarette production went from 5 614 830 million pieces in 1996 to 5 573 464 million pieces in 2000 (United States Department of Agriculture, 2001). If public health is winning, it is winning very slowly. Fifty years of obstruction and obfuscation has maintained industry profits and seen a steady increase in global mortality (Peto 1994). To be effective, tobacco control policy must be comprehensive and global.

Making tobacco policy is not the same as implementing it and the time lag between the two processes is often decades. Tobacco use is, and will remain, one of the most difficult health issues facing society in the twenty-first century. It is worth reflecting on the history of the major infectious diseases and the disappearance from developed countries within a decade or less of smallpox, measles, diphtheria, tetanus, whooping cough, rubella, and scarlet fever. These diseases were conquered by the discovery, and use, of penicillin and vaccines that both worked and were used. Some of these diseases persist in developing countries for reasons related to social organization and money but NOT to organized opposition, which explains the slow progress against the tobacco epidemic. The single reason for the dominance of the tobacco problem is that someone is selling it, whereas no one is selling diphtheria or tuberculosis. This fact is unique to tobacco which has been, until very recently, the subject of a 50-year campaign of denial. By contrast, there was never a serious suggestion that asbestos did not cause asbestosis or that drunken driving was merely a pleasurable habit.

That the environment has changed is due to the effects of litigation, mainly within the United States, which has led to the arrival in the public domain of over thirty three million documents which revealed what the tobacco industry knew and when it knew it. The outcome of this process has been, at least in the case of Philip Morris (newly named Altria), a policy reversal which led to the admission set out in the following paragraph, which is a quote from their web site (Philip Morris USA, 2002).

> Cigarette Smoking and Disease in Smokers: We agree with the overwhelming medical and scientific consensus that cigarette smoking causes lung cancer, heart disease, emphysema and other serious diseases in smokers. Smokers are far more likely to develop serious diseases, like lung cancer, than non-smokers. There is no 'safe' cigarette. These are and have been the messages of public health

authorities worldwide. Smokers and potential smokers should rely on these messages in making all smoking-related decisions.

This volte-face, accompanied as it is by a worldwide decline in the credibility of the industry, means that policy-makers are working in a completely different environment and that the task of proving the seriousness of the situation is less complicated, is more related to its magnitude, can focus on what needs to be done, and is much less of a debate. It does not mean that suggestions to governments go unopposed, or that the objective of market expansion has been abandoned by the industry.

This chapter will deal primarily with the cigarette, which is the most widely used and best-studied product. It should be noted that the remarkable mix of tobacco products that are smoked and chewed often in bizarre mixtures mostly in developing countries, pose singular difficulties, as they are usually regional, based on cottage industries and frequently not subject to tax, counting or inclusion in national statistics. The policy options available to deal with these are usually national and profoundly difficult to resolve. The bidi rolling industry in India exemplifies this. The role of women in the bidi rolling industry in India has important implications for the health of women but also bears on the economic 'worth' of women (it affects dowry negotiations). Since this industry also uses child labour when a village family undertakes a contract to a manufacturer it is clear that no simple solution exists.

Key policy issues include prevention of initiation; management of addiction; regulation of the cigarette, the way it is sold, its nicotine content and its emissions; protection of non-smokers from secondhand smoke; public education and control of labelling and trademarks; disincentives to purchase (tax) and restrictions on sales to minors. Many of these topics are covered in detail in the relevant chapters. This chapter will summarize what is, in effect, modern comprehensive policy.

Prevention of initiation

Tobacco smoking is a *learned* habit. *Initiation* of smoking is a psycho-social phenomenon discussed in detail in Chapter 17. *Maintenance* is sustained by the development of *addiction* (see Chapter 8).

Prevention of initiation requires removal of all the positive stimuli to take up smoking and the provision of effective education which warns teenagers of the dangers of smoking without triggering a desire to experiment. This is not easy to do.

Removal of all forms of tobacco promotion is also not easy to do. Many countries have passed effective legislation to prohibit all forms of advertising down to and including point of sale advertising. This was achieved by straightforward legislation in Norway and Finland but in Australia (which is a federation) separate legislation (sometimes at state level, sometimes federal) was required for health warnings; broadcast media; billboards; print media; and point of sale. Sponsorship of sport was eliminated indirectly by prohibition of advertising of brand names, which also covered 'brand stretching' (or sale of other products using the brand name, and often trade mark) of the cigarette. Ultimately overall Federal legislation brought all these individual pieces together over two decades after the first law was passed for health warnings.

Not all countries have the power to totally abolish tobacco promotion. Both the United States and the European Union probably lack the powers to do so. No country can prohibit transnational advertising such as accompanies the Formula One Grand Prix, both car and motor cycle, although individual countries can prohibit exhibition of brand names but then face the possibility that such events will be moved elsewhere. International sports advertising is ubiquitous and uses sports of wide interest such as car and motor cycle racing, cricket, golf, and soccer.

Voluntary codes for advertising restriction have not been successful. However, if global advertising is to cease it can probably only be achieved by negotiation with the international tobacco industry under the sort of litigation-induced duress that brought about negotiations for a settlement in the United States in 1997 (Gray 1997). Such negotiations are only conceivable within a framework which envisages acceptance by both sides that the global tobacco market should shrink. Negotiation with the international television industry is another conceivable option but similarly difficult, though not impossible, to achieve.

The relationship between promotion and chemistry

While the contribution of advertising to initiation is undoubted, it is now evident (Wayne and Connolly 2002) that changes to cigarette design, particularly during the 1980s, led to the cigarettes intended for the 'young adult smoker' (YAS) and the 'first usual brand young adult smoker' (FUBYAS) being made significantly 'smoother' with characteristics of less 'harshness', greater 'mildness' and 'lightness', among other features. Camel, in particular, developed an advertising campaign using Joe Camel, the 'smooth character' in parallel with significant design changes that sent the cigarette's chemistry in the direction desired by YAS and FUBYAS. Thus the cigarette became easier to smoke and easier to learn to smoke, and, as it had higher yields of nicotine, it may have become more addictive. Between 1987 and 1993, Camel's market share among 18 year olds grew from 2.5% to 14%.

Competitive marketing

The market for cigarettes, and other forms of tobacco, is intensely competitive. While this persists abolition of promotion will remain extremely difficult. As a matter of policy, consideration needs to be given to replacing the open marketplace with a centralized, government controlled wholesale purchaser for cigarettes (Borland 2003), similar to the systems which operate in many countries for the purpose of purchasing pharmaceutical drugs. Such a body would then be in a position to specify what products it is willing to place on the retail market.

The role of packet labeling

The branded and trade-marked cigarette packet is a potent advertisement (Wakefield *et al.* 2000), whether featured on a billboard or as observable in almost any streetscape where a smoker, or a teenager, offers a friend a cigarette from a well-known packet. The packet is also a potent opportunity to give information ranging from explicit, research-based health warnings to the graphic and similarly explicit warnings pioneered by Canada. In the longer term a generic packet with suitable warnings is the only possible policy objective. This means abolition of trade marks, an objective that will not be easily attained.

Labelling with 'tar' and nicotine yields has been shown to be misleading in that the Federal Trade Commission (FTC) method of measurement does not represent the dose of smoke actually taken in by the smoker, and compensatory smoking is a frequent occurrence (Jarvis *et al.* 2001; Kozlowski *et al.* 2001; Benowitz 2001). For this reason alone use of these terms on the packet should be prohibited.

A second reason for abolishing these terms is the credible body of evidence suggesting that switching to low yield cigarettes has been seen by smokers as a viable alternative to quitting (Weinstein 2001). Further they have been used as justification for the use of terms such as 'Light' and 'Mild' (Pollay and Dewhirst 2002) which have, rightly, been prohibited by a number of countries.

The management of addiction-smoking cessation

This topic is covered in Chapter 39. There can be no doubt that modern techniques of counselling, associated with Nicotine Replacement Therapy (NRT) and more recently developed drugs can substantially increase quit rates. The current position is unsatisfactory in most countries in that NRT is more expensive and less available than the cigarette. A further problem is posed by the failure of the health professions to use available knowledge and therapy in a widespread way (Boyle *et al.* 2000).

This situation is regrettable and represents a seriously missed opportunity as cessation offers the most immediate return for health expenditure in terms of mortality reduction.

Harm reduction

While abstinence from smoking is clearly the optimal approach, the concept of harm reduction is a logical approach to tobacco use (see Chapter 40). It can take three forms: reduction of risk by product switching; provision of nicotine to satisfy the addict's needs by other products such as a nicotine replacement therapy that is truly competitive with tobacco – which means it would presumably be addictive – and modification of the tobacco product itself (by regulatory means).

♦ Product switching can undoubtedly be used to reduce risk at a personal level, for example a change from the cigarette to low nitrosamine smokeless tobacco. At a population level the value of this as a policy depends significantly on the national environment. In the United States there are many suitable lower risk products and much opinion supports product switching but, however, switching to another product that supports and maintains nicotine addiction leaves the smoker vulnerable to reversion to cigarettes. Further the tobacco industry has seen the marketing opportunities provided by product switching and has provided same name smokeless tobacco products 'for when you can't smoke' and the possibility exists of the design of 'starter' smokeless tobacco products that might act as a gateway to smoking. Clearly the smokeless tobacco products used in Asia are totally unsuitable for reduction of risk, as they carry high risks of oro-pharyngeal cancers (Boffetta *et al.* 2008).

♦ Competitive nicotine replacement therapy could theoretically work, as well as switching to low nitrosamine smokeless tobacco and is very low risk apart from the serious potential to maintain nicotine dependence. However the pharmaceutical industry has not so far provided such a product for the probable reason that national regulators have given no indication that such a product would be acceptable and it is extremely likely that an addictive nicotine replacement therapy will only be produced when a major government asks for it. This is unlikely to happen while the international Tobacco Control movement remains divided on the issue.

♦ The first attempt to reduce the harmfulness of the cigarette was the policy of reducing tar and nicotine yields. This was logical at the time (the late 1960s) and should have been more successful than it was. Tar and nicotine reduction was subverted by the changes in design of the modern cigarette described by Hoffmann (Hoffmann *et al.* 2001). These changes involved increases in tobacco specific nitrosamines (TSNAs) which have been associated with increases in the relative and absolute risk of adenocarcinoma of the lung (Gray 2006). Together with other design changes (Kozlowski *et al.* 2001) which contributed to compensatory smoking the modern, low-yield cigarette, has not proven substantially less dangerous than its predecessor of 30–50 years (Thun and Burns 2001). The fact that the low-yield programme was not successful is no reason not to persist with attempts to regulate the content of cigarette smoke.

Two areas of regulation attract interest. Control of smoke levels of carcinogens and toxins, and control of the driver to inhalation, nicotine.

Control of carcinogens and toxins

The policy objective is to reduce as far as practical the levels of known carcinogens and toxins in smoke. Such regulatory control is best focussed on smoke content (the emissions) rather than the constituents of the cigarette even though certain substances, such as nitrosamines, may be best controlled at source – the nitrate levels in tobacco and the curing process. It does not seem sensible for governments to take responsibility for the design of the cigarette as the legal liability for design effects should remain with the manufacturer. While it is obvious that the ventilated filter is a serious problem there are ways of controlling emissions that are likely to lead to the industry abandoning it. Certainly removing tar, nicotine, and carbon monoxide measures from the packet would reduce the incentive to use filter ventilation.

Hoffmann has listed 15 major toxins and 69 carcinogens known to be in cigarette smoke (Hoffmann and Hoffmann 2001). Clearly these substances and certain other toxicants are prime candidates for reduction. A system has been proposed, based on analysis of cigarettes actually on the market now, by the Tobacco Regulation Study Group (TobReg) of the World Health Organization (WHO) whereby upper limits would be established for specified carcinogens and toxins in the emissions of tobacco smoke (WHO study group on tobacco product regulation, 2007). It is currently proposed to do the same for smokeless tobacco.

Such a regulatory system is practical now as some brands already on the market meet these criteria. There can be no justification for the continued marketing of cigarettes that are unnecessarily dangerous. If this form of regulation were to limit the number of brands available substantially, no harm would be done, cigarettes could still be sold profitably, and the harmfulness of cigarettes should be reduced. This in no way suggests that the cigarette could be 'safe' but it should certainly be less dangerous. Such an approach has been taken, successfully, to motor car exhausts.

Control of nicotine

Nicotine yields are currently measured by the FTC system, or something analogous. This system does not represent actual smoking patterns. A comparison of actual smoking patterns with the FTC method (Hoffmann and Hoffmann 2001) showed that smokers actually inhale between approximately one and a half to two and a half times as much nicotine, carbon monoxide, benz(a) pyrene, and 4-(methylnitrosamine)-1-(3-pyridyl)-1-butanone (NNK) than would be inhaled if the cigarette was smoked according to the FTC parameters.

Clearly, if nicotine dose is to be regulated, a better measuring system is needed. For regulatory purposes a simple measure of the amount of nicotine in the cigarette tobacco should suffice. However, if the smoker is to be informed of the dose he or she is getting, something much more complex would be needed.

Until now the dose given to the smoker has been determined by the cigarette manufacturer. The result is the carefully engineered (Kozlowski *et al.* 2001) modern cigarette which is smoked in a compensatory way. The degree of compensation occurring with this cigarette has not been meaningfully compared with the degree of compensatory inhalation that occurred three and more decades ago. It is probably greater. Clearly compensatory smoking delivers greater amounts of carcinogens and toxins to the lung and one object of regulation should be to reduce this.

The intricacies of nicotine policy are discussed elsewhere (see Chapter 8) and require consideration of nicotine in cigarettes and nicotine available in other forms. It is enough to canvass here the possible options for the cigarette. The first policy requirement is that nicotine becomes the object of regulation. The options then become:

♦ **Increase the amount of nicotine.**

Providing a 'satisfying' amount of nicotine (which may mean an increase) has the advantage that it could be presumed to reduce compensation and therefore carcinogen/toxin dose (Russell 1976). The disadvantage is that it does nothing to reduce (and may enhance) dependence on the cigarette as a source of nicotine. Regulatory authorities are unlikely to be comfortable with this approach after several decades of struggle to reduce the dose.

♦ **Allow the status quo**

This has the disadvantage of leaving decision-making to the tobacco industry, leaves today's level of compensatory smoking, and does nothing to reduce the addictiveness of the cigarette.

♦ **Reduce the amount of nicotine**

First proposed in 1994 (Benowitz and Henningfield 1994) this has the potential to reduce the addictiveness of the cigarette and the disadvantage that compensatory smoking might increase. It could only be done in parallel with a determined attempt to provide more widely available and efficacious NRT which might, used separately or together with cigarettes, replace the cigarette as the prime delivery system for nicotine. Clearly a major requirement would be a concerted comprehensive public education campaign. This option has possibilities in the long term but remains in the realm of the theoretical until nicotine levels in cigarettes are more universally captured by regulatory systems. The possibility of 'more efficacious' NRT being, or becoming, addictive, also needs to be faced.

Real control of dose and compensation

The above discussion of carcinogens/toxins and nicotine is aimed at reducing the amounts of the substances available per unit dose of smoke and need to be based on some form of standard measuring technique. The current FTC system is unsatisfactory and TobReg has preferred the Canadian 'intense' system and has phrased its recommended upper limits in amounts per milligram of nicotine. This takes some account of the smokers' practice of compensating and also provides a larger quantum of smoke for measurement.

Secondhand smoke-the role of the smoke-free environment

The issue of exposure to secondhand smoke has more public health significance than is indicated by its direct effects on health. Since early publications indicating that such exposure was associated with increased disease risk (Colley *et al.* 1974; Harlap and Davies 1974; Hirayama 1981; Trichopoulos *et al.* 1981; Chilmonczyk *et al.* 1993) the non-smoking public has been a significant force in supporting reduction of such exposures. To a considerable degree, smokers have been compliant with attempts to restrict smoking opportunities and have even been shown to favour smoke-free workplaces (Hocking *et al.* 1991) and public places.

The policy of reduction of exposure to secondhand smoke has several important effects. The most important is that it contributes to reduction in smoking and in smoking rates (Chapman *et al.* 1999). The second is that it can be expected to reduce disease in those susceptible, particularly, to asthma. The third is reduction in lost work-time (Borland *et al.* 1997). An important factor in the establishment of the smoke-free environment has been successful litigation by employees suffering compensable diseases induced by secondhand smoke (Chapman 2001; Stewart and Semmler 2002). In Australia in 1997, 28% of smokers did not smoke at home (Borland *et al.* 1999). The insurance industry is an important ally in this area, as court cases involving the tobacco industry have been extremely expensive and settling out of court can be cheaper.

Further, after successful litigation, insurance of workplaces where employees are exposed to smoke becomes more expensive and may even be unobtainable.

Taxation policy

Tax policy is a proven and long-established part of overall policy as it can be a strong disincentive to initiation. Cost also influences the amount smokers smoke, and contributes importantly to quitting (Manley *et al.* 1993). Taxes should be high to be as large a deterrent as possible, and may be responsible for a significant proportion of total government tax revenues. For example, they provided, in 1994–1995 4.34% of total tax in Argentina, 3.38% in Australia, 2.79% in China, and 2.43% in India (Sunley *et al.* 2000). Earmarking of a proportion of tax for health purposes is sensible and may be popular. Increasing tax to a point where it equals three quarters to two thirds of the price of cigarettes is regarded as achievable and appropriate (Chaloupka *et al.* 2000). Regular increases in excess of inflation are desirable and should be on every public health workers list of annual priorities.

Public education

There is a clear relationship between levels of consumer information and tobacco use, so the process of public education is an important element of comprehensive policy. In its simplest form, the provision of a health warning on the packet, provides a basis for further and more specific education campaigns. All available means should be used, including mass media (Friend and Levy 2002; Wakefield and Chaloupka 2000), and the best programmes should be based on relevant research in the population in question. Major educational interventions such as technical reports have important if short-lived effects (Kenkel and Chen 2000).

Availablility

Sales to children, aged 16–18 are prohibited in many countries. Such prohibition is sensible but is rarely policed. Attempts are underway in the Unites States to remedy this. Until these attempts are shown to fail the policy remains important and should be seriously considered by developing countries.

What works

What works is all of the above, together, as part of a comprehensive, planned, regularly reinforced exercise based on research within the society in which it is delivered, and policy initiatives should be regularly evaluated (see Chapter 37).

Clearly, everything cannot be done in every country at the same time but the fact that tobacco consumption is falling only slowly and that the manufacturers are successfully shifting their focus, and their recycled dishonest arguments, to developing countries can only be described as scandalous. Implementation if the Framework Convention on Tobacco Control, introduced as a treaty by the WHO needs to be supported vigorously by all countries. In particular, those countries where tobacco products are manufactured bear responsibility for what is exported, and countries that do not have local manufacture should avoid it and can more readily assert controls on what is allowed on to their market.

References

Benowitz, N.L. (2001). Compensatory smoking of low yield cigarettes. In: Anonymous *Risks Associated with Smoking Cigarettes with Low Machine-measured Yields of Tar and Nicotine*, pp. 39–63. Bethesda MD: US Department of Health and Human Services, National Institutes of Health, National Cancer Institute.

Borland, R. (2003). A strategy for controlling the marketing of tobaccco products: a regulated market model. *Tobacco Control*, **12**(4): 374–382.

Benowitz, N.L. and Henningfield, J.E. (1994). Establishing a nicotine threshold for addiction. The implications for tobacco regulation. *N. Engl. J. Med*, **331**:123–125.

Boffetta, P., Hecht, S., Gray, N., Gupta, P., and Straif, K. (2008). Smokeless tobacco and cancer. *Lancet Oncol.*, **7**:667–675.

Borland, R., Cappiello, M. and Owen, N. (1997). Leaving work to smoke. *Addiction*, **92**:1361–1368.

Borland, R., Mullins, R., Trotter, L. and White, V. (1999). Trends in environmental tobacco smoke restrictions in the home in Victoria, Australia. *Tob. Control*, **8**:266–271.

Boyle, P., Gandini, S., Robertson, C., Zatonski, W., Fagerstrom, K., Slama, K., *et al.* (2000). Characterisics of smoker's attitudes towards stopping. *Eur. J. Public Health*, **10**:5–14.

Chaloupka, F.J., Hu, T., Warner, K.E., Jacobs, R. and Yurekli, A. (2000). The taxation of tobacco products. In: Anonymous *Tobacco Control in Developing Countries*, pp. 237–272. Oxford: Oxford University Press.

Chapman, S. (2001). Australian bar worker wins payout in passive smoking case. *BMJ*, **322** (7295):1139.

Chapman, S., Borland, R., Scollo, M., Brownson, R.C., Dominello, A. and Woodward, S. (1999). The impact of smoke-free workplaces on declining cigarette consumption in Australia and the United States. *Am. J. Public Health*, **89**:1018–1023.

Chilmonczyk, B.A., Salmun, L.M., Megathlin, K.N., Neveux, L.M., Palomaki, G.E., Knight, G.J., *et al.* (1993). Association between exposure to environmental tobacco smoke and exacerbations of asthma in children. *N. Engl. J. Med*, **328**:1665–1669.

Colley, J.R., Holland, W.W. and Corkhill, R.T. (1974). Influence of passive smoking and parental phlegm on pneumonia and bronchitis in early childhood. *Lancet*, **2**:1031–1034.

Friend, K. and Levy, D.T. (2002). Reductions in smoking prevalence and cigarette consumption associated with mass-media campaigns. *Health Educ. Res*, **17**:85–98.

Gray, N. (1997). The global settlement – a global view. *J. Surg. Oncol.*, **66**:79–80.

Gray, N. and Boyle, P. (2002). Regulation of cigarette emissions. *Ann. Oncol*, **13**:19–21.

Harlap, S. and Davies, A.M. (1974). Infant admissions to hospital and maternal smoking. *Lancet*, **1**: 529–532.

Hirayama, T. (1981). Non-smoking wives of heavy smokers have a higher risk of lung cancer: a study from Japan. *Bull. World Health Organ 2000*, **78**:940–942.

Hocking, B., Borland, R., Owen, N. and Kemp, G. (1991). A total ban on workplace smoking is acceptable and effective. *J. Occup. Med*, **33**:163–167.

Hoffmann, D. and Hoffmann, I. (2001). The changing cigarette: chemical studies and bioassays. In: Anonymous *Risks Associated with Smoking Cigarettes with Low Machine-measured Yields of Tar and Nicotine*, pp. 159–191. Bethesda: US Department of Health and Human Services, National Institutes of Health, National Cancer Institute.

Hoffmann, D., Hoffmann, I. and El-Bayoumy, K. (2001). The less harmful cigarette: a controversial issue. a tribute to Ernst L. Wynder. *Chem. Res. Toxicol.*, **14**:767–790.

Jarvis, M.J., Boreham, R., Primatesta, P., Feyerabend, C. and Bryant, A. (2001). Nicotine yield from machine-smoked cigarettes and nicotine intakes in smokers: evidence from a representative population survey. *J. Natl. Cancer Inst*, **93**:134–138.

Kenkel, D. and Chen, l. (2000). Consumer information and tobacco use. In: P. Jha and F.J. Chaloupa (eds) *Tobacco Control in Developing Countries*, pp. 177–236. Oxford: Oxford University Press.

Kozlowski, L.T. and O'Connor, R.J. (2002). Cigarette filter ventilation is a defective design because of misleading taste, bigger puffs, and blocked vents. *Tob. Control*, **11**:i40–i50.

Kozlowski, L.T., O'Connor, R.J. and Sweeney, C.T. (2001). Cigarette design. In: Anonymous *Risks Associated with Smoking Cigarettes with Low Machine-measured Yields of Tar and Nicotine*, pp. 13–37. Bethesda MD: US Department of Health and Human Services, National Institutes of Health, National Cancer Institute.

Manley, M., Glynn, T.J. and Shopland, D. (1993). *The Impact of Cigarette Excise Taxes on Smoking among Children and Adults: Summary Report of a National Cancer Institute Expert Panel*. Bethesda MD: National Cancer Institute.

Peto, R. (1994). Smoking and death: the past 40 years and the next 40 years. *BMJ*, **309**:937–939.

Philip Morris USA. (2002). Health Issues for Smokers. Philip Morris USA. Available at: http://www.philipmorrisusa.com/DisplayPageWithTopic.asp?ID=60

Pollay, R.W. and Dewhirst, T. (2002). The dark side of marketing seemingly 'Light' cigarettes: successful images and failed fact. *Tob. Control*, **11**:I18–I31.

Russell, M.A. (1976). Low-tar medium-nicotine cigarettes: a new approach to safer smoking. *Br. Med J*, 1:1430–1433.

Stewart, B.W. and Semmler, P.C. (2002). Sharp v Port Kembla RSL Club: establishing causation of laryngeal cancer by environmental tobacco smoke. *Med J. Aust*, **176**:113–116.

Sunley, E.M., Yurekli, A. and Chaloupa, F.J. (2000). The design, administration, and potential revenue of tobacco excises. In: P. Jha and F.J. Chaloupa (eds) *Tobacco Control in Developing Countries*, pp. 409–426. Oxford: Oxford University Press.

Thun, M.J. and Burns, D.M. (2001). Health impact of 'reduced yield' cigarettes: a critical assessment of the epidemiological evidence. *Tob. Control*, 10 Suppl 1:14–11.

Trichopoulos, D., Kalandidi, A., Sparros, L. and MacMahon, B. (1981). Lung cancer and passive smoking. *Int. J. Cancer*, **27**:1–4.

United States Department of Agriculture. (2001). Tobacco World Markets and Trade. United States Department of Agriculture. Available at: http://www.fas.usda.gov/tobacco/circular/2001/0109/index.htm

Wakefield, M. and Chaloupka, F. (2000). Effectiveness of comprehensive tobacco control programmes in reducing teenage smoking in the USA. *Tob. Control*, **9**(2):177–186.

Wakefield, M., Morley, C., Horan, J.K. and Cummings, K.M. (2000). The cigarette pack as image: new evidence from tobacco industry documents. *Tob. Control*, 11 Suppl.1:I73–180.

Wayne, G.F. and Connolly, G.N. (2002). How cigarette design can affect youth initiation into smoking: Camel cigarettes 1983–93. *Tob. Control*, 11 Suppl.1:I32–139.

Weinstein, N.D. (2001). Public understanding of risk and reasons for smoking a low-yield product. In: Anonymous *Risks Associated with Smoking Cigarettes with Low Machine-measured Yields of Tar and Nicotine*, pp. 193–235. Bethesda MD: US Department of Health and Human Services, National Institutes of Health, National Cancer Institute.

WHO study group on tobacco product regulation. (2007). *Technical report series no. 95*, Geneva.

Chapter 39

Treatment of tobacco dependence

Robyn L. Richmond and Nicholas Zwar

Introduction

Tobacco use and dependence is for many people a chronic relapsing condition which they struggle to overcome over many years and which, in the words of the United States Clinical Practice Guideline 'often requires repeated intervention and multiple attempts to quit' [1]. This is primarily, though not entirely, associated with the addictive properties of nicotine. The neuropharmacology of nicotine and addiction has been comprehensively described in Chapter 8 in this book, while the genetics of nicotine addiction has been comprehensively covered in Chapter 8. Our intention in this chapter is not to repeat any of this material but to provide an overview of the principles of treatment of tobacco dependence.

The aim of treatment of tobacco dependence has been and remains to assist people to stop using tobacco products completely. This has been based on the fact that there is no safe level of tobacco smoking and every cigarette does harm [2]. Though cessation is the gold standard of treatment of tobacco dependence, the role of harm reduction strategies is expanding and is discussed in Chapter 40 in this book.

Key reasons for providing treatment for tobacco use and dependence are that, though unassisted quitting remains the most common method, rates of success are low (approximately 3–5% per year) [3] compared to evidence-based assistance strategies such as counselling and smoking cessation pharmacotherapies [4, 5]. A further reason is that the evidence on the benefits of cessation is clear, that successful quitting can result in an increase in life expectancy of up to 10 years [6].

General principles of treatment of tobacco dependence described in more detail later are [1]:

- Tobacco use should be identified and treatment offered to every tobacco user seen in a health care setting.
- Tobacco users who are willing to make a quit attempt should be encouraged to make use of evidence-based quitting strategies such as counselling and medications.
- Tobacco users can be offered a variety of counselling approaches such as individual, telephone quitlines, and group-based programmes as all have been shown to assist cessation.
- Tobacco users should be encouraged to use counselling and medication in combination as the combination is more effective than either alone.
- Professional and social support during the quit attempt are both of assistance in quitting.
- Tobacco users who are unwilling to quit should be offered motivational treatments.

Role of health professionals in the treatment of tobacco dependence

Health professionals have an important role to play in the treatment of tobacco dependence though it is important that this is seen as part of a comprehensive strategy for tobacco control. The strategy should also include public health measures such as legislation and regulation to restrict sale and advertising, restriction on use in public places, tax on tobacco products, and social marketing [7].

There is evidence that advice from health professionals is effective in encouraging smoking cessation. A Cochrane review examined evidence from 41 trials involving approximately 31 000 smokers [4]. The most common setting for advice was primary care. The pooled data from 17 trials revealed a small but significant increase in the cessation rate of about 2.5% at six months or more of follow-up compared to no advice (or usual care). Brief advice was defined as smoking cessation advice provided during a single consultation lasting less than 20 minutes plus up to one follow-up visit. This equates to one extra quitter for every 40 patients provided brief advice. In 11 trials where the intervention was more intensive, the estimated effect was higher. Further evidence that spending more time has a greater effect comes from the meta-analysis for the US Clinical Practice Guideline [8]. In this meta-analysis, minimal duration counselling (up to three minutes) was found to result in an abstinence rate of 13.4% at six months (2.5% higher than controls); low intensity (3–10 minutes) in an abstinence rate of 16.0% (5% higher than controls); and higher intensity (more than 10 minutes) in an abstinence rate of 22.1% (11% higher than controls).

A Cochrane Review of randomized trials of smoking cessation interventions delivered by nurses and involving at least six months follow-up also show a benefit [9]. Intervention provided by other health professionals such as psychologists, pharmacists, and dentists can also be effective [8]. The major effect of advice from health professionals is to motivate a quit attempt (three- to five-fold increase). It is important to remember that combining brief advice with other effective interventions such as pharmacotherapy can considerably reduce the number needed to treat.

Most of the studies examining physician advice were conducted in community settings, however smoking cessation interventions delivered to hospitalized patients can also be effective as admission to hospital can be a teachable moment for tobacco users. A Cochrane review concluded that at least one month of follow-up after discharge is needed to achieve an increase in abstinence at six months after the start of the intervention, compared to usual care [10].

Clinical practice guidelines for smoking cessation

Clinical practice guidelines are defined as 'systematically developed statements to assist practitioner and patient decisions about appropriate health care for specific clinical circumstances' [11]. Guidelines that promote interventions of proven benefit have the potential to improve health outcomes and consistency of care [12].

Given the potential health gain and cost-effectiveness of smoking cessation interventions [13], and the evidence that dissemination of guidelines can be an effective strategy for influencing clinical practice [12], there has been interest around the world in developing clinical practice guidelines for smoking cessation. The treatobacco.net website has links to 29 national or international guidelines. The majority are national guidelines but there are some on specific topics such a pregnancy or designed for particular health professionals such as primary care physicians or nurses.

Table 39.1 The 5 As for brief intervention

Ask about tobacco use	Identify and document tobacco use status for every patient at every visit
Advise to quit	In a clear, strong and personalized manner urge every tobacco user to quit
Assess willingness to make a quit attempt	Is the tobacco user willing to make a quit attempt at this time?
Assist in quit attempt	For the patient willing to make a quit attempt, use counselling and pharmacotherapy to help him or her quit
Arrange follow-up	Schedule follow-up contact, preferably the first week after the quit date

The 5As – a general description

A common approach in many clinical practice guidelines from around the world is the 5As approach of the US Clinical Practice Guideline [8]. It has been demonstrated in a randomized trial that this approach, when implemented, leads to increased cessation [14]. The 5As provide an easy to remember framework for identifying people who are tobacco users and structuring smoking cessation support. Table 39.1 from the US Clinical Practice Guideline summarizes the 5As for brief intervention. This chapter is structured around the 5As.

Figure 39.1 summarizes, in the form of a flow chart, the identification and treatment process for smokers using the 5As approach for brief intervention.

Step 1: Ask and identify the smoker

Asking about tobacco use is a key step to effective intervention and health professionals should consistently identify and document use of tobacco at every opportunity. The United States Clinical Practice Guideline recommends recording tobacco use as a vital sign along with blood pressure, pulse, weight, temperature, and respiratory rate [8].

Smoking status should be documented as current-smoker, former- or never-smoked. For current-smokers the frequency should be categorized as daily, weekly, or irregular. The amount (number per day) and year of commencement of cigarette smoking (or other tobacco use) should also be documented. For ex-smokers the quit date should be recorded.

The meta-analyses conducted for the development of the US Clinical Practice Guideline [8] found that having a screening system in place to identify smoking status leads to a substantially higher rate of clinician intervention and a small increase in the abstinence rate at six months follow-up. Instituting such a system in practice is therefore highly recommended.

Step 2: Advise

All tobacco users should be advised to quit in a way that is clear and unambiguous but also supportive and non-confrontational, personalized, and non-judgemental [8,15]. The need to quit can be linked to the patient's current health or illness to help the tobacco user recognize the personal importance of cessation. The health benefits of quitting can also be highlighted. Other ways to personalize the benefits of cessation are to discuss the importance of smoking as a risk factor for future illness, not exposing others (including children) to environmental smoke, importance as a role model to children and adolescents and saving money.

There is evidence that advising smokers repeatedly that they should quit, especially in consultations unrelated to smoking, can damage patient–doctor rapport [16]. A strategy to avoid this is to ask permission to discuss the subject of smoking [17].

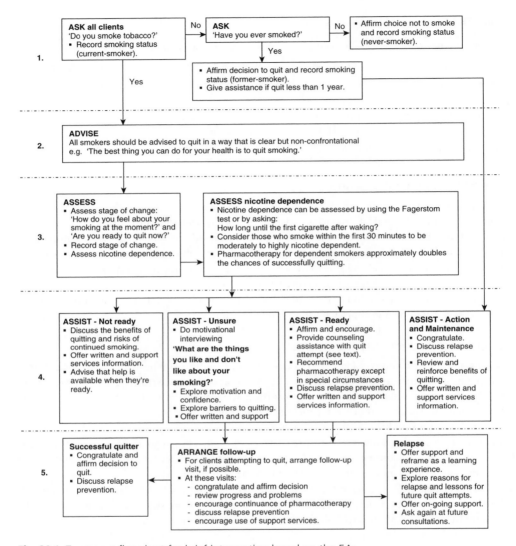

Fig. 39.1 Treatment flowchart for brief intervention based on the 5As.

Adapted from: Zwar N, Richmond R, Borland R *et al.* (2004). Smoking cessation guidelines for Australian General Practice. Canberra, Commonwealth Department of Health and Ageing [15].

All smokers should be offered written information about smoking and smoking cessation and the option of further assistance from support services such as referral to a telephone Quitline.

Step 3: Assess the smoker

The majority of smokers report wanting to quit and over 40% have made a quit attempt in the preceding year [18]. The process of stopping smoking (Stage of Readiness to Change) [19] involves a series of stages from thinking about quitting to making a quit attempt is a useful framework to identify a smoker's interest in quitting and to provide the appropriate support for the level of interest in quitting. Cessation is explained as a process, rather than a single discrete event and smokers cycle through the stages of being ready, quitting and relapsing on an average of three to four times, before achieving long term success [15].

Smokers will be in different stages of readiness when the physician sees them at different times, so readiness needs to be periodically re-evaluated (see Fig. 39.2).

However, there is increasing evidence that the likelihood of success in a quit attempt is unrelated to the smoker's expressed interest in quitting in the period leading up to the attempt: unplanned quit attempts are as likely (or even more likely) to be as successful as planned attempts [23]. This means that there is benefit in encouraging all smokers to consider quitting whenever the opportunity arises.

Willingness to quit can be assessed using a non-judgmental question [21] such as '*How do you feel about your smoking at the moment?*' Where needed, the response can be clarified by asking the smoker whether they are willing to make a quit attempt at this time or in the near future (e.g. the next 30 days).

Assessment also includes examining barriers to quitting, triggers for smoking (e.g., social situations, stress, negative emotions), social support, and the smoker's experiences in previous quit attempts. Assessing previous use of pharmacotherapy is helpful to determine if it was used optimally and what problems occurred. The implications of other physical health, mental health, and other drug dependencies also need to be assessed.

Assessing nicotine dependence

Most tobacco users become nicotine dependent. The neuropharmacology of nicotine and addiction has been covered in Chapter 8 in this book, while the cognitive effects of nicotine and withdrawal have been discussed by Balfour *et al.* Assessment of nicotine dependence will help predict whether the smoker is likely to experience nicotine withdrawal on stopping smoking. The American Psychiatric Association's Diagnostic and Statistical Manual of Mental Disorders (DSM-IV) states that nicotine dependence and withdrawal can develop with all forms of tobacco. Features of nicotine dependence include: smoking more heavily, smoking soon after waking, smoking when ill, difficulty refraining from smoking, reporting the first cigarette of the day to be the most difficult to give up and smoking more in the morning than in the afternoon.

The modified Fagerström Test for Nicotine Dependence is a validated tool to assess nicotine dependence [24] (Table 39.2).

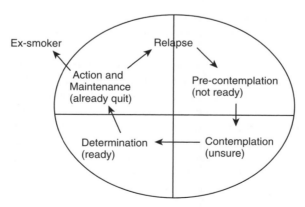

Fig. 39.2 Stages of readiness to stop smoking [20–22].

Table 39.2 Fagerström test for nicotine dependence [24]

Questions	Answers	Score
1. How soon after waking up do you smoke your first cigarette?	Within 5 minutes	3
	6–30 minutes	2
	31–60 minutes	1
2. Do you find it difficult to abstain from smoking in places where it is forbidden?	Yes	1
	No	0
3. Which cigarette would you hate to give up?	The first one in the morning	1
	Any other	0
4. How many cigarettes a day do you smoke?	10 or less	0
	11–20	1
	21–30	2
	31 or more	3
5. Do you smoke more frequently in the morning than in the rest of the day?	Yes	1
	No	0
6. Do you smoke even though you are sick in bed for most of the day	Yes	1
	No	0

Score: 1–2   very low dependence
     3–4   low dependence
     5   medium dependence
     6–7   high dependence
     8+   very high dependence

Patients who are nicotine dependent tend to smoke soon after waking so time to first cigarette is a useful quick assessment of nicotine dependence. Most dependent smokers have their first tobacco within thirty minutes of waking.

Step 4: Assist

The assistance provided is based on the assessment process described above in Step 3. The deliverable components for each readiness group (*not ready, unsure,* and *ready to quit now*), come from the Smokescreen Programme [21, 22].

Not ready smokers are not seriously considering quitting in the next six months. Smokers like these, who are unwilling to try to quit smoking, should be provided with brief advice to increase their motivation, such as pointing the benefits of quitting and the risks of continued smoking. They can be offered written information and the offer of further help at future visits.

Unsure smokers are uncertain or ambivalent about their smoking and are seriously considering quitting in the next six months. Smokers who are uncertain about quitting may be encouraged to make an attempt with *motivational interviewing* (MI). MI is a collaborative counselling technique based on a therapeutic partnership that acknowledges and explores a smoker's ambivalence about smoking and is a style of intervention that is effective in terms of provider and client satisfaction [25].

This is a method to prepare people for change and is particularly appropriate for those who are unsure and ambivalent about change and who may have concerns about quitting based on previous relapse [25, 26]. Motivation is a psychological state characterized by an eagerness or readiness to change and is dynamic and fluctuating and is not a constant trait.

Intervention delivered by a health professional enhances motivation and increases the likelihood that the smoker will try and quit [1, 27]. Smokers who receive such advice and assistance to stop smoking are more satisfied with their health care than those who do not [1, 28, 29]. It has been shown to be effective in increasing future quit attempts [16, 30].

Motivational interviewing includes a set of techniques designed to uncover ambivalence about smoking and to encourage and heighten readiness to change and enable behaviour change [1, 31, 32]. With MI the therapist/doctor explores the smoker's conflicting views about the good things about smoking and the less good things. MI is not confrontational or coercive as these approaches lead to patient resistance and reduce the probability of change. It identifies a patient's fears and difficulties and helps to resolve their issues and is a way of talking to smokers while they are struggling with behaviour change. The techniques of MI are designed to draw out the motivators or reasons of change within an individual [25, 33].

The principle of MI is to highlight the discrepancies between smoking and the smoker's own belief system. In MI there is recognition that smoking is a concern or problem and that the smoker would be better off quitting, and there is a belief that he/she will be able to quit (self-efficacy). When ambivalence about smoking has been revealed, the clinician supports change and commitment to non-smoking.

Motivational interventions are most likely to be effective when the physician is empathic, promotes patient autonomy, avoids arguments and supports the patient's self-efficacy [8]. Smokers who are unsure about quitting can be motivated to change by helping them to weigh up the pros and cons of smoking [21].

Motivation is the smoker's determination to quit smoking, become actively involved in the process of quitting, make sacrifices to achieve his/her goal, and explore the costs and benefits of quitting in a process of decisional balance. There are four steps in MI:

♦ Ask: What are the good things about smoking?
♦ Ask: What are the things you don't like about smoking?
♦ Summarize your understanding of the smoker's pros and cons and explore how much of a concern the negatives are for the smoker.
♦ Ask: Where does this leave you now?

Ready smokers are willing to quit in the next 30 days and have usually made a quit attempt within the last year. These patients can be assisted with their quit attempt. This involves the clinician helping the patient develop problems-solving skills and providing social support [8].

Box 39.1 Guiding principles of motivational interviewing

The four guiding principles [25] that underlie MI are:

♦ Express empathy by using open-ended questions, reflective listening and normalizing concerns

♦ Develop discrepancy. Cognitive dissonance is where the patient has simultaneously conflicting arguments between present behaviour (smoking) and goals (wants to quit) which generate emotional discomfort designed to assist with re evaluating motives and beliefs about smoking.

♦ Roll with resistance. Reflect back to the smoker when resistance is expressed.

♦ Support self-efficacy. With the smoker, identify and build on previous successes at quitting.

Growing out of a number of clinical trials, meta-analyses and the range of evidence-based clinical guidelines for smoking cessation; there are a number of principles and strategies to guide the clinician in delivering effective smoking cessation treatment, and these are presented in Box 39.2 and described in detail below.

Advice about quitting can be offered by many **different clinicians** including doctors, nurses, psychologists, dentists, social workers, smoking cessation specialists, and pharmacists. A multi-channel delivery approach in a variety of settings can increase the opportunities for giving the message of smoking cessation. Training improves the rates of clinical intervention with smokers [1, 35, 36]. Clinicians should foster a system change offering a **clinic-wide non-smoking environment**. This involves training staff and providing resources for smoking cessation in the waiting room. Clinicians intervene more with smoking patients when they have a clinic system that encourages identification of smokers and assessment and documentation of patients' smoking status [1]. Further, clinician training increases the likelihood of providing effective tobacco dependence treatments [1].

Cognitive behavioural therapy

Many clinical trials have shown that cognitive behavioural therapy in adult smokers improves cessation rates [37, 38]. There is a strong dose–response association between the intensity of tobacco dependence intervention and its effectiveness with an advantage of intensive advice over minimal advice [1]. Brief cognitive advice from health professionals of around 3 minutes decreased

Box 39.2 Evidence-based clinical approaches to reduce tobacco use

+ **All patients** entering primary care settings and other health care settings should be **asked about their smoking**. At the minimum, smokers should be encouraged and advised to make a quit attempt.

+ Advice about quitting can be offered by many **different clinicians** including doctors, nurses, dentists, psychologists, and pharmacists.

+ **Motivational interviewing** is a useful technique to assist smokers who are ambivalent about change to weigh up the pros and cons of smoking.

+ **Cognitive behavioural therapy** to stop smoking delivered by health professionals in a consultation setting has a significant effect on quit rates. Group or individual CBT is equally effective. Behavioural therapy offered to people with medical problems related to their smoking is highly effective.

+ **Intensive smoking cessation counselling** is more effective than brief intervention [1].

+ **Proactive** telephone counselling services, or Quitlines, and web-based interventions have a broad reach into the smoking population.

+ **Pharmacotherapies** increase the likelihood of abstinence and should be used as an adjunct to cognitive behavioural therapy.

+ **Sudden cessation**, also referred to as cold turkey, is as successful as gradual reduction in smoking [34].

+ **Follow up** increases the quit rate.

the proportion of smokers by 2% each year, while increasing the intensity of advice improves effectiveness and decreases the percent of smokers between 3% to 5% [39].

The elements of counselling and behavioral therapy include [8, 40]:

♦ review of smoking history and motivation to quit
♦ help in the identification of high-risk situations
♦ generation of problem solving strategies to deal with high-risk situations
♦ providing social support as part of treatment
♦ helping smokers obtain social support outside of treatment

Cognitive behavioral therapy offered in a **group or individually** is equally effective and success increases with treatment intensity and duration [1, 41]. The counselling components should include practical counselling consisting of problem solving and skills training, and social support included as part of treatment [1]. Group techniques, which focus on skills training and provide mutual support can also be effective in assisting smoking cessation. The meta-analysis for the United States Clinical Practice Guideline found an odds ratio of 1.3 (95% CI 1.1–1.6) with an abstinence rate of 13.9% at six months follow-up [8]. Group programmes are not appealing to all smokers but are likely to be helpful for those that do [42].

Intensive smoking cessation counselling is more effective than brief treatment [1]. There is a strong dose–response association between intensity of intervention and abstinence [1]. More intensive counselling for 10 minutes of more with further reinforcement telephone contact or multiple visits (four or more) increases the chances of smoking cessation by 55% at 6 months [1, 43]. Multiple visits of smoking cessation counselling, either face-to-face or by phone, combined with anti-smoking medications increases the likelihood of successful smoking cessation, with two or more session significantly enhancing treatment outcome, and more than eight sessions producing the highest abstinence rates [1]. However, cognitive behavioral counselling and pharmacotherapy treatments on their own are effective [1]. Among those smokers identified as not ready to quit, intense smoking cessation counselling increases satisfaction with overall healthcare [28, 44].

Self-help interventions for smoking cessation in the form of booklets, brochures, manuals, and CDs provide behavioural methods for smokers and are also available for use with other media such as video and computer [45]. On their own, these materials show marginal effect compared to no intervention [45].

Telephone counselling

Quitline telephone counselling services include proactive telephone counselling and call backs. Telephone counselling is an opportunity to deliver intensive, specialist delivered intervention which has the potential to reach a large number of smokers [1]. Telephone counselling, also known as Quitline, is provided through state or national services available in many countries (e.g., United Kingdom, Australia, United States, New Zealand). There is evidence that pro-active telephone counselling, where the counsellor initiates one or more calls to provide support or help avoid relapse is an effective intervention [1]. The meta-analysis for the United States Clinical Practice Guideline reported abstinence rate of 13% at six months follow-up [1]. Pro-active counselling is more effective than self-help intervention [46]. The evidence for reactive counselling, where the smoker initiates the call for assistance, is less clear and there is a lack of randomized studies. The impact of 'self help' intervention is smaller and less certain than pro-active counseling [8]. Adding Quitline counselling to pharmacotherapy and minimal intervention increases abstinence rates [1, 47].

Telephone counselling is effective if there is promotion of the service through the media [48]. For example, the Scottish Smokeline service and the English Quitline Services were advertised in the media and resulted in abstinence rates at 12 months of 24% and 15.6%, respectively [49, 50].

Like Quitlines, **web-based** smoking cessation interventions have the potential to reach a large number of smokers. They include proactive email prompts to smokers [51, 52]. Research will identify the best components of websites offering tobacco treatment.

Smoking cessation pharmacotherapies

Tobacco users who are willing to make a quit attempt should be encouraged to make use of evidence-based quitting strategies such as counselling and medications [8]. In the absence of contraindications, pharmacotherapy should be offered to all motivated smokers who have evidence of nicotine dependency. Smoking cessation pharmacotherapies are a useful adjunct to cognitive behavioural therapy and increase likelihood of abstinence [1].

Choice of pharmacotherapy is based on clinical suitability and patient choice [15]. The algorithm in Fig. 39.3 describes the range of pharmacotherapies to treat tobacco dependence.

Nicotine replacement therapy

The aim of nicotine replacement therapy (NRT) is to replace some of the nicotine from cigarettes without the harmful constituents found in tobacco smoke. NRT reduces withdrawal symptoms associated with nicotine addiction, allowing the smoker to focus on the psychosocial aspects of quitting [15]. Meta-analyses of the evidence on the efficacy of NRT published by the Cochrane Library [54] and United States Public Health Service [8] conclude that NRT is effective. The effect sizes (difference in abstinence rate between intervention and control groups) for different forms of NRT ranged from 5% to 12%, but no form of NRT (patch, gum, lozenge, microtab, and inhaler) was significantly better than another. In the meta-analysis of 47 studies by Fiore *et al.* the effect sizes from 7% to 17% comparing various forms of NRT to placebo at 6 months follow-up [8].

Highly dependent smokers (20 or more cigarettes per day) benefit more from 4 mg than 2 mg gum and there may be a small benefit of higher dose patches across the range of 15–42mg in 16 hour or 24 hour patches [54, 55]. Slower and rapid onset nicotine delivery systems have been combined in a number of studies, such as the transdermal patch for a steady background supply of nicotine, supplemented by gum for immediate relief of craving [56, 57]. A meta-analysis showed that combination therapy almost doubles cessation rates at 12 months, compared to one form of therapy [8]. Pre-treatment NRT, where patients who are reluctant to abruptly quit using NRT in the standard way start using NRT while they reduce smoking and then progress to a quit attempt, is also of value [58].

Nicotine replacement therapy can be used safely in people with stable cardiovascular disease but should be used with caution in people with recent myocardial infarction, unstable angina, severe arrhythmias, and recent cerebrovascular accident. NRT should be considered when a pregnant woman is otherwise unable to quit, and when the likelihood and benefits of cessation outweigh the risks of NRT [15]. Intermittent dosage forms are preferred in pregnancy due to the possible risks to the foetus of continuous exposure to nicotine. Common adverse effects with NRT depend on the dosage form. For patch they include skin erythema, allergy, and sleep disturbance; for gum, lozenge and microtab dyspepsia, and nausea; and for inhaler mouth and throat irritation [15].

Bupropion sustained release Originally developed as an antidepressant, bupropion is a non-nicotine, oral therapy which reduces the urge to smoke and symptoms from nicotine withdrawal. Bupropion doubles the cessation rate compared to placebo over 12 months. Data from two randomized, controlled trials showed 9% and 19% of smokers had not smoked for the 12 months

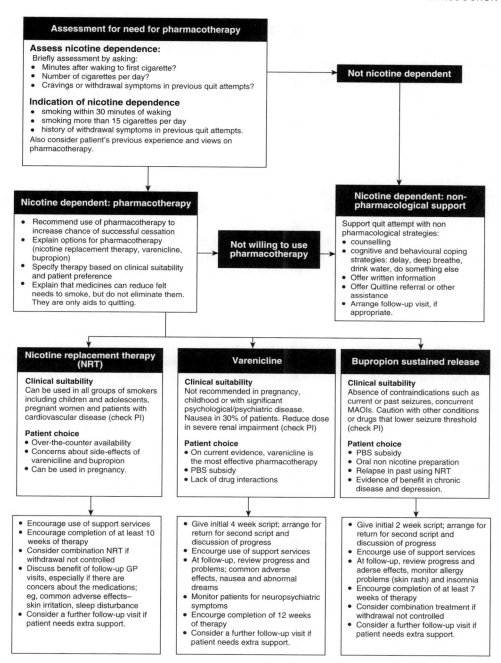

Assessment for need for pharmacotherapy

Assess nicotine dependence:
Briefly assessment by asking:
- Minutes after waking to first cigarette?
- Number of cigarettes per day?
- Cravings or withdrawal symptoms in previous quit attempts?

Indication of nicotine dependence
- smoking within 30 minutes of waking
- smoking more than 15 cigarettes per day
- history of withdrawal symptoms in previous quit attempts.
Also consider patient's previous experience and views on pharmacotherapy.

Not nicotine dependent

Nicotine dependent: pharmacotherapy
- Recommend use of pharmacotherapy to increase chance of successful cessation
- Explain options for pharmacotherapy (nicotine replacement therapy, varenicline, bupropion)
- Specify therapy based on clinical suitability and patient preference
- Explain that medicines can reduce felt needs to smoke, but do not eliminate them. They are only aids to quitting.

Not willing to use pharmacotherapy

Nicotine dependent: non-pharmacological support
Support quit attempt with non pharmacological strategies:
- counselling
- cognitive and behavioural coping strategies: delay, deep breathe, drink water, do something else
- Offer written information
- Offer Quitline referral or other assistance
- Arrange follow-up visit, if appropriate.

Nicotine replacement therapy (NRT)

Clinical suitability
Can be used in all groups of smokers including children and adolescents, pregnant women and patients with cardiovascular disease (check PI)

Patient choice
- Over-the-counter availability
- Concerns about side-effects of vareniciline and bupropion
- Can be used in pregnancy.

Varenicline

Clinical suitability
Not recommended in pregnancy, childhood or with significant psychological/psychiatric disease. Nausea in 30% of patients. Reduce dose in severe renal impairment (check PI)

Patient choice
- On current evidence, varenicline is the most effective pharmacotherapy
- PBS subsidy
- Lack of drug interactions

Bupropion sustained release

Clinical suitability
Absence of contraindications such as current or past seizures, concurrent MAOIs. Caution with other conditions or drugs that lower seizure threshold (check PI)

Patient choice
- PBS subsidy
- Oral non nicotine preparation
- Relapse in past using NRT
- Evidence of benefit in chronic disease and depression.

- Encourage use of support services
- Encourage completion of at least 10 weeks of therapy
- Consider combination NRT if withdrawal not controlled
- Discuss benefit of follow-up GP visits, especially if there are concers about the medications; eg, common adverse effects– skin irritation, sleep disturbance
- Consider a further follow-up visit if patient needs extra support.

- Give initial 4 week script; arrange for return for second script and discussion of progress
- Encourge use of support services
- At follow-up, review progress and problems; common adverse effects, nausea and abnormal dreams
- Monitor patients for neuropsychiatric symptoms
- Encourge completion of 12 weeks of therapy
- Consider a further follow-up visit if patient needs extra support.

- Give initial 2 week script; arrange for return for second script and discussion of progress
- Encourge use of support services
- At follow-up, review progress and aderse effects, monitor allergy problems (skin rash) and insomnia
- Encourge completion of at least 7 weeks of therapy
- Consider combination treatment if withdrawal not controlled
- Consider a further follow-up visit if patient needs extra support.

Fig. 39.3 Algorithm of treatment of tobacco with pharmacotherapies [53].

following placebo and bupropion therapy, respectively [41, 59]. Bupropion has been shown to be effective in a range of patient populations, including smokers with depression, cardiac disease, and respiratory diseases including chronic obstructive pulmonary disease [60]. It has also been shown to improve short-term abstinence rates for people with schizophrenia [61].

Bupropion is contraindicated in patients with a history of seizures, eating disorders, and patients taking monoamine oxidase inhibitors. It should be used with caution in people taking medications that can lower seizure threshold, such as antidepressants and oral hypoglycemic agents [62, 63]. The most clinically important adverse effect is seizures (0.1% risk). Common adverse effects are insomnia, headache, dry mouth, nausea, dizziness, and anxiety [53, 60].

Varenicline Varenicline binds with high affinity at the $\alpha4\beta2$ nicotinic acetylcholine receptor, where it acts as a partial agonist to alleviate symptoms of craving and withdrawal. At the same time, it blocks nicotine from binding to the $\alpha4\beta2$ receptor, thus reducing the intensity of the rewarding effects of smoking [53]. In two randomized double blind clinical trials, with identical study designs, varenicline was compared to both bupropion and to placebo. All three groups received brief behavioural counselling. Varenicline produced a continuous abstinence rate from week 9 through to one year of 21.9% (compared to 8.4% in the placebo group [p <0.001] and 16.1% in the bupropion group [$p = 0.057$]), and 23% (10.3% in the placebo group [p <0.001] and 14.6% in bupropion group [$p = 0.004$]), respectively [64, 65]. The abstinence rate for varenicline was significantly better than both bupropion and placebo long term.

There has been one published open label study comparing varenicline to nicotine replacement therapy, which showed a benefit for varenicline at the end of the treatment period. However, this did not reach statistical significance for the primary outcome measure of continuous abstinence from week 9 through 52 [66]. Prolonged use of varenicline has also been shown to reduce relapse, however the effect was small and not statistically significant by the one year follow-up point [67].

Nausea is the most common adverse effect with varenicline and in these studies it was reported in almost 30% of smokers, although less than 3% discontinued treatment due to nausea [65, 66]. Abnormal dreams were also more common in the varenicline group (13.1%) than either the bupropion (5.9%) or placebo groups (3.5%). The effectiveness and safety of varenicline has not been studied in patients with psychiatric conditions. Postmarketing, there have been reports of mood changes, depression, behaviour disturbance, and suicidality possibly associated with varenicline [68] and prescribers have been advised to monitor patients for emergence of these problems.

Nortriptyline The tricyclic antidepressant nortriptyline has been shown to approximately double cessation rates compared to placebo (OR=2.1) [61, 62]. A recent systematic review shows that the use of nortriptyline for smoking cessation resulted in higher prolonged abstinence rates after at least six months, compared to placebo treatment [69]. The efficacy of nortriptyline does not appear to be affected by a past history of depression; it is, however, limited in its application by its potential for serious side-effects including dry mouth, constipation, nausea, sedation, and headaches, and a risk of arrhythmia in patients with cardiovascular disease [63].

Possible future options There are a number of tobacco cessation therapies and nicotine vaccines in development. The selective type 1 cannabinoid receptor antagonist rimonabant and the nicotine receptor partial agonist cytisine have demonstrated some efficacy, and cytisine in marketed in parts of Europe, but further evidence is need on their role in smoking cessation.

Given that the currently available first line medications are equally efficacious, choice should be based on clinical suitability and patient preference.

Step 5: Arrange follow-up

Monitor smoking status After providing advice to quit, smoking status of patients should be monitored during follow-up visits particularly within the first week after quitting [1]. Follow-up has been shown to increase the likelihood of successful long-term abstinence [1, 70, 71]. As relapse frequently occurs early in the quitting process [8], follow-up contact should occur soon after the quit date, preferably during the first week [72–74] with a second follow-up recommended within the first month [1, 8] and follow-up phone calls from counsellors increases quitting [45].

Guidelines for clinician follow-up contact include:

♦ affirm abstinence and discuss benefits of not smoking
♦ monitor progress and discuss lapses if they have occurred
♦ monitor use of pharmacotherapy
♦ prepare for relapse prevention such coping strategies for high risk situations stress, negative emotional states, alcohol, social environment and weight gain
♦ encourage social support and use of support services such as the Quitline
♦ continue to enquire about smoking to encourage further quit attempts.

Relapse prevention The risk of relapse or return to smoking is more likely in the first week after a quit attempt [72, 73] with the majority of relapses occurring in the first six months. One third of ex-smokers may relapse even after non-smoking for 12 months. After two years the probability of relapse decreases to about 4% [75]. Relapse to smoking commonly occurs among those who have not planned to cope with cravings or triggers to smoke. Common triggers for relapse are alcohol and negative emotional states such as interpersonal conflict, anger, frustration, and anxiety. Smokers should be assessed for their readiness to make a quit attempt and offered more intense tobacco treatment, such as more visits to the clinician or specialist smoking cessation clinic, combination pharmacotherapy, and pro-active counselling from Quitline [1].

Recommended strategies to prevent relapse are:

♦ identify high-risk smoking situations and important smoking triggers
♦ plan coping strategies in advance
♦ consider lifestyle changes that may reduce the number of high-risk situations encountered, e.g. stress management, abstinence from alcohol, or reduction in alcohol consumption
♦ encourage patients to have a plan for how to deal with a slip to prevent it becoming a full relapse.

Quiting smoking without assistance Despite the availability of counselling support and pharmacotherapies many attempts to cease tobacco use occur without the use of evidence-based aids to cessation. Most quit attempts are unsupported and have a high rate of relapse. In the United States of the 17 million adults who attempted cessation in 1991 only 7% were still abstinent one year later [8].

Specialist smoking cessation clinics Intensive smoking cessation interventions are offered in outpatient clinics in hospitals. These are offered in group of individual sessions from specialist smoking cessation counsellors with adjunctive pharmacotherapies and self-help resources. Clinics report high success rates of between 22% and 32% [76–78]. Smokers attending clinics are a highly motivated and self-selected group compared with those attending their general practitioner and community-based programmes. Many smoking cessation clinics are engaged with research on treatment of tobacco dependence.

Special high risk groups There are specific populations that have a high burden from use of tobacco, including: women, adolescents, those with psychiatric morbidities, those who misuse substances, and those with medical co-morbidities which are commonly related to tobacco use, and prisoners. Evidence-based interventions in guidelines are effective among these groups at elevated risk. Some of treatments found to be effective among these population groups are described in Table 39.3.

Table 39.3 Smoking cessation treatments for specific sub-populations at high risk **from** tobacco use

Population group	Treatment for the specific group
Women including pregnant smokers	◆ First line pharmacotherapies: NRT, varenicline and bupropion [64] ◆ Cognitive behavioural intervention [79] ◆ Proactive telephone counselling [80] ◆ Follow-up to monitor progress and deal with problems encountered which may include weight gain, depression, hormonal changes [1, 15, 80] ◆ Pregnant women should be offered intense cognitive behavioural intervention (problem solving, social support) by their physician and proactive telephone counselling [1, 81] ◆ Self-help material in the form of booklets should supplement intervention [82, 83] ◆ The US Guidelines 2008 did not make a recommendation on use of pharmacotherapy during pregnancy, although trials of NRT reported safety of use during pregnancy [84, 85]
Adolescents	◆ Nicotine dependence is established rapidly [86, 87] ◆ Clinicians (doctors and dentists) should ask about smoking and provide a strong anti-smoking message. Cognitive behavioural counselling (self-monitoring and coping skills) increases successful abstinence [1, 88] ◆ Motivational interviewing [89, 90] ◆ Counselling sessions in a group [91] ◆ Social influence strategies [91] ◆ Monitor progress by following-up ◆ Adolescents prefer unassisted methods to stop smoking rather than intervention programmes [92] ◆ Pharmacotherapies have not been shown to promote long-term quitting [93, 94]
Those with psychiatric morbidities such as schizophrenia, depression, and suicidal ideation	◆ Bupropion [95, 96], nortriptyline [1, 96], and NRT [97, 98] ◆ Intensive smoking cessation counselling [71, 99, 100] ◆ Motivational interviewing [79, 101] ◆ Intense relapse prevention combined with NRT (patch, gum, inhaler) [79, 101] Self-help resources [102, 103] ◆ Follow-up [102, 103] ◆ As stopping smoking and nicotine withdrawal may exacerbate the patient's psychiatric condition and may affect the use of psychiatric medications, the doctor should closely monitor these patients during a quit attempt [104, 105]
Those with medical co-morbidities (e.g. cancer, coronary heart disease, chronic obstructive pulmonary disease, diabetes, and asthma) associated with and exacerbated by tobacco use	◆ Cognitive behavioural counselling [79, 99, 106] ◆ Motivational interviewing [107] including use of the medical condition as a teachable moment [108] ◆ Clinician counselling is effective among men at risk of cardiovascular disease [34] Physical activity [109] ◆ NRT [79] and bupropion [79, 110]

Table 39.3 (continued) Smoking cessation treatments for specific sub-populations at high risk **from** tobacco use

Population group	Treatment for the specific group
Those who misuse substances	◆ Varenicline [1]
Those from low socioeconomic backgrounds such as prisoners	◆ Offered advice to quit at all consultations with the doctor ◆ Motivational interviewing [1] ◆ Provide pharmacotherapy (NRT) [1] ◆ Proactive telephone counselling [1] Follow up [1] ◆ As many have limited education, booklets of advice to quit should be appropriate for the reading age of the patient.

Enhancers and barriers to quitting

Enhancers to quitting There are a number of factors that lead to successful abstinence. These include: high motivation to quit, ready to stop smoking, moderate to high belief that the quit attempt will be successful, and a social network at home and work that is supportive of non-smoking [1].

Barriers to quitting and some solutions Characteristics that are likely to lead to unsuccessful attempts at quitting include: high dependence on nicotine and heavy smoking of more than 20 cigarettes per day, depression, substance use, high levels of stress, and living with other smokers [82, 111]. Some smokers suffer depression which should be addressed at the time of quitting. Use of an antidepressant such as bupropion or nortriptyline may assist in a quit attempt as an adjunct to intensive smoking cessation counselling over several visits. A common problem encountered by smokers when attempting to quit is withdrawal symptoms. Nicotine replacement therapy will assist the smoker to overcome these symptoms by replacing the nicotine in a lower dose to that of the cigarette. Many new ex-smokers lapse during the process of long term quitting. Such lapses should be reframed as learning experiences and the lapser should be encouraged to continue in the process of abstinence. Intensive smoking cessation counselling from an expert smoking cessation or Quitline counsellor may be enhanced with pharmacotherapy or a change or combination of pharmacotherapies. Reassurance should be given as it may take many attempts at quitting before abstinence is achieved. Many smokers complain of weight gain when quitting. Some solutions include increasing physical activity and a healthy diet, and a combination of nicotine replacement therapies.

Barriers to offering smoking cessation advice Barriers raised by doctors to engaging in greater efforts to provide smoking cessation advice include: perception of lack of effect; lack of time; lack of smoking cessation skills; reluctance to raise the issue due to perceived patient sensitivity about smoking; and perceived lack of patient motivation [112].

Enhancing opportunities of clinician's offer of smoking cessation advice Training of clinicians in evidence-based smoking cessation techniques enhances delivery of effective tobacco dependence treatments [1]. Training should be directed to health professionals as well as students [113]. Medical and dental schools offer education in tobacco control and are instilling smoking cessation treatment as good clinical practice [113, 114].

Cost-effectiveness of smoking cessation interventions Smoking cessation interventions are cost-effective compared to a number of medical interventions such as the treatment of high blood pressure, high cholesterol, mammography, and Pap smears [115, 116]. Intervening with smokers is a good return on the time invested by clinicians [1], which can result in lower rates of absenteeism in the workplace [117, 118].

Smoking cessation among hospitalized patients and pregnant women is cost-effective as it reduces medical costs in the short term and the number of future bouts in hospital [119, 120]. Additionally smoking cessation among pregnant women results in fewer low birthweight babies and perinatal deaths, and fewer physical, behavioural, and cognitive problems [121].

Conclusions

Tobacco dependence is a chronic condition that often requires repeated assessment, intervention and multiple attempts to quit. This chapter has described the many principles underlying treatments for tobacco dependence that have been elucidated in Guidelines for smoking cessation. A common thread in Guidelines is the use of the 5As consisting of asking about smoking, advising on quitting, assessing nicotine dependence, and stage of readiness to change, assisting with smoking cessation using a range of components of interventions, and follow up to monitor progress. There are many effective components of treatments for smokers that produce long-term permanent abstinence. Cognitive behavioural counselling and pharmacotherapy increase the likelihood of cessation and clinicians should recommend these treatments to smokers. A multipronged approach is important to assist smokers to quit including reinforcement of non-smoking from several clinicians using a variety of evidence-based smoking cessation techniques.

References

1. Fiore, M.C., Jaen, C.R., Baker, T.B. *et al.* (2008). *Treating Tobacco Use and Dependence: 2008 Update.* Clinical Practice Guideline. US Department of Health and Human Services, Public Health Service.

2. US Department of Health and Human Services (1981). *The Health Consequences of Smoking. A Report of the Surgeon General.* US Department of Health and Human Services, Public Health Office, Office on Smoking and Health.

3. Doran, C.M., Valenti, L., Robinson, M. *et al.* (2006). Smoking status of Australian general practice patients and their quit attempts. *Addictive Behaviours*, **31**:758–66.

4. Stead, L.F., Bergson, G., Lancaster, T. *et al.* (2008). *Physician advice for smoking cessation. Cochrane Database of Systematic Reviews*, Issue 2. Art. No.: CD000165. DOI: 10.1002/14651858.CD000165.pub3.

5. Foulds, J., Steinberg, M.B., Williams, J.M. *et al.* (2006). Developments in pharmacotherapy for tobacco dependence: past, present and future. *Drug and Alcohol Review*, **25**(1):59–71.

6. Doll, R., Peto, R., Boreham, J. *et al.* (2004). Mortality in relation to smoking: 50 years' observations on male British doctors. *British Medical Journal*, **328**:1519.

7. World Health Organization (2003). *WHO Framework Convention on Tobacco Control*. Geneva, Switzerland.

8. Fiore, M.C., Bailey, W.C., Cohen, S.J. *et al.* (2000). *Treating Tobacco Use and Dependence. Clinical Practice Guideline*. Rockville, MD: US Department of Health and Human Services. Public Health Service, June.

9. Rice, V.H. and Stead, L.F. (2008). *Nursing Interventions for Smoking Cessation. Cochrane Database of Systematic Reviews*, Issue 1. Art. No.: CD001188. DOI: 10.1002/14651858.CD001188.pub3.

10. Rigotti, N., Munafo', M.R., and Stead, L.F. (2007). *Interventions for Smoking Cessation in Hospitalised Patients. Cochrane Database of Systematic Reviews*, Issue 3. Art. No.: CD001837. DOI: 10.1002/14651858.CD001837.pub2.

11 Field, M.J. and Lohr, K.N. (eds) (1990). *Clinical Practice Guidelines: Directions for a New Program*. Washington DC: National Academy Press.

12. Woolf, S.H., Grol, R., Hutchinson, A. *et al.* (1999). Potential benefits, limitations and harms of clinical guidelines. *British Medical Journal*, **318**:527–30.

13. Parrot, S., Godfrey,C., Raw, M. *et al.* (1998). Guidance for commissioners on the effectiveness of smoking cessation interventions. *Thorax*, 53:S1–38.

14. Katz, D.A., Muehlenbruch, D.R., Brown, R.L. *et al.* (2004). AHRQ Smoking Cessation Guideline Study Group. Effectiveness of implementing the agency for healthcare research and quality smoking cessation clinical practice guideline: a randomized, controlled trial. *Journal of the National Cancer Institute*, **96**(8):594–603.

15. Zwar, N., Richmond, R., Borland, R. *et al.* (2004). *Smoking Cessation Guidelines For Australian General Practice*. Canberra: Commonwealth Department of Health and Ageing, Canberra.

16. Butler, C.C., Rollnick, S., Cohen, D. *et al.* (1999). Motivational consulting versus brief advice for smokers in general practice: a randomized trial. *British Journal of General Practice*, **49** (445):11–616.

17. Butler, C.C. and Rollnick, S. (2002). Treatment of tobacco use and dependence. (Letter) *New England Journal of Medicine*, **347**(4):294–5.

18. Centers for Disease Control and Prevention (1997). Cigarette smoking among adults – United States 1995. *Morbidity and Mortality Weekly Report*, **46** (51):1217–20.

19. Prochaska, J.O. and Velicer, W.F. (1997). The transtheoretical model of health behavior change. *American Journal of Health Promotion*, **12**:38–48.

20. Prochaska, J.O. and DiClemente, C.C. (1983). Stages and processes of self-change in smoking: towards and integrative model of change. *Journal of Consulting and Clinical Psychology*, **51**:390–395.

21. Richmond, R., Webster, I., Elkins, L. *et al.* (1991). *Smokescreen for the 1990s: A stop Smoking Programme for General Practitioners to use with Smokers*. NSW Department of Health. 2nd Edition.

22. Richmond, R.L. and Mendelsohn, C.P. (1998). Physicians' views of programs incorporating stages of change to reduce smoking and excessive alcohol consumption. *American Journal of Health Promotion*, **12**(4):254–7.

23. West, R. and Sohal, T. (2006). 'Catastrophic' pathways to smoking cessation: findings from national survey. *British Medical Journal*, **332**:458–6.

24. Heatherton, T.F., Kozlowski, L.T., Frecker, R.C. *et al.* (1991). The Fagerstrom test for nicotine dependence: a revision of the Fagerstrom Tolerance Questionnaire. *British Journal of Addiction*, **86**:1119–1127.

25. Miller, W.R. and Rollnick, S. (2002). *Motivational Interviewing: Preparing People For Change* (2nd edn). New York, Guilford Press.

26. Rollnick, S., Butler, C.C., and Stott, N. (1997). Helping smokers make decisions: the enhancement of brief intervention for general medical practice. *Patient Education and Counselling*, **31**(3):191–203.

27. Rennard, S. and Daughton, D. (2000). Smoking cessation. *Chest*, **117**:360S–4S.

28. Barzilai, D.A., Goodwin, M.A., Zyzanski, S.J. *et al.* (2001). Does health habit counselling affect patient satisfaction? *Preventive Medicine*, **33**:595–9.

29. Quinn, V.P., Stevens, V.J., Hollis, J.F. *et al.* (2005). Tobacco-cessation services and patient satisfaction in nine nonprofit HMOs. *American Journal of Preventive Medicine*, **29**:77–84.

30. Steinberg, M.L., Ziedonis, D.M., Krejci, J.A. *et al.* (2004). Motivational interviewing with personalized feedback: a brief intervention for motivating smokers with schizophrenia to seek treatment for tobacco dependence. *Journal of Consulting and Clinical Psychology*, **72**:23–8.

31. Carpenter, M.J., Hughes, J.R., Solomon, L.J. *et al.* (2004). Both smoking reduction with nicotine replacement therapy and motivational advice increase future cessation among smokers unmotivated to quit. *Journal of Consulting and Clinical Psychology*, **72**:371–81.

32. Rollnick, S., Miller, W.R., and Butler, C.C. (2008). *Motivational Interviewing in Health Care: Helping Patients Change Behavior*. New York, The Guilford Press.

33. Dunn, C. and Rollnick, S. (2003). *Lifestyle Change* (Rapid Reference Series) C.V. Mosby, London, England.

34. Law, M. and Tang, J. (1995). An analysis of the effectiveness of interventions intended to help people stop smoking. *Archives of Internal Medicine*, **155**:1933–41.

35. Bao, Y., Duan, N., and Fox, S.A. (2006). Is some provider advice on smoking cessation better than no advice? An instrumental variable analysis of the 2001 National Health Interview Survey. *Health Services Research*, **41**:2114–35.

36. Carr, A.B. and Ebbert, J.O. (2007). Interventions for tobacco cessation in the dental setting. A systematic review. *Community Dental Health*, **24**:70–4.

37. Kottke, T., Battista, R., DeFriese, G. *et al.* (1988). A comparison of sustained-release bupropion and placebo for smoking cessation. *New England Journal of Medicine*, **259**: 2882–9.

38. Silagy, C. and Stead, L. (2002). *Physician Advice for Smoking Cessation (Cochrane Review)*. In: The Cochrane Library, Issue 1, Oxford: Update Software.

39. NHSCRD (National Health Service Centre for Reviews and Dissemination) (1998). Smoking cessation: what the health service can do. Effectiveness Matters, 3(1): [http://www.york.ac.uk/inst/crd/em31.htm].

40. Lancaster, T. and Stead, L.F. (2005). *Individual Behavioral Counseling for Smoking Cessation. The Cochrane Database of Systematic Reviews*, Issue 2.

41. Hurt, R., Sachs, D., Glover, E. *et al.* (1997). A comparison of sustained-release bupropion and placebo for smoking cessation. *New England Journal of Medicine*, **337**:1195–202.

42. Stead, L. and Lancaster, T. (2002). *Group behavior therapy programmes for smoking cessation*. Cochrane Review. In: The Cochrane Library, Issue 1, Oxford: Update Software.

43. Lancaster, T. and Stead, L.F. (2002). *Individual behavioral counselling for smoking cessation*. Cochrane Review. In: The Cochrane Library, Issue 1, Oxford: Update Software.

44. Conroy, M.B., Majchrzak, N.E., Regan, S. *et al.* (2005). The association between patient-reported receipt of tobacco intervention at a primary care visit and smokers' satisfaction with their health care. *Nicotine & Tobacco Research*, **7** Suppl 1:S29–34.

45. Lancaster, T. and Stead, L.F. (2002). *Self-help interventions for smoking cessation*. Cochrane Review. In: The Cochrane Library, Issue 1, Oxford: Update Software.

46. Borland, R., Segan, C.J., Livingstone, P.M. *et al.* (2001). The effectiveness of callback counseling for smoking cessation: a randomised trial. *Addiction*, **96**:881–9.

47. Stead, L.F., Perera, R., and Lancaster, T. (2006). *Telephone counselling for smoking cessation*. Cochrane Database of Systematic Reviews, Issue 3. Art. No.: CD002850. DOI: 10.1002/14651858.CD002850.pub2.

48. Ossip-Klein, D., Giovino, G., Megahed, N. *et al.* (1991). Effects of a smokers' hotline: results of a 10 county self-help trial. *Journal of Consulting and Clinical Psychology*, **59**:325–32.

49. Platt, S., Tannahil, A., Watson, J. *et al.* (1997). Effectiveness of antismoking telephone helpline: Followup survey. *British Medical Journal*, **314**:1371–5.

50. Owen, L. (2000). Impact of a telephone helpline for smokers who called during a mass media campaign. *Tobacco Control*, **9**:148–54.

51. Walters, S.T., Wright, J.A., and Shegog, R. (2006). A review of computer and Internet-based interventions for smoking behavior. *Addictive Behaviors*, **31**:264–77.

52. Lenert, L., Munoz, R.F., Perez, J.E. *et al.* (2004). Automated e-mail messaging as a tool for improving quit rates in an internet smoking cessation intervention. *Journal of the American Medical Informatics Association*, **11**:235–40.

53. Zwar, N., Richmond, R., Borland, R. *et al.* (2007). *Smoking cessation pharmacotherapy: an update for health professionals*. Melbourne: Royal Australian College of General Practitioners.

54. Stead, L.F., Perera, R., Bullen, C. *et al.* (2008). *Nicotine replacement therapy for smoking cessation. Cochrane Database of Systematic Reviews*, (1):CD000146.

55. Hughes, J.R., Lesmes, G.R., Hatsukami, D.K. *et al.* (1999). Are higher doses of nicotine replacement more effective for smoking cessation? *Nicotine and Tobacco Research*, **1**(2):169–74.

56. Kornitzer, M., Boutsen, M., Dramaix, M. *et al.* (1995). Combined use of nicotine patch and gum in smoking cessation: placebo controlled trial. *Preventive Medicine*, **24**:41–47.

57. Puska, P., Korhonen, H.J., Vartiainen, E. *et al.* (1995). Combined use of nicotine patch and gum compared with gum alone in smoking cessation: a clinical trial in North Karelia. *Tobacco Control*, **4**:231–5.

58. Shiffman, S. and Ferguson, S.G. (2008). *Nicotine patch therapy prior to quitting smoking: a meta-analysis*, **103**:557–63.

59. Jorenby, D.E., Leischow, S.J., Nides, M.A. *et al.* (1999). A controlled trial of sustained-release bupropion, a nicotine patch, or both for smoking cessation. *New England Journal of Medicine*, **340**:685–91.

60. Richmond, R. and Zwar, N. (2003). *Therapeutic review of bupropion sustained release. Drug Alcohol Review*, **22**:203–20.

61. Evins, A.E., Cather, C., Deckersbach, T., Freudenreich, O., Culhane, M.A., Olm-Shipman, C.M. *et al.* (2005). A double-blind placebo-controlled trial of bupropion sustained-release for smoking cessation in schizophrenia. *J Clin Psychopharmacol*, **25**:218–25.

62. Hughes, J.R., Stead, L.F., and Lancaster, T. (2005). Nortriptyline for smoking cessation: a review. *Nicotine Tobacco Res*, **7**:491–9.

63. Hughes, J.R., Stead, L.F., and Lancaster, T. (2007). Antidepressants for smoking cessation. *Cochrane Database of Systematic Reviews*, Issue 1. Art. No.: CD000031. DOI: 10.1002/14651858.CD000031.pub3.

64. Gonzales, D., Rennard, S.I., Nides, M., Oncken, C., Azoulay, S., Billing, C.B. *et al.* (2006). Varenicline, an $\alpha4\beta2$ nicotinic acetylcholine receptor partial agonist, vs sustained-release bupropion and placebo for smoking cessation. *J Am Med Assoc*, **296**:47–55.

65. Jorenby, D.E., Hays, J.T., Rigotti, N.A., Azoulay, S., Watsky, E.J., Williams, K.E. *et al.* (2006). Efficacy of varenicline, an $\alpha4\beta2$ nicotinic acetylcholine receptor partial agonist, vs placebo or sustained-release bupropion for smoking cessation. *J Am Med Assoc*, **296**:56–63.

66. Aubin, H.J., Bobak, A., Britton, J.R., Oncken, C., Billing, Jr. C.B., Gong, J. *et al.* (2008). Varenicline versus transdermal nicotine patch for smoking cessation: results from a randomized open-label trial. *Thorax*, **63**:717–24.

67. Tonstad, S., Tønnesen, P., Hajek, P., Williams, K.E., Billing, C.B., and Reeves, K.R. (2006). Effect of maintenance therapy with varenicline on smoking cessation. *J Am Med Assoc.*, **296**:64–71.

68. Cahill, K., Stead, L.F., and Lancaster, T. (2008). Nicotine receptor partial antagonists for smoking cessation. *Cochrane Database of Systematic Reviews*, 3:CD006103.

69. Wagena, E.J., Knipschild, P., and Zeegers, M.P. (2005). Should nortriptyline be used as a first-line aid to help smokers quit? Results from a systematic review and meta-analysis. *Addiction*, **100**:317–26.

70. Richmond, R.L., Austin, A., and Webster, I.W. (1986). Three year evaluation of a program by general practitioners to help patients stop smoking. *BMJ*, **292**:803–06.

71. Richmond, R.L., Makinson, R.J., Kehoe, L.A., Giugni, A.A., and Webster, I.W. (1993). One year evaluation of three smoking cessation interventions administered by general practitioners. *Addictive Behaviors*, **18**:187–99.

72. Hughes, J.R. (1994). *Nicotine withdrawal, dependence and abuse*. In T. Widiger, A. Frances, H. Pincus *et al.* (eds) *DSM-IV Sourcebook*. Vol 1, 109–16. Washington DC. American Psychiatric Association.

73. Kenford, S.L., Fiore, M.C., Jorenby, D.E. *et al.* (1994). Predicting smoking cessation. Who will quit with and without the nicotine patch. *JAMA*, **271**:589–94.

74. Brown, R.A., Lejuez, C.W., Kahler, C.W. *et al.* (2005). Distress tolerance and early smoking lapse. *Clin Psychol Rev*, **25**:713–33.

75. North, D., Barham, P., Glasgow, H., Glover, M. *et al.* (2002). *Guidelines for Smoking Cessation*. New Zealand National Advisory Committee on Health and Disability.

76. Foulds, J. (1996). Strategies for smoking cessation. *Br Med Bull*, **52**:157–73.

77. Croghan, I., Offord, K., Evans, R. *et al.* (1997). Cost-effectiveness of treating nicotine dependence: the Mayo Clinic experience. *Mayo Clini Proc.*, **72**:917–24.

78. Benton, B., Robinson, G., and Martin, P. (1989). The Wellington Hospital smoking cessation clinic. *NZ Med J.*, **102**:613–5.

79. Ludvig, J., Miner, B., and Eisenberg, M.J. (2005). Smoking cessation in patients with coronary artery disease. *Am Heart J*, **149**:565–72.

80. Miller, N., Frieden, T.R., Liu, S.Y., *et al.* (2005). Effectiveness of a large-scale distribution programme of free nicotine patches: a prospective evaluation. *Lancet*, **365**:1849–54.

81. Rigotti, N.A., Park, E.R., Regan, S. *et al.* (2006). Efficacy of telephone counselling for pregnant smokers: a randomized controlled trial. *Obstet Gynecol*, **108**:83–92.

82. Windsor, R.A., Cutter, G., Morris, J. *et al.* (1985). The effectiveness of smoking cessation methods for smokers in public health maternity clinics: a randomized trial. *Am J Public Health*, **75**:1389–92.

83. Windsor, R.A., Woodby, L.L., Miller, T.M. *et al.* (2000). Effectiveness of Agency for Health Care Policy and Research clinical practice guideline and patient education methods for pregnant smokers in Medicaid maternity care. *Am J Obstet Gynecol*, **182**:68–75.

84. Wisborg, K., Henriksen, T.B., Jespersen, L.B. *et al.* (2000). Nicotine patches for pregnant smokers: a randomized controlled study. *Obstet Gynecol*, **96**: 967–71.

85. Kapur, B., Hackman, R., Selby, P. *et al.* (2001). Randomized, double-blind, placebo-controlled trial of nicotine replacement therapy in pregnancy. *Curr Ther Res Clin Exp*, **62**:274–8.

86. DiFranza, J.R., Savageau, J.A., Fletcher, K. *et al.* (2007). Symptoms of tobacco dependence after brief intermittent use: the Development and Assessment of Nicotine Dependence in Youth-2 study. *Arch Pediatr Adolesc Med*, **161**:704–10.

87. DiFranza, J.R., Rigotti, N.A., McNeill, A.D. *et al.* (2000). Initial symptoms of nicotine dependence in adolescents. *Tob Control*, **9**:313–9.

88. Garrison, M.M., Christakis, D.A., Ebel, B.E. *et al.* (2003). Smoking cessation interventions for adolescents: a systematic review. *Am J Prev Med*, **25**:363–7.

89. Sussman, S., Sun, P., and Dent, C.W. (2006). A meta-analysis of teen cigarette smoking cessation. *Health Psychol*, **25**:549–57.

90. Colby, S.M., Monti, P.M., O'Leary Tevyaw, T. *et al.* (2005). Brief motivational intervention for adolescent smokers in medical settings. *Addict Behav*, **30**:865–74.

91. Horn, K., Dino, G., Kalsekar, I. *et al.* (2005). The impact of Not On Tobacco on teen smoking cessation: end-of-program evaluation results, 1998–2003. *J Adolesc Res*, **20**:640–61.

92. Centers for Disease Control and Prevention (2006). Use of cessation methods among smokers aged 16–24 years – United States, 2003. *MMWR*, **55**:1351–4.

93. Moolchan, E.T., Robinson, M.L., Ernst, M. *et al.* (2005). Safety and efficacy of the nicotine patch and gum for the treatment of adolescent tobacco addiction. *Pediatrics*, **115**:e407–14.

94. Muramoto, M.L., Leischow, S.J., Sherrill, D. *et al.* (2007). Randomized, double-blind, placebo-controlled trial of 2 dosages of sustained-release bupropion for adolescent smoking cessation. *Arch Pediatr Adolesc Med*, **161**:068–74.

95. Tashkin, D., Kanner, R., Bailey, W. *et al.* (2001). Smoking cessation in patients with chronic obstructive pulmonary disease: a double-blind, placebo-controlled, randomised trial. *Lancet*, **357**:1571–5.

96. Wagena, E.J., Knipschild, P.G., Huibers, M.J. *et al.* (2005). Efficacy of bupropion and nortriptyline for smoking cessation among people at risk for or with chronic obstructive pulmonary disease. *Arch Intern Med*, **165**:2286–92.

97. Evins, A.E., Cather, C., Rigotti, N.A. *et al.* (2004). Two-year follow-up of a smoking cessation trial in patients with schizophrenia: increased rates of smoking cessation and reduction. *J Clin Psychiatry*, **65**: 307–11. quiz 452–303.

98. Evins, A.E., Mays, V.K., Rigotti, N.A. *et al.* (2001). A pilot trial of bupropion added to cognitive behavioral therapy for smoking cessation in schizophrenia. *Nicotine Tob Res*, **3**:397–403.

99. Christenhusz, L., Pieterse, M., Seydel, E. *et al.* (2007). Prospective determinants of smoking cessation in COPD patients within a high intensity or a brief counselling intervention. *Patient Educ Couns*, **66**:162–6.

100. Sussman, S. (2002). Smoking cessation among persons in recovery. *Subst Use Misuse*, **37**:1275–98.

101. Wagena, E.J., van der Meer, R.M., Ostelo, R.J. *et al.* (2004). The efficacy of smoking cessation strategies in people with chronic obstructive pulmonary disease: results from a systematic review. *Respir Med*, **98**: 805–15.

102. Stevens, V.J., Glasgow, R.E., Hollis, J.F. *et al.* (1993). A smoking-cessation intervention for hospital patients. *Med Care*, **31**:65–72.

103. Miller, N.H., Smith, P.M., DeBusk, R.F. *et al.* (1997). Smoking cessation in hospitalized patients. Results of a randomized trial. *Arch Intern Med*, **157**:409–15.

104. Killen, J.D., Fortmann, S.P., Schatzberg, A. *et al.* (2003). Onset of major depression during treatment for nicotine dependence. *Addict Behav*, **28**:461–70.

105. Hughes, J.R. (1993). Pharmacotherapy for smoking cessation: unvalidated assumptions, anomalies, and suggestions for future research. *J Consult Clin Psychol*, **61**:751–60.

106. Ockene, J., Kristeller, J.L., Goldberg, R. *et al.* (1992). Smoking cessation and severity of disease: the Coronary Artery Smoking Intervention Study. *Health Psychol.*, **11**:19–26.

107. McClure, J.B., Westbrook, E., Curry, S.J. *et al.* (2005). Proactive, motivationally enhanced smoking cessation counselling among women with elevated cervical cancer risk. *Nicotine Tob Res.*, **7**:881–9.

108. Suplee, P.D. (2005). The importance of providing smoking relapse counselling during the postpartum hospitalization. *J Obstet Gynecol Neonatal Nurs*, **34**:703–12.

109. Fowler, B., Jamrozik, K., Norman, P. *et al.* (2002). Improving maximum walking distance in early peripheral arterial disease: randomised controlled trial. *Aust J Physiother.*, **48**:269–75.

110. Tonstad, S., Farsang, C., Klaene, G., *et al.* (2003). Bupropion SR for smoking cessation in smokers with cardiovascular disease: a multicentre, randomised study. *Eur Heart J*, **24**:946–55.

111. Han, E.S., Foulds, J., Steinberg, M.B., *et al.* (2006). Characteristics and smoking cessation outcomes of patients returning for repeat tobacco dependence treatment. *Int J Clin Pract.*, **60**:1068–74.

112. Zwar, N.A. and Richmond, R.L. (2006). Role of the general practitioners in smoking cessation. *Drug and Alcohol Rev*, **25**:21–6.

113. Richmond, R., Zwar, N., Taylor, R. *et al.* (2009 in Press). Teaching about tobacco in medical schools: a worldwide study. *Drug and Alcohol Rev.*,

114. Gordon, J., Albert, D., Crews, K. *et al.* (2009 in Press). Tobacco Education in Dentistry and Dental Hygiene. *Drug and Alcohol Rev.*,

115. Shearer, J. and Shanahan, M. (2006). Cost effectiveness analysis of smoking cessation interventions. *Aust N Z J Public Health.*, **30**:428–34.

116. Cornuz, J., Gilbert, A., Pinget, C. *et al.* (2006). Cost-effectiveness of pharmacotherapies for nicotine dependence in primary care settings: a multinational comparison. *Tob Control.*, **15**:152–9.

117. Halpern, M.T., Dirani, R., and Schmier, J.K. (2007). Impacts of a smoking cessation benefit among employed populations. *J Occup Environ Med.*, **49**:11–21.

118. Sindelar, J.L., Duchovny, N., Falba, T.A. *et al.* (2005). If smoking increases absences, does quitting reduce them? *Tob Control*, **14**:99–105.

119. Mohiuddin, S.M., Mooss, A.N., Hunter, C.B. *et al.* (2007). Intensive smoking cessation intervention reduces mortality in high-risk smokers with cardiovascular disease. *Chest*, **131**:446–52.

120. Lightwood, J., Fleischmann, K.E., and Glantz, S.A. (2001). Smoking cessation in heart failure: it is never too late. *J Am Coll Cardiol*, **37**:1683–4.

121. Lightwood, J.M., Phibbs, C.S., and Glantz, S.A. (1999). Short-term health and economic benefits of smoking cessation: low birth weight. *Pediatrics*, **104**:1312–20.

Chapter 40

Tobacco harm reduction

Dorothy Hatsukami and Mark Parascandola

Introduction

According to Orleans and Slade (1993) and Giovino (2002) there are four main targets for tobacco control: the Agent, the Vector, the Host, and the Environment. The majority of recent tobacco control efforts have been aimed at the Host (tobacco prevention and cessation programmes), the Environment (policies such as smoking bans, increased taxes, anti-smoking media campaigns, advertisement bans, pictorial warning labels), and the Vector (tobacco law suits). Relatively little attention has been focused on the Agent (the tobacco product), until recently. A range of new tobacco products have been introduced on the market with claims, implied or explicit, that they may reduce the users toxicant exposure or risk. The potential benefits and risks of these products have been actively debated among scientists and the tobacco control community, and in the policy arena. The controversial nature of this area is fueled, in part, by the concerns over the negative public health effects that resulted from prior attempts at tobacco harm reduction with the introduction of low-yield cigarettes (National Cancer Institute 2001). At the same time, the World Health Organization through the Framework Convention on Tobacco Control has proposed a reduction of tobacco toxicants in all tobacco products (Burns et al. 2008). The wide variability of toxicant levels in cigarettes (Counts et al. 2005) and in smokeless tobacco (Stepanov et al. 2005, 2008) observed in the tobacco products of most countries and the demonstrated capability of tobacco companies to reduce levels of tobacco toxicants to a specific maximal level as observed in Sweden suggest that it is feasible to implement policies to reduce toxicant levels in tobacco products.

Given the ongoing harm caused by tobacco products, re-examining a harm reduction approach to reduce tobacco-related mortality and morbidity is critically important. A high prevalence of smoking exists in many countries. Currently, over 44 million people in the United States smoke (Centers for Disease Control and Prevention 2007) and about 1.3 billion worldwide smoke cigarettes (Mackay et al. 2006). These numbers are associated with 435 000 tobacco-caused deaths per year in the United States (Centers for Disease Control and Prevention 2005) and almost 5 million per year worldwide with a projected 10 million deaths per year if current trends in smoking continue through 2020 (Mackay et al. 2006). For those who initiate tobacco use, tobacco cessation is the only known way to significantly reduce morbidity and mortality. However, because of the highly addictive nature of nicotine delivered through cigarette smoking, the majority of smokers who try to quit either on their own or through the use of behavioral and pharmacological treatments, fail to achieve abstinence (Fiore et al. 2008; Gilpin & Pierce 2002; US Department of Health & Human Services 2000). Furthermore, In recent years, the rate of decrease in the prevalence of US adult smoking has slowed significantly (Giovino 2002) and has remained at about 21% from 2004 to 2006 (Giovino 2007). Even in countries such as Ireland, which has a significant tobacco control programme (e.g., comprehensive smoke-free worksite policies, high cigarette price, and bans on tobacco advertising and promotion), a plateau in smoking prevalence has been observed (Warner 2007). This reduced rate of decline in smoking has been attributed to a plateau in smoking cessation success (Giovino 2002), leading some researchers to believe that the remaining population of smokers are either unable to quit or uninterested in making a quit attempt in the immediate future (Etter *et al.* 1997; Velicer *et al.* 1995; Warner & Burns 2003; Wewers *et al.* 2003). An appreciable number of these smokers may be experiencing mental health disorders (Warner 2007). According to results of the National Co-morbidity Survey, approximately 44.3% of the cigarettes consumed in the US are smoked by individuals with mental illness (Lasser *et al.* 2000). Although the level of interest in quitting among this vulnerable population is similar to a general population of smokers (Fiore *et al.* 2008), the rate of abstinence in some of the co-morbid populations is low (Hall 2007). The difficulty or lack of interest in quitting leaves many smokers continuing to use a highly deadly product. Therefore, it is important to consider and be open to alternative ways to reduce mortality and morbidity that complement and do not compromise current tobacco control measures. In 1998, the United Nations Focal Point on Tobacco or Health issued a report that concluded that 'to attain a substantial reduction in tobacco-caused death and disease in exiting smoker and future generations, it is important to adopt a triadic approach: a) tobacco-use prevention; b) smoking cessation; and c) reduction of exposure to tobacco toxins in people who are unable or unwilling to completely abstain from tobacco (UN Focal Point on Tobacco or Health 1998).

Ethical principles of harm reduction

The contemporary harm reduction movement originated in the substance abuse arena in the early 1980s. Early advocates of harm reduction criticized 'prohibitionist' responses to drug use and argued that criminalization and marginalization of drug users have detrimental effects (Berridge 1999). Instead, they argued that the primary focus should be on reducing the aggregate harm associated with drug use, rather than on the reduction or elimination of drug use as an end in itself (Reuter & Caulkins 1995). Examples where harm reduction interventions have been implemented include methadone programmes for heroin addicts and needle exchange to prevent HIV transmission (CDC 2005). While harm reduction approaches are not incompatible with abstinence, they are often contrasted with programmes primarily aimed at prevention or cessation of drug use. The International Harm Reduction Association currently defines harm reduction (in the context of illicit drug use) as encompassing 'policies and programs which attempt primarily to reduce the adverse health, social and economic consequences of mood altering substances to individuals drug users, their families and their communities' (International Harm Reduction Association 2009). Harm reduction approaches aim to reduce harm while, at the same time, respecting the individual choices of the drug user without making 'moralistic' judgments (Marlatt 1996; Riley & O'Hare 2000).

The fundamental values of harm reduction are closely aligned with those of public health. Scholars of public health cite four key principles in the ethical evaluation of public health interventions and programmes: maximizing conditions for health (improving morbidity and mortality), minimizing harms and burdens (the potential benefits of an intervention must be balanced against any associated risks), distributive justice (the risks and benefits of an intervention should be equitably distributed throughout the population), and respect for autonomy (Childress *et al.* 2002; Kass 2001). Public health efforts are often framed in harm reduction terms, or as relative improvements in health outcomes, because it is rare that an adverse exposure or outcome can be eliminated entirely. For example, a primary goal of the United States government's Healthy People 2010 document, for instance, is to 'increase quality and years of life (US Department of Health and Human Services 2000).

One of the key challenges, however, for both public health and harm reduction efforts is finding an appropriate balance among multiple values, which at times may appear to be in conflict (Guttman & Salmon 2004). For example, large-scale public health interventions sometimes raise concerns about conflicts between individual autonomy and maximizing health benefits to the population, such as in classic debates over disease quarantines. Public health organizations have adopted codes of ethics that recognize the need to balance population benefits with burdens to individual liberty (Thomas *et al.* 2002) and there is a substantial literature from ethicists and legal scholars on how to address this balance (Beauchamp & Steinbock 1999; Gostin 2000). In the tobacco control field, there have been calls for greater attention to human rights as a central ethical concept (Fox & Katz 2005). Nevertheless, in pursuing tobacco harm reduction, it is important to recognize the autonomy of tobacco users to make choices about their health, while, at the same time, working towards reducing the morbidity and mortality associated with tobacco use, both at the individual and population level. Thus, while it can be argued that consumers have a right to information about the relative risks of different tobacco products, there is also a public health interest in ensuring that such information is not used by tobacco manufacturers in product marketing or presented in a manner that is misleading to consumers.

While there are some parallels with harm reduction in other arenas, tobacco harm reduction poses some unique challenges. First, cigarettes and other tobacco products are heavily marketed by a large multinational industry with a well-document history of deceiving consumers regarding the health effects of its products. Second, previous attempts to promote tobacco harm reduction through reducing machine-measured tar and nicotine levels did not lead to public health benefits and may have increased harm by leading some smokers to continue smoking rather than quitting (National Cancer Institute 2001). Third, while other types of harm reduction interventions aim to reduce indirect or unintended harms associated with an activity or behaviour (such as infection caused by use of shared needles), with tobacco it is the product itself under normal conditions of use, particularly in the form of cigarettes, that confers the greatest risk.

Components associated with the assessment of harm reduction

The Institute of Medicine in the commissioned report, *Clearing the Smoke: Assessing the Science Base for Tobacco Harm Reduction*, concluded that 'for many disease attributable to tobacco use, reducing risk of disease by reducing exposure to tobacco toxicants is feasible' (Stratton, *et al.*, 2001). This conclusion was, in part, based on the dose–response relationship between toxicant exposure and risk for disease (e.g., Burns 2003; Jimenez-Ruiz *et al.* 1998; Menotti *et al.* 2001; Thun *et al.* 1995; Wynder & Stellman 1979). Burns (1997), using data from the American Cancer Society Cancer Prevention Study I, also suggested that significant and sustained reductions may lead to reduced premature mortality with the greatest benefit occurring the earlier the onset and magnitude of reduction. The IOM report also concluded that 'potential reduced exposure products ... have not been evaluated comprehensively enough to provide a scientific basis for concluding that they are associated with reduced risk for disease compared to conventional products'. Developing the science base for harm reduction will require extensive, broad-based, and multidisciplinary research.

The assessment of population harm of a tobacco product involves examining a range of variables, including the extent of toxicity of the product, intensity of use, and prevalence of use (MacCoun & Reuter 2001; Stratton & Institute of Medicine [US]. Committee to Assess the Science Base for tobacco harm reduction 2001). Furthermore, intensity of use and prevalence of use have factors that mediate or moderate their impact. Figure 40.1 illustrates these components.

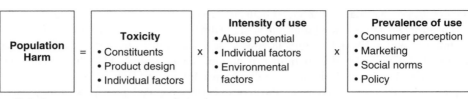

Fig. 40.1 Components to assess population harm.

Toxicity is associated with the amounts of toxicants in the product. The first stage in assessing a product's potential for exposure reduction involves examining the amount and type of constituents in the tobacco and in smoke compared to the most highly used conventional tobacco products, standardized products, or light or ultralight products. Product design features, such as cigarette ventilation (World Health Organization 2007), may also contribute to the extent of exposure to toxicants. Constituent analysis and product design analysis is accompanied by *in vitro* and *in vivo* toxicological analysis to determine if levels of specific constituents or introduction of new constituents have led to higher, similar, or lower levels of toxicity compared to existing marketed or standard testing products. Human puff smoking profiles, based on actual human smoking patterns, can be used to estimate the yields of toxicants that will potentially be delivered to humans.

However, the ultimate method to assess product toxicity is to examine the effects of the product in humans. Producing standardized methods of exposure in humans to assess the toxicity profile of a product compared with other products may be difficult. The only way this could conceivably be achieved is through controlled smoking topography (i.e., though controlling actual human smoking topography in a laboratory setting) which is then correlated with biomarkers of actual exposure or harm in the user. Valid biomarkers are related to tobacco-caused pathophysiology and distinguish tobacco users vs. non-tobacco users, demonstrate reduction as a result of cessation and a dose-response curve (cross-sectionally or as a result of reduction). Ideally, these biomarkers should also be predictive of disease (See Hatsukami *et al.* 2006 for review). Critical for the assessment of toxicant exposure is the use of exposure biomarkers, which are measures of constituents or the metabolites of these constituents in the body. Only biomarkers with short-half lives (e.g., nicotine, carbon monoxide) can be used in these human laboratory smoking topography studies because of the short duration of these trials. Toxicity may also be influenced by individual differences in bodily response to toxicants (e.g., for cancer, the extent of metabolic activation, of DNA adduct formation, repair and apoptosis and consequent gene mutation and growth of transformed cells) (Hecht and Hatsukami, in press).

Intensity or pattern of use determines the extent of exposure to toxicants. Intensity of use includes amount and topography of product use (e.g., number of cigarettes, puff duration, puff number, interpuff interval), whereas pattern of use includes temporal topography such as smoking more in the morning, smoking only during breaks at work or reserving most cigarettes until after work. Intensity or pattern of tobacco use may be moderated by the nicotine content or free nicotine levels of the product (Henningfield *et al.* 1997), product design (National Cancer Institute 2001; World Health Organization 2007), and route of delivery (which may determine amount and speed of nicotine delivery). These characteristics of a product can determine the abuse potential of the product. In addition to these product characteristics, individual factors such as nicotine metabolism (e.g., Ho & Tyndale 2007; Johnstone *et al.* 2006; Malaiyandi *et al.* 2005; Mwenifumbo & Tyndale 2007; Rao *et al.* 2000; Strasser *et al.* 2007) and dependence (Benowitz 2008), environmental factors such as bans on tobacco use and product price (Bonnie *et al.* 2007), and social factors such as extent of tobacco use within an individual's social network (e.g., Mueller *et al.* 2007) can contribute extent and pattern of use of the product.

The toxicity of the product and intensity and possibly pattern of product use will determine the extent of human exposure to the toxicants. The extent of toxicant exposure to these products can be determined by conducting clinical trials. In these clinical trials unlike the laboratory studies, biomarkers with longer half-lives such as cotinine (metabolite of nicotine) and carcinogen biomarkers (e.g., total NNAL) have been the most frequently used in studies. These biomarkers are reflective of exposure to specific constituents and are either measures of these tobacco or smoke constituents or their metabolites (e.g., 4-methylnitroasmino)-1-(3-pyridyl)-butanol [NNAL] and its glucuronides [NNAL glucs], metabolites of 4-methylnitroasmino)-1-(3-pyridyl)-butanone [NNK]; 1-hydroxypyrene [1-HOP] for pyrene; N'-nitrosonornicotine and its glucuronides for NNN; mercapturic acids of acrolein, butadiene, and benzene; see Carmella *et al.* (2009) or measures of complex mixtures (e.g., urine mutagenecity). In addition to biomarkers of exposure, biomarkers of effect can be used which includes biomarkers assessing biologically effective dose (toxicant levels in critical target tissue or organs, e.g., 4-aminobiphenyl hemoglobin adducts), injury such as early biochemical or histological effects (e.g., lipoproteins, white cells, C-reactive protein, fibrinogen, homocysteine, macrophages), or early health effects (e.g., hypertension, deterioration in lung function; Hatsukami *et al.* 2006). Exposure reduction or reductions in biomarkers of effect do not necessary connote health risk reduction. Therefore, when a product demonstrates substantial reduction in exposure and biological effects compared to conventional products or standard cigarettes, then assessments of health risk reduction resulting from the use of the products would need to be determined, particularly if the product is considered to have harm reduction potential. However, actual reduction in risk to health from switching to a PREP or in comparison with existing products may take a long period of time to determine, necessitating the need for biomarkers of exposure or effect that are associated with health risk or studying a population where clinical outcomes can be easily assessed.

To date, few biomarkers for health risk exist. The types of studies that need to be conducted is illustrated in studies that examined how levels of total NNAL, a biomarker for NNK, which is classified by International Agency for Research on Cancer as a potent carcinogen, is predictive of lung cancer (Church *et al.* 2009; Yuan *et al.* 2009). These studies used a prospective cohort, nested case-control design. Levels of total NNAL and cotinine were assessed in smokers who eventually were diagnosed with lung cancer vs. matched smokers who were not diagnosed with lung cancer. The results showed that increasing levels of NNAL were associated with increasing risk for lung cancer, even when adjusting for intensity and duration of smoking. One study found that smokers with the highest tertile total NNAL and cotinine levels showed a 8.5-fold lung cancer risk (95% CI, 3.7–19.5) compared to smokers in the lowest tertile total NNAL and cotinine levels (Yuan *et al.* 2009). Despite these two valuable studies, the level of reduction in total NNAL required for significant reduction in disease risk among long-term smokers is unknown. Data from a longitudinal study would suggest that at least a 50% reduction in cigarette smoking among smokers who smoked > 15 cigarettes per day (average of about 20 cigarettes per day to less than 10 cigarettes per day) may result in a 25% reduction in lung cancer compared to persistent heavy smokers (Godtfredsen *et al.* 2005). Interestingly, no significant reductions in fatal or nonfatal myocardial infarction, first hospitalization for chronic obstructive pulmonary disease or in all-cause mortality were observed among reducers vs. nonreducers (Godtfredsen, Holst *et al.* 2002; Godtfredsen *et al.* 2003; Godtfredsen, Vestbo *et al.* 2002). It is entirely possible that smokers would have to reduce the extent of exposure to less than five cigarettes per day, but even this level confers significant risk for disease (Bjartveit & Tverdal 2005). A more systematic study examining the extent of toxicant exposure reduction that is required for significant reduction in disease risk is needed. What is also critical for exposure and risk assessments is a panel of biomarkers that reflect the various diseases associated with tobacco use.

Prevalence or uptake of the product or the impact of a product on the uptake of other tobacco products can have a significant effect on population harm. According to the model introduced previously in Fig. 40.1 for assessing population harm, evaluating prevalence of use is an equally important component along with toxicity and intensity of use. Prevalence of use is affected not only by the abuse potential of the product (whether it is likely to promote addiction) but also by such factors as media exposure, advertising, and promotion of tobacco products, product claims and packaging and consumer perception of these claims, price as well as tobacco control measures such as smoking bans and anti-smoking campaigns and social norms (Bonnie *et al.* 2007; Hatsukami & Severson 1999; Lynch & Bonnie 1994; National Cancer Institute 2008; NIH 2006; Warner 2006; Wyckham 1999). Additionally, the introduction of a novel product may affect overall tobacco product use patterns in the population. Some scientists and tobacco control leaders have voiced significant concern about the potential for adverse consequences associated with novel nicotine and tobacco products marketed for harm reduction. These concerns include reduction in cessation rates, increased experimentation by children, or dual product use along with conventional cigarettes (Joseph *et al.* 2004; Martin *et al.* 2004). Examination of all these components is critical to determining whether changes in any one of these factors can affect population harm.

In summary, harm reduction involves the impact of the product in reducing mortality and morbidity of the population as a whole. Harm reduction is determined by the toxicity of the product, the intensity of use and therefore the extent of exposure to toxicants and resulting effect on health risk and how many people completely switch from a more deadly product to the less harmful product. If the product results in only a minor reduction in exposure to toxicants and health effects, the product abuse potential is high, and consumers perceive the product to be safer and show willingness to switch to the product, then the likelihood of population harm is high. On the other hand, if the product produces a substantial reduction in health risks compared to other marketed tobacco products, the abuse potential is moderate to high and consumers switch completely to the product, and there is no unintended consequences such as an overall increase in use of tobacco product, then the population health risk or harm may tend towards being lower.

Tobacco harm reduction approaches: potential reduced exposure products and a continuum of risk

A continuum of risk has been described for the various nicotine-containing products that have been marketed or proposed for tobacco harm reduction (Gray *et al.* 2005; Hatsukami, Joseph *et al.* 2007; Zeller *et al.* 2009). On the continuum of individual or perhaps even population risk, combustible products are considered to be the most hazardous tobacco product. Combusted potential reduce exposure products (PREPs) that reduce one or more toxicants are unlikely to significantly contribute to a reduction in the death and disease from tobacco use because of the number of complex mixtures of tobacco constituents associated with the combustion of tobacco products (Chapman 2007; Gray *et al.* 2005; Hatsukami, Joseph *et al.* 2007; Joseph *et al.* 2004; Martin *et al.* 2004; Royal College of Physicians 2007). Lower on the continuum of risk are the cigarette-like delivery devices that heat the tobacco product rather than combust them. Extensive evaluation has been conducted on these devices, primarily by the tobacco companies. One device (manufactured by Phillip Morris) in particular has been tested using a series of different methods including specific instructions for use or ad libitum use, use in a residential environment (Feng *et al.* 2006; Roethig *et al.* 2005; Roethig *et al.* 2007) or use of the product in the natural environment (Frost-Pineda *et al.* 2008; Roethig *et al.* 2008). A panel of carcinogen exposure and effect biomarkers and in one of the studies, cardiovascular risk factors (Roethig *et al.* 2008) have been used to assess the extent of reduction of the biomarkers as a result of switching to the electrically heated cigarette smoking system. The results across the studies showed significant reductions in nicotine equivalents (18–71% with the greatest reductions in residential studies) and biomarkers of carcinogen exposure such as total NNAL (25–73%), carboxyhemoglobin (23–93%), 3-hydroxypropylmercapturic acid for acrolein exposure (25–57%), S-phenylmercapturic acid for benzene exposure (49–85%) and urine mutagenicity (53–81%). A biomarker for pyrene, 1-hyrdoxypyrene, showed an increase of 17.5% at the end of the experimental phase but a reduction of 2.7% across the treatment weeks (Frost-Pineda *et al.* 2008) while other studies showed reductions from 53% to 72%. Reductions were observed for some cardiovascular risk factors but not for others (Roethig *et al.* 2008). These results demonstrate some promise in reducing exposure (although not necessarily health risks), however, one of the key issues for this device is whether consumers would readily use it.

Another tobacco harm reduction approach that has received a great deal of attention and debate is the substitution of cigarettes with lower nitrosamine, oral non-combusted tobacco products or smokeless tobacco. This approach is one of the most controversial potential methods to reduce tobacco harm. Most public health officials agree that smokeless tobacco is associated with less disease risk than smoking cigarettes. The relative risk of disease associated with smokeless tobacco use has been estimated to be at least 90% less than cigarette smoking (Rodu & Cole 1994, 1999). If smokers completely switched to smokeless tobacco use, then the relative risk of disease should theoretically be dramatically reduced (Bates *et al.* 2003; Fagerstrom & Schildt 2003; Foulds *et al.* 2003; Levy *et al.* 2004). In Sweden, the increased uptake of smokeless tobacco or snus has been used to explain the decrease in cigarette smoking among men with a consequent decrease in lung cancer mortality (Foulds *et al.* 2003), although others have suggested that the reduction in smoking in Sweden may have been due to strong tobacco control measures rather than the availability of snus (Tomar *et al.* 2003).

Whether or not this 'Swedish' experience will translate to other populations is unknown. Some public health researchers believe that reduced population harm is unlikely to occur, for example, in other countries such as the United States because of competitive marketing of both cigarettes and smokeless tobacco products and the potential of dual use of smokeless tobacco and cigarette products, the gateway effect in which smokeless tobacco users are at higher risk for cigarette smoking and the high toxicity of most US smokeless tobacco products compared to snus sold in Sweden (for a review see, Hatsukami, Ebbert *et al.* 2007; Hatsukami *et al.* 2004). Nonetheless, there are advocates for the use of smokeless tobacco as a substitute for cigarettes or as a cessation aid, particularly among those who are heavily addicted to nicotine (e.g., Bates *et al.* 2003; Ramstrom & Foulds 2006; Rodu & Cole 1994, 1999).

The rationale provided for the use of oral tobacco products is their potentially higher concentrations and faster delivery of nicotine than the existing medicinal nicotine products, and therefore greater satisfaction for the smoker. An additional benefit to the user is the widespread availability and lower cost of oral tobacco products. Yet to date, no clinical trial data exist to support the use of smokeless tobacco as a smoking cessation tool, or more importantly, to support the use of a product with fast and high nicotine delivery. Cross-sectional survey data from Sweden show that a higher rate of smoking cessation occurred among the men who began snus use after the onset of daily smoking (secondary snus users) compared to male daily smokers who never became daily snus users (88% vs. 56%; OR 5.7, 95% CI 4.9–8.1). Among male smokers who used a single smoking cessation aid, 66% of snus users quit smoking completely compared to 47% on nicotine gum (OR 2.2, 95% CI 1.3–3.7) and 32% on nicotine patch (OR 4.2, 95% CI 2.1–8.6) (Ramstrom & Foulds 2006). Similar observations were found in the small number of women using snus. National Health Interview Survey data from the United States show that male smokers who had smoked at least 100 cigarettes in their lifetime and who currently were daily snuff users were three to four times more likely to quit smoking or to have quit within the past year compared to male smokers who had never used snuff (Tomar 2002). However, in a recent United States study, researchers found men's smoking cessation rate was no higher than women's even with the greater preponderance of smokeless tobacco use in men (Zhu *et al.* 2009).

It is difficult to decipher if the findings from any of these studies reflect the characteristics of the population who is interested in using smokeless tobacco products or the effects of the products themselves. The best way to address this question would be a randomized clinical trial that compared oral tobacco products to nicotine replacement products. Although no medicinal nicotine control group was included, one small-scale study provided smokers ($n = 63$) with Skoal Bandits and a lecture on the health effects of tobacco as methods for cessation. At one year, 31% of men and 19% of women reported four weeks of cessation (Tilashalski *et al.* 1998). It is notable that among the 16 abstainers, 13 of them still used ST at one-year follow-up. Additionally, there were six other subjects who quit smoking without using smokeless tobacco products. Although the results of this pilot study appear promising, the continued use of the smokeless tobacco product is of concern because of the higher toxicity and abuse potential of these products compared to medicinal nicotine products. Therefore, if tobacco products are to be used to help smokers quit smoking, then it would be prudent to wean the user off them onto a safer product such as medicinal nicotine or to no products at all.

The product that has the least risk on the continuum is medicinal nicotine, which is essentially stripped from all constituents except nicotine. The highly regulated medicinal nicotine products have extensive safety data, but in the United States, these products are only used as a short-term cessation tool. Other countries in Europe, however, have approved use of these products for withdrawal relief, reduction of cigarette use, and even pre-treatment prior to cessation. Nonetheless, relatively speaking, for some countries the limited advertising and indications for the use of medicinal nicotine is in sharp contrast to the freely advertised tobacco products for use in any situation except cessation and use throughout the individual's lifetime. Furthermore, tobacco products can be made to be extremely addictive, can come in a multitude of flavours, and can be packaged and priced to be within the cost range of many consumers. In order to shift consumers unable to function without nicotine to safer products, a number of policies must be considered including equating the regulatory rules for tobacco and medicinal nicotine products, making medicinal products more accessible including unit cost of the product compared tobacco products, educating consumers about the relative risks of products and providing greater incentives for manufacturers to develop safer and better products that have greater appeal to the consumer (e.g., Gray *et al.* 2005; Henningfield & Slade 1998; Zeller *et al.* 2009). One caveat for advocating for the prolonged use of nicotine replacement products is the relatively few studies that have focused on primarily examining the health risks from these products. Studies have reported increase in cardiovascular risk factors and foetal toxicity associated with medicinal nicotine products (Benowitz 1998). Although no cancer risk has been associated with medicinal nicotine (Kozlowski 2007), recent studies show that in some oral medicinal product users, levels of NNN are similar to or higher at one or more time points than observed during baseline smoking. In nicotine patch users, only low levels of NNN were observed in the majority of the quitters (Stepanov *et al.* 2009). Nicotine or its metabolite, nornicotine, may be nitrosated endogenously to form significant amounts of NNN, particularly when nicotine is ingested orally, in some individuals. NNN along with NNK is one of the most carcinogenic tobacco-specific nitrosamines for humans (International Agency for Research on Cancer 2004) and has been associated with oesophageal and oral cancer in animals (Hecht 1998). Clearly, further research is needed in this area. However, these findings do not negate the premise that the medicinal nicotine products are the safest of all nicotine-containing products.

Tobacco harm reduction approaches: regulation and the reduction of tobacco toxicants

Tobacco product regulation has been considered as one of several tobacco control strategies. Currently, Article 9 in the World Health Organization Framework Convention for Tobacco Control states that each Party shall 'adopt and implement effective legislative, executive and administrative or other measures for testing and measuring [the contents and emissions of tobacco product and for the regulation of contents and emissions]'. In the United States, the Family Smoking Prevention and Control Act (Public Law 111–31): 1) grants FDA authority to require changes in current and future tobacco products to protect public health, such as the reduction or elimination of harmful ingredients, additives, and constituents; and 2) empowers FDA to reduce nicotine yields to any level other than zero (reserved to Congress). This means that the FDA could reduce nicotine to minimal levels, including levels that do not lead to addiction.

As described earlier, two main reasons highlight the urgency for research and policies in this area: 1) the wide variability of toxicant levels across currently marketed cigarette and smokeless tobacco brands and the existing capabilities of the tobacco companies to reduce the levels of these toxicants (Burns *et al.* 2008; Counts *et al.* 2005; Richter *et al.* 2008); and 2) the variability in nicotine levels across brands of cigarette and ST and the lack of oversight in the amount of nicotine in tobacco products.

The World Health Organization Study Group on Tobacco Product Regulation (TobReg) has proposed a regulatory strategy that would mandate the lowering of toxicant levels. The goal of this regulatory strategy would be to reduce the levels of selected toxic constituents per mg nicotine measured under standardized conditions (e.g., Health Canada intense smoking regimen) in the smoke of cigarettes allowed on the market. A secondary goal would be to prevent the introduction into a market of cigarettes with higher levels of smoke toxicants than brands that are already on the market (Burns *et al.* 2008). TobReg identified several cigarette toxicants targeted for regulation based on their carcinogenic and toxic activities in animals and humans, the concentrations in cigarette smoke and the potency of toxicity, the variability of toxicants across cigarette brands, the potential for the toxicant to be lowered in cigarette smoke with the existing technology, and 'the need to have constituents that represent the different phases of smoke (gas and particulate), different chemical classes, and toxicities that reflect heart and lung disease as well as cancer' (Burns *et al.* 2008). These toxicants include acetaldehyde, formaldehyde, benzene, 1,3-butadiene, acrolein, benzo(a)pyrene, carbon monoxide, NNN, and NNK. Modest reductions were recommended initially with the goal of further reductions with expanded knowledge and the development of new technologies. TobReg has also targeted the following toxicants for disclosure and monitoring: acrylonitrile, 4-aminobiphenhyl, 2-aminonaphthalene, cadmium, catechol, crotonaldehyde, hydrogen cyanide, hydroquinone, and nitrogen oxides. The study group also recommended tracking of nicotine yields per cigarettes and the ratio of tar to nicotine ratios to ensure that levels of nicotine are not increasing in these products. Furthermore, TobReg recommended that statements to consumers about the relative ranking of brands by toxicant levels should be prohibited, as they may mislead consumers into believing that these data constitute evidence that one brand is safer than another.

Nicotine content could also be an important target for regulations aimed at protecting public health. Mandated disclosure of nicotine yields and other ingredients that affect nicotine delivery would allow for stronger oversight over manufacturers' manipulation of nicotine delivery in the product. For example, one study, using data obtained from the State of Massachusetts under state reporting regulations, found that nicotine yield in cigarettes has been increasing over several years

(Connolly *et al.* 2007), which may contribute to greater dependence on cigarettes and difficulties in quitting smoking. Prior proposals for cigarettes have included maintaining high levels of nicotine while reducing tar (or toxicant) levels (Russell 1976). This strategy was proposed because cigarette smokers smoke cigarettes to achieve a specific level of nicotine and therefore, if nicotine levels in the tobacco products are high, then the smokers is unlikely to engage in compensatory tobacco use which may lead to higher levels of toxicant exposure. However, the primary concern regarding this approach would be the development and maintenance of dependence on cigarettes. Another strategy to reduce tobacco harm is to gradually reduce the nicotine content in tobacco products to non-addictive levels (Benowitz & Henningfield 1994) with or without reducing toxicant levels. Such a measure would reduce experimental smokers from becoming addicted to tobacco and would help current-smokers quit smoking. Although the proposal to reduce nicotine in cigarettes has been met with skepticism because of concerns over compensatory smoking behaviour (Jarvis & Bates 1999) and the emergence of a black market (Shatenstein 1999), this policy measure was considered to be technically feasible by the American Medical Association and the British Medical Association (Henningfield *et al.* 1998). Furthermore, in recent years, studies have been conducted that demonstrate that reduction in nicotine content in the cigarette itself, rather than through ventilated filters, does not result in any compensatory smoking behaviour (Benowitz *et al.* 2007; Benowitz *et al.* 2006; Rose & Behm 2004) or increased exposure to toxicants (Benowitz *et al.* 2007; Benowitz *et al.* 2006). Switching to reduced nicotine cigarettes can also lead to tobacco abstinence among smokers who were recruited for their lack of interest in quitting (Benowitz *et al.* 2007) and smokers who were interested in quitting (Hatsukami *et al.* 2010). Therefore, the harm reduction associated with reduced nicotine cigarettes may not be a result of reduced toxicant exposure, but a result of reducing the prevalence of smoking. The public health impact of this approach has been estimated to be equivalent to the impact of sanitation efforts in reducing death and disease, despite any mortality increases due to compensatory smoking or the emergence of a black market; and the prevalence of smoking was projected to decline from 23% to 5% (Tengs *et al.* 2005). To date, the optimal method to gradually reduce nicotine in cigarettes or other tobacco products and the period of time required for this reduction is unknown. Furthermore, the threshold dose for nicotine addiction is also unknown.

Summary and conclusion

Tobacco harm reduction can be considered as one approach to reduce tobacco-caused mortality and morbidity, but should not be considered as the primary approach. To date the only known method for reducing population harm is to eliminate the use of tobacco products through prevention or cessation. Yet, in order to assess the potential public health impact of novel products being introduced onto the market, it is essential to continue to monitor and study the evolving characteristics of tobacco products. Some new products are advertised with either explicit or implicit claims of reduced exposure or health risks which are not evidence-based and which may mislead consumers into thinking they are using 'safer' or 'safe' products. In addition, some of these novel products are advertised to be used in situations where smokers cannot smoke which may contribute to sustained dependence and continued use of tobacco products. However, some of these products may lead to reduced health risks if smokers were able to completely switch to using these products and may lead to eventual cessation of all tobacco products.

A meeting of tobacco control scientists and policy-makers predominantly from the United States was convened recently to develop a strategy and blueprint for tobacco harm reduction (Zeller *et al.* 2009). Four principles were identified as the basic foundation for the recommendations that evolved from the dialogue process: 1) 'The primary goal of tobacco control is to reduce mortality and morbidity associated with tobacco use', 2) 'Tobacco free should be the norm', 3) 'Achieving the primary goal might entail continued use of selected nicotine-containing products if to do so would deter the use of more toxic tobacco products', and 4) 'Any company marketing nicotine-containing products needs to be accountable for the toxicity of its products and must bear the burden of proof for any product claims.' The vision from this group was one in which 'virtually no one uses combustible tobacco products'. Combustible products were considered to be the most hazardous of tobacco products and to lead to the greatest proportion of tobacco-caused mortality and morbidity. In order to achieve this long-term goal, two short-term goals needed to be met which included the establishment of a public health-based regulatory control over all tobacco products and to shift tobacco users who continued to use tobacco products towards the least harmful products (e.g., medicinal nicotine) through policies and education.

Significant challenges remain to pursuing tobacco harm reduction as a public health strategy. There is a lack of evidence supporting the effectiveness, at both the individual and population level, of any specific harm reduction intervention. While theoretical and ethical principles provide a framework for pursuing harm reduction, data is needed to be able to assess the risks and benefits of any harm reduction intervention. Public health seeks to improve population health while respecting the autonomy of individual to make informed decisions about their own health. In the case of tobacco harm reduction, potential benefits must be weighed against the risks of adverse consequences, such as increased population harm from a new product or deceptive advertising that undermines individual autonomy.

Determining approaches that will reduce individual risk and population harm is complex in nature and will require examining not only the product itself but also how people use the product, individual, and environmental factors that influence product use, and how the introduction of the product will influence the use of other tobacco products. Critical to determining the feasibility of the harm reduction approach is the need for research that will provide measures and methods for tobacco product evaluation which includes assessment of toxic constituents, toxicological assays, biomarkers of exposure and effect, clinical trials, consumer perception, and surveillance. Additionally, future research should address the potential for nicotine reduction as well as tobacco toxicant reduction as a potential avenue for reducing tobacco related harm.

References

Bates, C., Fagerstrom, K., Jarvis, M.J., Kunze, M., McNeill, A. and Ramstrom, L. (2003). European Union policy on smokeless tobacco: a statement in favour of evidence based regulation for public health. *Tob Control*, **12**(4):360–7.

Beauchamp, D.E. and Steinbock, B. (1999). *New Ethics for the Public's Health*. New York: Oxford University Press.

Benowitz, N. (1998). *Nicotine Safety and Toxicity*. New York: Oxford University Press.

Benowitz, N. (2008). Clinical pharmacology of nicotine: implications for understanding, preventing, and treating tobacco addiction. *Clin Pharmacol Ther*, **83**(4):531–41.

Benowitz, N., Hall, S.M., Stewart, S., Wilson, M., Dempsey, D. and Jacob, P., 3rd. (2007). Nicotine and carcinogen exposure with smoking of progressively reduced nicotine content cigarette. *Cancer Epidemiol Biomarkers Prev*, **16**(11):2479–85.

Benowitz, N. and Henningfield, J.E. (1994). Establishing a nicotine threshold for addiction. The implications for tobacco regulation. *N Engl J Med*, **331**(2):123–5.

Benowitz, N., Jacob, P., 3rd and Herrera, B. (2006). Nicotine intake and dose response when smoking reduced-nicotine content cigarettes. *Clin Pharmacol Ther*, **80**(6):703–14.

Berridge, V. (1999). Histories of harm reduction: illicit drugs, tobacco, and nicotine. *Subst Use Misuse*, **34**(1):35–47.

Bjartveit, K. and Tverdal, A. (2005). Health consequences of smoking 1-4 cigarettes per day. *Tob Control*, **14**(5):315–20.

Bonnie, R. J., Stratton, K. and Wallace, R. B. (Eds.). (2007). *Ending the Tobacco Problem A Blueprint for the Nation*. Washington, DC: The National Academies Press.

Burns, D. (1997). Estimating the benefits of a risk reduction strategy., Poster presented at the Society for Research on Nicotine and Tobacco 3rd Annual Scientific Conference. Nashville.

Burns, D. (2003). Epidemiology of smoking-induced cardiovascular disease. *Progress in Cardiovascular Disease*, **46**(1):11–29.

Burns, D., Dybing, E., Gray, N., Hecht, S., Anderson, C., Sanner, T., *et al.* (2008). Mandated lowering of toxicants in cigarette smoke: a description of the World Health Organization TobReg proposal. *Tob Control*, **17**(2):132–41.

Carmella, S.G., Chen, M., Han, S., Briggs, A., Jensen, J., Hatsukami, D.K. *et al.* (2009). Effects of smoking cessation on eight urinary tobacco carcinogen and toxicant biomarkers. *Chem Res Toxicol*, **22**(4):734–41.

CDC. (2005). Access to Sterile Syringes. IDU/HIV Prevention. http://www.cdc.gov/idu/facts/aed_idu_acc. htm

Centers for Disease Control and Prevention. (2005). Annual smoking-attributable mortality, years of potential life lost, and productivity losses – United States, 1997–2001. *MMWR*, **54**: 625–8.

Centers for Disease Control and Prevention. (2007). Cigarette smoking among adults – United States, 2006. *MMWR*, **56**:1157–61.

Chapman, S. (2007). *Public Health Advocacy and Tobacco Control: Making Smoking History*. Oxford; Malden, MA: Blackwell Pub.

Childress, J.F., Faden, R.R., Gaare, R.D., Gostin, L.O., Kahn, J., Bonnie, R.J. *et al.* (2002). Public health ethics: mapping the terrain. *J Law Med Ethics*, **30**(2):170–8.

Church, T.R., Anderson, K.E., Caporaso, N.E., Geisser, M.S., Le, C.T., Zhang, Y., *et al.* (2009). A prospectively measured serum biomarker for a tobacco-specific carcinogen and lung cancer in smokers. *Cancer Epidemiol Biomarkers Prev*, **18**(1):260–6.

Connolly, G.N., Alpert, H.R., Wayne, G.F. and Koh, H. (2007). Trends in nicotine yield in smoke and its relationship with design characteristics among popular US cigarette brands, 1997–2005. *Tob Control*, **16**(5):e5.

Counts, M.E., Morton, M.J., Laffoon, S.W., Cox, R.H. and Lipowicz, P.J. (2005). Smoke composition and predicting relationships for international commercial cigarettes smoked with three machine-smoking conditions. *Regul Toxicol Pharmacol*, **41**(3):185–227.

Etter, J., Paernegger, T. and Ronchi, A. (1997). Distributions of smokers by stage: international comparison and association with smoking prevalence. *Prev Med*, **26**:580–5.

Fagerstrom, K.O. and Schildt, E.B. (2003). Should the European Union lift the ban on snus? Evidence from the Swedish experience. *Addiction*, **98**(9):1191–5.

Feng, S., Roethig, H.J., Liang, Q., Kinser, R., Jin, Y., Scherer, G. *et al.* (2006). Evaluation of urinary 1-hydroxypyrene, S-phenylmercapturic acid, trans,trans-muconic acid, 3-methyladenine, 3-ethyladenine, 8-hydroxy-2'-deoxyguanosine and thioethers as biomarkers of exposure to cigarette smoke. *Biomarkers*, **11**(1):28–52.

Fiore, M.C., Jaen, C.R., Baker, T.B., Bailey, W.C., Benowitz, N.L., Curry, S.J. et al. (2008). *Treating Tobacco Use and Dependence: 2008 Update*. Rockville, MD: US Department of Health and Human Services. Public Health Service.

Foulds, J., Ramstrom, L., Burke, M. and Fagerstrom, K. (2003). Effect of smokeless tobacco (snus) on smoking and public health in Sweden. *Tob Control*, **12**(4):349–59.

Fox, B.J. and Katz, J.E. (2005). Individual and human rights in tobacco control: help or hindrance? *Tob Control*, **14**(suppl_2):ii1–2. http://tobaccocontrol.bmj.com

Frost-Pineda, K., Zedler, B.K., Oliveri, D., Liang, Q., Feng, S. and Roethig, H.J. (2008). 12-Week clinical exposure evaluation of a third-generation electrically heated cigarette smoking system (EHCSS) in adult smokers. *Regul Toxicol Pharmacol.*

Gilpin, E.A. and Pierce, J.P. (2002). Demographic differences in patterns in the incidence of smoking cessation: United States 1950–1990. *Ann Epidemiol*, **12**(3):141–50.

Giovino, G.A. (2002). Epidemiology of tobacco use in the United States. *Oncogene*, **21**(48):7326–40.

Giovino, G.A. (2007). The tobacco epidemic in the United States. *Am J Prev Med*, **33**(6 Suppl):S318–26.

Godtfredsen, N.S., Holst, C., Prescott, E., Vestbo, J. and Osler, M. (2002). Smoking reduction, smoking cessation, and mortality: a 16-year follow-up of 19,732 men and women from The Copenhagen Centre for Prospective Population Studies. *Am J Epidemiol*, **156**(11):994–1001.

Godtfredsen, N.S., Osler, M., Vestbo, J., Andersen, I. and Prescott, E. (2003). Smoking reduction, smoking cessation, and incidence of fatal and non-fatal myocardial infarction in Denmark 1976-1998: a pooled cohort study. *J Epidemiol Community Health*, **57**(6):412–6.

Godtfredsen, N.S., Prescott, E. and Osler, M. (2005). Effect of smoking reduction on lung cancer risk. *JAMA*, **294**(12):1505–10.

Godtfredsen, N.S., Vestbo, J., Osler, M. and Prescott, E. (2002). Risk of hospital admission for COPD following smoking cessation and reduction: a Danish population study. *Thorax*, **57**(11):967–72.

Gostin, L.O. (2000). *Public Health Law: Power, Duty, Restraint.* Berkeley, New York: University of California Press; Milbank Memorial Fund.

Gray, N., Henningfield, J.E., Benowitz, N.L., Connolly, G.N., Dresler, C., Fagerstrom, K. *et al.* (2005). Toward a comprehensive long term nicotine policy. *Tob Control*, **14**(3):161–5.

Guttman, N. and Salmon, C.T. (2004). Guilt, fear, stigma and knowledge gaps: ethical issues in public health communication interventions. *Bioethics*, **18**(6):531–52.

Hall, S.M. (2007). Nicotine interventions with comorbid populations. *Am J Prev Med*, **33**(6 Suppl):S406–13.

Hatsukami, D., Benowitz, N.L., Rennard, S.I., Oncken, C. and Hecht, S.S. (2006). Biomarkers to assess the utility of potential reduced exposure tobacco products. *Nicotine Tob Res*, **8**(4):600–22.

Hatsukami, D., Ebbert, J.O., Feuer, R.M., Stepanov, I. and Hecht, S.S. (2007). Changing smokeless tobacco products new tobacco-delivery systems. *Am J Prev Med*, **33**(6 Suppl):S368–78.

Hatsukami, D., Joseph, A.M., Lesage, M., Jensen, J., Murphy, S.E., Pentel, P.R. *et al.* (2007). Developing the science base for reducing tobacco harm. *Nicotine Tob Res*, **9** Suppl 4:S537–53.

Hatsukami, D., Kotlyar, M., Hertsgaard, L.A., Zhang, Y., Carmella, S.G., Jensen, J. et al. (2010). Reduced nicotine content cigarettes: Effects on toxicant exposure, dependence and cessation. *Addiction*, **105** (2): 343–55.

Hatsukami, D., Lemmonds, C. and Tomar, S.L. (2004). Smokeless tobacco use: harm reduction or induction approach? *Prev Med*, **38**(3):309–17.

Hatsukami, D. and Severson, H.H. (1999). Oral spit tobacco: addiction, prevention and treatment. *Nicotine Tob Res*, **1**(1):21–44.

Hecht, S.S. (1998). Biochemistry, biology, and carcinogenicity of tobacco-specific N-nitrosamines. *Chem Res Toxicol*, **11**(6):559–603.

Hecht, S.S. and Hatsukami, D. (in press). Tobacco induced cancers and their prevention. In W. K. Hong, R. C. Bast, D. W. Kufe, R. R. Weischselbaum, W. N. Hait, R. Pollock, J. F. Holland & E. Frei (eds) *Cancer Medicine, Edition 8.* Hamilton, Ontario, Canada: BC. Decker, Inc.

Henningfield, J., Benowitz, N.L., Slade, J., Houston, T.P., Davis, R.M. and Deitchman, S.D. (1998). Reducing the addictiveness of cigarettes. Council on Scientific Affairs, *American Medical Association. Tob Control*, **7**(3):281–93. http://tc.bmjjournals.com/cgi/content/full/7/3/281.

Henningfield, J., Fant, R.V. and Tomar, S.L. (1997). Smokeless tobacco: an addicting drug. *Adv Dent Res*, **11**(3):330–5.

Henningfield, J. and Slade, J. (1998). Tobacco-dependence medications: public health and regulatory issues. *Food Drug Law J*, **53** suppl:75–114.

Ho, M.K. and Tyndale, R.F. (2007). Overview of the pharmacogenomics of cigarette smoking. *Pharmacogenomics J*, **7**(2):81–98.

International Agency for Research on Cancer. (2004). Tobacco smoke and involuntary smoking. In *IARC Monographs on the Evaluation of Carcinogenic Risks to Humans* (Vol. 83). Lyon, France: IARC.

International Harm Reduction Association. (2009). What is harm reduction? [Electronic Version]. Retrieved April 20, 2009 from http://www.ihra.net/Whatisharmreduction.

Jarvis, M.J. and Bates, C. (1999). Eliminating nicotine in cigarettes. *Tob Control*, **8**(1):106–7; author reply 7–9.

Jimenez-Ruiz, C., Kunze, M. and Fagerstrom, K. (1998). Nicotine replacement: a new approach to reducing tobacco-related harm. *Eur Resp J*, **11**(2):263–4.

Johnstone, E., Benowitz, N., Cargill, A., Jacob, R., Hinks, L., Day, I., *et al.* (2006). Determinants of the rate of nicotine metabolism and effects on smoking behavior. *Clin Pharmacol Ther*, **80**(4):319–30.

Joseph, A.M., Hennrikus, D., Thoele, M.J., Krueger, R. and Hatsukami, D. (2004). Community tobacco control leaders' perceptions of harm reduction. *Tob Control*, **13**(2):108–13.

Kass, N.E. (2001). An ethics framework for public health. *Am J Public Health*, **91**(11):1776–82.

Kozlowski, L.T. (2007). Effect of smokeless tobacco product marketing and use on population harm from tobacco use policy perspective for tobacco-risk reduction. *Am J Prev Med*, **33**(6 Suppl):S379–86.

Lasser, K., Boyd, J.W., Woolhandler, S., Himmelstein, D.U., McCormick, D. and Bor, D.H. (2000). Smoking and mental illness: A population-based prevalence study. *JAMA*, **284**(20):2606–10.

Levy, D.T., Mumford, E.A., Cummings, K.M., Gilpin, E.A., Giovino, G., Hyland, A., *et al.* (2004). The relative risks of a low-nitrosamine smokeless tobacco product compared with smoking cigarettes: estimates of a panel of experts. *Cancer Epidemiol Biomarkers Prev*, **13**(12):2035–42.

Lynch, B. S. and Bonnie, R. J. (Eds.). (1994). *Growing Up Tobacco Free: Preventing Nicotine Addiction in Children*. Washington, DC: National Academy Press.

MacCoun, R.J. and Reuter, P. (2001). *Drug War Heresies: Learning from Other Vices, Times, and Places*. Cambridge, UK; New York: Cambridge University Press.

Mackay, J., Eriksen, M. and Shafey, O. (2006). *The Tobacco Atlas* (Second edn). Atlanta, Georgia: American Cancer Society.

Malaiyandi, V., Sellers, E.M. and Tyndale, R.F. (2005). Implications of CYP2A6 genetic variation for smoking behaviors and nicotine dependence. *Clin Pharmacol Ther*, **77**(3):145–58.

Marlatt, G.A. (1996). Harm reduction: come as you are. *Addict Behav*, **21**(6):779–88.

Martin, E.G., Warner, K.E. and Lantz, P.M. (2004). Tobacco harm reduction: what do the experts think? *Tob Control*, **13**(2):123–8.

Menotti, A., Blackburn, H., Kromhout, D., Nissinen, A., Adachi, H. and Lanti, M. (2001). Cardiovascular risk factors as determinants of 25-year all-cause mortality in the seven countries study. *Eur J Epidemiol*, **17**:337–46.

Mueller, L.L., Munk, C., Thomsen, B.L., Frederiksen, K. and Kjaer, S.K. (2007). The influence of parity and smoking in the social environment on tobacco consumption among daily smoking women in Denmark. *Eur Addict Res*, **13**(3):177–84.

Mwenifumbo, J.C. and Tyndale, R.F. (2007). Genetic variability in CYP2A6 and the pharmacokinetics of nicotine. *Pharmacogenomics*, **8**(10):1385–402.

National Cancer Institute. (2001). *Risks associated with smoking cigarettes with low machine-measured yields of tar and nicotine*. Smoking and Tobacco Control Monograph No. 13 (Vol. NIH Pub. No. 02-5074). Bethesda, MD: US Department of Health and Human Services, National Institutes of Health, National Cancer Institute.

National Cancer Institute. (2008). *The role of the media in promoting and reducing tobacco use*. Tobacco Control Monograph No. 19 (Vol. NIH Pub. No. 07-6242). Bethesda, MD: US Department of Health and Human Services, National Institutes of Health, National Cancer Institute.

NIH. (2006). NIH State-of-the-Science Conference Statement on Tobacco Use: Prevention, Cessation, and Control. *Annals of Internal Medicine*, **145**:839–44.

Orleans, C. and Slade, J. (1993). *Nicotine Addiction: Principles and Management.* New York: Oxford University Press.

Ramstrom, L.M. and Foulds, J. (2006). Role of snus in initiation and cessation of tobacco smoking in Sweden. *Tob Control*, **15**(3):210–14.

Rao, Y., Hoffmann, E., Zia, M., Bodin, L., Zeman, M., Sellers, E.M. *et al.* (2000). Duplications and defects in the CYP2A6 gene: identification, genotyping, and in vivo effects on smoking. *Mol Pharmacol*, **58**(4):747–55.

Reuter, P. and Caulkins, J.P. (1995). Redefining the goals of national drug policy: recommendations from a working group. *Am J Public Health*, **85**(8 Pt 1):1059–63.

Richter, P., Hodge, K., Stanfill, S., Zhang, L. and Watson, C. (2008). Surveillance of moist snuff total nicotine, pH, moisture, un-ionized nicotine, and tobacco-specific nitrosamine content. *Nicotine & Tobacco Reseach*, **10**(11):1645–52. http://www.informaworld.com.floyd.lib.umn.edu/10.1080/14622200802412937.

Riley, D. and O'Hare, P. (2000). Harm reduction: policy and practice. *The Prevention Researcher*, **7**(2):4–8.

Rodu, B. and Cole, P. (1994). Tobacco-related mortality. *Nature*, **370**(6486):184.

Rodu, B. and Cole, P. (1999). Nicotine maintenance for inveterate smokers. *Technology*, **6**:17–21.

Roethig, H.J., Feng, S., Liang, Q., Liu, J., Rees, W.A. and Zedler, B.K. (2008). A 12-month, randomized, controlled study to evaluate exposure and cardiovascular risk factors in adult smokers switching from conventional cigarettes to a second-generation electrically heated cigarette smoking system. *J Clin Pharmacol*, **48**(5):580–91.

Roethig, H.J., Kinser, R.D., Lau, R.W., Walk, R.A. and Wang, N. (2005). Short-term exposure evaluation of adult smokers switching from conventional to first-generation electrically heated cigarettes during controlled smoking. *J Clin Pharmacol*, **45**(2):133–45.

Roethig, H.J., Zedler, B.K., Kinser, R.D., Feng, S., Nelson, B.L. and Liang, Q. (2007). Short-term clinical exposure evaluation of a second-generation electrically heated cigarette smoking system. *J Clin Pharmacol*, **47**(4):518–30.

Rose, J.E. and Behm, F.M. (2004). Effects of low nicotine content cigarettes on smoke intake. *Nicotine Tob Res*, **6**(2):309–19.

Royal College of Physicians. (2007). *Harm Reduction in Nicotine Addiction. Helping People Who Can't Quit.* London: Royal College of Physicians.

Russell, M.A. (1976). Low-tar medium-nicotine cigarettes: a new approach to safer smoking. *Br Med J*, **1**(6023):1430–3.

Shatenstein, S. (1999). Eliminating nicotine in cigarettes. *Tob Control*, **8**(1):106; author reply 7–9.

Stepanov, I., Carmella, S.G., Han, S., Pinto, A., Strasser, A.A., Lerman, C., *et al.* (2009). Evidence for endogenous formation of N'-nitrosonornicotine in some long-term nicotine patch users. *Nicotine Tob Res*, **11**(1):99–105.

Stepanov, I., Hecht, S.S., Ramakrishnan, S. and Gupta, P.C. (2005). Tobacco-specific nitrosamines in smokeless tobacco products marketed in India. *Int J Cancer*, **116**(1):16–9.

Stepanov, I., Jensen, J., Hatsukami, D. and Hecht, S.S. (2008). New and traditional smokeless tobacco: comparison of toxicant and carcinogen levels. *Nicotine Tob Res*, **10**(12):1773–82.

Strasser, A.A., Malaiyandi, V., Hoffmann, E., Tyndale, R.F. and Lerman, C. (2007). An association of CYP2A6 genotype and smoking topography. *Nicotine Tob Res*, **9**(4):511–18.

Stratton, K., Shetty, P., Wallace, R., and Bondurant, S. (eds) (2001). *Clearing the Smoke: Assessing the Science Base for Tobacco Harm Reduction.* Washington, D.C.: Institute of Medicine, National Academy Press. http://www.nap.edu/catalog/10029.html

Tengs, T.O., Ahmad, S., Savage, J.M., Moore, R. and Gage, E. (2005). The AMA proposal to mandate nicotine reduction in cigarettes: a simulation of the population health impacts. *Prev Med*, **40**(2):170–80.

Thomas, J.C., Sage, M., Dillenberg, J. and Guillory, V.J. (2002). A code of ethics for public health. *Am J Public Health*, **92**(7):1057–9.

Thun, M., Day-Lally, C., Calle, E., Flanders, W. and Heath, C. (1995). Excess mortality among cigarette smokers: changes in a 20-year interval. *Am J Public Health*, **85**(9):1223–30.

Tilashalski, K., Rodu, B. and Cole, P. (1998). A pilot study of smokeless tobacco in smoking cessation. *Am J Med*, **104**(5):456–8.

Tomar, S.L. (2002). Snuff use and smoking in US men: implications for harm reduction. *Am J Prev Med*, **23**(3):143–9.

Tomar, S.L., Connolly, G.N., Wilkenfeld, J. and Henningfield, J.E. (2003). Declining smoking in Sweden: is Swedish Match getting the credit for Swedish tobacco control's efforts? *Tob Control*, **12**(4):368–71.

US Department of Health & Human Services. (2000). *Reducing Tobacco Use: A Report of the Surgeon General*. Atlanta, Georgia: US Department of Health and Human Services, Centers for Disease Control and Prevention, National Center for Chronic Disease Prevention and Health Promotion.

US Department of Health and Human Services. (2000). Healthy People 2010 (Vol. Conference ed. 2 vols). Washington, DC: US Department of Health and Human Services. http://www.healthypeople.gov/.

UN Focal Point on Tobacco or Health. (1998). *Social and Economic Aspects of Reduction of Tobacco Smoking by Use of Alternative Nicotine Delivery Systems (ANDS)*. Geneva: United Nations.

Velicer, W.F., Fava, J.L., Prochaska, J.O., Abrams, D.B., Emmons, K.M. and Pierce, J.P. (1995). Distribution of smokers by stage in three representative samples. *Prev Med*, **24**(4):401–11.

Warner, K.E. (2007). Charting the science of the future where tobacco-control research must go. *Am J Prev Med*, **33**(6 Suppl):S314–7.

Warner, K. E. (Ed.). (2006). *Tobacco Control Policy, Robert Wood Johnson Foundation*. San Francisco, CA: Jossey-Bass.

Warner, K.E. and Burns, D.M. (2003). Hardening and the hard-core smoker: concepts, evidence, and implications. *Nicotine Tob Res*, **5**(1):37–48.

Wewers, M.E., Stillman, F.A., Hartman, A.M. and Shopland, D.R. (2003). Distribution of daily smokers by stage of change: Current Population Survey results. *Prev Med*, **36**:710–20.

World Health Organization. (2007). *The Scientific Basis of Tobacco Product Regulation*. Report of a WHO Study Group. Geneva, Switzerland: World Health Organization.

Wyckham, R.G. (1999). Smokeless tobacco in Canada: deterring market development. *Tob Control*, **8**(4):411–20.

Wynder, E. and Stellman, S. (1979). Impact of long-term filter cigarette usage on lung and larynx cancer risk: a case-control study. *J Natl Cancer Inst*, **62**:471–7.

Yuan, J.M., Koh, W.P., Murphy, S.E., Fan, Y., Wang, R., Carmella, S.G. *et al.* (2009). Urinary levels of tobacco-specific nitrosamine metabolites in relation to lung cancer development in two prospective cohorts of cigarette smokers. *Cancer Res*, **69**(7):2990–5.

Zeller, M., Hatsukami, D. and the Strategic Dialogue Group (2009). The strategic dialogue on tobacco harm reduction: A vision and blueprint for action in the United States. *Tob Control*, **18**:324–332.

Zhu, S.H., Wang, J.B., Hartman, A., Zhuang, Y., Gamst, A., Gibson, J. T. *et al.* (2009). Quitting Cigarettes Completely or Switching to Smokeless: Do U.S. Data Replicate the Swedish Results? *Tob Control*, **18**:82–87.

Chapter 41

Influencing politicians to implement comprehensive tobacco control: the power of news media

Simon Chapman

At the centre of comprehensive tobacco control programmes lie evidence-based strategies capable of reaching entire populations through tobacco tax, legislation, regulation, and well-funded mass reach public information campaigns. The Framework Convention on Tobacco Control (FCTC) [1] sets out the most complete articulation of what nations need to do to reduce tobacco consumption and the disease it causes. While the FCTC is the most complete statement of the tasks facing tobacco control, its key elements have been at the core of efforts to reduce tobacco use since the UICC first set them out in the historic 1980 document 'Guidelines for Smoking Control' [2].

In the 30 years since, the history of tobacco control has seen pioneering examples of political leadership in a handful of nations where comprehensive tobacco control was trailblazed. Leaders in nations such as Sweden, Finland, Thailand, Canada, Australia, and parts of the United States of America were the first to write into law proposals that had hitherto been seen as radical, and raised the ire of transnational tobacco corporations and many other industries which had benefited from tobacco advertising and sponsorship or which feared that smoke-free legislation would cause smokers to abandon restaurants and bars.

The actions of these pioneering politicians set in train rapid bandwagon effects, so that today comprehensive tobacco control programmes have become more common as politicians in less adventurous parliaments have been able to point to the growing normality of laws advertising bans, bold pack warnings, and smokefree indoor air legislation. Nations with negligible tobacco control legislation such as Indonesia are today in the minority and considered international tobacco control 'basket cases' [3].

Despite it being easier today for governments to act, regrettably many still do not, or instead to the dismay of public health community, they introduce tepid control measures implemented over long time frames. Moreover, nations which have already introduced the majority of the FCTC's provisions, still have millions of tobacco users and tobacco use is still the leading cause of death. In such nations, we are now witnessing efforts to expand the meaning of comprehensive tobacco control to embrace policies such as plain 'generic' packaging [4], laws that require all tobacco retail displays to be under the counter, and radical hikes in tobacco tax. If the recommendations of the World Health Organisation's TobReg Committee [5] get traction, we will also see widespread efforts to regulate tobacco itself.

So while tobacco control has made enormous leaps in the past decade, the need for potent advocacy remains as important as it has always been in the intertwined goals of raising public concern about the urgency tobacco control and convincing politicians to take action. Without political support, there is no hope for strong tobacco control law and policy. There is thus no more important task in tobacco control than in securing political support.

Below, I provide a brief practitioners' guide to some fundamental principles of tobacco control advocacy in its core tasks of convincing politicians to act and supporting them when they do. I have set these out at length in two books [6–7], which readers should consult for fuller expositions.

Throughout my career I have had professional and personal dealings with many health ministers from both progressive and conservative sides of politics. Politicians, particularly health ministers, are of absolutely cardinal importance of the passage of tobacco control legislation. If a health minister is not interested in tobacco control, or sees it as a political liability, that legislation will not progress. The central task of tobacco control advocacy is therefore how to persuade health ministers of the importance of tobacco control and to then try to extend that influence to the health minister's cabinet colleagues, without whose support legislation will not pass. If the government's political majority relies on the votes of a small number of independent politicians, these too will be critical to your efforts.

The importance of news media

A simple yet vital lesson about influencing politicians is to understand the centrality of the news media in their lives. Like many people, a politician's first waking moment everyday involves listening to the early morning news coverage on the clock radio alarm that wakes them up and then plays in their home as they get ready for work. Politicians also spent many hours in hotel rooms, with their main companion is the television set, again often in the form of news programmes. From the moment of waking, politicians are exposed more than any of us to how the news media is covering issues relevant to their portfolio. A newspaper is read at the breakfast table; news is consumed on the car radio on the way to work; and on arrival at work, the politician's press secretary will provide a briefing about opportunities and threats which are happening in the news media that day.

Many public health advocates put great energy into trying to secure face-to-face appointments with health ministers so that they can 'put their case' for a particular proposal. But if a health minister has never encountered the issue in the news previously, it is likely that low priority will be given to meeting with people representing an issue that is not the subject of news coverage. Politicians and their staff devote a great amount of effort to trying to get difficult issues out of news pages, and to climbing aboard issues they believe will advantage them politically.

Tobacco control advocates' tasks are therefore bound up with both keeping tobacco control in the news as an unavoidable issue for politicians while at the same time doing all that can be done to avoid framing the politicians who need to take action as the problem. As discussed below, like everyone else, politicians tend not to be attracted to people or movements who are constantly critical of them, preferring to assist and deal with people who can frame them in a good light. Here, tobacco control advocates can almost always frame the challenges of tobacco control as being about the need to control the tobacco industry and its beneficiaries. Attacking the politicians who are the ones you need to take political decisions is generally a step of the very last resort, and one that generally destines a proposal to be considered by a future government.

It follows from this that potent public health advocates need to make the business of news making part of their core business and in doing so, to acquire a thorough knowledge and instinctive understanding the way in which news organizations operates and the nature of newsworthiness. Information about the size of the audience and readership of different media at different times of the day is basic, as is familiarity with news routines and deadlines. Advocates need to also know the predilections of interests of journalists in all news media. Some will have particular interest in tobacco control. Others will be hostile toward it will therefore require careful attention.

Perhaps the most basic lesson but I have learned in my 30-year career in public health advocacy is the importance of standing back from the 'text' of news, and trying to understand the power of its subtexts. For example, a story about a new research report on smoking in bars, and the concentration of particles inhaled by bar staff, is likely to be deemed newsworthy not because of the scientific particulars of the story, the journal in which it was published, or anything to do with the quality of the research. Journalists are typically not trained in science or epidemiology, and do not run a research 'quality meter' over potential research stories in deciding to run them. What they do react to though, is the subtext of such research which here is bound up with the injustice of bar staff having to endure working conditions that other workers have long been protected from when smoking has been banned from other workplaces. The force and news values of the story lie in its implied injustice and implications for those responsible [8], not in the details of the exposure.

Politicians and their staff are also inexpert in science and epidemiology, and tend to react to stories in the same way as journalists. Advocates need to develop ways of seeing that anticipate and harness these very ordinary human ways of understanding news.

Ten basic questions for planning advocacy strategy[1]

The following ten questions should be considered by all advocates before embarking on an advocacy campaign.

1 What are your public health objectives with this issue?

Put simply, what do you want to change or preserve? All proposed advocacy strategies need then to be interrogated for their relevancy to achieving these objectives. Anyone engaging in advocacy needs to be clear about the overall public health aims and objectives of the advocacy work in which they are engaged. Failure to understand and constantly reflect on these objectives can mean embarking on strategies which consume much unproductive energy and contribute little to advancing the real public health goals with which advocates should be finally concerned. Advocacy is a *strategy* within public health, and like the adoption of any strategy, decisions about advocacy should result from a disciplined analysis of the problem being addressed. Advocacy is not an end in itself. Failure to understand this can lead to situations where advocacy objectives override the public health objectives that they were originally designed to meet.

2 Can a 'win–win' outcome be first engineered with decision-makers?

Politicians and other key decision-makers are naturally keen to avoid being seen to be pressured into making decisions, and would much prefer to be seen to be leading initiatives rather than being pressured into adopting them. Wherever possible, advocates should try to first work with government to affect a marriage of interests. I have long been in the habit of providing relevant politicians with copies of material and press releases that are about to be issued, in a spirit of not wanting to 'blindside' them, leaving an uninformed when a journalist calls for comment. I am almost always thanked for doing this.

When obdurate government intransigence is the root problem, criticism is generally unavoidable but will often close doors. In such circumstances, it is important to divide your advocacy voices into the moderates who will continue to work the 'inside route' with government and the vanguards who will take a critical public role in the media, setting the public agenda.

---

[1] This is an edited version of Chapman, S. (2004). Advocacy for public health: a primer. *Journal of Epidemiology and Community Health* **58**:361–5.

3 Who do the key decision-makers answer to, and how can these people be influenced?

In all democracies, key health decision-makers remain answerable to those who appoint or elect them. Political parties hang onto power by virtue of winning marginal seats in elections. If those marginal electorates vote differently at the next election, governments can fall. Health ministers are answerable to political cabinets and health bureaucrats are answerable to health ministers who will not relish their portfolio being criticized. Business executives are answerable to boards of directors. Advocates therefore need to study ways of accessing and influencing those whom key decision makers worry about or who endorse their policies.

4 What are the strengths and weaknesses of your and your opposition's position?

You, your opposition, and the positions both are advocating require ruthless auditing for the ways in which they are perceived by those whose support and influence is being courted. What you learn here will be critical both to your own presentation and to the tack you take in discrediting your opponents. Know your opposition inside out and keep all manner of antennae alert for feedback about your own organization's public reception. Rehearse the worst questions you could face, and practice putting forward your own most compelling points. Go to every interview with a maximum of three points you want to make, regardless of what you are asked.

5 What are your media advocacy objectives?

Your advocacy objectives must always serve your agreed public health objectives, and not be confused as ends in themselves (such as relentlessly pursuing media exposure with dubious connection to your agreed goals). Media advocacy objectives can include causing a neglected issue to become discussed or a much discussed issue to be discussed *differently*; discrediting one's opponents; introducing pivotally compelling facts and perspectives into a debate; or introducing different voices in ways calculated to enhance the authenticity or power of an argument.

6 How will you frame what is at issue?

Political debate is largely about multiple definitions of the same events and accordingly, advocates need to ensure that the way they define what is at issue in a health debate becomes the dominant definition circulating in the community. Framing strategy is the core skill of media advocacy. For example, in the debate about plain packaging, the tobacco industry will seek to frame tobacco packaging as sacrosanct, inviolable territory, the commercial intellectual property of each company. Those pushing for the adoption of plain packaging will describe the same packaging as the last bastions for tobacco companies to promote their products to young smoker. The tobacco industry seeks to frame tobacco advertising as freedom of speech, while tobacco control advocates try to reframe it as the highly researched effort at attracting children to smoking that will lead many of them into years of addiction and eventual disease. If the industry's definition dominates, controls on advertising are unlikely.

7 What symbols or word pictures can be brought into this frame?

The news media's demands for brevity require that we maximize every opportunity to leave a lasting impression with media audiences. Many public health issues appear arcane, technical, and impenetrable to ordinary people and unlikely to excite public or political interest. To gain their attention and to locate public health issues in shared value frameworks, the perspicacious and evocative use of analogy and metaphor is important. Think of how the change you want has parallels and precedents in other widely embraced areas of public life. Associate your cause with the same values that underlie these accepted issues.

Advocates also need to appreciate the dramaturgical dimension to news gathering. Significantly, journalists refer to those appearing in the news as 'talent' and audiences often assess news 'performance' through criteria like believability, trustworthiness, and how likeable those in the news were. Decide which 'role' you want to play and how you will seek to cast your opposition.

8 What sound bites can be used to convey 6 and 7?

The length of time given to newsmakers to speak in the media continues to shrink. In Australia and the United States today, the average length that a person interviewed on the news speaks for is just seven seconds [9]. Often, these 'sound bites' are the only statements reported and so assume critical importance. The larger the audience for a news bulletin, the more truncated is the time devoted to each item. Those who disdain and eschew such news media should be disqualified as serious advocates. Every interview with a journalist should plan to inject at least one sound bite into the conversation. These are pithy, memorable, and repeatable summations that can come to epitomize a debate. A memorable example: 'a non-smoking section of a restaurant is like a non-urinating section of a swimming pool'.

9 Can the issue be personalized?

A senior Sydney journalist once told me, unforgettably, that 'experts are fine, but they are not actually a living thing'. Journalists hunger for ways to locate health stories within stories about real people who are affected by a health problem [9]. Experts are typically stock embellishments to the 'real' human story that is crafted to address the concerns and interests of ordinary readers. If journalists try to ground the story via an ordinary citizen's perspective, involving consumers in advocacy will be important as you will be seen as having both expertise and authenticity.

Don't assume that tobacco control stories are all about experts and scientists. All tobacco control stories are ultimately about reducing disease in people who would otherwise die avoidable deaths. Try to bring them into the story.

10 How can large numbers of people be quickly organized to express their concerns?

Statements from 'the usual suspects' who always speak up for an issue risk being marginalized by politicians as predictable and unimportant. Efforts to build vocal constituencies for issues who are willing to speak out at strategically important times should therefore be given high priority. Newspaper letters pages are seen as key barometers of community concern. All politicians talk of the impression they gain from the reaction (or lack of it) of their electorate to issues in the news. Internet tools such as distribution lists, list servers, and chat rooms permit instant mass dissemination of 'action alerts' to hundreds and sometimes thousands of people: email templates that describe a problem, provide key pieces of information, outline suggested courses of action, and equip recipients with relevant facts and data. Within minutes, thousands of people can be mobilized to write letters to politicians and newspapers, call radio stations, vote in online opinion polls, or petition decision-makers.

Finally, advocacy for tobacco control takes time. Governments typically do not regard this area with the urgency with which they routinely treat acute health crises, where the number of people affected compared to those affected by tobacco can be much smaller. In Australia, governments first acted to control tobacco advertising in 1976, when direct radio and television advertising was banned. It took until 1994 for all sporting sponsorship by tobacco companies to end, and until 2004 for the exempted Formula One Grand Prix to stop running tobacco sponsored cars. The time it took between banning smoking in public halls and cinemas until smoking was banned in sites where smoke was most concentrated (bars) took even longer. These time spans are typical and hold special challenges for tobacco control advocates. The need to constantly refresh messages and avoid journalists believing that issue has gone stale, is utmost here.

References

1. Roemer, R., Taylor, A., and Lariviere, J. (2005). Origins of the WHO Framework Convention on Tobacco Control. *Am J Public Health*, **95**:936–8.
2. Gray, N. and Daube, M. (1980). *Guidelines for smoking control*. Geneva: UICC.
3. Reynolds, C. (1999). The fourth largest market in the world. *Tobacco Control*, **8**:89–91.

4. Freeman, B., Chapman, S., and Rimmer, M. (2008). Review: The case for plain packaging of tobacco products. *Addiction*, **103**:580–90.

5. Burns, D.M., Dybing, E., Gray, N., Hecht, S., Anderson, C., Sanner, T. *et al.* (2008). Mandated lowering of toxicants in cigarette smoke: a description of the World Health Organization TobReg proposal. *Tobacco Control*, **17**:132–41.

6. Chapman, S. and Lupton, D. (1994). *The Fight for Public Health: principles and practice of public health media advocacy*. London: British Medical Journal Books.

7. Chapman, S. (2007). *Public Health Advocacy and Tobacco Control: Making Smoking History*. Oxford: Blackwell.

8. Iyengar, S. (1991). *Is Anyone Responsible?: How Television Frames Political Issues*. Chicago: University of Chicago Press.

9. Chapman, S., Holding, S., Ellerm, J., Heenan, R., Fogarty, A., Imison, M. *et al.* (2009). The structure of Australian TV reportage on health and medicine: a guide for health workers. *Med J Aust*, **191**: 620–24.

Chapter 42

Origins and status of the WHO Framework Convention on Tobacco Control

Vera Luiza da Costa e Silva and Douglas Bettcher

Introduction

Although tobacco use was first identified as a public health problem in the mid-twentieth century, the tobacco epidemic only gained global attention many years later. Governments and the public health community postponed their reaction due to their inability to fully identify and understand the multi-sectoral dimensions and actions needed for effective tobacco control.

From the 1950s well into the 1990s, the scientific community rarely studied tobacco product design, contents, or emissions. The tobacco industry's marketing strategies were not well known and only a handful of countries were making serious attempts to regulate the products and the industry. Proposals on how to best to counteract the epidemic were in the early development stages in most countries. The industry's subversive tactics were evident [1] and the scientific community had to be cognizant that tobacco products are legally manufactured, traded, and used around the world and are subject to the same rights and rules of every legal good.

Globalization has opened the door for the tobacco industry to promote its products in new markets. This has shifted the epidemic from developed to developing countries. Over the later part of the twentieth century, significant increases in smoking were identified, especially among males. The epidemic was rapidly spreading to increasingly vulnerable groups such as women, youth, and finally the poor. The need for concerted national and international regulatory efforts became evident. Scientific studies in multiple countries and populations demonstrated that tobacco products caused consumer dependence, which in turn increased tobacco-related disease and ultimately death caused by tobacco use. In the 1990s, tobacco was accountable for about 3.9 million deaths and the death toll was over 4.9 million by the year 2000 with 4.1% of Disability Adjusted Life Years (DALYs)[1] (59.1 million) worldwide [2].

National tobacco control laws that have taken strong measures during this period of time proved to be powerless to address the transnational aspects of tobacco control such as: marketing and promotion; smuggling; regulation; and product design [3]. Other areas that needed international attention included tax and price interventions and strategies to monitor tobacco industry interference on public health policies.

Disturbingly, the largest private tobacco companies were transnational and had developed corporate strategies and operations that focused on global market penetration [1]. Furthermore, long-term consequences of the liberalization of tobacco-related trade and investment were

---

[1] DALYs = Disability Adjusted Life Years: The sum of years of potential life lost due to premature mortality and the years of productive life lost due to disability.

considered to significantly increase the burden of death and disease caused by tobacco, particularly in developing countries. Controlling the rapid globalization of tobacco consumption in an era of trade liberalization was therefore also daunting [4].

A new tactic was urgently needed to control the epidemic and empower countries to address the cross-border and transnational nature of the tobacco epidemic. Additional consideration was needed to establish mechanisms, means, and technical cooperation which would empower national governments to engage in tobacco control strategies [5, 6].

WHO reaction to the smoking epidemic

After a World Health Assembly (WHA) resolution in 1970, the World Health Organization (WHO) initiated a crusade to introduce tobacco control at the country level. Only after the passage of 16 WHA resolutions did Member States begin to adjust their views concerning the public health threat of tobacco [7]. After the 1970s, the tobacco industry quickly advanced their agenda to undermine tobacco control policies and regulations, notably discrediting the WHO [8].

The idea of a framework convention that utilized international law and that would include protocols to further public health was a catalyst for tobacco regulation. The so-called framework convention/protocol approach to international lawmaking allowed States to proceed incrementally. First, the proposed framework convention would establish the general norms and institutions of the regime – for example, its objective, principles, basic obligations, and institutions. Then, the protocols build on the parent agreement through the elaboration of additional (or more specific) commitments and institutional arrangements. Examples of the framework convention/protocol approach, the Vienna Convention on Ozone Depletion/Montreal Protocol and the Framework Convention on Climate Change/Kyoto Protocol, were considered as useful models to frame the tobacco control convention [9].

Although the WHA endorsed the idea of a tobacco control approach via an international treaty in 1996, an institutional commitment to the WHO Framework Convention on Tobacco Control (WHO FCTC) only surfaced in 1998 when Gro Harlem Brundtland took office as Director General of the WHO and created the Tobacco Free Initiative (TFI) as a cabinet project [10].

In May 1999, the Fifty-Second WHA paved the way for multilateral negotiations concerning the WHO FCTC and possible related protocols. Later on that year, a World Bank publication, *Curbing the Epidemic*, was released. This critical report provided both empirical and economic validation for the WHO FCTC [11]. The premier WHO Treaty whose key purpose was providing a global response to the tobacco epidemic negotiated under the WHO was forthcoming.

The WHO Framework Convention on Tobacco Control

The draft of WHO FCTC was negotiated during the six subsequent meetings of the Intergovernmental Negotiation Body that was created with a mandate to finalize a legally binding instrument that would be submitted to the WHA. The conclusion of the negotiating process and the unanimous adoption of the WHO FCTC, in full accordance with WHA resolutions in May 2003, represented a milestone for the promotion of public health and provided new legal dimensions for international health cooperation.

The WHO FCTC provides a good example of a Global Public Good (GPG), an economic tool that was created to discuss and analyse national governance. It establishes a rubric of coordinated action among states, which will bring about a significant health improvement not otherwise efficiently obtainable by states acting on their own (Taylor *et al.* 2003) [12].

The WHO FCTC became legally effective in February 2005, 90 days after the deposit of the fortieth instrument of ratification, approval, acceptance, accession, or formal confirmation was made by the 40th Party to the Treaty at the United Nation depositary.

Specific features make the WHO FCTC a unique Treaty:

1. The Treaty is entirely supported by empirical evidence, making it an evidence-based international legal instrument that promotes public health while weighing important social, economic, scientific, and political considerations.
2. In contrast to previous drug control treaties it represents a paradigm shift in developing regulatory strategy for an addictive product. The treaty addresses demand reduction and supply elements simultaneously, both as part of a comprehensive strategy.
3. The Treaty starts with a preambular paragraph, which states that the Parties to the Treaty are determined to give priority to their right to protect public health; a principle that reaffirms the right of all people to the highest standard of health independent of other aspects.
4. The WHO FCTC includes a provision that addresses liability, a novel aspect of an international treaty that focuses specifically on the tobacco industry.
5. The Treaty is designed to act as a global complement to, not a replacement for, national and local tobacco control programmes and activities. In this regard, it has a complex multisectoral and transdisciplinary nature and focuses on international collaboration while still incorporating provisions for country-level implementation.
6. As the first treaty negotiated under the auspices of WHO, the WHO FCTC negotiation and implementation process serves as a prototype for the development of other international health regulations that also rely on a multisectoral approach [13].
7. The treaty includes a financial component to support the resource needs for implementation of the WHO FCTC in low- and middle-income countries.

The Treaty provisions [14]:

In contrast to other international laws, the WHO FCTC is a comprehensive Treaty with many provisions that establish core elements for its implementation. The Treaty is composed of 11 parts including 38 articles that address all tobacco control elements agreed upon by WHO Member States as a comprehensive tobacco control roadmap (Table 42.1).

The *Preamble* outlines health principles and key factors fundamental to the need for an international instrument on tobacco control. Examples are:

- The recognition of the spreading epidemic;
- Serious concerns about the impact of all forms of advertising, promotion, and sponsorship aimed at encouraging the use of tobacco products; and
- The determination of Parties to give priority to the right to protect public health.

The *Introduction* includes the use of terms and defines the relationship between the WHO FCTC and other agreements and legal instruments.

The *Objective*, 'to protect present and future generations from the devastating health, social, environmental and economic consequences of tobacco consumption and exposure to tobacco smoke by providing a framework for tobacco control measures to be implemented by the Parties at the national, regional and international levels in order to reduce continually and substantially the prevalence of tobacco use and exposure to tobacco smoke', underscores the multifaceted nature and dimensions of tobacco control.

The *Guiding principles* emphasize the Treaty's key values such as strong political commitment to develop and support comprehensive multisectoral measures and coordinated responses at all levels. Another example of the Treaty's implementation further encourages the essential participation of civil society in achieving the objective of the Convention and its protocols.

Table 42.1 Structure of the WHO Framework Convention on Tobacco Control

Preamble

Part I – *Introduction*

Part II – *Objective, Guiding Principles and General Obligations*

Part III – *Demand Reduction Measures*

- ◆ price and tax measures to reduce the demand for tobacco, and
- ◆ non-price measures to reduce the demand for tobacco
  - protection from exposure to tobacco smoke;
  - regulation of the contents of tobacco products;
  - regulation of tobacco product disclosures;
  - packaging and labeling of tobacco products;
  - education, communication, training, and public awareness;
  - tobacco advertising, promotion, and sponsorship; and,
  - demand reduction measures concerning tobacco dependence and cessation.

Part IV – *Supply Reduction Measures*

- ◆ illicit trade in tobacco products;
- ◆ sales to and by minors; and,
- ◆ provision of support for economically viable alternative activities.

Part V – *Protection of the Environment*

Part VI – *Liability*

Part VII – *International Cooperation and Communication*

Part VIII – *Institutional Arrangements and Financial Resources*

Part IX – *Settlement of Disputes*

Part X – *Development of the Convention*

Part XI – *Final Provisions*

The *General obligations* outline the overarching responsibilities of the Parties. The obligation is included to establish or reinforce and finance a national coordinating mechanism or focal points for tobacco control. Parties are further obligated to protect policies from commercial and other vested interests of the tobacco industry per Article 5.3.

Part III and *Part IV* contain the core elements of the Treaty. It is within these key portions that the presence of a demand as well as supply mechanisms are implemented for cost-effective tobacco control measures [15]. If an important impact on tobacco consumption is to be realized the core elements of the WHO FCTC should be adopted by Member States. Implementation of these core measures include but are not limited to demand-oriented cost-effective measures referring to smoke-free places and health warnings. Tax and price measures are proposed in conjunction with supply measures like illicit trade of tobacco products. The Treaty further proposes the inclusion of a product regulation area as well as support for economically viable alternative activities.

Part V addresses the need for the protection of the environment and the health of persons who cultivate or manufacture tobacco products while *Part VI* deals with international cooperation and technical and legal assistance in criminal and civil liability, including compensation.

Part VII provides insight into one of the more important facets of international law, cooperation, and communication. This portion includes strategies for Party cooperation which may be directly or indirectly implemented to strengthen a Member State's capacity to fulfill the obligations. Part VII also addresses the need for the establishment of programmes for national, regional, and global surveillance of different aspects of tobacco consumption and exposure to tobacco smoke. This part of the Treaty also emphasizes the obligation of the Parties in reporting and exchanging information.

From *Part VIII* to *Part XI*, the Treaty addresses institutional and financial arrangements which initiates the machinery of the Treaty and further illuminates many areas related to the development of the convention and other procedural issues.

Developments after the Treaty entered into force

The Conference of the Parties (COP) is the established governing body of the WHO FCTC and is comprised of all Parties to the Convention. The COP meets regularly and monitors the implementation of the Convention and promotes the decisions necessary to advance its effective implementation. The COP may also adopt protocols, annexes, and amendments to the Convention [16].

The first meeting of the COP took place in early 2006. The Conference adopted its Rules of Procedure and Financial Rules and established the permanent Convention Secretariat within the WHO HQ. Further, the COP in meetings in 2007/2008, adopted: implementation guidelines for Article 5.3 (Protection of public health policies with respect to tobacco control from commercial and other vested interests of the tobacco industry); Article 8 (Protection from Exposure to Second Hand Smoke); Article 11 (Packaging and labeling of tobacco products); and Article 13 (Tobacco advertising, promotion, and sponsorship). These guidelines promote a global roadmap based on tobacco control best policies. The COP also created an Intergovernmental Negotiation Body (INB) to negotiate the first protocol to the convention, on illicit trade in tobacco products [17], which as discussed above will become a treaty in its own right. Since its inception, the COP has hold three sessions and is in the view of submitting the draft protocol for consideration on its fourth session in 2010. Four draft guidelines or progress reports will be also submitted to COP4: Guidelines on Articles 9 & 10: 'Regulation of the contents of tobacco products' and 'Regulation of tobacco product disclosures'; Article 12: 'Education, communication, training and public awareness'; Article 14: 'Demand reduction measures concerning tobacco dependence and cessation'; and Articles 17 & 18: 'Provision of support for economically viable alternative activities' and 'Protection of the environment and the health of persons'. http://www.who.int/fctc/en/ accessed on February, 10th 2010

Many Parties engaged in meeting their obligations by submitting the reports on the implementation of the Treaty that have been summarized by the Secretariat in conjunction with the COP [18]. These reports are submitted according to phases and groups of questions with Phase 1 (Group 1 questions) being submitted by Parties within 2 years of entry into force, Phase 2 (Group 2 questions) within 5 years and Phase 3 (Group 3 questions) being reported within 8 years of entry into force of the WHOFCTC for each Party. http://www.who.int/fctc/reporting/en/ last accessed on February, 10th 2010

As of the 1 July 2009, the Treaty had 165 Parties covering with its provisions a major fraction of world's population.

The global network developed over the period of the negotiations of the WHO FCTC has been important in preparing for the implementation of the Convention at country level. Furthermore, the negotiation process has brought tobacco control to the forefront of the political agenda in many Member States which has led to the adoption of many of the provisions regionally and nationally [19]. This network includes Intergovernmental Organizations and Non-Governmental Organizations, both observers to the COP after approval of their submissions to become official observers. According to the decisions of WHO Member States, the WHO through the TFI initiated its support to the implementation of the Treaty by releasing publications that proposed basic practical steps for the establishment of tobacco control programmes at country level, such as the publication of *Building Blocks for Tobacco Control: a Handbook* [20], a milestone in the capacity building process for countries. A technical assistance package (*MPOWER*) on selected demand reduction provisions of the WHO Framework Convention was further prepared to facilitate the Treaty implementation [21].

Conclusion

The WHO FCTC is public health history in the making and has become a landmark for the future of global public health with major implications for the WHO's health goals. It represents a milestone for the global promotion of public health policies and provides new legal dimensions for international health cooperation. It corroborates the critical roles of international law in preventing disease and promoting health. While the WHO FCTC represents one huge stride forward, it is but a single step in controlling the tobacco epidemic. The success or failure of the Treaty remains highly dependent on country level implementation, and on how international, regional, and national players from different sectors employ it.

> Without question, the WHO Framework Convention on Tobacco Control is the most powerful tool we have, as an international community, to reduce the global disease burden. As we all know, tobacco use is the single greatest preventable cause of death in the world today. Today, this first WHO treaty is at a critical moment in its evolution, where action is required to ensure its status as a living document with a long lifespan.
>
> Margaret Chan, Director General World Health Organization
> Opening statement for the third session of the Conference of the Parties to the WHO Framework Convention on Tobacco Control – Durban, South Africa 17 November 2008

If tobacco control measures are not ramped up by taking effective actions at country level up to one billion people in this century will needlessly perish. Effective implementation of the WHO FCTC has the capacity to save millions of lives in the future.

References

1. Yach, D. and Bettcher, D (2000). Globalisation of tobacco industry influence and new global responses. *Tob. Control*, **9**:206–216.
2. World Health Organization (2002). *World Health Report 2002 – Reducing Risks, Promoting Healthy Lives*. Geneva: WHO.
3. Yach, D. and Wipfli, H. (2006). A century of smoke. Annals of Tropical Medicine & Parasitology 100:5&6, 465–479.
4. World Health Organization (2001). Confronting the tobacco epidemic in an era of trade liberalization WHO/NMH/TFI/01.4, WHO.
5. Da Costa e Silva, V.L. and Nikogosian, H. (2003). Convenio marco de la OMS para el control del tabaco: la globalizacion de la salud publica.[WHO Framework Convention on Tobacco Control: the globalization of public health.] Prevencion del Tabaquismo [Prevention of tobacco addiction], **5**:71–5.
6. Bettcher, D., DeLand, K., Schlundt, J., González-Martín, F., Bishop, J., Hammide, S. *et al.* (in press). International public health instruments S. 4 Public health law and ethics, Oxford Textbook of Public Health 2009.

7. WHO FCTC Secretariat: The History of the World Health Organization Framework Convention on Tobacco Control (WHO FCTC) (Da Costa e Silva VL and David AM, eds.), April 2009, (in press).

8. Zeltner, T., Kessler, A., Martiny, A. and Randera, F. (2000). *Tobacco Company Strategies to Undermine Tobacco Control Activities at the World Health Organization*. Geneva: World Health Organization.

9. WHO (1999). Technical Briefing Series Framework Convention on Tobacco Control: The Framework/ Protocol Approach (Bodansky, D, ed.) WHO/NCD/TFI/99.1, World Health Organization.

10. World Health Organization: The WHO response to the tobacco epidemic, http://www.who.int/ tobacco/about/en/index.html Accessed 03 July 2009.

11. The World Bank (1999). Curbing the Epidemic: The Economics of Tobacco Control (Jha, P, ed.). The World Bank: Washington DC.

12. Taylor, A.L., Bettcher, D.W., and Peck, R. (2003). International law and the international legislative process: the WHO Framework Convention on Tobacco Control. In R. Smith, R. Beaglehole, D. Woodward, and N. Drager (eds) *Global Public Goods for Health: Health Economic and Public Health Perspectives*, pp. 212–32. Oxford University Press, Oxford.

13. Bettcher, D., DeLand, K., Schlundt, J., González-Martín, F., Bishop, J., Hammide, S. *et al.* (in press). International public health instruments in SECTION 4 Public health law and ethics, Oxford Textbook of Public Health 2009.

14. WHO Framework Convention on Tobacco Control World Health Organization (2003).

15. FAO Corporate Depository: Issues in the Global Tobacco Economy, Rome (2003). http://www.fao. org/docrep/006/y4997e/y4997e0l.htm Accessed 30 June 2009.

16. Conference of the Parties to the WHO Framework Convention on Tobacco Control http://www.who. int/fctc/cop/en/ Accessed 30 June 2009.

17. Guidelines on the Implementation of the WHO FCTC: http://www.who.int/fctc/guidelines/en/ Accessed 30 June 2009.

18. Reporting for the Implementation of the WHO FCTC: Summary Analysis of Parties Reports. http:// www.who.int/fctc/reporting/summary_analysis/en/index.html Accessed 01 July 2009.

19. Gostin, L. (2007). Global regulatory strategies for tobacco control. *JAMA*, 7 November —Vol 298, No. 17.

20. World Health Organization (2004). Building Blocks for Tobacco Control. A Handbook (Da Costa e Silva VL and David AM, eds). WHO: Geneva, Available at: http://www.who.int/tobacco/resources/ publications/tobaccocontrol_handbook/en/. Accessed 01 July 2009.

21. MPOWER 2009 flyer. Available at: http://www.who.int/tobacco/mpower/flyer/en/index.html. Accessed 01 July 2009.

Chapter 43

WHO—coordinating international tobacco control

Raman Minhas and Douglas Bettcher[1]

Introduction

The globalization of commerce has left the public health community increasingly vulnerable to the subversive tactics and potentially disastrous exploits of the tobacco industry. The tobacco industry has indeed demonstrated its unique ability to manipulate the various drivers of globalization in order to infiltrate previously inaccessible markets and pursue aggressive global product-distribution strategies. The tobacco industry makes use of targeted marketing campaigns and sponsorship strategies as well as promotional schemes billed as 'corporate social responsibility' in order to amplify the global spread of tobacco use. The tobacco industry's efforts are not without resistance – the international public health community, led by the World Health Organization (WHO), as well as other governmental and non-governmental institutions, remain committed to the containment of the tobacco epidemic. This commitment was evinced by the entry into force in 2005 of the landmark global public health Treaty, the WHO Framework Convention on Tobacco Control (WHO FCTC). With the establishment of this legally binding instrument addressing a wide range of tobacco supply and demand measures, the fight against the global spread of tobacco use driven by the tobacco industry's exploitation of globalization is now rooted in a set of baseline international norms.

The purpose of this chapter is to (i) outline the manner by which the tobacco industry manipulates globalization in its attempt to derail public health programmes combating tobacco consumption; and (ii) describe WHO's efforts in formulating counteractive measures to protect public health interests from that of the tobacco industry. Specifically, this chapter will focus on measures taken in relation to the WHO FCTC's provisions concerning the mitigation of tobacco industry interference and the strengthening of a global regulatory framework for tobacco products.

Globalization and the tobacco industry

An impressive and growing body of evidence demonstrates that the globalization of commerce has expansive implications for public health, particularly in the context of tobacco[1]. The various drivers of globalization, including trade liberalization, increasing cross-border flows of capital, goods, and services, and the development and transfer of novel technologies, have resulted in a greater threat to public health owing to the expansion of the global tobacco market. The dissolution

[1] The authors are staff members of the World Health Organization. The authors alone are responsible for the views expressed in this publication and they do not necessarily represent the decisions or the stated policy of the World Health Organization.

of previously steadfast economic barriers has not gone unnoticed by transnational tobacco companies. The tobacco industry, dominated by a small number of multinational corporations, continues to exploit globalization to achieve broad dissemination of their products in previously unattainable markets. This unique feature of the globalization of tobacco, driven by the efforts of the tobacco industry to achieve market penetration in developing countries and transitional market economies, is a significant contributor to the increased risk and occurrence of tobacco-related diseases worldwide [2]. Given the current situation where most of the world's smokers live in developing countries [3], attempts by the industry to expand global tobacco trade and infiltrate such markets risks potentially disastrous effects on public health.

Transnational tobacco companies present a distinctive element in the expansion of the global tobacco epidemic. The 'vector' of tobacco-related death and disease is not encompassed within a microscopic pathogen, but rather an affluent machinery familiar with both the multi-faceted nature of globalization and the manner by which an escalating economic framework can be maneuvered to increase market presence. The current globalized climate, then, is ripe for the tobacco industry to increase market share and devise unique strategies to circumvent global tobacco control policies proffered by public health organs such as WHO.

The current recipe for globalization is being uniquely stirred by multinational tobacco corporations through a number of carefully designed strategies. Expanding market opportunities in Africa and Asia continue to be at the forefront of the tobacco industry's global vision [4]. However, exploitation of trade liberalization and direct foreign investment represent only a subset of the tactics employed by tobacco conglomerates in pursuing growth in developing countries while contributing to the globalization of the tobacco epidemic [5]. Detailed analyses of internal industry documents demonstrate a history of deceitful industry practices including denying the harmful effects of tobacco use and the addictive powers of nicotine, refuting the harmful effects of second-hand smoke and altering cigarette design features in order to enhance their addictive potential [6]. Transnational tobacco companies have also been documented as having engaged in practices aimed at influencing the development of tobacco control policy. Through the use of financial, scientific, and political processes, these companies have attempted to subvert global tobacco control and advocacy efforts such as those coordinated by the WHO and its civil society partners [7]. More recently, the industry has taken to initiating novel strategies in order to propagate its product and communicate misleading health messages. With the advent of innovative streams of global communications, tobacco companies launch targeted marketing campaigns, particularly to women and youth, in efforts to provoke the global spread of tobacco use. Such campaigns employ the internet, cable and satellite television, music, sports, and entertainment as conduits in a myriad of advertising and sponsorship strategies in order to appeal to young people and expand a growing consumer base [8]. Furthermore, the industry persists in heavily investing in the development of modified or novel tobacco products in order to continue to attract new customers and to maintain existing nicotine addiction [9]. In addition, the role of tobacco companies in fueling the illicit trade of tobacco products has been highlighted as a practice which exploits porous national boundaries in a globalized environment, resulting in conditions which amplify the global spread of tobacco use [10]. Finally, recent industry initiatives touted under the guise of 'corporate social responsibility' have been promoted by big tobacco as socially conscious campaigns designed to improve the health and well-being of its consumers and the community at large. These programmes have been largely discredited as attempts to simply elevate tobacco industry perception among the public and policy-makers – a perception which continues to be challenged as tobacco control rises as a priority issue on the global public health agenda [11].

The tobacco industry's initiatives to enervate tobacco control presents an cumbersome obstacle for the transmission of WHO's global public health interventions. The industry clearly introduces a unique and variable factor in the growth of the tobacco epidemic – an element unseen in the underlying biological and epidemiological facets of infectious disease control. In the area of tobacco control, then, WHO and other public health bodies need not only be armed with the requisite level of science necessary to combat tobacco-related death and disease, but also must be acutely aware of the motivations and tendencies of a dynamic force. This realization precludes the industry from operationalizing its objectives in a vacuum. Thus, the industry's efforts are not without resistance, and the following section of this chapter highlights some of the approaches driven by WHO in combating industry initiatives designed to proliferate global tobacco use.

WHO and tobacco control

Despite incessant attempts by tobacco multinationals to shift expanding global market trends in their favour, public health professionals worldwide remain committed to the containment of the tobacco epidemic. WHO, in particular, has adopted and promoted robust, evidence-based measures aiming to reduce tobacco-related morbidity and mortality. Tobacco control strategies must be grounded in the pillars of a comprehensive tobacco control policy, namely the tripartite objectives of preventing initiation of tobacco use, protecting individuals from exposure to tobacco smoke, and promoting cessation among smokers. Concomitantly, the monitoring of tobacco industry marketing and activities, and the regulation of the contents and emissions of tobacco products form an integral part of any multifaceted tobacco control action plan [12]. These latter two elements reveal many instances where the tobacco industry has squarely endeavoured to profit from the elements of gobalization while compromising global public health. WHO's approaches to tobacco industry monitoring and tobacco product regulation will form the basis for discussion later in this chapter. The following section, however, describes the major vehicle through which WHO has performed, and continues to advance, global coordination in the area of tobacco control: first, through the building of global norms via the negotiation WHO Framework Convention on Tobacco Control, and second, through technical assistance provided to Contracting Parties to the WHO FCTC in implementing the provisions of the Treaty.

WHO Framework Convention on Tobacco Control [13]

The entry into force of the WHO FCTC [14] in 2005 marked an historic shift in the manner by which public health solutions are derived in the global arena. The construction and adoption of this scientifically anchored, international, legal instrument represented WHO's first foray into coordinating an institutionalized global action aimed at improving population health. The development of an international treaty-based approach to tobacco control demonstrated the conviction of the international community in mounting a global effort, grounded in legally binding norms, to combat the tobacco epidemic. After adoption of the WHO FCTC by the World Health Assembly in 2003, the interim secretariat role related to the Framework Convention was held by the WHO Tobacco Free Initiative (WHO TFI). WHO TFI remained in this official capacity until 2006 when, in accordance with Article 24 of the Treaty, the Conference of Parties established the *Convention Secretariat to the WHO FCTC (CSF)*. Subsequently, the 59th World Health Assembly adopted resolution WHA59.17 agreeing to host the permanent secretariat of the Convention within WHO. During the period until CSF became fully operational in mid-2007, WHO TFI continued to act as the interim secretariat of the WHO FCTC. Though no longer performing the Treaty's secretariat function, WHO continues to support Contracting Parties in a technical capacity in fulfilling their obligations under the WHO FCTC. As it stands, the WHO FCTC provides an effective mechanism in establishing a global governance structure in the area of tobacco, providing a platform for multilateral commitment to resist industry exploitation of trade liberalization and globalization [15].

The WHO FCTC represents an incremental process of international law which facilitates the erection of subsequent legally binding commitments through the negotiation of implementing protocols containing detailed obligations [16]. The WHO FCTC itself establishes baseline international norms addressing a wide range of supply (i.e. elimination of the illicit trade of tobacco products and restriction of sales to and by minors) and demand measures (price and tax measures, protection from exposure to environmental tobacco smoke) related to tobacco [17]. Uniquely, the WHO FCTC also contains provisions which transcend traditional supply and demand controls and assign a mandate to directly regulate and monitor the tobacco industry. Recognizing that the development and implementation of tobacco control policy by WHO operates in the shadow of the industry's attempts to subvert its public health function [18], Article 5.3 of the WHO FCTC directs Parties to protect tobacco control policies from the commercial and vested interests of the tobacco industry. Furthermore, Articles 9–11 of the Treaty, which call for the development of global standards regulating the contents, emissions, design, and labelling of tobacco products, acknowledge the need for an international regulatory framework under which the tobacco industry is kept from functioning in a state of insulation.

WHO's commitment to the effective global implementation of the WHO FCTC, then, has not simply materialized as reactive measures aiming to inject effective tobacco control policies at country-level. Rather, the aforementioned provisions of the WHO FCTC add a proactive element to tobacco control serving to impede innovative attempts by the tobacco industry to influence health policy or strengthen the addictiveness of products in a distended global market. These proactive sets of provisions, namely Article 5.3 and Articles 9–11, will be the focus of the following sections.

Protecting tobacco control policy and regulating the industry

As noted earlier, attempts by the tobacco industry to interfere with the development and implementation of tobacco control policies continue to severely impair global efforts to reduce tobacco-related morbidity and mortality. Additionally, the tobacco industry has a documented history of altering cigarette design characteristics and constituents in efforts to augment the initiation and maintenance of smoking addiction. Underscored by expanding economic borders, the tobacco industry is capitalizing on an increasingly globalized environment to foster its interference activities and infiltrate previously untapped markets with innovative or altered tobacco products.

In light of these specific industry practices, WHO not only provides technical assistance to WHO Member States in implementing the evidence-based provisions of the WHO FCTC to reduce tobacco consumption, but also employs mechanisms ingrained in the Treaty to provide global leadership in the areas of tobacco industry interference and tobacco product regulation. The following sections highlight the industry interference (Article 5.3) and product regulation provisions (Articles 9–11) of the WHO FCTC, and illustrate WHO's efforts to protect tobacco control policy from the vested interests of the industry, as well as install a global regulatory environment for the design and manufacture of tobacco products.

Industry interference—WHO FCTC Article 5.3

The tobacco industry's obstruction of health policy continues to be one of the greatest threats to the WHO FCTC's implementation and enforcement. The entrenchment of tobacco control in higher income countries catalysed a strategy shift which now sees big tobacco supporting policies augmenting globalization, in efforts to encumber weaker regulatory environments particularly in the developing world [19].

These initiatives to build and sustain 'tobacco-friendly environments' [20] through the use of a vast array of tactics designed to hamper the institutionalization of tobacco control have been explored in-depth [21]. A large body of evidence demonstrates that tobacco companies integrate a spectrum of practices to interfere with tobacco control, including:

- interfering with WHO FCTC ratification
- litigious action directed at governments
- demanding a seat at government negotiating tables
- promoting voluntary regulation
- drafting and distributing tobacco-friendly sample legislation
- subverting legislation and exploiting loopholes
- promoting and funding 'youth smoking prevention' programmes
- challenging government timelines for implementing laws
- attempting to bribe legislators
- gaining favour by bankrolling government health initiatives on other issues
- providing funds directly to government regulatory bodies
- pushing corporate social responsibility PR efforts
- defending trade at the expense of health [22, 23].

Tobacco industry strategies to influence policy and thwart effective regulation have not been limited to national or regional levels. Attempts by the industry to engage the enabling environment conferred by globalization has even rendered international public health policy making machinery vulnerable. Expert analyses of tobacco industry internal documents demonstrate a myriad of operations undertaken to debilitate WHO's development and implementation of global tobacco control policies and programmes [24]. These analyses, subsumed in the 2000 report of the WHO committee of experts entitled, *Tobacco industry strategies to undermine tobacco control activities at the World Health Organization*, concluded that 'the evidence shows that tobacco companies have operated for many years with the deliberate purpose of subverting the efforts of WHO to address tobacco issues. ... That tobacco companies resist proposals for tobacco control comes as no surprise, but what is now clear is the scale, intensity and most importantly, the tactics, of their campaigns' [25].

Recognizing the potential frailty of global tobacco control efforts in light of pervasive industry ventures, the 54th World Health Assembly unanimously adopted WHA Resolution 54.18, calling for transparency in tobacco control [26]. This resolution, *inter alia*, called on WHO to 'continue to inform Member States of activities of the tobacco industry that have a negative impact on tobacco control efforts' [27]. In response, WHO consistently draws global attention to tobacco industry activities and informs its Member States of novel and sophisticated strategies to derail tobacco control [28]. As an example, in 2007 WHO convened a group of international, industry monitoring experts to discuss tobacco industry interference in tobacco control and relevant public health policies of WHO and its Member States [29]. The outcome of this meeting, entitled *Tobacco Industry Interference with Tobacco Control*, underscored that 'effective tobacco control and the commercial success of the tobacco industry are fundamentally incompatible' [30].

These activities also accord with the principles of WHO FCTC. The preamble of the Treaty, for example, recognizes 'the need to be alert to any efforts by the tobacco industry to undermine or subvert tobacco control efforts and the need to be informed of activities of the tobacco industry that have a negative impact on tobacco control efforts' [31]. Furthermore, the importance of shielding public health policy development from the tobacco industry is also entrenched in the substantive provisions of the WHO FCTC. Recognition by the negotiators of the WHO FCTC of the destabilizing activities of the industry led to the inclusion of Article 5.3 in the Treaty – a provision which represents a momentous step international public health. Article 5.3 of the WHO FCTC, which aims to protect public health policy from the vested interests of the tobacco industry, provides internationally accepted credence to the view that the tobacco epidemic is propelled by more than merely biological, chemical, or behavioural elements. This was a view echoed by the third session of the Conference of Parties (COP) to the WHO FCTC in November 2008, when guidelines expanding upon the *General Obligations* contained in Article 5.3 were unanimously adopted by the Contracting Parties to the WHO FCTC. The Article 5.3 guidelines emphasize the fundamental and irreconcilable conflict between the tobacco industry's interests and public health policy interests [32], and espouse a number of recommendations essential in addressing tobacco industry interference in public health policy development, including:

(1) Raise awareness about the addictive and harmful nature of tobacco products and about tobacco industry interference with Parties' tobacco control policies.

(2) Establish measures to limit interactions with the tobacco industry and ensure the transparency of those interactions that occur.

(3) Reject partnerships and non-binding or non-enforceable agreements and partnerships with the tobacco industry.

(4) Avoid conflicts of interest for government officials and employees.

(5) Require that information collected from the tobacco industry be transparent and accurate.

(6) Denormalize and regulate activities described as 'corporate social responsibility' by the tobacco industry.

(7) Do not give privileged treatment to tobacco companies.

(8) Treat State-owned tobacco companies in the same way as any other tobacco industry [33].

In striving to further distend the schism between public health and the tobacco industry, WHO also supported the development of the WHO FCTC Article 5.3 guidelines concerning tobacco industry interference. In light of the specific recommendations adopted by the third session of the Conference of Parties to the WHO FCTC, and recognizing that the prevention of tobacco industry interference in public health policy development is pivotal, WHO continues to assist Member States in the implementation of the WHO FCTC Article 5.3 Guidelines. Meanwhile, the industry will likely continue to conceptualize unfamiliar methods to advance its economic interests. It is of paramount importance, then, that WHO ensures that such activities are expounded, communicated, and countered. The invariable monitoring of the industry is crucial for the success of tobacco control policies, as the information gained serves to provide a basis for formulating counteractive measures with the ultimate aim of advancing public health [34].

Tobacco product regulation – WHO FCTC Articles 9 and 10

In addition to well-documented political and financial strategies, industry designs to interfere with tobacco control have preyed on a historically weak regulatory framework for tobacco products to communicate misleading health messages and manufacture an array of harmful tobacco products. Whereas potentially hazardous chemical products such as medicines, pesticides, and food additives undergo strict toxicological analyses by institutionalized regulatory agencies in order to determine safety and risk, the regulation of tobacco products does not currently demand equivalent standards.

The devastating public health consequences resulting from the deceptive marketing of 'light' and 'low-tar' cigarettes provides one example of the industry's capacity to exploit a tethered tobacco product regulatory framework [35]. For decades, cigarette manufacturers employed the results of a flawed testing protocol measuring the tar, nicotine, and carbon monoxide content in cigarettes, namely the Cambridge Filter Method (also known as the ISO/FTC Test Method), in order to claim reduced health risks of 'light', 'ultra-light', 'mild', and 'low-tar' cigarettes [36]. Despite knowledge that this test method is insufficient to measure the biological or epidemiological impact of cigarette products and does not provide meaningful information about the relative health risks of different brands of cigarettes, the tobacco industry shaped the testing results to characterize its brands with the aforementioned misleading descriptors [37]. Numerous population-based studies have demonstrated the destructive public health consequences of having permitted such descriptive terms to remain on tobacco product packaging [38]. With the support of WHO and the global tobacco community, the United States Federal Trade Commission rescinded its guidance in 2008 which had allowed tobacco companies to make factual statements about tar and nicotine yields based on a single standardized test method [39].

The use of misleading descriptors illustrates merely one scenario whereby the tobacco industry has contributed to the tobacco epidemic through scientific distortion. Previously classified industry documents have revealed numerous instances of intentional and baseless discrediting of scientific evidence in order to misinform the public and policy-makers regarding the harmful nature of the contents and emissions of tobacco products [40, 41]. Coupled with expanding global markets facilitating the entry of novel or modified tobacco products in areas of the world previously unaffected, the absence of a regulated environment for tobacco products poses a grave threat for the future of tobacco control. The need to install a global regulatory framework for the design and manufacture of tobacco products has been at the forefront of WHO's assistance to Member States in implementing a comprehensive tobacco control strategy.

Tobacco product regulation is defined by WHO as the governmental oversight and enforcement of how tobacco products are manufactured (ingredients and emissions), distributed, packaged, and labelled in order to promote public health protection [42]. The product regulation provisions of the WHO FCTC, Articles 9–11, provide the basis for the regulation of tobacco product contents, emissions, design, and labelling:

- Article 9: provides for the adoption of guidelines on the testing and measuring of contents and emissions of tobacco products [43]
- Article 10: provides the parameters for the regulation of tobacco product disclosures [44]
- Article 11: provides parameters for packaging and labelling of tobacco products [45]

The need to link Articles 9 and 10 to effective communications mechanisms to convey the deadly effects of tobacco products is clear. WHO has undertaken a number of programmes and initiatives over the past decade in order to support not only the negotiations of Articles 9–11 of the WHO FCTC, but also the development of the guidelines for the implementation of Articles 9 and 10. The first session of the Conference of Parties to the WHO FCTC saw the formation an intersessional Working Group composed of interested Parties and invited experts to develop guidelines for the implementation of Articles 9 and 10 [46]. As the guideline development process has progressed through the second and third sessions of COP, WHO, through the WHO Tobacco Free Initiative (WHO TFI), has actively supported the process via its role as the Secretariat and coordinating body of two entities aiming to assist Member State implementation of the product regulation provisions of the WHO FCTC: an expert Study Group on tobacco production regulation; and a global network of laboratories for tobacco product testing.

In its efforts to provide a scientific basis to inform the negotiations of the product regulation provisions of the WHO FCTC, WHO, in its first foray into this area of work, established the *ad hoc* Scientific Advisory Committee on Tobacco Product Regulation (SACTob) to provide sound scientific information concerning issues related to the regulation of tobacco products [47]. SACTob, which held its first meeting in 2000, grounded its scientific recommendations on leading research in the field of tobacco products and served as the basis for negotiations and subsequent consensus reached on the language of these three articles of the WHO FCTC [48]. In November 2003, the WHO Director-General formalized the status of SACTob from an *ad hoc* scientific advisory committee to an expert Study Group, the WHO Study Group on Tobacco Product Regulation (WHO TobReg). The creation of WHO TobReg signified an important milestone in the manner by which global tobacco product regulation can combat tobacco consumption and its adverse effects. WHO TobReg, whose membership is drawn from national and international experts on product regulation, tobacco dependence treatment, and laboratory analysis of tobacco contents, emissions, and design, facilitates a forum for the deliberation of this complex area of tobacco control [49]. The WHO Study Group on Tobacco Product Regulation provides scientifically sound recommendations to WHO concerning effective, evidence-based means to fill regulatory gaps in tobacco control. It also provides support and expertise to the WHO Tobacco Laboratory Network (WHO TobLabNet) to strengthen global capacity in tobacco product testing [50].

Created in April 2005 by WHO, WHO TobLabNet seeks to act as the primary global source of laboratory support, methods development, and scientific information in the areas of tobacco product testing and research on product contents and emissions [51]. Commonplace in the area of communicable diseases, WHO TobLabNet represents the first such laboratory network in the area of non-communicable diseases prevention and control in the WHO structure. WHO TobLabNet is a global network of government, academic, and independent laboratories providing support as Member States aim to strengthen national and regional capacity for the testing and research of the contents and emissions of tobacco products, pursuant to Article 9 of the WHO FCTC. WHO TobLabNet aims to:

- establish global tobacco testing and research capacity to test tobacco products for regulatory compliance
- to provide developing countries tools to effectively regulate tobacco products
- to research and develop harmonized standards for contents and emissions testing
- to provide a forum for exchange of information related to tobacco research and testing standards and results
- to inform risk assessment activities related to the use of tobacco products
- to develop harmonized reporting of such results so that data can be transformed into meaningful trend information that can be compared across countries and over time [52].

Collectively, the advisory role and technical expertise of WHO TobReg and WHO TobLabNet enables WHO to assist Member States in achieving a coordinated regulatory framework for tobacco products in accordance with the WHO FCTC. The significance of the contribution of both entities spearheaded by WHO TFI is evinced by the recognition afforded by the Conference of the Parties, which, at its third session, invited WHO TobLabNet to conduct a global validation of scientific testing methods for priority constituents of cigarette contents and emissions [53]. WHO continues to support Member States in providing the scientific and technical assistance required to meet the obligations under the WHO FCTC related to tobacco product regulation.

A solidified regulatory environment will only serve to confine the tobacco industry's reach and will foster more effective global tobacco control.

Acknowledgements

The authors would like to acknowledge the following people for their contributions towards the chapter: Stella Bialous, Piyali Kundu, Leigh Hansen, and Candice Pillion.

References

1. Bettcher, D., Subramanian, C., Guindon, E. *et al.* (2001). *Confronting the Tobacco Epidemic in an Era of Trade Liberalization.* Available at: http://whqlibdoc.who.int/hq/2001/WHO_NMH_TFI_01.4.pdf (accessed 7 July 2009)

2. Taylor, A.L. and Bettcher, D.W. (2001). WHO Framework Convention on Tobacco Control: a global 'good' for public health. *Bulletin of the World Health Organization*, **78**(7):920.

3. WHO (World Health Organization) (2008). *WHO Report on the Global Tobacco Epidemic, 2008: The MPOWER package.* WHO, Geneva.

4. Bettcher, D., Subramanian, C., Guindon, E. *et al.* (2001). Confronting the Tobacco Epidemic in an Era of Trade Liberalization. *World Health Organization Publication.*

5. Gilmore, A. and McKee, M. (2005). Exploring the impact of foreign direct investment on tobacco consumption in the former Soviet Union. *Tobacco Control*, **14**:13–21.

6. Detels, R., Beaglehole, R., Lansang, M.A., and Gulliford, M. (2009). *Oxford Textbook of Public Health*, 5th edition. Section 10: Prevention and control of public health hazards. 10.1, Tobacco.

7. Ibid.

8. Ibid.

9. World Health Organization (2008). *Evolution of the Tobacco Industry Positions on Addiction to Nicotine.* Available at: http://www.who.int/tobacco/publications/evolution_tob_ind_pos_add_nicotine/en/index. html (accessed 7 July 2009).

10. *Supra*, at note 6.

11. Ibid.

12. Ibid.

13. For a more detailed discussion of the WHO Framework Convention on Tobacco Control, please see chapter on the WHO FCTC authored by Dr Vera da Costa e Silva.

14. World Health Organization (2003). *Preamble: WHO Framework Convention on Tobacco Control.* A56/8. Available at: http://www.who.int/tobacco/framework/WHO_FCTC_english.pdf (accessed 7 June 2009).

15. Taylor, A.L. and Bettcher, D.W. (2001). WHO Framework Convention on Tobacco Control: a global 'good' for public health. *Bulletin of the World Health Organization*, **78**(7):920.

16. *Supra*, at note 6.

17. Shibuya, K., Ciecierski, C., Guindon, E., *et al.* (2003). WHO Framework Convention on Tobacco Control: development of an evidence based global public health treaty. *BMJ*, **327**:154–7.

18. World Health Organization (2001). *World Health Assembly Resolution 54.18: Transparency in Tobacco Control.* Available at: http://www.who.int/tobacco/framework/wha_eb/wha54_18/en/index.html (accessed 7 July 2009)

19. McDaniel, P., Intinarelli, G. and Malone, R. (2008). *Tobacco Industry Issues Management Organizations: Creating a Global Corporate Network to Undermine Public Health.* Available at: http://www. globalizationandhealth.com/content/pdf/1744-8603-4-2.pdf (accessed 7 July 2009).

20. Ibid.

21. Ibid.

22. World Health Organization (2008). *Tobacco Industry Interference with Tobacco Control*. Available at: http://www.who.int/tobacco/resources/publications/9789241597340.pdf (accessed 7 July 2009).

23. Corporate Accountability International: *Dirty Dealings: Big tobacco's Lobbying, Pay-offs, and Public Relations to Undermine National and Global Health Policy*. Available at: http://www.stopcorporateabuse. org/sites/default/files/Dirty_Dealings.pdf (accessed 9 July 2009).

24. World Health Organization Committee of Experts on Tobacco Industry documents (2000). *Tobacco industry Strategies to Undermine Tobacco Control Activities at the World Health Organization*. Available at: http://www.who.int/tobacco/en/who_inquiry.pdf (accessed 9 July 2009).

25. Ibid.

26. World Health Organization (2001). *World Health Assembly Resolution 54.18: Transparency in Tobacco Control*. Available at: http://www.who.int/tobacco/framework/wha_eb/wha54_18/en/index.html (accessed 7 July 2009)

27. Ibid.

28. World Health Organization (2004). *Tobacco Industry and Corporate Social Responsibility ... An Inherent Contradiction*. Available at: http://www.who.int/tobacco/communications/CSR_report.pdf (accessed 7 July 2009).

29. *Supra*, at note 22.

30. Ibid.

31. World Health Organization (2003). WHO Framework Convention on Tobacco Control. *A56/8*. Available at: http://www.who.int/tobacco/framework/WHO_FCTC_english.pdf (accessed 7 June 2009).

32. Elaboration of guidelines for implementation of Article 5.3 of the Convention. Available at: http://apps. who.int/gb/fctc/PDF/cop3/FCTC_COP3_5-en.pdf (accessed 7 July 2009).

33. WHO FCTC Conference of the Parties (2008). *Decision FCTC/COP3(7): Guidelines for implementation of Article 5.3*. Available at: http://www.who.int/fctc/guidelines/article_5_3.pdf (accessed 7 July 2009)

34. World Health Organization. *Building blocks of tobacco control. A handbook. Chapter 13: Countering the tobacco industry*. Available at: http://www.who.int/tobacco/resources/publications/tobaccocontrol_ handbook/en/ (accessed 7 July 2009).

35. NCI Expert Committee, National Cancer Institute (2001). *Risks Associated with Smoking Cigarettes with Low Machine-Yields of Tar and Nicotine*. Smoking and Tobacco Control Monograph 13. Available at: http://cancercontrol.cancer.gov/tcrb/monographs/13/ (accessed 7 July 2009)

36. Ibid.

37. Ibid.

38. Warner, K.E. and Slade, J. (2001). Low tar. High toll. *American Journal of Public Health*, **82**: 17–18. See also, Diane C, et al. (2001). Changing the future of tobacco marketing by understanding the mistakes of the past: lessons from Lights. *Tobacco Control*; **10**(Suppl I): i43–i44.

39. Rescission of Federal Trade Commission Guidance Concerning the Cambridge Filter Method For Testing the Tar and Nicotine Yields of Cigarettes. Available at: http://www.ftc.gov/os/2008/11/ P944509cambridgefiltermethodfrn.pdf (accessed 7 July 2009).

40. Glantz, S.A., Slade, J., Bero, L.A., Hanauer, P., and Barnes, D.E. (1996). *The Cigarette Papers*. University of California Press, Berkeley, CA.

41. Bero, L.A. (2005). Tobacco industry manipulation of research. *Public Health Rep*, **120**: 200–08.

42. *Supra*, at note 6.

43. World Health Organization (2003). WHO framework convention on tobacco control. *A56/8*. Available at: http://www.who.int/fctc/en/ (accessed 7 July 2009).

44. Ibid.

45. Ibid.

46. *Supra*, at note 6.

47. Ibid.

48. World Health Organization Technical Report Series, 945 (2007e). *The scientific basis of tobacco product regulation*. Available at: http://www.who.int/tobacco/global_interaction/tobreg/9789241209458.pdf (accessed 7 July 2009)

49. Ibid.

50. Tobacco Free Initiative, World Health Organization. *WHO Tobacco Laboratory Network (TobLabNet)*. Available at: http://www.who.int/tobacco/global_interaction/toblabnet/history/en/index.html (accessed 7 July 2009)

51. Ibid.

52. Ibid.

53. Elaboration of guidelines for implementation of Articles 9 and 10 of the WHO Framework Convention on Tobacco Control. Available at: http://apps.who.int/gb/fctc/PDF/cop3/FCTC_COP3_6-en.pdf (accessed 7 July 2009).

Index